Problem Solving in Emergency Radiology

Problem Solving in Emergency Radiology

Stuart E. Mirvis, MD, FACR
Professor
Department of Diagnostic Radiology and Nuclear Medicine
University of Maryland School of Medicine
Baltimore, Maryland

Wayne S. Kubal, MD
Professor of Medical Imaging
Department of Medical Imaging
University of Arizona
Tucson, Arizona

Kathirkamanathan Shanmuganathan, MD
Professor of Radiology
Department of Diagnostic Radiology and Nuclear Medicine
University of Maryland School of Medicine
Baltimore, Maryland

Jorge A. Soto, MD
Professor of Radiology
Boston University School of Medicine
Vice Chairman
Department of Radiology
Boston Medical Center
Boston, Massachusetts

Joseph S. Yu, MD
Professor of Radiology and Orthopedic Surgery
Vice Chair of Academic Affairs and Education
The Ohio State University Wexner Medical Center
Columbus, Ohio

1600 John F. Kennedy Blvd.
Ste 1800
Philadelphia, PA 19103-2899

PROBLEM SOLVING IN EMERGENCY RADIOLOGY   ISBN: 978-1-4557-5417-5
Copyright © 2015 by Saunders, an imprint of Elsevier Inc.

Notices

Knowledge and best practice in this field are constantly changing. As new research and experience broaden our understanding, changes in research methods, professional practices, or medical treatment may become necessary.

Practitioners and researchers must always rely on their own experience and knowledge in evaluating and using any information, methods, compounds, or experiments described herein. In using such information or methods they should be mindful of their own safety and the safety of others, including parties for whom they have a professional responsibility.

With respect to any drug or pharmaceutical products identified, readers are advised to check the most current information provided (i) on procedures featured or (ii) by the manufacturer of each product to be administered, to verify the recommended dose or formula, the method and duration of administration, and contraindications. It is the responsibility of practitioners, relying on their own experience and knowledge of their patients, to make diagnoses, to determine dosages and the best treatment for each individual patient, and to take all appropriate safety precautions.

To the fullest extent of the law, neither the Publisher nor the authors, contributors, or editors assume any liability for any injury and/or damage to persons or property as a matter of products liability, negligence or otherwise, or from any use or operation of any methods, products, instructions, or ideas contained in the material herein.

Library of Congress Cataloging-in-Publication Data

Problem solving in emergency radiology / section/associate editors, Stuart Mirvis, Wayne S. Kubal, Kathirkamanathan Shanmuganathan, Jorge A. Soto, Joseph S. Yu.
    p. ; cm.
  Includes bibliographical references and index.
  ISBN 978-1-4557-5417-5 (hardcover : alk. paper)
  I. Mirvis, Stuart E., editor of compilation. II. Kubal, Wayne Scott, editor of compilation. III. Shanmuganathan, K. (Kathirkamanathan), editor of compilation. IV. Soto, Jorge A., editor of compilation. V. Yu, Joseph, editor of compilation.
  [DNLM: 1. Diagnostic Imaging. 2. Emergencies. WN 180]
  RC78
  616.07'57--dc23   2013046612

Senior Content Strategist: Don Scholz
Content Development Specialist: Julia Rose Roberts
Publishing Services Manager: Anne Altepeter
Project Manager: Ted Rodgers
Designer: Steven Stave

To Linda, for her patience and understanding, and Zack,
who always makes me smile
Stuart Mirvis

To my parents, Fred and Lillian,
who gave me the love and support to believe that all things are possible
Wayne Kubal

To my parents and sister, Nalayini Shan, who are always available
for moral support and advice when required
Kathirkamanathan Shanmuganathan

To my wife, Ana; my daughter, Andrea; and my son, Alejandro
Jorge Soto

To Cynthia and Sarah, the two anchors of my life
Joseph Yu

Foreword

Today's emergency departments (EDs) are emergency diagnostic centers. Of the 130 million patients who currently visit an ED each year in the United States, nearly half will have some type of imaging performed, making it clear that imaging has become an indispensable tool for diagnosing acute conditions and traumatic injuries in this setting. But it is computed tomography (CT) imaging in particular that has thrust imaging to the forefront of emergent care. The diagnostic use of CT in the ED increased 330% between 1996 and 2007, from 3% to 14% of all patient visits. There was a widespread increase in the use of CT for the 20 most common ED chief complaints. Within this context, the matured specialties of emergency medicine and trauma surgery, and modern health care in general, have placed great emphasis on contemporaneous imaging interpretation. Together, these forces have transformed the radiologist's role from minor participant to major player in care delivery and in so doing have given birth to the ascendant specialty of emergency radiology. Indeed, the need to provide coordinated radiologic care contemporaneous to the ED patient visit has never been greater. This is why this book is such an important and timely contribution to the specialty.

Radiologists who provide coverage of ED imaging require a broad fund of knowledge spanning most imaging modalities and organ systems. Although historically such practice has been characterized as *general radiology*, this term is now anachronistic and anathema to practicing emergency radiologists. Instead, the required interpretational expertise is defined by the common conditions affecting acutely ill or traumatized patients. Epidural hematoma, cervical spine fracture, aortic injury, liver laceration, stroke, aortic dissection, pulmonary embolus, pneumonia, appendicitis, diverticulitis, bowel obstruction, ectopic pregnancy, tubo-ovarian abscess, osteomyelitis, and the like define the field of emergency radiology.

Equally important, the skills required for optimal radiologic care in the ED extend well beyond interpretational expertise, particularly if that expertise is largely defined by a single organ system or imaging modality. Surely no one is convinced that optimal care for a severely traumatized patient transferred from an outside institution is achieved by seeking interpretations from multiple organ-based subspecialties remote from the ED. Contemporaneous clinical consultation, appropriateness oversight, examination protocol optimization, resource triage, image and radiation dose management across organ systems, and using the range of imaging modalities are required to optimize ED patient outcomes; these define the role of an emergency radiologist.

When such requirements are coupled with the 24/7 operations and time-sensitive obligations inherent in caring for ED patients, the most common legacy approaches to ED coverage often fall short in achieving a consistent standard of care, let alone an optimal one.

Analogous to the critical role emergency medicine plays in delivering clinical care and coordinating diverse medical and surgical specialties in the ED, emergency radiology sections are postured to resolve the care fragmentation that typically plagues imaging services provided by remote silos of organ- and modality-based radiology specialties. For better or worse, such change in radiology practice remains mostly evolutionary rather than revolutionary.

Dedicated emergency radiology sections first emerged in a few academic medical centers during the 1980s and 1990s. Although this care model was initially met with institutional inertia, in the past decade it has been more widely adopted, especially in large medical centers or multihospital systems with sufficient ED visits and/or Level 1 trauma services. Despite the growth in adoption of dedicated emergency radiology sections, resident and fellow interpretations remain a mainstay of "after-hours" coverage for many radiology departments with training programs. At smaller-scale institutions and in private practice, the growth in ED imaging, coincident with advances in computing technology and network speeds, resulted in a different course. During the 1980s and 1990s most community radiology practices provided coverage of after-hours ED imaging from home using web-based viewers rather than sophisticated teleradiology solutions. As the demand for this imaging dramatically increased during the mid to late 1990s, a commercial market emerged for outsourced teleradiology services. By 2007 a majority of private practice radiology groups used such services.

Although today's approach to coverage of ED imaging remains heterogeneous, it appears certain that greater emphasis will continue to be placed on the value, timeliness, and coordination of radiologic care provided. Advocating for optimal radiologic care of the ED patient has been the core mission of the American Society of Emergency Radiology (ASER). Founded in 1988, ASER has worked to advance the quality of diagnosis and treatment of acutely ill or injured patients by means of medical imaging and to enhance teaching and research in emergency radiology. In the quarter century since its founding, ASER has grown from its 8 founders (Drs. Gordon C. Carson, John H. Harris, Jr., Alan Klein, Jack P. Lawson, James J. McCort, Stuart E. Mirvis, Charles F. Mueller, and Robert A. Novelline) and 16 charter members to more than 900 members. ASER and its members have worked tirelessly to establish emergency radiology as a specialty within organized radiology. A successful peer-reviewed journal (*Emergency Radiology*), annual society meetings, a core educational curriculum for radiology trainees, a high-quality website (www.erad.org), and equal representation alongside other radiology specialties in important professional venues (for example, the Radiological Society of North America [RSNA], the American Roentgen Ray Society [ARRS], and the American College of Radiology [ACR]), are testaments to the Society's success. International members also have made significant contributions to ASER and have helped disseminate the practice of emergency radiology at the global level. New emergency radiology societies have been established outside the United States, most recently in Europe and Asia. For ASER leaders and many practicing emergency radiologists in the United States and abroad, the past 2 to 3 years have symbolized a tipping point toward the realization of our greater ambitions: full recognition as a specialty within the pantheon of radiology.

At this pivotal time for emergency radiology, it is important that a single text captures the core knowledge that defines this modern specialty. *Problem Solving in Emergency Radiology* represents the most up-to-date and comprehensive contribution from many leading authors in this field. Supported by ASER and edited by Dr. Mirvis, this text draws upon a large variety of expertise across the broad range of emergency imaging topics. Using a "head-to-toe" organizational approach, with sections based on anatomic regions and subdivision by traumatic and nontraumatic presentations, the text is well organized for rapid access to any relevant topic and easily serves as a companion to the ASER core curriculum. Most important, the book achieves

its most lofty goal, which is to more clearly define and broadly disseminate the body of knowledge that defines emergency radiology practice today. Given Dr. Mirvis's lifelong devotion to and stature within the field of emergency radiology, from founding member of ASER to leading international authority on trauma and noteworthy journal editor, there is no better steward of this worthy ambition.

This book will have broad appeal to many audiences. It will prove an invaluable resource to any practicing radiologist providing coverage of emergency department imaging, regardless of whether or not the radiologist self-identifies as an emergency radiologist. It is required reading for every diagnostic radiology resident or fellow and will be of great interest to emergency medicine physicians, trauma surgeons, and the many other physicians and care providers who consult on patients in the ED. Dr. Mirvis and colleagues have assembled what is sure to become the new reference text on emergency radiology.

Stephen Ledbetter, MD, MPH
Chief of Radiology
Brigham and Women's Faulkner Hospital
Boston, Massachusetts

Preface

Problem Solving in Emergency Radiology is one of a series of texts published by Elsevier starting in 2007 that are intended to provide core reviews of major areas of diagnostic imaging, focusing on what the authors believe are the most relevant, up-to-date concepts in the areas of their expertise, as well as to provide practical knowledge to help in negotiating complex cases and unusual imaging presentations of acute pathologic conditions and in distinguishing actual from "pseudo" pathologic conditions.

This text is divided into five sections representing major anatomic areas. Each section was prepared by a coeditor, including Joseph S. Yu, MD (Musculoskeletal Emergencies), Stuart E. Mirvis, MD, FACR (Thoracic Emergency Radiology), Wayne S. Kubal, MD (Spine Emergencies, Craniocerebral and Orbital-Maxillo-Facial Emergencies), and Kathirkamanathan Shanmuganathan, MD (Blunt Abdominal and Retroperitoneal Trauma) and Jorge A. Soto, MD (Nontraumatic Abdominal Emergencies) sharing the work of the section on Abdominal Emergencies. The book starts with overview chapters on strategies for computed tomography radiation reduction in the acute care setting by Aaron Sodickson, MD, PhD, and image management in emergency radiology by Martin L. Gunn, MBChB, FRANZCR, and Jeffrey D. Robinson, MD. Both chapters have general application in all aspects of emergency imaging. There are 88 contributors to the text, offering a wide spectrum of information covering a huge number of topics in emergency radiology.

The goal of this text is to bring together in one book both traumatic and nontraumatic imaging findings of emergency radiology. Some of our goals were to provide an update on imaging techniques, to review the evolving scoring (grading) systems for trauma and nontraumatic conditions, to present recent terminology, to offer a generous quantity of up-to-date imaging with postprocessing enhancement, to show and discuss confusing variants that simulate pathologic conditions and atypical presentations of common emergency pathologic conditions, and to expose the reader to rarely encountered emergency imaging diagnoses.

One difficulty encountered in multiauthored textbooks is maintaining a consistent writing style and a similar level of detail in coverage of the subject. Different writing styles, chapter length limitations, and multiple chapter contributors create this variation. It is our hope that readers can navigate these differences in chapter structure to glean the core information provided within. The chapters review major regional imaging anatomy, clinical concepts germane to the topic, and the application of various imaging modalities and their strengths and limitations where appropriate. The authors attempt to provide a basic foundation for imaging emergent pathologic conditions to address the needs of radiologists in training, as well as to provide advanced concepts, detailed information, subtle findings, and challenging cases for the more seasoned radiologist.

In addition to imaging specialists, physicians specializing in emergency medicine, critical care and internal medicine, and emergent surgical conditions will find an understandable, clinically relevant, timely, and comprehensive text to gain new or refresh prior knowledge that is essential to diagnosis and planning treatment of acutely ill or injured patients.

Stuart E. Mirvis, MD, FACR

Contributors

Stephan W. Anderson, MD
Associate Professor of Radiology, Boston Medical
    Center, Boston, Massachusetts

Krystal Archer-Arroyo, MD
Assistant Professor, Diagnostic Radiology and
    Nuclear Medicine, University of Maryland School
    of Medicine, Baltimore, Maryland

Alexander B. Baxter, MD
New York University School of Medicine,
    New York, New York

Mark Bernstein, MD
Trauma and Emergency Radiology, NYU School
    of Medicine, NYU Langone Medical Center/
    Bellevue Hospital Center, New York, New York

Sanjeev Bhalla, MD
Professor of Radiology, Mallinckrodt Institute of
    Radiology, Washington University School of
    Medicine, St. Louis, Missouri

Uttam K. Bodanapally, MD
Assistant Professor, Department of Diagnostic
    Radiology and Nuclear Medicine, University
    of Maryland School of Medicine, Baltimore,
    Maryland

Syed Ahmad Jamal Bokhari, MD
Professor of Radiology and Surgery, Yale University
    School of Medicine, New Haven, Connecticut

Ritu Bordia, MBBS
NYU School of Medicine, New York, New York

Alexis Boscak, MD
Assistant Professor, Diagnostic Radiology and
    Nuclear Medicine, University of Maryland School
    of Medicine, Baltimore, Maryland

Kim Caban, MD
Assistant Professor of Clinical Radiology, University
    of Miami Miller School of Medicine, Miami,
    Florida

Giovanna Casola, MD, FACR, FRCPC
Professor of Radiology, University of California,
    San Diego, San Diego, California

Felix S. Chew, MD
Professor and Section Head of Musculoskeletal
    Radiology, University of Washington, Attending
    Radiologist, Harborview Medical Center, Seattle,
    Washington

Suzanne T. Chong, MD, MS
Assistant Professor and Director, Division of
    Emergency Radiology, Department of Radiology,
    University of Michigan Health System, Ann Arbor,
    Michigan

Christine B. Chung, MD
Professor of Radiology, University of California,
    San Diego, San Diego, California

Stephanie L. Coleman, MD, MPH
Radiology Resident, Boston Medical Center, Boston,
    Massachusetts

John M. Collins, MD, PhD
Assistant Professor of Radiology, The University
    of Chicago, Chicago, Illinois

Gary Danton, MD, PhD
Assistant Professor of Clinical Radiology, Director
    of Radiology Residency Program, University of
    Miami Miller School of Medicine, Director of
    Radiology Services at Jackson Memorial Hospital,
    Miami, Florida

Anthony M. Durso, MD
Assistant Professor of Radiology, University of
    Miami Miller School of Medicine, Miami, Florida

Georges Y. El-Khoury, MD, FACR
Department of Radiology and Orthopaedics,
    University of Iowa Hospitals and Clinics, Iowa
    City, Iowa

Maxwell D. Elia, MD
Resident in Department of Ophthalmology and
    Visual Science, Yale University School of Medicine,
    New Haven, Connecticut

Kathleen R. Fink, MD
Assistant Professor of Radiology, Harborview
    Medical Center, University of Washington,
    Seattle, Washington

Thorsten R. Fleiter, DrMed
Associate Professor, Diagnostic Radiology and
 Nuclear Medicine, University of Maryland School
 of Medicine, Baltimore, Maryland

Rachel F. Gerson, MD
Radiologist, Highline Medical Center, Partner, iRAD
 Medical Imaging, Burien, Washington

James H. Grendell, MD
Chief, Division of Gastroenterology, Hepatology,
 and Nutrition, Department of Medicine,
 Winthrop—University Hospital, Mineola,
 New York, Professor of Medicine, State University
 of New York at Stony Brook School of Medicine

Martin L. Gunn, MBChB, FRANZCR
Associate Professor of Radiology,, University of
 Washington, Seattle, Washington

Nidhi Gupta, MD
Assistant Professor, Musculoskeletal Division,
 Department of Radiology, Ohio State University,
 Columbus, Ohio

Tudor H. Hughes, MD
Professor of Clinical Radiology, Radiology Resident
 Program Director, Vice Chair of Education, UC
 San Diego Health Services, San Diego, California

David Y. Hwang, MD
Department of Neurology, Yale University School
 of Medicine, New Haven, Connecticut

Jon A. Jacobson, MD
Professor of Radiology, Director, Division of
 Musculoskeletal Radiology, University of
 Michigan, Ann Arbor, Michigan

Bruce R. Javors, MD
Professor of Clinical Radiology (Retired), Albert
 Einstein College, Bronx, New York, Attending
 Radiologist (Retired), Winthrop—University
 Hospital, Mineola, New York

Jamlik-Omari Johnson, MD
Department of Radiology and Imaging Sciences,
 Emory University School of Medicine, Atlanta,
 Georgia

Michele H. Johnson, MD
Department of Diagnostic Radiology, Yale University
 School of Medicine, New Haven, Connecticut

Douglas S. Katz, MD, FACR
Professor of Clinical Radiology, State University of
 New York at Stony Brook School of Medicine,
 Stony Brook, New York, Director of Body Imaging
 and Vice Chair of Clinical Research and Education,
 Department of Radiology, Winthrop—University
 Hospital, Mineola, New York

Daniel Kawakyu-O'Connor, MD
Assistant Professor of Imaging Sciences, University
 of Rochester Medical Center, Rochester, New York

Ania Z. Kielar, MD
Assistant Professor of Medical Imaging, University
 of Ottawa, Director of Abdominal and Pelvic
 Imaging, The Ottawa Hospital, Ottawa, Canada

Wayne S. Kubal, MD
Professor of Medical Imaging, Department of
 Medical Imaging, University of Arizona, Tucson,
 Arizona

Russ Kuker, MD
Assistant Professor of Clinical Radiology, University
 of Miami Miller School of Medicine, Miami,
 Florida

Flora Levin, MD
Assistant Professor, Department of Ophthalmology
 and Visual Science, Yale University School of
 Medicine, New Haven, Connecticut

Ken F. Linnau, MD, MS
Assistant Professor of Radiology, University of
 Washington, Seattle, Washington

Peter S. Liu, MD
Assistant Professor of Radiology and Vascular
 Surgery, University of Michigan Medical Center,
 Ann Arbor, Michigan

Patrick McLaughlin, FFR, RCSI
Emergency Radiologist, Vancouver General Hospital,
 University of British Columbia, Vancouver,
 Canada

F.A. Mann, MD
Medical Imaging, Swedish Medical Center, Seattle, Washington

Carrie P. Marder, MD, PhD
Acting Instructor in Radiology (Neuroradiology section), University of Washington, Seattle, Washington

Michael B. Mazza, MD
Assistant Professor of Radiology, University of Michigan, Ann Arbor, Michigan

Vincent M. Mellnick, MD
Assistant Professor, Mallinckrodt Institute of Radiology, Washington University School of Medicine, St. Louis, Missouri

David M. Melville, MD
Assistant Professor of Radiology, University of Arizona, Tucson, Arizona

Christine Menias, MD
Professor of Radiology, Mayo Clinic School of Medicine, Scottsdale, Arizona

Arash Meshksar, MD
Clinical Fellow in Medical Imaging, University of Arizona, Tucson, Arizona

Monique Anne Meyer, MD
Assistant Professor of Radiology, University of Louisville School of Medicine, Louisville, Kentucky

Lisa A. Miller, MD
Assistant Professor, Department of Diagnostic Radiology and Nuclear Medicine, University of Maryland School of Medicine, Baltimore, Maryland

Stuart E. Mirvis, MD, FACR
Professor, Department of Diagnostic Radiology and Nuclear Medicine, University of Maryland School of Medicine, Baltimore, Maryland

Felipe Munera, MD
Professor of Radiology, University of Miami School of Medicine, Medical Director of Radiology Services, University of Miami Hospital, Miami, Florida

Refky Nicola, MS, DO
Assistant Professor, Department of Imaging Sciences and Emergency Medicine, University of Rochester Medical Center, Rochester, New York

Savvas Nicolaou, MD, FRCR
Emergency Radiologist, Vancouver General Hospital,, University of British Columbia, Vancouver, Canada

Diego B. Nunez, MD, MPH
Professor of Diagnostic Radiology, Yale University School of Medicine, Vice Chair, Yale New Haven Hospital, New Haven, Connecticut

Howard J. O'Rourke, MD
Clinical Assistant Professor of Radiology, University of Iowa Hospitals and Clinics, Iowa City, Iowa

Michael N. Patlas, MD, FRCPC
Associate Professor of Radiology, Director, Division of Trauma/Emergency Radiology, McMaster University, Hamilton, Canada

Jason E. Payne, MD
Assistant Professor of Radiology, The Ohio State University Wexner Medical Center, Columbus, Ohio

Alexandra Platon
Department of Radiology, Emergency Radiology Unit, University Hospital of Geneva, Geneva, Switzerland

Pierre-Alexandre Poletti
Associate Professor, Department of Radiology, Emergency Radiology Unit, University Hospital of Geneva, Geneva, Switzerland

Colin Shiu-On Poon, MD, PhD, FRCPC
Adjunct Assistant Professor of Radiology, Yale University School of Medicine, New Haven, Connecticut

Valeria Potigailo
Neuroradiology Fellow, The University of Chicago Pritzker School of Medicine, Chicago, Illinois

Thomas Ptak, MD, PhD, MPH
Assistant Professor of Radiology, Harvard Medical School, Associate Radiologist, Massachusetts General Hospital, Boston, Massachusetts

Shamir Rai
Department of Radiology, University of British
    Columbia, Vancouver, Canada

Constantine A. Raptis, MD
Assistant Professor of Radiology, Mallinckrodt
    Institute of Radiology, Washington University
    School of Medicine, St. Louis, Missouri

Jeffrey D. Robinson, MD
Assistant Professor of Radiology, University of
    Washington, Seattle, Washington

Alan Rogers, MD
Assistant Professor of Radiology, The Ohio State
    University Wexner Medical Center, Columbus, Ohio

Michael F. Rolen, MD
Chief Resident, Department of Diagnostic
    Radiology, Yale University School of Medicine,
    New Haven, Connecticut

Luigia Romano
Director, Emergency Radiology Department,
    Cardarelli Hospital, Naples, Italy

Mariano Scaglione
Director of Diagnostic Imaging, Pineta Grande
    Medical Center, Castel Volturno, Italy

Thomas M. Scalea, MD, FACS
Physician in Chief, R. Adams Cowley Shock
    Trauma Center, University of Maryland Medical
    Center, Francis X. Kelly Distinguished Professor
    of Trauma, University of Maryland School of
    Medicine, Baltimore, Maryland

Joseph L. Schindler, MD
Department of Neurology, Yale University School
    of Medicine, New Haven, Connecticut

Javier Servat, MD
Assistant Professor of Ophthalmology and Visual
    Science, Department of Ophthalmology and
    Visual Science, Yale University School of Medicine,
    New Haven, Connecticut

Kathirkamanathan Shanmuganathan, MD
Professor of Radiology, Department of Diagnostic
    Radiology and Nuclear Medicine, University of
    Maryland School of Medicine, Baltimore, Maryland

Lewis K. Shin, MD
Assistant Professor of Diagnostic Radiology, VA Palo
    Alto Health Care System, Stanford University
    Medical Center, Palo Alto, California

Waqas Shuaib, MD
Department of Radiology and Imaging Sciences,
    Emory University School of Medicine, Atlanta,
    Georgia

Clint W. Sliker, MD
Associate Professor, Department of Diagnostic
    Radiology and Nuclear Medicine, University
    of Maryland School of Medicine, Baltimore,
    Maryland, Attending Radiologist, Trauma and
    Emergency Radiology Section, Diagnostic Imaging
    Department, University of Maryland Medical
    Center and R. Adams Cowley Shock Trauma
    Center, Baltimore, Maryland

Aaron Sodickson, MD, PhD
Section Chief of Emergency Radiology, Brigham
    and Women's Hospital, Medical Director of CT,
    Brigham Radiology Network, Associate Professor
    of Radiology, Harvard Medical School, Boston,
    Massachusetts

Jorge A. Soto, MD
Professor of Radiology, Boston University School
    of Medicine, Vice Chairman, Department of
    Radiology, Boston Medical Center, Boston,
    Massachusetts

Daniel Souza, MD
Staff Radiologist, Brigham and Women's Faulkner
    Hospital, Instructor of Radiology, Harvard Medical
    School, Boston, Massachusetts

Leena Tekchandani, MD
Clinical Instructor of Radiology, State University
    of New York at Stony Brook School of Medicine,
    Stony Brook, New York, Resident Physician,
    Department of Radiology, Winthrop—University
    Hospital, Mineola, New York

Anuj M. Tewari, MD
Assistant Professor, Department of Radiology
    and Imaging Sciences, Emory University School
    of Medicine, Atlanta, Georgia

Hamid Torshizy, MD
Fellow, Division of Musculoskeletal Radiology,
  University of California, San Diego, San Diego,
  California

Jennifer W. Uyeda, MD
Clinical Assistant in Abdominal and Interventional
  Radiology, Massachusetts General Hospital,
  Boston, Massachusetts

Xin Wu, MD
Resident Physician in Diagnostic Radiology,
  New York University Medical Center, New York,
  New York

Joseph S. Yu, MD
Professor of Radiology and Orthopedic Surgery,
  Vice Chair of Academic Affairs and Education,
  The Ohio State University Wexner Medical Center,
  Columbus, Ohio

Sarah M. Yu
Department of Radiology, The Ohio State University
  Wexner Medical Center, Columbus, Ohio

William B. Zucconi, DO
Assistant Clinical Professor of Radiology, Yale
  University School of Medicine, New Haven,
  Connecticut

Contents

SECTION V   MUSCULOSKELETAL EMERGENCIES

Strategies for Reducing Radiation Exposure From Multidetector Computed Tomography in the Acute Care Setting

Aaron Sodickson

Acknowledgments

All figures and much of the text in this chapter have been reprinted with permission from: Sodickson A. Strategies for reducing radiation exposure in multi-detector row CT. *Radiol Clin North Am.* 2012;50(1):1-14; and Sodickson A. Strategies for reducing radiation exposure from multidetector computed tomography in the acute care setting. *Can Assoc Radiol J.* 2013;64(2):119-129.

■ SYNOPSIS

Many tools and strategies exist to enable reduction of radiation exposure from computed tomography (CT). The common CT metrics of x-ray output—the volume CT dose index ($CTDI_{vol}$) and dose length product (DLP)—are explained and serve as the basis for monitoring radiation exposure from CT scans. Many strategies to dose optimize CT protocols are explored that, in combination with available hardware and software tools, allow robust, diagnostic-quality CT scans to be performed with a radiation exposure appropriate for the clinical scenario and the size of the patient. Specific emergency department (ED) example protocols are used to demonstrate these techniques.

■ INTRODUCTION

Radiation exposure has received much attention of late in the medical literature and lay media. It is commonly recognized that CT has tremendously advanced our diagnostic capabilities in the ED and broadly throughout medicine. These diagnostic benefits have combined with widespread availability and rapidity of scanning to produce marked increases in CT use, estimated at approximately 69 million CT scans per year in the United States.[1] However, rapidly increasing use has heightened concerns about the collective radiation exposure to the population as a whole and about the high levels of cumulative exposure that may occur in patients undergoing recurrent imaging for chronic conditions or persistent complaints.[2-4]

CT has received the greatest scrutiny because of its relatively high radiation dose per examination. Although it constitutes about 17% of all medical imaging procedures, it produces approximately half of the population's medical radiation exposure, with nuclear medicine contributing approximately one quarter of the collective dose to the population and fluoroscopy and conventional x-ray examinations accounting for the remainder.[5,6] Yet even in relatively young patients (in whom the radiation risks are thought to be larger), the risks for mortality related to the underlying disease or condition have been found in general to be far greater than the estimated risks for radiation-induced cancer mortality from CT.[7]

There are many possible strategies for reducing radiation exposure to the population as a whole and to individual patients.[8] Once the decision is made to perform a CT scan, many imaging strategies can reduce the radiation dose while maintaining appropriate diagnostic quality for the clinical task at hand. There have been tremendous advances in CT technology in recent years that allow high-quality examinations to be performed at progressively lower radiation dose. The common practice of porting CT protocols from older to newer scanners often fails to take maximal advantage of these new technologies. Routine optimal scan acquisition requires that radiologists invest the effort to understand their technology and to implement dose-optimized protocols, ideally in collaboration with CT manufacturers, CT technologists, and medical physicists. This is admittedly a daunting task for many radiologists, who often view their primary role as diagnosticians and interpreters of images and often have little detailed training in CT technology.

This chapter will describe several practical opportunities to reduce radiation exposure from CT, with emphasis on how CT protocols can be modified to reduce dose while maintaining diagnostic quality. Specific implementation of these strategies is highly dependent on the available technology, and there is no replacement for hands-on training at the scanner.

■ REDUCING RADIATION EXPOSURE: BEFORE THE SCAN

The most effective way to reduce radiation exposure is to avoid performing the examination. Before a scan is performed, many measures can be taken to control use, with the goal of reducing low-yield examinations that will not contribute significantly to the care of the patient. It is admittedly often challenging to prospectively determine which examinations these will be. Nonetheless, scrutiny of examination appropriateness is vital. In optimal circumstances this can rely on well-validated clinical decision rules such as those for pulmonary embolus or for head or cervical-spine imaging in trauma.[9-11] These rules may be integrated into predefined imaging algorithms in the effort to standardize the imaging approach in specific clinical scenarios or patient populations. Alternatively, these algorithms or expert panel appropriateness criteria may be incorporated into decision support advice during computerized physician order entry.[12-14]

Duplicative and recurrent imaging are natural targets for radiation dose reduction.[15,16] Ordering physician awareness of duplicate imaging may be achieved via review of the medical record or in automated fashion as part of decision support tools.[17] In certain circumstances, interventions to eliminate unnecessary repeat imaging can be highly effective in reducing use. As an example, during interhospital patient transfers, importation to a picture archiving and communication system (PACS) of outside hospital imaging examinations via image transfer networks or from CD has been found to significantly reduce CT use (by 16% at our institution), primarily by eliminating unnecessary repeat scans.[18-20]

Defensive medicine and self-referral of diagnostic imaging have both been implicated as significant contributors to imaging use.[21,22] Effectively addressing these systemic issues will require higher-level attention in our health care delivery system.

■ UNDERSTANDING THE X-RAY OUTPUT METRICS CTDI$_{VOL}$ AND DLP

To understand and monitor radiation exposures from CT scans, a basic understanding is first needed of the radiation exposure metrics commonly used in CT. The CTDI$_{vol}$ and the DLP are well-calibrated and standardized measures of x-ray tube output.[23,24] They are measured in cylindrical acrylic phantoms of standard diameter—either a 16-cm "head" phantom or a 32-cm "body" phantom. A 100-mm long ionization chamber connected to an electrometer is placed inside a hole in either the center or periphery of the CTDI phantom, and measurements are made (with the CT table stationary) under a particular CT exposure to yield CTDI$_{100}$ measurements. The CTDI$_{vol}$ is a weighted sum of these

central and peripheral measurements, along with a geometric correction to account for the pitch of a helical scan:

$$CTDI_{vol} = \left(\frac{2}{3}CTDI_{100,\,periph} + \frac{1}{3}CTDI_{100,\,center} \right)\Big/pitch$$

The CTDI$_{vol}$ reported by the CT scanner is most commonly the average value over the entire length of the scan (although some scanner models report the maximum value). DLP is simply the average CTDI$_{vol}$ times the z-axis extent of the CT exposure from head to foot, so that a doubling in z-axis coverage at fixed CTDI$_{vol}$ will result in a doubling of the DLP.

CTDI$_{vol}$ and DLP depend heavily on the selected scan parameters, including the peak kilovoltage (kVp) and the tube current-time product mAs (which relates to the tube current in milliamperes [mA], rotation time, and pitch as mAs = [mA × rotation time]/pitch). They capture intrinsic scanner factors, including x-ray source efficiency, filtration and collimation. As such, they are reliable metrics of x-ray tube output or x-ray flux but do not accurately represent the radiation dose to a particular patient, primarily because they do not take into consideration the size of the patient.[25]

Limitations of Patient Dose Estimates from CTDI$_{vol}$ and DLP

CTDI$_{vol}$ (measured in milligray [mGy]) is commonly used to approximate patient organ doses. However, this is accurate for only a narrow range of patient sizes closely approximating the size of the CTDI phantom, and the actual organ dose a patient receives depends greatly on the size of the patient.[26-28] CTDI$_{vol}$ overestimates organ dose to large patients because subcutaneous soft tissues attenuate the incident x-rays, essentially shielding the internal organs. Conversely, CTDI$_{vol}$ underestimates organ dose to small patients because more of the incident x-rays reach the internal organs. There are several methods to correct these dose estimates by incorporating patient size information.[28]

The DLP is often used to estimate overall effective dose to the patient through the use of multiplicative conversion k factors derived by Monte Carlo simulations.[24,29] In this approach the DLP for a particular anatomic region is multiplied by the k factor derived for the same anatomic region to arrive at an estimated effective dose in millisieverts (mSv). Effective dose is a single number intended to reflect the uniform whole-body exposure that would be expected to produce the same overall risk of radiation-induced cancer as the partial-body exposure of the CT scan. It is calculated as a weighted sum of the absorbed doses to the exposed organs, where the weighting factors depend on the relative sensitivity of the organs to developing radiation-induced cancer. However, effective dose has substantial limitations in accuracy when applied to individual patients because the weighting factors used represent population averages and do not incorporate the known dependence of radiation sensitivity on age or sex.[30] Further, the commonly used k-factor method assumes a "typical" size patient and does not incorporate the substantial impact of patient size.[31]

Review CTDI$_{vol}$ and DLP on Every Scan

Current CT scanners have the ability to produce a "patient protocol" or "dose report screen capture" and to include these as a separate series in each examination. Although formats and content vary between manufacturers and scanner models, all at minimum contain the CTDI$_{vol}$ and DLP. Some contain additional scan parameters, and some specify whether the 16-cm head phantom or the 32-cm body phantom is used for the reporting.

California has recently enacted legislation to require inclusion of such information in the radiology report,[32] and other regulatory efforts are under way.[33] Regardless of reporting practices or requirements, however, it is crucially important for radiologists to review the CTDI$_{vol}$ and DLP for every scan they interpret. This allows radiologists to gain familiarity with typical values and to develop a sense of how these metrics ought to vary with patient size. Identification of outliers is important for quality control efforts to direct CT protocol modifications or to target technologist interventions as needed. In addition, diagnostic reference levels are becoming more commonplace and represent recommended values of CTDI$_{vol}$ or DLP expected to be adequate for diagnostic-quality examinations in the majority of patients (to be exceeded only in the largest of patients).[34,35] Radiologists, technologists, and medical physicists should all have a sense of how their scans compare to these reference values.

■ REDUCING RADIATION EXPOSURE: DURING THE SCAN

During the scan the key intervention is to design dose-optimized CT protocols that find the sweet spot of the lowest exposure appropriate for the particular clinical scenario, while still providing a robust, diagnostic-quality examination. These measures are the primary focus of this chapter.

■ CT PROTOCOL STRATEGIES TO REDUCE RADIATION EXPOSURE

Once the decision has been made to perform a CT scan, there are many available strategies to reduce radiation exposure.[36,37]

Use Size-Dependent Protocols

CT images are created from the small fraction of incident x-rays that successfully pass through the body and reach the detector array, with image noise varying as the square root of the x-ray flux. Large patients absorb more of the incident x-rays than small patients, so in order to maintain the desired image quality, greater x-ray tube output is needed in large patients compared to small patients. As a result, CT protocols should vary technique according to the size of the patient. The pediatric radiology community was the leader in the

concept of "child-sizing" CT protocols to avoid excessive pediatric exposures, but the general principle holds for adult patients as well, and many methods exist to rationally adjust scan parameters to patient size.[38,39]

Understand and Enable Scanner Dose-Reduction Tools

The most widely available and most important method to adjust CT technique for patient size is automated tube current modulation (TCM), also called dose modulation. TCM techniques adjust the x-ray tube output to the patient's anatomy to maintain a desired level of image quality, as shown in Figure 1-1.[40,41] In longitudinal or z-axis TCM the x-ray tube output is varied along the z-axis (from head to foot) of the patient, with greater mAs used in areas with more tissue to traverse, such as the shoulders or the pelvis, and lower mAs used in regions containing less attenuating material, such as the lungs.

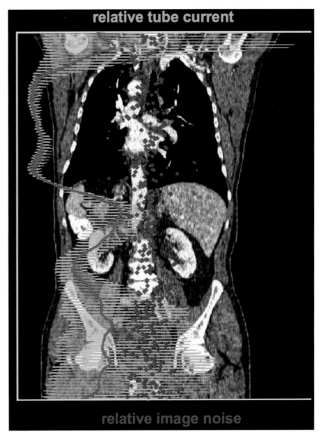

Figure 1-1 Tube-current modulation schemes adjust the x-ray tube output *(green)* as a function of position to maintain a desired image quality, in this case a relatively constant level of image noise *(red)*. Longitudinal tube current modulation (TCM) *(thick green line)* adjusts x-ray flux along the craniocaudal z-axis. Note the lower tube current through the lungs, compared to the more attenuating shoulders and pelvis. Axial or in-plane TCM adjusts tube current as the gantry rotates around the patient *(light green line)*. Note the much greater tube current required to penetrate through the shoulders in a lateral versus a frontal projection. (Modified from Kalendar WE. *Computed tomography*. 3rd ed. Erglangen, Germany: Publicis Publishing; 2011; with permission.)

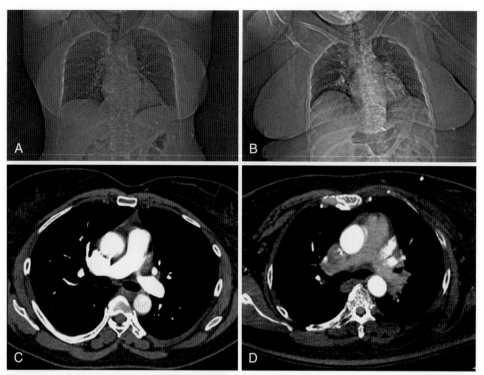

Figure 1-2 Clinical effect of automatic tube current modulation (CareDose4D, Siemens AS+ scanner; Forscheim, Germany). A 180-pound patient (**A**) underwent a CT pulmonary angiogram (**C**), and a 325-pound patient (**B**) underwent a dissection CT angiogram (**D**), both with the same kVp of 120 and quality reference mAs value of 200 (but with different contrast timing delays for the different clinical indications). For the smaller patient the average effective mAs was automatically adjusted to 276, for a $CTDI_{vol}$ of 18.7 mGy, whereas for the larger patient the average effective mAs was adjusted to 628, for a $CTDI_{vol}$ of 42.4 mGy. To maintain comparable image quality for both patients, automatic tube current modulation appropriately varied the x-ray tube output by a factor of 2.3 between the two patients. (Reprinted with permission from Elsevier from Sodickson A. Strategies for reducing radiation exposure in multi-detector row CT. *Radiol Clin North Am.* 2012;50(1):1-14.)

Axial or in-plane modulation adjusts the x-ray tube output as the gantry rotates around the patient, typically increasing mAs for lateral projections, where there is more tissue to penetrate, and decreasing mAs for frontal projections, where there is less tissue to penetrate. Depending on the manufacturer, this in-plane mAs variation can be derived using orthogonal scout views or using heuristic estimation methods from a single scout view, or it can be derived "online" using the angular variation of attenuation observed during the previous gantry rotation to determine the mAs variation during the next rotation.

Electrocardiographic-modulation TCM schemes are used for cardiac-gated scans, in which the x-ray tube output is substantially decreased or eliminated during portions of the cardiac cycle where data are not needed. Typically, full x-ray tube output is used during the relatively motion-free diastolic portion of the cardiac cycle and is decreased during the more motion-prone systolic portion of the cardiac cycle.

Appropriate use of automatic TCM results in substantial decreases in $CTDI_{vol}$ and DLP for smaller patients as compared to larger patients. Large patients require more x-ray tube output to yield enough x-rays passing all the way through the patient to reach the detectors and create a diagnostic-quality scan. Figure 1-2 shows an example of the clinical effects of TCM.

For scans of the abdomen and pelvis, $CTDI_{vol}$ varies severalfold between the largest and smallest adult patients. However, as illustrated in the schematic of Figure 1-3, the actual patient doses vary by a smaller factor because of the shielding effect of the soft tissues.[26,42] Additional techniques are needed to size-correct the $CTDI_{vol}$ to obtain reasonably accurate patient doses.[28,43]

It is important to understand manufacturer-specific TCM methodology and configuration parameters to ensure appropriate and expected functionality. All of the CT manufacturers use either one or two CT projection radiographs (named the *scout, surview, scanogram,* or *topogram* depending on the manufacturer) to plan the TCM by measuring the patient's attenuation as a function of position. All approaches allow the user to select a desired level of image quality as a starting point, but the image quality metric varies by manufacturer. This may be a selectable sample image containing the desired level of image noise, or it may be a quality reference mAs value, where an increased value produces higher radiation exposure and an overall reduction in image noise. Alternatively, it may be a noise index (which roughly equates to the standard deviation of a region of interest expected in a water phantom of similar overall attenuation as the patient), in which case an increased value has the reverse effect of increased image noise by virtue of lower radiation exposure. If the noise index is used, it is important to understand how radiation exposure will vary if reconstructed slice thickness or reconstruction kernel is changed in the protocol, because some

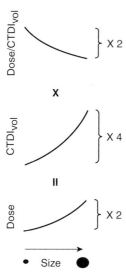

Figure 1-3 Schematic representation of x-ray tube output and organ dose as a function of patient size, for a typical range of adult sizes during abdomen/pelvis scans. *Top,* For a given x-ray tube output $CTDI_{vol}$, internal organ doses decrease with increasing patient size because of shielding effects. However *(middle)*, appropriately used automatic tube current modulation schemes adjust $CTDI_{vol}$ to patient size to maintain desired image quality. The result *(bottom)* of these competing geometric factors is that organ doses are larger for larger patients, but to a lesser degree than the raw $CTDI_{vol}$ values would predict. (From Sodickson A, Turner AC, McGlamery K, et al. Variation in organ dose from abdomen-pelvis CT exams performed with tube current modulation: evaluation of patient size effects. Radiographic Society of North America 2010 annual meeting; Chicago, IL; with permission.)

scanner models increase exposure when thinner image reconstructions or sharper reconstruction kernels are planned. There is also substantial variability between manufacturers in how radiation exposure is adjusted to the size of the patient. Some scanners strive to maintain the desired level of image noise until a predefined maximum milliampere (mA) is reached, whereas others permit somewhat greater image noise in large patients to blunt the degree of the radiation dose increase as patient size increases.

Because the implementation details of the CT manufacturers' TCM schemes are quite varied, it is vitally important that radiologists, technologists, and medical physicists be well educated about the exact operations of their particular scanners' TCM methods to realize the desired dose-saving and image-quality benefits. If used incorrectly—such as by selecting an inappropriate image quality constraint—these techniques can paradoxically result in undesired and inappropriate increases to patient dose. This is thought to have played a role in some of the recent high-profile medical errors in CT perfusion for stroke.[44]

Reduce the Number of Passes

It is important to critically examine the value of each pass in a given CT protocol. For example, for routine contrast-enhanced scans of the abdomen and pelvis for undifferentiated abdominal pain, many practices have historically performed additional pyelographic phase scans of the kidneys and bladder with the rationale that

they provide additional "free" information. Although some radiologists have anecdotally discovered a small number of incidental transitional cell carcinomas, these additional exposures through the kidneys and bladder each typically add approximately 30% of the dose of the full abdomen/pelvis scan (because each covers approximately 30% of the full scan range), resulting in a combined 60% dose increase for very low incremental clinical yield. These extra passes should be eliminated in routine use unless there is a compelling clinical reason to keep them in a particular case.

The development of rapid multidetector scanners in the mid-1990s led to a proliferation of multiphase CT applications incorporating imaging at different time points during intravenous (IV) contrast administration to provide additional information about the enhancement characteristics of certain organs or lesions. Depending on the specific clinical question, it is often possible in these protocols to eliminate or at least substantially reduce radiation exposure of one or more of the phases, such as an initial noncontrast or a delayed postcontrast phase. In protocols for mesenteric ischemia or gastrointestinal bleeding, for example, some might argue to eliminate the noncontrast phase, thereby diverting this additional radiation exposure. The relatively recent advent of dual-energy CT systems creates another opportunity to eliminate the noncontrast pass in certain multiphase applications by allowing virtual noncontrast images to replace the original noncontrast acquisition.[45,46]

In certain circumstances it may also be possible to combine different contrast phases. For example, CT urography may be performed with a split-bolus technique, in which a portion of the IV contrast is administered and allowed enough time to pass into the renal collecting system before the remainder of the contrast is administered with usual nephrographic phase timing, resulting in combined nephrographic and excretory phase imaging from one rather than two CT exposures.[47]

One of the highest-dose examinations common in the ED is for aortic dissection. Traditional aortic dissection CT angiography (CTA) examinations often include three passes. First is a noncontrast scan of the chest to assess for intramural hematoma by demonstrating crescentic peripheral high attenuation against the less-dense blood pool. This is often followed by a cardiac-gated contrast-enhanced CTA scan of the chest, which is then followed by a delayed scan of the chest, abdomen, and pelvis to assess for branch vessel involvement. Although this approach was designed to answer all possible questions about the aorta, and thus makes sense for complex aortas, it is worth reconsidering the approach for emergency department use.

In an ED setting, dissection CTA may be considered a "screening" examination, typically performed to exclude a low pretest probability of this potentially fatal condition. As a result, the yield for acute aortic dissection is often quite low (on the order of 1% to 2% at our institution). Of the positive scans with acute findings, very few demonstrate isolated intramural hematoma without a visible intimal flap. In addition, these are often tachycardic patients in whom cardiac gating works poorly but typically results in a higher dose than a nongated scan.

As a result, we have adopted the imaging algorithm for aortic dissection shown in Figure 1-4. The vast majority of patients have a nongated contrast-enhanced CT angiogram of the chest alone. Elimination of the initial noncontrast chest scan and of the delayed scan through the chest, abdomen, and pelvis yields typical dose savings exceeding 75% compared to the gold-standard approach.

In this algorithm a multipass protocol may be performed for patients with a high pretest probability of disease, such as those with known aortic dissection and concern for extension. However, the vast majority of patients in the low pretest probability category have the single-pass protocol including a nongated chest CTA scan. If this scan is normal, the workup ends. If dissection is present, the scan is extended through the abdomen and pelvis to assess visceral extension. In our practice, an emergency radiologist is available 24 hours a day 7 days a week to monitor these scans live at our ED CT scanner, which allows this decision to be made instantaneously during real-time monitoring of the scan, so that the extended scan range can be included with the same contrast injection. In a different practice model where a radiologist is not immediately available to make this decision, the scan may be extended through the abdomen and pelvis or the patient may be subsequently reinjected with a small amount of additional contrast material to assess distal extent of dissection.

If the single-pass protocol is indeterminate, additional steps may be taken depending on the cause of the indeterminate result. If crescentic peripheral soft tissue along the wall of the aorta raises concern for isolated intramural hematoma without a defined intimal flap, a delayed postcontrast chest CT scan may be performed 5 to 10 minutes later, after the iodine has cleared the circulating blood pool, as demonstrated in Figure 1-4. In general, aortic root pulsation artifact can be readily differentiated from aortic root dissection, but in cases where it is truly impossible to differentiate, or where there is concern for a type A dissection extending into the coronary arteries, a repeat injection may be performed for cardiac-gated chest CTA.

Reduce Duplicate Coverage

When scanning adjacent body regions, there is often substantial overlap in coverage regions, which results in unnecessary additional radiation exposure. In the example of Figure 1-5 a patient undergoing a trauma "pan-scan" has substantial coverage overlap between the head and cervical spine scans, the cervical spine and chest scans, and the chest and abdomen/pelvis scans.

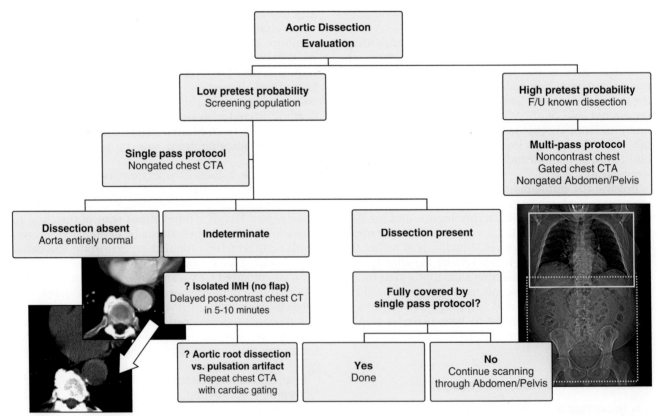

Figure 1-4 Dose-reducing aortic dissection imaging algorithm. Most patients undergo the single-pass protocol, with negative results. If dissection is present during real-time monitoring, the scan is immediately extended through the abdomen and pelvis to assess distal extent (*dotted box on planning topogram at right*). Any concern for isolated intramural hematoma (IMH) prompts a delayed postcontrast scan (*images at left*). Pulsation artifact can typically be differentiated from type A dissection, but if needed, a repeat injection of intravenous contrast could theoretically be performed. (Modified with permission from Elsevier from Sodickson A. Strategies for reducing radiation exposure in multi-detector row CT. *Radiol Clin North Am.* 2012;50(1):1-14.)

It should be understood that there is also additional unseen overlap due to z-overscanning, in which the CT scanner exposes an additional area above and below the prescribed range to acquire enough data to reconstruct the top and bottom images. This additional exposure can be substantial but can be significantly reduced on some newer scanners equipped with adaptive collimation systems that minimize the unnecessary additional irradiation.[48]

These areas of prescribed duplicate coverage may be greatly reduced with technologist training or eliminated entirely with combined protocols that image adjacent body regions with a single helical acquisition. The greatest overlap typically occurs between the chest and the abdomen/pelvis scans because chest scans traditionally extend below the posterior costophrenic sulci or adrenal glands, and abdominal scans typically extend above the diaphragm, often with an additional buffer to ensure full scan coverage. In the trauma setting it is often not necessary to image this overlap region twice. A simple improvement is to instruct the technologists to end the chest scan above the diaphragm, with only enough overlap to ensure complete coverage. Another solution is to perform adjacent scan parts in a single continuous acquisition, although in this situation care must be taken to ensure timing for the appropriate phase of contrast.[49,50] For example, a portal venous phase is most commonly used to detect solid abdominal organ injuries, whereas an earlier arterial phase is preferable to assess aortic injury in the chest. With rapid scanners a single-pass acquisition may thus require a compromise in scan timing or a larger bolus of IV contrast.

Reduce mAs when Possible

Image noise requirements and thus radiation exposure requirements depend on the diagnostic task at hand and the clinical question to be answered. It is possible to tolerate increased levels of image noise when assessing intrinsically high-contrast structures, where the tissue or pathologic condition of interest is of substantially different attenuation than the surrounding structures. Evaluation of the lung, CTA, and renal stones are the prototypical examples where reduced mAs may be used, allowing the radiologist to differentiate a high-density structure of interest from the background despite an increase in image noise. Conversely, low-dose imaging may be quite detrimental in inherently "low-contrast" applications such as liver lesion detection, in which the attenuation of the target abnormality is similar to that of the background.

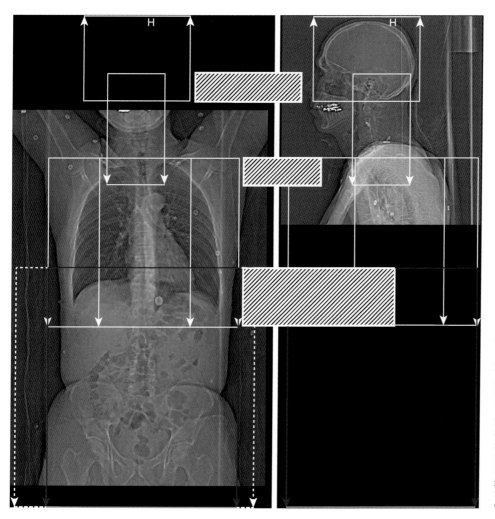

Figure 1-5 Overlap between adjacent scan regions in a trauma "pan-scan" of the head, cervical spine, chest, abdomen, and pelvis. Thin-line boxes denote separately prescribed scan parts, with cross-hatched regions indicating areas of overlap that may be reduced with technologist directives or protocol modifications that combine adjacent parts into a single scan. (Reprinted with permission from Elsevier from Sodickson A. Strategies for reducing radiation exposure in multi-detector row CT. *Radiol Clin North Am.* 2012;50(1):1-14.)

Pulmonary nodules stand out against the background air-filled lungs, so scans performed specifically for this reason may be performed at substantially lower dose than those designed for detailed assessment of mediastinal soft tissues. In CTA, successful IV contrast administration creates high-density vascular enhancement against a soft tissue or air background. In ureter CT, high-density renal stones are easy to visualize against the soft tissue density background even at a greatly reduced dose.[51] However, it is important to clearly define the scope of the desired scan. We have not tremendously reduced the mAs in our routine ED ureter CT scans because it is not uncommon to find alternate diagnoses accounting for symptoms when no stones are found.

As a general strategy, practices may systematically reduce dose by incrementally decreasing mAs for select protocols or clinical indications in order to gradually approach the threshold above which diagnostic confidence is maintained despite noisier images. In seeking the lower end of this comfort zone, incremental 10% to 20% reductions in mAs are reasonable step sizes because these will result in relatively minor increases in image noise on the order of 5% to 10%.

Optimize Intravenous Contrast Infusions

Any intervention that increases the inherent contrast-to-noise ratio between the target and the background can enable further x-ray tube output reduction by offsetting the increased noise with an increase in the inherent image contrast. For vascular examinations, careful attention to optimizing IV contrast infusion parameters[52] may routinely increase vascular enhancement, thus increasing the inherent contrast-to-noise ratio and enabling subsequent reduction in x-ray tube output.

Reduce kVp for CTA

Iodine attenuates lower-energy x-rays far more strongly than higher-energy x-rays, resulting in higher Hounsfield units at lower kVp for the same underlying concentration of iodine, as shown in Figure 1-6. At the same time, lowering kVp substantially reduces radiation exposure if mAs is unchanged. This combination of increased enhancement at lower dose is an ideal synergy for contrast-enhanced CTA examinations, and in

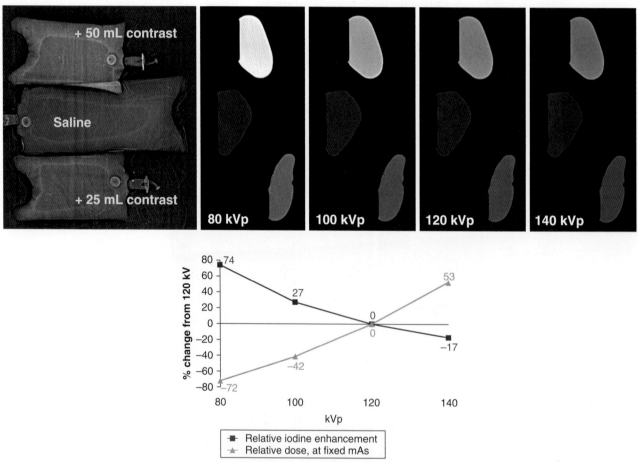

Figure 1-6 Impact of reducing kVp in vascular examinations. *Top left,* A homemade phantom consisting of a central bag of saline and two peripheral bags of saline containing different iodine concentrations. *Top right,* Images were obtained with fixed mAs at different kVp values from 80 to 140 on a Siemens Sensation 64 scanner. The graph at bottom shows relative iodine enhancement *(red line)* at each kVp and relative changes in CTDI$_{vol}$; *orange line,* normalized to the values at 120 kVp. For vascular examinations in small enough patients, lowering kVp increases iodine enhancement while decreasing dose. (Reprinted with permission from Elsevier from Sodickson A. Strategies for reducing radiation exposure in multi-detector row CT. *Radiol Clin North Am.* 2012;50(1):1-14.)

patients who are small enough, may be used to improve image quality, to reduce radiation exposure, to reduce administered IV contrast volume, or any combination of the three.[53]

Figure 1-7 demonstrates the use of these methods to optimize CT pulmonary angiograms. We used an approximate size threshold of 175 pounds, below which we used 100 kVp and a reduced volume and flow rate of IV contrast material.[53] To maintain constant image noise, one would technically need to increase x-ray tube output (mAs) at lower kVp because a greater fraction of the lower-energy x-rays is absorbed. However, we instead left our TCM reference mAs unchanged and tolerated the associated increase in image noise in these scans, relying on the kVp reduction to preserve or increase vascular enhancement despite a concurrent reduction in total IV contrast volume.

It is important to note that low kVp imaging should not be performed indiscriminately for patients of all sizes because the increase in image noise is simply too great in very large patients. Attempting to correct for this noise increase by increasing mAs is only possible to a point because inherent engineering system limits come into play in the form of a maximum achievable x-ray

tube current mA. When performing CTA examinations with reduced kVp, approximate size thresholds are thus needed and will depend on the scanner capabilities. This threshold may be chosen based on patient weight or body mass index, physical dimensions, or measures of patient attenuation.[54,55] A recent new development is automated selection of kVp by the CT scanner based on the topogram-measured attenuation of the patient (analogous to TCM of mAs values), which has the advantage of directly detecting patient attenuation and adjusting the CT technique to maintain an image quality criterion of choice while ensuring that fundamental CT system limits are respected.[56,57]

External Shielding—Should It Be Used?

A common question is whether bismuth breast shields should be used to reduce dose to these relatively radiation-sensitive organs. Proponents point to substantive dose reductions to the breast from use of overlying shields, whereas opponents argue that the shields introduce noise and artifacts, and that similar dose reductions and image quality can be achieved by lowering the

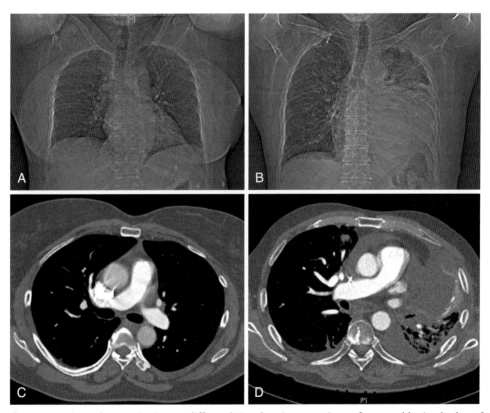

Figure 1-7 CT pulmonary angiography examinations at different kVp values in two patients of comparable size, both performed using automated tube current modulation (TCM; Care Dose4D) with reference mAs of 200 on a Siemens AS+ scanner. Patient in **A** and **C** was scanned at 120 kVp using an intravenous (IV) contrast infusion of 75 mL iopromide 370 (Bayer, Berlin, Germany) at 5 mL/sec, followed by a 40-mL saline flush at 5 mL/sec. Patient in **B** and **D** was scanned at 100 kVp using an IV contrast infusion of 50 mL iopromide 370 at 4 mL/sec, followed by a 40 mL saline flush at 4 mL/sec. Automated tube current modulation detects similar attenuation for both patients, resulting in an average effective mAs of 276 for **C** and 272 for **D**. However, the decrease to 100 kVp results in a 42% reduction in CTDI$_{vol}$ from 18.6 to 10.7 mGy. Although **D** is slightly noisier than **C**, image quality remains excellent despite the 33% decrease in administered IV contrast. These high-flow-rate contrast infusions work well for breath-hold scan durations less than 9 to 10 seconds but require accurate triggering at the beginning of the contrast-enhancement curve—we use automated bolus tracking with a region of interest in the main pulmonary artery and a trigger value of 80 HU above unenhanced blood. (Reprinted with permission from Elsevier from Sodickson A. Strategies for reducing radiation exposure in multi-detector row CT. *Radiol Clin North Am.* 2012;50(1):1-14.)

overall scan mAs. For these reasons the American Association of Physicists in Medicine recommends against their use.[58] Nonetheless, if overlying shields are used, it is vitally important to use them correctly. The shields must be placed after the planning scout views. Because all manufacturers use the scout images to plan TCM, placement of shields before the scouts causes the scanner to compensate by increasing x-ray output to penetrate the additional detected attenuation. For the same reason, shields should not be used on scanners with real-time adjustments of the axial TCM because this too will result in an undesired increase in exposure to the patient.

Special Considerations in Trauma Imaging

Trauma CT imaging can impart substantial dose to the patient[59] because of the combined effects of large anatomic coverage (often head through pelvis or greater), frequent use of multiphase imaging in the abdomen and pelvis, and often substantial overlap between adjacent scan parts. Nonetheless, many of the strategies outlined earlier can be applied to trauma imaging.

Size-dependent CT protocols including automated TCM should be incorporated into trauma scanning. The arms should be raised whenever possible during torso imaging because this accomplishes improved image quality and lower radiation dose by removing unwanted attenuating material from the scan region.[60]

Reducing the number of passes can be accomplished by reserving delayed imaging of the abdomen and pelvis to only those patients in whom traumatic intra-abdominal injury is identified on the initial pass. These delayed passes add no value in the absence of injury. This approach is practical only in settings where a radiologist is available to oversee trauma scans in real time.

Reducing duplicate coverage can in some situations be accomplished by combining adjacent scan regions into a single scan, if attention is paid to optimizing the combined technique with an eye toward both radiation dose and image quality. To address the most substantial area of overlap between the chest and the abdomen, there has recently been a growing effort to develop novel multiphasic IV contrast infusions that enable combined arterial and portal venous phase scanning in a single CT pass through the chest, abdomen, and pelvis.[61] This approach may work well in trauma imaging to screen patients with a relatively low probability of solid organ injury but is likely not optimal for high-risk patients, who benefit from both arterial and portal venous phase scanning.[62]

Reducing mAs (by lowering reference mAs or raising noise index) may be incorporated particularly when multiple passes are used in the abdomen and pelvis. Some practices maximize image quality during a single phase of scanning—typically the portal venous phase—but tolerate more noise on additional phases, including arterial imaging of high-contrast vascular structures or delayed passes primarily intended to detect changes in configuration of extravasated contrast material. Reduced kVp should also be considered for arterial phase imaging in nonobese patients to maximize conspicuity of vascular structures despite lower radiation dose.

■ REDUCING RADIATION EXPOSURE: AFTER THE SCAN

Postprocessing Methods to Decrease Noise

There are a variety of postprocessing methods that can be used to reduce image noise. These methods can be used to improve image quality for a given acquisition. Conversely, the scans may be performed with reduced radiation exposure and postprocessing techniques used to lower image noise back to desired levels, assuming the postprocessed images are considered of adequate quality when judged on features beyond simply noise levels. In this way these postprocessing methods may be used in synergy with the acquisition strategies listed earlier.

Reconstruct With Smoother Kernels

Use of smoother kernels reduces image noise, as in the noticeable difference between images reconstructed using a soft tissue algorithm versus a bone algorithm. The inevitable tradeoff is in the loss of fine edge detail. Nonetheless, this may be a helpful strategy to salvage noisy images such as those obtained in obese patients.[63]

Reconstruct at Larger Slice Thickness

Image noise is proportional to the square root of the number of x-rays contributing to image creation. Because the number of x-rays scales with slice thickness, image noise is thus proportional to the square root of the slice thickness, if all other parameters are unchanged in image acquisition and reconstruction. For this reason, 1-mm thick images will contain twice as much noise as 4-mm thick images if reconstructed from the same raw data and with the same reconstruction algorithm. One should thus use caution in moving to thinner and thinner slices if they are not truly needed for the diagnostic task at hand.

Iterative Reconstruction

There has been substantive recent effort from all the major CT manufacturers to develop a class of advanced postprocessing methods loosely grouped under the name *iterative reconstruction*.[64-67] Theoretically, iterative reconstruction transforms back and forth between the raw data "projection-space" and the image domain with successive steps of filtered back projection (converting raw data to images) and forward projection (converting images back to raw data). During each iteration the newly simulated raw data are compared to the acquired raw data, and nonlinear processing is used to correct differences related to image noise and artifacts, until a close-enough match is achieved.

However, because this theoretical approach would require tremendous computer processing power, most manufacturers have implemented more rapid shortcut algorithms designed to achieve similar ends. Implementation details vary between manufacturers but generally involve a variety of algorithms to shift some of the iterative "correction steps" into the raw data or image domains, combined with advanced modeling of the CT acquisition system and nonlinear image filtering to reduce noise in homogeneous regions while attempting to preserve anatomic edge information.

The somewhat different noise texture of the resultant images may require some acclimatization on the part of radiologists. However, if resultant image quality is deemed satisfactory, the noise-reduction effect may enable substantial reductions in radiation dose.

AFTER THE SCAN: CAPTURING AND MONITORING RADIATION DOSES

The commonly available dose-screen reports are helpful for scan-by-scan monitoring but are not routinely database accessible for large-scale quality improvement and dose-monitoring efforts.[68] Ongoing implementations of standardized Digital Imaging and Communication in Medicine (DICOM) radiation dose structured reports (DICOM RDSR)[69] promise to help these efforts prospectively after widespread adoption. In the meantime, efforts are underway to extract patient- and examination-specific exposure information through other means from historical examinations available on PACS.[70-72]

Combining the magnitudes of recorded radiation exposure metrics with knowledge of the anatomic region scanned and of the size of the patient will ultimately enable patient-centric longitudinal dose monitoring and radiation risk estimation. Integration of this information into the electronic medical record or incorporation into point-of-care decision support tools may ultimately prove beneficial in risk-benefit decision making and in improving understanding of the magnitude of risk by both physicians and patients.

SUMMARY

Many tools and strategies exist to enable reduction of radiation exposure from CT. Available hardware and software tools continue to evolve, and it is vitally important to learn exactly what tools are available on one's CT system and how to configure these tools properly to achieve safe and effective results. Numerous CT protocol optimization strategies have been outlined, which may be used in synergy with one another and with the available technology to create robust, high-quality CT protocols with radiation exposure appropriate for the clinical setting and the size of the patient. Successful implementation requires primary engagement of the radiologist, ideally in collaboration with CT manufacturers, CT technologists, and medical physicists.

References

1. IMV Medical Information Division. *Benchmark Report CT 2007*. Des Plaines, IL: IMV Medical Information Division; 2007.
2. Brenner DJ, Hall EJ. Computed tomography—an increasing source of radiation exposure. *N Engl J Med*. 2007;357(22):2277-2284.
3. Sodickson A, Baeyens PF, Andriole KP, et al. Recurrent CT, cumulative radiation exposure, and associated radiation-induced cancer risks from CT of adults. *Radiology*. 2009;251(1):175-184.
4. Berrington de Gonzalez A, Mahesh M, Kim KP, et al. Projected cancer risks from computed tomographic scans performed in the United States in 2007. *Arch Intern Med*. 2009;169(22):2071-2077.
5. Mettler FA, Bhargavan M, Faulkner K, et al. Radiologic and nuclear medicine studies in the United States and worldwide: frequency, radiation dose, and comparison with other radiation sources—1950-2007. *Radiology*. 2009;253(2):520-531.
6. Fazel R, Krumholz HM, Wang Y, et al. Exposure to low-dose ionizing radiation from medical imaging procedures. *N Engl J Med*. 2009;361(9): 849-857.
7. Zondervan RL, Hahn PF, Sadow CA, et al. Body CT scanning in young adults: examination indications, patient outcomes, and risk of radiation-induced cancer. *Radiology*. 2013;267(2):460-469.
8. Amis ES, Butler PF, Applegate KE, et al. American College of Radiology white paper on radiation dose in medicine. *J Am Coll Radiol*. 2007;4(5):272-284.
9. Wells PS, Anderson DR, Rodger M, et al. Excluding pulmonary embolism at the bedside without diagnostic imaging: management of patients with suspected pulmonary embolism presenting to the emergency department by using a simple clinical model and d-dimer. *Ann Intern Med*. 2001;135(2): 98-107.
10. Stiell IG, Wells GA, Vandemheen K, et al. The Canadian CT head rule for patients with minor head injury. *Lancet*. 2001;357(9266):1391-1396.
11. Stiell IG, Wells GA, Vandemheen KL, et al. The Canadian C-spine rule for radiography in alert and stable trauma patients. *JAMA*. 2001;286(15): 1841.
12. Khorasani R. Can radiology professional society guidelines be converted to effective decision support? *J Am Coll Radiol*. 2010;7(8):561-562.
13. American College of Radiology. *ACR Appropriateness Criteria*. http://www.acr.org/secondarymainmenucategories/quality_safety/app_criteria.aspx. Accessed June 8, 2011.
14. Raja AS, Ip IK, Prevedello LM, et al. Effect of computerized clinical decision support on the use and yield of CT pulmonary angiography in the emergency department. *Radiology*. 2012;262(2):468-474.
15. Griffey RT, Sodickson A. Cumulative radiation exposure and cancer risk estimates in emergency department patients undergoing repeat or multiple CT. *AJR Am J Roentgenol*. 2009;192(4):887-892.
16. Birnbaum S. Radiation safety in the era of helical CT: a patient-based protection program currently in place in two community hospitals in New Hampshire. *J Am Coll Radiol*. 2008;5(6):714-718.e5.
17. Wasser EJ, Prevedello LM, Sodickson A, et al. Impact of a real-time computerized duplicate alert system on the utilization of computed tomography. *JAMA Intern Med*. 2013;173(11):1024-1026.
18. Sodickson A, Opraseuth J, Ledbetter S. Outside imaging in emergency department transfer patients: CD import reduces rates of subsequent imaging utilization. *Radiology*. 2011;260(2):408-413.
19. Flanagan PT, Relyea-Chew A, Gross JA, et al. Using the Internet for image transfer in a regional trauma network: effect on CT repeat rate, cost, and radiation exposure. *J Am Coll Radiol*. 2012;9(9):648-656.
20. Lu MT, Tellis WM, Fidelman N, et al. Reducing the rate of repeat imaging: import of outside images to PACS. *AJR Am J Roentgenol*. 2012;198(3): 628-634.
21. Massachusetts Medical Society. *Investigation of defensive medicine in Massachusetts*. www.massmed.org/defensivemedicine. Published 2008. Accessed September 9, 2011.
22. Levin DC, Rao VM. The effect of self-referral on utilization of advanced diagnostic imaging. *AJR Am J Roentgenol*. 2011;196(4):848-852.
23. McNitt-Gray MF. AAPM/RSNA physics tutorial for residents: topics in CT. Radiation dose in CT. *Radiographics*. 2002;22(6):1541-1553.
24. American Association of Physicists in Medicine. *The Measurement, Reporting and Management of Radiation Dose in CT. Report 96. AAPM Task Group 23 of the Diagnostic Imaging Council of CT Committee*. College Park, MD: American Association of Physicists in Medicine; 2008.
25. McCollough CH, Leng S, Yu L, et al. CT dose index and patient dose: they are not the same thing. *Radiology*. 2011;259(2):311-316.
26. Turner AC, Zhang D, Khatonabadi M, et al. The feasibility of patient size-corrected, scanner-independent organ dose estimates for abdominal CT exams. *Med Phys*. 2011;38(2):820-829.
27. Huda W, Vance A. Patient radiation doses from adult and pediatric CT. *AJR Am J Roentgenol*. 2007;188(2):540.
28. *American Association of Physicists in Medicine Report 204: Size-Specific Dose Estimates (SSDE) in Pediatric and Adult Body CT Examinations*. College Park, MD: American Association of Physicists in Medicine; 2011.
29. Shrimpton P. Assessment of patient dose in CT. National Radiological Protection Board PE/1/2004. Chilton, UK. http://www.msct.eu/PDF_FILES/Appendix%20paediatric%20CT%20Dosimetry.pdf. Published 2004. Accessed March 29, 2013.

30. National Research Council (U.S.). *Committee to Assess Health Risks From Exposure to Low Level of Ionizing Radiation. Health Risks From Exposure to Low Levels of Ionizing Radiation: BEIR VII, Phase 2.* Washington, DC: National Academies Press; 2006.

31. McCollough CH, Christner JA, Kofler JM. How effective is effective dose as a predictor of radiation risk? *AJR Am J Roentgenol.* 2010;194(4):890–896.

32. Padilla A, Alquist EK. California Senate Bill 1237. http://www.leginfo.ca.gov/pub/09-10/bill/sen/sb_1201-1250/sb_1237_bill_20100929_chaptered.html. Published 2010. Accessed February 25, 2014.

33. Center for Drug Evaluation and Research. Radiation Dose Reduction. *White paper: initiative to reduce unnecessary radiation exposure from medical imaging.* http://www.fda.gov/Radiation-EmittingProducts/RadiationSafety/RadiationDoseReduction/ucm199994.htm. Accessed December 24, 2010.

34. Bongartz G, Golding SJ, Jurik AG, et al. *European Guidelines for Multislice Computed Tomography.* http://www.msct.eu/CT_Quality_Criteria.htm. Published March 2004. Accessed June 8, 2011.

35. The American College of Radiology. *ACR Practice Guideline for Diagnostic Reference Levels in Medical X-ray Imaging.* www.acr.org/SecondaryMainMenuCategories/quality_safety/guidelines/med_phys/reference_levels.aspx. Published 2008. Accessed September 9, 2011.

36. Kalra MK, Maher MM, Toth TL, et al. Strategies for CT radiation dose optimization. *Radiology.* 2004;230(3):619.

37. McCollough CH, Primak AN, Braun N, et al. Strategies for reducing radiation dose in CT. *Radiol Clin North Am.* 2009;47(1):27–40.

38. The Alliance for Radiation Safety in Pediatric Imaging. Image gently. http://www.pedrad.org/associations/5364/ig/index.cfm?page=614. Accessed May 26, 2011.

39. Strauss KJ, Goske MJ, Kaste SC, et al. Image gently: ten steps you can take to optimize image quality and lower CT dose for pediatric patients. *AJR Am J Roentgenol.* 2010;194(4):868.

40. Kalendar WA. *Computed Tomography.* ed 3 Erlangen, Germany: Publicis Publishing; 2011.

41. McCollough CH, Bruesewitz MR, Kofler JM. CT dose reduction and dose management tools: overview of available options. *Radiographics.* 2006;26(2):503–512.

42. Sodickson A, Turner AC, McGlamery K, et al. Variation in organ dose from abdomen-pelvis CT exams performed with tube current modulation (TCM): evaluation of patient size effects. Scientific abstract at: Radiographic Society of North America 2010 annual meeting; November 28-December 3, 2010; Chicago, IL.

43. Israel GM, Cicchiello L, Brink J, et al. Patient size and radiation exposure in thoracic, pelvic, and abdominal CT examinations performed with automatic exposure control. *AJR Am J Roentgenol.* 2010;195(6):1342.

44. FDA. Safety investigation of CT brain perfusion scans: update 11/9/2010. http://www.fda.gov/medicaldevices/safety/alertsandnotices/ucm185898.htm. Accessed June 6, 2011.

45. Chandarana H, Godoy MCB, Vlahos I, et al. Abdominal aorta: evaluation with dual-source dual-energy multidetector CT after endovascular repair of aneurysms—initial observations. *Radiology.* 2008;249(2):692–700.

46. Vlahos I, Godoy MCB, Naidich DP. Dual-energy computed tomography imaging of the aorta. *J Thorac Imaging.* 2010;25(4):289–300.

47. Chow LC, Kwan SW, Olcott EW, et al. Split-bolus MDCT urography with synchronous nephrographic and excretory phase enhancement. *AJR Am J Roentgenol.* 2007;189(2):314.

48. Deak PD, Langner O, Lell M, et al. Effects of adaptive section collimation on patient radiation dose in multisection spiral CT. *Radiology.* 2009;252(1):140.

49. Ptak T, Rhea JT, Novelline RA. Radiation dose is reduced with a single-pass whole-body multi-detector row CT trauma protocol compared with a conventional segmented method: initial experience. *Radiology.* 2003;229(3):902.

50. Nguyen D, Platon A, Shanmuganathan K, et al. Evaluation of a single-pass continuous whole-body 16-MDCT protocol for patients with polytrauma. *AJR Am J Roentgenol.* 2009;192(1):3.

51. Poletti PA, Platon A, Rutschmann OT, et al. Low-dose versus standard-dose CT protocol in patients with clinically suspected renal colic. *AJR Am J Roentgenol.* 2007;188(4):927.

52. Bae KT. Intravenous contrast medium administration and scan timing at CT: considerations and approaches. *Radiology.* 2010;256(1):32.

53. Sodickson A, Weiss M. Effects of patient size on radiation dose reduction and image quality in low-kVp CT pulmonary angiography performed with reduced IV contrast dose. *Emerg Radiol.* 2012;19(5):437–445.

54. Menke J. Comparison of different body size parameters for individual dose adaptation in body CT of adults. *Radiology.* 2005;236(2):565.

55. Luaces M, Akers S, Litt H. Low kVp imaging for dose reduction in dual-source cardiac CT. *Int J Cardiovasc Imaging.* 2009;25(S2):165–175.

56. Grant K, Schmidt B. CARE kV: Automated dose-optimized selection of x-ray tube voltage. White paper. Siemens. http://www.medical.siemens.com/siemens/en_US/gg_ct_FBAs/files/Case_Studies/CarekV_White_Paper.pdf. Published 2011. Accessed September 9, 2011.

57. Yu L, Li H, Fletcher JG, et al. Automatic selection of tube potential for radiation dose reduction in CT: a general strategy. *Med Phys.* 2010;37(1):234–243.

58. AAPM position statement on the use of bismuth shielding for the purpose of dose reduction in CT scanning. http://www.aapm.org/publicgeneral/BismuthShielding.pdf. Published 2012. Accessed February 25, 2014

59. Winslow JE, Hinshaw JW, Hughes MJ, et al. Quantitative assessment of diagnostic radiation doses in adult blunt trauma patients. *Ann Emerg Med.* 2008;52(2):93–97.

60. Brink M, de Lange F, Oostveen LJ, et al. Arm raising at exposure-controlled multidetector trauma CT of thoracoabdominal region: higher image quality, lower radiation dose. *Radiology.* 2008;249(2):661–670.

61. Loupatatzis C, Schindera S, Gralla J, et al. Whole-body computed tomography for multiple traumas using a triphasic injection protocol. *Eur Radiol.* 2008;18(6):1206–1214.

62. Boscak AR, Shanmuganathan K, Mirvis SE, et al. Optimizing trauma multidetector CT protocol for blunt splenic injury: need for arterial and portal venous phase scans. *Radiology.* 2013;268(1):79–88.

63. Modica MJ, Kanal KM, Gunn ML. The obese emergency patient: imaging challenges and solutions. *Radiographics.* 2011;31(3):811–823.

64. Thibault, Jean-Baptiste. Veo: CT model-based iterative reconstruction. http://www.gehealthcare.com/dose/pdfs/Veo_white_paper.pdf. Accessed December 21, 2012.

65. Siemens. SAFIRE: Sinogram Affirmed Iterative Reconstruction. https://www.medical.siemens.com/siemens/en_INT/gg_ct_FBAs/files/brochures/SAFIRE_Brochure.pdf. Accessed December 21, 2012.

66. Irwan R, Nakanishi S, Blum A. AIDR 3D: Reduces dose and simultaneously improves image quality. http://www.toshiba-medical.eu/upload/TMSE_CT/White%20Papers/White%20Papers/Toshiba_White%20paper%20CT_nov 11.pdf. Accessed December 21, 2012.

67. Philips. iDose4 iterative reconstruction technique. http://www.healthcare.philips.com/pwc_hc/main/shared/Assets/Documents/ct/idose_white_paper_452296267841.pdf. Accessed December 21, 2012.

68. Sodickson A, Khorasani R. Patient-centric radiation dose monitoring in the electronic health record: what are some of the barriers and key next steps? *J Am Coll Radiol.* 2010;7(10):752–753.

69. Digital Imaging and Communication in Medicine (DICOM) Supplement 127: CT radiation dose reporting (dose SR). DICOM Standards Committee. ftp://medical.nema.org/medical/dicom/final/sup127_ft.pdf. Published 2007. Accessed February 25, 2014

70. Cook TS, Zimmerman SL, Steingall SR, et al. Informatics in radiology: RADIANCE: an automated, enterprise-wide solution for archiving and reporting CT radiation dose estimates. *Radiographics.* 2011;31(7):1833–1846.

71. Sodickson A, Warden GI, Farkas CE, et al. Exposing exposure: automated anatomy-specific CT radiation exposure extraction for quality assurance and radiation monitoring. *Radiology.* 2012;264(2):397–405.

72. Shih G, Lu ZF, Zabih R, et al. Automated framework for digital radiation dose index reporting from CT dose reports. *AJR Am J Roentgenol.* 2011;197(5):1170–1174.

CHAPTER **2**

Image Management in Emergency Radiology

Martin L. Gunn and Jeffrey D. Robinson

■ BACKGROUND

Imaging of Patients at Outside Facilities Before Transfer

Early and timely transfer of injured patients to a trauma center capable of definitive care has been shown to decrease mortality. Although long-standing national guidelines from the American College of Surgeons Committee on Trauma recommend simple clinical parameters and radiography to identify patients who benefit from transfer to a Level I or II trauma center, these are not uniformly followed. In fact, in one large study over 50% of severely injured patients received computed tomography (CT) scans before transfer from an outlying hospital. The use of CT in this group was not found to increase morbidity or mortality. The exact reason for noncompliance with these national guidelines is unclear. Concerns about medicolegal liability, expectations of the receiving institutions, a desire by the sending physician to establish a diagnosis before transfer, and local cultural and insurance status have been postulated as reasons.

With such a large proportion of patients receiving outside imaging, access to, and management of, outside images and outside reports by the receiving hospital has become an important issue for emergency departments (EDs) and emergency radiology providers.

Repeat Imaging at the Receiving Hospital

A large proportion of outside imaging is repeated when trauma patients transfer to a major trauma center. Repeat CT rates at the receiving hospital vary, but most studies have found a repeat rate approaching 60%, resulting in an overall repeat imaging cost of almost $3000 per patient. Factors associated with an increased rate of repeat imaging include higher injury severity score, longer stay at the outside hospital, and inability to access the outside imaging. Inadequacy of outside examinations, inability to upload to a picture archiving and communication system (PACS), and "administrative reasons" have all been used to justify repeat imaging. Repeating outside imaging also increases radiation exposure but has not been found to improve patient outcomes.

Techniques Used to Transfer Images Between Facilities

Compact Discs

Traditionally, images were transferred between facilities by sending "hard copy film": sending either radiographs or printed cross-sectional images with the patient. Presently, the most common transmission method is using CDs. In a recent national survey, 67% of facilities reported that a substantial majority of outside imaging studies arrived via CD. However, several problems complicate the use of CDs for image transfer. The images can only arrive with the patient, precluding teleconsultation when transfer decisions are based on imaging findings. Patients who undergo CT at an outside facility have been found to have an average of 90 minutes longer length of stay before transfer. Part of this delay may be due to the time taken to "burn" the CD before transfer. Once the patient and CD arrive, some institutions may be unable, or unwilling, to upload the outside CDs to their PACS system due to incompatibility or concerns about security. In addition, viewing CDs using the poor or unfamiliar navigation tools that are included with the images may be time consuming. Moreover, CDs may be lost in transit.

When outside CDs can be uploaded to a receiving institution's PACS, the rate of repeat diagnostic imaging can be reduced. In a study by Sodickson et al, the implementation of a CD importation process and PACS uploading software resulted in a 17% reduction in the rate of subsequent diagnostic imaging (including a 16% reduction in CT) within 24 hours of the importation attempt. Similar results have been found by others. Incompatible CD storage formats have caused PACS uploading problems in the past, but it appears that this is becoming less of a problem, perhaps due to a wide variety of CD-upload software programs that have recently become available. Conformance with the Portable Data for Imaging framework of the Integrating the Healthcare Enterprise (IHE) consortium may contribute to the decrease in incompatibility.

Electronic Image Transfer

Electronic transfer of ED patient images is not a new concept. One of the earliest scientific reports dates back to 1990, when a telephone link was used to transfer CT images of the head. In this study the number of patients ultimately transferred was reduced by 43%. However, in recent years there has been a rapid rise in the use of Internet-based technologies for remote viewing and interpretation of emergency radiologic images. These technologies are ideally suited for image transfer for emergency patients because they offer several potential benefits, as outlined in Box 2-1. These include the ability to send images before, during, or after patient transfer, greater compatibility with the recipient hospital's PACS system than CDs or film, ability to resend further images after a patient arrives, easier sharing of outside radiology reports, and transfer of images and reports from the tertiary care center back to the community for future reference.

The IHE consortium has implemented a framework for the electronic exchange of health care information between health care providers. The framework dedicated to image and report exchange is the Cross-Enterprise Document Sharing for Imaging (XDS-I).

Ways to Share Images Electronically

As storage, PACS, network, and image-sharing architecture continue to evolve, several different interrelated formats have emerged that provide new ways to share images for transferring patients.

Picture Archiving and Communication Systems With Vendor Neutral Archives

Recent advances in PACS architecture allow some PACS systems to access images that may originate on more than one archive. A vendor neutral archive (VNA) acts as single large storage archive for images that may come from several different PACS vendors or sources. Storage and indexing of these images uses nonproprietary formats. This archive can be accessed by radiologists and physicians using viewers from any number of PACS vendors. This archive may be sited locally or in the "cloud" (i.e., a data center that is located remotely and accessed via the Internet). Health care organizations with multiple sites of practice are ideally suited to the use of VNAs. Images and reports from one site are available across the organization, allowing for seamless transfer and access to radiologic images and medical records. However, because image sharing is at the organizational level, true image sharing for most regional trauma systems is not fully supported.

Virtual Private Networks

A virtual private network (VPN) is a way of connecting two separate computer networks together across the Internet. Usually a VPN is established as a point-to-point connection using encryption. It appears as a private network link to the users. In the ED transfer patient setting, Digital Imaging and Communication in Medicine (DICOM) images from one PACS system (or even a CT or magnetic resonance scanner) in one location are "pushed" down a VPN Internet "tunnel" to another site, arriving at the recipient hospital. Images may then be manually registered and uploaded to the receiving hospital's PACS system. Most VPN systems involve agreements between individual hospitals, forming a hub-and-spoke infrastructure (Fig. 2-1). This format generally limits the ability to query a remote PACS for images and prevents two nonhub hospitals from sharing images without passing them through the hub.

Cross-Enterprise Document Sharing for Images

Properly implemented, XDS-I.b is a standards-based approach that is a scalable means for multiple institutions across a large geographic region (also known as an *XDS-I affinity domain*) to share radiologic images and reports for emergency patients. The essentials of an XDS-I system are summarized in Figure 2-2. The XDS registry forms the fundamental component of this system. An XDS registry catalogs information about the images and reports available at the various connected PACS/radiology information system (RIS) systems across the

---

Box 2-1   Potential Benefits of Electronic Image Sharing for Emergency Radiology

Ability to Send Images Before or During Patient Transfer
- Potential to reduce unnecessary patient transfers where management decisions are based on radiologic findings
- Access to subspecialty image interpretations
- Receiving hospital can fully assess the nature of injuries before the patient arrives and appropriately mobilize resources (surgeons, operating rooms, interventional radiologists)
- Avoiding transfer delays while images are burned to CD

Simple Transfer of Outside Images to Receiving Hospital's Picture Archiving and Communication System
- Low risk of incompatible images
- Hospital-wide concurrent viewing of images by multiple clinical services
- Familiar viewing and navigation tools for outside imaging studies
- Reduced rate of repeat imaging at the receiving facility

Ability to Resend Images After Patient Arrives
- Ability to perform retrospective reconstruction of multiplanar reformats, volume-rendered images, or thin-section images by the outside facility as requested by the receiving hospital after the patient arrives, for diagnostic clarification or surgical planning
- Limited potential for images to get "lost" compared to CD or printed film

Sharing of Outside Image Reports, with the Potential for Real-Time Updates
- Reduced potential for report discrepancies and medicolegal risk
- Supports quality improvement initiatives

Transfer of Tertiary Referral Center Images to Community Hospital
- Baseline imaging available to community hospital for comparison and follow-up

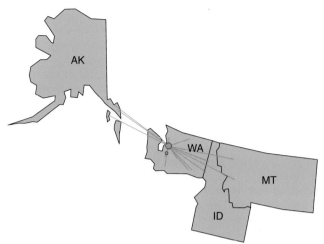

Figure 2-1 Regional image transfer in the Pacific Northwest. Map (not to scale) of a four-state region showing image part of the image transfer network. This network uses a hub-and-spoke approach, with unidirectional image "pushes" to the central hub *(large orange circle)* at Harborview Medical Center in Seattle. However, because some multisite practices participate in this network, they can route images from their outlying clinics via their own network to Seattle even if there is no direct connection between Seattle and the clinic. An example of this smaller hub is shown south of Seattle.

network. The registry stores patient demographics and information ("metadata") about the images and reports (e.g., imaging procedure type, modality, date, anatomic region) but does not store images or reports. The registry is connected to all consumers and sources of images. XDS sources or repositories are the locations where the images are stored, which could be a number of radiology department PACS databases, cloud storage, VNAs, or a combination of these. A hospital receiving a trauma patient in transfer (in the role of a consumer) can query the XDS registry, find the images at the outside facility, and either view them using a Web PACS viewer or initiate image transfer to the receiving hospital. This "federated" approach for image storage has several advantages. It is easily scalable, can support image query, retrieve, and image "push," and with proper security, facilitates transfer of images between any two sites on the affinity domain.

Cloud-Based Image Sharing
Over the last decade, several commercially available systems have emerged that use large external data centers (cloud storage) to store radiologic images. The architecture of these systems varies considerably. These systems may support image transfer and uploading (from PACS, modalities, or CDs) to the cloud by either patients or radiology departments and transfer of images to

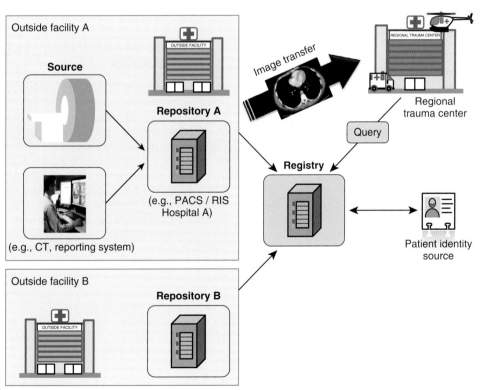

Figure 2-2 Use of the Integrating the Healthcare Enterprise (IHE) cross-enterprise document sharing model for image exchange. Images and reports are generated (e.g., by computed tomography [CT] scanners, voice recognition software) and saved locally on a document "repository" (in most cases, this is a picture archiving and communication system [PACS] archive). Catalog information ("metadata") about the study is stored centrally on a Cross-Enterprise Document Sharing for Imaging (XDS-I) registry. Consumers (e.g., a regional trauma center) can query this registry to determine what images and documents are available within the region, and if sufficient privileges are obtained, retrieve images from the repository at one of many participating outside facilities. In this example the images are transferred from "Outside facility A" to the "Regional Trauma Center." A patient identity source may be connected to the registry to match up images and documents with the correct patient across many repositories.

another facility connected to the cloud. Access to the system is usually via a Web interface. Some systems support normalization of outside patient demographics and imaging data using automated routing rules, simplifying image storage in the receiving hospital system's PACS archive by using local formats and accession numbers. Most vendors charge by the volume of transferred images and a small subscription fee.

■ PROBLEM SOLVING: REMAINING COMPLIANT WITH INFORMATION SECURITY STANDARDS

The Health Information Technology for Economic and Clinical Health (HITECH) Act was passed in 2009 as part of the American Recovery and Reinvestment Act. This act promotes the electronic exchange of patient information to improve the quality of health care and is a component of Medicare incentives ("meaningful use"). The HITECH Act also strengthened the privacy and security regulations of the Health Insurance Portability and Accountability Act of 1996. Whenever images are stored and transferred, federal regulations specify the security and privacy standards that should be implemented. Although these standards (and interpretation of these standards) are evolving, it is vital to recognize that electronic information sharing must comply with the Federal Information Processing Standards.

■ PROBLEM SOLVING: WORK-FLOW CHALLENGES WITH OUTSIDE IMAGES

Unfortunately, often patients arrive at a tertiary hospital's ED with images but no outside report. A survey of American Society of Emergency Radiology (ASER) members in 2011 by Robinson and McNeeley found that of 91% of respondents whose sites receive transfer patients, more than half of all transferred studies were not accompanied by an outside report, and when an outside report was available, more than half of respondents stated that 75% of them were unsigned preliminary reports. Limited access to outside reports causes both work-flow and potential medicolegal challenges. Many trauma centers offer abbreviated informal ("curbstone" or "curbside") opinions for outside imaging, and in some cases formal second opinion interpretations are also offered.

■ PITFALL: INFORMAL CONSULTATIONS

Informal consultations between physicians usually go undocumented or are only briefly documented in the medical record. The medicolegal implications of these abbreviated outside image interpretations are unclear. However, it is generally believed that in most cases when a radiologist reviews an outside imaging study he or she establishes a physician-patient relationship. If a radiologist's opinion leads to clinical decision making, the radiologist may be legally responsible for the decisions that are made. Lack of accurate documentation poses the greatest problem for the radiologist: when there is

no documentation, the radiologist's opinion may be inaccurately recollected at a later time, or even worse the radiologist's opinion may be misrepresented in the medical record by the consulting physician.

The risk of harm with informal consultations might be greater for outside image interpretations than local studies for several reasons. First, the quality of the outside study might be below that of the receiving hospital's standard. Second, the images may be reviewed on film or using unfamiliar viewing software, and this review might be brief. Third, two differing interpretations of a single study might be generated (one each from the sending facility and the receiving facility). This risk is compounded when outside reports are unavailable or in preliminary status.

■ PITFALL: DISCREPANCIES BETWEEN OUTSIDE INTERPRETATIONS AND RECEIVING HOSPITAL INTERPRETATIONS

Two studies evaluating imaging reports of transferred patients found the discrepancy rate between the sending and receiving facilities to be about 12%. The clinical impact of these discrepancies has not been evaluated, but in the study by Sung et al these discrepancies resulted in a judged upgrade in clinical severity in 30%, a downgrade in 44%, and no change in 26%. The majority (70%) of discrepancies were interpretive rather than observational.

■ OUTSIDE IMAGE INTERPRETATION: THE PROCESS

At our facility, physicians are offered a formal second opinion report whenever a patient is transferred to our ED with outside imaging that has no final outside report or when we have a significant discrepancy with an outside report. In all cases we make a considerable effort to obtain any outside interpretations that are available, usually by phoning the outside facility and requesting a facsimile. However, because of the speed with which decisions must be made and the fact that many patients transfer in the evening and overnight, second-opinion formal interpretations are made before a final outside interpretation is available. The second-opinion reports are complete reports, provided after careful review of the entire study. They are available on the PACS, RIS, and electronic medical record systems throughout our enterprise. In order to seek reimbursement from the Centers for Medicare and Medicaid Services (CMS) and other insurers, we use structured reports that contain the components shown in Table 2-1.

Reimbursement of Outside Image Interpretation

Although local carrier approaches will differ, professional fee reimbursement can be obtained for indicated outside image interpretations from both CMS and private insurers provided adequate documentation is submitted. In the study by Jeffers et al approximately 70%

Table 2-1 Components of an Outside Imaging Report

Component of Report	Description or Component
Justification	Reason why the image interpretation was requested by the referring physician
Outside report	Whether an outside final, preliminary, or no outside report was available at the time of review
Image acquisition details	Where and when the study was acquired
Clinical indication	Indication for the outside study
Technique/procedure	Description of the scan range, phases, image reconstruction technique, number of views (radiographs), use of intravenous or oral contrast administration
Image quality	Description of any limitations of the outside study compared to a local study
Findings	Same format as local radiology study
Impression	Same format as local radiology report
Discrepancy	Whether the outside facility's report (if available) differs from our hospital's interpretation, with a list of the discrepancies
(Communication)	If necessary, a record of how the findings were conveyed by the radiologist to the requesting physician

of submitted claims were reimbursed on initial submission in Boston, Massachusetts. Claims are usually submitted using the same Current Procedural Terminology (CPT) code that would be used for the same examination performed locally, but with a -26 (professional services only) modifier. A -77 modifier (repeat service by another physician) may be necessary in some situations. At present there is no means to claim the technical component for local image processing (e.g., reformatting) of studies obtained at outside facilities. Three-dimensional reformations generated on the in-house workstation, however, can be submitted.

■ SUMMARY

Liberal use of CDs and Internet-based image exchange technologies is recommended to avoid the delays, costs, and radiation exposure associated with repeat imaging when patients transfer between facilities. When outside images are reviewed at the receiving hospital, radiologists should consider issuing formal, written interpretations. At present, when there is demonstrable medical necessity, reimbursement can be obtained for these reports.

Selected Reading

Berlin L. Curbstone consultations. *AJR Am J Roentgenol.* 2002;178(6):1353–1359. http://dx.doi.org/10.2214/ajr.178.6.1781353.

Berlin L. Curbstone consultations. *AJR Am J Roentgenol.* 2011;197(1):W191. http://dx.doi.org/10.2214/AJR.10.5499.

Boland GW. The impact of teleradiology in the United States over the last decade: driving consolidation and commoditization of radiologists and radiology services. *Clin Radiol.* 2009;64(5):457–460. http://dx.doi.org/10.1016/j.crad.2008.11.010. discussion 461-452.

Celso B, Tepas J, Langland-Orban B, et al. A systematic review and meta-analysis comparing outcome of severely injured patients treated in trauma centers following the establishment of trauma systems. *J Trauma.* 2006;60(2):371–378. http://dx.doi.org/10.1097/01.ta.0000197916.99629.eb. discussion 378.

Clunie D. Portable Data for Imaging Framework. from http://www.ihe.net/Technical_Framework/index.cfm#radiology; 2009.

Emick DM, Carey TS, Charles AG, et al. Repeat imaging in trauma transfers: a retrospective analysis of computed tomography scans repeated upon arrival to a Level I trauma center. *J Trauma Acute Care Surg.* 2012;72(5):1255–1262. http://dx.doi.org/10.1097/TA.0b013e3182452b6f.

Flanagan PT, Relyea-Chew A, Gross JA, et al. Using the Internet for image transfer in a regional trauma network: effect on CT repeat rate, cost, and radiation exposure. *J Am Coll Radiol.* 2012;9(9):648–656. http://dx.doi.org/10.1016/j.jacr.2012.04.014.

Gupta R, Greer SE, Martin ED. Inefficiencies in a rural trauma system: the burden of repeat imaging in interfacility transfers. *J Trauma.* 2010;69(2):253–255. http://dx.doi.org/10.1097/TA.0b013e3181e4d579.

Haley T, Ghaemmaghami V, Loftus T, et al. Trauma: the impact of repeat imaging. *Am J Surg.* 2009;198(6):858–862. http://dx.doi.org/10.1016/j.amjsurg.2009.05.030.

Integrating the Healthcare Enterprise. Cross-enterprise Document Sharing for Imaging. Retrieved 3/6/2013, from http://wiki.ihe.net/index.php?title=Cross-enterprise_Document_Sharing_for_Imaging; 2013.

Jeffers AB, Saghir A, Camacho M. Formal reporting of second-opinion CT interpretation: experience and reimbursement in the emergency department setting. *Emerg Radiol.* 2012;19(3):187–193. http://dx.doi.org/10.1007/s10140-011-1016-x.

Kalia V, Carrino JA, Macura KJ. Policies and procedures for reviewing medical images from portable media: survey of radiology departments. *J Am Coll Radiol.* 2011;8(1):39–48. http://dx.doi.org/10.1016/j.jacr.2010.07.007.

Lee T, Latham J, Kerr RS, et al. Effect of a new computed tomographic image transfer system on management of referrals to a regional neurosurgical service. *Lancet.* 1990;336(8707):101–103.

Lu MT, Tellis WM, Fidelman N, et al. Reducing the rate of repeat imaging: import of outside images to PACS. *AJR Am J Roentgenol.* 2012;198(3):628–634. http://dx.doi.org/10.2214/AJR.11.6890.

MacKenzie EJ, Rivara FP, Jurkovich GJ, et al. A national evaluation of the effect of trauma-center care on mortality. *N Engl J Med.* 2006;354(4):366–378. http://dx.doi.org/10.1056/NEJMsa052049.

McNeeley MF, Gunn ML, Robinson JD. Transfer patient imaging: current status, review of the literature, and the Harborview experience. *J Am Coll Radiol.* 2013. http://dx.doi.org/10.1016/j.jacr.2012.09.031.

Mohan D, Barnato AE, Angus DC, et al. Determinants of compliance with transfer guidelines for trauma patients: a retrospective analysis of CT scans acquired prior to transfer to a Level I trauma center. *Ann Surg.* 2010;251(5):946–951. http://dx.doi.org/10.1097/SLA.0b013e3181d76cb5.

National Institute of Standards and Technology. (2010, 3/11/2013). Information Technology Laboratory Homepage. Retrieved 3/21/2013, 2013, from http://www.nist.gov/itl/

Onzuka J, Worster A, McCreadie B. Is computerized tomography of trauma patients associated with a transfer delay to a regional trauma centre? *CJEM.* 2008;10(3):205–208.

Prior F, Ingeholm ML, Levine BA, et al. Potential impact of HITECH security regulations on medical imaging. *Conf Proc IEEE Eng Med Biol Soc.* 2009:2157–2160. http://dx.doi.org/10.1109/IEMBS.2009.5332507.

Robinson JD, McNeeley MF. Transfer patient imaging: a survey of members of the American Society of Emergency Radiology. *Emerg Radiol.* 2012;19(5):447–454. http://dx.doi.org/10.1007/s10140-012-1047-y.

Sodickson A, Opraseuth J, Ledbetter S. Outside imaging in emergency department transfer patients: CD import reduces rates of subsequent imaging utilization. *Radiology.* 2011;260(2):408–413. http://dx.doi.org/10.1148/radiol.11101956.

Sung JC, Sodickson A, Ledbetter S. Outside CT imaging among emergency department transfer patients. *J Am Coll Radiol.* 2009;6(9):626–632. http://dx.doi.org/10.1016/j.jacr.2009.04.010.

CRANIOCEREBRAL ORBITAL-MAXILLO-FACIAL EMERGENCIES

CHAPTER **3**

Craniocerebral Trauma

Traumatic Brain Injury

Monique Anne Meyer
and Wayne S. Kubal

Traumatic brain injury (TBI) occurs when an external mechanical force results in tissue and cellular damage within the brain that may lead to permanent or temporary impairment of cognitive, physical, or psychosocial functions and a diminished or altered state of consciousness. There are two types of TBI: closed and penetrating. Closed TBI is an injury to the brain caused by movement of the brain within the skull. Causes may include falls, a motor vehicle crash, or being struck by or with an object. Penetrating TBI is an injury to the brain caused by a foreign object entering the skull. Causes may include firearm injuries or being struck with a sharp object. The simplest form of TBI is concussion, which may be defined as transient impairment of neurologic function with or without loss of consciousness occurring at the time of injury. About 75% of TBIs that occur each year are concussions or other forms of mild TBI.

TBI is one of the leading causes of disability and death in the Western world. According to the Centers for Disease Control and Prevention's (CDC's) report *Traumatic Brain Injury in the United States: Emergency Department Visits, Hospitalizations, and Deaths, 2002-2006*, it has been estimated that at least 1.7 million people sustain a TBI in the United States per year. Of those individuals, about 52,000 die, 275,000 are hospitalized, and 1.365 million are treated and released from the emergency department (ED). The number of people with TBI who are not seen in a hospital or ED or who receive no care is unknown. TBI is a contributing factor to a third (30.5%) of all injury-related deaths in the United States.

The CDC data reveal that the leading causes of TBI are falls (35.2%), motor vehicle accidents (17.3%), collisions with moving or stationary objects (16.5%), and assaults (10%). Falls cause half (50%) of the TBIs among children ages 0 to 14 years and 61% of all TBIs among adults ages 65 years and older. Among all age-groups, motor vehicle crashes and traffic-related incidents were the second leading cause of TBI (17.3%) and resulted in the largest percentage of TBI-related deaths (31.8%). In every age-group, TBI rates are higher for males than for females with males ages 0 to 4 years having the highest rates of TBI-related ED visits, hospitalizations, and deaths.

TBI is heterogeneous in terms of pathophysiology, clinical presentation, and outcome, with case fatality rates ranging from less than 1% in mild TBI and up to 40% in severe TBI. A large proportion of patients with moderate to severe TBI are young adults; consequently, these patients often face decades of disability, with associated emotional, social, and financial difficulties. Approximately 5.3 million Americans are living with a TBI-related disability.

A severe TBI not only affects the life of an individual and his or her family, but it also has a large societal and economic toll. The estimated economic cost of TBI in 2010, including direct and indirect medical costs, is estimated to be approximately $76.5 billion. The cost of fatal TBIs and TBIs requiring hospitalization, many of which are severe, account for approximately 90% of the total of TBI medical care costs.

The mortality from TBI is related to the severity of brain injury as determined by the Glasgow Coma Scale (GCS). The GCS is used to provide a uniform approach to the clinical assessment of patients with acute head trauma and is the most frequently used means of grading the severity of injury within 48 hours. GCS is the sum of three components: eye opening, motor response, and verbal response. Persons with a GCS score of 3 to 8 are classified with a severe TBI, those with scores of 9 to 12 are classified with a moderate TBI, and those with scores of 13 to 15 are classified with a mild TBI (Box 3-1).

Patients with TBI have also been classified into mild, moderate, and severe grades by the Brain Injury Interdisciplinary Special Interest Group of the American Congress of Rehabilitation Medicine based on a period of loss of consciousness, loss of memory for events immediately before or after the trauma, changes in mental status, and focal neurologic deficits. Mild head injury is defined as a traumatically induced physiologic disruption of brain function manifested by one of the following: any period of loss of consciousness; any loss of memory for events immediately before or after the accident; any alteration in mental state at the time of the accident (e.g., feeling dazed, disoriented, confused); or focal neurologic deficits, which may or may not be transient. However, the severity of the injury does not exceed the following: loss of consciousness of 30 minutes; after 30 minutes, an initial GCS score of 13 to 15; and posttraumatic amnesia not greater than 24 hours. Additional criteria for defining mild TBI include GCS score greater than 12; no abnormalities on computed tomography (CT) scan; no operative lesions; and length of hospital stay less than 48 hours. Moderate TBI is defined as length of stay at least 48 hours, GCS score of

Box 3-1 Glasgow Coma Scale

The Glasgow Coma Scale (GCS) defines the severity of a traumatic brain injury (TBI) within 48 hours of injury.

Eye Opening
- Spontaneous = 4
- To speech = 3
- To painful stimulation = 2
- No response = 1

Motor Response
- Follows commands = 6
- Makes localizing movements to pain = 5
- Makes withdrawal movements to pain = 4
- Flexor (decorticate) posturing to pain = 3
- Extensor (decerebrate) posturing to pain = 2
- No response = 1

Verbal Response
- Oriented to person, place, and date = 5
- Converses but is disoriented = 4
- Says inappropriate words = 3
- Says incomprehensible sounds = 2
- No response = 1
  The severity of TBI according to the GCS score (within 48 hours) is as follows:
- Severe TBI = 3-8
- Moderate TBI = 9-12
- Mild TBI = 13-15

9 to 12, operative intracranial lesion, and abnormal CT findings. Severe TBI is usually self-evident at the time of presentation.

■ IMAGING MODALITIES

The goals of emergency imaging of TBI are to allow life-threatening injuries to be rapidly diagnosed and treated, to explain the findings on neurologic examination, and to establish a prognosis for the patient.

Computed Tomography

Noncontrast CT is the first imaging test performed in the ED setting for the evaluation of head trauma. The goal of emergency imaging is to depict lesions that need emergency neurosurgical treatment or that may alter therapy. When trauma is evaluated with CT, images are reviewed in brain, subdural, and bone settings at the workstation. Wide window settings aid in separating high-density blood from the high density of bone. Bone windows aid in the evaluation of fractures. Coronal and sagittal reformatted images should be provided to increase accuracy of interpretation and decrease misses.

CT perfusion allows the noninvasive evaluation of tissue perfusion. CT perfusion is performed by continuous scanning of a single slice or contiguous slices after the administration of iodinated contrast. The passage of the contrast bolus through the brain is analyzed to measure the time to peak density, the mean transit time,

the cerebral blood volume, and the cerebral blood flow. CT perfusion can provide prognostic information about patients with severe TBI but is not widely used in the setting of acute TBI.

Magnetic Resonance Imaging

Magnetic resonance imaging (MRI) is reserved for showing lesions that could explain clinical symptoms and signs that are not explained by prior CT or to help define abnormalities seen on CT. Due to its superior contrast resolution for soft tissues, MRI is far more sensitive than CT in detecting all the different stages of hemorrhage, diffuse axonal injury (DAI), and ischemia. Standard sequences such as T1 weighted, T2 weighted, and fluid-attenuated inversion recovery (FLAIR) are usually performed as part of the examination. Detecting acute subarachnoid hemorrhage (SAH) is difficult if FLAIR imaging is not performed. The absence of beam-hardening artifact with MRI enables better visualization of the inferior frontal and temporal lobes and posterior fossa.

Gradient-recalled echo (GRE) sequences are especially sensitive to multiple blood breakdown products and are capable of depicting areas of microhemorrhage not well depicted on CT. Susceptibility-weighted imaging (SWI) is a high-spatial-resolution three-dimensional (3-D) gradient-echo magnetic resonance (MR) technique involving phase postprocessing that accentuates the paramagnetic properties of blood products such as deoxyhemoglobin, intracellular methemoglobin, and hemosiderin. When this technique is used, a mask is created to enhance the phase differences between susceptibility artifacts and surrounding tissues. The contrast-to-noise ratio is optimized by multiplying the mask and magnitude images. A minimal-intensity projection is created to facilitate differentiation between veins and focal lesion. The phase images are sensitive for depiction of regions of local alteration of the magnetic field (i.e., susceptibility) caused by various substances, such as hemorrhage and iron and other metals. SWI is three to six times more sensitive than conventional GRE sequences for the detection of small hemorrhages in DAI. A potential pitfall in SWI interpretation is that the signal intensity of veins depends on blood oxygenation. Veins are hypointense compared to arteries. The magnetic properties of intravascular deoxygenated hemoglobin and the resultant phase differences with adjacent tissues cause signal loss. To prevent misregistration of vessel versus focal lesions, the thickness of the minimal-intensity projection should be adjusted to the brain size to minimize partial volume effects, particularly in neonates.

Perfusion MRI methods exploit signal intensity changes that occur with the passage of a gadolinium-based contrast agent. As the contrast agent passes in high concentration through the microvasculature, susceptibility-induced T2 relation occurs in the surrounding tissues, which is seen as a decrease in signal intensity. The decrease in signal intensity is assumed to be linearly related to the concentration of gadolinium-based contrast agent in the microvasculature. The changes in the signal intensity of the tissues are quantitatively related to the local concentration of gadolinium-based contrast agent and are converted into a curve of concentration versus time. By applying tracer kinetics to the concentration-time curve of the first passage of the bolus of contrast agent, relative cerebral blood volume and cerebral blood flow maps are calculated.

The use of diffusion-weighted imaging (DWI) and diffusion tensor imaging (DTI) in assessment of patients with TBI is widely gaining acceptance. DWI is based on the random motion of water molecules, also known as *brownian motion*. This motion is affected by the intrinsic speed of water displacement depending upon the tissue properties and type (i.e., gray matter, white matter, cerebral spinal fluid [CSF]). DWI can detect changes in the rate of microscopic water motion. Water molecules within the ventricles diffuse freely, whereas water molecules within the cells have their diffusion restricted. Water molecules within the extracellular space have an intermediate diffusion. When there is movement of water from the extracellular space to the intracellular space, the overall diffusion within that volume of tissue becomes more restricted. This restricted diffusion correlates with cytotoxic edema and allows for the early detection of ischemic changes.

Apparent diffusion coefficient (ADC) is a measure of diffusion. This measure has been used as an indicator of edema. Recently it has been shown that the use of mean ADC in the whole brain is the best predictor of outcome among all degrees of TBI.

DTI incorporates pulsed magnetic field gradients into a standard MRI sequence that characterizes the local diffusivity (the magnitude of diffusion) of water. The fiber structure of the central nervous system can be evaluated using DTI by observing restricted water diffusion. In healthy white matter there is greater diffusion along the long axis of the axonal bundles than along the radial axis because of hindrance from the myelin sheath. Two key measures associated with water diffusion are diffusivity and anisotropy (the direction of water diffusion). DTI is based on the fact that microscopic water diffusion in white matter tracts tends to occur in one direction rather than randomly, which is termed *anisotropy*. The degree of anisotropy in a white matter region can be viewed as a reflection of the degree of structural integrity of white matter. A number of different measures of anisotropy can be used; one of the more commonly used is fractional anisotropy. Fractional anisotropy is sensitive to changes in white matter integrity and provides pertinent information regarding the degree of white matter damage, including factors such as myelin sheath thickness and axonal membrane integrity. Given that white matter damage is a predominant feature in TBI, there is a resultant decrease in fractional anisotropy values in severe TBI.

MR spectroscopy (MRS) allows the chemical environment of the brain to be examined noninvasively. The metabolites detected by MRS are sensitive to hypoxia, energy dysfunction, neuronal injury, membrane turnover, and inflammation. MRS localization techniques can be divided into single voxel and multivoxels. The most common brain metabolites that are measured with proton (^{1}H) MRS include *N*-acetyl aspartate (NAA), creatine (Cr), choline (Cho), glutamate, lactate, and myoinositol. Water-suppressed localized proton MRS of the brain can be performed at long or short echo times. At long echo times the human brain reveals four major resonances: a peak at 3.2 ppm, arising mainly from tetramethylamines, especially choline-containing phospholipids; a peak at 3.0 ppm, arising from Cr, either alone or as phosphocreatine; a peak at 2.0 ppm, arising from *N*-acetyl groups, especially NAA; and a doublet peak at 1.3 ppm arising from the methyl resonance of lactate, which is normally barely visible above baseline. NAA, an amino acid synthesized in mitochondria, is a neuronal and axonal marker that decreases with neuronal loss or dysfunction. Cr is a marker for intact brain energy metabolism. Cho is a marker for membrane synthesis or repair, inflammation, or demyelination. Lactate accumulates as a result of anaerobic glycolysis and, in the setting of TBI, may be a response to the release of glutamate. Signals from important compounds such as myoinositol (3.56 ppm) and glutamate (2.1 to 2.4 ppm) are preferentially obtained with short echo time measurements. Specifically, glutamate and immediately formed glutamine are excitatory amino acid neurotransmitters released to the extracellular space after brain injury and play a major role in neuronal cell death. *Myo*-inositol, an organic osmolyte located in astrocytes, increases as a result of glial proliferation. When interpreting MRS, comparisons are made with the Cr peak because it tends to be the most stable in a variety of conditions. The normal NAA peak is nearly twice the height of the Cr peak, whereas the normal Cho peak is only slightly smaller than the Cr peak (Fig. 3-1).

The expression of lactate in the brain is usually an expression of a pathologic condition. These include impairment of the oxidative metabolism or infiltration of macrophages and inflammatory cells. All these conditions take place after TBI. Studies have consistently found large increases in Cho level and diffuse decreases in NAA level in the brains of TBI patients. The diffuse elevation of Cho level after TBI may reflect membrane disruption, increased cell membrane turnover, and/or astrocytosis. The findings of widespread low levels of NAA in TBI should be interpreted as due to permanent neuro-axonal damage or in acute conditions such as TBI, might also depend on potentially reversible axonal dysfunction to postinjury mitochondrial impairment (see Fig. 3-1). Reduced NAA (or NAA/Cr, NAA/Cho) level is apparent within the first 24 hours of injury, possibly as early as 8 hours after TBI.

■ CLASSIFICATION OF INJURY

Traumatic brain injuries may be separated into two major categories: primary injury and secondary complications. Primary injury and its primary complications are directly related to immediate impact damage, whereas secondary complications result from the primary injury over time. Primary injuries are considered irreversible, whereas secondary injuries are potentially preventable with efficient triage and stabilization.

Primary Injury

The primary brain injury is the physical damage to the parenchyma (tissue, vessels) that occurs during a traumatic event, resulting in shearing and compression of

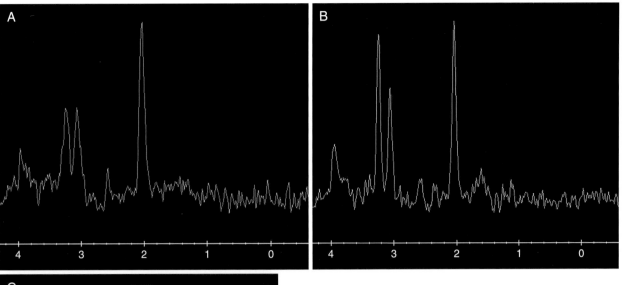

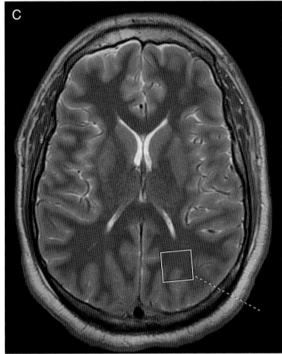

Figure 3-1 Magnetic resonance spectroscopy (MRS). A, Normal MRS. The *N*-acetyl aspartate (NAA) peak at 2.0 ppm is twice the height of the creatine peak at 3.0 ppm, whereas the normal choline peak at 3.2 ppm is the same height as the creatine peak. **B,** MRS was obtained 12 days following traumatic brain injury (TBI). The NAA peak at 2.0 ppm is mildly depressed. A normal NAA peak would be approximately twice the height of the creatine (Cr) peak seen at 3.0 ppm. The most striking abnormality is the increased choline (Cho) peak seen at 3.2 ppm. **C,** Axial T2-weighted image indicates the voxel sampled (*box*) for the MRS. There is a normal imaging appearance of the left occipital lobe. MRS often shows metabolic abnormalities in portions of the brain that are structurally normal. (Kubal WS. Update imaging of traumatic brain injury. *Radiol Clin North Am.* 2012;50:15-41.)

the surrounding brain tissue. Two different mechanisms are principally responsible for primary injury: (1) direct contact between the skull and an object and (2) inertial injury resulting from the differential accelerations between white and gray matter.

Secondary Complications

The secondary brain injury is the result of a complex process, following and complicating the primary brain injury in the ensuing hours and days. Secondary complications are temporally removed from the original trauma and result in brain injury, including increased intracranial pressure (ICP), hypoxia, infection, infarction, and herniation. Numerous secondary brain insults, both intracranial and extracranial or systemic,

may complicate the primarily injured brain and result in secondary complications. Secondary, systemic brain insults are mainly ischemic in nature. In recent years, increased recognition, ICP and cerebral perfusion pressure (CPP) monitoring, and early respiratory and circulatory support have decreased the extent of secondary complications and improved outcomes among TBI patients. In addition, implementation of and adherence to guidelines advocating a structured and systemic approach to TBI patients have also improved outcomes.

Scalp and Skull Injury

Close examination of the scalp soft tissues should be one of the first steps in interpreting a trauma head CT. Identification of soft tissue injury helps the radiologist to pinpoint the site of impact, or the "coup" site. This site should be carefully inspected for the presence of an underlying skull fracture, as well as evidence of soft tissue laceration and foreign bodies.

Fractures of the skull and of the skull base can lead to several complications, including CSF leakage, neurovascular damage, meningitis, facial palsy, deafness, carotid dissection, and carotid cavernous fistula. Fractures can also serve as an indication of adjacent hematomas and can indicate the possibility of associated delayed complication, even if no initial hematoma is present. CT, including coronal and sagittal reconstructions, is the best method for the detection of skull fractures.

Extra-Axial Injuries

We will discuss four types of extra-axial fluid collections: epidural hematoma (EDH), subdural hematoma (SDH), subdural hygroma, and subarachnoid hemorrhage (SAH). Pneumocephalus, intracranial air, can occur in any of these four locations, as well as in the brain parenchyma, referred to as a *pneumatocele.*

The imaging appearance of posttraumatic fluid collections is best understood in relation to the meningeal layers covering the brain. The three meningeal layers are the dura mater, arachnoid mater, and pia (Fig. 3-2). The pia is the deepest layer, covering the brain surface and lining the cortical gyri. It also lines the perivascular space, the Virchow-Robin space, which communicates with the subarachnoid space. This space normally contains a small amount of CSF. The arachnoid is superficial to the pia and is attached to the pia via innumerable arachnoid trabeculations. The subarachnoid space is the space between the arachnoid and pia.

The subdural space lies between the inner layer of the dura and the arachnoid. Bridging cortical veins transverse the subdural space. Because the dura is firmly attached to the skull and the arachnoid is attached to the cerebrum, most brain motion occurs across the subdural space, placing the bridging cortical veins at risk for tear.

The dura is composed of two layers: an outer periosteal layer and an inner meningeal layer that forms the dural reflections such as falx cerebri and tentorium cerebelli. The periosteal and meningeal layers are tightly bound to each other and to the skull. The dura surrounds and supports the venous sinuses. The two leaves of the dura separate only to enclose the venous sinuses. The potential space between the periosteal layer of the dura and the inner table of the skull is the epidural space. Running within the epidural space are branches of the middle meningeal artery. The periosteal layer is tightly adherent to the margins of the cranial sutures; therefore epidural fluid collections do not cross the suture margins.

Epidural Hematoma

EDHs are caused by contact forces that are of high magnitude and short duration. The potential space between the inner table of the skull and the dura is the epidural space. At the moment of impact the dura may be stripped away from the inner table, and extravasated blood from injured meningeal vessels, diploic

veins, or dural sinuses fill the newly created space. EDHs are more common in adolescents because the dura is not as firmly attached to the skull as it is in older people. EDHs are usually biconvex in configuration because of firm adherence of the dura to the inner table and its attachment to the sutures. The most common cause of EDH is head trauma with skull fracture (adjacent skull fracture is present in greater than 90% of cases) in the temporoparietal region crossing the vascular territory of the middle meningeal artery. Arterial EDHs are far more common than venous EDHs in the supratentorial region. Venous EDH is most often noted in the pediatric population and carries a lower incidence of skull fracture. In addition, skull fracture may not be present in children due to the increased plasticity of the calvaria. Venous EDHs that are associated with skull fractures typically occur infratentorially from injury to the transverse sinus or sigmoid sinuses. Venous EDHs are associated with a better prognosis, as they rarely increase in size because the pressure exerted by extravasated venous hemorrhage is insufficient to cause further stripping of the dura from the skull. Venous EDHs often involve a basilar fracture extending to the torcular Herophili or the transverse sinus. These hematomas are uncommon (15%) as compared with arterial EDHs (85%).

Symptoms after injury are directly related to the mass effect from the EDH. The "classic" presentation is a lucid interval as the lesion expands before causing midline shift and deterioration; however, fewer than 20% of the patients demonstrate this presentation. Expanding high-volume EDHs can produce a midline shift and subfalcine herniation of the brain. Compressed cerebral tissue can also impinge on the third cranial nerve, resulting in ipsilateral pupillary dilation with contralateral hemiparesis or extensor motor response.

EDHs are not limited by the falx and tentorium. The CT appearance of both arterial and venous EDHs is that of a high attenuation, biconvex, extra-axial collection. Low attenuation regions within the collection may represent areas of active bleeding within the EDH. CT findings that are associated with an adverse clinical outcome in patients with an EDH include pterional location of the skull fracture, EDH thickness greater than 1.5 cm, EDH volume greater than 30 mL, location within the lateral aspect of the middle cranial fossa, associated midline shift greater than 5 mm, and the presence of active bleeding within the EDH. Because of their high density, acute EDHs are usually well seen in CT. MRI can also show these collections; however, it is typically less sensitive for the identification of the associated skull fractures. MRI is useful for evaluation of associated injuries that may be present.

Chronic EDHs reveal low density and peripheral enhancement, and they may be concave. Chronic EDHs should be distinguished from other epidural masses such as infection, inflammation, or tumor and from subdural lesions such as empyema.

Small EDHs may be managed conservatively. Acute EDHs isolated to the anterior aspect of the middle cranial fossa constitute a subgroup of traumatic EDHs with a benign natural history. It is postulated that they arise from

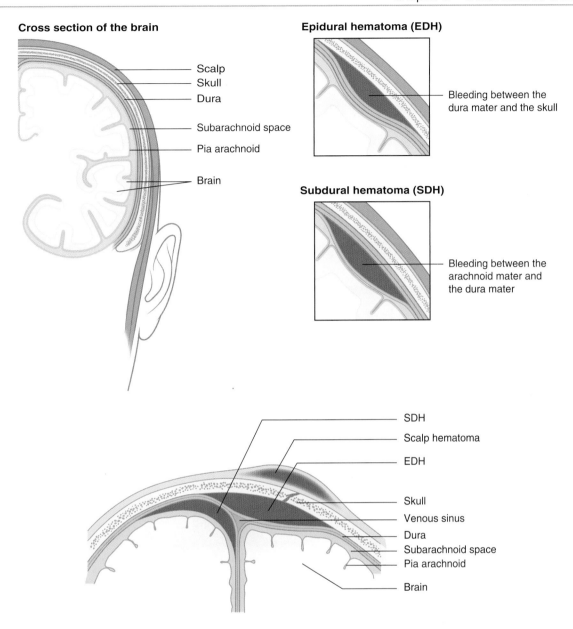

Cross section of the brain

- Scalp
- Skull
- Dura
- Subarachnoid space
- Pia arachnoid
- Brain

Epidural hematoma (EDH)

Bleeding between the dura mater and the skull

Subdural hematoma (SDH)

Bleeding between the arachnoid mater and the dura mater

- SDH
- Scalp hematoma
- EDH
- Skull
- Venous sinus
- Dura
- Subarachnoid space
- Pia arachnoid
- Brain

Figure 3-2 The three meningeal layers are the dura matter, arachnoid matter, and pia. The pia is the deepest layer, covering the brain surface and lining the cortical gyri. The subarachnoid space is the space between the arachnoid and pia. The subdural space lies between the inner layer of the dura and the arachnoid. Bridging cortical veins transverse the subdural space. The dura is composed of two layers: an outer periosteal layer and an inner meningeal layer that forms the dural reflections such as falx cerebri and tentorium cerebelli. The potential space between the periosteal layer of the dura and the inner table of the skull is the epidural space.

venous bleeding because disruption of the sphenoparietal sinus. Emergency surgical decompression is nearly always needed for larger EDHs, hematomas associated with active bleeding, and hematomas associated with substantial mass effect. The surgical goal is to alleviate mass effect from the EDH before secondary injury occurs.

Subdural Hematoma

Hemorrhage in the potential space between the pia-arachnoid and the dura is termed a *subdural hematoma*. Hemorrhage may originate from cerebral veins, venous sinuses, or adjacent cerebral contusions. Acute SDHs are typically the result of significant head injury and are caused by the shearing of bridging veins. SDH can be seen in both the coup and contrecoup locations, with the contrecoup location being more common. The most common locations are along the cerebral convexities, the falx cerebri, and tentorium cerebelli. SDHs may cross suture lines but not dural reflections, such as the falx and tentorium. Older adults and infants are particularly susceptible to this injury because their bridging veins are stretched due to age-associated cerebral and cerebellar volume loss. Because of the

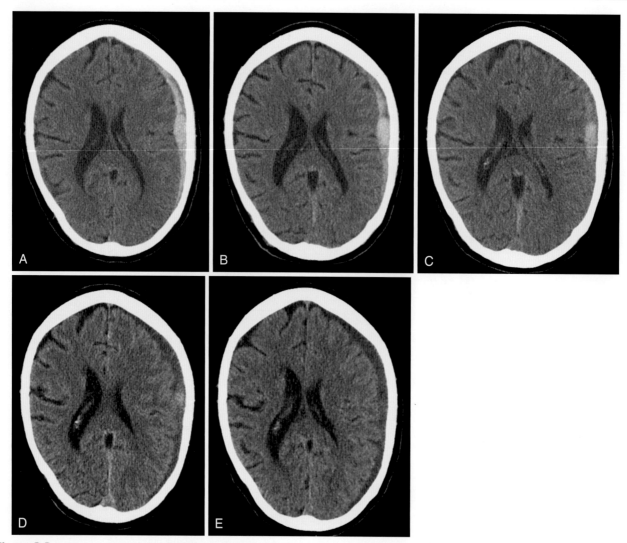

Figure 3-3 Evolving subdural hematoma (SDH). **A,** Initial noncontrast computed tomography (CT) shows a mildly heterogenous but predominantly hyperdense left SDH. **B,** CT obtained 4 days after the initial study shows the SDH to be slightly less dense. **C,** CT obtained 7 days after the initial study shows that portions of the SDH are now isodense to brain. **D,** CT obtained 13 days after the initial study shows only a small focus of hyperdensity within the subdural collection. **E,** CT obtained 19 days after the initial study shows the entire subdural collection to be hypodense compared to brain. (Kubal WS. Update imaging of traumatic brain injury. *Radiol Clin North Am.* 2012;50:15-41.)

loose connection between the arachnoid and the dura, an SDH spreads over a considerable area and usually has a crescent configuration overlying the convexity of the brain.

Small SDHs may be missed because of high-convexity locations, beam-hardening artifacts, or narrow window settings. A wider window (width, 200; level 70) helps to differentiate acute hemorrhage from bone. MRI is more sensitive than CT in the detection of small SDHs and tentorial or interhemispheric SDHs. A potential pitfall is an ossified cerebral falx, which contains bone marrow with a high T1 signal, which may mimic an SDH on MRI.

SDHs may be classified as simple or complicated. Simple SDHs are without associated brain injury, and complicated SDHs occur with parenchymal injury. Lesions occurring at the time of injury are acute, 3 days to 3 weeks are subacute, and greater than 3 weeks are chronic. Acutely, these collections usually have a uniform high density on CT, although approximately 40% are heterogeneous in density. Causes of low-density regions within an acute SDH include unclotted blood in an

early stage of hematoma development, serum extruded into the early phase of clot retraction, and CSF within the subdural space because of an arachnoid tear. Occasionally the acute SDH may be isodense or hypodense due to underlying anemia. As the SDH becomes subacute to chronic, the collection becomes isodense to brain in the subacute phase and hypodense to brain in the chronic phase (Fig. 3-3). During the subacute period an isodense phase can occur, and the collection can be difficult to detect on noncontrast CT but more conspicuous on MRI (Fig. 3-4). MRI can be useful in indicating the chronicity of the SDH by showing blood in different oxidation states. Imaging clues to the presence of an isodense SDH are abnormally thick cortex, white matter buckling, and the presence of mass effect.

By CT, chronic SDHs may not be distinguishable from subdural hygromas (Fig. 3-5). However, the walls of hygromas do not enhance. Subacute to chronic subdural lesions enhance because of vascularization of the subdural membranes, which are formed between 1 and

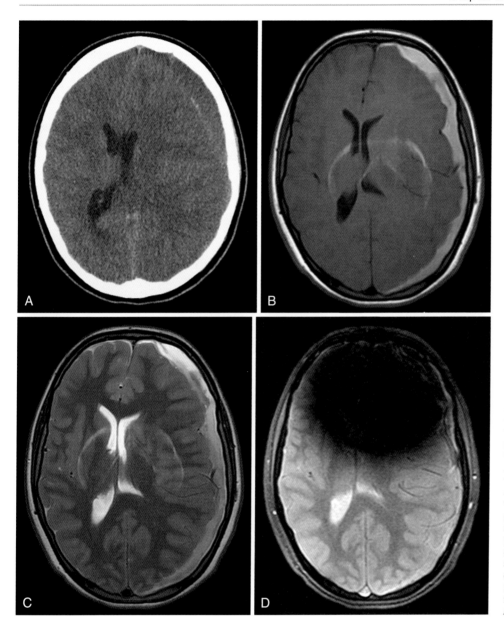

Figure 3-4 Isodense subdural hematoma (SDH). A, Noncontrast computed tomography (CT) shows shift of the midline structures toward the right. There is an isodense extra-axial collection in the frontoparietal region consistent with a subacute SDH. It can be recognized by the mass effect it has on the adjacent brain parenchyma. **B,** Noncontrast axial T1-weighted magnetic resonance imaging (MRI) shows the extent of the extra-axial collection better than does CT. Note the artifact within the center of this image; it is from the patient's dental hardware. **C,** Axial T2-weighted MRI shows mild heterogeneity within the panhemispheric SDH. Also noted are cortical veins traversing the subdural space. **D,** Axial gradient-recalled echo (GRE) shows a large bifrontal artifact from the patient's dental hardware. GRE sequences are very sensitive to the susceptibility artifact from a metal or blood breakdown products. (Kubal WS. Update imaging of traumatic brain injury. *Radiol Clin North Am.* 2012;50:15-41.)

3 weeks after injury. Repeated episodic bleeding within an SDH results in fibrous septations and compartments within the hematoma (Fig. 3-6). Subacute and chronic hematomas may also display layering with dependent cells and cellular debris and an acellular supernatant.

The prognosis for patients with SDH is variable and is related to the extent of the primary underlying brain injury rather than the SDH itself.

Subdural Hygroma
Collections of fluid within the subdural space that have imaging characteristics similar to CSF are termed *hygromas.* They can result from trauma and can occur acutely as a tear in the arachnoid membrane with CSF collecting in the subdural space or result from the chronic degeneration of an SDH.

In subdural hygroma the collection is between the dura and the arachnoid, forcing the arachnoid inward along with the cortical veins. In patients with volume loss the cortical veins on the surface of the brain are seen extending across and within the fluid collection. With MRI one might see high protein, which reveals itself as high signal intensity on FLAIR and small amounts of residual hemorrhage on gradient echo imaging.

Subarachnoid Hemorrhage
Traumatic SAH is the result of injury to small, bridging cortical vessels on the pia or arachnoidal leptomeninges that cross the subarachnoid space. Hemorrhage from an intracerebral hematoma may decompress directly into the subarachnoid space or dissect into the ventricular system. The most frequent location of traumatic SAH is the convexity, followed by the fissures and basal cistern (Fig. 3-7). SAH may induce cerebral vasospasm, which is more likely to occur when SAH is accompanied by SDH, intraventricular hemorrhage, cerebral contusion, or intracerebral hemorrhage. Aneurysmal SAH can typically be differentiated from traumatic SAH based on the

distribution of the hemorrhage. Aneurysmal SAH tends to be distributed centrally, commonly involving the suprasellar, interpeduncular, and prepontine cisterns, whereas posttraumatic SAH has a peripheral distribution.

On CT, acute SAH presents as high attenuation within the subarachnoid space. It is important to differentiate true SAH from pseudo-SAH present in diffuse cerebral edema. In diffuse cerebral edema the elevated ICP causes an increase in the density of the subarachnoid

space (pseudo-SAH), which may be the result of decreased CSF in the subarachnoid space or engorgement and dilatation of the small pial vessel in the subarachnoid space. With MRI, FLAIR images are needed to detect small areas of acute or subacute SAH. A pitfall of the FLAIR sequence is that it does not differentiate between abnormalities that appear increased in signal intensity such as hemorrhage, inflammatory exudate, neoplastic leptomeningeal infiltration, vascular slow flow, and hyperoxygenation during sedation or anesthesia. Subacute and chronic SAH are difficult to detect on CT because SAH is typically isodense to CSF on CT.

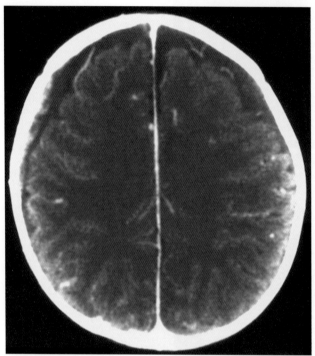

Figure 3-5 Subdural hematoma (SDH) shows bridging veins. Axial contrast-enhanced computed tomography (CT) shows bifrontal, low-density, extra-axial fluid collections compatible with chronic SDH. A more acute component is also present on the right. Note the enhancing bridging veins. (Kubal WS. Update imaging of traumatic brain injury. *Radiol Clin North Am.* 2012;50:15-41.)

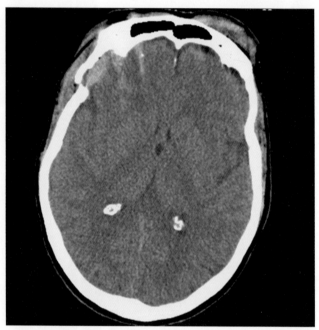

Figure 3-7 Subarachnoid hemorrhage (SAH) and frontal contusion. Noncontrast axial computed tomography (CT) shows a small forehead hematoma and dense material that conforms to the right frontal cortical sulci. This appearance is typical of CT for posttraumatic, peripheral SAH.

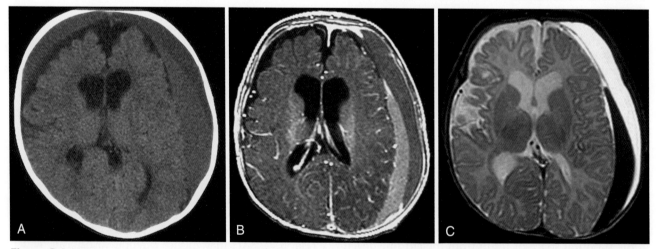

Figure 3-6 Multicomponent subdural hematoma (SDH). A, Noncontrast computed tomography (CT) shows bilateral SDHs; the left SDH shows differing densities between the two components. **B,** T1-weighted contrast enhanced magnetic resonance imaging (MRI) shows a multicomponent left extra-axial fluid collection with enhancement of the membrane walls. **C,** Axial T2-weighted MRI shows a multicomponent left SDH. SDHs may form membranes within the collection that separate components of differing ages and differing oxidation states. This information is important to the surgeon attempting to drain the SDH. (Kubal WS. Update imaging of traumatic brain injury. *Radiol Clin North Am.* 2012;50:15-41.)

Subacute and chronic SAH is best detected on MRI. Subacute hemorrhage is best detected with FLAIR imaging with altered signal intensity within the CSF, and chronic blood products are best detected on GRE and SWI with weighted images appearing as areas of decreased signal intensity.

Communicating hydrocephalus may result as a chronic sequela of prior SAH. As SAH is cleared from the CSF, the blood is phagocytized and transferred to the arachnoid villi. The arachnoid villi become distended and filled with phagocytes. They may become obliterated by the proliferation of connective tissue ("scarring"), causing impaired absorption of CSF.

Intra-Axial Injuries

Contusions
Contusion is bruising of the brain caused by direct contact and occurs when the brain surface rubs across the rough inner table of the calvaria. Capillary injury and edema are the result. The most common locations for brain contusions are the anterior and inferior surfaces of the frontal lobes as well as the temporal and occipital lobes. The differential acceleration of the brain relative to the calvaria in the setting of trauma results in abrasion and impaction of the brain along the inner table. Both coup and contrecoup injuries can be associated with intra-axial hemorrhage.

Most cerebral contusions are subtle on initial CT scanning but tend to become larger and more obvious during the first 3 days post trauma because of progression of edema and hemorrhage (Fig. 3-8). Nonhemorrhagic contusions are best seen acutely with MRI on DWI. Many superficial contusions initially are hemorrhagic, reflecting the rich vascular supply of the cortex. On T2-weighted MRI, an acute contusion has a central dark signal representing deoxyhemoglobin with surrounding hyperintensity representing edema. As the

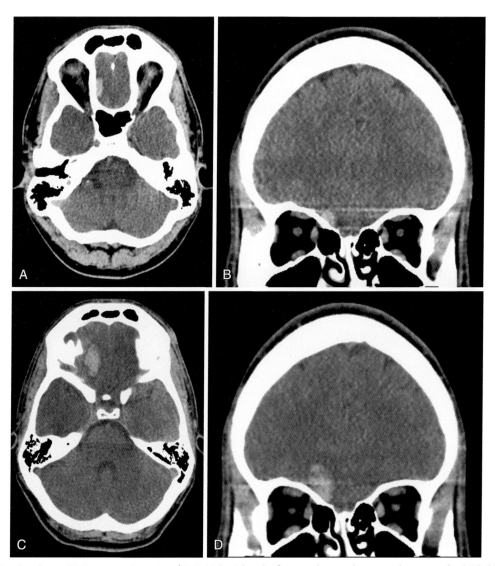

Figure 3-8 Enlarging frontal lobe contusion. **A** and **B**, Initial axial and reformatted coronal computed tomography (CT) shows a small area of contusion in the inferior right frontal lobe. This contusion was likely caused by the movement of the frontal lobe over the irregularities of the anterior cranial fossa. **C** and **D**, Axial and reformatted coronal CT scans obtained 7 hours after the initial CT show enlargement of the right frontal lobe contusion and the development of subtle edema around the hematoma. (Kubal WS. Update imaging of traumatic brain injury. *Radiol Clin North Am.* 2012;50:15-41.)

contusion becomes subacute, it appears hyperintense on T1, representing evolution of the blood products to methemoglobin with increased surrounding vasogenic edema. Subacute contusions and hematoma can mimic brain abscess, infarct, or neoplasm if history of trauma is unknown, as it often demonstrates ring enhancement following intravenous contrast administration. Chronic contusion may present itself as an area of encephalomalacia or area of hemosiderin best seen on GRE and SWI sequences because they are of decreased signal intensity (Fig. 3-9).

Intraparenchymal Hematoma

Traumatic intraparenchymal hematoma may be the result of shear-induced hemorrhage due to rupture of small intraparenchymal blood vessels or coalescence of multiple cortical contusions. Rarely, approximately 1 to 4 days following the onset of the initial trauma, delayed intracerebral hematomas can occur in areas that previously demonstrated focal contusions on CT or MRI. These delayed hematomas tend to occur in multiple lobar locations and are associated with a poor prognosis.

There is a linear relationship between CT attenuation and hematocrit. The increased attenuation of whole blood is based primarily on its protein concentration rather than iron. Therefore acute hematomas are increased in density as compared to the adjacent brain parenchyma. After extravasation, density progressively increases for approximately 72 hours secondary to clot formation and retraction. After the third day the density of the clot decreases and progressively becomes more isodense over the following 2 weeks. If contrast is given, intraparenchymal hemorrhage is often associated with a peripheral rim of enhancement from approximately 6 days to 6 weeks after the initial event. This finding of peripheral enhancement could be confused with abscess, infarct, or neoplasm.

Diffuse Axonal Injury

DAIs or shear injuries are the most common cause of significant morbidity and mortality after head trauma. DAI is responsible for coma and poor outcomes in most patients with significant closed head injury. Unfortunately, CT underestimates their extent because most individual lesions are small and initially nonhemorrhagic. At the time of injury the stress induced by rotational acceleration/deceleration movement of the head causes some regions of the brain to accelerate or decelerate faster than other regions of the brain, resulting in axonal injury. Portions of the brain where tissue density differs and tissue abuts rigid structures such as the falx are affected most commonly. The most common locations for these injuries are as follows: cerebral hemisphere (gray-white junction), basal ganglia, splenium of the corpus callosum, and dorsal midbrain. Shearing injuries of the brainstem are found only in severe trauma and are nearly always associated with multiple other white matter hemorrhages. The severity of the DAI is related to the magnitude of the rotational acceleration.

Classically, patients with DAI present with a history of immediate loss of consciousness. Results of CT in these patients may be normal; to explain the patient's neurologic status, MRI is obtained. CT is not as sensitive as MRI in detecting DAI. On CT one may visualize focal punctate regions of high density that may be surrounded by a collar of low-density edema. On CT it is difficult to detect nonhemorrhagic shearing injury early in its course. Both hemorrhagic and nonhemorrhagic shearing injuries can be detected by MRI, typically as high signal intensity on T2-weighted/FLAIR images.

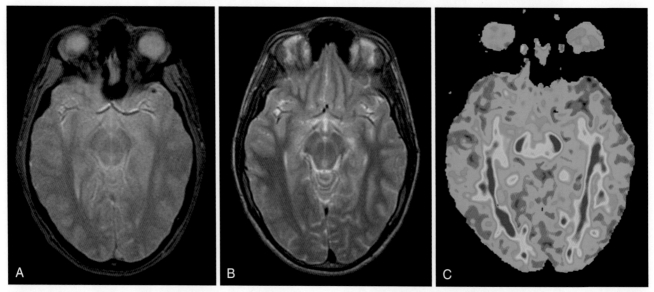

Figure 3-9 Temporal contusion. The patient suffered a deceleration injury several months before the magnetic resonance (MR) examination. **A,** Axial gradient-recalled echo (GRE) image shows a small focus of hemosiderin in the anterior left temporal lobe. **B,** Axial T2-weighted image appears nearly normal; there may be a small focus of T2 prolongation within the left anterior temporal lobe. **C,** Fractional anisotropy map shows increased blue signal indicating loss of anisotropy within the left anterior temporal lobe. Note that the extent of white matter abnormality within the temporal lobe is considerable larger than that defined by either the GRE or the T2-weighted sequence. (Kubal WS. Update imaging of traumatic brain injury. *Radiol Clin North Am.* 2012;50:15-41.)

Lesions may be ovoid or elliptic, with the long axis parallel to fiber bundle directions. Gradient echo images are extremely sensitive for the detection of microhemorrhage. Regions of acute DAI can also be depicted as high signal intensity on DWI and dark regions on ADC maps because of restricted diffusion caused by acute cell death (Fig. 3-10). SWI and GRE demonstrate more lesions compared to T2-weighted/FLAIR images, with SWI being even more sensitive than conventional GRE. Sensitive detection of DAI is important to predicting clinical outcome. SWI also detects prognostically important microhemorrhages in the brainstem, which may go undetected on conventional MRI.

DTI is an ideal tool for investigating the progression of atrophy in TBI because of its sensitivity to abnormalities in the microstructure of white matter, which is extensively disrupted after TBI. DTI can be performed in the acute phase of DAI. DAI leads to axonal disruption and can result in decreased fractional anisotropy (see Fig. 3-9). DTI studies have demonstrated a relationship of decreased fractional anisotropy with motor deficits and cognitive disorders in patients with DAI.

Brainstem Injuries

Primary and secondary injury of the brainstem can occur. Primary contusion of the brainstem is usually

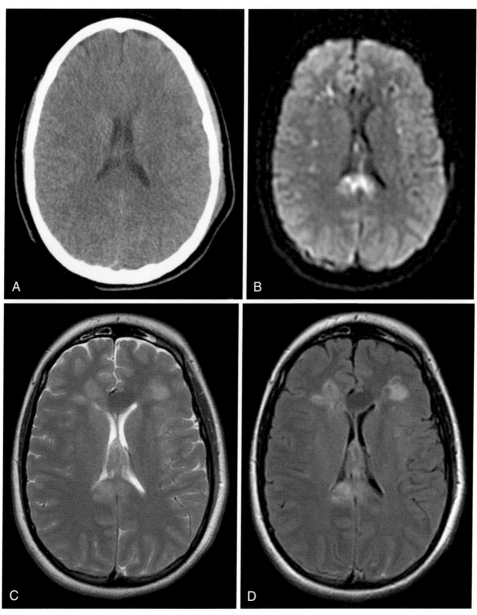

Figure 3-10 Nonhemorrhagic diffuse axonal injury (DAI) involving the splenium of the corpus callosum. A, Axial noncontrast computed tomography (CT) is nearly normal but shows subtle subarachnoid hemorrhage (SAH) within the left sylvian fissure and subtle hypodensity within the corpus callosum. **B,** Axial diffusion-weighted imaging (DWI) shows restricted diffusion within the splenium of the corpus callosum and scattered smaller foci of restricted diffusion seen at the gray-white junction. Findings are compatible with DAI. **C and D,** Axial T2-weighted and fluid-attenuated inversion recovery (FLAIR) images show T2 prolongation within the splenium of the corpus callosum and scattered foci of T2 prolongation within the splenium of the corpus callosum and scattered foci of T2 prolongation at the gray-white junction of the frontal lobes. (Kubal WS. Update imaging of traumatic brain injury. *Radiol Clin North Am.* 2012;50:15-41.)

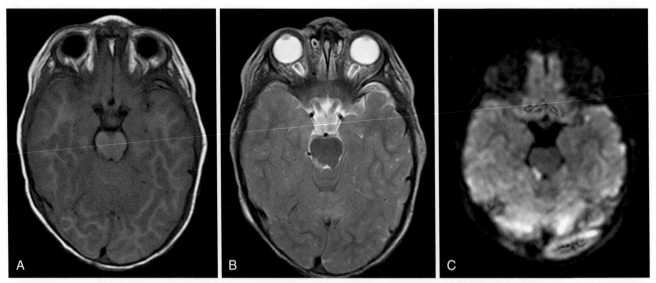

Figure 3-11 Brainstem contusion. **A,** Axial T1-weighted magnetic resonance imaging (MRI) shows a subtle area of low signal intensity involving the left posterior lateral aspect of the pons. **B,** Axial T2-weighted MRI shows a small area of high signal intensity involving the left posterior lateral aspect of the pons. **C,** Axial diffusion-weighted imaging (DWI) shows a small area of restricted diffusion involving the right posterior lateral aspect of the pons. Findings are compatible with a nonhemorrhagic contusion likely caused by impact against the tentorial incisura. (Kubal WS. Update imaging of traumatic brain injury. *Radiol Clin North Am.* 2012;50:15-41.)

the result of impact of the brainstem with the ipsilateral tentorium, which can result in hemorrhagic or nonhemorrhagic contusion. The location is characteristic, occurring in the posterior lateral aspect of the pons (Fig. 3-11). The distinction between a contusion and DAI may be important for long-term prognosis because outcome from DAI is less favorable. Shearing injuries of the brainstem are found only in severe trauma. They are nearly always associated with other white matter hemorrhages.

Compression of the midbrain by transtentorial herniation can result in lateral translation of the brainstem so great that the contralateral cerebral peduncle is compressed against the tentorial edge. This phenomenon is called a *Kernohan notch* and results in ipsilateral motor weakness, also known as a *false localizing sign*. It is associated with high intensity on T2WI in the midbrain from compression and occlusion of perforating arteries at the tentorial notch. Prolonged and progressive transtentorial herniation leads to stretching and eventual rupture of the perforating arteries and venules in the brainstem, causing punctate hemorrhages, also known as *Duret hemorrhages*. Duret hemorrhages are typically in the central pons, which distinguishes them from direct traumatic hemorrhagic contusions. Compression related to Duret hemorrhage may compromise the cardiorespiratory centers, resulting in death (Fig. 3-12). Disruption of the brainstem can lead to decorticate posture, respiratory center depression, and death. The brainstem, like the rest of the brain, can also undergo secondary ischemic injury.

Brain Swelling (Fig. 3-13) and Herniation

The skull is a fixed structure that allows no compensation for expansion of brain tissue. The cranial cavity is compartmentalized by inelastic dural folds and bony ridges. The inward reflections on the dura (which include the falx cerebri, tentorium cerebelli, and the falx

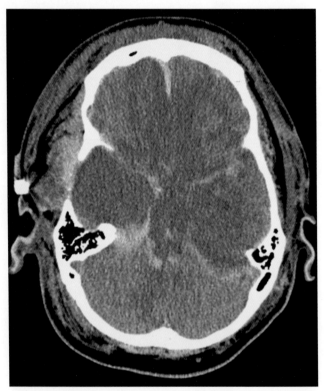

Figure 3-12 Subarachnoid hemorrhage (SAH), Duret hemorrhage. Axial noncontrast computed tomography (CT) shows diffuse SAH and a small hemorrhage within the central pons. The central pontine hemorrhage likely represents Duret hemorrhage. Incidentally noted is a right temporal craniotomy. (Kubal WS. Update imaging of traumatic brain injury. *Radiol Clin North Am.* 2012;50:15-41.)

cerebelli) protect and stabilize the brain against excessive movement.

Intracranial volume is constant and described by the Monro-Kellie doctrine: Intracranial volume = Brain volume + CSF volume + Blood volume, with the intracranial

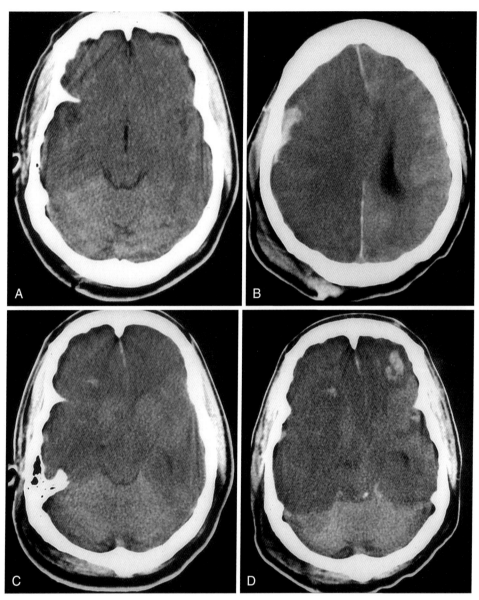

Figure 3-13 Delayed hemorrhage and herniation. A, Patient presents with trauma. Initial computed tomography (CT), although mildly degraded by patient motion, appears normal. **B** and **C,** Patient's clinical condition deteriorated and a second CT was obtained after approximately 24 hours. Two images from the second CT show extensive brain swelling manifested by decreased density within the frontal lobes bilaterally and the right temporal lobe. There is compression of cortical sulci and narrowing of the quadrigeminal plate cistern. Several areas of hemorrhage are also noted in the right frontal lobe. **D,** Patient's condition continued to deteriorate, and another CT was obtained approximately 34 hours after the initial trauma. The CT findings have progressed. The brain swelling has increased to the point at which the quadrigeminal plate cistern is completely effaced. New areas of hemorrhage are now present within the left frontal lobe. The patient died shortly after this study. (Kubal WS. Update imaging of traumatic brain injury. *Radiol Clin North Am.* 2012;50:15-41.)

components almost being noncompressible. Increase in one intracranial volume leads to a decrease/compression of another. Normal ICP is 5 to 15 mm Hg. The pressure components include CPP, mean arterial pressure (MAP), and ICP, which maintain the relationship of CPP = MAP − ICP. If ICP increases, the MAP must increase to maintain CCP. If there is no increase of the MAP, then an increase in ICP results in a decreased CPP, which in turn leads to the cascade effect of decreased CPP leading to tissue ischemia, tissue ischemia leads to edema and further swelling, edema leads to further increases in ICP, and further increases in ICP can lead to tissue death. A CPP below 50 mm Hg should be avoided. A low CPP may jeopardize regions of

the brain with preexisting ischemia, and improvement of the CPP may help to avoid cerebral ischemia. The CPP should be maintained at a minimum of 60 mm Hg in the absence of cerebral ischemia and at a minimum of 70 mm Hg in the presence of cerebral ischemia. Cerebral ischemia is considered the single most important secondary event affecting outcome following severe TBI. Therefore it is critically important for patients with both diffuse and focal cerebral swelling to be carefully monitored in an attempt to prevent secondary brain injury. Patients with persistent swelling have a short survival and high mortality. The Brain Trauma Foundation recommends that ICP should be monitored on all salvageable patients with severe TBI and abnormal CT scan findings. Also, ICP monitoring is indicated in patients with severe TBI with normal CT scan findings if two or more of the following features are noted at admission: 40 years of age or older, unilateral or bilateral motor posturing, or systolic blood pressure less than 90 mm Hg. Based on physiologic principles, potential benefits of ICP monitoring include earlier detection of intracranial mass lesions, guidance of therapy, and avoidance of indiscriminate use of therapies to control ICP, such as drainage of CSF with reduction of ICP and improvement of CPP, and determination of prognosis.

Brain edema refers to swelling within the tissues due to the accumulation of fluid (cytotoxic and vasogenic), which may occur as a response to direct focal injury such as contusion or DAI. Vascular occlusion and pressure necrosis may lead to cerebral edema. Three effects of edema are visible on imaging: loss of gray-white differentiation, swelling of sulci, and mass effects. Cerebral swelling/edema is seen on CT as focal or diffuse areas of low attenuation with loss of normal gray-white differentiation. As more and more water enters into the tissues, the relative density of both gray and white matter decreases, as does the difference in density between the two tissues. There are signs of mass effect, including effacement of cortical sulci, cisterns, and ventricles. On MRI the brain shows an increase in edema; this is noted as areas of increased signal intensity on FLAIR and T2-weighted sequences. Subtle, early edema, such as that seen in association with mild contusion, may not be readily visible in the acute phase on T2-weighted sequences but is more likely to be visualized on DWI. DWI can detect subtle cytotoxic edema before it is seen on any other type of MR pulse sequence. Specifically, DWI is sensitive for showing restricted diffusion characteristic of cytotoxic edema seen in acute stroke. TBI produces cytotoxic edema as seen in contusions and DAI, but it also results in vasogenic edema with increased water diffusion and net flow toward the ventricles. These findings are more easily visualized after a day or two, when more significant edema has developed.

Brain herniation represents a shift of the brain through or across one compartment to another (separated by calvarial and/or dural boundaries) due to mass effect; cerebral edema or hematoma can displace a portion of the brain from its normal location in the setting of trauma. There are five basic patterns of herniation: inferior tonsillar and cerebellar herniation, superior vermian or upward herniation, temporal lobe or uncal herniation, central transtentorial herniation, and subfalcine herniation (Fig. 3-14).

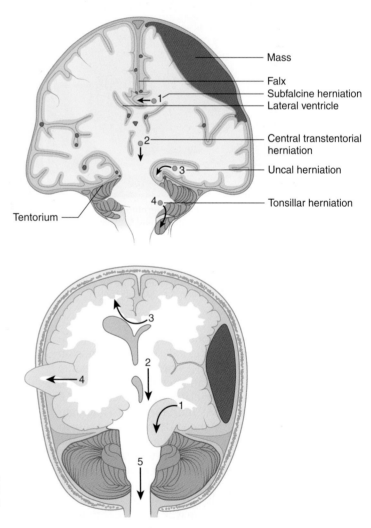

Figure 3-14 Herniations of the brain. Coronal diagram with subfalcine herniation, transtentorial herniation, uncal herniation, and tonsillar herniation (Meyer figure herniation patterns).

Tonsillar herniation, also called *downward cerebellar herniation,* occurs when the cerebellar tonsils move downward into/through the foramen magnum. Extension of cerebellar tonsils into the spinal canal may be seen in normal individuals or in Chiari malformations. Extension of 5 mm or more below the foramen magnum is considered abnormal. Tonsillar herniation is often coexisting with ascending transtentorial herniation. Tonsillar herniation can result in compression of the posterior inferior cerebellar arteries and may result in cerebellar infarction. It can also result in obstruction of CSF outflow from the fourth ventricle, resulting in hydrocephalus. Compression of brainstem nuclei can result in respiratory/cardiac failure, coma, and death.

Transtentorial herniation occurs when the brain traverses across the tentorium at the level of the incisura. Transtentorial herniation can be further subdivided into ascending and descending transtentorial herniations. Descending transtentorial herniation occurs when mass effect forces cerebral structures downward through the opening (incisura) of the tentorium. Structures typically involved in descending transtentorial herniation include the tentorium, uncus, parahippocampal gyrus, perimesencephalic cistern, mesencephalon, posterior cerebral artery and its branches, anterior choroidal artery, and the oculomotor nerve (cranial nerve III). Imaging findings of descending transtentorial herniations include asymmetry of the ambient cistern with ipsilateral ambient cistern widening and contralateral effacement. There is resultant widening of the contralateral temporal horn of the lateral ventricle. The herniated brain is forced medially and inferiorly beneath the tentorium into the perimesencephalic cistern with compression of the ipsilateral cerebral peduncle by the uncus. In severe cases there is obliteration of all basilar cisterns. To a variable extent the herniated temporal lobe can compress the oculomotor nerve, the posterior cerebral artery, the anterior choroidal artery, and the superior cerebellar artery. Compression of the oculomotor nerve against the tentorial edge produces exotropic, hypotropic eye position (down and outward), ipsilateral ptosis, and ipsilateral fixed pupillary dilatation. Compression of the posterior cerebral artery between the temporal lobe and tentorial edge can result in infarction of the occipital lobe but may also cause thalamic infarcts. The anterior choroidal artery originates from the distal internal carotid artery and traverses along the uncus dorsally. Occlusion of the anterior choroidal artery results in infarction of the structures in its vascular supply, which include the optic tract, temporal lobe, posterior limb of the internal capsule, the lateral aspect of the thalamus, cerebral peduncles, and midbrain.

Ascending transtentorial herniation is due to increased pressure in the posterior fossa forcing cerebellar structures upward through the tentorial incisura. Ascending transtentorial herniation is less common than descending transtentorial herniation. Imaging changes associated with ascending transtentorial herniation can be subtle and difficult to identify. Changes are often bilateral and symmetric with no asymmetry to help with identification. Also, the differing appearance of perimesencephalic cisterns with different gantry angles in CT may complicate imaging findings. Imaging characteristics of ascending herniation include the "spinning top" appearance of the midbrain. This is due to compression bilaterally on the posterolateral aspects of the midbrain as the posterior fossa squeezes through the incisura from below, compressing the midbrain from a bilateral location, and narrows the ambient cisterns. With increasing upward herniation the quadrigeminal cistern becomes effaced and the midbrain displaces anteriorly against the clivus. Increased mass effect may occlude the cerebral aqueduct, resulting in hydrocephalus and increased ICP. Direct compression of the vein of Galen and basal vein of Rosenthal can further aggravate parenchymal congestion and increase ICP. Midbrain compression may also be complicated by periaqueductal necrosis of the brainstem. Rapidly expanding lesions present with emergent clinical findings due to compression of brainstem nuclei: respiratory failure, coma, and death. These lesions are often coexistent with foramen magnum herniation. Compression of posterior cerebral and superior cerebellar arteries may lead to occipital or cerebellar infarction.

Uncal herniation is a subset of descending transtentorial herniations. The uncus/parahippocampus is displaced medially and inferiorly over the edge of the tentorium cerebelli into the suprasellar cistern (Fig. 3-15). On imaging there is truncation of the usual "star" configuration of the suprasellar cistern on the ipsilateral side of the herniation. There is often compression of one or both of the cerebral peduncles, which can appear flattened, and the midbrain can be rotated or tilted. Mass effect upon the third cranial nerve and compression of the ipsilateral cerebral peduncle causes a blown pupil with contralateral hemiparesis.

Subfalcine herniations occur as the brain pushes under the falx and crosses midline between the supratentorial compartments (see Fig. 3-15). On imaging, the ipsilateral cingulate gyrus is pushed down and under the midline falx with compression of the contralateral gyrus. There is also depression of the ipsilateral corpus callosum and elevation/compression of the contralateral corpus callosum. The anterior cerebral arteries and their branches are located between the falx cerebri and the adjacent gyri of the frontal and parietal lobes. Complications of subfalcine herniations include ipsilateral anterior cerebral artery infarction. This occurs as the cingulate sulcus extends under the falx, which carries along with it the anterior cerebral artery, which can become compressed against the falx and lead to infarction (Fig. 3-16). When located posteriorly there may be compression of the internal cerebral veins, vein of Galen, or the deep subependymal veins. Compression of these veins raises the pressure in the entire deep venous system, which further aggravates parenchymal congestion and increases ICP. Compression of the parafalcine cortex may lead to contralateral leg paresis.

Penetrating Injuries

Penetrating injuries to the head have a high morbidity and mortality. Penetrating injuries to the brain are caused by a foreign object entering the skull. Two major mechanisms of tissue damage are recognized: tissue crushing (or permanent cavitation) and temporary cavitation

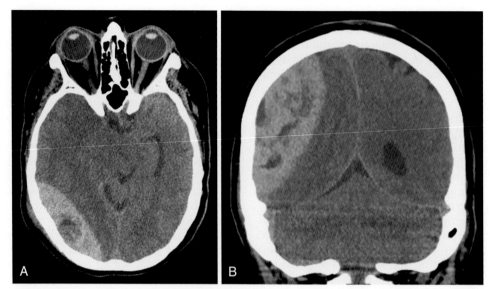

Figure 3-15 Epidural hematoma (EDH), subfalcine and uncal herniation. A, Noncontrast computed tomography (CT) demonstrates a high-density, biconvex, extra-axial fluid collection consistent with an acute EDH. The central area of decreased density within the collection is suggestive of unclotted blood from active hemorrhage, also known as the *swirl sign*. There is considerable mass effect with herniation of the uncus of the hippocampus medially into the suprasellar cistern. **B,** Coronal reformatted CT shows the extent of the EDH and the associated subfalcine herniation. (Kubal WS. Update imaging of traumatic brain injury. *Radiol Clin North Am.* 2012;50:15-41.)

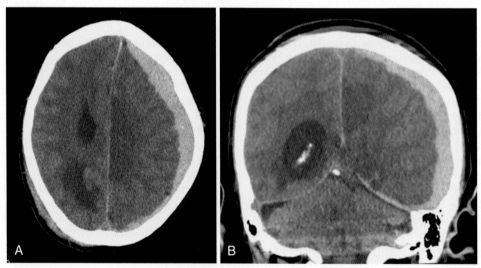

Figure 3-16 Subfalcine herniation, anterior cerebral artery infarct, acute subdural hematoma (SDH). A and B, Axial and reformatted coronal computed tomography (CT) show a left high-density extra-axial fluid collection compatible with an acute SDH. The hematoma is causing considerable mass effect and causing subfalcine herniation. The low density noted adjacent to the falx represents infarction involving a branch of the left anterior cerebral artery. The artery is compressed against the underside of the falx by the mass effect generated by the SDH.

(or tissue stretching). The projectile itself crushes the brain in its path, creating a permanent track of injury, known as a *laceration*. Projectiles traveling at higher velocities carry more kinetic energy and cause more damage. Close-range firearm injury is expected to be more severe because the maximum amount of initial kinetic energy is transferred to the brain tissue. Temporary cavitation is typically associated with projectile injuries in which the force of impact moves the tissue radially, creating a temporary cavity, the size of which will be related to the surface area exposed to the projectile. The tissue damage and temporary cavity are caused by the outward movement of the tissue, which stretches and tears parenchyma and produces localized blunt trauma and shear injury. Comminuted bone fragments themselves become secondary

missiles, increasing the extent of crushed tissue and therefore injury (Fig. 3-17). Advanced age, suicide attempts, associated coagulopathy, a low GCS score with bilaterally fixed and dilated pupils, and high ICP have been correlated with worse outcomes in patients with penetrating brain injuries. Cranial gunshot injury can be described based on the location of the bullet at the time of injury and degree of penetration of the cranial vault: superficial injuries, in which there is no intracranial penetration; penetrating injuries; and perforating injuries, in which the bullet has entered and exited the skull.

Vascular injury in penetrating brain injury can be the result of contact forces of the projectile or the shearing force of a pulsating temporary cavity, which can result in partial or complete transection of an arterial wall.

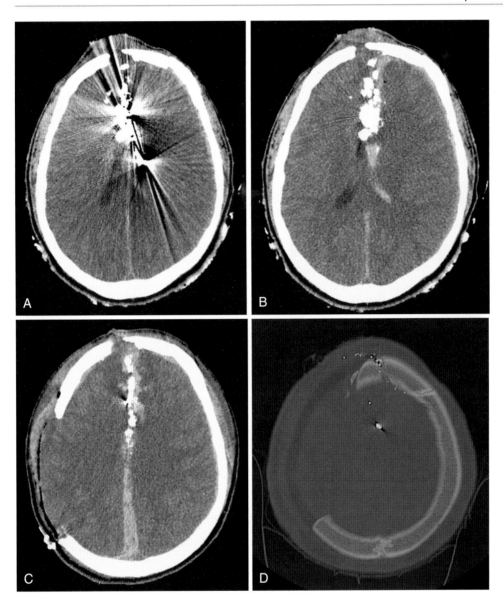

Figure 3-17 Gunshot injury to the brain. A and B, Noncontrast computed tomography (CT) shows gunshot injury to the frontal lobes with extensive intracranial bone and bullet fragments. There is intraventricular hemorrhage and subdural hemorrhage along the falx. C, Noncontrast CT obtained 1 day later shows a craniectomy with brain herniating through the craniectomy defect. There has been brain swelling, indicated by loss of cortical sulci and blurring of the gray-white margin. The parafalcine sudural hematoma (SDH) has increased in volume. D, Noncontrast CT shows that, after several additional surgical procedures, many but not all of the bone fragments and bullet fragments have been removed and the patient has received a right cranioplasty. (Kubal WS. Update imaging of traumatic brain injury. *Radiol Clin North Am.* 2012;50:15-41.)

Injury to a blood vessel can lead to dissection, acute hemorrhage, and pseudoaneurysm. Traumatic pseudoaneurysms are especially vulnerable to rupture and may result in delayed intracerebral hematoma, SAH, or both.

The initial imaging modality is noncontrast CT. Despite potential problems associated with streak artifact from metallic penetrating weapons, unenhanced CT of the brain with attention to the scout images remains the first imaging modality. Repeat imaging with the gantry angled may ameliorate this effect. CT angiography (CTA) can be performed if there is concern for associated vascular injury. CT findings of multilobar injury and intraventricular hemorrhage correlate with poor outcomes. Emergency MRI in these patients is probably contraindicated if there are metallic foreign bodies.

Brain Death

Brain death is the irreversible loss of function of the brain, including the brainstem. Current standards for making the diagnosis of brain death require identification of the suspected cause of coma, determination that the

coma is irreversible, performance of a clinical examination, and interpretation of the appropriate neurodiagnostic and laboratory data. Because brain death is a clinical diagnosis, laboratory and radiologic tests are indicated only when confounding variables must be ruled out or confirmatory evidence of brain death must be obtained, when the findings on clinical examination are equivocal, or a full examination cannot be performed.

The absence of cerebral blood flow is generally accepted as a sign of brain death, which can be demonstrated on radionuclide perfusion studies. Additional findings that can be seen on CT or MRI are severe brain edema with global hypoattenuation of brain, completely obscured corticomedullary differentiation, effaced brain sulci, and slitlike compressed ventricles (Fig. 3-18).

Axial minimal-intensity-projection SWI may demonstrate marked hypointensity of all deep, intramedullary, and sulcal dilated veins throughout both hemispheres. Hypointensity and prominence of veins on SWI likely result from a combination of low venous oxygen concentration due to increased or maximized oxygen extraction fraction, limited or absent brain perfusion due to increased

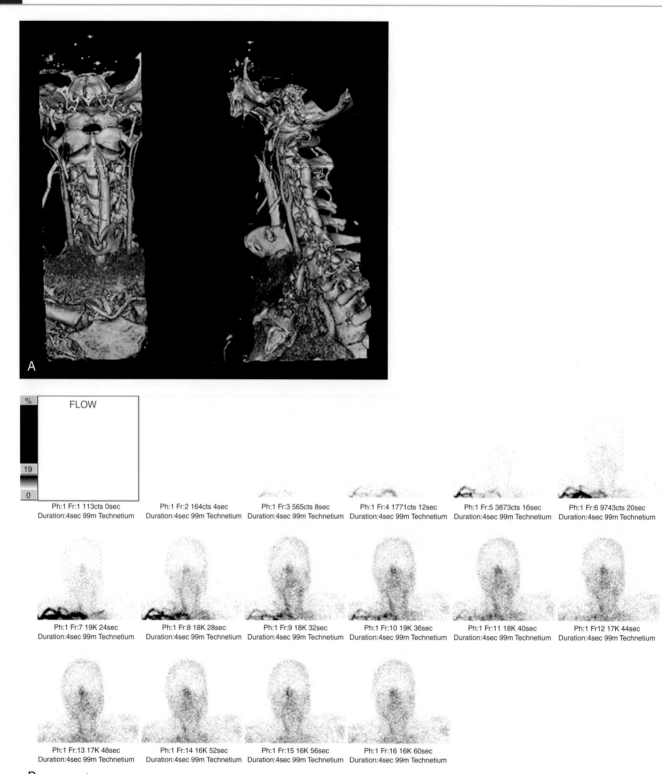

Figure 3-18 Absence of cerebral blood flow. **A,** Three-dimensional (3-D) reconstruction from a computed tomographic angiography (CTA) scan shows absence of the intracranial arteries. Subsequently a radionuclide perfusion study was performed for confirmation of absent cerebral perfusion. Following the intravenous administration of 26.0 mCi of technetium Tc 99m bicisate (Neurolite), immediate angiographic imaging was performed of the head. After 10 minutes, additional planar imaging was obtained followed by single-photon emission computed tomography (SPECT) imaging. **B,** Angiographic images show no evidence of cerebral perfusion. Delayed planar images after 10 minutes show no cerebral uptake of radiotracer.

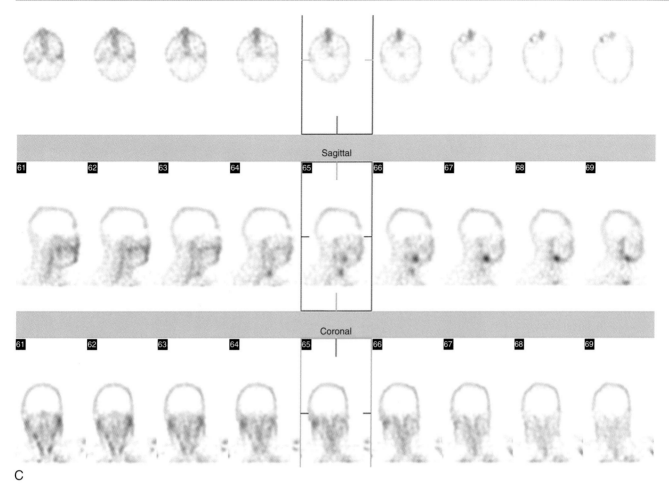

Figure 3-18, cont'd C, The additional SPECT, cross-sectional imaging, showed no brain perfusion. Of note, a tiny focus of radiotracer accumulation is seen in the right orbital region that is consistent with hematoma upon correlation with prior head CT.

ICP, resulting venous stasis, and venous dilatation due to injury-induced adenosine release.

■ SUMMARY

Both CT and MRI play important roles in the evaluation of TBI. CT is the mainstay initial imaging procedure. Overall patient treatment can be optimized using the diagnostic and prognostic information derived from current imaging techniques.

Skull Base and Temporal Bone Fractures
Colin Shiu-On Poon, John M. Collins, and Valeria Potigailo

Evaluation of skull base fractures can be daunting because of the complex anatomy and the multiple traumatic injuries that can occur in the same traumatic incident. Many of these fractures can be subtle and easy to miss. In addition, there are many normal fissures and foramina in the skull base that can mimic fractures, potentially resulting in false-positive and false-negative diagnosis.

The importance of detection of skull base fracture is to prevent complications and morbidity. Therefore, rather than merely focusing on fracture detection, a more clinically useful and practical approach for evaluation of skull base trauma is to consider the clinical importance of various types of fractures and their potential complications.

We will provide a practical approach to evaluation of skull base trauma. We will discuss the technical issues pertinent to imaging of skull base trauma. Examples of various types of skull base fractures will be presented, with inclusion of normal structures that can mimic fractures and result in misdiagnosis. Emphasis will be placed on a practical classification of fractures and their potential complications.

■ TECHNICAL ISSUES

CT is the primary modality for evaluation of traumatic skull base injury. Using modern multidetector volumetric CT technology, imaging typically provides isotropic spatial resolution of less than 0.7 mm. Images in axial, coronal, and sagittal planes are reconstructed from the volumetric data set. If necessary, additional oblique planes in any

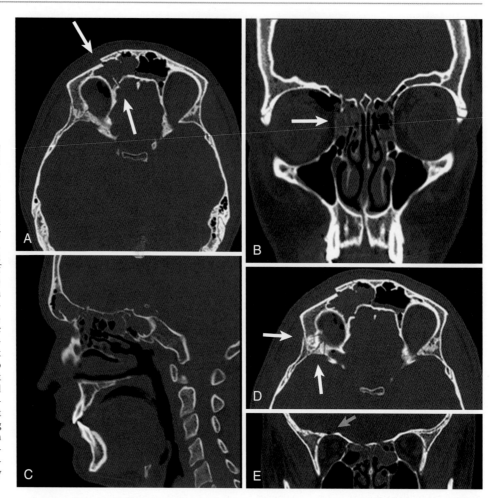

Figure 3-19 Anterior skull base fracture. A, Axial computed tomography (CT) bone window, **B,** Coronal CT bone window. **C,** Sagittal CT bone window. There is a moderately displaced comminuted fracture through the right frontal sinus involving both the anterior and posterior walls (*arrows* in **A**). The fracture extends posteriorly and medially along the right orbital roof into the ethmoid air cells (*arrow* in **B**) with involvement of the right fovea ethmoidalis and planum sphenoidale. **D,** Axial CT bone window. **E,** Coronal CT bone window. The fracture plane extends in a comminuted fashion through the right lamina papyracea and laterally into the right greater sphenoid wing at the level of the lateral orbital wall (*arrows* in **D**). A tiny focus of pneumocephalus is seen along the right orbital roof (*arrow* in **E**), indicating violation of the skull base. Attention to subtle pneumocephalus is important for evaluation of skull base fracture because this may be the only clue to an occult fracture.

orientation can be obtained. Image-viewing software now allows image reformation in any arbitrary planes, which can be useful for complex or subtle fractures. Conner and Flis have reported that the use of high-resolution multiplanar reformats results in improved detection rate (99%) of skull base fractures, although many fractures detected only on the high-resolution multiplanar reformats may have little clinical significance.

CT cisternogram can be used to detect and identify the site of CSF leak due to traumatic dural tear. This is usually performed sometime after trauma when patients present with persistent rhinorrhea or otorrhea. Through a lumbar puncture, iodinated contrast material is infused into the thecal sac. CT is performed when the contrast material reaches the intracranial subarachnoid space. CSF leak will manifest as direct contrast extravasation.

MRI can be useful for evaluation of soft tissue injuries or complications associated with skull base fractures, especially in the evaluation of intracranial injury. MR angiography can also be used for evaluation of vascular dissection and has the advantage of improved depiction of mural hematoma. However, it is less available than CT and may be more difficult to perform in an acute traumatic setting.

SKULL BASE FRACTURES

The skull base is made up of five bones: frontal, temporal, ethmoid, sphenoid, and occipital bones. For convenience, it can be grouped into four parts: the anterior skull base, central skull base, posterior skull base, and the temporal bone. We will discuss skull base fractures based on these divisions. The importance of evaluation of skull base fractures is to go beyond fracture detection and consider the potential complications associated with the fractures.

ANTERIOR SKULL BASE

The anterior skull base forms the floor of the anterior cranial fossa and roof of the nose. Centrally, it includes the cribriform plate and roof of the ethmoid sinus. The cribriform plate contains multiple perforations that transmit olfactory nerves from the nasal mucosa to the olfactory bulb. Laterally, the anterior skull base includes the orbital plate of frontal bone. The planum sphenoidale and lesser wing of the sphenoid bone form the posterior part of the anterior skull base.

Anterior skull base fractures are frequently associated with injury of the other maxillofacial structures, the paranasal sinuses and the orbits. Fractures often involve the forehead, orbital roof, ethmoidal complex, and cribriform plate (Figs. 3-19 to 3-21). Complications of anterior skull base fractures include CSF leak as a result of dural tear, injury of the olfactory tract, and orbital injury.

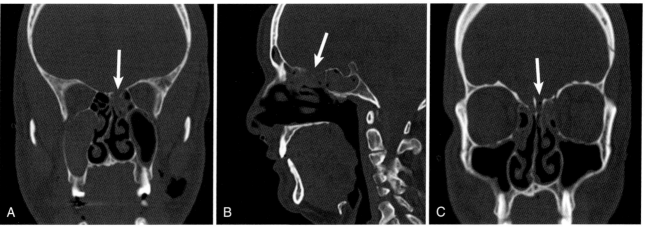

Figure 3-20 Anterior skull base fracture. A and B, Computed tomography (CT) images in bone window. C, Depressed fracture of the left fovea ethmoidalis (*arrows* in A and B). Punctate focus of air in the region of the left olfactory groove (*arrow* in C) with adjacent left fovea ethmoidalis and left orbital roof fracture.

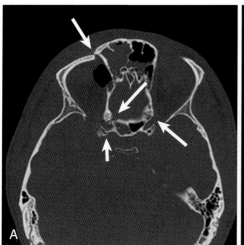
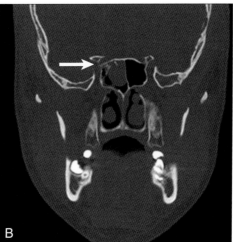

Figure 3-21 A, Axial computed tomography (CT) and, B, coronal CT show anterior skull base fractures (*anterior arrow* in A) through bilateral planum sphenoidale extending to the anterior clinoid processes and involving the optic struts bilaterally (*posterior arrows* in A & *arrow* in B). Disruption of the optic struts may result in violation of anterior dural attachment.

◼ CENTRAL SKULL BASE

The central skull base forms the floor of middle cranial fossa, roof of sphenoid sinus, and greater wing of sphenoid. It includes the sphenoid bone, basisphenoid, greater wing of sphenoid, and the portion of temporal bone anterior to the petrous ridge. Many normal foramina and fissures traverse the central skull base. These foramina and fissures transmit important structures (Table 3-1). Evaluation of central skull base fractures should include evaluation of involvement of these structures.

The majority of central skull base fractures involve the orbital surface of the greater wing of sphenoid, pterygoid process, and sphenoid sinus (Figs. 3-22 and 3-23). Complications that can be associated with central skull base fracture include CSF leak, cranial nerve injury, and vascular injury, including vascular dissection, pseudoaneurysm, and carotid-cavernous fistula.

◼ POSTERIOR SKULL BASE

The posterior skull base is the part of the skull posterior to the dorsum sellae and petrous ridge. It includes the occipital bone and the portion of temporal bone posterior to

Table 3-1 Foramina and Fissures of the Central Skull Base

Foramina and Fissures	Contents
Optic canal	CN II (optic nerve), ophthalmic artery
Superior orbital fissure	CN III, CN IV, CN V1, superior ophthalmic vein
Inferior orbital fissure	Infraorbital artery, vein, and nerve
Carotid canal	Internal carotid artery, sympathetic plexus
Foramen rotundum	CN VII, artery of foramen rotundum, emissary veins
Foramen ovale	CN VIII, lesser petrosal nerve accessory meningeal branch of maxillary artery, emissary vein
Foramen spinosum	Middle meningeal artery and vein, meningeal branch of CN VIII
Foramen lacerum	Forms cartilaginous floor of medial part of horizontal petrous internal carotid artery canal
Vidian canal	Vidian artery and vein

CN, Cranial nerve.

the petrous ridge. The posterior skull base also contains many foramina, fissures, and synchondroses (Table 3-2). The synchondroses and fissures in the posterior skull base may potentially be misinterpreted as fractures.

Injury to the posterior skull base (Fig. 3-24) can result in intracranial hematoma and parenchymal brain injury, dural tear, and CSF leak. The major dural venous sinuses run along the posterior skull base. Posterior skull base fracture can result in tear of the dural venous sinuses, resulting in formation of venous EDH. Venous sinus injury can also result in venous sinus thrombosis. Lower cranial nerves can be injured in posterior skull

base fracture. Occipital condylar fracture may result in hypoglossal nerve injury.

■ TEMPORAL BONE

Although part of the skull base, the temporal bone is often discussed as a separate entity. It includes the external auditory canal, middle ear, and inner ear. The middle ear contains the ossicles and tympanic membrane, which are the crucial structures for conductive hearing. The inner ear includes the otic capsule, which houses the cochlear, semicircular canals, vestibules, and cochlear nerve. The structures in the otic capsule provide the important function of sensorineural hearing and balance. In addition, the facial nerve traverses the temporal bone.

Temporal bone fractures have traditionally been classified as either longitudinal or transverse, reflecting whether the overall axis of the fracture runs parallel to, or cuts across, the long axis of the petrous pyramid. A longitudinal fracture is reportedly the most common of the two traditional classes, representing between 70% and 90% of temporal bone fractures. A longitudinal fracture begins in the squamous or mastoid temporal bone and extends anteromedially, often involving the anterosuperior external

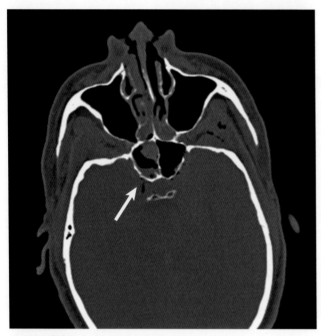

Figure 3-22 Central skull base fracture. Fractures through the posterior wall of the right sphenoid sinus and at the tuberculum sella. Foci of gas in the right cavernous sinus *(arrow)* indicate fracture involving this region and raise the concern of vascular injury. Subsequent catheter angiogram did not show any vascular injury in this region.

Table 3-2   Foramina and Fissures of the Posterior Skull Base.

Foramina and Fissures	Contents
Internal auditory canal	CN VII-VIII, labyrinthine artery
Jugular foramen	CN IX, CN X, CN XI, Jacobson nerve, Arnold nerve, jugular bulb, inferior petrosal sinus, posterior meningeal artery
Hypoglossal canal	CN XII
Foramen magnum	CN XI, vertebral arteries, medulla
Stylomastoid foramen	CN VII

CN, Cranial nerve.

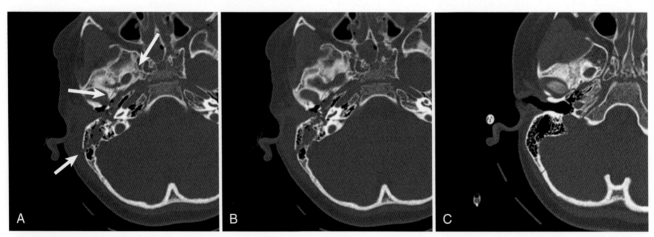

Figure 3-23 Central skull base fracture extending into temporal bone. A and **B,** A linear minimally displaced fracture extends through the posterior aspect of the greater wing of the right sphenoid bone (*middle arrow* in **A**) and runs across the foramen ovale (*anterior arrow* in **A**). It continues anteriorly and superiorly through the body of the sphenoid. A comminuted temporal bone fracture is also present (*posterior arrow* in **A**). **C,** The normal contralateral left greater wing of the sphenoid is shown for comparison (image is flipped horizontally for the purpose of comparison).

auditory canal, through the middle ear toward the petrous apex (Fig. 3-25). As a further refinement, anterior and posterior subtypes are recognized. The posterior subtype arises behind the external auditory canal, usually within the posterior squamous or mastoid region. It courses through the middle ear, often terminating at the foramen lacerum or foramen ovale. The anterior subtype arises anterior to the external auditory canal in the squamous portion of temporal bone, coursing in a more directly medial path, sometimes through the mandibular fossa, along the tegmen tympani toward the petrous apex. Both anterior and posterior subtypes are liable to involve the facial nerve canal at the level of the geniculate ganglion. The posterior subtype is more likely to involve the ossicular chain, whereas the anterior subtype may result in serious injury to the middle meningeal artery. Either subtype may occasionally involve the carotid canal. Longitudinal fractures in general spare the inner ear structures.

Transverse fractures represent between 10% and 30% of temporal bone fractures. These fractures course from the foramen magnum or jugular fossa, across the petrous pyramid, to terminate in the middle cranial fossa (Fig. 3-26). Transverse fractures have also been subdivided into medial and lateral subtypes. The medial subtype runs medial to the arcuate eminence, which is a subtle convexity of the petrous bone resulting from the arc of the superior semicircular canal. A medial subtype fracture will traverse the internal auditory canal and often results in serious injury to the seventh and eighth nerve complex. The lateral subtype runs lateral to the arcuate eminence, traversing the bony labyrinth. Both subtypes carry a high likelihood of sensorineural hearing loss. The middle ear and ossicular chain are mostly spared. As with longitudinal fractures, transverse fractures may also occasionally involve the carotid canal.

In practice, most temporal bone fractures are neither purely longitudinal nor purely transverse, and some are so complicated as to defy description. They can be referred to as mixed or complex fractures (Fig. 3-27).

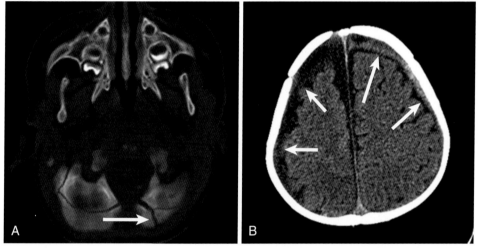

Figure 3-24 Posterior skull base fracture. **A,** Axial computed tomography (CT) of the skull base shows an acute-appearing left occipital bone fracture (*arrow*). **B,** Axial CT superior to the ventricles shows bilateral subdural hematomas (SDHs) (*arrows*). The left subdural collection contains densities of varying degrees, suggesting multiple stages of hematoma, which is suspicious for nonaccidental trauma.

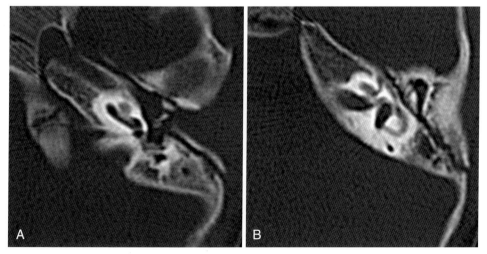

Figure 3-25 Longitudinal temporal bone fracture. **A** and **B,** Axial views showing a purely longitudinal fracture passing through the mastoids and middle ear cavity. (From Collins JM, et al. Multidetector CT of temporal bone fractures. *Semin Ultrasound CT MR.* 33:418-431.)

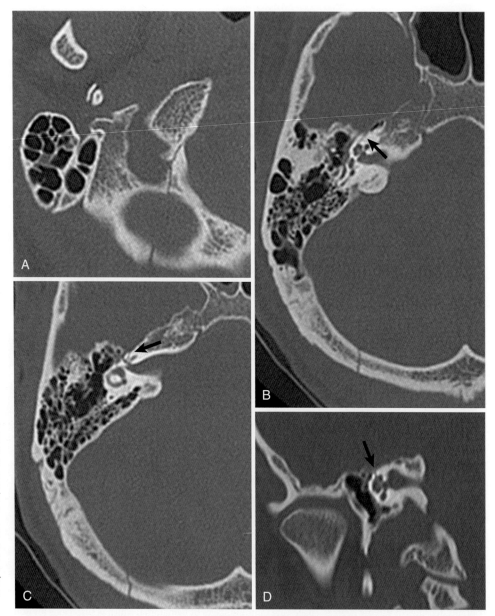

Figure 3-26 Predominantly transverse fracture. A to C, Axial views showing a skull base fracture with a predominantly transverse component involving the cochlea (*arrows* in **B** and **C**). The fracture parallels the tympanic segment of the facial nerve canal (**B**) and may cross the labyrinthine segment (**C**). This patient did manifest facial nerve palsy. **D**, Coronal view of the same fracture confirming cochlear involvement (*arrow*). (From Collins JM, et al. Multidetector CT of temporal bone fractures. *Semin Ultrasound CT MR.* 33:418-431.)

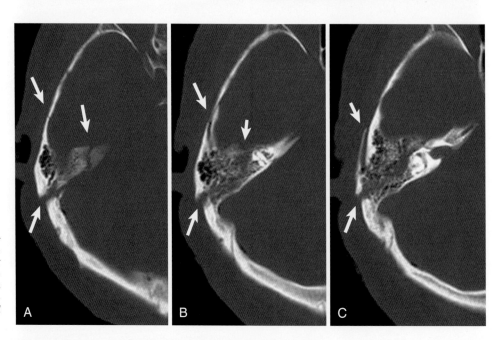

Figure 3-27 Complex, predominantly longitudinal fracture. A to C, Axial views showing a multiplanar fracture (*arrows*) with an overall longitudinal orientation. (From Collins JM, et al. Multidetector CT of temporal bone fractures. *Semin Ultrasound CT MR.* 33:418-431.)

Recently a new classification scheme has been proposed that may offer a more accurate prediction of the likelihood of serious or long-term complications. Fractures are segregated into those that violate the otic capsule and those that do not. Otic capsule–violating fractures involve the inner ear structures and are more likely to be associated with neuro-otologic (severe hearing loss, facial paralysis) and nonotologic (significant intracranial hemorrhage, CSF leak, meningitis) complications.

In evaluation of temporal bone fractures, radiologists should review carefully the integrity of the ossicular chain and inner ear structures, including the cochlear and semicircular canals, because these structures affect hearing. In addition, the course of the facial nerve should be reviewed carefully to exclude injury.

■ DIAGNOSTIC PITFALLS

The presence of small foci of intracranial air is an important clue to an underlying skull base fracture. Another important clue is abnormal fluid in the mastoid air cells, middle ear cavity, or paranasal sinuses. When these findings are present in the setting of acute trauma, the bone structures in these areas need to be scrutinized carefully.

Pseudofractures can present a challenge to evaluation of skull base trauma. Many normal fissures, canals, and channels are present in the skull base and temporal bones (Figs. 3-28 to 3-32). They can be misinterpreted as fractures. Comparison of the left and right sides may help, but some of these pseudofractures can present unilaterally.

■ COMPLICATIONS ASSOCIATED WITH SKULL BASE INJURY

Orbital Injury

It is important to evaluate for potential orbital injury when fractures of the anterior and middle skull base are present. Orbital injury can include direct trauma to orbital contents and retrobulbar hematoma, or indirect

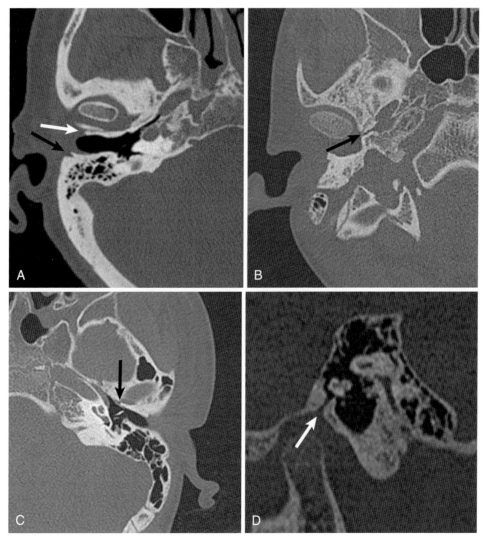

Figure 3-28 Intrinsic sutures. A, Axial views of the tympanosquamous *(white arrow)* and tympanomastoid *(black arrow)* fissures. **B,** Axial view of the petrosquamosal fissure *(black arrow)*. **C** and **D,** Petrotympanic (glaserian) fissure *(arrows)* on axial **(C)** and sagittal **(D)** views. On the sagittal view the petrotympanic fissure connects the tympanic cavity superiorly to the mandibular fossa inferiorly. (From Collins JM, et al. Multidetector CT of temporal bone fractures. *Semin Ultrasound CT MR.* 33:418-431.)

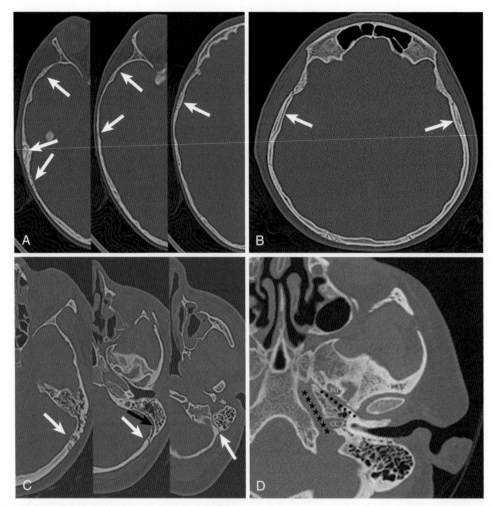

Figure 3-29 Extrinsic sutures. A, Axial views showing a highly serpentine temporoparietal (squamosal) suture *(arrows)*. **B,** Axial view in another patient showing much more linear bilateral temporoparietal sutures *(arrows)*. **C,** Axial images showing the occipitomastoid suture *(white arrows)*. Note the presence of a venous channel *(black arrow)*. **D,** Axial image showing the sphenopetrosal *(black dots)* and petrooccipital *(black stars)* sutures. *CC,* Carotid canal; *FO,* foramen ovale. (From Collins JM, et al. Multidetector CT of temporal bone fractures. *Semin Ultrasound CT MR.* 33:418-431.)

injury such as soft tissue edema or hematoma causing optic nerve impingement. Indirect injury can be subtle. The optic nerve traverses the optic canal, which is a very narrow space. Even a minimally displaced bone fragment or a small hematoma can potentially result in optic nerve impingement and visual loss if the injury is not treated promptly (Fig. 3-33). Axial and coronal plane CT offers the best assessment of the orbital apex.

Cranial Nerve Injury

All cranial nerves potentially can be injured in skull base trauma. Significant traumatic injury to the ethmoidal complex and cribriform plate can suggest the presence of olfactory nerve damage. Clival fracture may result in cranial nerve VI injury. Fractures through the temporal bones, particularly otic-violating fractures or transverse fractures, can result in injury of the facial nerve (Figs. 3-34; see Fig. 3-26). Fractures through any of the other foramina transmitting the cranial nerves can potentially result in injury of the corresponding nerve.

Dural Tear, Cerebrospinal Fluid Leak, and Encephalocele

Skull base fracture can result in dural tear and CSF leak, putting the patients at risk for meningitis. CSF leak may not be apparent at the time of trauma and can present as an early subacute complication. Eighty percent of CSF leaks present in the first 48 hours. CSF leak can be difficult to diagnose in an acute setting, but in a later stage, CT cisternogram can be used to identify the site of the dural tear and CSF leak. Recent literature has also demonstrated that CSF leak can be reliably detected using high-resolution CT without intrathecal contrast, when high-resolution imaging in multiple orthogonal planes is used.

CSF leak has the highest association with anterior skull base fracture. At the anterior skull base there is dense adhesion of the dura to the bone, which predisposes to injury. Common sites of injury include the posterior table of the frontal sinus, fovea ethmoidalis, and cribriform plate, particularly at the lateral lamella where the anterior ethmoidal artery enters the anterior skull base.

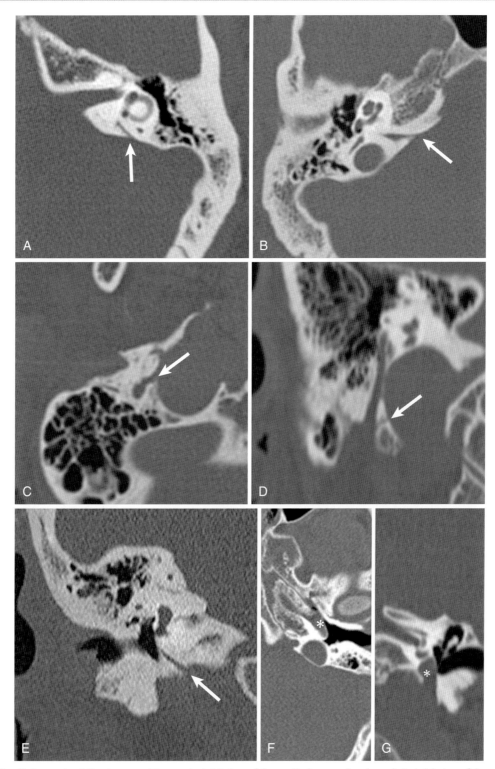

Figure 3-30 Small channels of the temporal bone. **A,** Axial view of the vestibular aqueduct (*arrow*). **B,** Axial view of the cochlear aqueduct (*arrow*). **C** and **D,** Mastoid canaliculus in axial (**C**) and coronal (**D**) views. **E,** Coronal view of the inferior tympanic canaliculus (*arrow*). **F** and **G,** Aberrant internal carotid artery *(white star)* traversing an enlarged inferior tympanic canaliculus on axial (**F**) and coronal (**G**) views. (From Collins JM, et al. Multidetector CT of temporal bone fractures. *Semin Ultrasound CT MR.* 33:418-431.)

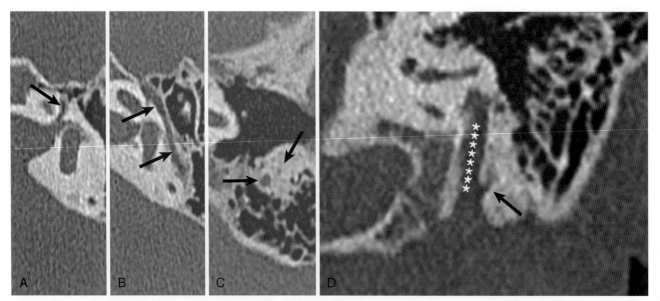

Figure 3-31 Facial nerve canal. A, Axial view of the labyrinthine segment *(arrow)*. B, Axial view of the tympanic segment *(arrow)*. C, Axial view of the mastoid segment *(horizontal arrow)*. Note the chorda tympani nerve *(angled arrow)*. D, Coronal view of the mastoid segment *(white stars)*. Again, note the origin of the chorda tympani nerve *(small black arrow)*. (From Collins JM, et al. Multidetector CT of temporal bone fractures. *Semin Ultrasound CT MR*. 33:418-431.)

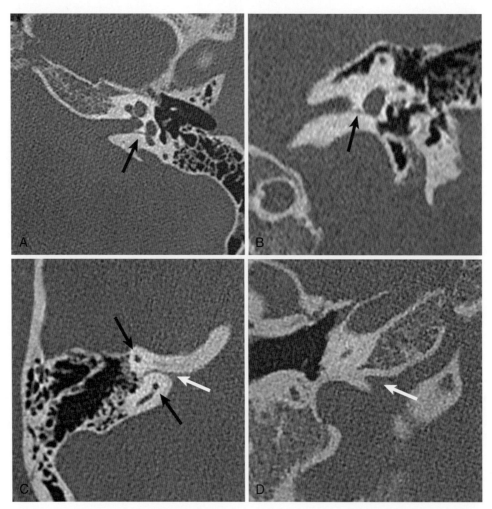

Figure 3-32 Small channels of the temporal bone continued. A and B, Singular canal *(arrows)* on axial (A) and coronal (B) views. C, Axial view of the petromastoid canal *(white arrow)* passing beneath the arch of the superior semicircular canal *(black arrows)*. D, Axial view of the glossopharyngeal sulcus *(arrow)*. (From Collins JM, et al. Multidetector CT of temporal bone fractures. *Semin Ultrasound CT MR*. 33:418-431.)

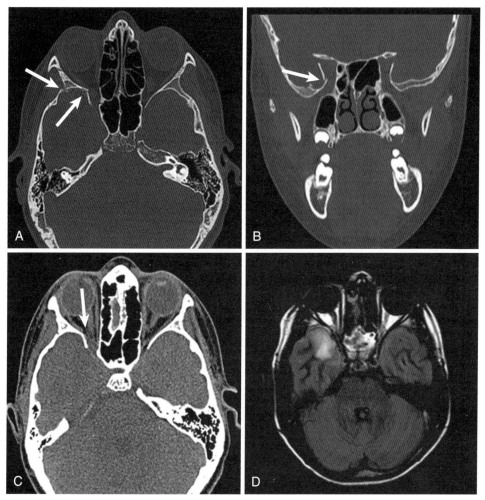

Figure 3-33 **A** and **B,** Fracture through the posterior lateral aspect of the right greater wing of the sphenoid (*arrows*) with associated full shaft width posterior displacement of the distal fragment at the level of the middle cranial fossa. **C,** Evaluation of the orbital contents demonstrates mass effect upon the right lateral rectus and subtle abutment of the right inferior rectus by the buckled posterior lateral orbital wall fracture (*arrow*). Evaluation of the optic nerve shows asymmetric obscuration of the perineural fat at the level of the orbital apex and subtle increased soft tissue is seen adjacent to the nerve as it enters into the optic canal in the region of the planum sphenoidale fracture. **D,** Abnormal signal is present along the anterior aspect of the right temporal lobe adjacent to the posterolateral sphenoid bone fracture, consistent with traumatic brain injury (TBI)/contusion.

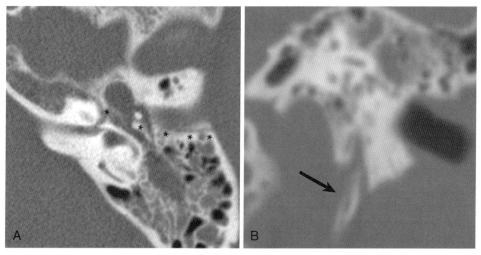

Figure 3-34 **Findings suggestive of facial nerve injury.** **A,** Axial view showing a curvilinear fracture (*black stars*) running through the mastoids, middle ear cavity, and directly into the region of the geniculate ganglion. **B,** Coronal view showing a fracture of the styloid process (*arrow*) that has been displaced into the region of the stylomastoid foramen. (From Collins JM, et al. Multidetector CT of temporal bone fractures. *Semin Ultrasound CT MR.* 33:418-431.)

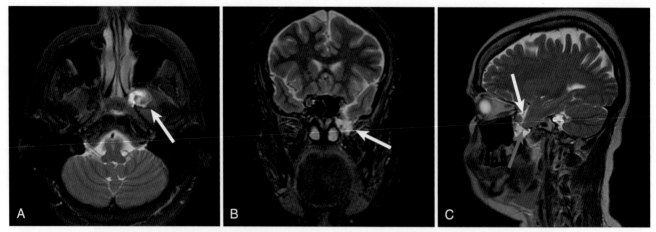

Figure 3-35 Central skull base fracture resulting in encephalocele. A to C, Axial, coronal, and sagittal T2-weighted images demonstrate left middle cranial fossa encephalocele (*arrows*) associated with sphenoid bone deficit.

A large dural defect can result in encephalocele (Fig. 3-35). Although CSF leak can be treated conservatively initially, a traumatic encephalocele usually requires urgent surgical repair.

Hearing Loss

Posttraumatic hearing loss may be conductive, sensorineural, or mixed; of immediate or delayed onset; and transient, fixed, or progressive.

Sensorineural hearing loss implies direct injury to the special sense organs of the inner ear, the cochlear nerve at any point from the internal auditory canal to the root entry zone, or the central auditory pathways, including the cochlear nuclei themselves. In the case of an otic-violating or transverse fracture through the bony labyrinth, the cause and nature of the hearing loss are readily apparent (see Fig. 3-26). In some cases, a fracture line may not be evident, but T1-weighted MRI images will demonstrate hyperintense signal in the labyrinthine structures indicative of hemorrhage. Overall, sensorineural hearing loss carries a worse prognosis than does conductive hearing loss.

Conductive hearing loss is believed to be the more common type following trauma. In some cases, the cause is simply obstructive, with fractures of the external auditory canal resulting in canal stenosis or blood and fluid filling the canal or middle ear (see Fig. 3-27). Hemotympanum, or hemorrhagic opacification of the middle ear, is particularly common following temporal bone fracture and may in fact be the initial finding that prompts a more careful search for a subtle fracture. Conductive hearing loss may also result from rupture of the tympanic membrane, with or without evidence of fracture. All of these processes result in transient hearing loss. Complete restoration of hearing is expected following resorption of any middle ear blood or debris and healing of the tympanic membrane.

Disruption of the ossicular chain is a more severe cause of traumatic conductive hearing loss (Figs. 3-36 and 3-37). Ossicles may be subluxed from their normal articulations or fractured, with subluxation being more common. Of the three ossicles, the incus is the least well supported and consequently the most likely to be subluxed. The malleus is firmly attached to the tympanic membrane and is further supported by four malleolar ligaments and the tensor tympani muscle. The stapes is firmly attached to the oval window and is further supported by the stapedius muscle. By contrast, the incus is supported only by its articulations with the malleus and stapes and by one ligament. Following trauma, the incudostapedial joint is the most common site of subluxation, followed by complete incus dislocation. Derangements of the incus are best appreciated on axial images. The incudomallear joint is easily assessed because it forms the classic "ice cream cone" appearance within the epitympanum on axial CT. The interface between the head of the malleus (ice cream) and the short limb of the incus (cone) should be razor thin. Any widening of this joint space, which may require comparison with the opposite side, or any offset of the malleus head relative to the incus, is suggestive of at least partial subluxation. The incudostapedial articulation is more difficult to assess given the smallness of the structures, but high-quality axial images may demonstrate a gap between the lenticular process of the incus and the capitulum of the stapes. A complete incus dislocation should be easy to diagnose with the displaced incus found somewhere in the middle ear cavity, or not found at all. Ossicular fracture is less common and most likely to affect the incus for reasons already mentioned. The stapes arch is also a common site of fracture. The long and lenticular processes of the incus are best appreciated on coronal imaging, along with the manubrium of the malleus. The stapes superstructure is best seen on axial images. Of note, any of these ossicular derangements may be seen in the absence of a temporal bone fracture.

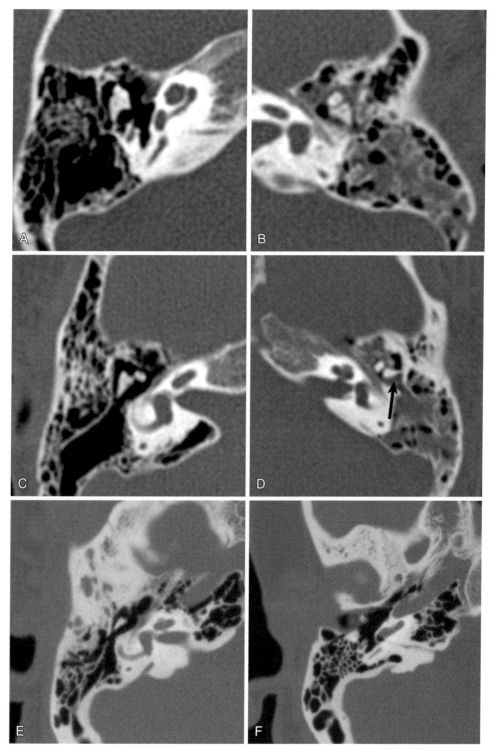

Figure 3-36 Ossicular derangements A, Axial view of a normal malleoincudal articulation. The joint space is nearly imperceptible. B, Axial view of a subtle malleoincudal dislocation. C, Axial view of a not-so-subtle malleoincudal dislocation with lateral translation of the head of the malleus. D, Axial view showing an apparently mild malleoincudal separation, but note the abnormal counterclockwise rotation of the short limb of the incus *(black arrow)*, indicating a more serious derangement. E and F, Complete malleus dislocation. Axial views showing (E) absence of the malleus in the epitympanum, with calcific material at the level of the tympanic membrane (F) possibly representing the dislocated malleus or simply dystrophic calcium. (From Collins JM, et al. Multidetector CT of temporal bone fractures. *Semin Ultrasound CT MR*. 33:418-431.)

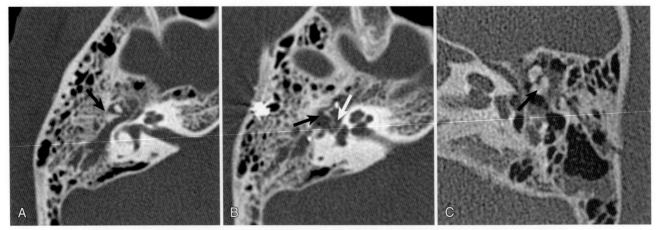

Figure 3-37 Ossicular derangements continued. **A** and **B,** Axial views of severe derangement of the incus following gunshot injury. The short process of the incus is abnormally rotated to almost 180 degrees (*black arrow* in **A**). **B,** Abnormal angulation of the long and lenticular processes of the incus suggesting fracture (*black arrow*), and dislocation of the lenticular process from the stapes head (*white arrow*). The stapes itself appears intact. **C,** Axial view of a longitudinal fracture coursing through the epitympanum with an associated cleft through the incus short process (*black arrow*) suggesting fracture. (From Collins JM, et al. Multidetector CT of temporal bone fractures. *Semin Ultrasound CT MR.* 33:418-431.)

Selected Reading

Biffl WL, Egglin T, Benedetto B, et al. Sixteen-slice computed tomographic angiography is a reliable noninvasive screening test for clinically significant blunt cerebrovascular injuries. *J Trauma.* 2006;60(4):745–751.

Biffl WL, Moore EE, Offner PJ, et al. Blunt carotid and vertebral arterial injuries. *World J Surg.* 2001;25:1036–1043.

Biffl WL, Rat Jr CE, Morre EE, et al. Treatment-related outcomes from blunt cerebrovascular injuries: importance of routine follow-up arteriography. *Ann Surg.* 2002;235(5):699–707.

Bosnell R, Giorgio A, Johansen-Berg H. Imaging white matter diffusion changes with development and recovery from brain injury. *Dev Neurorehabil.* 2008;11:174–186.

Botteri M, Bandera E, Minelli C, et al. Cerebral blood flow thresholds for cerebral ischemia in traumatic brain injury: a systemic review. *Crit Care Med.* 2008;36:3089–3092.

Cannon CR, Jahrsdoerfer RA. Temporal bone fractures: review of 90 cases. *Arch Otolaryngol.* 1983;109:285–288.

Castillo M. Whole-brain N-acetyl aspartate: a marker of the severity of mild head trauma. *Clin Med.* 2008;8:502–507.

Chavan GB, Babyn PS, Thomas B, et al. Principles, techniques, and applications of T2*-based MR imaging and its special applications. *Radiographics.* 2009;29:1433–1449.

Chokshi FH, Munera F, Rivas LA, et al. 64-MDCT angiography of blunt vascular injuries of the neck. *AJR Am J Roentgenol.* 2011;196(3):W309–W315.

Coburn MW, Rodriguez FJ. Cerebral herniations. *Appl Radiol.* 1998;27:10–16.

Connor SEJ, Flis A. The contribution of high-resolution multiplanar reformats of the skull base to the detection of skull-base fractures. *Clin Radiol.* 2005;60:878–885

Coronado VG, McGuire LC, Sarmiento K, et al. Trends in Traumatic Brain Injury in the U.S. and the public health response: 1995-2009. *J Safety Res.* 2012;43(4):299–307

Dahiya R, Keller JD, Litofsky NS, et al. Temporal bone fractures: otic capsule sparing versus otic capsule violating clinical and radiographic considerations. *J Trauma.* 1999;47:1079–1083.

Dubroff JG, Newberg A. Neuroimaging of traumatic brain injury. *Semin Neurol.* 2008;28:548–557.

Faul M, Xu L, Wald MM, et al. *Traumatic Brain Injury in the United States: Emergency Department Visits, Hospitalizations, and Deaths.* Atlanta, GA: Centers for Disease Control and Prevention, National Center for Injury Prevention and Control; 2010.

Galloway NR, Tong KA, Ashwal S, et al. Diffusion-weighted MR imaging improves outcome prediction in pediatric traumatic brain injury. *J Neurotrauma.* 2008;25:1153–1162.

Gentry L. Temporal bone trauma: current perspectives for diagnostic evaluation. *Neuroimaging Clin N Am.* 1991;1:319–340.

Greenberg SM, Vernooij MW, Cordonnier C, et al. Cerebral microbleeds: a guide to detection and interpretation. *Lancet Neurol.* 2009;8:165–174.

Haddad SH, Arabi YM. Critical care management of severe traumatic brain injury in adults. *Scand J Trauma, Resusc, Emerg Med.* 2012;20:12–27.

Ishman SL, Friedland DR. Temporal bone fractures: traditional classification and clinical relevance. *Laryngoscope.* 2004;114:1734–1741.

Kazim SF, Shamim MS, Tahir MZ, et al. Management of penetrating brain injury. *J Emerg Trauma Shock.* 2011;4(3):395–402.

Kohler R, Vargas MI, Masterson K, et al. CT and MR angiography features of traumatic vascular injuries of the neck. *AJR Am J Roentgenol.* 2011;196:W800–W809.

La Fata V, McLean N, Wise SK, et al. CSF leaks: correlation of high-resolution CT and multiplanar reformations with intraoperative endoscopic findings. *AJNR Am J Neuroradiol.* 2008;29:536–541.

Laine FJ, Shedden AI, Dunn MM, et al. Acquired intracranial herniation: MR findings. *AJR Am J Roentgenol.* 1995;165:967–973.

Liang W, Xiaofeng Y, Weiguo L, et al. Traumatic carotid cavernous fistula accompanying basilar skull fracture: a study on the incidence of traumatic carotid cavernous fistula in the patients with basilar skull fracture and the prognosis analysis about traumatic carotid cavernous fistula. *J Trauma.* 2007;63:1014–20.

Lloyd KM, DelGaudio JM, Hudgins PA. Imaging of skull base cerebrospinal fluid leaks in adults. *Radiology.* 2008;248(3):725–736.

Lovell M. The management of sports-related concussion: current status and future trends. *Clin Sports Med.* 2009;28:95–111.

Marino S, Ciurleo R, Bramanti P, et al. 1H-MR spectroscopy in traumatic brain injury. *Neurocrit Care.* 2011;14:127–133.

Offiah C, Twigg S. Imaging assessment of penetrating craniocerebral and spinal trauma. *Clin Radiol.* 2009;64:1146–1157.

Provenzale JM. Imaging of traumatic brain injury: a review of recent medical literature. *AJR Am J Roentgenol.* 2010;194:16–19.

Resnick DK, Subach BR, Marion DW. The significance of carotid canal involvement in basilar cranial fracture. *Neurosurgery.* 1997;40:1177–81.

Shenton ME, Hamoda HM, Schneiderman JS, et al. A review of magnetic resonance imaging and diffusion tensor imaging in mild traumatic brain injury. *Brain Imaging Behav.* 2012;6(2):137–92. http://dx.doi.org/10.1007/s11682-012-9156-5.

Tollard E, Galanaud D, Vincent Perlbarg V, et al. Experience of diffusion tensor imaging and 1H spectroscopy for outcome prediction in severe traumatic brain injury: preliminary results. *Crit Care Med.* 2009;37:1448–1455.

Verschuuren S, Poretti A, Buerki S, et al. Susceptibility-weighted imaging of the pediatric brain. *AJR Am J Roentgenol.* 2012;198:W440–W449.

Weissman JL, Curtin HD, Hirsch BE, et al. High signal from the otic labyrinth on unenhanced magnetic resonance imaging. *AJNR Am J Neuroradiol.* 1992;13:1183–1187.

York G, Barboriak D, Petrella J, et al. Association of internal carotid artery injury with carotid canal fractures in patients with head trauma. *AJR Am J Roentgenol.* 2005;184:1672–78.

Zayas JO, Feliciano YZ, Hadley CR, et al. Temporal bone trauma and the role of multidetector CT in the emergency department. *Radiographics.* 2011;31:1741–1755.

CHAPTER 4

Nontraumatic Brain Emergencies

Intracranial Hemorrhage
Arash Meshksar and Wayne S. Kubal

◼ NONTRAUMATIC INTRACRANIAL HEMORRHAGE

Initial Diagnosis

Although many cases of intracranial hemorrhage (ICH), including intra-axial and extra-axial hemorrhage, are due to trauma, this discussion will be limited to atraumatic intracranial hemorrhage. Abrupt onset of neurologic symptoms in any patient should be considered to be of vascular origin until proven otherwise. It is not possible to differentiate ischemic from hemorrhagic accidents based on the patient's symptoms alone. Neuroimaging is thus an essential initial step not only for determining the initial diagnosis, but also for determining the type, location, and underlying mechanism in patients with intracranial hemorrhage. Computed tomography (CT) and magnetic resonance imaging (MRI) are both very sensitive for detection of intracranial hemorrhage; however, due to easier accessibility, lower cost, and shorter imaging time, CT scan is preferred for the initial evaluation of patients with suspected acute hemorrhage. The task of the radiologist is to diagnose the hemorrhage based on initial noncontrast CT (NCCT) or MRI, analyze the pattern of hemorrhage, and make recommendations for further workup. Performing these tasks efficiently and accurately can improve patient outcome and can optimize work flow in a busy emergency radiology section.

The first point of analysis for the radiologist is to determine the location of the intracranial hemorrhage. Specifically, the radiologist needs to determine whether the hemorrhage is primarily a subarachnoid hemorrhage (SAH) or intraparenchymal hemorrhage (IPH). Although there is some overlap in the etiologies and workup of SAH and IPH, we will consider them separately.

Subarachnoid Hemorrhage

Subarachnoid hemorrhage is bleeding into the subarachnoid space. Atraumatic SAH usually occurs because of ruptured aneurysms. Nonaneurysmal perimesencephalic hemorrhage, vascular malformation, or less commonly

vasculitis and vessel dissection are additional causes of non-traumatic intracranial hemorrhage one should consider. There is a wide geographic variation in the incidence of atraumatic SAH. China reports an incidence of 2 cases per 100,000 population per year, whereas Finland reports the highest incidence at over 20 cases per 100,000 per year. In the United States the incidence is 9.6 to 14.0 cases per 100,000 according to different reports. That incidence translates to approximately 30,000 new cases annually. Risk factors for SAH include female sex, hypertension, smoking, alcohol use, and the abuse of drugs such as cocaine. It is the responsibility of the radiologist to meticulously search for the signs of SAH in patients investigated for headache and also determine the cause of the hemorrhage as early as possible. Computed tomography remains the cornerstone of diagnosis, having a sensitivity of approximately 98% to 100% in the first 12 hours after hemorrhage. Computed tomography sensitivity declines after this period with a sharp decline after 5 to 7 days. Lumbar puncture is often required in these patients to show xanthochromia and confirm the diagnosis. Negative predictive value of absence of xanthochromia to rule out SAH has been shown to be about 99%.

Magnetic resonance imaging can be an alternative to lumbar puncture in potential SAH cases with negative CT scan results. Bleeding into the subarachnoid space causes a change in relaxation time of the cerebral spinal fluid (CSF), which in turn causes T1 signal change. This change also causes insufficient nulling of the CSF signal by fluid-attenuated inversion recovery (FLAIR) and consequent hyperintensity of subarachnoid space. Even though the sensitivity of FLAIR imaging has been reported to be nearly the same as CT, the specificity remains lower than lumbar puncture for excluding SAH. Other disease entities such as meningitis, leptomeningeal spread of malignant disease, and meningeal enhancement after contrast administration also lead to increased subarachnoid signal on FLAIR sequence.

Aneurysm

Approximately 80% of patients with atraumatic SAH have aneurysm as the cause of hemorrhage (Fig. 4-1). The most common presenting symptom is headache that is usually described by the patient as the "worst headache of life." Other symptoms include vomiting, meningismus, and altered level of consciousness or even coma. Some patients experience milder symptoms (usually milder headache and nausea/vomiting) 2 to 8 weeks before the overt SAH. These symptoms can be caused by minor

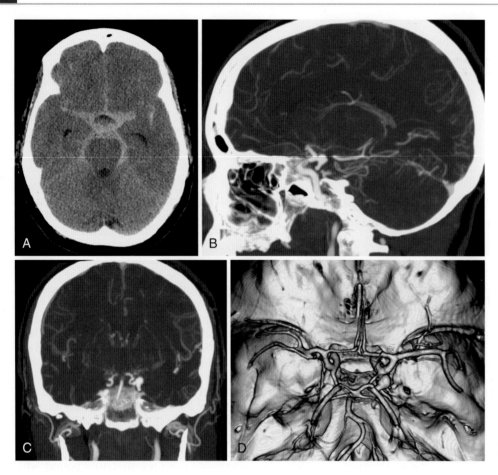

Figure 4-1 Diffuse subarachnoid hemorrhage (SAH). Noncontrast computed tomography (NCCT) (**A**) shows diffuse increased density in subarachnoid space, including the suprasellar cistern. Sagittal (**B**) and coronal (**C**) reformatted computed tomographic angiography (CTA) show a left posterior communicating artery aneurysm. Three-dimensional (3-D) reformatted CTA (**D**) confirms the left posterior communicating artery aneurysm and shows its relationship to the skull base and other neighboring vessels.

hemorrhages from an aneurysm leak, which is called a *sentinel or warning bleed.* Review of several large studies showed that about 20% among 1752 patients with SAH in those studies had a history of headache before the SAH event. Only 1% of patients presenting to the emergency department (ED) with headache have SAH. A high degree of suspicion and proper screening in patients with headache can detect those with a sentinel bleed, a potentially lifesaving diagnosis in this group of patients.

An accurate diagnosis of SAH based on initial CT scan requires knowledge of the common locations where the blood may accumulate after the incident. These areas include dependent areas of the CSF space, including the suprasellar cistern (aneurysm of anterior communicating artery), the deep sulci adjacent to the interhemispheric fissure (aneurysms of distal anterior cerebral artery), the interpeduncular cistern (aneurysms of posterior circulation), and the Sylvian fissure (aneurysm of middle cerebral artery [MCA] bifurcation). Sometimes the aneurysms can be visualized as lucent lesions within the hyperdense hemorrhagic material in CSF space or as curvilinear calcifications.

The description of the location of aneurysms mentioned earlier involves saccular aneurysms, which are the most common. It should be noted that infectious aneurysms (mycotic aneurysms) could also be the cause of SAH. These aneurysms can be located anywhere in the cerebral vasculature and can be suspected according to the patient's clinical setting and imaging findings.

Table 4-1 Computed Tomography Grading System for Prediction of Vasospasm After Subarachnoid Hemorrhage

Grade	Computed Tomography Appearance of Subarachnoid Hemorrhage
1	No visualized blood
2	Visualized layers of blood less than 1 mm thick
3	Visualized layers or focal clots more than 1 mm thick
4	Any thickness with intraventricular or intraparenchymal hemorrhage

Patients who survive the initial few hours after SAH are threatened by intracranial complications such as brain ischemia secondary to vasospasm, rebleeding, and hydrocephalus. A CT grading system known as the *Fisher scale* (Table 4-1) has been used for prediction of cerebral vasospasm in patients with SAH.

The odds ratio of cerebral vasospasm after SAH is estimated to be in orders of 1.2, 2.2, and 1.7 for grades 2, 3, and 4 compared to grade 1, respectively. Thus SAH patients with focal thick clots in the subarachnoid space or concomitant intraventricular hemorrhage (IVH)/IPH are at increased risk for vasospasm. Although the case fatality has decreased in industrialized nations over the past 25 years, SAH still carries a poor prognosis. Mortality rates vary widely across different reports, ranging from 8% to 67%. The median mortality rate from epidemiologic studies in the United States has been 32% versus

43% in Europe and 27% in Japan. Morbidity, including lifestyle restriction, persistent dependence, and cognitive impairment, ranges from 8% to 20% in survivors. The goal is early treatment of the source of hemorrhage.

Nonaneurysmal Perimesencephalic Hemorrhage

Nonaneurysmal perimesencephalic hemorrhage (NAPH) accounts for about 10% of SAH cases. The hemorrhage is characterized by accumulation of blood predominantly around the brainstem mostly ventral to the midbrain or pons or less commonly in the quadrigeminal plate cistern (Fig. 4-2, *A* and *B*). The diagnosis requires the exclusion of aneurysms or any other source of bleeding (see Fig. 4-2, *C* and *D*). The symptoms and clinical course in these patients are more benign than with aneurysmal rupture. Rebleeding and ischemia do not usually occur. The cause of the NAPH has not been fully determined. Some clues suggest that the origin of bleeding is venous as opposed to arterial in aneurysms. It has been shown that patients with this form of hemorrhage have an aberrant pattern of deep cerebral venous drainage much more frequently than patients with aneurysmal causes. Perimesencephalic hemorrhage often follows physical exertion. Some investigators believe that increased intracranial venous pressures secondary to increased intrathoracic pressure during exercise causes the hemorrhage. There is controversy regarding the best method to exclude an aneurysm as the etiology of perimesencephalic hemorrhage. Many experts advocate use of catheter angiography for this purpose. The remaining 10% of SAH cases are caused by a variety of pathologic conditions such as arteriovenous malformation (AVM), dissection, vasculitis, cavernous hemangioma, and unspecified causes.

Workup of Subarachnoid Hemorrhage After Initial Diagnosis

After the diagnosis of SAH has been made, the imaging workup should be directed toward determining the cause of the hemorrhage and providing information for subsequent treatment. Given the preponderance of aneurysmal ruptures as the cause of SAH (80% of cases), the next step in imaging workup is directed toward vascular imaging with the goal of detecting and defining possible intracranial aneurysm or aneurysms. Aneurysms may be detected with catheter digital subtraction angiography (DSA), computed tomographic angiography (CTA), or magnetic resonance angiography (MRA). Although DSA is still the gold standard, CTA is most commonly used for the initial evaluation. Magnetic resonance angiography has a limited role in the initial vascular evaluation of SAH patients because of longer acquisition time, higher cost, susceptibility to patient movement, and lower sensitivity. The sensitivity of MRA has been reported to be 74% to 98% for aneurysms larger than 3 mm.

The emergence of three-dimensional (3-D) rotational DSA and flat panel detectors as the newer technologies integrated into the DSA technique has made DSA even more sensitive in detecting small aneurysms that otherwise would not be detected because of overlapping vessels. Digital subtraction angiography provides the highest spatial resolution (0.125-mm pixel size) and is still the best modality for studying aneurysm relationship to the parent artery and to the neighboring perforator arteries, as well as measurement of the aneurysm neck and dome.

In many centers CTA has replaced DSA as the initial imaging modality. Computed tomography angiography has the advantage of being quick to obtain while the patient is in the CT scanner for initial screening and allows for interpretation by the emergency radiologist before activating either the endovascular or neurosurgical services. The accuracy of CTA has improved over the last few years with improvements in CT technology. The advent of multirow detector CTA has yielded a very good spatial resolution with a maximum pixel size of 0.35 mm. Administration of an average 50 to 80 mL of contrast medium is usually sufficient to obtain diagnostic-quality images. Computed tomography angiography has also been shown to be very accurate in providing information about the configuration of the aneurysm to allow for planning of endovascular therapy (Fig. 4-3; see Fig. 4-1). One important advantage of CTA over DSA is the ability to show the osseous and extraluminal structures, which helps the surgeon with surgery planning. It also configures the shape and size of the aneurysm dome and neck very well, which can help with planning endovascular treatment. Computed tomography angiography has an approximate overall sensitivity of 98% in detecting aneurysms as measured in a meta-analysis of multiple studies conducted in 2011. One important limitation of CTA is detection of aneurysms smaller than 3 mm located near the skull base. For detecting aneurysms smaller than 3 mm the sensitivity is reported to be between 77% and 86% in different studies.

To reduce the risk of missing aneurysms near the skull base, bone subtraction algorithms have been implemented that include simple subtraction of unenhanced from enhanced data and also selective bone removal or "matched masked bone elimination." These algorithms enhance visualization of aneurysms near the skull base and bony structures. A preliminary image called *bone mask* is acquired before contrast administration. After the contrast administration and acquisition of all images, the bone mask is spatially coregistered with the contrast-enhanced image and then subtracted from it. The final result is contrast-enhanced image with unenhanced structures, including bone, removed from it. The penalty is increased radiation dose to the patient because of the need to acquire precontrast and postcontrast images.

Recently the advent of dual-energy multirow CT scanners has enabled direct bone removal, hence obviating the need for additional radiation for acquiring bone mask and also obviating the problems with misregistration of precontrast and postcontrast images caused by patient movement. Dual-energy CT uses two orthogonally mounted tube arrays and detectors that operate simultaneously and can be set to different tube potentials (i.e., 80 and 140 kilovolts peak [kVp]), allowing CT acquisition with two different energy levels at the same time. The resultant data sets can be reformatted with the scanner software to extract maps of contrast-enhanced material without complex image registration. Some recent small studies have shown that dual-energy CTA is

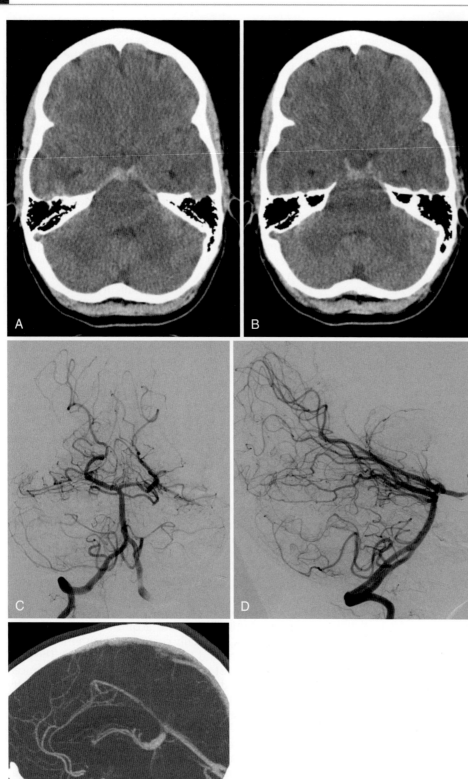

Figure 4-2 Nonaneurysmal perimesencephalic subarachnoid hemorrhage (SAH). Noncontrast computed tomography (NCCT) (**A** and **B**) shows a focal area of SAH in the prepontine cistern. No evidence of hemorrhage in other parts of cerebral spinal fluid (CSF) is seen. Anteroposterior (AP) (**C**) and lateral (**D**) digital subtraction angiography (DSA) show no arterial abnormality such as aneurysm or arteriovenous malformations (AVMs). CT venogram (CTV) (**E**) shows normal configuration of deep venous structures. The findings are highly suggestive of nonaneurysmal perimesencephalic SAH.

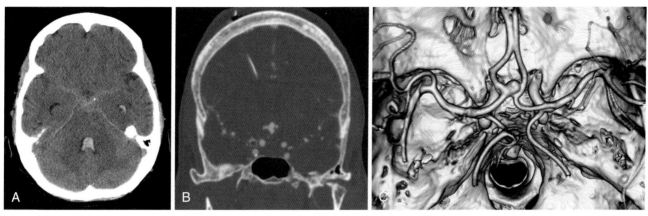

Figure 4-3 *Anterior communicating artery aneurysm in a patient with subarachnoid hemorrhage (SAH).* Axial source (**A**) and coronal reformatted (**B**) computed tomographic angiography (CTA) images show an anterior communicating artery aneurysm. Three-dimensional (3-D) reformatted CTA (**C**) confirms anterior communicating artery aneurysm and shows its relationship to the skull base.

more sensitive than the previous generation of CT scans in detecting small skull base aneurysms, but the sensitivity is still lower than DSA.

Reformatted CTA images in coronal and sagittal projections should be routinely obtained from the axial data set (see Figs. 4-1 and 4-3). In addition, 3-D reconstructed images targeted to areas of clinical concern can be very useful in clearing equivocal findings or providing spatial information about the aneurysms detected (see Fig. 4-3, *C*). Aneurysms usually arise at arterial branch points near the circle of Willis. Common supratentorial sites for aneurysms include the anterior communicating artery, the bifurcation of the MCA, and the posterior communicating artery. In the posterior fossa the most common site is the tip of the basilar artery. Each of these sites should be thoroughly interrogated by the interpreting radiologist. It is also important to carefully scrutinize the entire study even after finding a single aneurysm. Multiple aneurysms have been detected in up to 20% of patients presenting with nontraumatic SAH. When multiple aneurysms are detected, careful examination of the contour of each aneurysm may show a focal irregularity or "Murphy's tit" indicating the likelihood of recent aneurysmal rupture.

When evaluating the cerebral vessels it is also important to evaluate for a possible AVM. Arteriovenous malformations more commonly present with IPH or a mixed pattern of SAH and IPH/IVH rather than pure SAH (Fig. 4-4). After completing examination of the intracranial arteries, the radiologist should also evaluate the venous sinuses for patency. Venous sinus thrombosis is a potential, albeit unusual, cause of SAH (Fig. 4-5).

If careful analysis of the CTA shows no evidence for a vascular abnormality, the possibility of NAPH should be considered. If the SAH is limited to the basilar cisterns, the initial CTA shows no vascular abnormality, and the patient has a benign clinical course without rebleeding or vasospasm, some authors believe that the patient probably does not need further angiographic workup. Many centers are more conservative, nearly always performing a second vascular imaging study. In patients with widespread SAH or a more complicated clinical course, repeat vascular imaging with either CTA or catheter angiography has been shown to be of value. Combining eight angiographic series between 1985 and 1996 demon-

strated a 17% yield of previously undiagnosed aneurysm on the second angiogram. Even a third examination may show aneurysms undetected on the prior studies.

Intraparenchymal Hemorrhage

Intraparenchymal hemorrhage is bleeding into the parenchyma of the brain. Intraparenchymal hemorrhage may extend into the ventricles. It is not possible to differentiate ischemic from hemorrhagic accidents based on the patient's symptoms alone. Symptoms such as systolic blood pressure above 220 mm Hg, vomiting, sudden progression of symptoms, severe headache, decreased level of consciousness, and coma favor intracranial hemorrhage rather than ischemia; however, they are not specific. Intraparenchymal hemorrhage is the second most common cause of stroke after ischemic stroke and more than twice as common as SAH. According to a recent meta-analysis, the incidence of IPH is 24.6 per 100,000 persons, which has not decreased in the last 3 decades. Asian populations have a two times higher rate of IPH compared to other ethnic groups. Each year 40,000 to 50,000 people in the United States present with IPH. The rate is expected to double during the next 50 years in part as a result of the increasing age of the population. Intraparenchymal hemorrhage is more likely to result in death or major disability than cerebral infarction or SAH. The case fatality rate of patients with IPH in 1 month after the accident approaches 40%.

Intraparenchymal hemorrhage may result from a large and heterogeneous group of causes, including primary causes such as hypertension and amyloid angiopathy or secondary causes such as AVM, intracranial aneurysms, cavernous angiomas, dural venous sinus thrombosis, intracranial neoplasms, coagulopathy, vasculitis, drug use, and hemorrhagic ischemic stroke. Hypertensive and amyloid angiopathy causes account for 78% to 88 % of IPH cases; however, underlying vascular abnormalities must always be considered in the appropriate clinical circumstances because of the high risk for recurrent hemorrhage and the availability of treatment options.

Computed tomography scan is very sensitive for detecting acute IPH and is considered the procedure of choice for

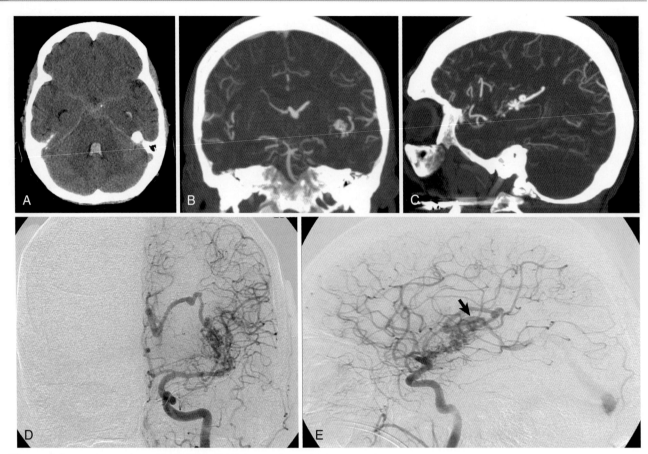

Figure 4-4 Arteriovenous malformation (AVM) in a patient with intraventricular hemorrhage (IVH) and subarachnoid hemorrhage (SAH). Noncontrast computed tomography (NCCT) (**A**) shows dense clot in the fourth ventricle and the temporal horn of the left lateral ventricle. SAH, more diffuse in the suprasellar cistern, is also present. Coronal (**B**) and sagittal (**C**) reformatted computed tomographic angiography (CTA) show an abnormal tangle of vessels in the left temporal lobe consistent with the nidus of an AVM. Anteroposterior (AP) (**D**) and lateral (**E**) views from the left carotid cerebral catheter angiogram confirm the AVM with an enlarged vein draining centrally. Lateral view of the angiogram (**E**) shows early venous drainage into the internal cerebral vein *(arrow)*. AVM in this patient has caused both SAH and IVH.

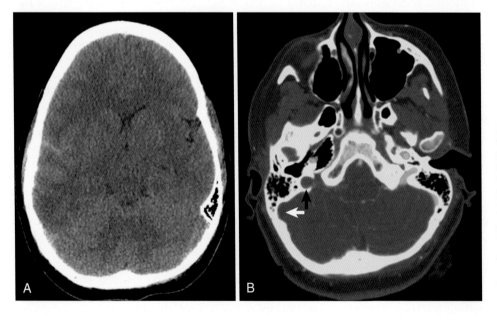

Figure 4-5 Venous sinus thrombosis. Noncontrast computed tomography (NCCT) (**A**) shows subtle curvilinear increased attenuation at the right parietal convexity in favor of subarachnoid hemorrhage (SAH) in a patient with no trauma. Computed tomographic angiography (CTA) (**B**) shows lack of filling of the right sigmoid sinus with contrast *(arrows)*. The left sigmoid sinus is normally filled and visualized with contrast. The findings are diagnostic of left sigmoid sinus thrombosis.

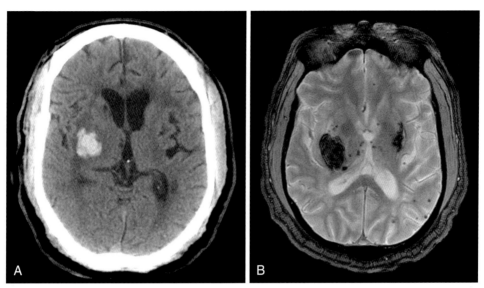

Figure 4-6 Right basal ganglia hematoma in a patient with a history of hypertension. Noncontrast computed tomography (NCCT) (**A**) shows a round well-defined hyperdense lesion in the right basal ganglia suggestive of acute nature of the hematoma. Gradient-recalled echo (GRE) magnetic resonance imaging (MRI) (**B**) shows decreased signal intensity and blooming effect in the corresponding area and confirms the diagnosis of hematoma. Another area with hypointense signal and blooming effect is seen in the left basal ganglia, which shows deceased density and volume loss on CT. The findings are suggestive of chronic resolved hematoma in this area. Multiple small foci of decreased signal intensity are seen in GRE image scattered in basal ganglia and posterior left parietal lobe, indicative of microbleeds.

initial imaging because of easy availability, fast imaging, and low cost compared to MRI. In the hyperacute and acute phases of IPH, CT shows a well-defined hyperdense lesion compared with the adjacent brain parenchyma (Fig. 4-6, A). The hematocrit, hemoglobin content, and degree of blood clot retraction determine the density of the lesion. In patients with severe anemia, reduced concentrations of hemoglobin causes the acute hematoma to appear less hyperdense than expected. In late subacute phase, progressive lysis of the red blood cells and proteolysis of the hemoglobin result in decreasing density of the lesion. The hematoma may appear isodense to the adjacent brain parenchyma. The hematoma is then progressively resorbed, and in the chronic phase it is typically seen as a smaller hypodense defect.

Magnetic Resonance Imaging Appearance of Hemorrhage

The appearance of hematoma on MRI depends on the state of hemoglobin, the magnetic field strength, and the pulse sequence used. The breakdown products of hemoglobin have different oxidation states of iron and, as such, have different magnetic properties. In the hyperacute stage the hemoglobin is still oxygenated and has no unpaired electrons. It is diamagnetic in this stage. The hematoma is isointense or mildly hyperintense on T1-weighted MRI and hyperintense on T2-weighted MRI, owing to the hemoglobin content. In the acute stage the hemoglobin is deoxygenated. Deoxyhemoglobin has few unpaired electrons and is paramagnetic. Consequently, the hemorrhage is isointense or hypointense on T1-weighted and hypointense on T2-weighted sequences (Fig. 4-7). In the early subacute phase, methemoglobin is paramagnetic and confined to the intracellular compartment, with a magnetic gradient between the intracellular and the extracellular compartments; the hemorrhage

is hyperintense on T1-weighted and hypointense on T2-weighted MRI. In the late subacute stage, methemoglobin is released by lysis of the red blood cells. This cancels the magnetic gradient between the intracellular and extracellular compartments and causes the hemorrhage to appear hyperintense on both T1- and T2-weighted MRI. Finally, in the chronic phase, because hemosiderin has many unpaired electrons and is superparamagnetic, the hemorrhage is isointense or hypointense on T1- and T2-weighted MRI. FLAIR sequence also shows the same characteristics of T2-weighted sequences. Gradient-recalled echo (GRE) sequence is a T2*-weighted sequence that is sensitive to static magnetic field inhomogeneity or to the T2* characteristics of the tissue. Gradient-recalled echo detects the paramagnetic effects of deoxyhemoglobin and methemoglobin. Gradient-recalled echo shows a core of heterogeneous signal intensity in hyperacute hematoma, reflecting the most recently extravasated blood that may still contain significant amounts of diamagnetic oxyhemoglobin. A hypointense rim surrounds the core that represents part of the hemorrhage that has had time to become more fully deoxygenated and paramagnetic. Table 4-2 summarizes the appearance of hematoma in CT and MRI according to the stage of the lesion in chronologic sequence.

The GRE sequence can also detect microbleeds that may not be visible on CT scan. Microbleeds are generally defined as round, punctate, hypointense foci less than 5 to 10 mm in size in brain parenchyma. They can be seen in 80% of patients with primary ICH (hypertension and amyloid angiopathy), 25% of patients with ischemic stroke, and 8% of elderly people. They correspond to hemosiderin-laden macrophages lying adjacent to the vessels and indicate prior extravasation of blood. Microbleeds have been suggested to be predictors of bleeding-prone angiopathy (see Fig. 4-6, B). Some studies

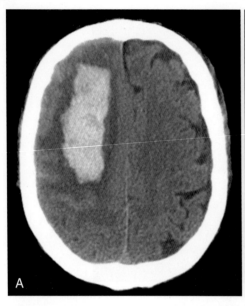
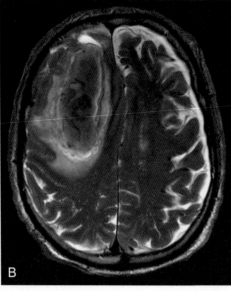

Figure 4-7 Intraparenchymal hematoma. Noncontrast computed tomography (NCCT) (**A**) shows a massive intraparenchymal hemorrhage (IPH) involving the right frontal and parietal region. T2-weighted magnetic resonance imaging (MRI) (**B**) shows decreased signal intensity in corresponding area. The hematoma is in acute stage (12 hours to 2 days). Hemoglobin is in deoxygenated stage showing paramagnetic characteristics, which causes decreased signal in the hematoma core. Vasogenic edema surrounding the hematoma is shown as area of increased signal intensity.

Table 4-2   Appearance of Hematoma on Computed Tomography and Magnetic Resonance Imaging According to Stage

Age/Stage	CT Scan	T1-Weighted MRI	T2-Weighted and FLAIR MRI	GRE MRI
Hyperacute (<12 hr)	Hyperdense	Isointense or mildly hyperintense	Hyperintense	Hypointense rim
Acute (12 hr to 2 days)	Hyperdense	Isointense or hypointense	Hypointense	Hypointense rim growing toward center
Early subacute (2-7 days)	Hyperdense	Hyperintense	Hypointense	Hypointense
Late subacute (8 days to 1 mo)	Isodense	Hyperintense	Hyperintense	Hypointense
Chronic (>1 mo)	Hypodense	Isointense or hypointense	Hypointense	Hyperintense core surrounded by hypointense rim

CT, Computed tomography; *FLAIR,* fluid-attenuated inversion recovery; *GRE,* gradient-recalled echo; *MRI,* magnetic resonance imaging.

have shown that patients with microbleeds may be at increased risk for ICH after anticoagulation or thrombolytic treatment; however, this is controversial and not confirmed in all studies.

Hematoma expansion occurs in approximately one third of acute primary IPH cases and is associated with high mortality, disability, and functional deterioration. An accurate and reliable method for predicting hematoma expansion is thus needed to determine the prognosis and further clinical management. Contrast material extravasation within the hematoma visualized in CTA, called the *spot sign*, is one of the most promising predictors of hematoma expansion. A recent multicenter prospective study, Predicting Hematoma Growth and Outcome in Intracerebral Hemorrhage Using Contrast Bolus CT (PREDICT), showed that the spot sign is an independent predictor of hematoma expansion in patients with IPH. Some investigators devised a spot sign scoring system that includes measurement of the number, size, and attenuation of the visualized spots. Table 4-3 shows the suggested scoring system. Spot sign scores of 0, 1, 2, and 3 independently predict a 2%, 33%, 50%, and 94% risk for hematoma expan-

Table 4-3   Calculation of Spot Sign Score

Spot Sign Characteristics	Points
Number of Spot Signs	
1-2	1
≥3	2
Maximum Axial Dimension	
1-4 mm	0
≥5 mm	1
Maximum Attenuation	
120-179	0
≥180	1

sion, defined as more than a 30% or 6-mL increase in hematoma volume. Radiologists should be careful not to include preexisting calcified areas as a spot sign. They are also advised to evaluate the source axial images carefully to avoid overcounting the spots because of contiguous vessel or enhancing parts falsely projecting as separate spots in different slices.

In all cases of ICH, clinical and imaging investigation should be made to rule out secondary causes such as AVMs, tumors, moyamoya disease, and cerebral vein thrombosis. Clinical symptoms suggesting a secondary cause include prodrome of headache or neurologic deficits before the onset of the accident or other clinical findings that suggest an underlying disease. Imaging findings suggestive of secondary causes include the presence of SAH and ICH at the same time, unusual shape of the hematoma, increased edema compared to the size of the hematoma, and visualization of a masslike lesion or abnormal vessels.

Magnetic resonance imaging including MR angiogram and venogram or CT with CT angiogram and venogram is reasonably sensitive at identifying secondary causes of hemorrhage. A catheter angiogram may be considered if clinical suspicion is high or noninvasive studies are suggestive of an underlying vascular cause. We will discuss each of the causes of ICH, including their pathophysiology and imaging appearance. We will then offer an imaging algorithm based on initial CT findings and clinical data.

Hypertension

Hypertensive ICH accounts for over 50% of cases. Hemorrhage occurs most commonly in the basal ganglia (55% to 62% within the lentiform nucleus and 10% to 26% within the thalamus) (see Fig. 4-6). Less common locations include the pons (5% to 10%) and the cerebellar hemispheres (6% to 10%). Over 90% of the patients are older than 45 years of age. Recently there has been a decrease in the incidence of hypertensive hemorrhage, likely secondary to more effective and more widespread control of systemic hypertension. The bleeding results from the rupture of small penetrating arteries. In 1868 Charcot and Bouchard described the cause of the bleeding as rupture of small points of dilatation in the walls of small arterioles (microaneurysms). Modern electron microscopic studies suggest that most of the bleeding occurs at or near the bifurcations of the affected arteries where degeneration of the media and smooth muscle causes these microaneurysms. Chronic hypertension also causes lipohyalinotic changes (or fibrinoid necrosis) in penetrating arteries that reduce the arterial wall compliance and increase the likelihood of rupture.

The imaging appearance on CT scan is a typical round dense mass in the basal ganglia and/or thalamus (see Fig. 4-6). Intraventricular hemorrhage can occur and is most commonly associated with thalamic hemorrhage. Intraventricular hemorrhage can lead to hydrocephalus because of impairment of the CSF circulation. Angiography studies, including CTA, MRA, and DSA, usually do not show any lesion in this type of hemorrhage, and thus performance of any of them is not recommended in typical hypertensive ICH patients.

Cerebral Amyloid Angiopathy

Although hypertension is the most common cause for IPH in elderly patients, cerebral amyloid angiopathy (CAA) has been implicated in as many as 15% of patients older than 60 years of age and almost 20% of patients 70 years of age and older (Fig. 4-8). The hemorrhage results from the rupture of small- and medium-sized arteries. Deposition of β-amyloid protein in the vessel walls has

been identified as a causative agent. This protein is essentially identical to the protein present within the senile plaques of Alzheimer disease. Possibly the deposition of these proteins within the aging brain predisposes to both ICH and dementia. Indeed, Alzheimer disease or senile dementia of the Alzheimer type is commonly observed in these patients. The locations of the bleeds are lobar, cortical, or subcortical as opposed to the basal ganglia location in hypertensive IPH. Most commonly, bleeds are seen in the frontal lobe, followed by the parietal, occipital, and temporal lobes. Hemorrhage into the deep gray matter or cerebellum is uncommon. Cerebral amyloid angiopathy should be considered as the cause of IPH in patients older than 55 years of age with hemorrhage in the lobar or cortical-subcortical location and evidence of prior macrohemorrhages or microhemorrhages. Patients with CAA are at substantial increased risk for recurrent hemorrhage, estimated at approximately 10% annually. On CT it is common to see multiple microhemorrhages and hematomas of varying ages. Magnetic resonance imaging including GRE and/or susceptibility-weighted imaging (SWI) is recommended as a further step in evaluation of patients suspected of CAA. Magnetic resonance imaging shows both acute and old hemorrhagic lesions that may include macrohemorrhages, microhemorrhages, and superficial siderosis in patients with CAA (see Fig. 4-8).

Susceptibility-weighted imaging is a 3-D, velocity-compensated, GRE sequence that combines magnitude (used in conventional GRE) with phase information to increase the visibility of microhemorrhages or small pathologic vessels. Microhemorrhages contain paramagnetic hemosiderin that causes large variations in local magnetic field and a local reduction in $T2^*$. Susceptibility-weighted imaging, with its unique sensitivity to blood products and hemorrhage, is well suited to detect imaging changes consistent with CAA. It should be noted that sensitivity of $T2^*$-weighted MRI to paramagnetic substances other than hemosiderin, including calcifications and iron deposits, gives rise to findings that resemble microhemorrhages. These artifacts are likely to be more of a problem when using more sensitive sequences such as SWI. Angiographic studies typically have normal results in patients with CAA. Once a diagnosis of CAA is made based on MRI findings, there is no need for further imaging workup in the initial phase of screening.

Arteriovenous Malformations

Brain AVMs are vascular malformations with arteriovenous shunting with no intervening capillary bed. Arteriovenous malformations consist of feeding arteries, a nidus, and draining veins. The feeding arteries and draining veins are microscopically enlarged and may show associated varices, areas of stenosis, or aneurysms. The nidus is a conglomeration of numerous small arteriovenous shunts with thin dysplastic walls. Most commonly AVMs bleed either from the nidus or from the most proximal portions of the draining veins. Arteriovenous malformations may be found anywhere between the subarachnoid space and the ventricles. The majority of the hemorrhages are intraparenchymal in location; however, deep-seated AVMs may bleed directly into the ventricles (Fig. 4-9). Noncontrast CT is usually unable to show an underlying

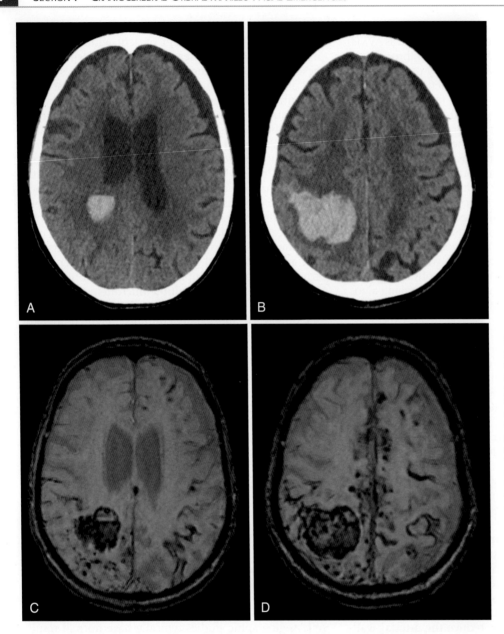

Figure 4-8 Amyloid angiopathy. Noncontrast computed tomography (NCCT) (**A** and **B**) shows a large right parietal intraparenchymal hematoma in an 87-year-old patient with no history of hypertension or malignancy. Gradient-recalled echo (GRE) magnetic resonance imaging (MRI) (**C** and **D**) demonstrates the hematoma as area of low signal intensity with blooming effect. Multiple microbleeds are seen surrounding the hematoma. The lobar-subcortical location of the hematoma, the presence of multiple microbleeds, and the lack of visualization of abnormal vessels are highly suggestive of cerebral amyloid angiopathy (CAA) as the cause of hemorrhage. Superficial siderosis on the left parietal gyri indicates prior bleeds in favor of a chronic process of amyloid angiopathy.

AVM, especially in cases of large IPH. In some cases CT may detect calcific densities and serpentine vessels in the AVM. Computed tomography angiography usually shows the large vessels of AVM, especially the draining veins (see Fig. 4-9, *C* and *D*); however, small AVMs may be missed even with CTA.

Magnetic resonance imaging represents a significant improvement in noninvasive imaging of AVMs. This is partly because of high sensitivity of MRI to flow in vascular structures. The feeding arteries and draining vessels are well shown in T2-weighted images as large signal-void structures described as "bags of black worms." In cases in which suspicion exists as to the cause of the signal voids, GRE sequences with very short time to echo (TE) show high signal in flow-bearing structures and can be confirmatory for the presence of vascular malformation. FLAIR may show increased signal intensity in adjacent brain parenchyma because of gliotic reaction. Recent studies have shown that time-of-flight

and contrast-enhanced MRA can depict AVMs and their architectural characteristics, including configuration of feeder and draining vessels and nidus size with a very good intermodality agreement when compared to DSA.

Diagnosis in the acute phase is made more difficult by vascular spasm and compression by the hematoma. In one series 6 of 29 patients with angiographically negative ICHs were shown to have AVMs at pathologic examination. In angiographically negative cases that do not go to surgery, follow-up evaluation with CTA, MRA, or DSA is recommended after the clot has resorbed. Diagnosis of the underlying AVM and potential associated aneurysm is extremely important because of the high rate of recurrent hemorrhage.

Aneurysms

Intracranial aneurysm rupture usually results in SAH. However, a significant number of IPHs result from aneurysm rupture (Figs. 4-10 and 4-11). In one series of 460

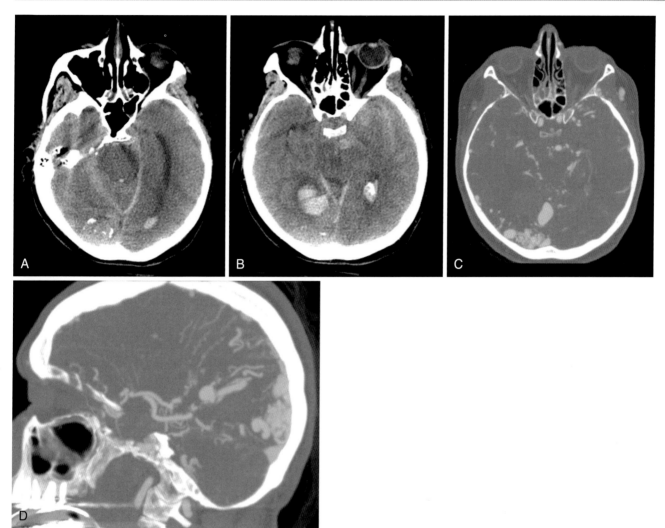

Figure 4-9 Arteriovenous malformation (AVM). Noncontrast computed tomography (NCCT) (**A** and **B**) shows intraventricular and intraparenchymal hemorrhages. A round area of increased density with punctate calcification is also present in the right occipital lobe abutting the dura. CT angiography (CTA) (**C**) shows abnormal vessels in the right occipital lobe, including multiple dilated venous channels consistent with AVM. Sagittal reformatted CTA (**D**) shows a dilated vein of Galen.

patients with dense SAH, 25% had an associated IPH. Specific aneurysm sites predispose to IPH. These sites should be carefully scrutinized during angiographic evaluation. The most common site is the MCA, where an upwardly pointing aneurysm may hemorrhage into the deep frontal lobe. Nearly as common are anterior communicating artery aneurysms, which may bleed into the gyrus rectus. Distal anterior cerebral artery aneurysms, usually arising at the origin of the pericallosal artery, are associated with hematomas of the corpus callosum or medial frontal lobe. Noncontrast CT may detect curvilinear calcification in the aneurysm wall, but diagnosis is usually made by CTA or DSA. As in the case of AVMs, identification of the aneurysm is made more difficult in the acute period by the mass effect of the hematoma, as well as potential vasospasm.

Cavernous Angiomas

Cavernous angiomas are defined as benign vascular hamartomas containing a mass of adjacent immature blood vessels constituting well-circumscribed sinusoidal vascular channels with a single layer of endothelium. On gross examination they look like "mulberry-like" nodules.

Because of their thin vascular walls and low intravascular pressures, cavernous angiomas are prone to recurrent microscopic hemorrhages, accounting for the blood seen in various stages of oxidation. Typically these lesions enlarge slowly and may present with seizures or progressive neurologic deficit. Less typically, overt hemorrhage may occur with a more sudden and dramatic neurologic presentation. In 25% of patients, cavernous angiomas are multiple. These lesions are often angiographically occult because the feeding arteries and draining veins are normal. Computed tomography scan may be normal in up to 50% of cases of uncomplicated cavernous angiomas, or it may show high-attenuation lesions with little or no surrounding edema. Magnetic resonance imaging, given its greater sensitivity to blood products in various stages, is a more sensitive modality and almost always diagnostic (Fig. 4-12). Use of SWI is even more sensitive than the conventional GRE sequence for detection of these lesions. Once MRI confirms the diagnosis of cavernous angioma, no further diagnostic imaging workup for the patient is required. ICHs due to cavernous angiomas are usually smaller and occur at younger ages when compared with

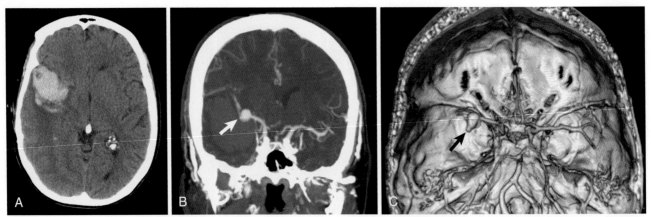

Figure 4-10 Aneurysm in a patient with intraparenchymal hematoma. Noncontrast computed tomography (NCCT) (**A**) shows a large right perisylvian intraparenchymal hemorrhage (IPH). Coronal reformatted CT angiography (CTA) (**B**) shows displacement of the right middle cerebral artery (MCA) by the hematoma and a right MCA aneurysm. Three-dimensional (3-D) reformatted CTA (**C**) shows a right MCA bifurcation aneurysm. Note the "Murphy's tit" *(arrow)* in both **B** and **C** pointing toward the hematoma, indicative of recent hemorrhage from the aneurysm.

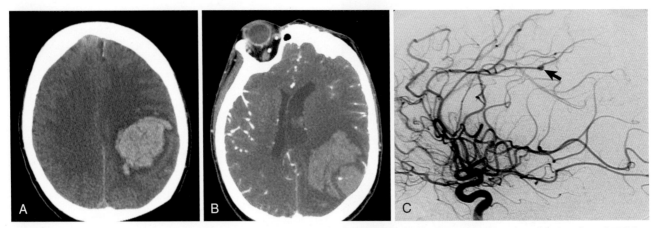

Figure 4-11 Mycotic aneurysm. Noncontrast computed tomography (NCCT) (**A**) shows a large intraparenchymal hemorrhage (IPH) in a patient with sepsis. CT angiography (CTA) (**B**) shows a small abnormal vessel within the hematoma. Lateral view of the arterial phase of a left internal carotid angiogram (**C**) shows a distal aneurysm *(arrow)* likely mycotic in cause.

ICH due to AVM. Cavernous angiomas may be associated with developmental venous anomalies. Developmental venous anomalies are caused by early arrest of medullary veins during development in the embryo, resulting in persistence of large embryonic deep white matter veins. They are described as a collection of small stellate veins converging into large collector veins draining into a dural sinus or an ependymal vein. Developmental venous anomalies are usually asymptomatic unless associated with other anomalies such as cavernous angiomas or cortical dysplasias.

Cerebral Venous Sinus Thrombosis

Cerebral venous sinus thrombosis (CVST) is an uncommon disorder affecting the venous side of the neurovasculature. It accounts for 1% to 2% of stroke cases in adults. The estimated incidence of CVST is 3 to 4 cases per million in adults. CVST can result in venous hypertension and parenchymal edema or infarction. Early ICH is seen in 40% of patients with CVST and is associated with poor outcome (Fig. 4-13). Clinical symptoms depend on the patient's age, presence of parenchymal involvement, and extent of thrombosis and include headache, seizures, focal neurologic deficit, and impaired level of consciousness. Clinical factors that may predispose to cerebral venous

thrombosis include dehydration, stasis due to localized neoplasm, infection, or coagulopathy as may be seen with oral contraceptive use. On NCCT the clot within the dural sinus or cortical vein may be seen as a high-attenuation lesion (cord sign). Contrast-enhanced CT or CTA will demonstrate nonfilling of the affected structure with enhancement of the surrounding dura (empty delta sign). Venous obstruction results in increased pressure, decreased local cerebral blood flow, and eventually venous infarction. Venous infarcts are more commonly hemorrhagic than arterial infarcts. Similar to arterial infarcts, venous infarcts show mass effect and involve the cortex in the pattern of cytotoxic edema. However, they do not conform to an arterial distribution. It is important to differentiate venous from arterial infarcts, because despite the hemorrhage, current management for cerebral venous thrombosis is anticoagulation in selected patients. Several reports have shown a favorable outcome to endovascular management, including direct thrombolysis and/or thrombus extraction.

Neoplasm

Bleeding can occur into either a metastatic or primary neoplasm. The most common lesion is a small bleed into a pituitary neoplasm. Of the remaining neoplasms,

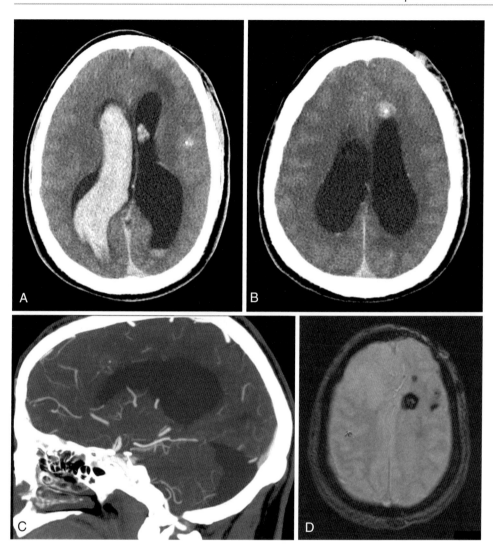

Figure 4-12 Multiple cavernous angiomas. Noncontrast computed tomography (NCCT) (**A** and **B**) shows a large intraventricular clot and multiple, nodular, parenchymal calcifications. Sagittal reformatted CT angiography (CTA) (**C**) shows no abnormal vessels associated with the nodular calcifications. Gradient-recalled echo (GRE) magnetic resonance imaging (MRI) (**D**) shows multiple, low-signal-intensity hemosiderin deposits consistent with multiple cavernous angiomas.

metastases are more likely to show hemorrhage than primary neoplasms. As reported in the literature, the incidence of intratumoral hemorrhage is 1% to 15%. Of the hemorrhages within metastases, approximately one third are macroscopic and two thirds are microscopic. Common intracranial metastases to hemorrhage include melanoma, choriocarcinoma, bronchogenic carcinoma, thyroid cancer, and renal cell carcinoma. The most common primary neoplasm to contain hemorrhage is glioblastoma. In the majority of patients, tumoral hemorrhage occupies only a portion of the neoplasm. Underlying mechanisms for tumoral hemorrhage include tumor necrosis, invasion of blood vessels by the tumor, and rupture of newly formed vessels. Unenhanced CT or MRI typically shows the hemorrhage within the tumor. Because most metastases and many primary neoplasms demonstrate considerable vasogenic edema, the presence of substantial vasogenic edema should suggest an underlying neoplasm. Significant enhancement of the lesion on contrast-enhanced CT or MRI early after the clinical symptoms is also highly suggestive of a neoplasm as the underlying cause (Fig. 4-14). The hemorrhage caused by tumor may also extend to other locations such as the subarachnoid or subdural space. In cases of large hemorrhage, identifying the tumor as the underlying cause may be very challenging acutely.

In these cases, performing follow-up imaging after resorption of the hematoma is recommended.

For additional discussion, see the subchapter Acute Presentation of Neoplasm.

Bleeding Disorders

Bleeding disorders account for a small, but significant, risk factor associated with intracranial hemorrhage. Aspirin therapy may slightly increase the baseline risk. Patients who are anticoagulated to a therapeutic range have a 7 to 10 times increased risk for ICH. Approximately two thirds of the hemorrhages in anticoagulated patients are intraparenchymal, with the remaining mostly subdural in location. Patients receiving urokinase or streptokinase for the treatment of acute myocardial infarction have a rate of intracranial hemorrhage of 1% to 2%. Patients receiving tissue plasminogen activator (t-PA) have a hemorrhage risk of less than 1%.

Other examples of bleeding disorders leading to ICH include thrombocytopenia due to congenital causes, use of certain drugs, or bone marrow diseases. Liver disease, congenital bleeding disorders such as hemophilia, and other factor deficiencies can also cause ICH. Neoplastic diseases such as leukemia are the other group of diseases causing coagulopathy. Because the pattern of hemorrhage

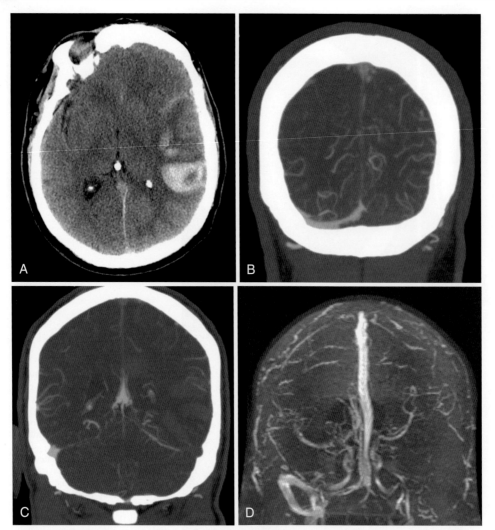

Figure 4-13 Venous sinus thrombosis with hemorrhagic venous infarct. Noncontrast computed tomography (NCCT) (**A**) shows left temporal intraparenchymal hemorrhage (IPH) and slight subarachnoid hemorrhage (SAH). Coronal reformatted CT angiography (CTA) (**B** and **C**) show thrombosis of the left transverse sinus. Coronal view of a two-dimensional time-of-flight magnetic resonance (MR) venogram (**D**) confirms the venous thromboses. IPH has developed secondary to venous infarct.

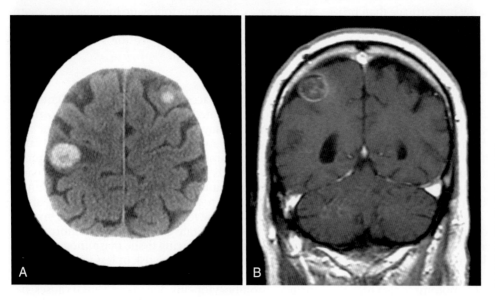

Figure 4-14 Hemorrhagic metastases. Noncontrast computed tomography (NCCT) (**A**) shows multiple intraparenchymal hematomas centered at the gray-white matter junction in a patient with lung cancer. Note the vasogenic edema surrounding the larger lesion. Magnetic resonance imaging (MRI) with contrast (**B**) shows the peripheral enhancement of one of the lesions.

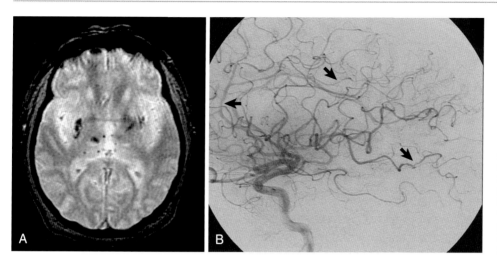

Figure 4-15 Vasculitis. Gradient-recalled echo (GRE) magnetic resonance imaging (MRI) (**A**) shows multiple hemosiderin deposits primarily in the basal ganglia. Lateral view of an arterial phase cerebral angiogram (**B**) shows multiple areas of arterial narrowing *(arrows)* consistent with diffuse vasculitis.

in patients with coagulation disorders overlaps many of the other patterns, history and laboratory tests are essential to making an accurate diagnosis.

Intracranial Vasculitis

Vasculitis includes a heterogeneous group of disorders characterized by nonatheromatous inflammation and necrosis of blood vessel walls. The abnormal vessels predispose to ICH. Computed tomography may show hemorrhage or infarction secondary to the vasculitis. To make the diagnosis an angiographic study is required. The spatial resolution of CTA and MRA may be insufficient to detect subtle disease; DSA remains the gold standard. The classic appearance of the vessels is caliber change; specifically, there are multifocal areas of smooth or irregularly shaped stenoses alternating with dilated segments (Fig. 4-15).

Drug Abuse

Drug abuse has become an important diagnostic consideration in young adults with intracranial hemorrhage. Both SAH and IPH have been related to cocaine abuse. The locations of the IPH associated with cocaine abuse are similar to the locations seen in hypertensive hematomas in older patients. Underlying lesions, such as congenital or mycotic aneurysm or AVM may bleed secondary to the acute transient surge in systemic blood pressure caused by the drug abuse. Vasculitis with narrowed and even occluded vessels is often present. Other drugs associated with ICH include amphetamines and phencyclidine.

Hemorrhagic Ischemic Stroke

Hemorrhagic ischemic stroke is defined as secondary hemorrhage within the area of ischemic infarction (Fig. 4-16). The hemorrhage can range from small petechial type to large hematomas. Hemorrhagic stroke accounts for approximately 15% of all strokes. Of these, two thirds show IPH and one third show SAH. The hemorrhagic components of infarcts are thought to be secondary and may not be present during the very early stages. Typically, bland infarcts transform into hemorrhagic infarcts within hours to weeks of clinical ictus. An embolus initially obstructs a proximal vessel, producing

ischemic insult to the brain and vascular endothelium. As the embolus is later lysed by endogenous factors, circulation is restored to the ischemic area. Autoregulation has maximally dilated the arterial tree, and the endothelium is chemically damaged, leading to leakage or gross extravasation of blood into the infarcted tissue. Most hemorrhagic infarcts resulting from thromboembolic disease primarily affect the gray matter, whereas hemorrhage in venous infarcts primarily affects the white matter.

Imaging Algorithm

According to the described causes and imaging findings, we suggest the following guidelines for imaging patients with atraumatic intracranial hemorrhage:

1. Noncontrast CT is the imaging procedure of choice for initial evaluation in patients with suspected ICH.
2. Computed tomography angiography is generally performed in all patients without a clear cause of hemorrhage who are surgical candidates.
3. Computed tomography angiography is not required for older, hypertensive patients who have hemorrhage in the basal ganglia, thalamus, cerebellum, or brainstem.
4. Magnetic resonance imaging is strongly considered in those patients with a suspected neoplasm, AVM, amyloid angiopathy, or cavernous angioma.
5. Digital subtraction angiography is considered in those patients who require angiographic evaluation and are potential vascular interventional candidates.
6. Digital subtraction angiography or MRA is recommended for patients who are not suitable candidates for CTA.

These guidelines correspond closely to those put forth by the American Heart Association. It is the responsibility of the radiologist to recognize the imaging and clinical findings that may suggest the underlying causes of ICH. Based on a provisional differential diagnosis, the radiologist can guide the imaging workup of these patients. Here are some common scenarios:

1. If the patient is elderly with a basal ganglia hemorrhage and hypertension, the IPH is likely hypertensive in cause, and no further imaging workup is required.
2. If the patient is elderly and normotensive with a lobar hemorrhage, the most likely cause is amyloid angiopathy. Computed tomography angiography

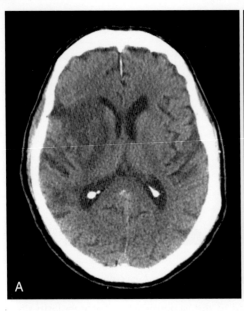 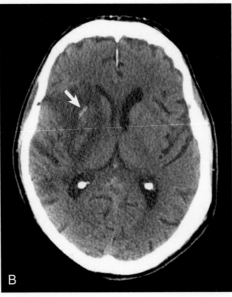

Figure 4-16 Hemorrhagic conversion of an infarct. Noncontrast computed tomography (NCCT) (**A**) shows a large area of low density in the right middle cerebral artery (MCA) territory consistent with a bland ischemic infarct. Follow-up CT (**B**) obtained 2 days later shows a linear area of increased density in the center of the lesion indicative of hemorrhagic conversion within the infarct (*arrow*).

should be performed if the patient is a candidate for emergent clot removal. Otherwise, we often perform MRI to evaluate for microhemorrhages, underlying neoplasm, or cavernous hemangioma.

3. If the patient is younger, or if the patient has a combination of IPH and either IVH or SAH, CTA assessment is useful to evaluate for intracranial aneurysm, vascular malformation, vasculitis, or dural venous sinus thrombosis. Repeat CTA or DSA should be considered if no cause is found.

4. If cytotoxic edema is present, infarct should be suspected. Arterial infarcts occupy an arterial distribution, whereas venous infarcts assume a nonarterial distribution. Also, recall that hemorrhagic arterial infarcts primarily affect the gray matter, whereas the hemorrhage in venous infarcts primarily affects the white matter.

Intracranial Infections
Carrie P. Marder and Kathleen R. Fink

Intracranial infections often present acutely, and the diagnostic evaluation begins in the ED. Correct diagnosis depends on a combination of clinical, laboratory, and radiologic investigations, with CSF analysis playing a central role. Imaging provides or narrows the differential diagnosis and occasionally identifies a particular entity or organism. Imaging is also crucial for identifying complications of infection.

This section emphasizes the overall strategy for emergent imaging of suspected intracranial infections, highlighting specific entities in which imaging aids diagnosis. Emergency imaging in immunocompromised patients and major complications of intracranial infections that might present in the ED are also considered.

■ IMAGING STRATEGY

Patients with suspected intracranial infection presenting with altered mental status, seizures, or focal neurologic deficits require emergent NCCT to exclude hydrocephalus, cerebral edema, mass lesions, hemorrhage, or impending brain herniation. Noncontrast CT is widely available, rapidly acquired, and well tolerated by critically ill patients. Once immediately life-threatening conditions have been excluded, contrast-enhanced MRI may be needed to detect subtle signs of infection or complications such as infarcts.

The American College of Radiology (ACR) Appropriateness Criteria contains many guidelines for appropriate imaging that are applicable to patients in the ED. Both NCCT and contrast-enhanced MRI of the head are usually appropriate for patients presenting with new headache and suspected meningitis or encephalitis, with the choice of test depending on local preference and availability. Contrast-enhanced CT may be a suitable alternative when MRI is unavailable or contraindicated, such as in patients with metal implants, severe claustrophobia, or severe renal dysfunction. Cerebrovascular complications of infection are frequent and may require evaluation with MRA or CTA and MR venography (MRV) or CT venography (CTV). Advanced techniques and nuclear medicine studies are reserved for problem solving and are not usually performed from the ED.

Uncomplicated rhinosinusitis generally does not require imaging. If there is suspicion for intracranial or orbital complications of rhinosinusitis, both NCCT and contrast-enhanced MRI of the head, orbits, and paranasal sinuses are usually appropriate (ACR Appropriateness Criteria, "Sinonasal Disease"). Evaluation for intracranial extension is best accomplished with contrast-enhanced MRI. If gadolinium is contraindicated, noncontrast MRI augmented with contrast-enhanced CT of the head and sinuses is recommended.

In immunocompromised individuals with new headache, MRI with or without contrast is usually appropriate

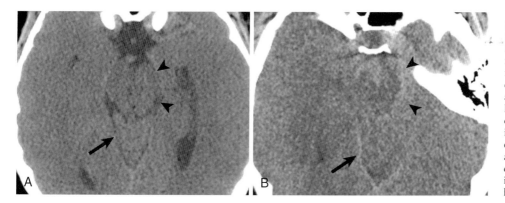

Figure 4-17 Bacterial meningitis: brain herniation after lumbar puncture (LP). Initial noncontrast computed tomography (NCCT) (A) showed no contraindication to LP with open ambient *(arrowheads)* and cerebellar cisterns *(arrow)*, but there were clinical signs of mass effect, including coma. NCCT after LP (B) demonstrates interval effacement of ambient *(arrowheads)* and superior cerebellar *(arrow)* cisterns, indicating worsening cerebral edema and herniation.

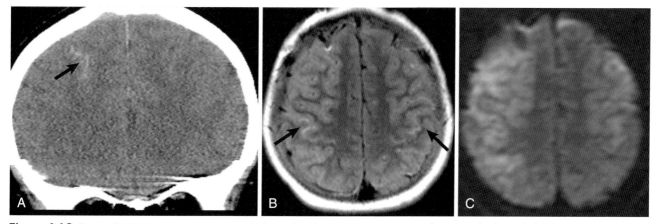

Figure 4-18 Pyogenic *(Streptococcus pneumoniae)* meningitis. Noncontrast computed tomography (NCCT) (A) shows hyperdense subarachnoid material *(arrow)*. Magnetic resonance imaging (MRI) fluid-attenuated inversion recovery sequence (FLAIR) (B) shows subarachnoid hyperintensity *(black arrows)*. Diffusion-weighted imaging (DWI) (C) demonstrates bilateral cortical infarctions, a complication of meningitis.

as the initial imaging test (ACR Appropriateness Criteria, "Headache"). Immunocompromised patients with rhinosinusitis are at high risk for intracranial or orbital complications, and imaging may be performed earlier than in immunocompetent patients.

MENINGITIS

Meningitis refers to inflammation of the pia and arachnoid membranes and may be classified based on cause and CSF profile. Pyogenic bacterial meningitis is characterized by CSF findings of neutrophilic pleocytosis, elevated protein level, low glucose level, and elevated opening pressure. Viral meningitis is characterized by CSF findings of lymphocytic pleocytosis with near normal protein and glucose levels, normal opening pressure, and absence of bacterial growth on cultures ("aseptic" meningitis). Granulomatous or chronic meningitis usually refers to chronic inflammation of the basal surfaces of the brain ("basilar" meningitis) and may be due to infectious causes, including tuberculosis or fungal infections, as well as noninfectious causes such as sarcoidosis. Cerebral spinal fluid findings include mild lymphocytosis, elevated protein level, and low glucose level.

The goals of imaging in suspected meningitis are primarily to exclude contraindications to lumbar puncture and to evaluate for complications such as hydrocephalus. Noncontrast CT is usually the first test, but not all patients with suspected meningitis require CT. Patients

with impaired consciousness, seizure, focal neurologic signs, immunocompromised state, and age older than 60 years are more likely to have positive imaging findings and benefit from NCCT.

Brain herniation is a dreaded complication of acute bacterial meningitis that occurs in up to 5% of patients and is associated with significant mortality. Because of the theoretical potential for lumbar puncture to cause brain herniation in a patient with cerebral edema, lumbar puncture should be avoided in patients with midline shift, effacement of the basilar cisterns, posterior fossa mass effect, or clinical signs of increased intracranial pressure, even if NCCT results are normal (Fig. 4-17).

Bacterial Meningitis

Imaging results are usually normal in meningitis, but cerebral edema, inflammatory material in the subarachnoid spaces, or leptomeningeal enhancement may suggest the diagnosis. Cerebral edema appears as narrowed or compressed sulci, ventricles, and basilar cisterns. Inflammatory material in the subarachnoid spaces appears as hyperdense or enhancing material on CT (Fig. 4-18), FLAIR signal hyperintensity (see Fig. 4-18), and enhancement or restricted diffusion on MRI. Leptomeningeal enhancement appears as thin linear enhancement closely apposed to the brain surface in a gyriform pattern.

Imaging also reveals complications of meningitis, including brain herniation, infarcts (see Fig. 4-18), hydrocephalus, extra-axial pus collections, ventriculitis, cerebritis, and cerebral abscess. Hydrocephalus may be the only abnormal finding in a patient with meningitis, particularly basilar meningitis.

Sterile subdural effusions occur with meningitis but generally resolve spontaneously. They are more common in children and appear identical to or slightly more proteinaceous than CSF on all imaging modalities. Sterile subdural effusions can be differentiated from prominent subarachnoid spaces by the presence of bridging vessels crossing the collection. Sterile subdural effusions sometimes develop internal septations and may become infected, resulting in subdural empyema (SDE).

Viral Meningitis and Encephalitis

Uncomplicated viral meningitis is usually diagnosed clinically and confirmed by CSF analysis. Imaging results may be normal or may show thin linear leptomeningeal enhancement. Viral meningitis is less likely than bacterial, fungal, or tuberculous meningitis to produce FLAIR signal hyperintensity in the subarachnoid space.

Viral meningitis may be complicated by encephalitis, as in cases of arthropod-borne viruses (arboviruses). Examples from this diverse group include the viruses causing eastern, western, or Venezuelan equine, West Nile, Japanese, St. Louis, California, Murray Valley, and tick-borne encephalitides. Magnetic resonance imaging results may be normal or may show areas of T2/FLAIR signal hyperintensity, restricted diffusion, or enhancement. Classically lesions are located in the basal ganglia and thalami bilaterally, an imaging pattern that strongly suggests arboviral encephalitis in any potentially exposed patient (Table 4-4). The differential diagnosis includes anoxic/hypoxic encephalopathy, toxic exposures, metabolic disorders, and other infections such as Creutzfeldt-Jakob disease. Other nonspecific patterns include involvement of the meninges, brainstem, spinal cord, cortical gray matter, and cerebral and cerebellar white matter. Involvement of the mesial temporal lobes may occur, sometimes resembling herpes simplex encephalitis. Involvement of the basal ganglia and thalami with relative sparing of the anterior portions of the temporal lobes helps to distinguish arboviral infections from herpes simplex virus (HSV).

Granulomatous Meningitis

Granulomatous or chronic meningitis preferentially involves the basilar cisterns, which become filled with a thick inflammatory exudate. Tuberculosis is a classic example, although bacterial meningitis may also present with a basilar pattern. Hydrocephalus is often an early clue. Isodense material in the basilar cisterns may be present, which may enhance following intravenous contrast (Fig. 4-19). Infarcts and tuberculomas also occur (see Fig. 4-19).

Tuberculomas are granulomatous lesions with a variable imaging appearance depending on the extent of central caseation. Classic CT findings include central calcification surrounded by an enhancing rim. On MRI,

Table 4-4 Characteristics of Viral Encephalitis by Entity

Viral Infection	Diagnostic Pearls
Enteroviruses	■ Normal or thin linear leptomeningeal enhancement
HSV	■ Bilateral medial temporal and inferior frontal lobes, sparing basal ganglia ■ With or without abnormal DWI, enhancement, hemorrhages ■ Mass effect initially, followed by atrophy over several weeks
VZV	■ Lesions at gray-white interface, white matter, gray matter ■ Vascular imaging may show vasculitis ■ May occur in the absence of rash
Arboviruses	■ Bilateral basal ganglia and thalami lesions ■ Can involve any brain area, including medial temporal lobes
HIV	■ Generalized cerebral atrophy ■ Symmetric periventricular white matter FLAIR hyperintensity with T1 isointensity
PML	■ Asymmetrical white matter signal abnormality in subcortical U fibers ■ Cerebellar crescent-shaped lesions ■ Minimal mass effect and enhancement, except with IRIS ■ May see "leading edge" of abnormal DWI and enhancement ■ Progresses on follow-up; may lead to atrophy long-term
CMV	■ Periventricular enhancement or calcification

CMV, Cytomegalovirus; *DWI,* diffusion-weighted imaging; *FLAIR,* fluid-attenuated inversion recovery; *HIV,* human immunodeficiency virus; *HSV,* herpes simplex virus; *IRIS,* immune reconstitution inflammatory syndrome; *PML,* progressive multifocal leukoencephalopathy *VZV,* varicella-zoster virus.

tuberculomas may be T2 hypointense or may appear targetlike, with a T2 hyperintense core surrounded by a low T2 rim. Enhancement may be solid, nodular, or ringlike.

Tuberculous abscesses are pus-containing encapsulated masses containing viable mycobacteria and occur more commonly in immunocompromised patients. Distinguishing a tuberculoma with central caseation from a tuberculous abscess is difficult by imaging. Tuberculous abscesses also resemble pyogenic abscesses on MRI, with rim enhancement and a central diffusion-restricted necrotic core. Magnetic resonance spectroscopy may assist in making the diagnosis.

Fungal infections, such as coccidiomycosis and cryptococcosis, also present as granulomatous meningitis, with similar findings of hydrocephalus and enhancing inflammatory material in the basilar cisterns. Coccidiomycosis, like tuberculosis, is associated with vasculitis and may cause infarcts. Uncommonly, enhancing parenchymal brain lesions may occur with severe disease.

■ PYOGENIC INFECTIONS

Epidural Abscess and Subdural Empyema

Epidural abscesses result from direct extension of adjacent infections, particularly sinusitis or otomastoiditis, and also occur after trauma or neurosurgical procedures.

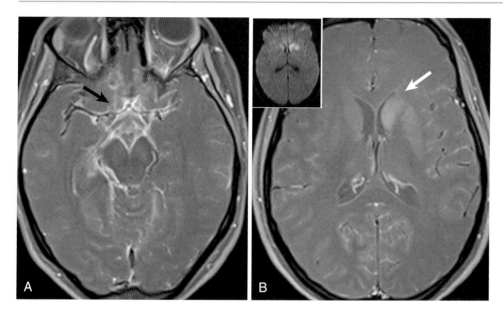

Figure 4-19 Tuberculous meningitis. Postcontrast T1-weighted magnetic resonance imaging (MRI) demonstrates thick enhancing material in the basilar cisterns (**A**, *black arrow*), consistent with granulomatous meningitis. Enhancing left caudate lesion (**B**, *white arrow*) with corresponding restricted diffusion (inset) was consistent with a subacute enhancing infarct from tuberculous vasculitis. Tuberculomas, on the other hand, do not generally show restricted diffusion.

Infected material collects between the dura and calvarium. Epidural abscesses are isodense or hypodense on CT and may contain gas. Magnetic resonance imaging better depicts these collections and usually shows intense enhancement of the dura.

Epidural abscesses may spread to the subdural space or underlying brain parenchyma. Coexistence of subdural and epidural collections is common. Magnetic resonance imaging may help differentiate them by delineating the relationship of the enhancing dura to the collection. Additionally, epidural abscesses are lentiform, freely cross dural reflections such as the falx, and are bounded by cranial sutures.

Subdural empyema results from head and neck infections, trauma, neurosurgical procedures, or complications of meningitis. Infected material collects between the dura and arachnoid membranes. Early recognition is vital for appropriate surgical management. Subdural empyema appears as hypodense or isodense crescentic collections on CT (Fig. 4-20). Magnetic resonance imaging is more sensitive, particularly FLAIR and diffusion-weighted imaging (DWI) sequences. Rim enhancement is typical (see Fig. 4-20). Restricted diffusion helps distinguish SDE from sterile subdural effusions. Complications of SDE include dural venous sinus thrombosis, cerebral edema, cerebritis, and cerebral abscess.

Cerebritis and Brain Abscess

Cerebritis refers to focal brain inflammation, which may be secondary to bacterial infection. Cerebritis commonly occurs adjacent to infected subdural or epidural collections. The imaging appearance is nonspecific, with focal low density on CT and T2/FLAIR hyperintensity on MRI. Enhancement is variable. Hemorrhage or restricted diffusion may occur. The differential diagnosis may include ischemia, neoplasm, or status epilepticus.

Cerebritis may develop into an abscess, which is suggested by a ring-enhancing mass with restricted diffusion. Cerebral abscess refers to a focal intraparenchymal pus collection with a surrounding capsule that results

from direct extension of local infection or hematogenous spread. Abscesses from blood-borne infections tend to be multiple and located at the gray-white junction, whereas abscesses arising from local spread are spatially related to the primary infection.

Regardless of cause, abscesses share common imaging features. On NCCT, abscesses appear as hypodense masses with surrounding vasogenic edema, sometimes with a hyperdense rim corresponding to the abscess capsule (Fig. 4-21). Magnetic resonance imaging also shows a localized mass with a T2-hyperintense necrotic core and a markedly T2-hypointense rim. The central core usually demonstrates markedly restricted diffusion.

On both CT and MRI, cerebral abscesses demonstrate thick smooth rim enhancement, sometimes with thinning of the medial wall. Focal wall rupture results in formation of a daughter abscess. In immunocompromised patients, ring enhancement may be absent and vasogenic edema may be mild, requiring a high index of suspicion for diagnosis.

Complications of cerebral abscess include mass effect and brain herniation. It is important to evaluate for intraventricular rupture of the abscess with resulting ventriculitis, because this is a marker of poor prognosis and requires aggressive treatment. Imaging findings of ventricular rupture include layering isodense debris in the lateral ventricles on CT, more evident on MRI FLAIR and DWI sequences, with enhancement of the ependymal (ventricular) lining (see Fig. 4-21).

■ SPECIFIC ENTITIES

Neurocysticercosis

Neurocysticercosis may involve brain parenchyma, ventricles, or subarachnoid spaces. The imaging appearance varies with location and stage of infection. Parenchymal neurocysticercosis is classified into four stages. In the vesicular stage, a thin-walled cyst forms containing the invaginated scolex, which may be visible on FLAIR and contrast-enhanced sequences. In the colloidal vesicular

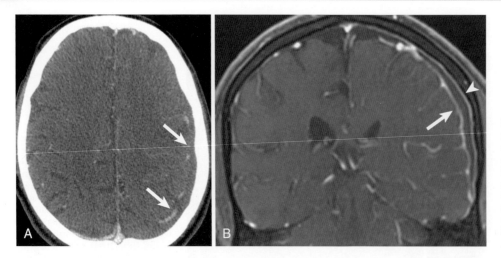

Figure 4-20 Subdural empyema (SDE). Contrast enhanced computed tomography (CT) (**A**) demonstrates an isodense collection displacing cortical veins *(arrows)*. Contrast-enhanced magnetic resonance imaging (MRI) (**B**) confirms the subdural location of the collection, between enhancing leptomeninges *(arrow)* and dura *(arrowhead)*.

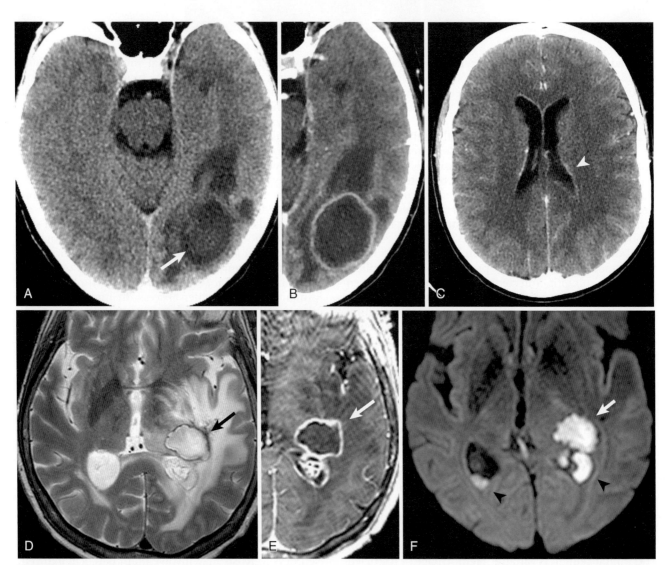

Figure 4-21 Brain abscesses complicated by ventriculitis in two patients. Noncontrast computed tomography (NCCT) (**A**) shows a mass lesion with extensive vasogenic edema *(arrow)*. Contrast-enhanced CT (**B**) shows ring enhancement of the mass. Subtle ependymal enhancement (**C**, *arrowhead*) indicates associated ventriculitis. Magnetic resonance imaging (MRI) of another patient demonstrates T2-hypointense rim (**D**, *arrow*), with associated ring enhancement (**E**). Diffusion-weighted imaging (DWI) demonstrates restricted diffusion of the central necrotic core (**F**, *arrow*) and the intraventricular debris *(arrowheads)*.

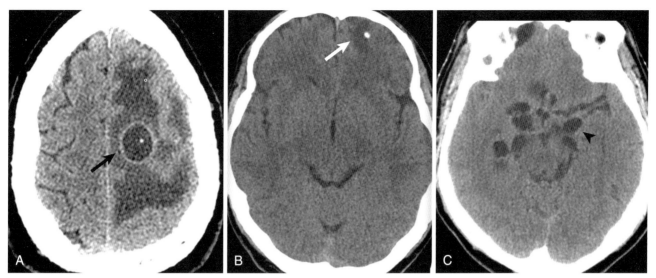

Figure 4-22 Neurocysticercosis. Noncontrast computed tomography (NCCT) in three cases. **A,** Colloidal vesicular phase with cyst, central scolex, and surrounding vasogenic edema *(arrow)*. **B,** Calcified nodular stage *(arrow)* with some residual edema. **C,** Subarachnoid (racemose) neurocysticercosis with multiple cysts along the subarachnoid spaces *(arrowhead)*.

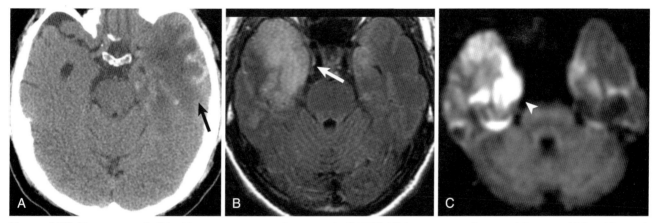

Figure 4-23 Herpes encephalitis. Noncontrast computed tomography (NCCT) (**A**) demonstrates edematous left temporal lobe with associated petechial hemorrhages *(black arrow)*. Fluid-attenuated inversion recovery (FLAIR) (**B**) and diffusion-weighted imaging (DWI) (**C**) in a second patient demonstrate edematous right anterior and mesial temporal lobe *(white arrow)* with associated restricted diffusion *(white arrowhead)*.

stage, the cyst degenerates and becomes proteinaceous, and the scolex may disappear (Fig. 4-22). In the granular nodular stage, the cyst retracts and vasogenic edema decreases, but enhancement persists. Finally, during the nodular calcified stage, edema and enhancement subside, leaving a small calcified nodule (see Fig. 4-22). Magnetic resonance imaging is best for identifying lesions in the vesicular, colloidal vesicular, and granular nodular stages. Computed tomography is excellent at detecting lesions in the nodular calcified stage, as is GRE MRI sequence.

Intraventricular neurocysticercosis may occur alone or in conjunction with other forms. Imaging findings include cystic lesions within the ventricles, commonly in the fourth ventricle. There may be associated obstructive hydrocephalus. Cysts are thin walled and contain CSF-like fluid. High-resolution heavily T2-weighted MRI sequences (MR cisternography) may help to visualize the cyst walls. Subarachnoid neurocysticercosis has a predilection for the basilar cisterns and appears as multilobular clusters of cystic lesions (racemose, or grapelike) (see Fig. 4-22). The scolex is often not visible.

Herpes Simplex Virus

Herpes simplex virus type 1 is the most common cause of acute viral encephalitis, and early diagnosis and treatment are critical. Recognizing the characteristic imaging features is important and sometimes precedes clinical suspicion of the disease. Infection usually begins in the anterior and medial aspects of the temporal lobe but may extend to the lateral temporal lobes, inferior frontal lobes, insular cortex, and cingulate gyrus. Findings may be unilateral or bilateral. Computed tomography results may be normal initially or may show low attenuation, mass effect, gyral enhancement, or hemorrhage (Fig. 4-23). Magnetic resonance imaging is more sensitive for early disease and better demonstrates edema (see Fig. 4-23). Restricted diffusion (see Fig. 4-23) may precede findings on other sequences. Hemorrhages and enhancement occur with disease progression, and encephalomalacia evolves over several weeks.

The differential diagnosis of HSV encephalitis includes ischemia, neoplasm, limbic encephalitis, and

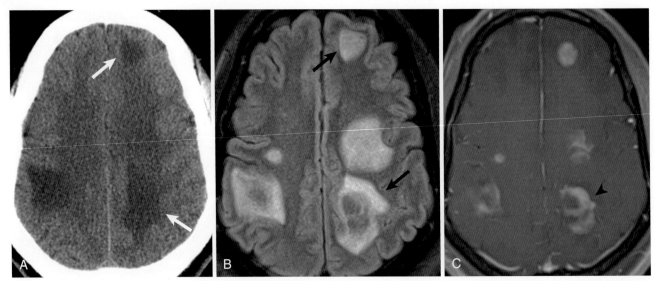

Figure 4-24 Acute disseminated encephalomyelitis (ADEM). Noncontrast computed tomography (NCCT) (**A**) demonstrates multiple lesions in the cerebral hemispheres at the gray-white junction (*white arrows*). Magnetic resonance imaging (MRI) fluid-attenuated inversion recovery sequence (FLAIR) (**B**) better demarcates the lesions (*black arrows*), which enhance (**C**). Open ring pattern of enhancement suggests demyelination (*black arrowhead*).

non-HSV viral infections such as Rasmussen encephalitis and arboviral encephalitis. Features favoring the diagnosis of HSV include bilaterality, involvement of the medial and lateral temporal lobes in a nonvascular distribution, and normal basal ganglia.

Acute Disseminated Encephalomyelitis

Acute disseminated encephalomyelitis (ADEM) is an inflammatory autoimmune demyelinating condition that typically begins abruptly several weeks following a viral illness or vaccination and follows a monophasic course lasting several weeks. Computed tomography results may be normal or may show nonspecific areas of low attenuation (Fig. 4-24), sometimes with peripheral enhancement. Magnetic resonance imaging is more sensitive, but results may also be normal initially. ADEM lesions have high T2/FLAIR and low T1 signal intensity and are typically multiple, bilateral, asymmetric, and located in the supratentorial white matter (see Fig. 4-24). Lesions may also occur in the deep gray nuclei, infratentorial white matter, spinal cord, and optic nerves. Lesions may be small and round or large and irregular, sometimes with a central T2-hyperintense portion creating a "fried egg" appearance. Mass effect and surrounding edema are typically absent, except with "tumefactive" and rare hemorrhagic forms. A peripheral incomplete ring of enhancement, the "open ring" sign, occurs in demyelinating lesions that partially abut white matter and cortex, in which case only the white matter edge enhances (see Fig. 4-24). Closed ring, solid, nodular, and gyral enhancement patterns also occur.

Acute disseminated encephalomyelitis lesions usually resolve or improve on follow-up, sometimes with residual gliosis. Clinical resolution may precede radiographic resolution. Relapsing forms of the disease exist but should be distinguished from protracted monophasic disease or incomplete treatment. The main differential diagnosis by imaging is multiple sclerosis (MS), although the clinical scenario is distinct between these two entities.

■ IMMUNOCOMPROMISED PATIENTS

Immune system compromise may affect humoral immunity or cell-mediated immunity and may be due to primary immune deficiency or secondary to infections such as human immunodeficiency virus (HIV), cancers such as leukemia, and medications such as chemotherapy and immunosuppressants. Neutropenic patients are particularly susceptible to bacterial and fungal infections. Immunocompromised patients in general are prone to frequent, severe, and long-lasting infections that may be caused by opportunistic pathogens such as progressive multifocal leukoencephalopathy (PML), cytomegalovirus, toxoplasmosis, cryptococcosis, and coccidiomycosis. Tuberculosis and syphilis are also increasingly common in immunocompromised patients.

Human Immunodeficiency Virus

Imaging findings in HIV may result from direct HIV infection of the central nervous system (CNS) or from opportunistic infections. Direct effects of HIV infection include generalized cerebral volume loss and symmetric confluent periventricular white matter disease without contrast enhancement or mass effect. Human immunodeficiency virus infection may resemble age-related volume loss and chronic microvascular ischemia, but progression is faster than expected. Human immunodeficiency virus encephalopathy may also resemble PML but can be differentiated by the periventricular distribution, symmetry, and isointensity on T1-weighted images.

Toxoplasmosis

Toxoplasmosis appears as one or more ring- or nodular-enhancing abscesses (Fig. 4-25). T2 signal is heterogeneous

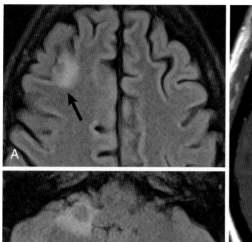
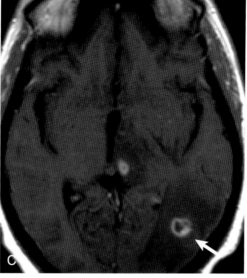

Figure 4-25 Toxoplasmosis in human immunodeficiency virus (HIV). Noncontrast computed tomography (NCCT) was normal (not shown). Magnetic resonance imaging (MRI) fluid-attenuated inversion recovery sequence (FLAIR) (**A** and **B**) demonstrates multiple small lesions *(black arrows)*. Contrast-enhanced MRI (**C**) in another patient demonstrates multiple small rim-enhancing lesions, one of which appears as an eccentric target sign *(white arrow)*.

and may vary according to abscess stage and treatment effects. The "eccentric target sign" refers to an enhancing nodule along the ring-enhancing wall of the lesion, a relatively specific but insensitive sign for toxoplasmosis. Typical abscess locations include the basal ganglia, thalami, and gray-white junction. Differentiating toxoplasmosis from lymphoma in a patient with acquired immunodeficiency syndrome (AIDS) remains problematic. Fludeoxyglucose F 18 positron emission tomography (FDG-PET), thallium-201 single-photon emission computed tomography (SPECT), and DWI sequence may be helpful, as is serial imaging showing response to antibiotics.

Progressive Multifocal Leukoencephalopathy

Progressive multifocal leukoencephalopathy is a progressive and frequently fatal demyelinating opportunistic infection caused by the JC virus, which directly infects the myelin-producing oligodendrocytes. A recently described subset of at-risk patients includes those with MS or Crohn disease treated with natalizumab. The diagnosis is established by demonstrating JC viral deoxyribonucleic acid (DNA) in the CSF, but characteristic MRI findings may first suggest the disease. Progressive multifocal leukoencephalopathy may resemble ADEM, but the two entities are usually distinguished clinically by immune status and onset and course of disease.

Progressive multifocal leukoencephalopathy appears as confluent subcortical white matter hypoattenuation on CT involving arcuate or U fibers, sparing the cortex (Fig. 4-26). Magnetic resonance imaging shows T2/FLAIR hyperintensity with progressive T1 hypointensity (see Fig. 4-26), classically lacking mass effect or enhancement. Scant peripheral enhancement as well as restricted diffusion is sometimes observed at the "leading edge" of demyelination. Marked enhancement and mass effect usually imply coexistence of the immune reconstitution inflammatory syndrome (IRIS). Parietooccipital lobes and corpus callosum are typically affected, but periventricular white matter is relatively spared compared to

MS. Lesions may be multiple and asymmetric bilaterally, with increasing confluence and extension to new areas on follow-up. Infratentorial lesions also occur, sometimes in isolation, and cerebellar lesions often have a characteristic crescent-shaped morphologic structure.

Immune Reconstitution Inflammatory Syndrome

IRIS is a complication of highly active antiretroviral therapy (HAART) that occurs in the setting of severe AIDS-related immunodeficiency shortly after the initiation of therapy. The syndrome is characterized by an exaggerated inflammatory response to dead, latent, or viable organisms or self-antigens and may coexist with a variety of opportunistic infections, most commonly PML and cryptococcosis. The imaging findings might be confused with new or worsening opportunistic infection. The diagnosis is usually suspected when there is paradoxical clinical deterioration with imaging findings that are atypical for a given opportunistic infection. For example, in IRIS-PML, there may be greater than expected enhancement and/or mass effect.

◼ CEREBROVASCULAR COMPLICATIONS OF INFECTION

Intracranial vascular complications of infections may be arterial or venous and may occur in the setting of meningitis, head and neck infections, or systemic infections. Examples include infectious vasculitis, septic venous thrombophlebitis, septic emboli, septic (mycotic) aneurysms, and disseminated intravascular coagulation.

Infectious Vasculitis

Cerebral vasculitis may be primary and idiopathic or secondary to systemic vasculitis, drugs, or infections. Infectious cerebral vasculitis is potentially treatable; therefore infected patients with neurologic deficits warrant brain and cerebrovascular imaging. Pathogens known to cause

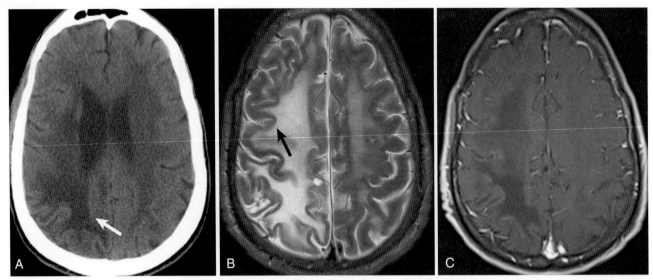

Figure 4-26 Progressive multifocal leukoencephalopathy (PML). Noncontrast computed tomography (NCCT) **(A)** demonstrates markedly hypodense white matter, particularly of the right parietal lobe *(white arrow)*. T2 magnetic resonance imaging (MRI) **(B)** shows markedly hyperintense white matter, extending to the cortical ribbon *(black arrow)*, with no enhancement **(C)** or restricted diffusion (not shown).

infectious cerebral vasculitis include pyogenic bacteria, tuberculosis, syphilis, varicella-zoster virus, and various fungi and parasites. Any cause of infectious basilar meningitis can lead to vasculopathy involving the vessels at the base of the brain. Vascular complications of pyogenic bacterial meningitis are common, and outcomes are poor, with a high risk for stroke (see Fig. 4-18). Definitive diagnosis of infectious vasculitis is based on CSF analysis in concert with clinical and radiologic signs.

The vascular imaging findings of infectious vasculitis include segmental vasoconstriction with a "sausages-on-a-string" appearance, vessel wall irregularity, smooth narrowing, dissection, occlusion, or aneurysm formation. There may be contrast enhancement of the vessel walls. Complications of vasculitis include infarcts and hemorrhages, including SAH. Multiple lesions at the gray-white interface are characteristic of varicella-zoster virus vasculopathy.

Septic Thrombophlebitis

Cerebral venous septic thrombophlebitis is an important pathway for the spread of head and neck infections and may also complicate meningitis. Septic thrombophlebitis can involve dural venous sinuses, cavernous sinuses, or cortical veins. Diabetic and immunocompromised patients presenting with coalescent mastoiditis or frontal or sphenoid sinusitis are at highest risk. Specific patterns include sigmoid sinus thrombosis secondary to coalescent mastoiditis (Fig. 4-27), superior sagittal sinus thrombosis secondary to frontal sinusitis, and cavernous sinus thrombophlebitis secondary to sphenoid sinusitis/osteomyelitis or orbital cellulitis.

Imaging signs of cavernous sinus thrombosis include filling defects, diminished enhancement, or an expanded contour of the cavernous sinus. Indirect findings may include proptosis, enlargement of the extraocular muscles, and enlargement, nonenhancement, or filling defects within the superior ophthalmic veins.

Occasionally, gas bubbles are present in the cavernous sinus due to dehiscence of the sphenoid sinus walls related to osteomyelitis. Secondary arterial complications involving the cavernous internal carotid artery may occur, including arteritis, thrombosis, and aneurysm formation.

Imaging signs of dural venous thrombosis include a hyperdense venous sinus on NCCT, abnormal flow voids on noncontrast MRI, absence of the normal flow-related signal on noncontrast MRV, and filling defects on contrast-enhanced CTV or MRV. Obstructive dural venous sinus thrombosis may lead to secondary complications of venous hypertension, including venous infarction, vasogenic edema, parenchymal hemorrhages, ischemic or hemorrhagic infarcts, or isolated convexal SAH.

Cortical vein thrombosis may be occult or may appear on NCCT as a hyperdense, serpiginous cortical structure corresponding to the thrombosed vein, which does not opacify on CTV. Magnetic resonance imaging may show abnormal susceptibility on GRE sequence. Secondary complications related to venous hypertension are similar to those of dural venous sinus thrombosis.

Septic Emboli, Septic Aneurysms, and Disseminated Intravascular Coagulation

Infectious endocarditis and systemic sepsis from any cause can lead to intracranial complications from septic emboli, septic (mycotic) aneurysms, or complex clotting disorders such as disseminated intravascular coagulation. Septic emboli may lead to multiple cerebral infarctions, microhemorrhages, and microabscesses (Fig. 4-28). The imaging findings on NCCT include loss of gray-white differentiation or hypoattenuation corresponding to acute infarcts. Magnetic resonance imaging may show multifocal areas of FLAIR signal hyperintensity and/or restricted diffusion at the gray-white interface, often associated with small areas of abnormal susceptibility on GRE

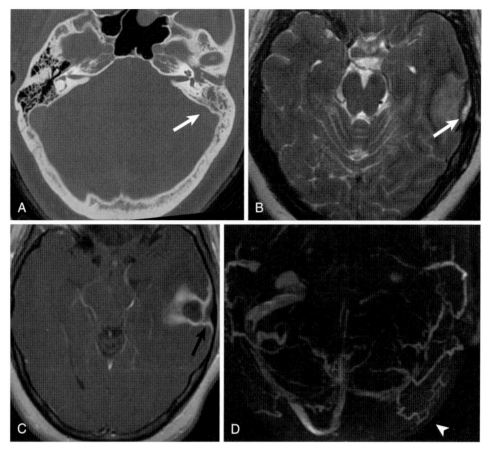

Figure 4-27 Septic thrombophlebitis. Noncontrast computed tomography (NCCT) (**A**) demonstrates opacified mastoid air cells *(arrow)*. Magnetic resonance imaging (MRI) T2-weighted sequence (**B**) demonstrates small hyperintense epidural abscess *(arrow)* with associated cerebritis within the adjacent temporal lobe. Postcontrast T1-weighted sequence (**C**) shows a rim-enhancing parenchymal abscess and epidural collection *(black arrow)*. Noncontrast MR venogram (MRV) (**D**) shows absence of flow-related signal in the left transverse and sigmoid sinuses *(white arrowhead)*, consistent with venous sinus thrombosis.

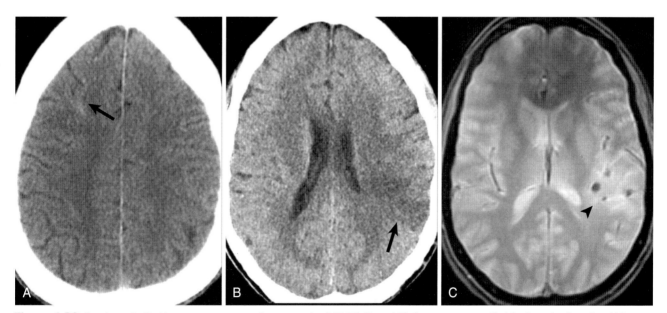

Figure 4-28 Septic emboli. Noncontrast computed tomography (NCCT) (**A** and **B**) demonstrates small right frontal subarachnoid hemorrhage (SAH) (**A**, *black arrow*) and small left cortical infarct (**B**, *black arrow*). Magnetic resonance imaging (MRI) T2*-weighted sequence demonstrates a cluster of small microhemorrhages (**C**, *arrowhead*).

images (see Fig. 4-28). Contrast-enhanced images show multiple peripherally enhancing lesions at the gray-white interface. Multifocal SAH isolated to the cerebral convexities is another presentation of septic emboli, possibly secondary to focal arteritis or rupture of small vessels at the sites of embolic occlusion. Convexal SAH may be visible on NCCT as peripheral areas of hyperdensity within the cerebral sulci or as subarachnoid space FLAIR signal hyperintensity on MRI.

Septic aneurysms may form in association with septic emboli or as a consequence of systemic sepsis or spread from local head and neck infections. Rupture of a septic aneurysm may result in diffuse SAH indistinguishable from saccular aneurysm rupture, or a more localized presentation of SAH confined to a sylvian fissure or a cerebral convexity. On angiography, septic aneurysms often appear irregular in shape and arise in abnormal locations, usually more distally in the vascular tree compared to saccular aneurysms.

Disseminated intravascular coagulation usually occurs in the setting of systemic sepsis and may also result in multiple cerebral infarcts and hemorrhages, including multifocal convexal SAH. Infarcts and hemorrhages result from the systemic cascade of microclot formation, consumption of platelets and clotting factors, and bleeding complications in multiple organ systems. The imaging findings are nonspecific and may share overlapping features with septic emboli.

SUMMARY

Imaging plays an important role in the emergent evaluation of CNS infections. Noncontrast CT is an important initial study for patients with suspected brain infection, and MRI plays a complementary role. Leptomeningeal enhancement, extra-axial collections, cerebritis, encephalitis, and enhancing lesions may confirm suspected intracranial infection or may raise the possibility of infection as an unsuspected cause of a patient's neurologic status. Specific imaging appearances may predict a particular cause, such as tuberculosis or HSV encephalitis. Additionally, imaging is vital to exclude complications of CNS infections, including hydrocephalus, brain herniation, cerebral edema, infarcts, and other vascular abnormalities.

Stroke

Michele H. Johnson, David Y. Hwang, and Joseph L. Schindler

DEFINITION OF STROKE

Acute ischemic stroke is the most common nontraumatic neurologic diagnosis of exclusion in the ED. The origin of the term *stroke* referred to any "sudden neurologic deficit"; as such, the word historically encompasses a wide variety of causes. Acute ischemic stroke develops secondary to intracranial vascular occlusion that results in

ischemic parenchymal injury. The clinical deficit is determined by the anatomic distribution of the parenchymal injury. Vascular occlusion may be embolic, resulting from cardiac or cervical vascular disease. Alternatively, occlusion may result from focal thrombosis, often associated with underlying stenosis or dissection. Global ischemia as seen in hypotension or anoxic injury results in ischemia/infarction in the watershed or border zones between major vascular territories. An understanding of acute ischemic stroke diagnosis, triage and management, and the critical role of emergent neuroimaging is important for the emergency radiologist on the front lines.

IMAGING TOOLS AND OPTIONS

The key imaging modality for assessment of the patient with stroke is the head NCCT. It is fast and readily available in most EDs. Modern scanners can accommodate patients of all sizes, from infants to bariatric patients. There is robust radiation dose reduction software to protect the most vulnerable of patients. Noncontrast CT permits rapid diagnosis of hemorrhage. When no hemorrhage is identified, a careful assessment for the earliest signs of acute ischemic stroke must be performed. Noncontrast CT may demonstrate a nonvascular cause of the neurologic deficit, such as tumor or infection, and exclude the diagnosis of acute ischemic stroke. Clinical evaluation may suggest an alternative source of neurologic deficit, such as seizures and/or a postictal state. Vascular imaging is often employed for evaluation of cervical or intracranial vessel patency and is best correlated with clinical findings to exclude stroke mimics.

STROKE CENTERS AND CURRENT TREATMENT OPTIONS

Before neuroimaging, the initial clinical assessment involves the confirmation of the time of symptom onset and a neurologic examination. Up to 30% of patients will have neurologic symptoms that mimic acute ischemic stroke. Central to the emergent clinical assessment is the performance of the National Institutes of Health Stroke Scale (NIHSS), which quantifies the severity of the stroke. The NIHSS is a 15-item impairment scale assessing level of consciousness, language, orientation, visual loss, strength, sensation, and incoordination. Higher scores are associated with a greater volume of potentially infarcted brain and are associated with a less favorable prognosis, although lower scores may be equally disabling. NIHSS scores greater than 10 may suggest large vessel occlusion. Right hemispheric strokes tend to have lower scores because NIHSS is highly dependent on language. Posterior circulation infarcts tend to have lower scores because cranial nerves and gait are not emphasized in the scoring. History, time of onset, neurologic examination, and neuroimaging (NCCT) are critically reviewed to determine the risk and benefits of treatment options and make recommendations to the family.

Intravenous (IV) t-PA remains the only Food and Drug Administration (FDA)-approved drug for the acute treatment for stroke patients, although nationally only

4% of stroke sufferers receive this medication. A number of reasons exist for this statistic. First, most patients do not arrive in the ED within the IV t-PA narrow therapeutic window. IV t-PA is FDA approved for administration within 3 hours after symptom onset (ictus); however, it is endorsed by the American Heart Association to be given in selected circumstances up to 4½ post ictus. Secondly, even for those who arrive in time, many still do not receive IV treatment because of inability to deliver the medication in a timely manner.

These factors led to the recommendation for the establishment of primary stroke centers from a multidisciplinary group of specialists called the Brain Attack Coalition. Stroke centers coordinate the safe and timely administration of IV t-PA to patients who are deemed candidates via a multidisciplinary stroke team that includes radiologists. Stroke center protocols define roles and establish inclusion and exclusion criteria for IV t-PA administration.

The risk for symptomatic intracerebral hemorrhage following IV t-PA administration was 6% in the original National Institute of Neurological Disorders and Stroke (NINDS) study. Many ED physicians are uncomfortable providing this recommendation without neurologic expertise. Because of the limited availability of specialty expertise and stroke centers, TeleStroke was originated in the late 1990s, and since then approximately 27 networks, many of them academic medical centers, have provided video consultations to outlying hospitals. The American Heart Association has recommended the use of telemedicine for acute stroke when neurologic expertise is not available. The telemedicine stroke assessment, including performing the NIHSS and review of neuroimaging, has been demonstrated to be both reliable and effective. In fact, a study comparing the use of telephone and telemedicine in assessing acute stroke patients demonstrated better sensitivity and specificity for accuracy of stroke diagnosis and appropriateness of administering IV t-PA through the use of telemedicine.

■ RELEVANCE OF IMAGING IN STROKE

Noncontrast CT represents the primary imaging decision point for triage and management in acute stroke. The goal of imaging in stroke is the determination of ischemic versus hemorrhagic causes of sudden nontraumatic neurologic deficit. Once hemorrhage is excluded and a clinical decision about t-PA administration is made, the patient with suspected acute stroke (without underlying mass or other pathologic condition) will often go on to noninvasive extracranial and intracranial vascular imaging, most commonly using CTA. Alternatively MRA may be added, particularly when acute stroke MRI is performed (see later discussion). Magnetic resonance imaging for acute stroke includes diffusion, apparent diffusion coefficient (ADC) map, FLAIR, and GRE or susceptibility-weighted sequences. Imaging modality selection may vary with availability and the time of onset of the neurologic deficit. Noncontrast CT is most commonly employed in the setting of acute ischemic stroke under consideration for IV or intra-arterial

Table 4-5   Key Terminology

Acute ischemic stroke	Injury resulting from abrupt arterial occlusion leading to cell death
Ictus	The onset of acute neurologic symptoms; often defined by the last time of normal neurologic status (last seen normal)
Infarct core	The central zone of acute infarction where cellular death occurs
IV t-PA	t-PA given IV is the standard of care for treatment of acute ischemic stroke within 3.0-4.5 hours of onset
Lacunar stroke	Small infarct in the end arteries usually within the basal ganglia
Mechanical thrombectomy (IA therapy)	Transcatheter mechanical methods for clot removal, including suction devices and stent retrievers
NIH Stroke Scale	Clinical 15-item impairment scale designed to assess stroke severity
Penumbra	The peripheral zone of acute infarction where tissue is at risk for permanent ischemic injury and cellular death if revascularization is not achieved
Transient ischemic attack	Brief acute neurologic deficit with rapid return to baseline; often precedes acute ischemic stroke
Wake-up stroke	Acute neurologic deficit recognized upon awakening with no definite time of onset

IA, Intra-arterial; *IV,* intravenous; *NIH,* National Institutes of Health; *t-PA,* tissue plasminogen activator.

therapies, whereas subacute and chronic or recurrent stroke symptoms may be more completely evaluated by MRI. Both CT and MR perfusion are available for patient assessment but are not currently validated as entrance criteria for treatment with IV or intra-arterial therapies.

■ LANGUAGE AND GEOGRAPHY OF STROKE: KEY TO PROTOCOLS AND TRIAGE

The emergency radiologist must be familiar with the language and geography of stroke and the role of each imaging tool in the assessment and triage of patients with acute, subacute, and chronic stroke (Table 4-5).

■ BRIEF PATHOPHYSIOLOGY OF ACUTE ISCHEMIC STROKE

Pathologically, impairment of local cerebrovascular perfusion leads to neuronal contraction, cytotoxic edema, cellular death, and inflammatory infiltration. Tissue ischemia and the influx of water molecules lead to the decreased density of ischemic tissue on NCCT and some of the earliest signs of stroke, including loss of gray-white differentiation. The influx of water results in further injury to the cell, resulting in restriction of the

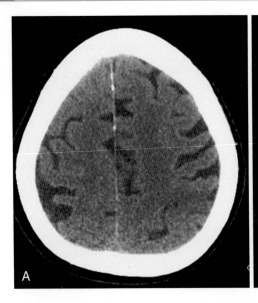
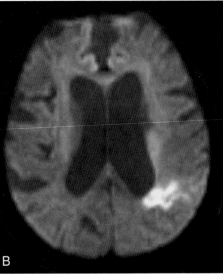

Figure 4-29 A, Axial noncontrast computed tomography (NCCT) demonstrates hypodensity in the posterior parietal cortex on the left with loss of gray-white matter differentiation and sulcal effacement. **B,** Diffusion-weighted magnetic resonance imaging (MRI) demonstrates restricted diffusion corresponding to the region of gray-white matter differentiation loss on NCCT.

ability of water molecules to move freely within the cell. When the diffusion capacity of water within the tissue is restricted, there is increased signal within the area of infarction on diffusion-weighted MRI sequences.

■ EARLIEST SIGNS OF ACUTE ISCHEMIC STROKE ON NONENHANCED COMPUTED TOMOGRAPHY

One of the earliest signs of stroke on CT relates to the loss of gray-white matter differentiation caused by the influx of water into the cell (i.e., cytotoxic edema) (Fig. 4-29). Gray matter is more susceptible to ischemic injury than white matter due to its higher metabolic rate. In MCA territory infarction, subtle decease in density at the gray-white junction may be seen at the insular ribbon, lentiform nucleus, or peripheral cortex. Similar early gray-white junction hypodensities involving the cortical and subcortical regions can be seen with anterior cerebral, posterior cerebral, or vertebrobasilar territory infarction. These hypodensities are initially subtle and poorly defined over the first 3 hours post ictus, becoming more hypodense and more clearly defined over time. As cytotoxic edema progresses and vasogenic edema ensues, sulcal effacement occurs as a consequence of acute ischemia (see Fig. 4-29). Occasionally the effacement of sulci may precede visualization of loss of gray-white differentiation. Acute lacunar infarction can be subtle and may not be apparent on CT for several hours to a day, dependent upon size and location.

The hyperdense artery sign is often sought after as an early sign of stroke caused by hyperdense thrombus within a major artery, first described in the proximal MCA (Fig. 4-30). This sign may precede other early signs of stroke. It is an inconstant finding and may be absent in the face of angiographically defined major vessel occlusion. It is important to compare the density of the hyperdense vessel to other circle of Willis branches to avoid undercalling or overcalling this finding.

Involvement of more than one third of the MCA territory on NCCT within the 0- to 6-hour time window is associated with large areas of infarction with increased risk for hemorrhagic transformation and poorer outcomes following IV t-PA administration. In an effort to quantify the extent of early signs of infarction on NCCT, the Alberta Stroke Program Early CT Score (ASPECTS) was proposed as a 10-point CT-based scoring system for MCA ischemia with good intraobserver agreement. An ASPECTS score of greater than 7 correlates with a poorer outcome and higher risk for hemorrhagic transformation, analogous to the one-third MCA territory rule (2).

■ EARLIEST SIGNS OF ACUTE ISCHEMIC STROKE ON MAGNETIC RESONANCE IMAGING

The earliest signs of infarction on MRI relate to alterations in local cerebral blood flow and cerebral tissue perfusion. Restricted diffusion, increased signal intensity within the zone of ischemia/infarction, is the hallmark of acute ischemia on MRI, caused by the influx of water molecules into the cell in the form of cytotoxic edema. Diffusion restriction on diffusion-weighted MRI sequences may be identified as early as minutes to 2 hours following the onset of ischemia/infarction. The ADC sequence demonstrates decreased signal intensity matching the region of increased signal intensity on the diffusion-weighted sequence. It is important to use the ADC to confirm true diffusion restriction because T2 signal effects ("T2 shine-through") may mimic restricted diffusion (see Fig. 4-30).

Loss of the normal flow void within a major vessel indicates occlusion or near occlusion on MRI (Fig. 4-31). Loss of the flow void may be associated with other signs of early ischemia such as restricted diffusion, sulcal effacement, or flow-related enhancement.

Flow-related enhancement is seen on FLAIR sequences as high signal intensity within vessels where occlusive vascular disease causes distal reduced (i.e., slow) flow. This may be seen early, before the onset of sulcal effacement,

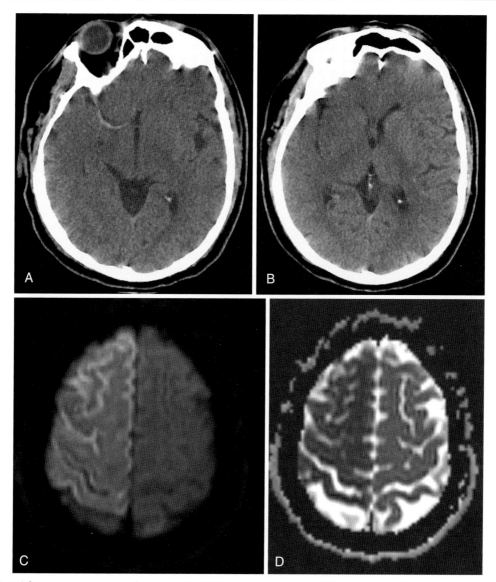

Figure 4-30 A, Axial noncontrast computed tomography (NCCT) in a patient with left hemiparesis and a hyperdense right middle cerebral artery (MCA) sign. **B**, Hypodensity on axial NCCT is identified in the insular ribbon and in the lentiform nucleus consistent with early right MCA territory infarct. **C**, Diffusion-weighted magnetic resonance imaging (MRI) shows high-signal-intensity restricted diffusion in the high right frontal and parietal regions consistent with MCA and anterior cerebral artery (ACA) infarction. **D**, Low signal intensity on the apparent diffusion coefficient (ADC) map confirms the restricted diffusion high right frontal and parietal region, confirming MCA and ACA infarction.

and can be helpful when the occluded vessel is distal to the circle of Willis (Fig. 4-32). Diffusion/perfusion mismatch exists when the region of abnormal perfusion is greater than the ischemic core as defined by the area of restricted diffusion. The difference is the ischemic penumbra or "tissue at risk" that may go on to complete infarction should revascularization not occur (see Fig. 4-32).

■ GEOGRAPHY OF ISCHEMIC STROKE

Familiarity with the major arterial vascular territories of the brain is important for diagnosis of acute ischemic stroke and can help exclude those lesions that often involve more than one arterial vascular territory (or are not confined to a single arterial territory), such as venous infarction, tumor, or infection. The pattern

of vascular territorial involvement in cerebral infarction may provide a clue to the cause of the ischemia. The clinical symptoms and infarct severity relate to the ischemic core and the penumbral tissue at risk. Single vascular territory infarction is often caused by occlusion of a major vessel due to focal thrombosis or embolus. Infarction of multiple major vascular territories in the same hemisphere may be due to a large vessel occlusion. Multiple bilateral infarcts and/or both supra tentorial and infratentorial infarcts suggest an embolic cause such as from atrial fibrillation or bacterial endocarditis.

Hypotension and anoxia may result in watershed or border-zone infarctions that involve regions of the brain supplied by distal branches of major vascular territories. Perfusion reserve may be more limited because these border zones are particularly vulnerable to reduced perfusion pressure. Ischemic changes

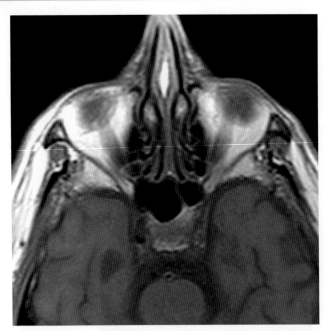

Figure 4-31 T1-weighted axial magnetic resonance imaging (MRI) demonstrates normal flow void in the right internal carotid artery and absence of the flow void on the left due to left internal carotid occlusion.

in nonarterial territories, particularly adjacent to dural venous sinuses, suggest venous infarction due to cortical vein or dural venous sinus thrombosis.

■ IMAGING CORRELATES OF ACUTE STROKE SYNDROMES

Acute anterior circulation stroke syndromes result from occlusion of major or medium-sized anterior circulation branches. Noncontrast CT has high specificity with lower sensitivity for identification of early infarct. Detection is in part dependent upon time of onset and availability of collaterals. Vascular imaging using CTA can demonstrate the vascular occlusion and inform treatment decisions (Fig. 4-33).

Acute posterior circulation stroke syndromes result from occlusion of major or medium-sized posterior circulation branches and/or small perforating branches that supply valuable real estate in the brainstem or deep gray structures. Noncontrast CT is limited in the assessment of early posterior circulation infarction because of intrapetrous artifact and limited spatial resolution of tiny basilar perforator infarctions. Subacute infarctions are more easily identified on NCCT because of both hypodensity and associated mass effect. Magnetic resonance imaging is critical for the confirmation of early posterior circulation stroke (Fig. 4-34).

Lacunar stroke is caused by arterial or perforator domain infarction, often within the basal ganglia, and may be similar in appearance to prominent Virchow-Robin (perivascular) spaces. Although NCCT may demonstrate the abnormality, MRI is much more sensitive for determination diagnosis and acuity. Imaging in the setting of transient ischemic attack is largely performed to exclude hemorrhage and to assess for evidence of prior ischemic infarction. Vascular imaging is performed to look for extracranial and intracranial vascular disease that may be responsible for the acute symptoms. Although this imaging assessment may be performed in the ED, the complete laboratory and imaging risk factor assessment is most commonly performed in a less urgent fashion.

Pediatric stroke deserves specific mention because a high percentage of pediatric stroke patients experience a delay in diagnosis. Early identification of the stroke syndrome supplemented with early imaging may improve diagnostic accuracy and clinical outcome. Noncontrast CT is commonly the first imaging study; however, hyperacute MRI may supplant the CT to eliminate the radiation dose in a vulnerable population. Magnetic resonance imaging also permits better visualization of the posterior fossa and is a more effective survey for nonischemic pathologic conditions (Fig. 4-35).

Venous infarction is a result of occlusion of a cortical vein, a dural venous sinus, or, more rarely, a deep cerebral vein. Dehydration or underlying infection, such as meningitis or mastoiditis, may result in venous occlusion and venous infarction. The most important clue to the diagnosis is the nonarterial territorial distribution of the infarction. Often venous infarction is associated with hemorrhage. Missed diagnosis may delay treatment, which usually includes anticoagulation.

■ EVOLUTION OF ACUTE THERAPIES AND CURRENT STROKE TRIALS

As previously discussed, a central goal of acute ischemic stroke neuroimaging in the ED is not only to aid in determining whether a given patient is a candidate for IV t-PA but also to help decide whether a patient may be a candidate for acute catheter-based therapy. Since the initial publication of PROACT II (Prolyse in Acute Cerebral Thromboembolism II), which established intra-arterial recombinant prourokinase as a potential treatment option for MCA occlusion up to 6 hours following onset of symptoms, the field of acute neurointervention for stroke secondary to large vessel disease has rapidly evolved. Many generations of catheter-based devices for mechanical thrombectomy (e.g., Merci, Penumbra, Solitaire, Trevo) that can be used up to 8 hours following anterior circulation stroke (and perhaps longer time windows for severe posterior circulation stroke) have subsequently been developed over the past decade, many with impressive reported recanalization rates.

However, despite the challenges of performing large multicenter randomized controlled trials for such interventions, with many neurologists and neurointerventionalists initially lacking clinical equipoise, three major studies published simultaneously in 2013 (IMS-III, SYNTHESIS, and MR RESCUE) overall failed to show an outcome benefit for intra-arterial mechanical thrombectomy, regardless of whether patients received t-PA or whether advanced neuroimaging was performed in an attempt to assess the ischemic penumbra. Rather than implying that catheter interventions for ischemic stroke are wholesale ineffective, these studies have established new equipoise among the stroke research community and have thus created consensus that further studies are necessary to determine exactly

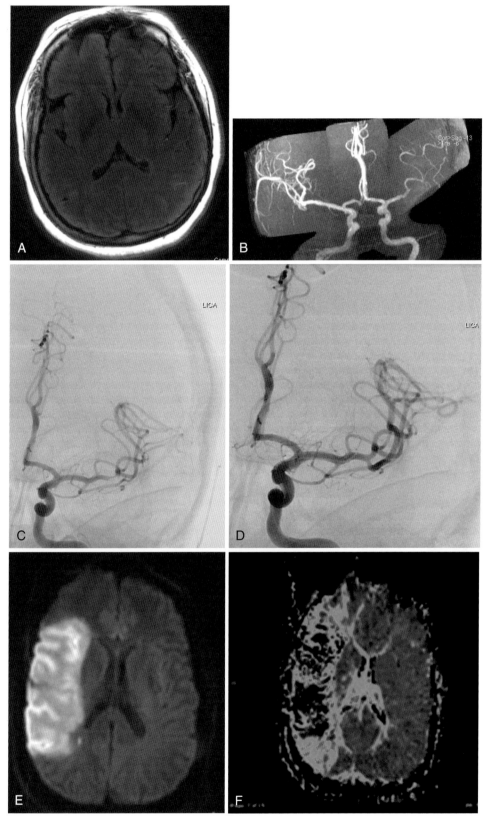

Figure 4-32 A, Fluid-attenuated inversion recovery (FLAIR) images demonstrate flow-related enhancement in the left middle cerebral artery (MCA) territory correlating with slow flow in the sylvian branches. B, Coronal magnetic resonance angiography (MRA) maximum intensity projection (MIP) image demonstrates left inferior M2 branch occlusion with a paucity of branches visible in the MCA territory. C, Anteroposterior (AP) left internal carotid artery digital subtraction angiography (DSA) confirms the inferior M2 branch occlusion. D, AP left internal carotid artery DSA following the thrombectomy demonstrates recanalization of the inferior M2 branch. E, Diffusion-weighted MRI demonstrates restricted diffusion in the right MCA territory. Hypodensity on the apparent diffusion coefficient (ADC) map (not shown) confirms ischemia/infarction. F, MR perfusion shows prolongation of the mean transit time involving the MCA territory and both the anterior and posterior watershed zones. This finding represents a mismatch between the diffusion and perfusion images and demonstrates the penumbra (i.e., the tissue at risk).

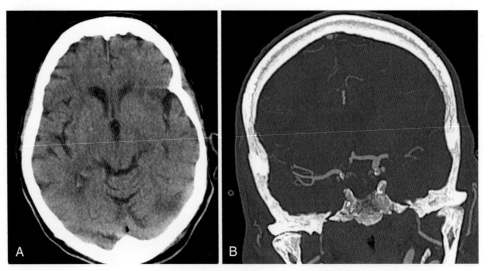

Figure 4-33 A, This patient presents with new-onset aphasia and mild right hemiparesis. On noncontrast computed tomography (NCCT) there is loss of the anterior aspect of the insular ribbon on the left with adjacent hypodensity frontally. In addition, there is sulcal prominence and hypodensity in the posterior temporal region on the left. B, Computed tomographic angiography (CTA) in the coronal plane demonstrates occlusion of the midsegment of the M1 on the left with patency of the M1 bifurcation.

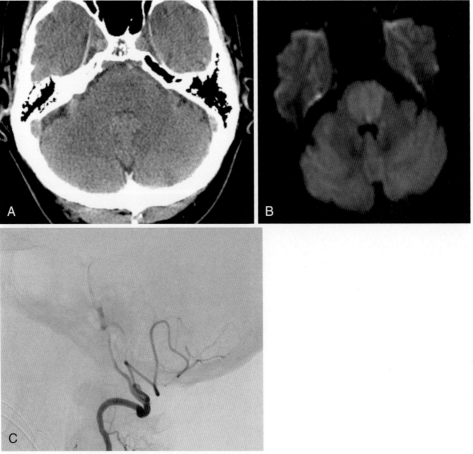

Figure 4-34 A, This patient with sudden collapse presents with a hyperdense basilar artery sign and questionable hypodensity in the mid pons seen on noncontrast computed tomography (NCCT). B, Diffusion-weighted magnetic resonance imaging (MRI) demonstrates mild diffusion restriction in the pons. The apparent diffusion coefficient (ADC) map (not shown) shows hypodensity in the pons consistent with ischemia/infarction. C, Lateral left vertebral artery digital subtraction angiography (DSA) demonstrates basilar occlusion with clot in the mid and distal basilar arteries.

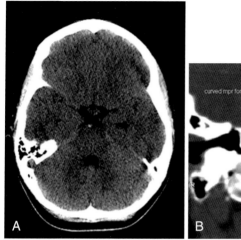
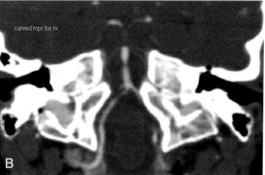
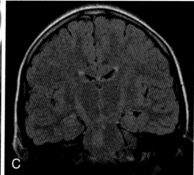

Figure 4-35 **A,** Noncontrast computed tomography (NCCT) in a 14-year-old with nausea, vomiting, and mutism reveals a hyperdense basilar artery without definite hypodensity in the pons. **B,** Curved reformatted coronal computed tomographic angiography (CTA) demonstrates occlusion of the distal basilar segment with opacification of the posterior cerebral arteries likely via the posterior communicating arteries. **C,** Coronal fluid-attenuated inversion recovery (FLAIR) image demonstrates hyperintensity in the right hemipons, consistent with ischemia/infarction.

Table 4-6   Selected Acute Ischemic Stroke Clinical Trials Currently Enrolling at Major Stroke Centers

Name of Trial	Intervention Being Tested
CLOTBUST-ER	Transcranial ultrasonography in conjunction with IV t-PA
DIAS-4	IV desmoteplase for thrombolysis up to 9 hours following stroke onset
GAMES-RP	IV glyburide as agent to prevent cerebral edema following large MCA stroke
ICTuS	Endovascular hypothermia in conjunction with IV t-PA
SWIFT PRIME	Solitaire mechanical thrombectomy device

IV, Intravenous; *MCA,* middle cerebral artery; *t-PA,* tissue plasminogen activator.

how best to select patients who will benefit from acute neurointervention.

The field of acute stroke therapy outside of IV t-PA continues to evolve, and prompt referral of all acute stroke patients with high NIHSS scores to a comprehensive stroke center for enrollment in important clinical trials examining newer-generation mechanical thrombectomy devices as well as promising non–catheter-based therapies remains critical and time sensitive. Table 4-6 summarizes a selection of ongoing multicenter acute ischemic stroke clinical trials (clinicaltrials.gov).

■ CONCLUSIONS AND OBSERVATIONS

Emergent neuroimaging is pivotal in the diagnosis, triage, and management of acute ischemic stroke. The emergency radiologist is a valuable member of the stroke team. Familiarity with the earliest imaging signs of infarction on CT and MRI, as well as the clinical diagnostic considerations, will improve diagnostic accuracy. With early diagnosis there is the potential for earlier treatment and better outcomes. The phrase "Time Is

Brain" is the most compelling rallying cry for rapid imaging diagnosis and assessment in the setting of acute ischemic stroke.

Acute Presentation of Neoplasm
Alexander B. Baxter and Xin Wu

Intracranial tumors and other masses that can mimic tumors are encountered frequently in the emergency setting. This section summarizes the more common intracranial masses, with emphasis on neoplasm, and addresses several diagnostic problems that can arise in patients presenting with CT findings of either a mass or secondary phenomenon such as hemorrhage, hydrocephalus, and edema.

■ CLINICAL PRESENTATION AND IMAGING APPROACH

Acute symptoms of intracranial neoplasms reflect generalized increased intracranial pressure, local tumor infiltration, or brain compression. These symptoms are often nonspecific and include headache, new-onset seizure, focal weakness, sensory disturbance, and altered personality. Some patients may be completely asymptomatic with tumors that are incidentally detected on CT scans obtained for head trauma. The most immediately available imaging study, nonenhanced CT, serves to rapidly identify or exclude most intracranial lesions. The detection rate is low; CT examination results obtained in the emergency setting for indications such as altered mental status, headache, and head trauma with normal Glasgow coma scale score will usually be normal.

Headache is so common that an intracranial mass will be identified in less than 0.2% of patients presenting with this symptom. Unfortunately, headache may be the sole presenting symptom for serious conditions, and imaging strategies are necessary. Although patients with an established or typical headache syndrome (migraine, cluster, tension) are rarely imaged in the ED, the patient with a new or persistent headache and no previous history should be studied, usually by nonenhanced CT. Headache due to increased intracranial pressure occurs daily, is worse early in the morning or in the evening, worse with Valsalva, and can be associated with nausea or vomiting. Headache associated with neurologic deficit or depressed sensorium is also suspicious enough to merit imaging, absent an established history of migraine. Findings to be sought include parenchymal mass, focal edema, hyperdense venous sinus or cerebral veins, hydrocephalus, and hemorrhage.

Seizure indicates a cortical abnormality, a metabolic disturbance, or both. In children most seizures are either idiopathic or developmental; fewer than 3% are due to an underlying tumor. In young adults, posttraumatic and metabolic causes predominate. New-onset seizures in the middle years are more likely to be due to primary brain neoplasm or metastatic disease, with posttraumatic injuries and drug withdrawal common as well. In older adults, cortical injuries due to prior infarct and metastatic disease are the most frequent causes of a first seizure.

Acute focal neurologic deficits, including localized weakness or numbness, can be due to acute arterial or venous infarct, hemorrhage, neoplasm, or post-seizure paralysis. Subacute or insidious onset favors neoplasm over infarct, but presentations may overlap. Computed tomography in this setting can exclude hemorrhage and allow presumptive treatment of infarct or can reveal an intracranial mass that could explain the patient's symptoms. Although many intracranial masses are true neoplasms, infectious, vascular, demyelinating, and traumatic conditions can have confounding appearances (Table 4-7).

Most primary brain neoplasms are sporadic, but some are associated with defined genetic syndromes. Patients with neurofibromatosis type 1 have an increased incidence of optic pathway gliomas. Those with neurofibromatosis type 2 characteristically develop intracranial schwannomas, meningiomas, and ependymomas. The finding of bilateral eighth nerve schwannomas is diagnostic of this condition. Other syndromes carrying an increased risk for brain neoplasm include tuberous sclerosis (multiple hamartomas), von Hippel-Lindau syndrome (hemangioblastoma), Gorlin syndrome (medulloblastoma), Li-Fraumeni syndrome (choroid plexus carcinoma), Turcot syndrome (malignant glioma and medulloblastoma), and *RB1* germline mutations (bilateral retinoblastoma and pineal tumors).

■ TOOLS FOR DISCRIMINATION

Several characteristics of intracranial masses are useful for identification and categorization. The most valuable of these are the pattern of edema, location of the mass,

Table 4-7 Differential Diagnosis by Location, Patient Age, and Cause

Location	Adult	Pediatric	Nonneoplastic
Intraparenchymal	Low-grade glioma High-grade glioma Metastasis Lymphoma	PNET Juvenile pilocytic astrocytoma	Abscess/cerebritis Toxoplasmosis (HIV) Arteriovenous malformation Cavernous malformation Hypertensive hemorrhage
Extraparenchymal	Meningioma Dural/calvarial metastasis Plasmacytoma	Calvarial neuroblastoma	Arachnoid cyst Epidermoid Epidural hematoma Subdural hematoma Empyema
Intraventricular / periventricular	Central neurocytoma Ependymoma	Choroid plexus papilloma Germinoma (pineal)	Hemorrhage Third ventricle colloid cyst
Cerebellar and fourth ventricle	Hemangioblastoma Metastasis Choroid plexus tumor	Medulloblastoma (PNET) Juvenile pilocytic astrocytoma Ependymoma	Hemorrhage
Cerebellopontine angle	CN VIII Schwannoma		Arachnoid cyst Epidermoid
Skull base, sella, and perisellar	Pituitary adenoma Craniopharyngioma (middle age) CN V schwannoma Metastasis Meningioma Chondrosarcoma	Craniopharyngioma (adolescent)	Aneurysm Rathke cleft cyst Cavernous sinus thrombosis

CN, Cranial nerve; *HIV*, human immunodeficiency virus; *PNET*, primitive neuroectodermal tumor.

number of lesions, patient age, contrast enhancement, necrosis, and CT density.

Edema Pattern

Vasogenic edema, a consequence of increased cerebrovascular capillary permeability, may be due to three factors: increased hydrostatic pressure (malignant hypertension), tight junction dysfunction due to local production of vascular endothelial growth factor (neoplasm), and hypoxic damage due to endothelial cells (high-altitude cerebral edema). On CT, low-attenuation vasogenic edema preferentially involves the white matter, sparing the cortex and basal ganglia. It is typically associated with abscess, metastatic or aggressive primary brain tumors, and some meningiomas. White

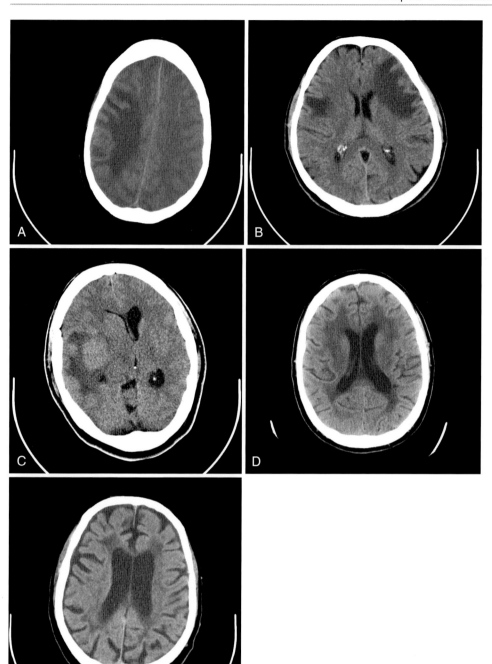

Figure 4-36 Vasogenic edema. Diminished white matter attenuation with preservation of cortical density. **A**, Dural metastasis from breast carcinoma. **B**, Multiple metastases from lung carcinoma. **C**, Right middle cranial fossa meningioma. **D**, Small vessel ischemic or chronic hypertensive change in older patients. **E**, White matter lesions of multiple sclerosis (MS) can mimic vasogenic edema.

matter changes due to small vessel ischemic or hypertensive disease, as well as demyelinating lesions in severe MS, can have a similar appearance (Fig. 4-36).

In contrast, cytotoxic edema results when hypoxic, ischemic, or metabolic cellular injury leads to failure of membrane sodium-potassium adenosine triphosphate (ATP) pumps and consequent cellular swelling, disruption, and death. Because glial and neuronal cells in gray and white matter are similarly involved, low-attenuation CT changes do not favor the white matter, and differentiation of gray and white matter is lost. This pattern is most commonly seen with venous or arterial cerebral infarcts and in the setting of global hypoxic ischemic or metabolic injury (Fig. 4-37).

Lesion Location and Patient Age

The most useful discriminators for establishing the identity of an intracranial mass are its location and the age of the patient. Intraparenchymal masses include primary glial and neuronal neoplasms, metastases, lymphoma, nonneoplastic masses such as infarcts, AVMs, cavernous malformations, bacterial abscesses, and toxoplasmosis. Some neoplasms are more commonly found in the posterior fossa (hemangioblastoma, juvenile pilocytic

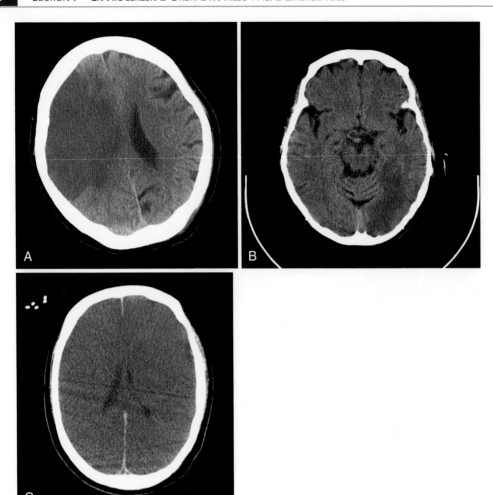

Figure 4-37 Cytotoxic edema. Diminished gray and white matter attenuation. **A,** Subacute right middle cerebral artery (MCA) distribution infarct. **B,** Subacute left posterior cerebral artery distribution infarct. **C,** Diffuse anoxic injury.

astrocytoma, metastatic gastrointestinal and genitourinary tumors), and within or adjacent to the ventricles (central neurocytoma, ependymoma, choroid plexus tumors) (see Table 4-7).

Extraparenchymal convexity masses arise from the skull and meninges, the majority of which are meningiomas, arachnoid cysts, and dural or calvarial metastases. Primary pituitary adenomas and benign neoplasms such as craniopharyngioma and developmental cysts may be found in the sella and suprasellar cistern. Masses involving the suprasellar and parasellar regions can arise from the meninges (planum sphenoidale meningioma), the blood vessels (aneurysm), and the cartilage of the skull base (chondrosarcoma). Primary nasopharyngeal carcinoma can extend superiorly to involve the central skull base. Salivary gland neoplasms can involve the skull base via perineural extension to the cavernous sinus and foramen ovale. Louis Armstrong's nickname, SATCHMO, is an acronym permitting recall of the most common sellar and suprasellar masses (sarcoid/sellar adenoma, aneurysm, teratoma/tuberculosis, craniopharyngioma, hypothalamic glioma/hamartoma of tuber cinereum/histiocytosis X, meningioma, metastasis, optic glioma).

Determining whether a mass is intraparenchymal or extraparenchymal on axial NCCT is not always obvious, and imaging in the sagittal and coronal planes can be helpful. Useful findings that indicate an extraparenchymal mass include a broad dural attachment, inward displacement of cortical vessels, and pockets of CSF (CSF cleft sign). Meningiomas, in particular, may be associated with hyperostosis of the adjacent calvarium or an enhancing dural "tail" extending from the mass (Fig. 4-38).

Contrast Enhancement

High-grade primary neoplasms, metastases, and abscess almost invariably result in blood-brain barrier disruption and consequent accumulation of contrast in the extracellular space at the margins of the mass. "Ring-enhancing" masses include primary and metastatic neoplasm, abscesses, subacute infarcts, subacute contusions, acute demyelinating disorders, and radiation change (Box 4-1).

Hemorrhage

Solitary intracerebral hemorrhage in the adult population is most commonly due to hypertensive vascular disease, and it usually involves the basal ganglia, pons, or cerebellum. Amyloid angiopathy in older adults, rupture of an occult AVM, and venous infarct

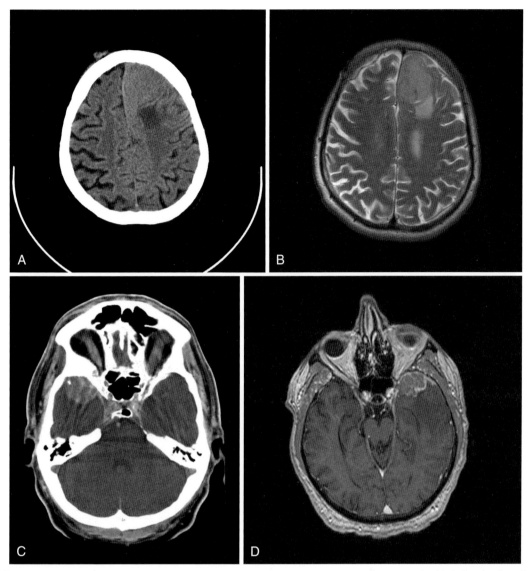

Figure 4-38 Meningiomas showing features of extraparenchymal mass. A, Computed tomography (CT) showing broad dural attachment to anterior falx with compression of cortical sulci and focal vasogenic edema. **B,** Corresponding T2-weighted magnetic resonance imaging (MRI) showing small cerebral spinal fluid cleft. **C,** Right sphenoid wing meningioma with hyperostosis. **D,** Postgadolinium T1-weighted MRI with enhancing dural "tail" extending from lateral aspect of mass.

Box 4-1   Differential Diagnosis of Ring-Enhancing Cerebral Lesions (MAGIC DR)

Metastasis
Abscess
Glioma
Infarct (subacute)
Contusion (subacute)
Demyelinating disease
Radiation necrosis/resolving hematoma

---

can all cause "lobar" or hemispheric bleeds (see Fig. 4-8 and related section). To exclude an occult hemorrhagic neoplasm, contrast-enhanced MRI should be considered for unusual intracerebral hemorrhages that do not fit one of these patterns or in which an underlying vascular abnormality cannot be identified.

Some malignancies are more likely to result in hemorrhagic metastases to the brain than others. Although they do not have the greatest tendency to bleed, the most common hemorrhagic metastases are due to primary lung and breast carcinomas because they are by far the most common metastatic neoplasms. Neoplasms with a propensity for hemorrhage include choriocarcinoma, thyroid carcinoma, melanoma, and renal cell carcinoma (Fig. 4-39). These can be remembered using the mnemonic CT-MR. Less common causes of acute multifocal hemorrhages include herpes encephalitis and leukemic blast crisis.

■ COMMON INTRACRANIAL NEOPLASMS

Intracranial masses can be organized by cause, the most common categories being neoplastic, vascular, infectious, traumatic, and noninfectious inflammatory. Neoplasms

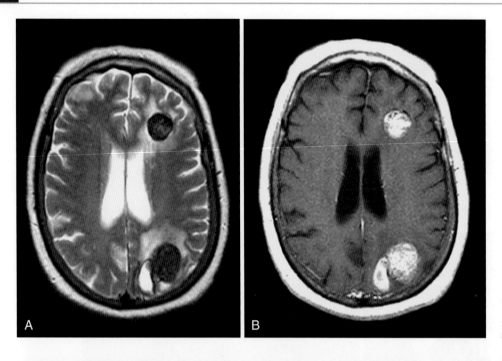

Figure 4-39 Renal cell carcinoma metastases. T2-weighted (A) and T1-weighted (B) magnetic resonance imaging (MRI) showing subacute hemorrhage.

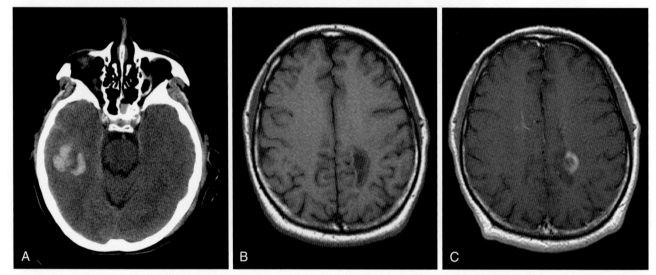

Figure 4-40 Mimics of neoplasm. A, Contusion in characteristic inferior temporal location. B, Tumefactive multiple sclerosis (MS) has low signal on T1-weighted magnetic resonance imaging (MRI). C, There is ringlike enhancement on corresponding postgadolinium image.

are primary, arising from neurons, glial cells, meninges, or nerve sheaths; metastatic; or hematologic (leukemia and lymphoma). True nonneoplastic masses include vascular malformations, abscesses, and hematomas. Other conditions that can mimic tumors include infarcts, contusions, radiation necrosis, and tumefactive MS (Fig. 4-40).

Most primary brain neoplasms are gliomas, which comprise astrocytomas, oligodendrogliomas, ependymomas, and mixed tumors. All of these tumors can vary in their aggressiveness. Although low-grade tumors may be histologically relatively benign, they usually require definitive biopsy and treatment to ensure the best possible prognosis. Unresected or recurrent portions of low-grade tumor may also undergo later malignant transformation; a low-grade astrocytoma may recur as an anaplastic astrocytoma or glioblastoma.

Glioma

The most common parenchymal glioma is the astrocytoma, which can be further characterized into pilocytic astrocytoma, xanthoastrocytoma, low-grade fibrillary astrocytoma, mixed oligodendroglioma/astrocytoma, anaplastic astrocytoma, and glioblastoma.

In children and young adults, low-grade astrocytomas are the most common glial tumors. Their incidence peaks in the third or fourth decade of life, and patients usually present with seizure. Most low-grade astrocytomas are infiltrative, do not make blood vessels, and appear as nonenhancing areas of low CT attenuation or increased T2 signal (Fig. 4-41). In children the most common subtype is juvenile pilocytic astrocytoma, which is often infratentorial or can arise along the optic pathway. They may have a characteristic cyst and

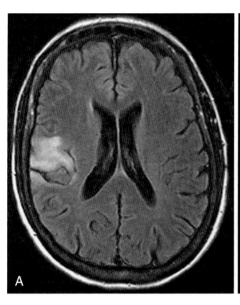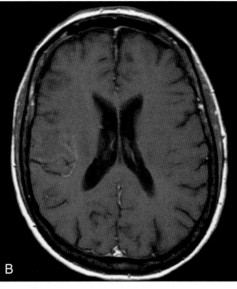

Figure 4-41 Low-grade astro-cytoma. These tumors reflect abnormally increased local numbers of glial cells without neo-vascularity or necrosis. **A,** Fluid attenuation inversion recovery (FLAIR) magnetic resonance imaging (MRI) shows an area of increased focal signal and mild sulcal enlargement in the right frontal cortex and subcortical white matter. **B,** There is no intravenous contrast enhancement on T1-weighted image.

nodule appearance that can be similar to that of a hemangioblastoma (Fig. 4-42). Recurrences tend to be local, although conversion to malignant or high-grade astrocytoma is not uncommon.

High-grade astrocytomas include anaplastic astrocytomas and glioblastoma multiforme (Fig. 4-43). They can arise de novo or from malignant degeneration of a previously diagnosed lower-grade astrocytoma. Pathologically, high-grade astrocytomas are characterized by neovascularity without necrosis, whereas necrosis is the hallmark of glioblastomas. In adults, anaplastic astrocytomas occur in the fourth or fifth decade, whereas glioblastomas occur in the sixth or seventh decade. These tumors also account for 10% to 20% of brain malignancies in children.

On MRI, high-grade astrocytomas are heterogeneous, with poorly defined margins and variable, sometimes ringlike enhancement. They can have significant surrounding edema, sometimes with enough mass effect to cause herniation. Astrocytomas arise in the white matter and can cross the corpus callosum to affect both hemispheres (Fig. 4-44). Because tumor cells migrate along white matter tracts, they can have significant pathologic extension beyond the radiographic margins demonstrated on CT and MRI. Metachronous deposits and subarachnoid/intraventricular spread can occur with high-grade astrocytomas. Prognosis for malignant astrocytomas remains poor, with less than 50% survival at 2 years for pediatric patients. For adults, median survival for anaplastic astrocytoma is 3 years, and 1 year for glioblastoma.

Oligodendrogliomas, tumors arising from pure oligodendrocyte populations or mixed oligodendrocyte/astrocyte populations, make up about 20% of all gliomas. Low-grade oligodendrogliomas are frequently radiologically indistinguishable from low-grade astrocytomas (Fig. 4-45). However, they are more likely to calcify and have a greater propensity to hemorrhage and present with symptoms of acute headache, lethargy, and hemiparesis. Although not completely curative, chemotherapy has lengthened mean survival time for low-grade oligodendrogliomas to as long as 16 years. As with low-grade astrocytomas, low-grade oligodendrogliomas can undergo malignant transformation.

Ependymomas account for 6% of pediatric CNS tumors. Childhood ependymomas, located in the ventricles (usually the fourth), may extend through foramina or cause hydrocephalus. Ependymomas in adults are more likely to arise in the lateral ventricles. In contrast, choroid plexus neoplasms usually arise in the lateral ventricles in children and in the fourth ventricle in adults (Fig. 4-46).

Meningioma

Meningioma is the most common extra-axial intracranial mass. Women are more likely to have meningiomas than men, and some patients may have multiple meningiomas. Most of these masses are slow growing, are asymptomatic, and are discovered incidentally on autopsy. In symptomatic patients the incidence of meningiomas is approximately 2 per 100,000. Symptoms are either nonspecific, such as headache or dizziness, or they may be related to tumor location and compression of cerebral cortex. For example, tumors at the convexities may cause seizures or progressive hemiparesis, whereas tumors at the skull base may cause compressive cranial neuropathies. Of these masses, 5% are histologically aggressive, and 2% are frankly malignant.

Meningiomas are usually round, well-marginated extra-axial masses that are recognized by their dural-based location and the manner in which they compress the underlying brain. A characteristic sign is a dural tail in which the enhancing meningioma merges into the normal meninges. Because meningiomas are extra-axial, cortical vessels and small CSF pockets can be interposed between the meningioma and the underlying brain, the CSF cleft sign. Meningiomas typically demonstrate homogeneous and avid enhancement with contrast. Although most do not elicit much inflammatory response, some may show extensive vasogenic edema (Fig. 4-47).

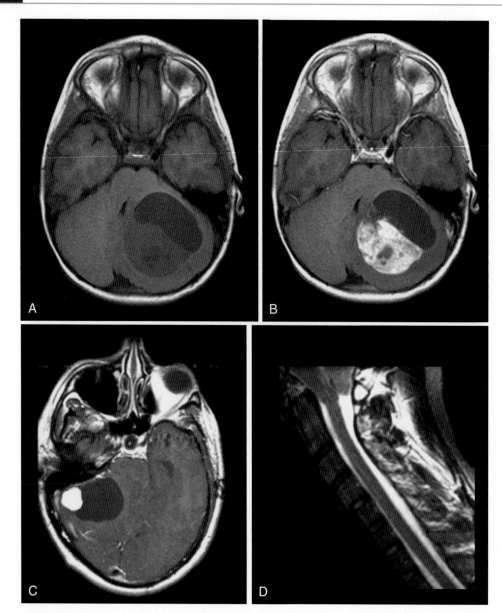

Figure 4-42 Juvenile pilocytic astrocytoma (JPA). T1-weighted magnetic resonance imaging (MRI) with (**A**) and without (**B**) gadolinium shows left cerebellar enhancing JPA with associated cyst and compression of the fourth ventricle. **Cerebellar hemangioblastoma in a patient with Von Hippel Lindau syndrome.** (C) Axial post-gadolinium MRI shows as right cerebellar cyst with enhancing nodule, compression of brainstem and effacement of the fourth ventricle (**D**) Tonsillar herniation is evident on T2-weighted cervical spine MRI.

Primitive Neuroectodermal Tumors/ Medulloblastoma

Primitive neuroectodermal tumors account for 7% of intracranial neoplasms. Supratentorial primitive neuroectodermal tumors are complex hemispheric, suprasellar, or pineal masses with minimal surrounding edema. They enhance heterogeneously and frequently contain calcifications, hemorrhage, and necrosis. In the posterior fossa, medulloblastomas are CT-dense masses that arise from the roof of the fourth ventricle, with variable enhancement and restricted diffusion on MRI (Fig. 4-48). These tumors can disseminate in the CSF and cause "dropped metastases."

Schwannoma

Schwannomas are extra-axial masses arising from neuronal axons of peripheral and cranial nerves that account for 6% of all intracranial neoplasms. The eighth cranial nerve is involved in 95% of all schwannomas, and these are located in the internal auditory canal or cerebellopontine angle (Fig. 4-49). On CT, schwannomas are isodense or slightly hyperdense to brain, and they demonstrate avid enhancement. The surrounding bone may show smooth scalloping, reflecting slow growth. Schwannomas can also arise from cranial nerves V and VII, appearing as cavernous sinus and temporal bone masses, respectively (see Fig. 4-49).

Pituitary Adenoma

Pituitary adenomas account for 5% of all intracranial neoplasms. They can be divided by size into microadenomas (<10 mm) or macroadenomas. Pituitary macroadenomas can extend upward into the sella. Rarely, the lesions can invade the skull base and simulate a malignant neoplasm. On CT examination the masses are isodense with gray matter and may demonstrate cysts, necrosis, hemorrhage, or calcifications. On MRI,

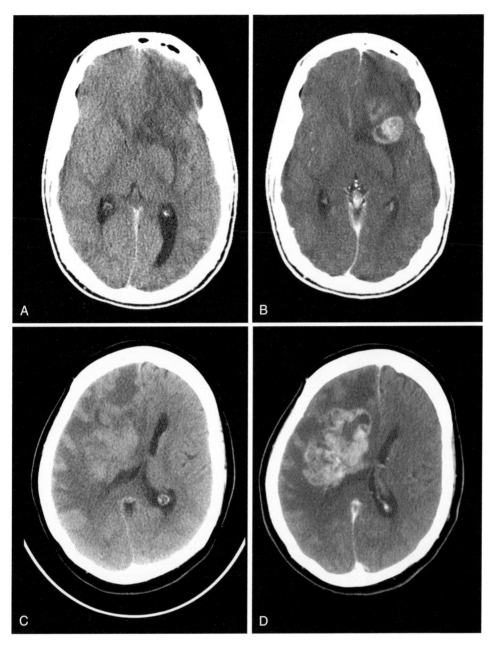

Figure 4-43 High-grade gliomas. A and **B,** Anaplastic astrocytoma. Enhancing nodule (**B**) within a larger area of abnormal brain with mild subfalcine herniation. These often arise in preexisting low-grade astrocytomas and are characterized by vascular proliferation without necrosis. **C** and **D,** Glioblastoma. A highly aggressive tumor with necrosis. Glioblastomas may be multifocal, extend across the corpus callosum, and spread via the subarachnoid space.

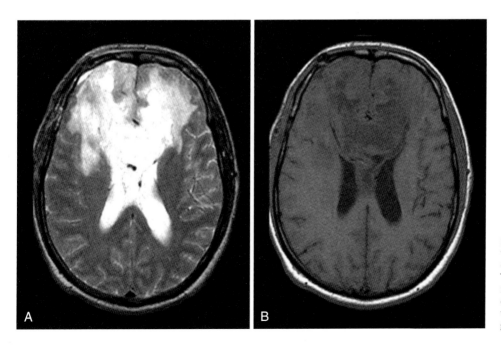

Figure 4-44 Glioblastoma with transcallosal tumor extension. T2-weighted (**A**) and T1weighted (**B**) magnetic resonance imaging (MRI). Thickening of the corpus callosum genu, as well as extensive associated vasogenic edema.

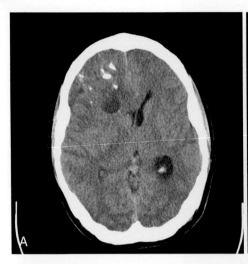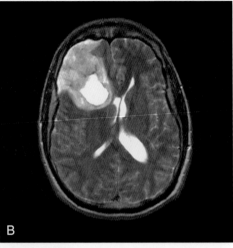

Figure 4-45 Oligodendroglioma. A, Computed tomography (CT) with calcifications indicating relatively slow growth. **B,** T2-weighted image with large cyst.

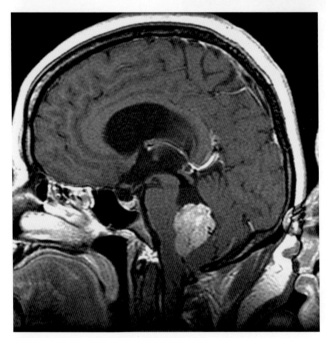

Figure 4-46 Ependymoma. Sagittal T1-weighted image in an adult with a fourth ventricular enhancing mass and secondary hydrocephalus.

microadenomas can be identified as lesions that enhance more slowly than the remainder of the pituitary gland (Fig. 4-50). The primary treatment modality is surgical resection, with medical treatment as an alternative.

Craniopharyngioma

Craniopharyngiomas are benign, cystic, sellar, and suprasellar masses that are derived from the Rathke pouch. The two subtypes are adamantinomatous, which presents in childhood, and papillary, which presents in adulthood as a solid, noncalcified mass. Pediatric patients with adamantinomatous craniopharyngioma may suffer morning headache, visual defect, and short stature related to growth hormone deficiency. These masses are frequently large (>5 cm), heterogeneous, multicystic, and partially calcified. There is often enhancement of cyst walls and heterogeneous enhancement of solid nodules (Fig. 4-51).

Craniopharyngiomas can be suprasellar, intrasellar, or a combination of the two.

Lymphoma

The incidence of primary CNS lymphomas, most prevalent in the fourth and fifth decades of life, has increased dramatically since the AIDS epidemic began in the 1980s. After toxoplasmosis, CNS lymphoma is the second most common CNS mass lesion affecting AIDS patients and is considered an AIDS-defining illness. The incidence of primary CNS lymphoma has also nearly tripled in immunocompetent patients, which may partially reflect improved imaging techniques and physician awareness.

The pathogenesis of primary CNS lymphomas may be related to viral infection. Association with Epstein-Barr virus or cytomegalovirus infection is especially strong in AIDS-related cases. Most lymphomas involve the supratentorial brain. These tumors typically enhance with contrast and are located in and around the basal ganglia and ependymal surfaces. Lymphoma is usually hyperdense on CT, reflecting its high nuclear-to-cytoplasmic ratio. Two features of lymphoma are very rapid growth and striking initial response to steroid therapy. Necrosis and hemorrhage are particularly common in AIDS-related lymphoma (Fig. 4-52). Secondary CNS lymphomas, those relating to systemic lymphomas, are uncommon and tend to involve the dura and leptomeninges more commonly than primary CNS lymphomas.

Other Neoplasms

Choroid plexus tumors may occur in very young patients (younger than 2 years of age) and can be subcategorized based on grading, ranging from choroid plexus papilloma (World Health Organization [WHO] grade I) to atypical choroid plexus papilloma (WHO grade II), and choroid plexus carcinoma (grade III). Although surgery is the primary modality of treatment for low-grade tumors, high-grade choroid plexus carcinomas are often chemoresponsive. Radiation therapy may improve survival but is carefully reserved because of its potential for side effects in a young patient population (Fig. 4-53).

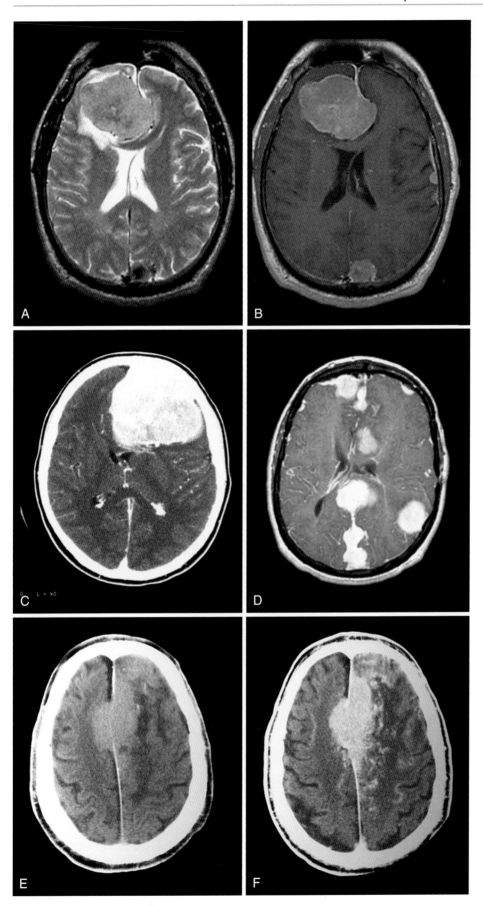

Figure   4-47 Meningioma.
T2-weighted (**A**) and T1-weighted (**B**)
postgadolinium images of three separate meningiomas. The anterior mass
arises from the falx, displaces cortical
vessels, and traps cerebral spinal fluid
(CSF) (CSF cleft sign). The left parietal
mass (**B**) has an enhancing dural tail.
C and **D**, Multiple meningiomas in a
patient with neurofibromatosis type
2 showing broad dural attachment,
vascular displacement, and enhancing dural tails. Precontrast (**E**) and
postcontrast (**F**) computed tomography (CT) of falcine meningioma with
extensive vascular recruitment and
vasogenic edema.

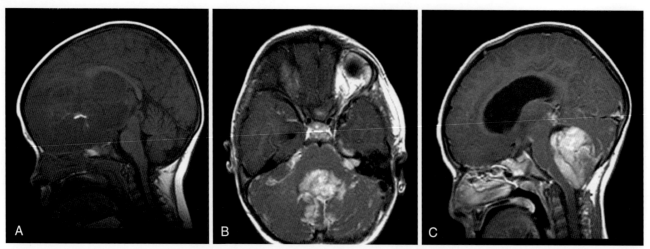

Figure 4-48 Primitive neuroectodermal tumor. A, Primitive neuroectodermal tumor. Sagittal T1-weighted image reveals large low-signal-intensity frontal lobe mass in a young child. **B** and **C,** Medulloblastoma. T1-weighted postgadolinium images show enhancing posterior fossa mass in a child with extensive subarachnoid tumor spread.

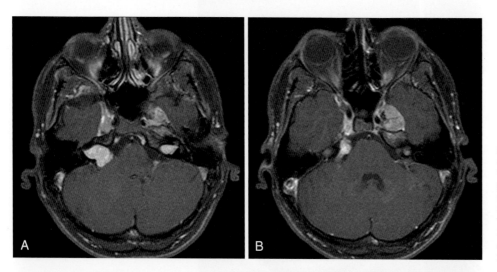

Figure 4-49 Cranial nerve schwannoma in neurofibromatosis type 2. T1-weighted postgadolinium magnetic resonance imaging (MRI). **A,** Bilateral cranial nerve VIII schwannomas expand the internal auditory canals. **B,** Right cisternal and left cavernous sinus cranial nerve V schwannomas.

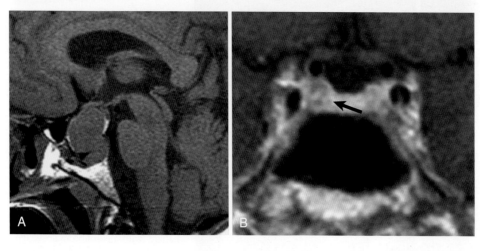

Figure 4-50 Pituitary adenoma. A, T1weighted image. Infrasellar and suprasellar macroadenoma with waist at diaphragma sellae. **B,** T1-weighted postgadolinium image. Right-sided microadenoma showing delayed contrast enhancement.

Germ cell tumors consist of pure germinomas and nongerminomatous germ cell tumors such as embryonal yolk sac tumors, choriocarcinomas, endodermal sinus tumors, and malignant teratomas. They tend to be midline tumors in suprasellar or pineal locations. They can be diagnosed with serum or CSF markers such as α-fetoprotein and β-human chorionic gonadotropin.

On MRI, germ cell tumors appear as heterogeneous, T2-bright, contrast-enhancing masses, frequently with cystic components. Radiation, in conjunction with chemotherapy, is the preferred treatment modality. Pure germinomas have a long-term survival rate greater than 90%, whereas nongerminomatous germ cell tumors have a 60% to 70% overall survival rate (Fig. 4-54).

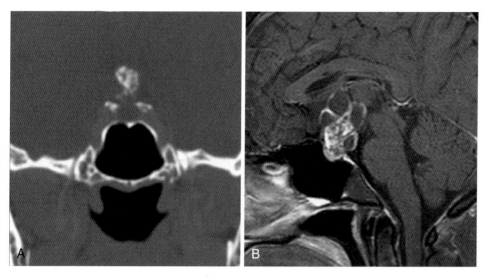

Figure 4-51 Craniopharyngioma. A, Computed tomography (CT) shows suprasellar calcification. B, T1-weighted postgadolinium magnetic resonance imaging (MRI) shows cysts and mural enhancement.

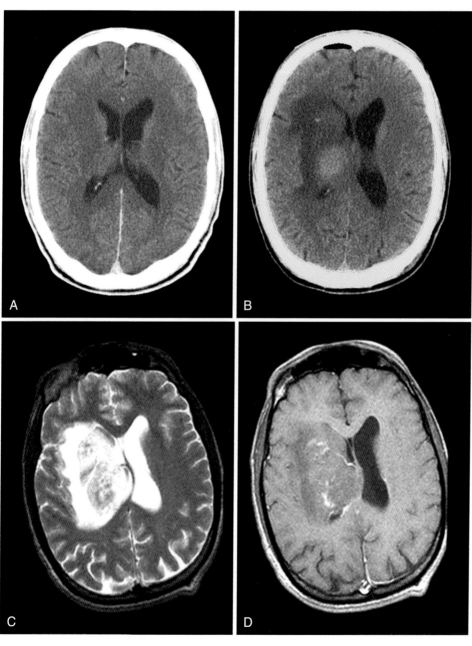

Figure 4-52 Primary central nervous system (CNS) lymphoma. A and B, Computed tomography (CT). Rapid (1 month) growth of right thalamic hyperdense mass. C, and D, T2-weighted (C) and T1-weighted (D) postgadolinium magnetic resonance imaging (MRI). There is incomplete enhancement and moderate vasogenic edema.

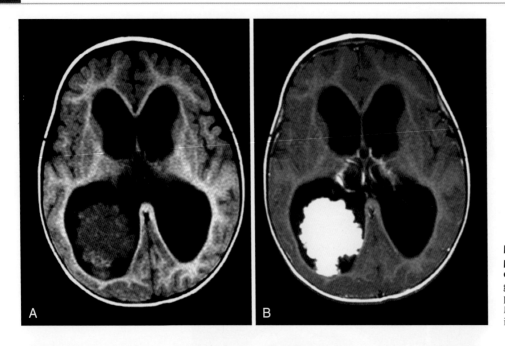

Figure 4-53 Choroid plexus papilloma with chronic hydrocephalus. T1-weighted pregadolinium (**A**) and T2-weighted postgadolinium (**B**) images. Marked enhancement of lobulated intraventricular mass.

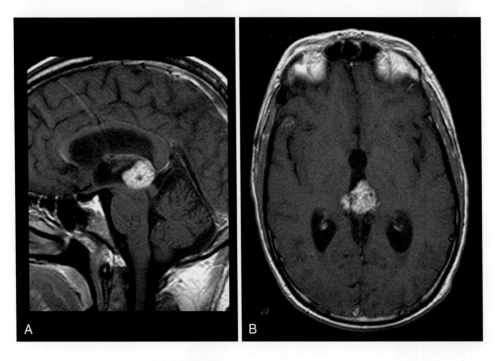

Figure 4-54 Germinoma. Sagittal (**A**) and axial (**B**) T1-weighted postgadolinium images show enhancing pineal region mass with mild hydrocephalus. Other masses that occur in this location include pinealomas, pineal carcinomas, and tectal gliomas.

■ NONNEOPLASTIC MASSES

Cavernous malformations appear on nonenhanced CT as fuzzy calcified nodules and can mimic hyperdense metastases. Arteriovenous malformations can also be mistaken for small tumors but on careful inspection show enlarged feeding arteries or draining veins. Unruptured aneurysms are typically intracisternal, located near the circle of Willis, and have smooth margins. Cavernous malformations have a pathognomonic "popcorn" or "mulberry" MRI appearance. Both AVMs and aneurysms are reliably diagnosed by CTA.

Brain abscesses can be associated with direct extension of sinus or mastoid infection or can arise from embolic deposition of bacteria or parasites (toxoplas-

mosis). Patients with right-to-left circulatory shunts are at increased risk, as are immunocompromised individuals and patients with left-sided endocarditis. Osler-Weber-Rendu syndrome (hereditary hemorrhagic telangiectasia) may present with brain abscess due to the multiple pulmonary arteriovenous fistulas that characterize this condition.

Epidermoid and arachnoid cysts are two common extra-axial masses that can both occur in the cerebellopontine angle. Epidermoid cysts are congenital ectodermal inclusion cysts, whereas arachnoid cysts are formed when a duplicated portion of arachnoid tissue fails to communicate with the ventricular system and forms a simple CSF-containing cyst (Fig. 4-55).

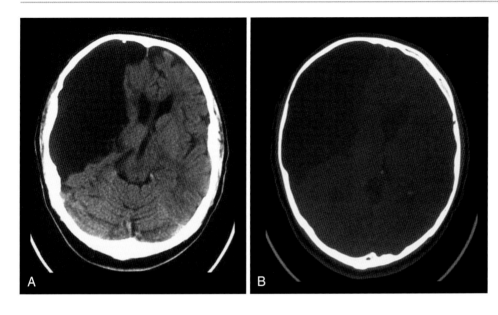

Figure 4-55 Arachnoid cyst. A, Large right frontal arachnoid cyst with cerebral spinal fluid (CSF) attenuation. **B,** There is remodeling of the calvarium.

■ PROBLEM SOLVING

Common diagnostic problems in evaluating the patient with abnormal head CT findings indicating a possible tumor include distinguishing neoplasm from infarct, abscess, vascular malformation, and tumefactive MS. Other problems include the differentiation of toxoplasmosis from lymphoma in patients with AIDS, the evaluation of a CSF-density extra-axial mass, and differentiation of meningiomas from dural metastatic disease.

Neoplasm Versus Infarct

Acute infarcts are often undetectable on CT; the purpose of the CT is to exclude hemorrhage or establish an alternative diagnosis. Subacute embolic or arterial thrombotic infarcts are hypodense to brain parenchyma, involve both gray and white matter, and lie within an arterial vascular distribution territory. Venous infarcts also involve both gray and white matter, are often superficial, and may be hemorrhagic.

Primary brain neoplasms involve both gray and white matter depending on size and location, but they are more likely to extend along white matter tracts and sometimes cross the corpus callosum. They are often associated with varying degrees of vasogenic edema. Metastatic nodules and inflammatory masses are typically well defined, occur near the gray-white junction, and elicit pronounced vasogenic edema, a focal area of which may be the only indication of metastasis or abscess visible on an NCCT examination. This finding should prompt further evaluation with contrast-enhanced MRI or CT.

Primary Versus Metastatic Brain Neoplasm

Metastases constitute 50% of all brain masses. To distinguish a primary intracranial neoplasm from a metastasis, consider the number and location of nodules. As elsewhere in the body, multiple intracranial lesions indicate metastatic disease. However, about half of all intracranial metastases are solitary. Metastases tend to occur at the gray-white junction because of the increased arterial blood flow, whereas primary gliomas usually are seen in the deep white matter, and primary brain lymphoma is often periventricular. Generally metastases are round, well-circumscribed masses that cause more vasogenic edema than similarly sized primary neoplasms. They enhance and will not demonstrate restricted diffusion on MRI unless they are very cellular, distinguishing them from abscesses and infarcts.

Neoplasm Versus Infection

Distinguishing an intracranial neoplasm and a focal pyogenic infection may be difficult, especially because the appearance of an infection will evolve depending on the stage. Early cerebritis lacks the well-defined, enhancing capsule displayed by late abscesses, and it appears as low CT attenuation change with variable enhancement (more prominent on MRI). In contrast to primary high-grade tumors, abscesses tend to have a smooth inner wall and may have small satellite abscesses. On MRI, abscesses typically have low-signal-intensity T2 rims and central diffusion restriction.

Neoplasm Versus Tumefactive Multiple Sclerosis

Tumefactive MS lesions are solitary lesions greater than 2 cm that can mimic neoplasms. Like glioblastoma and lymphoma, tumefactive MS affects the white matter and can cross the corpus callosum. However, tumefactive MS lesions tend to demonstrate little mass effect and edema for their size. Furthermore, they usually demonstrate an incomplete ring of enhancement. Because MS involves the perivenular space, dilated veins can be seen in the middle of a tumefactive MS lesion on MRI or post-contrast CT imaging. A true neoplasm would displace or invade into the course of these vessels. Tumefactive MS lesions tend to have decreased perfusion; true neoplasms demonstrate increased perfusion.

Toxoplasmosis Versus Lymphoma in Immunocompromised Patients

The appearance of CNS lymphoma on contrast-enhanced studies varies depending on the immune status of the patient; lymphoma in immunocompetent patients usually enhances homogenously, whereas in immunocompromised patients ring enhancement is the rule. Although this may mimic the eccentric target pattern of enhancement seen in acquired toxoplasmosis, toxoplasmosis lesions tend to be hypodense on NCCT and will usually show ring enhancement if larger than 1 cm. Perfusion imaging may also be helpful in distinguishing lymphoma, which demonstrates increased perfusion, from toxoplasmosis, which demonstrates decreased perfusion. A solitary mass or the presence of ependymal spread will support the diagnosis of lymphoma.

Meningioma Versus Dural Metastasis

Dural metastases and meningiomas can be difficult to distinguish because they can both show dural tails, dense enhancement, and high attenuation on CT. One useful differentiating factor is multifocality, which indicates metastatic disease. Dural metastases are more likely hemorrhagic and can extend to the skull, appearing as permeative, lytic, or sclerotic lesions. Although meningiomas can also cause osseous remodeling and hyperostosis, the adjacent involved bone tends to have a well-defined zone of transition. Meningiomas commonly demonstrate internal calcifications. Neuroblastoma and prostate and breast carcinoma can commonly metastasize to the dura; knowledge of underlying malignancy is an important discriminator.

Epidermoid Versus Arachnoid Cyst

Although epidermoid and arachnoid cysts both measure nearly CSF density and can be nearly identical in appearance on CT imaging, several features aid in distinguishing the two. Epidermoid cysts tend to insinuate into cisterns and encase neurovascular structures, whereas arachnoid cysts displace structures and cause bony remodeling. Magnetic resonance imaging signal intensity within an arachnoid cyst is simple CSF and is therefore completely suppressed on FLAIR sequences, whereas epidermoid cysts show higher signal intensity. The best sequence to differentiate the two entities is DWI, which will show restricted diffusion for epidermoid cysts but not for arachnoid cysts. This distinction is important because most arachnoid cysts do not require intervention, but epidermoid cysts often require surgical excision.

Selected Reading

Alberts MJ, Latchaw RE, Selman WR, et al. Recommendations for comprehensive stroke centers: a consensus statement from the Brain Attack Coalition. *Stroke.* 2005;36:1597–1616.

American College of Radiology Appropriateness Criteria. http://www.acr.org/Quality-Safety/Appropriateness-Criteria.

Barber PA, Zhang J, Demchuk AM, et al. Why are stroke patients excluded from TPA therapy? An analysis of patient eligibility. *Neurology.* 2001;56:1015–1020.

Broderick JP, Palesch YY, Demchuk AM, et al. Endovascular therapy after intravenous t-PA versus t-PA alone for stroke. *N Engl J Med.* 2013;368:893–903.

Chimowitz MI. Endovascular treatment for acute ischemic stroke—still unproven. *N Engl J Med.* 2013;368:952–955.

Chow FC, Marra CM, Cho TA. Cerebrovascular disease in central nervous system infections. *Semin Neurol.* 2011;31:286–306.

Ciccone A, Valvassori L, Nichelatti M, et al. Endovascular treatment for acute ischemic stroke. *N Engl J Med.* 2013;368:904–913.

Connolly ES Jr, Rabinstein AA, Carhuapoma JR, et al. Guidelines for the management of aneurysmal subarachnoid hemorrhage: a guideline for healthcare professionals from the American Heart Association/American Stroke Association. *Stroke.* 2012;43:1711–1737.

DeAngelis LM. Brain tumors. *N Engl J Med.* 2001;344:114–123.

Delgado Almandoz JE, Yoo AJ, Stone MJ, et al. Systematic characterization of the computed tomography angiography spot sign in primary intracerebral hemorrhage identifies patients at highest risk for hematoma expansion: the spot sign score. *Stroke.* 2009;40:2994–3000.

Demchuk AM, Dowlatshahi D, Rodriguez-Luna D, et al. Prediction of haematoma growth and outcome in patients with intracerebral haemorrhage using the CT-angiography spot sign (PREDICT): a prospective observational study. *Lancet Neurol.* 2012;11:307–314.

Fischer U, Arnold M, Nedeltchev K, et al. NIHSS score and arteriographic findings in acute ischemic stroke. *Stroke.* 2005;36:2121–2125.

Flaherty ML, Woo D, Haverbusch M, et al. Racial variations in location and risk of intracerebral hemorrhage. *Stroke.* 2005;36:934–937.

Fleming AJ, Chi SN. Brain tumors in children. *Curr Probl Pediatr Adolesc Health Care.* 2012;42:80–103.

Gupta RK, Soni N, Kumar S, et al. Imaging of central nervous system viral diseases. *J Magn Reson Imaging.* 2012;35:477–491.

Hand PJ, Kwan J, Lindley RI, et al. Distinguishing between stroke and mimic at the bedside: the Brain Attack Study. *Stroke.* 2006;37:769–775.

Huynh TJ, Demchuk AM, Dowlatshahi D, et al. Spot sign number is the most important spot sign characteristic for predicting hematoma expansion using first-pass computed tomography angiography: analysis from the PREDICT study. *Stroke.* 2013;44:972–977.

Kidwell CS, Jahan R, Gornbein J, et al. A trial of imaging selection and endovascular treatment for ischemic stroke. *N Engl J Med.* 2013;368:914–923.

Kidwell CS, Wintermark M. Imaging of intracranial haemorrhage. *Lancet Neurol.* 2008;7:256–267.

Koeller KK, Sandberg GD. Armed Forces Institute of Pathology. From the archives of the AFIP. Cerebral intraventricular neoplasms: radiologic-pathologic correlation. *Radiographics.* 2002;22:1473–1505.

Koeller KK, Smirniotopoulos JG, Jones RV. Primary central nervous system lymphoma: radiologic-pathologic correlation. *Radiographics.* 1997;17:1497–1526.

Lansberg MG, Bluhmki E, Thijs VN. Efficacy and safety of tissue plasminogen activator 3.0 to 4.5 hours after acute ischemic stroke: a metaanalysis. *Stroke.* 2009;40:2438–2441.

Levine SR, Gorman M. Telestroke" the application of telemedicine for stroke. *Stroke.* 1999;30:464–469.

Linn J, Bruckmann H. Differential diagnosis of nontraumatic intracerebral hemorrhage. *Klin Neuroradiol.* 2009;19:45–61.

Loevner LA. Imaging features of posterior fossa neoplasms in children and adults. *Semin Roentgenol.* 1999;34:84–101.

Lu L, Zhang LJ, Poon CS, et al. Digital subtraction CT angiography for detection of intracranial aneurysms: comparison with three-dimensional digital subtraction angiography. *Radiology.* 2012;262:605–612.

Martin PJ, Young G, Enevoldson TP, et al. Overdiagnosis of TIA and minor stroke: experience at a regional neurovascular clinic. *QJM.* 1997;90:759–763.

Mohan S, Jain KK, Arabi M, et al. Imaging of meningitis and ventriculitis. *Neuroimaging Clin N Am.* 2012;22:557–583.

Morgenstern LB, Hemphill JC 3rd, Anderson C, et al. Guidelines for the management of spontaneous intracerebral hemorrhage: a guideline for healthcare professionals from the American Heart Association/American Stroke Association. *Stroke.* 2010;41:2108–2129.

Nieuwkamp DJ, Setz LE, Algra A, et al. Changes in case fatality of aneurysmal subarachnoid haemorrhage over time, according to age, sex, and region: a meta-analysis. *Lancet Neurol.* 2009;8:635–642.

Okahara M, Kiyosue H, Yamashita M, et al. Diagnostic accuracy of magnetic resonance angiography for cerebral aneurysms in correlation with 3D-digital subtraction angiographic images: a study of 133 aneurysms. *Stroke.* 2002;33:1803–1808.

Post MJ, Thurnher MM, Clifford DB, et al. CNS-immune reconstitution inflammatory syndrome in the setting of HIV infection, 1: overview and discussion of progressive multifocal leukoencephalopathy-immune reconstitution inflammatory syndrome and cryptococcal-immune reconstitution inflammatory syndrome. *AJNR Am J Neuroradiol.* 2012;34(7):1297–1307.

Provenzale JM, Hacein-Bey L. CT evaluation of subarachnoid hemorrhage: a practical review for the radiologist interpreting emergency room studies. *Emerg Radiol.* 2009;16:441–451.

Ricard D, Idbaih A, Ducray F, et al. Primary brain tumours in adults. *Lancet.* 2012;379:1984–1996.

Romijn M, Gratama van Andel HA, van Walderveen MA, et al. Diagnostic accuracy of CT angiography with matched mask bone elimination for detection of intracranial aneurysms: comparison with digital subtraction angiography and 3D rotational angiography. *AJNR Am J Neuroradiol.* 2008;29:134–139.

Schwamm LH, Holloway RG, Amarenco P, et al. A review of the evidence for the use of telemedicine within stroke systems of care: a scientific statement from the American Heart Association/American Stroke Association. *Stroke.* 2009;40:2616–2634.

Smith AB, Smirniotopoulos JG, Rushing EJ. From the archives of the AFIP: central nervous system infections associated with human immunodeficiency virus infection: radiologic-pathologic correlation. *Radiographics.* 2008;28:2033–2058.

Sobri M, Lamont AC, Alias NA, et al. Red flags in patients presenting with headache: clinical indications for neuroimaging. *Br J Radiol.* 2003;76:532–535.

Tenembaum S, Chitnis T, Ness J, et al. Acute disseminated encephalomyelitis. *Neurology.* 2007;68(16 Suppl 2):S23–S36.

van Asch CJ, Luitse MJ, Rinkel GJ, et al. Incidence, case fatality, and functional outcome of intracerebral haemorrhage over time, according to age, sex, and ethnic origin: a systematic review and meta-analysis. *Lancet Neurol.* 2010;9:167–176.

van der Schaaf IC, Velthuis BK, Gouw A, et al. Venous drainage in perimesencephalic hemorrhage. *Stroke.* 2004;35:1614–1618.

van Gijn J. Cerebral vasoconstriction, headache and sometimes stroke: one syndrome or many? *Brain.* 2007;130:3060–3162.

van Gijn J, van Dongen KJ, Vermeulen M, et al. Perimesencephalic hemorrhage: a nonaneurysmal and benign form of subarachnoid hemorrhage. *Neurology.* 1985;35:493–497.

Wada R, Aviv RI, Fox AJ, et al. CT angiography "spot sign" predicts hematoma expansion in acute intracerebral hemorrhage. *Stroke.* 2007;38:1257–1262.

Westerlaan HE, van Dijk JM, Jansen-van der Weide MC, et al. Intracranial aneurysms in patients with subarachnoid hemorrhage: CT angiography as a primary examination tool for diagnosis—systematic review and meta-analysis. *Radiology.* 2011;258:134–145.

Wintermark M, Sanelli PC, Albers GW, et al. Imaging recommendations for acute stroke and transient ischemic attack patients: a joint statement by the American Society of Neuroradiology, the American College of Radiology and the Society of NeuroInterventional Surgery. *J Am Coll Radiol.* 2013;10:828–832.

Zhang LJ, Wu SY, Niu JB, et al. Dual-energy CT angiography in the evaluation of intracranial aneurysms: image quality, radiation dose, and comparison with 3D rotational digital subtraction angiography. *AJR Am J Roentgenol.* 2010;194:23–30.

CHAPTER 5

Face and Neck Emergencies

Midfacial Trauma

Ken F. Linnau

■ INDICATIONS AND RATIONALE FOR REPAIR

The overt physical manifestation of facial trauma often causes acute psychologic distress and long-term psychologic sequelae in addition to the loss of facial organ function. The use of modern surgical repair procedures, including internal reduction, microplate fixation, and the use of bone and allograft material has led patients to expect near normal if not normal appearance and function following the repair of midfacial injuries. The maxillofacial surgeon strives to restore both the physiologic function of the face and the anatomic form of an individual to resemble as closely as possible the appearance of the patient before the insult. Swelling of the facial soft tissues usually limits reliable clinical evaluation of the injuries and precludes immediate repair in the acute posttrauma period. Associated injuries such as cranial or facial hemorrhage, head injury, cervical spine injury, or major trauma to other body regions may require more immediate attention and treatment before midfacial injury repair. Most surgeons believe that the optimal time for internal fixation of midfacial injuries is approximately 7 to 10 days after the injury, when the initial swelling has subsided but before early fibrous tissue formation and tissue contraction. Anatomically correct realignment of displaced fracture fragments is most easily achieved before early bone healing occurs. To avoid refracture or osteotomy for movement and subsequent fixation of displaced facial skeletal segments, it is important that surgical procedures are performed in a timely fashion. The final configuration of the facial soft tissues will depend on the anatomic position of the underlying facial skeleton, and only then will soft tissue healing occur in the normal configuration. Incompletely reduced facial fractures may result in cicatricial contracture with permanent thickening, shortening, and displacement of the facial soft tissue structures, potentially requiring multiple reoperations. Delayed or secondary repair of both bone and soft tissue defects is more challenging with less favorable results compared to primary reconstruction. Reoperation through scar tissue that has resulted from previous surgical procedures increases the risk for iatrogenic complication

such as lid retraction or ectropion (Table 5-1). Early comprehensive surgical repair is therefore advocated, which requires high-resolution high-quality imaging to supplement clinical examination and allow for precise operative planning.

■ THE BUTTRESS SYSTEM OF THE FACE

The facial anatomy is very complex and at times overwhelming. It is therefore useful to categorize facial injury by distinct facial region, including the nose, the orbit, the maxilla, the mandible, and the zygoma. From the surgical perspective, the soft tissues of the face, including the dermis, connective tissues, and muscles, are layered over a deep supporting latticelike system of bony buttresses (Fig. 5-1). The integrity of this honeycomb-like bony grid is instrumental for satisfactory aesthetic results after midfacial microplate surgery. Using the buttress concept in evaluating facial injury can therefore facilitate fracture description and conceptualization and aid in preopera-

Table 5-1 Common Deformities Resulting From Untreated or Poorly Reduced Midfacial Injuries

Deformity	Description
Enophthalmos, exophthalmos	Abnormal globe position due to abnormal orbital volume post injury
Saddle nose	Nasal deformity due to ischemic septal necrosis from unrecognized nasal septum hematoma
Telecanthus	Malposition of the medial canthal ligament with lateral displacement and rounding of the inner canthus
Shortened midface	Upward "telescoping" of the maxilla on itself can be caused by exaggerated reduction of Le Fort I or II injuries
"Dish face" deformity	Flattened and widened midface due to posterior and lateral displacement of the paired midfacial components (especially zygoma)
"Facies equina" deformity	Elongated face due to downward displacement of the palatoalveolar complex and forward rotation of the mandible

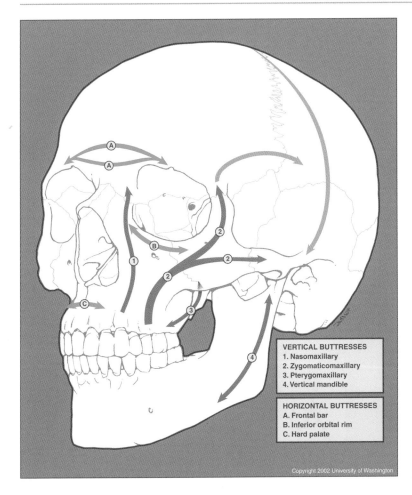

VERTICAL BUTTRESSES
1. Nasomaxillary
2. Zygomaticomaxillary
3. Pterygomaxillary
4. Vertical mandible

HORIZONTAL BUTTRESSES
A. Frontal bar
B. Inferior orbital rim
C. Hard palate

Figure 5-1 Buttress anatomy of the face. (From Linnau KF, Stanley RB, Hallam DK, et al. Imaging of high-energy midfacial trauma: what the surgeon needs to know. *Eur J Radiol.* 2003;48(1):17-32, with permission.)

tive decision making. The strongest midfacial buttresses (see Fig. 5-1) are vertically oriented in response to physiologic loads on the system exerted by similarly directed masticatory forces. Weaker horizontally and sagittally oriented buttresses reinforce the system. The buttress system is therefore less resistant to external direct impact from the front or side, which may lead to traumatic disruption of one buttress and weakening of the entire lattice with subsequent collapse. This collapse, however, is not altogether a random process but occurs in characteristic fracture patterns (Fig. 5-2). Familiarity with the major buttresses of the face allows the radiologist to more easily detect facial injury and conduct a structured step-by-step image evaluation without overlooking subtle facial injury.

■ IMAGING TECHNIQUE

Imaging evaluation of maxillofacial injury aims to depict the location and displacement of facial fractures and to define soft tissue injury that potentially compromises respiration, vision, mastication, and lacrimal system function. Today multidetector computed tomography (MDCT) has become the imaging modality of choice for evaluation of apparent or suspected facial injuries, nearly completely replacing facial radiography. Particularly in the polytrauma setting, rapid submillimeter MDCT image acquisition has proven to be very efficient owing to highly accurate isotropic pixel resolution of

thin-collimation computed tomographic (CT) images that allow real-time multiplanar reformations (MPRs) without moving the patient. To facilitate injury depiction and aid operative planning, three-dimensional (3-D) image reconstruction is frequently used at major trauma centers. Some surgeons advocate intraoperative CT scanning to monitor the repair.

At Harborview Medical Center, trauma patients with obvious or suspected facial injuries undergo helical scanning of the entire skull extending from the vertex to the mandibular angle. Using the same data set, head CT images for intracranial and brain evaluations and maxillofacial CT images are reconstructed. Asymmetric patient positioning in the scanner gantry, which is not uncommon in severely injured polytrauma patients, is retrospectively corrected by aligning image reconstruction with the standard craniometric reference planes (Frankfurt horizontal plane, also referred to as the *orbitomeatal plane, auriculoinfraorbital plane,* or *eye-ear plane*) used for surgical planning and repair of facial fractures. For facial evaluation, 0.6-mm-thick slices in the axial, sagittal, and coronal plane are routinely generated in bone and soft tissue algorithm. If midfacial injury is detected, the same data set is used to subsequently create shaded-surface-3-D rendered images of the facial skeleton to aid surgical planning. In the setting of orbital injury, sagittal reformations are aligned along the optic nerve. Although not part of the midfacial skeleton, the vertically oriented portion of the mandible (ramus) functions as the most

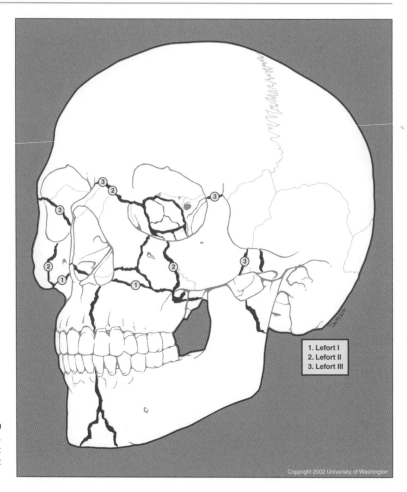

1. Lefort I
2. Lefort II
3. Lefort III

Figure 5-2 Fracture patterns commonly seen in severe midfacial trauma. (From: Linnau KF, Stanley RB, Hallam DK, et al. Imaging of high-energy midfacial trauma: what the surgeon needs to know. *Eur J Radiol.* 2003;48(1): 17-32, with permission.)

posterior vertical buttress of the facial skeleton and comes into play in severely comminuted midfacial fracture repair. It is therefore essential for surgical planning to include the entire mandible in the initial facial CT evaluation.

Patterns of Injury

Facial fractures can involve multiple regions or bones of the face, and it is often difficult to classify facial fractures on the basis of the bones involved alone. Facial fractures can at times be overwhelming but may be categorized by classic fracture patterns, including, nasal, naso-orbitoethmoid (NOE), zygomaticomaxillary complex (ZMC), orbital, and maxillary Le Fort fractures. The role of the emergency radiologist is to recognize these fracture patterns, summarize the injuries detected, and alert clinical providers of unexpected findings and potential complications.

Nasal Bone and Naso-orbitoethmoid Fractures

Nasal fractures are very common owing to the prominence of the nasal dorsum and the relatively weak bony support. Young men in their second and third decades are most commonly affected. Potential sequelae of nasal fracture include airway obstruction, cosmetic deformity, and cerebrospinal fluid leak. Hematoma in the nasal septum may lead to necrosis of its cartilaginous portion

with ensuing saddle nose deformity. An associated anterior maxillary spine fracture can be the hallmark to indicate disruption of the cartilaginous portion of the nasal septum.

Naso-orbitoethmoid complex injuries occur during high-energy impactions when the nasal bones, which are more resistant to frontal impact, fail and expose the delicate ethmoid air cells behind them (Fig. 5-3). The nasal bones then telescope into the deep face, involving the medial orbital wall. An increased intercanthal distance (telecanthus) and flattening of the nasal dorsum or disruption of the medial canthal ligament insertion (positive eyelid traction test) should raise suspicion for NOE fracture. Naso-orbitoethmoid fractures are clinically classified according to integrity of the central fragment, where the medial canthal ligament inserts.

Zygomaticomaxillary Complex Fractures

The zygoma forms the cornerstone of the facial frame, and its strong bone defines the projection or depth of the malar eminence of the cheek. The zygoma is related to the surrounding craniofacial skeleton through two critical arcs of the external facial contour. First, the horizontal external arc curves from the lacrimal fossa along the inferior orbital rim over the malar eminence to the zygomatic arch. Second, the vertical arc also crosses over the malar eminence

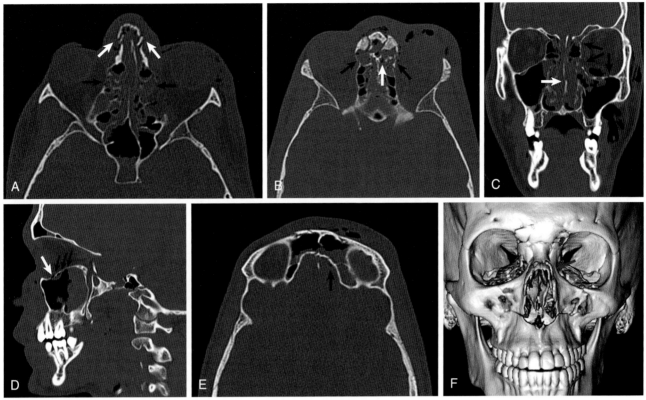

Figure 5-3 Naso-orbitoethmoid (NOE) injury. A, Axial computed tomographic (CT) image of a 21-year-old man who was assaulted shows comminuted fractures of the nasal bone bilaterally *(white arrows)*, with posterior displacement of the dorsum of the nose. The walls of the anterior and middle ethmoid air cells are disrupted *(black arrows)* and are telescoping posteriorly along the lamina papyracea, indicative of NOE injury. **B,** More cephalad axial CT image at the crista galli illustrates disrupted anterior ethmoid air cells *(black arrows)* and fracture extension through the cribriform plate *(white arrow)*. **C,** On the coronal CT image, disruption of the very thin medial orbital wall and floor (lamina papyracea) is easily appreciated *(black arrows)*. Comminuted fracture of the bony nasal septum without septal hematoma is present *(white arrow)*. **D,** Sagittally reformatted CT image illustrates a small orbital floor fracture *(white arrow)* with preservation of the upward convex curve of the orbital floor posterior to the globe *(black arrows)*. **E,** There is a small amount of pneumocephalus *(black arrow)* in the anterior cerebral fossa deep to associated fractures of the inner and outer table of the frontal sinus. **F,** The shaded-surface rendered three-dimensional (3-D) reformation gives a quick overview of the injury extent and illustrates the intact lateral zygomaticomaxillary buttress. The NOE injury shows a single fracture of the central fragment *(red arrow)*, suggestive of intact medial canthal ligament (type I injury).

and defines the course of the lateral facial buttress from the maxilla to the lateral frontal bone. The zygoma thus becomes a central part of the zygomaticomaxillary (lateral) vertical buttress of the face (see Fig. 5-1). Sutural attachments of the zygoma include the frontal bone (zygomaticofrontal suture), the maxilla (zygomaticomaxillary suture), the arch of the temporal bone (zygomaticotemporal suture), and the greater wing of the sphenoid (zygomaticosphenoid suture), which should not be mistaken for fractures. Because the zygoma forms a portion of the lateral orbital wall and lateral orbital floor, orbital fractures are frequent components of ZMC injuries (Fig. 5-4). In addition, fractures may cross the infraorbital canal, injuring the infraorbital nerve with subsequent cheek paresthesia. Postoperative spatial location of the zygoma will play a major role in reconstruction to reestablish correct facial height as well as width and projection (depth) of the face at this level. Careful anatomic realignment of all portions of the articulation of the zygoma to the surrounding craniofacial skeleton and stabilization of the zygoma in this position are mandatory for satisfactory aesthetic surgical repair.

Orbital Fractures

The orbit is a complex, conically shaped compartment composed of multiple bones contained within the buttress system of the midface. In practice the orbit consists of the medial orbital wall, the orbital floor, the lateral orbital wall, and the orbital roof (Fig. 5-5). Collapse of the walls puts the orbital soft tissue organs at risk for injury. Fortunately, the thick superior orbital rim of the frontal bone and the strong lateral and inferior orbital rim of the zygoma enclose the orbital aperture in a ringlike fashion, protecting areas of relative weakness in the middle portion of the orbit (i.e., the very thin medial wall and orbital floor). The posterior orbital third is again composed of relatively thick bone that protects the vital soft tissue structures at the orbital apex (optic nerve, ophthalmic artery, carotid siphon, cavernous sinus). The orbital roof, floor, and medial wall are concave relative to each other, producing the greatest diameter of the orbit approximately 15 mm posterior to the inferior orbital rim. The globe is situated at this level of the orbital floor, which then inclines upward and inwardly in a convex curve behind the eyeball (see Fig. 5-3, *D* and Fig. 5-5) to create a relative retrobulbar constriction to maintain the position of the retrobulbar soft tissues. Reconstruction of the orbital walls can begin only

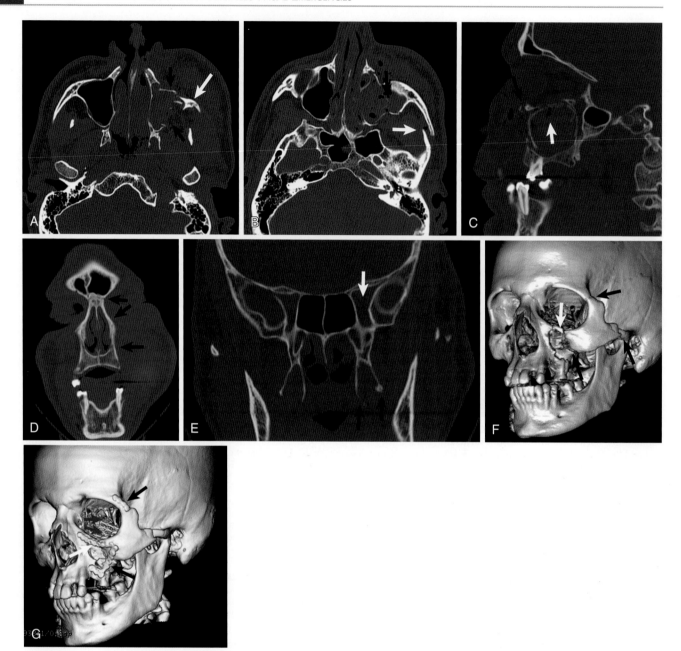

Figure 5-4 Zygomaticomaxillary (ZMC) injury with associated orbital blow-out fracture. A, Axial computed tomographic (CT) image of a 40-year-old man who was involved in a high-speed motor vehicle crash shows a ZMC injury with loss of projection (posterior and lateral displacement) of the left malar eminence *(white arrow)*. The anterior and lateral walls of the left maxillary sinus are fractured *(black arrows)*. **B,** Owing to the posterior displacement of the zygoma, the zygomatic arch is fractured with overriding apposition *(white arrow)*. Comminuted bone fragments from the injured orbital floor are noted in the blood-filled left maxillary sinus *(black arrow)* on this axial CT image. **C,** The extent of the orbital blow-out injury is better appreciated on sagittal CT reformations, which show disruption of the inferior orbital rim *(black arrow)* and severe comminution of the thin orbital floor *(white arrow)*, which has lost its retrobulbar upward convex slope. The orbital roof remains intact. **D,** The anterior coronal CT image demonstrates bilaterally intact vertical medial (nasomaxillary) buttress *(black arrows)*, which makes Le Fort injury unlikely. **E,** Bilaterally intact medial and lateral plates of the pterygoid process *(black arrows)* on the posterior coronal CT reformation confirm that no Le Fort injury is present. The integrity of the orbital apex *(white arrow)* is reassuring. **F,** The shaded-surface rendered three-dimensional (3-D) reformation summarizes the ZMC injury pattern with disruption of the vertical zygomaticomaxillary buttress *(black arrows)* and inferior orbital rim *(white arrow)*, resulting in posterior and lateral displacement of the zygoma. **G,** The immediate postoperative 3-D CT image shows restoration of zygomatic projection with microplate fixation of the vertical zygomaticomaxillary buttress *(black arrows)* and horizontal infraorbital rim *(white arrow)*. The lamina papyracea (orbital floor and medial orbital wall) has been reconstructed with allograft material *(red arrows)* to maintain correct globe position.

after the vertical and horizontal buttresses and thus the outer ring of the orbit have been restored and stabilized. This ring then serves as an anchor point for bone grafts or alloplastic implants that may replace the fragmented bone in the middle third of the orbit. Re-creation of the upward convexity of the normal orbital roof, the concave anterior orbital floor, the convex posterior floor, and the obtuse angle of the transition of the floor to the medial orbital wall (lamina papyracea) are surgically challenging (see Figs. 5-4 and 5-5), commonly leading to undercorrection or overcorrection with altered orbital volume. Orbital volume changes exceeding 1.5 mL (approximately 5% of

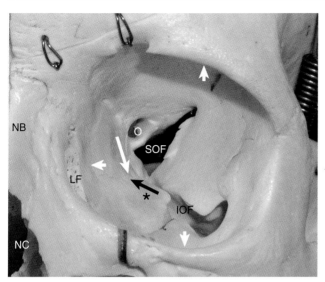

Figure 5-5 Photograph of dry bone preparation of the normal left orbit. Orbital roof, floor, and medial wall are concave relative to each other anteriorly *(short white arrows)*. More posteriorly, orbital floor inclines upward, creating retrobulbar constriction *(asterisk)*. Medial orbital wall *(long white arrow)* and orbital floor *(black arrow)* meet at an obtuse angle without sharp demarcation. Characteristics of orbital shape need to be recreated surgically to restore correct orbital volume. *IOF,* Inferior orbital fissure; *LF,* lacrimal fossa; *NB,* nasal bone; *NC,* nasal cavity; *O,* optic foramen; *SOF,* superior orbital fissure. (From Linnau KF, Stanley RB, Hallam DK, et al. Imaging of high-energy midfacial trauma: what the surgeon needs to know. *Eur J Radiol.* 2003;48(1):17-32, with permission.)

the normal orbital volume) may lead to an asymmetry in globe position that is aesthetically noticeable (enophthalmos or less commonly exophthalmos). With CT the convexity of the orbital floor is best appreciated on sagittal reformations, whereas coronal reconstructions allow accurate evaluation of the thin orbital floor and medial orbital wall integrity. Because the orbital axis is oblique, reconstructions parallel to the optic nerve are optimal. Orbital trauma may be isolated, such as a blow-out fracture, or more commonly, associated with complex midfacial fracture patterns, including NOE, ZMC, and Le Fort fractures (Figs. 5-6 and 5-7; see Fig. 5-4).

Mandible Fractures

Midfacial fracture repair often begins with the placement of arch bars and maxillomandibular fixation (MMF) wires to maintain accurate interdigitation of the maxillary and mandibular teeth. If the strong bone of the horseshoe-shaped mandible remains entirely intact or is accurately reconstructed from condyle to condyle, the desired functional relationship between the bite plane (that is the imaginary surface anatomically relating the cranium to the occluding surfaces of the teeth) and the skull base is accomplished (see Fig. 5-1). In this way the mandible can serve as a platform for maxillary reconstruction, particularly in the setting of highly comminuted Le Fort fractures (see Fig. 5-7, *E*). The intact mandibular ramus buttress in anatomic position thereby guarantees correct posterior vertical dimension because the posterior midfacial buttress, composed of the plates of the pterygoid process, is not

accessible to surgical repair. Similarly, anatomic position of the body and angle of the mandible guarantee the width of the lower aspect of the midface to avoid an overly rounded postoperative frontal facial appearance. Mandibular integrity is of particular importance if a displaced sagittal split fracture of the hard palate alters the maxillary width.

Frontal Bone Fractures

The frontal bone is composed of a strong osseous ridge, which forms the upper margin of the face and owing to its strength is often referred to as the *frontal bar*. It is able to sustain large forces before fracturing. If this strong osseous ridge is uninjured or adequately restored, the maxillofacial surgeon may use it as a starting point for midfacial reconstruction. Deep to the most superficial cortex of the frontal bone lies the frontal sinus, which is bound by anterior and posterior bony walls commonly referred to as *anterior and posterior tables*. The posterior table separates the sinus from the anterior cranial fossa. When both tables of the frontal sinus are fractured in the setting of facial injury, a compound (open) skull fracture involving the central nervous system (CNS) results (see Fig. 5-7) and requires at the minimum antibiotic treatment to prevent CNS complications such as meningitis, encephalitis, brain abscess, and cavernous sinus thrombosis. A key finding to detect involvement of the posterior table is pneumocephalus, which can be subtle and should be actively sought by the radiologist (see Fig. 5-3, *E*). Posterior propagation of frontal bone fractures may manifest as CNS rhinorrhea.

Maxilla and Le Fort Fractures

Centrally in the middle of the face lies the paired maxilla, housing the upper teeth and contributing to the walls of the nasal cavity, oral cavity, and orbit. The maxilla is part to three vertically oriented facial buttresses, which developed as a response to the forces of the masticatory muscles (see Figs. 5-1 and 5-4). Most medially lies the nasomaxillary (nasofrontal) buttress connecting to the medial frontal bone at the level of the glabella. The bifurcated zygomaticomaxillary buttress lies more laterally and extends from the alveolar process over the malar eminence of the zygoma to the zygomatic process of the frontal bone at the level of the lateral orbital rim. The posterior (pterygomaxillary) vertical buttress of the midface, which is surgically not accessible, extends from the posterior wall of the maxillary sinus (maxillary tuberosity) to the medial and lateral plates of the pterygoid process of the sphenoid bone. The inferior orbital rim, zygomatic arch, and palatoalveolar complex provide secondary horizontal buttress support.

The three classic fracture patterns of the maxilla were originally described by Le Fort based on his exemplary cadaver studies. The common feature of Le Fort maxillary fractures is the involvement of the pterygoid plates of the sphenoid bones, resulting in separation of the midface from the skull base. In clinical practice,

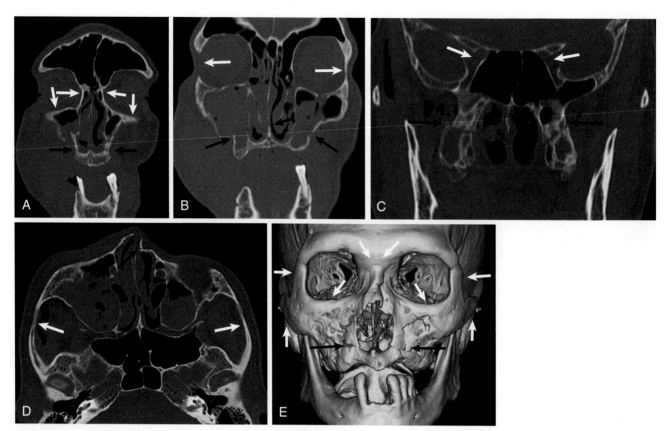

Figure 5-6 Le Fort I. A, Coronal computed tomographic (CT) image of a 60-year-old man who was assaulted shows horizontally oriented bilateral maxillary fractures just above the hard palate *(black arrows)*, suggestive of Le Fort I injury. The bilateral medial facial buttress and bilateral inferior orbital rims are intact *(white arrows)*, which makes Le Fort II or III unlikely. **B,** Horizontally oriented fractures through the maxilla and the bony nasal septum *(black arrows)* are shown more posteriorly on coronal CT. The bilateral lateral orbital walls of the lateral zygomaticomaxillary buttress remain intact *(white arrows)*, excluding Le Fort III injury. **C,** Bilateral horizontal fracture through the pterygoid process of the sphenoid *(black arrows)* on coronal CT confirms complete separation of the midface from the cranium, bilateral Le Fort I. The orbital apex bilaterally is normal *(white arrows)*. **D,** Bilaterally the zygomatic arch remains uninjured *(white arrows)* on axial CT, excluding Le Fort III fractures. There is a mildly comminuted associated left nasal fracture *(black arrow)*. **E,** Shaded-surface rendered three-dimensional (3-D) image confirms horizontally oriented bilateral Le Fort I injury of the maxilla just above the hard palate *(black arrows)* without involvement of the upper midface and zygomatic arch *(white arrows)*, excluding Le Fort II and III.

midfacial fractures tend to be asymmetric, and each side can be described as a separate hemi–Le Fort fracture to facilitate communication among providers (see Figs. 5-2 and 5-7).

The Le Fort I fracture pattern involves the maxilla and nasal septum at the level of the inferior aspect of the piriform aperture, thereby creating a free-floating hard palate and alveolar process, which are separated from the remainder of the midface (see Fig. 5-6). The Le Fort II, or pyramidal, fracture pattern separates the nasal region from the cranium by extension through the nasal bridge and inferior orbital rim. The zygomatic bone remains attached to the skull base in pyramidal fractures (see Fig. 5-7). The Le Fort III fracture pattern causes complete craniofacial disjunction through fracture through the nasofrontal suture, lateral orbital rim, and zygomatic arch (see Fig. 5-7). All Le Fort fracture patterns include posterior fracture of the pterygoid process.

Reconstruction of the midfacial buttress system begins with stabilization of the frontal bar, to which the more gracile displaced midfacial structures are then suspended. Through stepwise top-to-bottom reconstruction of the buttresses, the vertical dimension of the midface is restored with careful attention to avoid overreduction, which can result in telescoping and shortening of the midface. Given the high incidence of concurrent facial fractures such as NOE or frontal bone injury, surgical repair of these injuries is usually complex. Of particular concern are concomitant fractures of the hard palate, dentoalveolar units, and posterior fracture extension toward the orbital apex and optic nerve.

Complex Facial Fractures

Panfacial fractures or facial smash injuries (see Fig. 5-7) are sustained during high-energy trauma with simultaneous injury of multiple regions of the face, often as part of accompanied multisystem trauma. For these injuries no universally accepted calcification system exists. Sequelae of maxillofacial reconstruction are common in these patients (see Table 5-1). To integrate treatment plans and better evaluate patient outcomes, a comprehensive facial fracture severity scoring system, which is not specific to a particular facial region, has been proposed for panfacial injury.

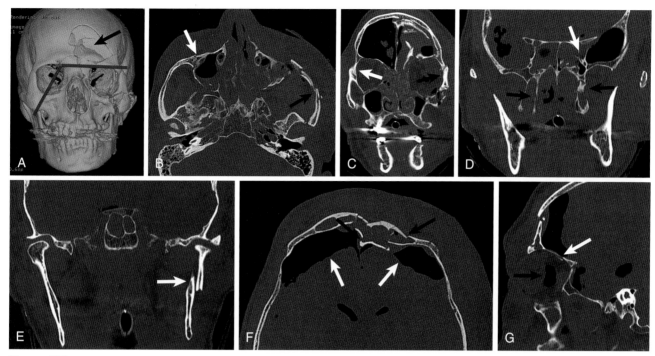

Figure 5-7 *Panfacial injury including left hemi–Le Fort III and right hemi–Le Fort II fractures* (see also Fig. 5-2). **A,** Facial shaded-surface rendered three-dimensional (3-D) computed tomographic (CT) reformations of a 54-year-old man who was assaulted shows panfacial injuries. With severe injury, 3-D reformations are helpful to appreciating major injury patterns. In this patient right hemi–Le Fort II *(oblique red line)* and left hemi–Le Fort III *(horizontal red line)* injuries are suspected. A compound left frontal skull fracture is also present *(black arrow)*. **B,** Axial CT at the level of the zygomatic arch shows right disruption of the infraorbital rim *(white arrow)*, in keeping with right hemi–Le Fort II. On the left side the zygomatic arch is disrupted *(black arrow)*, in keeping with left hemi–Le Fort III. **C,** Coronal CT image of the orbit confirms an intact right lateral orbital wall *(white arrow)*, in keeping with right hemi–Le Fort II. The left lateral orbital wall is fractured *(black arrow)*, in keeping with left hemi–Le Fort III. Also noted are large bilateral pneumocephalus, frontal bone fractures, and left orbital fractures. **D,** The coronal CT image through the pterygoid processes confirms the presence of bilateral fractures *(black arrows)*. Specifically, a left hemi–Le Fort III and a right hemi–Le Fort II are present. There is an associated sphenoid sinus fracture with fracture fragments impinging on the left orbital apex *(white arrow)*. **E,** Coronal CT shows displaced fracture of the left mandibular ramus *(white arrow)*, which will be repaired before midfacial reconstruction to restore the most posterior vertical buttress of the face. **F,** Axial CT of the frontal bar confirms substantially comminuted both-table frontal sinus fracture *(black arrows)* with a large amount of pneumocephalus, creating a "Mount Fuji sign" *(white arrows)* and extending into the bilateral lateral ventricles, indicative of dural injury. **G,** Sagittal CT reformation outlines the fracture involvement of the orbital roof *(white arrow)*. Retrobulbar soft tissue emphysema is present *(black arrow)*. Frontal bone fracture and pneumocephalus are again visualized.

Traumatic Craniocervical Vascular Injuries

Clint W. Sliker

Neither blunt nor penetrating traumatic craniocervical arterial injuries are common, but both are very significant groups of injuries encountered in the practice of trauma and emergency radiology because both are associated with high mortality. Penetrating neck trauma is associated with a mortality ranging from 2% to 10% with most early death resulting either directly or indirectly from arterial injury that leads to exsanguination, airway compromise, or stroke. Mortality is high in patients with blunt arterial injuries (BAIs) as well, ranging from 8% to 38%. Although mortality in patients with BAIs frequently can be attributed to other severe coexisting injuries; injury-specific mortality secondary to stroke is common. The key to reducing morbidity and mortality in patients with both penetrating arterial injuries (PAIs) and BAIs is rapid diagnosis and treatment.

As with most vascular disease, craniocervical arterial injuries can be diagnosed with a number of different imaging modalities, including digital subtraction angiography (DSA), magnetic resonance angiography, duplex Doppler sonography, and multidetector computed tomographic angiography (CTA). Each diagnostic option has its own particular merits and limitations. However, of the group, CTA has the greatest overall practical utility when evaluating the acutely injured patient in that it is noninvasive, quick, readily available in most contemporary emergency departments (EDs), and easily integrated into established diagnostic algorithms. In addition, multidetector CTA has been shown to be a useful tool that can have a positive clinical impact when used to evaluate patients for either penetrating or blunt craniocervical arterial injuries.

Craniocervical arterial injuries are varied in morphologic and physiologic manifestations. Manifestations of injury include minimal intimal injury (i.e., intimal irregularity), intramural hematoma (Figs. 5-8 and 5-9), raised intimal flap (see Fig. 5-9), pseudoaneurysm (Fig. 5-10), intraluminal thrombus, occlusion (Fig. 5-11; see Fig. 5-9), complete or partial transection with active hemorrhage

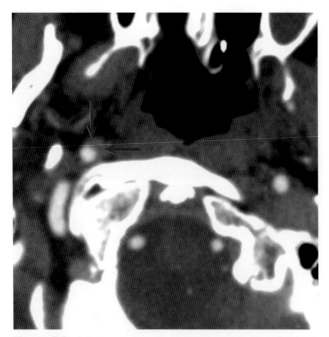

Figure 5-8 Right internal carotid artery distal cervical segment high-attenuation acute intramural hematoma *(arrows)* in a 65-year-old woman who was in a motor vehicle collision.

(Fig. 5-12), and arteriovenous fistula (AVF) (Fig. 5-13). Both blunt and penetrating mechanisms can result in any of the various types of injury, although, in my experience, active hemorrhage tends to be more frequently encountered in patients with PAI.

■ BLUNT CERVICAL ARTERIAL INJURIES

Blunt injury may occur anywhere along the length of the carotid and vertebrobasilar arterial systems, but clinically significant injuries tend to occur in the cervical segments of the internal carotid and vertebral arteries. Vascular injury may occur as the consequence of a direct blow to the vessel. However, the main cause of blunt injury is thought to be stretching of the artery to the point of mechanical failure. The predominant mechanism is thought to be hyperextension and contralateral rotation of the head, which stretches the internal carotid artery over the transverse processes of C1 and C2, or cervical spine subluxation/dislocation that stretches the vertebral artery over fixed spinal structures. Arteries may also be stretched by craniocervical distraction or crushed between bone fragments at sites of craniofacial or cervical spine fracture. Reflecting the complex mechanisms

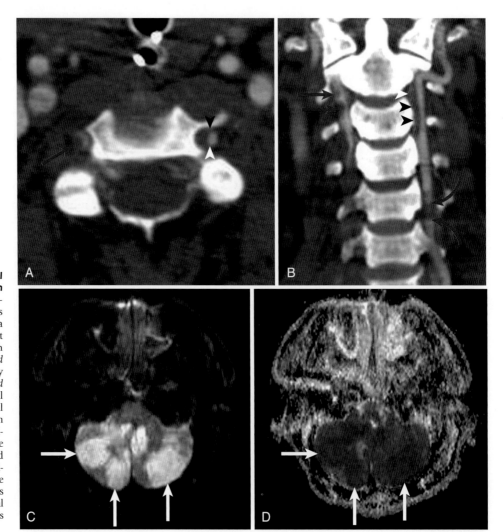

Figure 5-9 Thin-slab coronal maximum intensity projection (MIP). A and **B,** Computed tomographic angiography (CTA) images of a 39-year-old man who was in a motorcycle crash demonstrate a right vertebral artery intimal flap with probable adherent thrombus *(red arrows)* and two left vertebral artery injuries: segmental occlusion *(curved arrows)* and eccentric intramural hematoma narrowing the arterial lumen *(arrowheads).* Traumatic brain and solid organ injury contraindicated antithrombotic therapy at the time of CTA. Diffusion-weighted **(C)** and apparent diffusion coefficient **(D)** brain magnetic resonance imaging (MRI) performed 7 days later confirms diminished signal of bilateral cerebellar acute infarcts *(white arrows).*

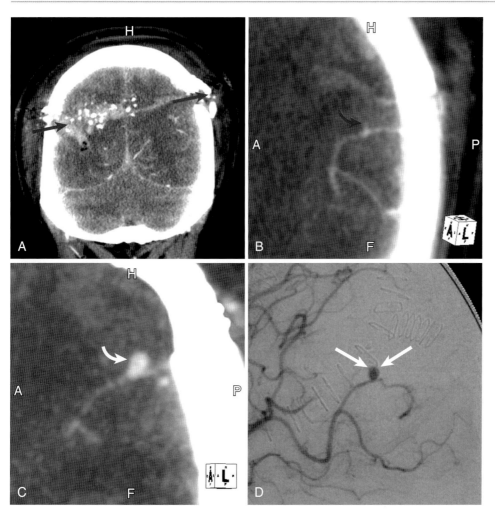

Figure 5-10 Enlarging pseudoaneurysm following transcranial gunshot wound. A, Coronal thin-slab maximum intensity projection (MIP) and oblique thin-slab volume-rendered admission brain computed tomographic angiography (CTA) demonstrate the wound track *(red arrows)*. **B,** Shows a left middle cerebral artery distal branch small pseudoaneurysm *(curved red arrow)* near the exit wound. **C,** Five-day follow-up CTA MIP image demonstrates interval enlargement of the pseudoaneurysm *(curved white arrow)*. **D,** Digital subtraction angiography (DSA) confirmed pseudoaneurysm *(white arrows)*.

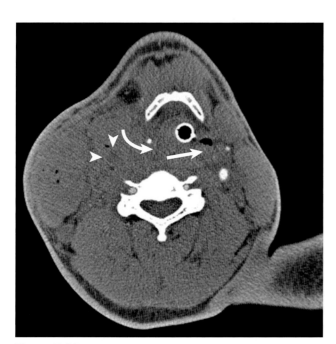

Figure 5-11 Zone II stab wound. The track *(straight arrow)* of a right-sided zone II stab wound crosses the occluded right common carotid artery *(arrowheads)* through the posterolateral hypopharynx *(curved arrow)*. Common carotid artery and hypopharyngeal injuries were confirmed at surgical exploration.

of injury experienced by many multitrauma patients, multivessel injuries (i.e., more than one carotid and/or vertebral artery segment injured) are common and diagnosed in 18% to 38% of patients with BAI (see Fig. 5-9).

Clinical signs of BAI include active arterial hemorrhage from an open wound, mouth, nose, or ears; an expanding neck hematoma, cervical bruit, especially in patients younger than 50 years; pulsatile tinnitus; pulsatile exophthalmos; Horner syndrome or oculosympathetic paresis; fixed neurologic deficits, either lateralizing or central, that are incongruent with the findings of neurologic imaging; transient ischemic attack; and neuroimaging findings of cerebral infarction that are unexplained by hypotension, intracranial herniation, or anoxia. Many patients come to the ED with clinical signs of injury. However, in 56% to 86% of patients, BAI typically *does not manifest until after a clinically silent interval* that usually lasts several hours but may last several months.

In both symptomatic patients and asymptomatic patients with BAI, treatment improves patient outcome. Twenty-six percent to 57% of patients with untreated BAI may experience BAI-specific stroke (see Fig. 5-9), whereas only 0% to 4% of patients in whom injury is treated suffer stroke, resulting in decreased injury-specific mortality. Although both surgical repair and endovascular intervention have roles in the treatment

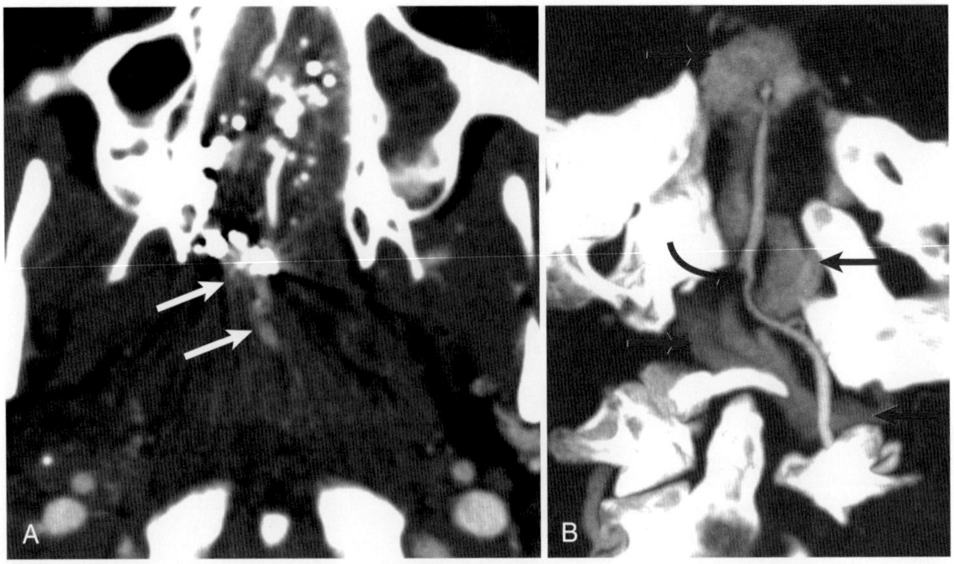

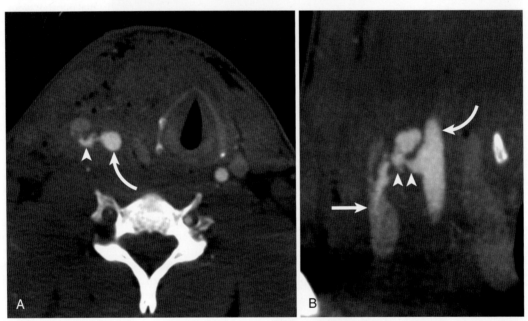

Figure 5-12 Computed tomographic angiography (CTA) demonstrating active arterial hemorrhage in two different patients. A, Active hemorrhage *(white arrows)* into the nasopharynx following facial gunshot wound. B, Posterior fossa and upper cervical active hemorrhage *(red arrows)* associated with craniocervical distraction injury following a motor vehicle collision. The exact site of arterial transection was not identified. The right vertebral artery V₄ segment is occluded *(curved arrow)*.

Figure 5-13 Axial image **(A)** and coronal maximum intensity projection (MIP) image **(B)** from computed tomographic angiography (CTA) demonstrate a right common carotid artery–to–internal jugular vein arteriovenous fistula (AVF) following zone II gunshot wound. Fistulous tract *(arrowheads)* connects the common carotid artery *(curved arrows)* with the internal jugular vein *(straight arrow)*.

of BAI in select patients, the current mainstays of treatment are anticoagulation and antiplatelet therapy, either alone or in combination.

Injury Grading

Based on the various imaging manifestations of injury, Biffl and colleagues devised a BAI injury scale for blunt carotid artery injuries that they later applied to blunt vertebral artery injuries. In the Biffl blunt arterial injury scale (also known as the Denver scale), grade I injuries include those with minimal intimal irregularity or intramural hematoma (see Fig. 5-8) causing less than 25% luminal stenosis. Grade II injuries (see Fig. 5-9) exhibit a raised intimal flap, an intraluminal thrombus, or an intramural hematoma causing 25% or more luminal compromise.

Grade III injuries are pseudoaneurysms. Grade IV injuries (see Fig. 5-9) are arterial occlusions. Grade V injuries (see Fig. 5-12) are arterial transections with active hemorrhage or hemodynamically significant AVFs. The highest possible grade is attributed to each injury, and in patients with more than one BAI, each is graded separately. Although initially devised to characterize injuries diagnosed with DSA, the Biffl grading system can be readily applied to BAI diagnosed with multidetector CTA. In addition to providing prognostic information, injury grading is a practical means of simplifying injury characterization and communication within the context of the varied imaging appearances of BAI. Moreover, though the efficacy of several currently accepted therapeutic options relative to others remains unsettled, some institutions, such as mine, tailor therapy based on injury grade.

Blunt arterial injury grading has particular value in the instance of blunt carotid artery injuries because Biffl and coworkers demonstrated a general linear relationship in the grade of blunt carotid injury and frequency of injury-related strokes: 3%, 11%, 33%, 44%, and 100% with injury grades I, II, III, IV, and V, respectively. The relationship between grade of blunt vertebral artery injury and frequency of stroke is nonlinear, with higher rates of stroke associated with injury grades II (40%) and IV (33%) (see Fig. 5-9), whereas grades I and III are associated with stroke in 19% and 13% of patients, respectively. Mortality rates are generally proportionate to the stroke rates for each injury grade. Note that Biffl and coworkers did not publish data for grade V blunt vertebral artery injuries, although I have diagnosed three grade V vertebral artery injuries in my practice, all of which were the likely cause of patient mortality. Blunt arterial injuries are not static lesions and may either regress or progress in grade over the course of as little as 1 week, leading to changes in management, which highlights the need for routine imaging follow-up at 7 to 10 days.

Multidetector Computed Tomographic Angiography— Accuracy and Clinical Utility

Initially multidetector CTA showed promise as a means to accurately diagnose BAI, relative to the accepted reference standard, DSA, with 16-channel CTA having a reported sensitivity of 98%. However, subsequent studies provided less favorable results with sensitivities ranging from 29% to 64%, which were not improved with advancing 32- and 64-channel technology. Clearly, multidetector CTA cannot be considered to be diagnostically equivalent to DSA when used to diagnosis BAI.

Despite its diagnostic limitations in regard to accuracy, multidetector CTA is still a valuable tool when used to evaluate patients for BAI. Not only does CTA have practical advantages over other diagnostic options, including DSA, but it has also been shown to be a more cost-effective tool when used as the primary means to diagnose BAI. The cost-effectiveness relative to DSA, MRA, and sonography can be realized whether patients are acutely symptomatic or asymptomatic.

For clinical utility, multidetector CTA is probably most useful when used to diagnose BAI in the context of screening. Recall that treatment of BAI while asymptomatic improves patient outcomes. From 56% to 86% of patients with BAI do not exhibit symptoms from hours to months after injury is sustained. Early identification of asymptomatic BAI may alter the initial treatment plan in up to 68% of patients. It has been reported repeatedly that screening select groups of blunt trauma patients for BAI allows diagnosis and treatment of patients before onset of symptoms, usually related to ischemia, and improves patient outcomes. Adoption of a structured BAI screening program based on the use of multidetector CTA can significantly increase the frequency of BAI diagnosed at a given institution. More important clinically, BAI-specific stroke and mortality rates are significantly lower in screened populations relative to unscreened populations. Though screening with DSA may also yield clinically significant improvement in BAI-specific mortality, primary use of CTA rather than DSA still results in improved patient outcomes with fewer injury-specific strokes, presumably because of more-rapid access to CTA.

To achieve the benefits of any screening program, there must be a high-risk patient population to target for screening. A number of specific injury patterns or clinical findings have been reported as risk factors for BAI and therefore indications to screen for arterial injury. In general, they suggest that the patient was subjected to those injury mechanisms that may cause BAI, and they are readily identified early in patients' clinical course. Among the more widely reported risk factors are Glasgow Coma Scale score less than 6, diffuse axonal injury, skull base fractures involving the central skull base or carotid canal, Le Fort II or Le Fort III facial fractures, major thoracic injuries (Abbreviated Injury Scale score greater than 3), and cervical spine injury manifesting as fracture or subluxation. Blunt arterial injury may be diagnosed in nearly two thirds of patients with established "high-risk" criteria, yet up to 20% of asymptomatic BAI will go still go undiagnosed. To identify more of those "missed" BAIs, complex skull fractures, scalp degloving injury, and mandible fractures can also trigger screening. As a practical matter, clinical judgment and recognition of injury mechanism, rather than a specific injury or clinical sign, are of paramount importance in identifying patients who may harbor BAI. Accordingly, irrespective of specific screening criteria, all patients who may have been subjected to hyperextension in the craniocervical region, especially with rotation, distraction, or crush/direct impact, should have multidetector CTA of the head and neck to evaluate for BAI.

■ PENETRATING NECK TRAUMA

The neck is an anatomically complex region with multiple vital structures located in a small region. When penetrating trauma to the neck violates the platysma, multiple structures that require early treatment can be injured, including the vascular system, aerodigestive tract, and spine. Arterial injuries occur in 15% to 25% of patients with penetrating neck trauma, whereas laryngotracheal and esophageal injuries occur in 1% to 7% and 0.9% to 6.6%, respectively.

Consequently, despite the extreme clinical importance of the major neck arteries, the diagnostic evaluation of neck-penetrating arterial injuries can only be approached in the context of the neck as a whole.

Although any penetrating object may violate multiple tissue planes and anatomic compartments, the extent of damage from penetrating trauma depends greatly upon the nature of the projectile or sharp object. Low-energy trauma, such as a knife stab wound or nail-gun injury, is generally associated with less extensive injuries resulting from direct impact against a given anatomic structure. With high-energy penetrating trauma, such as a gunshot wound from a shotgun or high-velocity hunting rifle, injuries result from direct impact, as well as tissue cavitation resulting from a shock wave and/or secondary missile formation (e.g., bone fragments). The situation can be further complicated when there are multiple, comingled penetrating wound tracks.

Surgically accessible PAIs are frequently treated with surgical repair, which also affords the opportunity to inspect, and potentially repair, other vital structures in the region of the wound track. Some difficult-to-access or surgically-inaccessible PAIs can be addressed with endovascular treatment.

Diagnosis and Treatment—Influence of Clinical Examination and Anatomy

Clinical decisions regarding the appropriate initial steps taken in both diagnosis and treatment of patients with penetrating trauma violating the platysma are based upon the clinical examination findings of any "hard" or "soft" signs of clinically significant penetrating neck injuries. Hard clinical signs—those strongly suggestive of a significant injury—include brisk, active bleeding from the wound; an expanding or pulsatile neck hematoma; cervical bruit or thrill (especially in a young patient); massive hemoptysis or hematemesis; shock refractory to intravenous fluids; and air bubbling from the wound. Soft clinical signs—those weakly suggestive of a significant injury—include venous oozing from the wound, nonexpanding and nonpulsatile neck hematoma, minor hemoptysis, dysphonia, dysphagia, and subcutaneous emphysema. Those presenting with hard signs of injury typically undergo immediate surgery to promptly diagnose and repair potentially fatal vascular or aerodigestive injuries. Patients with soft signs of penetrating neck injury generally can be evaluated with less invasive means, including diagnostic imaging and endoscopy. Most patients without any clinical signs of significant penetrating injury can usually be safely observed for 24 hours to look for delayed manifestations of injury, though 23% to 30% may harbor clinically significant, albeit acutely asymptomatic injuries, thereby suggesting that this population should be considered for diagnostic testing.

Management of penetrating neck injuries is also guided by the site of the entry wound based on the zonal anatomy of the neck. In the setting of penetrating neck trauma, the neck is divided into three zones (Fig. 5-14). Overlapping inferiorly with the thoracic inlet, zone I extends from the sternal notch and clavicles to the level of the cricoid cartilage superiorly. Zone II includes the region between the cricoid and the level of the mandibular angles. Finally, zone III extends from the mandibular angles to the skull base. To the surgeon, localization of the anatomic zone of injury is important because it may influence the approach he or she uses to treat any clinically significant injury. For example, many zone II injuries are accessible to the surgeon via an approach from the neck. In contrast, given the overlap with the thoracic inlet, zone I injuries frequently require combined thoracic and cervical approaches. Surgical access to zone III injuries may be either difficult or impossible due to facial structures and proximity to the skull base. Accessible injuries usually undergo direct surgical repair, though in very select patients, nonoperative management may be initially attempted. In regard to surgically inaccessible injuries, especially vascular, imaging-guided repair is frequently employed.

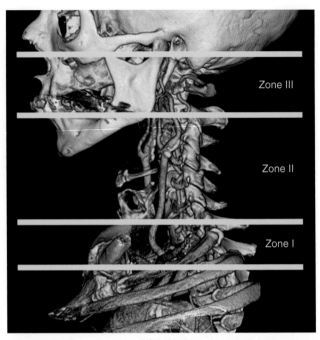

Figure 5-14 Multidetector computed tomographic angiography (CTA) volume-rendered image demonstrating the vascular zonal anatomy of the neck.

Multidetector Computed Tomographic Angiography—Accuracy and Clinical Utility

A number of studies report the accuracy of CTA for detecting clinically significant penetrating neck injuries. Because of the complexity of neck-penetrating trauma, the reference standards to which CTA was compared typically comprised the aggregate results of surgical exploration, DSA, esophagography, endoscopy, and clinical observation. Overall, results for CTA are excellent, regardless of the number of detectors, with sensitivities and specificities of 90% to 100% and 93.5% to 100%, respectively. Reflecting my clinical experience, reported false-positive results typically involved potential aerodigestive injuries.

The high accuracy of CTA for identifying significant injuries can greatly streamline the diagnostic evaluation of patients with penetrating neck injury. Importantly, in patients without indications for immediate surgery, reports in the medical literature suggest that negative neck exploration rates can be significantly reduced, albeit not eliminated entirely, when CTA is used to guide management decisions rather than the combination of clinical findings and anatomic zone of the entry wound. In regard to specific diagnostic tests, the use of CTA significantly reduces the need for DSA in this population. It is less clear if the use of CTA also leads to a significant reduction in the need for either esophagography or endoscopy, but the trend suggests that it does, which is supported by my experience. Finally, cervical spine fractures are common in patients with penetrating neck trauma, and CT is an integral part of evaluating cervical spine and facial fractures. Therefore, when CT scan protocols are constructed to account for and clearly display bony structures, as well as vascular and aerodigestive structures, multidetector neck CTA can be better used as a comprehensive diagnostic tool.

The key to both maximizing the diagnostic accuracy of CTA and realizing its full clinical utility when evaluating patients with penetrating neck trauma is the identification of the wound track (or tracks). Imaging manifestations of the track include gas, hemorrhage/edema (i.e., fat stranding), ill-defined fluid or hematoma, and either primary or secondary missile fragments, especially when caused by a thin, sharp object, such as a stiletto, or small caliber firearm. Imaging manifestations of the wound tract may be very subtle. Because it is common for wound tracks to extend through multiple anatomic zones and compartments, a thorough search for the signs of the track must be mounted both in close proximity to and remote from the entry wound. Viewing with an independent workstation allows for oblique multiplanar reconstructions, facilitates track identification.

Delineating the wound track can lead one to identify all vital structures that are injured or potentially injured by the penetrating object (see Figs. 5-10 and 5-11). Conversely, identification of the track may help one exclude injury to those structures spatially removed from the wound track. In most instances, when a specific injury is identified, the comprehensive examination provided by CTA allows definitive therapeutic plans to be made. Despite an otherwise normal appearance, when a vascular or aerodigestive structure is within the wound track, it is difficult to definitively exclude an injury to that structure. In those instances, further diagnostic testing or at times surgical exploration can be targeted to those areas at greatest risk for injury.

■ INTRACRANIAL VASCULAR INJURIES

Multidetector Computed Tomographic Angiography—Accuracy

The accuracy of CTA for specifically detecting intracranial arterial injuries has not yet been fully explored in the medical literature, and data are very limited. When used to diagnose cerebral aneurysms in patients with posttraumatic subarachnoid hemorrhage (SAH), multidetector CTA has reported sensitivities and specificities of 95% to 97.6% and 95.1% to 96.2%, respectively. However, because of the varying morphologic manifestations of BAI, it is uncertain if comparable accuracies can be achieved when CTA is used to evaluate for BAI. Still, given its practical advantages, multidetector CTA is a desirable first-line diagnostic option.

Arterial Injuries

Intracranial arterial injuries are much less common than cervical arterial injuries, but they remain a clinically significant group of injuries. Like cervical arterial injuries, they may lead to thromboembolic stroke. However, they pose a greater risk for hemorrhagic complications, especially from pseudoaneurysms, leading to hematoma that causes mass effect and subsequent cerebral injury. When

an arteriovenous malformation (AVM) occurs, neurologic complications may result from either vascular steal–associated ischemia or intracranial hemorrhage.

Blunt Arterial Injuries

Like cervical BAIs, intracranial BAIs tend to be associated with other injuries that result in either traction on the artery or impaction by a fracture fragment. In my experience, cavernous internal carotid segment injuries are more common and occur when fractures extend through the central skull base into the cavernous-sphenoid complex. Supraclinoid internal carotid artery or middle cerebral artery M1 segment injuries may occur as a consequence of acceleration-deceleration, a mechanism shared by diffuse axonal injury, which causes traction to be exerted upon the relatively fixed artery by the more mobile brain. Finally, the vertebral and basilar arteries can be stretched when there is a craniocervical distraction injury (see Fig. 5-12, *B*), or, rarely, the basilar artery can be entrapped in a clivus fracture. In general, given comparable clinical manifestations and considerable overlap of risk factors for both intracranial and cervical injuries, multidetector CTA of patients with potential BAI should include both the brain and neck.

Penetrating Arterial Injuries

The true incidence of intracranial PAI is uncertain. Though generally considered uncommon, the frequency of intracranial PAI may be high in some subsets of patients. For example, a recent study of war-related penetrating head trauma revealed a prevalence of 34%. Like BAI, intracranial PAI may occur anywhere within the intracranial circulation, but PAIs are more frequently diagnosed in the peripheral cerebral artery branches than in central arteries. Peripheral intracranial PAIs tend to be pseudoaneurysms, although AVFs are also commonly encountered. Although some may spontaneously regress, PAIs tend to be dynamic lesions that will worsen (e.g., pseudoaneurysm enlargement) over time (see Fig. 5-10), thereby increasing the risk for infarction or hemorrhage. Arteriospasm is a frequent associated finding, usually in or near the wound track, which may hinder either diagnosis or treatment of the injury itself. Accessible peripheral lesions may be treated surgically, but endovascular repair or occlusion of both peripheral and central injuries is a therapeutic option in many instances.

Indications for CTA in patients with penetrating head trauma are not uniformly defined. However, reported indications for cerebrovascular imaging of patients with penetrating head injury include penetrating injury through the pterional or orbitofrontal region, arterial injury demonstrated at surgical exploration, transcranial Doppler ultrasound findings of arteriospasm, and a spontaneous, unexplained decrease in either partial pressure of brain-tissue oxygenation or cerebral blood flow. In addition, given that arteriospasm may obscure an injury and that subtle injuries may increase in conspicuity over time, an initially CTA with negative findings should be followed with a repeat scan in 7 to 10 days.

Carotid-Cavernous Fistulas

A carotid-cavernous fistula (CCF), a subtype of AVF that results from abnormal direct communication between the internal carotid artery and cavernous sinus, is among the more common AVFs encountered in clinical practice. In penetrating trauma the fistulous communication occurs where the wound track crosses through the cavernous sinus into the cavernous segment of the internal carotid artery. Carotid-cavernous fistula secondary to blunt trauma likely occurs when shear stresses are transmitted through the connective tissue fibers within the cavernous sinus to the wall of the relatively fixed internal carotid artery, which occurs most frequently when a central skull base fracture extends into the cavernous sinus region. Complications of CCF include blindness or neurodeficits caused by either steal-induced ischemic infarction or venous hemorrhagic infarction. Posttraumatic CCFs are high-flow fistulas and rarely heal spontaneously. The longer the fistula goes without repair, the greater the chance of irreversible neurologic or ocular damage. Early treatment with endovascular techniques can improve clinical outcomes.

At times a CCF may be immediately apparent or may rapidly develop, although it usually takes several days for it to manifest clinically. Typical signs and symptoms include proptosis, chemosis, and orbital bruit, but it is not unusual for any one of these manifestations to be absent. It is important to consider that in severely injured multitrauma patients, especially those with severe craniofacial injuries, identifying signs and symptoms of CCF can be very challenging or impossible. Therefore a high level of suspicion is required by both the traumatologist and radiologist to ensure prompt diagnosis.

Computed tomography angiography signs of CCF (Fig. 5-15) mirror the complex morphologic and physiologic changes that occur as a result of the injury. Though CCF is difficult to definitively identify, CTA can demonstrate a full-thickness defect within the cavernous internal carotid artery. Reflecting the abnormal arterialization of intracranial venous flow, the cavernous sinus may bulge laterally; the cavernous sinus may exhibit asymmetrically intense enhancement relative to the contralateral sinus; the sphenoparietal, inferior petrosal, and/or superior petrosal sinuses may be enlarged and exhibit asymmetrically increased enhancement; and cortical veins may be enlarged. Orbital abnormalities reflect abnormally increased venous outflow from the cavernous sinus and corresponding elevation in intraorbital pressure. The superior ophthalmic vein is typically abnormal, exhibiting asymmetric enlargement (diameter greater than 4 mm), early enhancement, and tortuosity. Other common orbital findings include proptosis and extraocular muscle enlargement (medial or

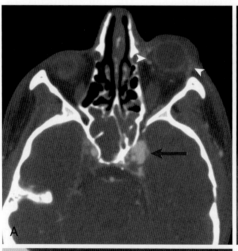 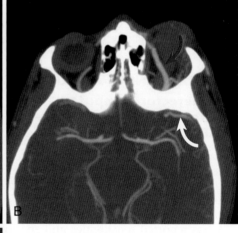

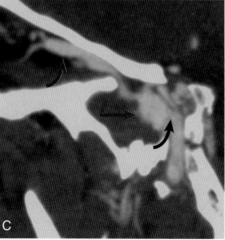

Figure 5-15 Carotid-cavernous fistula (CCF) in patient with central skull base fracture following motor vehicle collision. **A** and **B**, Axial images from computed tomographic angiography (CTA) demonstrate left-sided bulging cavernous sinus *(red arrow)*, enlarged superior ophthalmic vein *(curved red arrow)*, and asymmetrically enhancing sphenoparietal dural venous sinus *(curved white arrow)*. **C**, Sagittal maximum intensity projection (MIP) shows communication between the internal carotid artery and cavernous sinus *(curved black arrow)*, distended cavernous sinus *(red arrow)*, and dilated superior ophthalmic vein *(curved red arrow)*.

lateral rectus muscle diameter greater than 4 mm). Typically, but not universally, severe injuries to the orbit are ipsilateral to the CCF abnormalities, although they may manifest in the contralateral sinus and orbit as well. As with the clinical signs of injury, these abnormalities may be very subtle or absent soon after injury, and a repeat CTA several days later may reveal them.

Intracranial Venous Injuries

Blunt and penetrating trauma may both result in venous injuries. A penetrating wound track passing through a dural venous sinus or skull fracture crossing the site of dural sinus attachment may lead to venous sinus mural disruption and epidural hematomas. Posttraumatic cortical vein and dural venous sinus thrombosis can also occur. With blunt trauma, thrombosis may occur without an overlying fracture, but it is more typical when the sinus is crossed by a fracture. Forty percent of calvarial and skull base fractures crossing a point of dural venous sinus attachment or into the jugular foramen (Fig. 5-16) may be complicated by venous thrombosis. The clinical significance of a specific venous lesion may be difficult to predict, but up to 7% of patients with posttraumatic dural venous sinus thrombosis may experience venous infarction. In patients with risk factors for both venous and arterial injury, many of which are common to both injuries, evaluation for posttraumatic venous injury can be expedited by including cranial CT venography with CTA.

■ FACIAL AND EXTRACALVARIAL CRANIAL ARTERIAL INJURIES

Given the potential for associated neurologic injury, injuries to those arteries supplying the intracranial contents understandably garner the greatest attention in patients with histories of both blunt and penetrating trauma, but facial and extracalvarial cranial arterial injuries can be very significant as well. Both BAI and PAI can lead to death due to exsanguination or airway compromise either acutely or due to delayed rupture. Many such injuries may be clinically obvious, especially when located in

superficial locations, such as the scalp. Yet other lesions may not be clinically apparent due to extensive regional trauma or obscuration by bandages, cervical collars, or other support paraphernalia. Consequently, the radiologist must closely scrutinize the external carotid artery distribution (see Fig. 5-12, A) and other superficial structures for signs of acute vascular injury. Furthermore, in patients with craniofacial trauma, multidetector CTA should be performed so that superficial arterial branches, especially those in the distribution of the external carotid arteries, are imaged along with the other major cervical and intracranial arterial branches of the head and neck.

■ DIAGNOSTIC PITFALLS
Preexisting Arterial Abnormalities and Anatomic Variants

Among the more common abnormalities that may complicate interpretation of CTA for arterial injuries is noncalcified atherosclerotic plaque. Frequently the patient's age can be used as a discriminating factor because one would not expect plaque in a young patient, thereby pointing to acute injury rather than atherosclerosis. In older patients, noncalcified plaque can frequently be distinguished from intramural hematoma by its density, with plaque having low attenuation relative to the higher attenuation typical of acute intramural hematoma. In equivocal cases, magnetic resonance imaging (MRI) with fat-saturated T1-weighted images may be able to differentiate the two abnormalities.

Tortuous vessels are among the more commonly encountered normal variations. It is atypical for them to complicate interpretation of CTA, but areas of extreme tortuosity may mimic or obscure injuries when images are limited to those reconstructed in routine axial, coronal, and sagittal planes. Liberal use of an independent workstation to create off-axis multiplanar and 3-D reconstructions can be useful in this situation.

Variations in vessel size, especially hypoplasia and aplasia, can sometimes complicate interpretations of CTA for acute injury. At times an occlusive or stenotic injury may be mimicked, and it is important to recognize findings

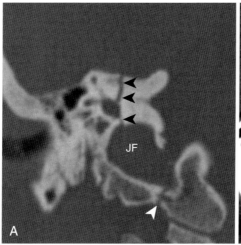
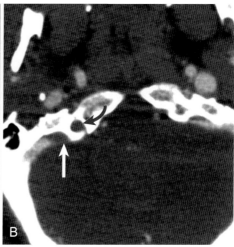

Figure 5-16 Basilar skull fracture and dural venous sinus thrombosis following motor vehicle collision. **A,** Sagittal temporal bone computed tomography (CT) demonstrates petrous temporal bone fracture *(black arrowheads)* extending through the jugular foramen *(JF)* into the basiocciput *(white arrowhead).* **B,** CT venogram demonstrates sigmoid sinus *(straight white arrow)* and jugular bulb *(curved red arrow)* thrombosis.

associated with normal variation, such as commensurate bony foramen aplasia/hypoplasia and contralateral arterial enlargement. At times, hypoplasia resulting in extremely small arterial size may make visualization of an artery difficult with CTA, especially in the presence of venous contamination. In this latter situation, DSA may be required to evaluate vascular integrity.

Artifact

Among the more common diagnostic pitfalls is metallic streak artifact when using multidetector CTA to evaluate patients with penetrating neck or craniofacial injuries, in which artifact from retained bullet or shrapnel fragments may completely obscure a particular artery. Though less of a problem in clinical practice, streak artifact emanating from either dental amalgam or surgical hardware may also compromise the diagnostic quality of CTA. In large patients, detail of the lower neck and thoracic inlet can be compromised by beam-hardening artifact from the patient's shoulders. When any of these situations in patients with high risk for either PAI or BAI is encountered, multidetector CTA should be followed by DSA.

■ DIGITAL SUBTRACTION ANGIOGRAPHY

Despite the advantages of multidetector CTA, there is still a role for the use of DSA in the diagnostic evaluation for both BAI and PAI of the head and neck. As already mentioned, DSA may be warranted in patients in whom the diagnostic quality of CTA images is hindered by normal variants or artifact. Technical limitations, such as timing of the contrast bolus, may limit the ability of CTA to identify or fully characterize some injuries, especially AVFs. Finally, particularly in the setting of BAI, multidetector CTA still has not matched the accuracy of DSA for detecting arterial injury in the head and neck. Consequently, in patients in whom clinical suspicion for an arterial injury is high and multidetector CTA results are negative for an injury, DSA should be performed to definitively exclude an injury.

Neck and Facial Infections

William B. Zucconi and
Diego B. Nunez

Infections of the face and neck represent a common cause of ED visits in both adult and pediatric populations. In the head and neck, clinical manifestations of infection often allow for a presumptive diagnosis. However, in the case of deep neck infection, the disease itself and its extent can escape accurate assessment on physical examination. In addition, common disease manifestations of regional swelling, erythema, and fever may be reduced or absent in patients with impaired immunity or in those who have received outpatient antibiotics (a significant percentage of patients presenting to the

ED with deep neck infection). In these patients, imaging studies are of critical importance in diagnosing and demarcating the anatomic extent of disease as well as directing patient management. Computed tomography remains the primary imaging modality with the greatest degree of utilization in the ED setting, but there are also indications for MRI and ultrasonography. Because deep neck infections have the potential to rapidly progress to severe and life-threatening situations such as airway compromise, mediastinitis, sepsis, and vascular complications, timely diagnosis and treatment are critical.

■ PROBLEM SOLVING AND GOALS FOR THE RADIOLOGIST

In this chapter we will review the contributions crosssectional imaging makes toward problem solving in the diagnosis and management of acute and/or complicated head and neck infection. When reviewing a positive case, a thorough search is performed for the origin of the infection. Most commonly it is a tonsillar source in the pediatric patient and a periodontal nidus in the adult. Alternate sites of primary infection include the oral cavity, the paranasal sinuses, and the tympanic/mastoid air spaces. Infection can spread from any superficial site and seed the deep spaces through the lymphatic or venous system, giving rise to lymphadenitis, nodal suppuration, and abscess. Once the infection is established, it may spread along or across the fascial planes and between deep neck spaces.

The full extent of the disease process must be described, including all anatomic spaces involved and the location of any potential abscess. If an abscess is identified, it should be described with respect to surgical landmarks such the carotid sheath, thyroid cartilage, and sternocleidomastoid muscle as an aid to the interventionalist or surgeon. The disease extent and the presence of abscess and other complications drive management decisions such as duration of treatment and whether or not a surgical course of action is warranted. For example, in patients with primary tonsillar infection in which the parapharyngeal, retropharyngeal, or prevertebral spaces are involved, a longer duration of antibiotic therapy is the standard. It is important to keep in mind that neck infection may coexist with other disease entities, such as preexisting cysts and congenital abnormalities, ulcerated mucosal tumor, or complications of head and neck radiation therapy. Acute tendonitis of the longus colli and necrotic or cystic nodal metastases can all be mistaken for an infectious process as well.

In the paragraphs to follow, we present a traditional overview of the anatomic compartments and basic facial demarcations of the neck followed by a simplified scheme that divides the neck into three broad regions corresponding to three common clinical scenarios.

■ ANATOMY

Beginning in the mouth, the oral cavity is differentiated from the oropharynx by the ringlike plane formed by the soft palate, the tonsillar pillars, and the circumvallate papillae that separate the oral tongue from its own base, or posterior third. The dental arches and the hard palate superiorly and the mylohyoid muscle inferiorly complete the boundaries of this space. It is particularly important to be familiar with the anatomy of the floor of the mouth. The mylohyoid muscle represents the anatomic floor and is shaped like two handheld fans meeting at the midline, forming a diaphragm attached to the medial aspect of the mandible. Above the mylohyoid muscle is the sublingual space, part of the oral cavity. The submandibular space is below the muscle, which is part of the anterior suprahyoid neck. Posteriorly, the free edge of the mylohyoid muscle is positioned at the level of the second or third molar tooth, straddled by the submandibular gland, where the two spaces communicate.

The deep face and neck is classically divided by the hyoid bone into the suprahyoid and infrahyoid segments. The suprahyoid segment extends superiorly to the skull base, and the layers of the deep cervical fascia divide this segment into five lateral spaces (parotid, masticator, mucosal, parapharyngeal, and carotid spaces), and two posterior midline spaces (retropharyngeal and prevertebral) behind the airway. A practical approach to the evaluation of a lesion in one of these lateral spaces is to establish its relationship with the parapharyngeal space, which is positioned in the center and surrounded by the other four lateral compartments. Because the parapharyngeal space predominantly contains fat, it provides the tissue contrast to do so. It has the shape of an inverted cone or pyramid that extends approximately 10 to 12 cm from the skull base to the hyoid bone. This space is limited by the masticator space anterolaterally, the mucosal pharyngeal space medially, the parotid space laterally, and the vascular compartment posteriorly. For example, a pharyngeal tonsillitis with abscess formation originates in the mucosal space and displaces the parapharyngeal space laterally. Conversely, a suppurative parotid sialoadenitis extends inward toward the parapharyngeal space, displacing it medially.

The anatomy and content of these spaces is relatively constant, allowing for consistent recognition and differentiation of disease processes that arise within. This often permits a reasonably accurate differential according to the space of origin and the extension of disease. Disease in the posterior midline spaces (retropharyngeal and prevertebral) may be differentiated by effects on the prevertebral muscles. Lesions arising in the retropharyngeal space may displace the longus colli muscles posteriorly, and lesions arising from the prevertebral space may displace these muscles anteriorly.

To simplify, we will divide the neck in three broad anatomic areas: (1) infections of the orbit and paranasal sinuses, (2) the lateral upper neck and floor of the mouth, and (3) the deep spaces surrounding the airway.

■ PROBLEM SOLVING IN COMPLICATED ORBITAL AND SINOGENIC INFECTIONS

Determine the following in a patient presenting with orbital cellulitis:
1. Is the lesion related to sinus infection, and if so, is it limited to the preseptal space or is there a postseptal component?
2. Is there evidence of a subperiosteal abscess?

3. Is there intracranial or other spread beyond the sinus?
4. Can the extent of the lesion compromise cranial nerve function or result in vascular complications?

Distinguishing between preseptal and postseptal infection in patients with sinogenic orbital cellulitis directs management with regard to use of intravenous antibiotics and need for surgical intervention. The orbital anatomy largely determines the propensity for sinus infection to spread to the orbit, particularly through the lamina papyracea. The periorbita, a fibrous circumferential membrane that thickens at the orbital margins in the shape of an arch contributes to the orbital septum; the barrier between the preseptal and postseptal spaces (Fig. 5-17). The periorbita also reinforces the osseous lining of the orbit as its periosteum and represents a strong barrier to the intraorbital spread of infection. When the thin ethmoid lamina is breached, the periorbita or orbital periosteum will initially contain the infectious process, forming a subperiosteal abscess that bulges toward the orbit (Fig. 5-18, A). Transgression of the periosteum allows wide intraorbital spread

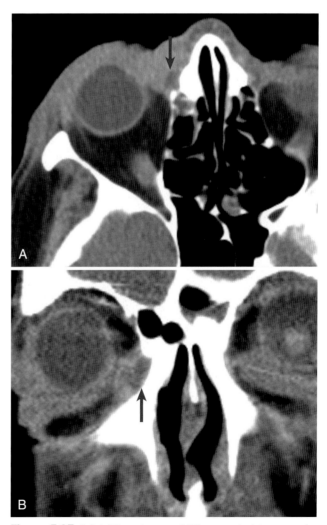

Figure 5-17 Axial (A) and coronal (B) computed tomography (CT). Complicated right-sided agar nasi sinusitis with a small adjacent preseptal abscess *(arrow)* and cellulitis presenting as pseudodacryocystitis.

of disease, resulting in intraconal or retrobulbar cellulitis, phlegmon, or abscess (Fig. 5-18, *B*).

Intracranial disease is most commonly a complication of frontal sinusitis through progressive osseous, meningeal, and parenchymal brain involvement, facilitated by valveless emissary veins. Magnetic resonance imaging plays a crucial role in diagnosing or excluding

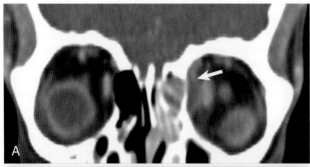
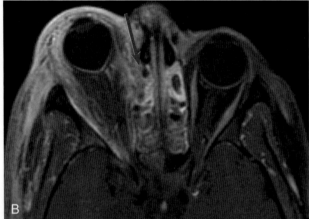
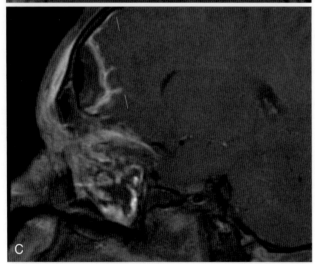

Figure 5-18 A, Coronal contrast-enhanced computed tomographic (CECT) image shows a left-sided subperiosteal orbital abscess *(white arrow)* due to ethmoid sinusitis. **B,** Axial postcontrast T1-weighted image with fat suppression in a different patient shows extensive (preseptal and postseptal) sinogenic orbital cellulitis with dehiscence of the anterior lamina papyracea *(red arrow)*, proptosis, and posterior tenting of the globe at the optic nerve insertion. **C,** Sagittal postcontrast T1-weighted image with fat suppression in the same patient as in **B** shows frontal sinusitis and an air-fluid level in an epidural abscess over the frontal pole. There is adjacent enhancement of the meninges *(arrowheads)*.

intracranial involvement. Dural enhancement, epidural or subdural empyema, leptomeningeal spread, and encephalitis with necrotizing parenchymal changes are all part of the spectrum of intracranial complications of frontoethmoidal sinusitis (Fig. 5-18, *C*). Frontal sinus disease may also spread superficially, in the form of a scalp abscess well known as a *Pott puffy tumor* (Fig. 5-19).

Ophthalmoplegia, cranial nerve deficits, and vascular lesions are severe complications of sinus infections. Specifically, ophthalmoplegia can occur when the spread of disease affects the intraorbital musculature function either by direct involvement or by compression from expanding lesions such as a mucocele. The latter, although typically a chronic condition, can present with acute oculomotor dysfunction or field defect when obstructed sphenoid and ethmoid compartments expand into the orbital apex or superior orbital fissure (Fig. 5-20). Additional complications can occur when sphenoid sinus infections spread to the adjacent cavernous sinus, resulting in either cranial nerve involvement or cavernous sinus thrombosis. Aggressive infections in this location can also result in epidural abscesses and mycotic pseudoaneurysm (Fig. 5-21).

■ PROBLEM SOLVING IN THE UPPER LATERAL NECK AND FLOOR OF MOUTH INFECTIONS

Determine the following in a patient with fever and lateral cervicofacial or submandibular swelling:

1. Is there evidence of a dental or salivary gland source of infection?
2. Do the changes reflect cellulitis, phlegmon, or abscess formation?
3. Is the abscess amenable to percutaneous drainage?
4. Does the infection extend beyond the space of origin (i.e., across the midline)?

We will address infections of the masticator space, oral cavity, and sublingual and submandibular spaces in addition to the parotid space. Cervicofacial swelling with signs of cellulitis and trismus often accompanies infectious processes of the oral cavity, the masticator space, and the salivary glands. Because the clinical examination in these patients is often limited by reduced range of jaw motion, cross-sectional imaging plays an important role in the workup.

Swelling of the masticator muscles and adjacent soft tissues is often a finding related to primary odontogenic infection (Fig. 5-22) that is overall the most common source in the adult patient. Periodontal infections and abscesses often resolve by spontaneously draining through the gingival tissues or are adequately controlled by tooth extraction. Complications can include osteomyelitis of the jaw and involvement of adjacent tissues. The disease can spread in any direction beyond the jaw with a dental source but is more frequent toward the oral cavity due to the relatively thinner cortex on the lingual side. This allows disease to access the sublingual space in the case of anterior tooth disease or submandibular and masticator space involvement in the case of posterior molar periodontitis. Some facial infections, particularly the polymicrobial odontogenic variety, can

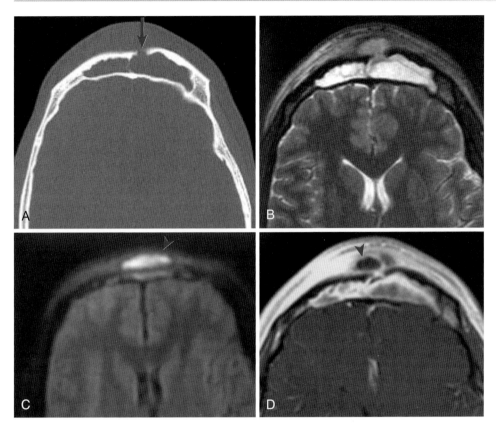

Figure 5-19 Pott puffy tumor. Axial computed tomographic (CT) image shows focal anterior dehiscence of the left frontal sinus wall (**A**; *arrow*), with scalp swelling. Magnetic resonance imaging (MRI) confirms subgaleal abscess on axial T2-weighted image (**B**) with restricted diffusion on axial diffusion-weighted imaging (**C**) corresponding to the collection on postcontrast T1-weighted image (**D**; *arrowheads*).

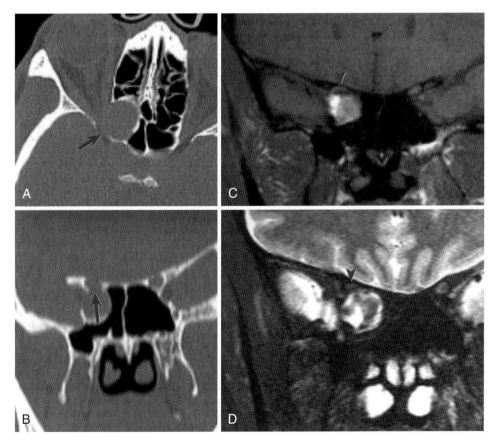

Figure 5-20 Posterior ethmoid mucocele. Axial (**A**) and coronal (**C**) computed tomographic (CT) images show an expanded, opacified posterior ethmoid air cell that is border forming to the optic canal. Note that the inferior and medial wall of the bony optic canal is demineralized *(arrows)*. Coronal T1-weighted (**B**), and T2-weighted (**D**) magnetic resonance imaging (MRI) show compression of the right optic nerve *(arrowheads)*. The mucocele contains mixed T1 and T2 signal intensities, indicating the varied protein concentration/ inspissation of the secretions.

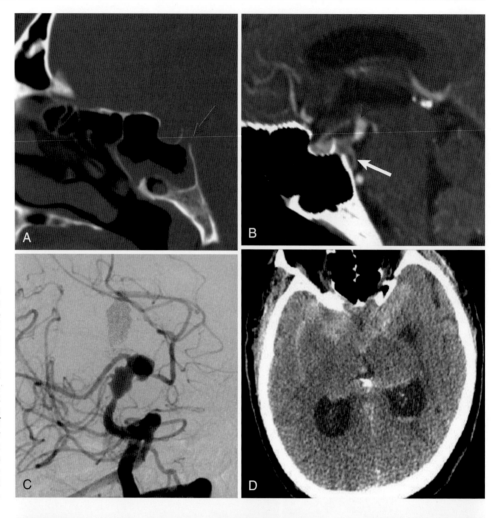

Figure 5-21 Sphenoid sinusitis complicated by epidural abscess and basilar artery pseudoaneurysm. A, Initial sagittal computed tomographic (CT) image shows sphenoid sinus disease with focal demineralization of the dorsum sellae *(arrow)* and adjacent retroclival soft tissue density (not shown). **B,** Sagittal reformat from a postcontrast head CT shows a retroclival abscess *(white arrow)* despite treatment of the sinusitis. Fullness of the basilar tip was also noted *(arrowhead)*. **C,** An irregular basilar artery aneurysm was confirmed with catheter angiography. **D,** The patient later succumbed to subarachnoid hemorrhage (SAH).

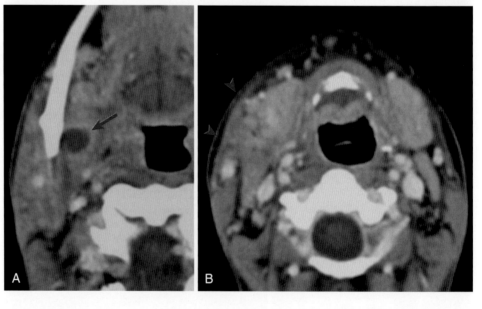

Figure 5-22 Odontogenic abscess. A, Postcontrast axial computed tomographic (CT) image shows abscess formation *(arrow)* following extraction of the third mandibular molar. **B,** The collection is situated along the inferior masticator space just posterior to the mylohyoid, allowing cellulitis and sialoadenitis in the submandibular space *(arrowheads)*.

have an aggressive behavior with rapid progression of phlegmonous change, deep space involvement, necrotizing infection, and airway compromise as seen in Ludwig angina (Fig. 5-23). As emphasized in the subsequent section, the airway should be a concern of the radiologist and the treating clinician in this region as well. An infection can gain access to and compromise the aerodigestive tract via the parapharyngeal space if the posteromedial mandibular cortex is breached. In addition, the stylomandibular tunnel may conduct primary parotid space infection to the parapharyngeal space. Depending on the relationship to the buccinator muscle insertion,

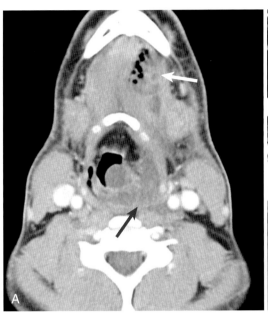 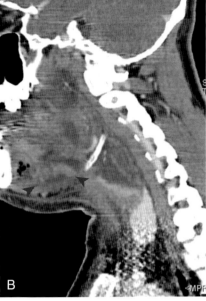

Figure 5-23 Ludwig angina. A, Axial postcontrast computed tomography (CT). Extensive, bilateral deep and superficial cellulitis with left-sided multilocular gas-containing sublingual abscess *(white arrow)*. Note associated phlegmon and abscess along the left posterior supraglottic and hypopharyngeal walls that compromise the airway *(red arrow)*. There is also lateral retropharyngeal fluid. B, Sagittal reformat shows the fluid collections surrounding the floor of mouth (mylohyoid; *red arrowheads*) with anterior sublingual gas locules.

if the outer or buccal cortex of the jaw is perforated, the infection can spread to the buccinator space and present clinically with cheek swelling. The buccinator space communicates freely to the periorbital and preseptal tissues, which, aside from permitting odontogenic preseptal cellulitis, allows access to the facial and angular veins, placing the cavernous sinus at risk for infectious thrombophlebitis.

Careful review of the images using bone windows is required to assess bone loss surrounding the dental roots, the pericoronal region in unerupted molars, and in the adjacent mandibular or maxillary cortex. Bone loss may be very subtle even in patients with florid surrounding soft tissue infection. To the extent possible, frank osteomyelitis should also be excluded.

The full extent of disease and the presence or absence of an abscess should be clearly stated in the radiology report. Appropriate window settings should also be used to look for signs of liquefaction as expected in abscess formation. To that end, differentiation between phlegmon and abscess is not always possible, particularly when it comes to predicting whether a lesion is amenable to percutaneous or surgical drainage. It has been estimated that with CT, accurate differentiation between abscess and phlegmon can be achieved in approximately 75% of patients. Due to better tissue characterization, MRI may be useful in determining the potential success of a drainage procedure (Fig. 5-24, *A* and *B*).

If a dental source is not identified, or if there are obvious signs of sialoadenitis, causes of salivary gland obstruction are sought. Ductal dilation or intraglandular sialectasis may be present due to an obstructive calculus, which is routinely identified on postcontrast imaging alone. Precontrast CT for the sole purpose of stone detection is not necessary. Purulent parotitis is a less common source of facial infection that may develop as a complication of sialolithiasis and sialoadenitis. In these patients, glandular enlargement with heterogeneous density should raise the possibility of suppuration and potential abscess formation (Fig. 5-24, *C* to *F*).

PROBLEM SOLVING AROUND THE AIRWAY

Determine the following in a patient presenting with difficulty swallowing:
1 Is there compromise of the airway, and at what level and extent?
2 Is there a tonsillar infection, and if so, is it complicated by peritonsillar or parapharyngeal abscess formation?
3 Is there spread of infection to the mediastinum or the vascular space?
4 If there is soft tissue swelling posterior to the airway, is the origin retropharyngeal or prevertebral? Is MRI warranted?

In patients with suspected deep neck infections and compromise of the airway, cross-sectional imaging plays a fundamental role. The airway is encircled by the mucosal space, which spans the entire length of the neck from the skull base to the chest, and is bounded posterolaterally by the middle layer of the deep buccopharyngeal fascia.

Infections in the mucosal space and its adjacent retropharyngeal and prevertebral spaces can produce significant narrowing of the airway, and assessment with cross-sectional imaging is an excellent problem-solving tool that can determine the origin, site, and extent of airway compromise.

The palatine tonsils are part of the lateral mucosal space of the oropharynx and are the most common origin of deep neck infection, particularly in children. Tonsillitis is a clinical diagnosis, but excluding abscess formation may require CT. In patients with positive findings, it is important to determine whether the abscess is limited to the tonsillar space confined by the pharyngeal constrictor muscles, or whether the muscle boundary has been transgressed, allowing infection to advance laterally into the parapharyngeal space (Fig. 5-25). The adjacent carotid sheath structures may also become involved, as in cases of Lemierre syndrome (Fig. 5-26).

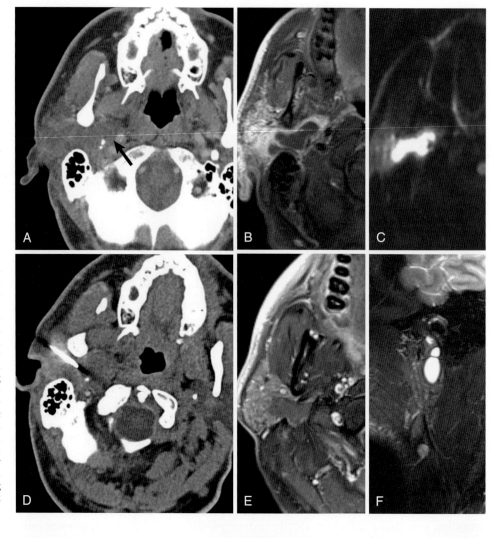

Figure 5-24 Deep parotid abscess. A, Contrast-enhanced axial computed tomography (CT) shows that the deep portion of the gland is swollen, effacing the parapharyngeal fat lateral to the carotid sheath (*black arrow;* compare to contralateral side). CT fails to demonstrate the abscess. **B,** Contrast-enhanced, fat-suppressed axial T1-weighted image clearly defines the rim-enhancing collection protruding through the stylomandibular tunnel into the parapharyngeal space. **C,** Diffusion-weighted imaging shows restricted diffusion within the collection (confirmed on apparent diffusion coefficient map, not shown). **D,** Based on magnetic resonance imaging (MRI), the collection was triangulated for CT-guided drainage. Several months after near-complete resolution, a noninflamed collection *(red arrows)* recurred (**E,** axial T1-weighted postcontrast and **F,** sagittal T2 weighted) immediately below the cartilaginous external auditory canal *(arrowhead),* raising the possibility of preexisting first branchial cleft cyst.

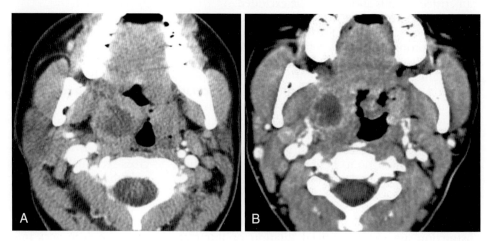

Figure 5-25 Tonsillar abscess. A, Abscess is medial to the parapharyngeal space. **B,** Parapharyngeal abscess.

A potentially severe infection of the mucosal space is acute inflammation of the epiglottis and supraglottic structures. It is a rare condition, but its potential for a fulminant clinical course has long been recognized particularly in children and more recently in the adult population. An enlarged epiglottis, enlarged aryepiglottic folds, or a swollen, bulging mucosa of the hypopharynx can easily obstruct the airway posteriorly. Radiography and CT can help in establishing the diagnosis and determining the extent of this condition (Fig. 5-27). The radiologist should also be cognizant of the risks and imaging features of aspiration in these patients.

Retropharyngeal abscesses occur mainly in children secondary to lymph node seeding from sinus or oropharyngeal infections resulting in suppurative adenitis and abscess formation (Fig. 5-28). This condition is

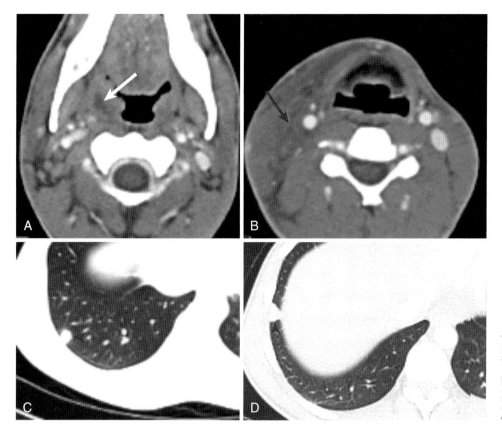

Figure 5-26 Lemierre syndrome. A, Contrast-enhanced axial computed tomographic (CT) image shows a right-sided tonsillar abscess *(white arrow)* and occlusive thrombophlebitis of the right internal jugular vein (B; *red arrow*). C and D, Example of several small noncavitary septic emboli *(arrowheads)*.

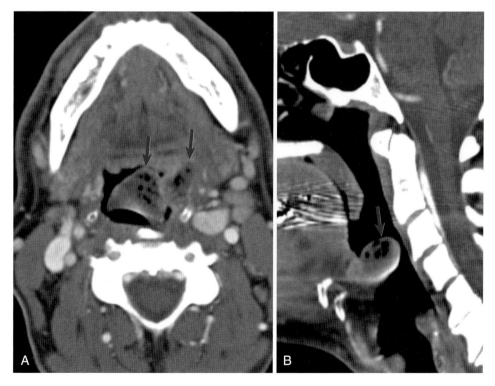

Figure 5-27 Emphysematous epiglottitis. Axial (A), and sagittal (B) post-contrast computed tomography (CT) demonstrates large gas-containing abscesses *(arrows)* along the ventral surface of the epiglottis extending into the left lateral hypopharyngeal mucosal space.

much less common in adults given the involution of retropharyngeal nodes after puberty. Occasionally a retropharyngeal abscess may be seen in adults after penetrating pharyngeal injuries.

Behind the parapharyngeal space and anterior to the cervical column is the prevertebral space, bound by the deep layer of the deep cervical fascia. By evaluating the prevertebral longus colli/capitis musculature, one may be able to distinguish retropharyngeal from prevertebral disease proper. In the former the prevertebral muscles may be pushed posteriorly with preserved signal characteristics on MRI provided the prevertebral

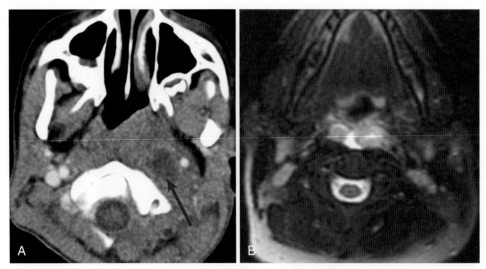

Figure 5-28 Left-sided retropharyngeal nodal abscess (**A**; *arrow*) medial to carotid sheath structures. The left internal jugular vein was congenitally small and compressed. T2-weighted magnetic resonance imaging (MRI; **B**) shows suppurative adenitis and retropharyngeal cellulitis.

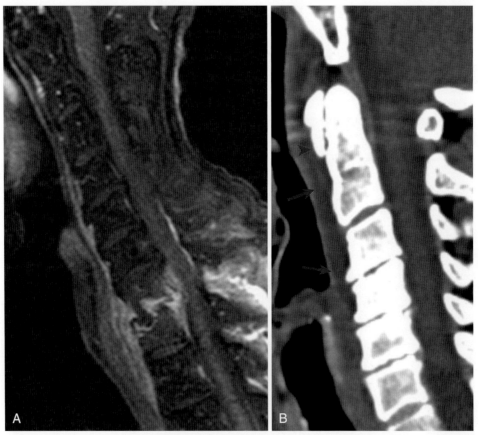

Figure 5-29 A, C7-T1 infectious spondylodiscitis with prevertebral effusion, edema, and epidural phlegmon compressing the thecal sac on fat-suppressed postcontrast sagittal T1-weighted image. **B,** Sagittal computed tomographic (CT) image on a different patient with a prevertebral effusion *(arrows)*, secondary to acute tendonitis of the longus colli. Note the tendinous calcification *(arrowhead)*.

fascia has not been violated. In prevertebral disease the longus colli/capitis muscles may be swollen and edematous, pushing the retropharyngeal and mucosal structures anteriorly. In these patients the vertebrae and intervertebral disc spaces must be carefully assessed for any signs of infectious discitis and osteomyelitis.

In this instance, extension of disease to the anterior epidural space or spinal canal must be excluded and can include epidural abscess with or without thecal sac and cord compression. Magnetic resonance imaging is best suited to recognize these potential causes and complications (Fig. 5-29).

Traumatic Orbital Emergencies

Michael F. Rolen and
Syed Ahmad Jamal Bokhari

Trauma to the eye is relatively common, accounting for approximately 3% of all ED visits and representing approximately 40% of monocular blindness in the United States. Many of these injuries occur in the context of motor vehicle collisions or sports-related trauma. Imaging plays a crucial role in the assessment of orbital trauma because it is often challenging to perform an adequate clinical examination on a severely injured patient who may be unable to cooperate or whose swollen eye prevents funduscopic evaluation.

Although the sensitivity of radiography for identifying fractures of the orbits is between 64% and 78%, plain films are not sensitive for soft tissue injury and thus are rarely performed today. Ultrasonography can be quite useful in evaluating the globe, with the added benefit of no ionizing radiation. However, due to the small amount of pressure placed on the globe by the transducer, ultrasonography is contraindicated in patients with suspected globe rupture. Magnetic resonance imaging also lacks ionizing radiation and, given its high contrast resolution, is superb for evaluating the orbital soft tissues. Magnetic resonance imaging is particularly sensitive in detecting subtle injuries of the globe and optic nerve and, unlike ultrasonography, can be used in patients with open-globe injury. However, MRI is contraindicated if there is a possibility of a metallic intraorbital foreign body, which could move in the presence of the magnet and possibly lead to vision loss. Other disadvantages of MRI that preclude it from being the initial study in patients with eye injury are its relative expense and the difficulty in performing the study emergently at most medical centers. Computed tomography is currently the initial and primary modality for imaging orbital trauma given its ready availability in most EDs, fast acquisition time, and ability to obtain thin axial sections (0.625 to 1.25 mm) with subsequent MPR. Because of its high spatial resolution, CT is excellent for identifying orbital fractures and metallic foreign bodies, the latter of which must be excluded before considering further evaluation with MRI. The disadvantage of CT lies in its use of ionizing radiation, with the lens being particularly susceptible. Thus the goal of the radiologist is to optimize the study in order to make an accurate diagnosis while minimizing the radiation exposure to the lens.

◼ ANATOMY

The orbit is a pyramidal space bounded by seven bones of the face and skull: the frontal, zygomatic, maxillary, lacrimal, ethmoid, sphenoid, and palatine. The globe lies anteriorly within this space and is a largely spherical structure with a diameter of approximately 24 mm. The wall of the globe is formed by three layers: an outermost fibrous layer composed of the sclera and cornea, a middle layer made up of the choroid and ciliary body,

and an innermost layer composed of the retina. Radially oriented zonular fibers connect the lens with the sclera. The lens divides the globe into a smaller anterior segment and a larger posterior segment, which are filled with aqueous and vitreous humor, respectively. The iris further subdivides the small anterior segment into an anterior and posterior chamber.

If a line is drawn between the anterior margin of the lateral and medial walls of the bony orbit on an axial CT in the midorbital plane, the normal globe should be bisected with 50% anterior to the line and 50% posterior to the line. In patients with traumatic exophthalmos, there is decreased orbital volume secondary to a blow-in fracture or retrobulbar hematoma, which displaces the majority of the globe anterior to the line. Conversely, traumatic enophthalmos is a consequence of increased orbital volume, such as that seen with a blow-out fracture. Because the intraorbital contents are allowed to occupy a larger volume by extruding through the fracture site, the globe is retracted such that the majority is displaced posterior to the line.

The six extraocular muscles lie posterior to the globe and form an intraorbital conical structure. Within this cone is the orbital fat, which also contains a few veins and lymphatics. The dural-covered optic nerve sheath courses through this fat centrally and joins the posterior globe to the brain. The optic nerve, ophthalmic artery, and small veins lie within the nerve sheath.

◼ ANTERIOR CHAMBER INJURIES

The two primary injuries involving the anterior chamber of the globe are traumatic hyphema and corneal laceration.

Traumatic Hyphema

Traumatic hyphema is bleeding into the anterior chamber secondary to disruption of blood vessels in the iris or ciliary body. Although hemorrhage from these vessels can occur in extravasation into either the anterior or posterior chamber, the term *hyphema* is reserved for bleeding into the anterior chamber whereas bleeding into the posterior chamber is referred to as *vitreous hemorrhage*.

On clinical examination, a blood-fluid level can be seen, which represents the extravasation of blood into the anterior chamber. A four-part grading system exists based on the amount of blood filling the anterior chamber, with grade I being less than one third and grade IV describing the total filling of the anterior chamber. Although CT can demonstrate increased attenuation in the anterior chamber because of hemorrhage, imaging in the context of clinical traumatic hyphema is performed primarily to evaluate for other related injuries (Figs. 5-30 and 5-31).

Corneal Laceration

Corneal lacerations are often seen in the context of penetrating trauma. The key finding on CT is decreased volume of the anterior chamber, which is readily apparent when compared with the nonaffected globe (see Fig. 5-30). An

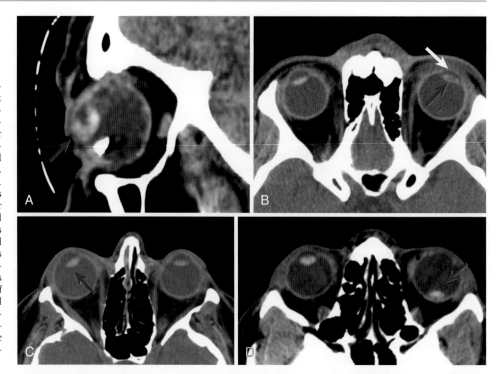

Figure 5-30 A, Traumatic hyphema. Sagittal noncontrast computed tomography (CT) demonstrates high-attenuation hemorrhage within the anterior chamber *(red arrow)*. Also note the triangular-shaped metallic foreign body and intraocular air within the vitrea. **B,** Corneal laceration and lens edema. Axial noncontrast CT demonstrates decreased volume of the anterior chamber of the right globe compared to the left *(white arrow)*. The right lens is also low in attenuation compared to the left, consistent with acute lens edema *(red arrow)*. **C,** Partial lens dislocation. Axial noncontrast CT shows angulation of the right lens *(red arrow)* due to tearing of the lateral zonular fibers. **D,** Complete lens dislocation. Axial noncontrast CT demonstrates posterior dislocation of the left lens *(red arrow)* that is seen layering dependently within the vitrea.

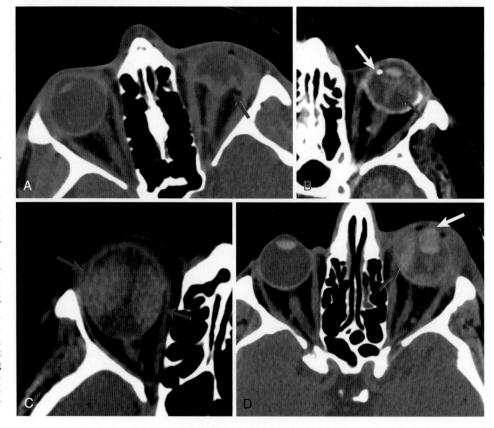

Figure 5-31 A, Globe rupture. Axial noncontrast computed tomography (CT) demonstrates abnormal posterior contour and volume loss of a ruptured left globe, known as the *mushroom sign (red arrow)*, with the ruptured globe being the cap and the optic nerve resembling the stalk of the mushroom. **B,** Retinal detachment. Axial noncontrast CT demonstrates a V-shaped high-attenuation collection in the posterior segment *(red arrow)*. Note the adjacent intraocular metallic foreign body near the medial aspect of the lens *(white arrow)*. **C,** Choroidal detachment. Axial noncontrast CT shows parallel biconvex high-attenuation collections *(red arrows)* due to tearing of the choroidal veins. **D,** Traumatic hyphema and choroidal detachment. Axial noncontrast CT demonstrates high-attenuation collections within the anterior chamber of the left globe consistent with hyphema *(white arrow)* and a convex high-attenuation collection along the medial wall of the posterior segment *(red arrow)*. Note the small foci of additional retinal and vitreous hemorrhage.

important mimic of corneal laceration is anterior subluxation of the lens because both present with decreased volume of the anterior chamber. Therefore it is important for the radiologist to assess the lens position when confronted with a decreased volume of the anterior chamber in order to differentiate these two entities.

■ LENS INJURIES

Injuries to the lens are often seen in the context of blunt trauma as deformation of the globe that results in posterior displacement of the cornea and anterior sclera with compensatory equatorial expansion of the globe. The increase in transverse diameter of the globe causes stretching of the zonular attachments that hold the lens in place, which can ultimately lead to partial or complete dehiscence.

Dislocation

In partial dislocation the zonular fibers tear on only one side while the contralateral fibers remain intact. The intact fibers act as a hinge, resulting in posterior angulation and protrusion of the affected side of the lens into the vitreous humor. As such, the lens takes on a more vertically angled appearance (see Fig. 5-30). A complete dislocation occurs when there is bilateral dehiscence of the zonular attachments. Although the lens can dislocate anteriorly, posterior subluxation is much more common given that the iris acts as a barrier that impedes anterior subluxation (see Fig. 5-30). It is important for the radiologist to be cognizant that not all lens dislocations are the result of trauma. Spontaneous lens dislocations can occur in the context of multiple systemic disorders, most commonly Marfan syndrome, Ehlers-Danlos syndrome, and homocystinuria. An important clue that suggests a nontraumatic cause is bilateral lens dislocation.

Traumatic Cataract

Not all lens injuries involve tearing of the zonular fibers. The normal lens lies within a thin capsule. When blunt or penetrating trauma disrupts this capsule, water is allowed to enter the lens, resulting in acute lens edema or a "traumatic cataract." On CT the affected lens will appear hypodense compared to the contralateral side, often with a Hounsfield unit (HU) difference of at least 30 HU (see Fig. 5-30). Just as bilateral lens dislocations suggest a systemic cause, bilateral lens edema suggests a nontraumatic cause, such as diabetes. The mechanism in diabetic patients begins with an elevated glucose level within the globe, which creates an osmotic gradient across the lens. Thus water is drawn into the lens, resulting in bilateral lens edema.

◼ OPEN-GLOBE INJURIES

Also known as a *ruptured globe*, an open-globe injury is often devastating, and these injuries are a major cause of blindness. The primary mechanism of injury involves perforation of the sclera, typically just posterior to the insertions of the extraocular muscles where the sclera is thinnest, with resultant extrusion of the vitreous. Although this diagnosis may be obvious on clinical examination, CT can be used in suspected cases of clinically occult open-globe injury, although the sensitivity of CT varies from 56% to 68%.

Findings of globe rupture on CT include an abnormal globe contour, posterior flattening, volume loss, scleral discontinuity, and the presence of intraocular air or foreign bodies (Fig. 5-32). The abnormal contour of the globe has been descriptively termed the *flat tire* or *mushroom sign*, particularly when posterior flattening and volume loss are present (see

Fig. 5-31). Although the presence of intraocular foreign bodies implies anterior perforation, it is also important for the radiologist to evaluate for evidence of concurrent posterior perforation (double perforation), as this is a poor prognostic sign because posterior perforations cannot typically be repaired. A more subtle CT finding of a torn sclera is a deep (expanded) anterior chamber where vitreous flows through a scleral defect, resulting in posterior volume loss and posterior migration of the lens. However, because the zonular attachments of the lens remain intact, the posterior displacement of the lens results in expansion of the anterior chamber, consistent with open-globe injury.

Just as with lens dislocations, not all contour abnormalities are the consequence of globe rupture. Nontraumatic lesions of the globe can be congenital (e.g., coloboma) or acquired (e.g., staphyloma) and may have an identical imaging appearance with open-globe injury. A posttraumatic orbital hematoma can also deform the globe, mimicking rupture. Other important pitfalls to avoid are iatrogenic changes in the globe related to prior ophthalmologic procedures. Perfluoropropane gas can be injected into the vitreous as means of a gas tamponade treatment for retinal detachment, resulting in low attenuation areas within the globe that have an identical appearance to traumatic intraocular air. Other iatrogenic mimics are ocular appliances such as low-attenuation silicone sponges and high-attenuation scleral buckles, both of which can indent the globe and be mistaken for open-globe injury in the presence of penetrating intraocular foreign bodies.

◼ OCULAR DETACHMENT

The wall of the globe is composed of three different layers: the retina (inner), choroid (middle), and sclera (outer). Fluid can accumulate within the potential spaces between these layers, resulting in retinal or choroidal detachment.

Retinal Detachment

The retina can become detached from the choroid in the setting of inflammation, neoplasm, or trauma. The majority of the retina is loosely attached to the choroid, although there are very firm attachments seen along its anterior margin, called the *ora serrata*, and posteriorly at the optic disc. Thus, when a tear in the retina allows vitreous fluid to accumulate in the subretinal space, the fluid collection assumes a V-shaped configuration, with the apex at the optic disc and the extremities at the ora serrata (see Fig. 5-31). If a subretinal fluid collection is seen in a child, it is important for the radiologist to raise concern for possible nonaccidental trauma.

Choroidal Detachment

The underlying cause of choroidal detachment is ocular hypotony, which can be inflammatory, iatrogenic, or traumatic in cause. The decreased ocular pressure results

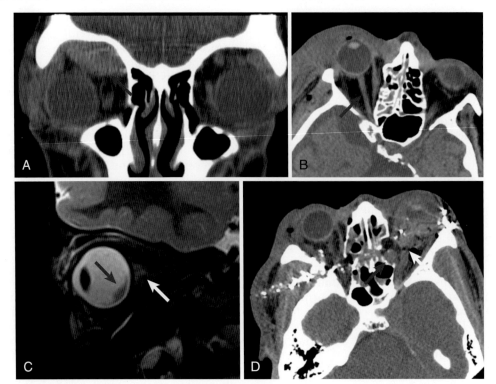

Figure 5-32 **A,** Retrobulbar hematoma. Coronal noncontrast computed tomography (CT) demonstrates a large intraconal collection *(red arrow)* that is high in attenuation compared to the low-attenuation intraorbital fat. **B,** Traumatic optic neuropathy (TON). Axial noncontrast CT demonstrates relative thinning and stretching of the right optic nerve *(red arrow)*, secondary to retrobulbar hematoma (not shown) and resulting in traumatic exophthalmos of the globe. **C,** TON and retinal hemorrhage. Sagittal T2-weighted magnetic resonance image (MRI) of the right orbit demonstrates increased signal edema in the optic sheath near its attachment with the posterior globe *(white arrow)*. There is also a layering collection of decreased T2 signal within the posterior globe, consistent with acute hemorrhage *(red arrow)*. **D,** Gunshot wound through bilateral orbits. Axial noncontrast CT demonstrates a linear trail of metallic and bony fragments traversing a ruptured left globe, ethmoid sinuses, and anterior aspect of the right orbital apex. There is complete transection of the left optic nerve *(white arrow)* and avulsion of the medial rectus muscle, which is enlarged and herniating through the lamina papyracea into the adjacent ethmoid sinus *(red arrow)*.

in decreased pressure in the potential space between the choroid and sclera. A transudate can then accumulate, known as a *serous choroidal detachment*. If there is tearing of the arteries and veins that tether the choroid to the sclera, a hemorrhagic choroidal detachment results, which is higher in attenuation than the serous variety. This distinction is important because serous detachments are usually more benign and often resolve spontaneously, whereas hemorrhagic detachments are associated with a poorer prognosis. Unlike the V-shaped configuration of retinal detachment, choroidal detachments assume a biconvex or lentiform configuration that extends from the level of the ora serrata to the vortex veins (see Fig. 5-31).

■ INTRAORBITAL FOREIGN BODIES

Detection and localization of ocular foreign bodies is an extremely important task because their presence can lead to infection, globe rupture, retinal toxicity, and vision loss. Fortunately, CT is sensitive for detecting both metallic and nonmetallic fragments and is often the first line of imaging performed, though its sensitivity varies with the specific content of the foreign body (Fig. 5-33).

Metal

Computed tomography has been shown to be very sensitive in identifying metallic foreign bodies, even those fragments that are less than 1 mm in size (see Figs. 5-30 and 5-31). This is an important issue because metallic fragments must be definitively ruled out before MRI. Failure to exclude intraorbital metal before MR imaging can result in globe perforation and blindness should the metallic fragment move in the presence of the high field–strength magnet. The removal of metallic foreign bodies is also important because many metals contain copper or iron, both of which can cause retinal toxicity and subsequent blindness. Potential pitfalls in the evaluation of intraorbital metallic foreign bodies are surgical devices, such as scleral bands, which can lead to a false-positive result. Conversely, false negatives can occur if there is eye or head movement during image acquisition.

Glass

Computed tomography is also the most sensitive imaging modality for the detection of intraocular glass. The detection rates of CT vary based upon the size of the fragment, the type of glass, and the location within the

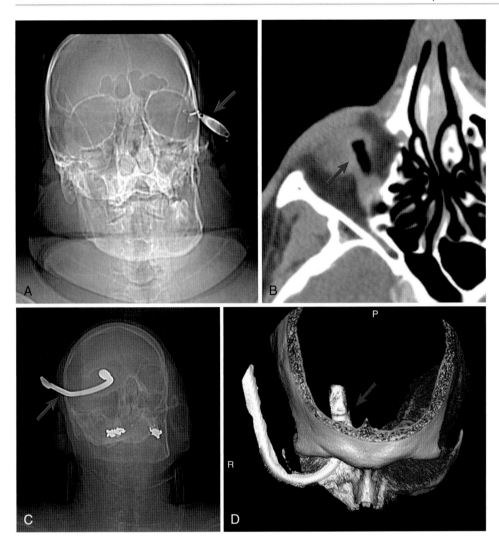

Figure 5-33 **A**, Fish hook in eye. Frontal computed tomographic (CT) scout image demonstrates a multipronged metallic fishing hook *(red arrow)* extending into the lateral aspect of the left orbit. **B**, Wooden foreign body. Axial noncontrast CT demonstrates a very low attenuation, intraorbital structure located just superior to the right globe *(red arrow)*, which mimics intraorbital air but has geometric margins. **C**, Coat hook in eye. Frontal CT scout image shows a large metallic hook projecting over the right orbit *(red arrow)*. **D**, CT three-dimensional (3-D) reconstruction of the same patient as in **C** demonstrates the intracranial extension of the hook through the right orbit *(red arrow)*.

orbit. Those fragments that are easiest to detect are 1.5 mm or greater in size, are composed of green beer-bottle glass, and are located within the anterior chamber. In contrast, the hardest fragments to detect are less than 0.5 mm in size, are composed of spectacle glass, and are located on the corneal surface. Unfortunately, case reports exist that have shown even relatively large 4-mm glass fragments have also evaded detection on CT.

Wood

Identifying wooden foreign bodies on CT can be challenging. Unlike the high-attenuating substances of metal and glass, wooden fragments are very low in attenuation due to their air-filled porous microstructure and thus can be mistaken for intraorbital air. In addition, the attenuation of wood can increase over time, which is thought secondary to fluid displacing air within the pores. On CT the key to distinguishing air from wood is that wooden fragments typically demonstrate a geometric margin (see Fig. 5-33). When there is clinical suspicion of intraocular wooden foreign body in the presence of negative or equivocal CT findings, MRI can be used for further investigation. On MRI the key finding is identifying evidence of inflammation in the area of concern using T2-weighted or contrast-enhanced sequences.

■ RETROBULBAR HEMATOMA

Hemorrhage within the retrobulbar space is relatively uncommon but when present can constitute an ophthalmologic emergency. Given the bony confines of the orbit, a retrobulbar hematoma can lead to a rise in intraorbital pressure. If the rise in orbital volume is small, compensatory proptosis and prolapse of intraorbital fat can ensue. However, if the intraorbital pressure rises rapidly, compression of the optic nerve or central retinal artery can occur, resulting in ischemia and blindness. Identifying a retrobulbar hematoma on CT is relatively straightforward because the normal low-attenuating intraconal fat contrasts with high-attenuating hemorrhage (see Fig. 5-32). Findings should be communicated immediately to the referring clinician because emergent decompression can be vision saving. First-line surgical intervention is lateral canthotomy, which can be performed at the bedside.

EXTRAOCULAR MUSCLE AVULSION

Complete or partial avulsion of the extraocular muscles is uncommon and presents as strabismus (misalignment of gaze). The most common extraocular muscles involved are the medial rectus and inferior rectus, likely related to their proximity to the relatively thin lamina papyracea and orbital floor, respectively. Fractures of these structures can result in entrapment or shearing of the adjacent extraocular muscle. Alternatively, avulsion can occur in the setting of direct penetrating trauma such as stab wounds. On CT the avulsed muscle may appear enlarged and retracted (see Fig. 5-32). In the absence of penetrating trauma, there will often be evidence of orbital fracture with herniation of intraorbital fat. The globe may also be subluxed within the bony orbit.

CAROTID-CAVERNOUS FISTULA

A clinical history of posttraumatic diplopia (double vision), proptosis (anterior bulging of the globe), chemosis (conjunctival swelling), and objective pulsatile tinnitus should prompt the radiologist to look for evidence of a CCF. These entities begin with a tear in the cavernous portion of the internal carotid artery. High-pressure arterial blood then enters the normally low-pressure cavernous sinus, and this increase in cavernous pressure leads to retrograde venous reflux. The superior and inferior ophthalmic veins can become engorged, thus increasing intraocular pressure, which in turn decreases retinal perfusion pressure, ultimately leading to blindness. This condition is illustrated and further discussed in the section on vascular trauma.

OPTIC NERVE INJURIES

Traumatic optic neuropathy (TON) is relatively uncommon and is seen in approximately 5% of patients with facial fractures. Clinically these patients may present with acute onset of monocular vision loss or more subtly with a relatively afferent pupillary defect. Traumatic optic neuropathy can result from either direct or indirect injury to the optic nerve.

Direct injuries are less common and usually are the result of a penetrating foreign body or blunt trauma that leads to fracturing of the orbital apex or optic canal. This type of injury can lead to subsequent shearing of the axons within the nerve sheath or laceration/transection of the optic nerve itself (see Fig. 5-32). Indirect injuries occur more frequently and result in compression and ischemia of the optic nerve (see Fig. 5-32). Causes of indirect injury include intraorbital hematoma, retrobulbar hemorrhage, vascular dissection, or edema within the nerve sheath.

As with all patients with orbital trauma, CT is the initial imaging study in patients with suspected TON. The radiologist should evaluate the orbit for foreign body, particularly those made of metal that may preclude further evaluation with MRI. In addition to an obvious nerve transection, the posterior segment of the globe and retrobulbar regions should also be inspected for evidence of hemorrhage, which may indicate indirect TON (see Fig. 5-32). It is important to evaluate for subtle fractures involving the orbital apex, especially the optic canal and anterior clinoid process. If CT is negative for metallic foreign body, but negative or equivocal for TON, MRI can be obtained to evaluate for signal changes within the optic nerve, particularly on T2-weighted and postcontrast T1-weighted sequences (see Fig. 5-32).

Nontraumatic Orbital Emergencies

Maxwell D. Elia, Javier Servat, Flora Levin, and Michele H. Johnson

Nontraumatic orbital emergencies commonly present with acute visual loss, pain, proptosis, and/or ophthalmoplegia. Alternatively, patients may present with a combination of local and systemic signs and symptoms. Infection, inflammatory disorders, neoplasms, and vascular lesions may each present emergently, and imaging may contribute to diagnosis and delineation of extent of the process or help to inform patient management. Imaging has little role in the assessment of "floaters" or retinal or choroidal detachments in the nontraumatic setting; however, associated pathologic conditions may be identified on routine orbital imaging. For example, although optic neuritis is a clinical diagnosis, the association with multiple sclerosis discovered on imaging can clarify the diagnosis and aid in treatment decision making. Computed tomography is the imaging method of choice in adults with acute nontraumatic ophthalmologic presentations suggesting space-occupying pathologic conditions. Modern CT scanners employ dose-reduction techniques to minimize radiation exposure. Rapid assessment of the orbit and its contents can be achieved with the added benefit of excellent visualization of adjacent structures such as the paranasal sinuses that may contribute to the disease process. Magnetic resonance imaging of the orbit can be extremely revealing in patients with nontraumatic orbital disease because of the exquisite tissue resolution and should be used preferentially in children when available to limit the radiation dose to the lens.

ORBITAL INFECTION AND INFLAMMATORY DISEASE

Orbital inflammation may arise from infection, autoimmune disease, vasculitis, and/or idiopathic orbital inflammatory syndrome (orbital pseudotumor). Although differentiating these entities typically requires clinical correlation, imaging can be helpful in determining the extent and character of orbital involvement. Infection is typically classified based upon its extent in relation to the orbital septum. For example, with regard to cellulitis, *preseptal* denotes involvement anterior to the orbital septum, and *orbital* denotes involvement posterior to the orbital septum.

Preseptal Cellulitis

These patients present with eyelid erythema and edema because the soft tissue infection involves the tissues anterior to the orbital septum. Despite the fact that the eyelid may be swollen shut, the globe is not involved, and vision, extraocular motility, and pupillary function are normal. Preseptal cellulitis typically arises from underlying sinus (ethmoid) disease, chalazion, dacryocystitis, or cutaneous trauma. Computed tomography imaging demonstrates soft tissue swelling and edema without intraorbital fat stranding or subperiosteal abscess (Fig.5-34).

Orbital Cellulitis

Orbital cellulitis refers to infection involving tissues posterior to the orbital septum. These patients present with pain, eyelid erythema, edema, proptosis, and pain with extraocular movements. Depending on the extent of orbital involvement, there may be additional symptoms, including visual loss, restriction of ocular motility, and pupillary abnormalities. In the majority of patients, orbital cellulitis arises as an extension from infection within periorbital structures, most commonly sinus or dental infection. Computed tomography reveals orbital fat stranding and may identify adjacent infection or abscess (Fig. 5-35). In the most severe cases, infection may extend to involve the cavernous sinus, with or without the development of cavernous sinus thrombosis. These patients will often develop complete ophthalmoplegia

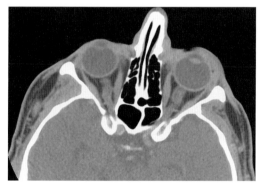

Figure 5-34 Preseptal cellulitis. Axial computed tomography (CT) with contrast demonstrates left preseptal soft tissue swelling with sparing of the intraorbital contents. Note the lack of intraorbital fat stranding.

with anesthesia in the cranial nerve V_1 and V_2 distribution, typical of cavernous sinus involvement (see Cavernous Sinus Syndrome).

Infectious Endophthalmitis

Infectious endophthalmitis is an infection that involves both the anterior and posterior chambers of the eye. Patients complain of pain and vision loss and have marked conjunctival injection on physical examination. Frequently a layering of white blood cells called a *hypopyon* is noted on ophthalmologic examination. Although the risk for endophthalmitis is higher among patients with a history of eye surgery, it may also arise endogenously from bacteremic or fungemic patients secondary to hematogenous dissemination. Infectious endophthalmitis is typically diagnosed clinically, with or without the use of ultrasound imaging. Computed tomography may reveal increased density of the vitreous cavity associated with inflammation of the sclera (see Fig. 5-35).

Necrotizing Fasciitis

Necrotizing fasciitis of the orbit is a potentially fatal infection, most commonly caused by group A streptococcus. In most cases patients are immunocompromised. Early presenting symptoms may include shock and anesthesia overlying the affected area, although overlying anesthesia progresses to severe pain. Urgent radiologic confirmation is imperative because patients almost always need rapid surgical intervention (Fig. 5-36).

Dacryocystitis

Dacryocystitis is an infection of the lacrimal sac, most commonly occurring as a result of nasolacrimal duct obstruction. With obstruction of the nasolacrimal duct, tears do not flow, and stasis leads to infection. Patients present with pain and erythema overlying the nasolacrimal sac, and purulent discharge is common. The nasolacrimal sac is dilated with rim enhancement on imaging, indicative of infection. Importantly, both CT and MRI can aid in distinguishing whether the obstruction is caused by an intrinsic lesion (such as a lacrimal sac tumor) or results from extrinsic compression (i.e., extension of a malignancy arising within the sinuses) (Fig. 5-37).

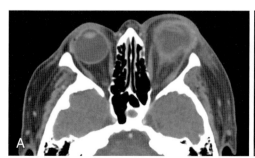
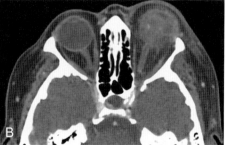

Figure 5-35 Orbital cellulitis and endophthalmitis. A and **B,** Axial contrast-enhanced computed tomographic (CT) scans at the level of the globe and optic nerve head demonstrate preseptal soft tissue swelling extending to involve the subcutaneous and temporalis region. Notable are the stranding within the intraorbital fat, proptosis, and heterogeneous increased density within the abnormally shaped globe. The sclera is thickened. Treatment required orbital exenteration.

THYROID EYE DISEASE

Thyroid eye disease (thyroid ophthalmopathy) typically presents with eyelid retraction, proptosis, and restriction of extraocular motility leading to diplopia. The disease is most commonly bilateral, although unilateral proptosis may be seen. In severe cases the orbital congestion and muscular edema that arise from inflammation of the extraocular muscles may induce optic neuropathy, leading to emergent presentation with visual field loss and pupillary abnormalities. Thyroid eye disease may arise in the absence of serum markers of thyroid abnormalities. Computed tomography is especially helpful in identifying the extraocular muscle enlargement. Additional CT findings include stranding within the orbital fat and fusiform enlargement of the extraocular muscles with sparing of the muscular origins and insertions. The clinical course is usually chronic and progressive rather than acute or rapidly progressive, an important differential consideration (Fig. 5-38). In rare cases, thyroid eye

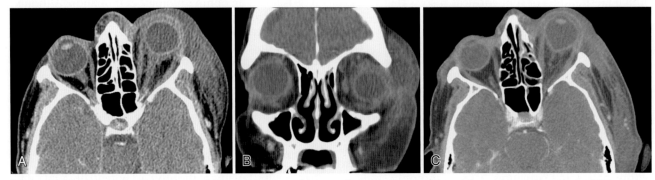

Figure 5-36 Necrotizing fasciitis. A and **B,** Axial and coronal images obtained at presentation to the emergency department (ED) demonstrate marked periorbital soft tissue swelling with soft tissue abscess in the temporalis region. **C,** 24 hours later there was increased extension of the scalp soft tissue swelling with abnormally shaped globe and increased density in the vitreous consistent with endophthalmitis. Treatment required orbital exenteration.

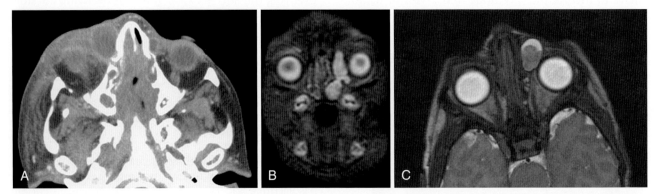

Figure 5-37 Dacryocystitis. A, Adult patient with painful mass involving the medial orbit and nose. Computed tomography (CT) demonstrates enhancing cystic mass arising from the nasolacrimal sac. **B** and **C,** In this pediatric patient with pain, erythema, and purulent discharge on the left, coronal T2-weighted magnetic resonance imaging (MRI) demonstrates bright signal intensity expansion of the nasolacrimal apparatus typical for dacryocystitis. Note the mixed signal intensity on the axial images consistent with inflammatory debris.

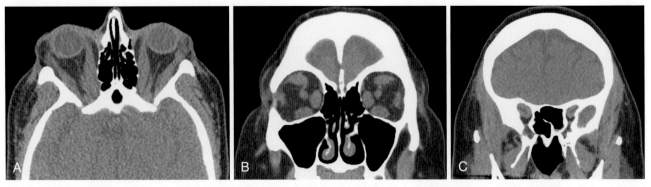

Figure 5-38 Thyroid eye disease. A, Axial noncontrast computed tomography (CT) through the orbit at the level of the medial and lateral rectus muscles demonstrates bilateral marked fusiform enlargement of the extraocular muscles with sparing of their insertions and origins. Note the bilateral proptosis. **B** and **C,** Coronal noncontrast CT scans through the retrobulbar orbit and through the orbital apex confirm the diffuse extraocular muscle involvement and the compromise of the optic nerve at the orbital apex with obliteration of the fat at the apex. This patient required orbital decompression to preserve vision.

disease may progress rapidly, making imaging particularly important because these cases are more likely to produce optic neuropathy. These cases of compressive optic neuropathy are more common in certain races, especially Asians, in whom the orbit tends to be shallower. Older men also have an increased tendency for more extensive disease.

■ IDIOPATHIC ORBITAL INFLAMMATORY SYNDROME

Idiopathic orbital inflammatory syndrome, also known as *orbital pseudotumor*, is an inflammatory disorder affecting only the tissues within the orbit resulting in painful proptosis, restriction of extraocular motility, and diplopia. Most commonly the inflammation can be diffuse with fat stranding and involvement of the extraocular muscles (myositis) and/or the lacrimal gland (dacryoadenitis). A distinguishing feature between idiopathic orbital inflammatory syndrome and thyroid eye disease is that idiopathic orbital inflammatory syndrome affects the tendons of the extraocular muscles, whereas these are spared in thyroid eye disease (Fig. 5-39). Thickening of the posterior sclera and the overlying Tenon capsule, identified on contrast-enhanced CT, may produce a "ring sign." There appears to be an increased incidence of ophthalmic complications, including idiopathic orbital inflammatory syndrome, in patients taking oral and intravenous bisphosphonates. These complications include eye pain secondary to scleritis, episcleritis, conjunctivitis, and uveitis. It may rarely manifest as a diffuse inflammatory process mimicking orbital cellulitis. Treatment of idiopathic orbital inflammatory syndrome includes high-dose steroids rather than antibiotics. Awareness of this entity in the differential diagnosis is imperative.

■ SARCOIDOSIS

Sarcoidosis may involve the orbit, although it most commonly involves the lung. Rarely, orbital findings may occur in the absence of systemic disease. Lacrimal gland inflammation, unilateral or bilateral, is the most common orbital manifestation, but inflammation from sarcoidosis may also affect the extraocular muscles or optic nerves. Chest x-ray examination and/or CT should also be considered in patients with clinical suspicion of sarcoidosis.

■ WEGENER GRANULOMATOSIS

Wegener granulomatosis is a small-to-medium–sized vessel vasculitis also known as *granulomatosis with polyarteritis*. It classically involves the paranasal sinuses (sinus mucosal inflammation), the lung (inflammatory lesions), and the kidney (glomerulonephritis). This small-vessel, necrotizing, granulomatous vasculitis involves the orbit in 20% to 50% of patients. Typically patients present with scleritis, episcleritis, or uveitis; however, more diffuse involvement may occur via direct extension from adjacent sinuses. The more diffuse form presents with decreased vision, strabismus, and diplopia caused by inflammatory mass effect within the orbit. Orbits and paranasal sinuses may be involved in isolation without renal or pulmonary involvement.

■ SILENT SINUS SYNDROME

Chronic inflammation from uncontrolled sinus disease can lead to erosion of the orbital floor, causing nontraumatic displacement of the globe into the maxillary sinus, causing resultant enophthalmos and diplopia. Noncontrast CT is the optimal imaging modality in patients with suspected silent sinus syndrome. The images reveal extensive sinus disease and complete erosion of the maxillary sinus.

■ CAVERNOUS SINUS SYNDROME

Cavernous sinus syndrome describes a clinical constellation of multiple unilateral cranial nerve palsies, including cranial nerves III, IV, V_1, V_2, and VI. This may occur as a result of AVF, tumors, cavernous sinus thrombosis, orbital inflammation, or orbital infection, including both bacterial and fungal infection. Proptosis may be present. The classic presentation of multiple cranial nerve palsies necessitates imaging of the orbits, sinus, and brain for assessment and differential diagnosis because vascular, inflammatory, infectious, and neoplastic lesions each require different therapeutic management. Increased density within the cavernous sinus on CT, expansion of the cavernous sinus with loss of the normal concave lateral margin, heterogeneity of signal intensity on MRI, and increased vascular flow voids are all findings indicating cavernous sinus pathologic changes.

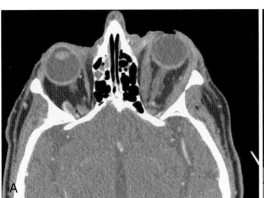
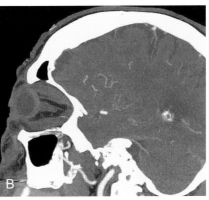

Figure 5-39 Idiopathic orbital inflammatory syndrome. A and **B,** Axial and sagittal noncontrast computed tomography (CT) through the orbit at the level of the rectus muscles demonstrates marked fusiform enlargement of the extraocular muscles with involvement of both insertions and origins. Note proptosis and fat stranding on the left.

NONINFECTIOUS UVEITIS/SCLERITIS

Uveitis is a term used to describe inflammation of the uvea, composed of the iris, ciliary body, and choroid. Uveitis may be isolated to a particular chamber of the eye, as in anterior or posterior uveitis, or it may affect the entire eye, as in panuveitis. The effects of the inflammatory diseases that cause uveitis lead to vision loss through the development of cataracts, cystoid macular edema, glaucoma, or retinal vasculitis. Occasionally metastatic disease, particularly hematologic malignancies, may mimic inflammatory uveitis (Fig. 5-40).

Although CT and MRI are not the modalities of choice for the initial diagnosis and management of patients with uveitis, patients may present with vision loss or eye pain, prompting radiologic evaluation. Most forms of uveitis are not identifiable by either CT or MRI. However, scleritis and panuveitis may be noted on contrast-enhanced CT, MRI, or ultrasonography as inflammation and thickening of the sclera. Magnetic resonance imaging and ultrasonography may also demonstrate exudative retinal detachment in some severe cases of uveitis.

CAROTID-CAVERNOUS FISTULA

Patients present with chemosis and proptosis with or without associated tinnitus, increased ocular pressure, and vision loss. In the absence of trauma these are dural AVFs between the distal dural branches of the external carotid artery and the cavernous sinus. These are referred to as *indirect fistulas* as opposed to the direct internal carotid artery–to–cavernous sinus fistula seen in the traumatic setting. Imaging demonstrates enlargement of the superior ophthalmic vein, enlargement of the cavernous sinus, and proptosis with stranding of the intraorbital fat and engorgement of the extraocular muscles.

LYMPHATIC MALFORMATIONS

Lymphatic malformations, also referred to as *lymphangiomas* or *venolymphatic malformations*, within the orbit occur as a result of vascular dysgenesis. The lesions typically present in the first decade of life, and they typically induce proptosis during periods of upper respiratory infection, as a result of stimulation of the lymphoid tissue. The bony orbit may be remodeled and expanded. Lymphangiomas

may spontaneously hemorrhage, causing acute proptosis. During periods of hemorrhage these lesions demonstrate fluid-fluid layering on CT and MRI (Fig. 5-41).

VENOUS MALFORMATIONS AND ORBITAL VARICES

Venous malformations, also known as *orbital varices*, also occur as a result of vascular dysgenesis. These low-flow lesions may cause proptosis that is accentuated during periods of Valsalva or when the head is in a dependent position. Valsalva during CECT will reveal enlargement of the venous varix when engorged. These rarely present acutely in the ED setting.

CAVERNOUS HEMANGIOMA

Orbital hemangiomas cause slowly progressive proptosis. They are the most common neoplasm of the orbit in adults, occurring more commonly in women. Magnetic resonance imaging demonstrates a homogeneously enhancing lesion with slow intralesional flow. Typically identification of these lesions does not necessitate emergent treatment unless vision is compromised.

NEOPLASTIC DISEASE

A wide range of tumors has been reported to metastasize to the orbit; the most common metastatic tumors are breast and lung. Orbital metastases typically present with pain and proptosis or enophthalmos. The two most common sites of metastasis within the orbit are the extraocular muscles and the bone marrow of the sphenoid bone; both areas have high blood flow and thus are predisposed to hematogenous spread. Imaging may reveal bony erosion, remodeling, or destruction; metastatic disease is the most common cause of lytic bony destruction of the orbit. Direct extension of tumors from the paranasal sinuses or orbital contents may also cause bone destruction (Figs. 5-42 and 5-43). Metastatic lesions are the most common intraocular tumors, typically affecting the choroid because of its rich vascular supply. Ocular choroidal deposits may be multiple and may be discovered incidentally in patients with widely metastatic cancers. Primary tumors of the orbit rarely present emergently except in the setting of intratumoral hemorrhage leading to pain and/or acute vision loss.

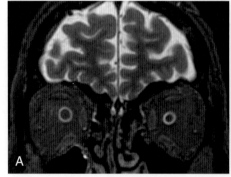 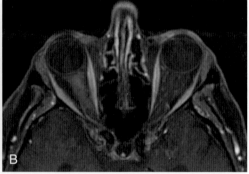

Figure 5-40 Lymphomatous uveitis. A, Coronal short tau inversion recovery (STIR) image demonstrates enlargement of the right optic nerve in this patient with non-Hodgkin lymphoma and acute vision loss. **B,** Axial contrast-enhanced T1-weighted fat-saturated image reveals patchy enhancement of the enlarged right optic nerve.

Breast cancer is the most common metastatic lesion of the orbit in women. It may present decades after original treatment. Patients typically present with restricted extraocular motility and enophthalmos. Although the tumor has infiltrated the orbit diffusely, it typically induces a fibrous response, pulling the globe into the orbit.

Bronchogenic carcinoma is the most common source of orbital metastatic disease in men. It presents with proptosis and reduced extraocular muscle motility.

Orbital lymphoma most commonly presents as a progressively enlarging orbital mass. These lesions commonly occur anterior in the orbit (most frequently in the lacrimal fossa) and most commonly are not painful. Orbital lymphomas vary histologically, but most commonly orbital lymphomas are either mucosa-associated lymphoid tissue lymphomas or chronic lymphocytic lymphoma. Orbital lymphoma typically occurs unilater-

ally. Cases of bilateral lymphoproliferative disease should raise suspicion of possible systemic disease, although, even in patients with bilateral involvement, local treatment may be sufficient. Magnetic resonance imaging is especially valuable in the diagnosis of orbital lymphoma, classically demonstrating infiltration of orbital structures without distortion or indentation of the globe.

Rhabdomyosarcoma is the most common primary orbital malignancy in children and may present as rapid unilateral proptosis, with or without ptosis or strabismus. Rhabdomyosarcoma typically affects children around age 10 years. Computed tomography and MRI are especially helpful in determining the burden of disease. Children with suspected rhabdomyosarcoma should have a chest x-ray examination to look for distant metastasis.

Neuroblastoma may metastasize to the orbit, inducing abrupt ecchymosis and proptosis sometimes referred to

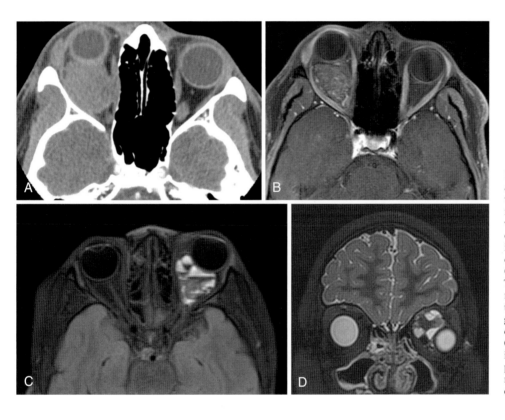

Figure 5-41 Lymphangioma and venolymphatic malformation. A, Contrast computed tomography (CT) in an adolescent patient with acutely worsening proptosis demonstrates a homogeneous mass, isodense with extraocular muscles displacing the globe anteriorly. **B,** Contrast-enhanced fat-saturated T1-weighted image reveals heterogeneous enhancement, expansion of the orbit, and displacement of the globe and optic nerve. Findings are consistent with a lymphangioma. **C** and **D,** Magnetic resonance image (MRI) in another child with proptosis reveals an expansile mass with fluid-fluid levels typical of venolymphatic malformation.

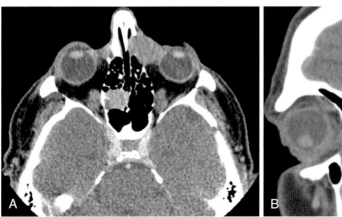
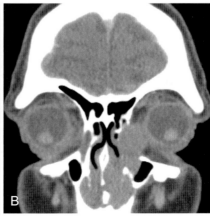

Figure 5-42 Plasmacytoma. A and **B,** Axial and coronal contrast-enhanced computed tomography (CECT) of the orbits and paranasal sinuses reveal a mass involving the left lateral nasal wall, ethmoid sinuses, and inferomedial orbit contiguous with the medial rectus muscle.

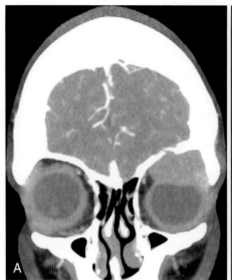
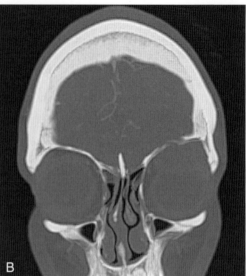

Figure 5-43 Adenoid cystic carcinoma of the lacrimal gland. A and **B,** Coronal computed tomography (CT) and soft tissue and bone windows from a CT angiogram demonstrate an expansile homogeneously enhancing mass lesion with bone destruction. Note the dehiscence of the orbital roof.

as *raccoon eyes*. Bony destruction is commonly noted on CT and MRI. Because orbital metastasis typically occurs late, identification of orbital neuroblastoma necessitates a full systemic evaluation.

■ PHYSIOLOGIC CALCIFICATIONS AND POSTSURGICAL CHANGES

The radiologist will identify various physiologic calcifications and surgical implants during the course of routine imaging. Familiarity with the appearance of these findings will help to differentiate them from orbital foreign bodies.

Scleral Buckle

Scleral buckle is a silicone band used to encircle the globe to repair some types of retinal detachment. Implanted directly on bare sclera, the scleral buckle compresses the equator of the globe closer toward the vitreous cavity, helping to bring the wall of the eye closer to the detached retina to aid in reattachment. Unless the scleral buckle becomes infected, it typically remains in place permanently.

Silicone Oil and Gas

To repair some retinal detachments, silicone oil or gas is instilled into the eye to tamponade the retina against the choroid. Oil is typically removed at a later date, and gas is gradually absorbed, but these may be detected on routine imaging.

Glaucoma Drainage Devices

Although medical management of glaucoma has improved, some patients still require surgical treatment to lower their eye pressure. These devices (Molteno, Baerveldt, Ahmed, and Eagle Vision) are made of either polypropylene or silicone. They include a plate that rests on the posterior sclera, ranging from 133 to 365 mm^2,

and a tube extending into the anterior chamber. Fluid is drained from the eye into the subconjunctival space. Although these may be noted incidentally, it is important to remember that all glaucoma implants increase the risk for endophthalmitis.

■ SUMMARY

Imaging of the orbit with CT in the setting of nontraumatic orbital emergencies is most helpful in the localization and characterization of intraorbital processes causing compromise of structure and/or function of the orbital contents. Awareness of the normal anatomy and pathologic conditions of the orbit and the clinical manifestations can improve diagnostic accuracy.

Selected Reading

Adesanya OO, Dawkins DM: Intraorbital wooden foreign body (IOFB): mimicking air on CT, *Emerg Radiol* 14:45–49, 2007.

Avery LL, Susarla SM, Novelline RA: Multidetector and three-dimensional CT evaluation of the patient with maxillofacial injury, *Radiol Clin North Am* 49(1):183–203, 2011.

Bonavolonta G, Strianese D, Grassi P, et al: An analysis of 2,480 space-occupying lesions of the orbit from 1976 to 2011, *Ophthal Plast Reconstr Surg* 29:79–86, 2013.

Bord SP, Linden J: Trauma to the globe and orbit, *Emerg Med Clin North Am* 26:97–123, 2008. vi-vii.

Burlew CC, Biffl WL, Moore EE, et al: Blunt cerebrovascular injuries: redefining screening criteria in the era of noninvasive diagnosis, *J Trauma Acute Care Surg* 72:330–335, 2012.

Capps EF, Kinsella JJ, Gupta M, et al: Emergency imaging assessment of acute, nontraumatic conditions of the head and neck, *Radiographics* 30:1335–1352, 2010.

Catapano J, Fialkov JA, Binhammer PA, et al: A new system for severity scoring of facial fractures: development and validation, *J Craniofac Surg* 21(4): 1098–1103, 2010.

Crespo AN, Chone CT, Fonseca AS, et al: Clinical versus computed tomography evaluation in the diagnosis and management of deep neck infection, *Sao Paulo Med J* 122(6):259–263, 2004.

De Wyngaert R, Casteels I, Demaerel P: Orbital and anterior visual pathway infection and inflammation, *Neuroradiology* 51:385–396, 2009.

Detorakis ET, Drakonaki E, Kymionis G, et al: Clinical and imaging findings in multifocal orbital vascular lesions: a case series, *Semin Ophthalmol* 24: 241–244, 2009.

DiCocco JM, Emmett KP, Fabian TC, et al: Blunt cerebrovascular injury screening with 32-channel multidetector computed tomography: more slices still don't cut it, *Ann Surg* 253:444–450, 2011.

Dunkin JM, Crum AV, Swanger RS, et al: Globe trauma, *Semin Ultrasound CT MR* 32:51–56, 2011.

Figueira EC, Francis IC, Wilcsek GA: Intraorbital glass foreign body missed on CT imaging, *Ophthal Plast Reconstr Surg* 23:80–82, 2007.

Gadre AK, Gadre KC: Infections of the deep spaces of the neck. In Bailey BJ, Johnson JT, editors: *Head and Neck Surgery: otolaryngology*, ed 4, Philadelphia, PA, 2006, Lippincott Williams & Wilkins, p 665–682.

Gonzalez-Beicos A, Nunez D: Imaging of acute head and neck infections, *Radiol Clin North Am* 50(1):73–83, 2012.

Gor DM, Kirsch CF, Leen J, et al: Radiologic differentiation of intraocular glass: evaluation of imaging techniques, glass types, size, and effect of intraocular hemorrhage, *AJR Am J Roentgenol* 177:1199–1203, 2001.

Hardjasudarma M, Rivera E, Ganley JP, et al: Computed tomography of traumatic dislocation of the lens, *Emerg Radiol* 1:180–182, 1994.

Inaba K, Branco BC, Menaker J, et al: Evaluation of multidetector computed tomography for penetrating neck injury: a prospective multicenter study, *J Trauma Acute Care Surg* 72:576–583, 2012.

Kruger JM, Lessell S, Cestari DM: Neuro-imaging: a review for the general ophthalmologist, *Semin Ophthalmol* 27:192–196, 2012.

Kubal WS: Imaging of orbital trauma, *Radiographics* 28:1729–1739, 2008.

Lane JI, Watson RE, Witte RJ, et al: Retinal detachment: imaging of surgical treatments and complications, *Radiographics* 23:983–994, 2003.

LeBedis CA, Sakai O: Nontraumatic orbital conditions: diagnosis with CT and MR imaging in the emergent setting, *Radiographics* 28:1741–1753, 2008.

Lento J, Glynn S, Shetty V, et al: Psychologic functioning and needs of indigent patients with facial injury: a prospective controlled study, *J Oral Maxillofac Surg* 62(8):925–932, 2004.

Linnau KF, Hallam DK, Lomoschitz FM, et al: Orbital apex injury: trauma at the junction between the face and the cranium, *Eur J Radiol* 48:5–16, 2003.

Linnau KF, Stanley RB, Hallam DK, et al: Imaging of high-energy midfacial trauma: what the surgeon needs to know, *Eur J Radiol.* 48(1):17–32, 2003.

Ludwig BJ, Foster BR, Saito N, et al: Diagnostic imaging in nontraumatic pediatric head and neck emergencies, *Radiographics* 30(3):781–799, 2010.

Lui A, Glynn S, Shetty V: The interplay of perceived social support and posttraumatic psychological distress following orofacial injury, *J Nerv Ment Dis* 197(9):639–645, 2009.

Mafee MF, Karimi A, Shah J, et al: Anatomy and pathology of the eye: role of MR imaging and CT, *Neuroimaging Clin N Am* 15:23–47, 2005.

Mahajan A, Crum A, Johnson MH, et al: Ocular neoplastic disease, *Semin Ultrasound CT MR* 32:28–37, 2011.

Malhotra A, Minja FJ, Crum A, et al: Ocular anatomy and cross-sectional imaging of the eye, *Semin Ultrasound CT MR* 32:2–13, 2011.

McKellop JA, Bou-Assaly W, Mukherji SK: Emergency head and neck imaging: infections and inflammatory processes, *Neuroimaging Clin N Am* 20(4):651–661, 2010.

Mehta N, Butala P, Bernstein MP: The imaging of maxillofacial trauma and its pertinence to surgical intervention, *Radiol Clin North Am* 50(1):43–57, 2012.

Novelline R, Liebig T, Jordan J, et al: Computed tomography of ocular trauma, *Emerg Radiol* 1:56–67, 1994.

Ozgen B, Oguz KK, Oguz CA: Diffusion MR imaging features of skull base osteomyelitis compared with skull base malignancy, *Am J Neuroradiol* 32:179–184, 2011.

Platnick J, Crum AV, Soohoo S, et al: The globe: infection, inflammation and systemic disease, *Semin Ultrasound CT MR* 32:38–50, 2011.

Rao AA, Naheedy JH, Chen JY, et al: A clinical update and radiologic review of pediatric orbital and ocular tumors, *J Oncol* 2013:975908, 2013.

Rudloe TF, Harper MB, Prabhu SP, et al: Acute periorbital infections: who needs emergent imaging? *Pediatrics* 125:e719–e726, 2010.

Schwab P, Harmon D, Bruno R, et al: A 55-year-old woman with orbital inflammation, *Arthritis Care Res* 64:1776–1782, 2012.

Segev Y, Goldstein M, Lazar M, et al: CT appearance of a traumatic cataract, *AJNR Am J Neuroradiol* 16:1174–1175, 1995.

Sliker CW: Blunt cerebrovascular injuries: imaging with multidetector CT angiography, *Radiographics* 28:1689–16708, 2008.

Steenburg SD, Sliker CW, Shanmuganathan K, et al: Imaging evaluation of penetrating neck injuries, *Radiographics* 30:869–886, 2010.

Vieira F, Allen SM, Stocks RM, et al: Deep neck infection, *Otolaryngol Clin North Am* 41(3):459–483, 2008.

Wang AC, Charters MA, Thawani JP, et al: Evaluating the use and utility of noninvasive angiography in diagnosing traumatic blunt cerebrovascular injury, *J Trauma Acute Care Surg* 72:1601–1610, 2012.

SPINE EMERGENCIES

CHAPTER **6**

Spinal Trauma

Cervical Spine Emergencies

Mark Bernstein, Alexander B. Baxter, and F.A. Mann

Each year in North America approximately 3 million patients are evaluated for spinal injury. Although the incidence of vertebral fracture and spinal cord injuries is low, the consequences of a missed injury or delayed diagnosis can be devastating. Although most cervical spine fractures are localized to a single vertebra, two or three noncontiguous injuries are often seen in high-energy trauma, occurring in up to 25% of patients.

Accurate diagnosis requires cooperation between clinician and radiologist, a reliable and repeatable approach to interpreting cervical spine computed tomography (CT), and the awareness that a patient may have a significant and unstable ligamentous injury despite normal imaging findings. This chapter reviews imaging modalities, approach to image evaluation, concepts of stability, and descriptions of common cervical spine injury patterns.

■ IMAGING APPROACH AND MODALITIES

Screening

Emergency physicians triage patients with suspected cervical spine injury into high- and low-risk groups, those who require imaging for confirmation and accurate evaluation and those who can be confidently discharged. Both the Canadian C-spine (Cervical Spine) Rule (CCR) and the National Emergency X-radiography Utilization Study (NEXUS) criteria provide guidelines for deciding which patient for whom imaging is not indicated (Table 6-1). Anyone with midline tenderness, focal neurologic deficit, altered sensorium, or a distracting injury requires CT imaging, as well as protection of the spine in a hard cervical collar. Other high-risk factors include age greater than 65 years and significant energy-transfer mechanism. Systematic use of validated clinical decision rules substantially reduces unnecessary cervical spine imaging in adult (CCR, NEXUS) and pediatric (NEXUS) victims of blunt trauma.

Because osseous displacement that occurs *at the moment of impact* can be subsequently reduced by recoil and muscle spasm, and because placement of a hard collar can mask instability by maintaining vertebral alignment, an apparently normal examination should be viewed with skepticism in any patient with neurologic deficit or persistent pain; significant ligamentous injury may be present despite normal CT findings. Magnetic resonance imaging (MRI) detects ligamentous edema with great sensitivity, but ligamentous edema alone does not necessarily indicate an unstable injury. Dynamic evaluation with delayed flexion and extension radiographs under neurosurgical supervision is the sine qua non for identification of unstable ligamentous injury, and patients with pain but without neurologic symptoms are generally discharged in a hard cervical collar. Flexion/extension radiographs are best performed 1 to 2 weeks after injury, after muscle spasm has had sufficient time to resolve.

Conventional Radiographs

Conventional radiographs of the cervical spine have been replaced by multidetector CT as the primary screening tool for detection and characterization of cervical spine trauma. In the initial imaging evaluation of cervical spine injury, the American College of Radiology (ACR) Appropriateness Criteria recommends conventional radiography only when CT is not available.

Computed Tomography

Multidetector CT with thin-section reconstruction and sagittal and coronal multiplanar reformations (MPRs) identifies the exact location and displacement of fractures and bone fragments and defines the extent of any potential spinal canal, neuroforaminal, or vascular compromise.

Computed Tomography Angiography

The aim of CT angiography (CTA) in the setting of acute cervical spine trauma is to detect asymptomatic vascular injury and prevent subsequent stroke with early anticoagulation. Vascular injury is present in greater than 20% of patients who are screened using the following criteria:

Diffuse axonal injury with Glasgow Coma Scale score of less than 6.

Skull base fracture extending to the carotid canal.

Le Fort II or III fracture.

Severe cervical spine fractures.

Cervical spine fractures involving a transverse foramen.

Table 6-1   Appropriate Patient Selection for Imaging

Canadian C-Spine Rule (CCR) Imaging Not Indicated	NEXUS Criteria (Low Risk) Imaging Not Indicated
Absence of high-risk factors, including: ■ Age >65 years ■ "Dangerous mechanism"* ■ Paresthesias in extremities Low-risk factors that allow safe assessment of range of motion, including: ■ Simple rear-end motor vehicle collision† ■ Sitting position in emergency department ■ Ambulatory at any time ■ Delayed onset of neck pain ■ Absence of midline cervical tenderness Able to actively rotate neck 45 degrees left and right	No midline cervical tenderness No focal neurologic deficits No intoxication or indication of brain injury No painful distracting‡ injuries Normal alertness

*"Dangerous mechanism" defined as fall from an elevation of 3 feet or five stairs, axial load to the head (e.g., diving), motor vehicle collision at high speed (>45 mph or >100 km/hr) or with rollover or ejection, collision involving a motorized recreational vehicle (e.g., all-terrain vehicle), or bicycle collision (M. Copass, personal communication, 2005).
†Simple rear-end motor vehicle collision excludes being pushed into oncoming traffic, being hit by a bus or a large truck, a rollover, and being hit by a high-speed vehicle (M. Copass, personal communication, 2005).
‡"Distracting" injuries identified by loss of two-point discrimination ≥ 4 mm (M. Copass, personal communication, 2005).
C-spine, Cervical spine; *NEXUS,* National Emergency X-radiography Utilization Study.

Approximately 20% of untreated patients in whom an asymptomatic cerebrovascular injury is detected will suffer a significant complication, usually embolic infarct or intracerebral hemorrhage. Less than 1% of medically treated patients will do so.

Magnetic Resonance Imaging

When available and following CT assessment of osseous spinal integrity, MRI is valuable in evaluation of patients with an acute neurologic deficit because it accurately identifies epidural hematoma, traumatic disk herniation, and spinal cord contusion. But the immediate clinical question in acute spine trauma is always "Does the patient require surgical decompression?" and evaluation of canal and neuroforaminal patency is adequately accomplished by CT alone.

Sagittal T2 and gradient-echo magnetic resonance (MR) sequences are of particular value in depicting patterns predictive of neurologic outcome: normal, single versus multilevel edema, spinal cord hemorrhage, and cord rupture.

■ IMAGE EVALUATION AND INTERPRETATION

An accurate clinical history that specifies injury mechanism and location of pain is essential for interpreting the significance of subtle findings, particularly in older patients with degenerative disk disease or prior injury. To avoid the common errors of observation failure and satisfaction of search, it is helpful to have a checklist in mind that ensures all important structures are examined and that common injury patterns are sought as outlined in the following subsections.

Transaxial Images
Examine the integrity and rotational alignment of each vertebral segment, facet joint articulations, cervical soft tissues, spinal canal diameter, and neuroforaminal patency (Fig. 6-1, *A* and *B*).

Midline Sagittal Images
Evaluate the prevertebral soft tissues, the thickness of which should be less than 5 mm at C2 or 15 mm at C5 (due to the normal esophagus). The anterior spinal line, posterior spinal line, and spinolaminar line should be continuous, and interspinous distances should be uniform. The dens-basion distance should be 9.5 mm or less, and a line drawn vertically along the dorsal body of C2 (posterior axial line) should be less than 5.5 mm posterior to the basion. The atlantodental interval should be less than 3 mm in adults. The C1-2 interspinous distance measured at the spinolaminal line should be less then 7.8 mm (see Fig. 6-1, *C*).

Parasagittal Images
The occipital condyles should be intact. The atlanto-occipital and atlantoaxial articulations should be congruent, and the facets should align normally, with the inferior articulating facet of the upper vertebral body posterior to the superior articulating facet of the adjacent lower vertebral body (see Fig. 6-1, *D*).

Coronal Images
The occipital condyles, C1, and C2 should be intact and aligned. The dens should be centered between the lateral masses of C1 (see Fig.6-1, *E*).

In addition to developing a repeatable approach, maintaining suspicion that a radiographically normal spine may still be injured, and appreciating the surgical decisions that must be made in the acute setting, familiarity with the appearance of common cervical spine fracture patterns and an understanding of spinal stability is invaluable.

■ CONCEPTS OF STABILITY

A stable spine is able to withstand physiologic loads without producing mechanical deformity, progressive neurologic injury, or worsening pain. These are biomechanical rather than anatomic concepts, and imaging studies predict stability only indirectly, by evaluating the condition of the vertebrae and their ligamentous supports. Stability at the craniocervical junction depends on the integrity of the transverse ligament, the tectorial membrane, and the alar and apical ligaments and their bony attachments.

Both clinically and radiologically, the three-column concept of Denis is most widely applied for evaluating thoracolumbar spine stability (Fig. 6-2). It is reasonable to extrapolate these concepts to the subaxial (C3-C7) cervical spine. In Denis's model the anterior column includes the anterior longitudinal ligament and the anterior vertebral body and disk. The middle column includes the posterior vertebral body cortex, posterior disk anulus, and the posterior longitudinal ligament. The posterior column includes the posterior bony arch, facets, and the posterior ligament complex (PLC) composed of the

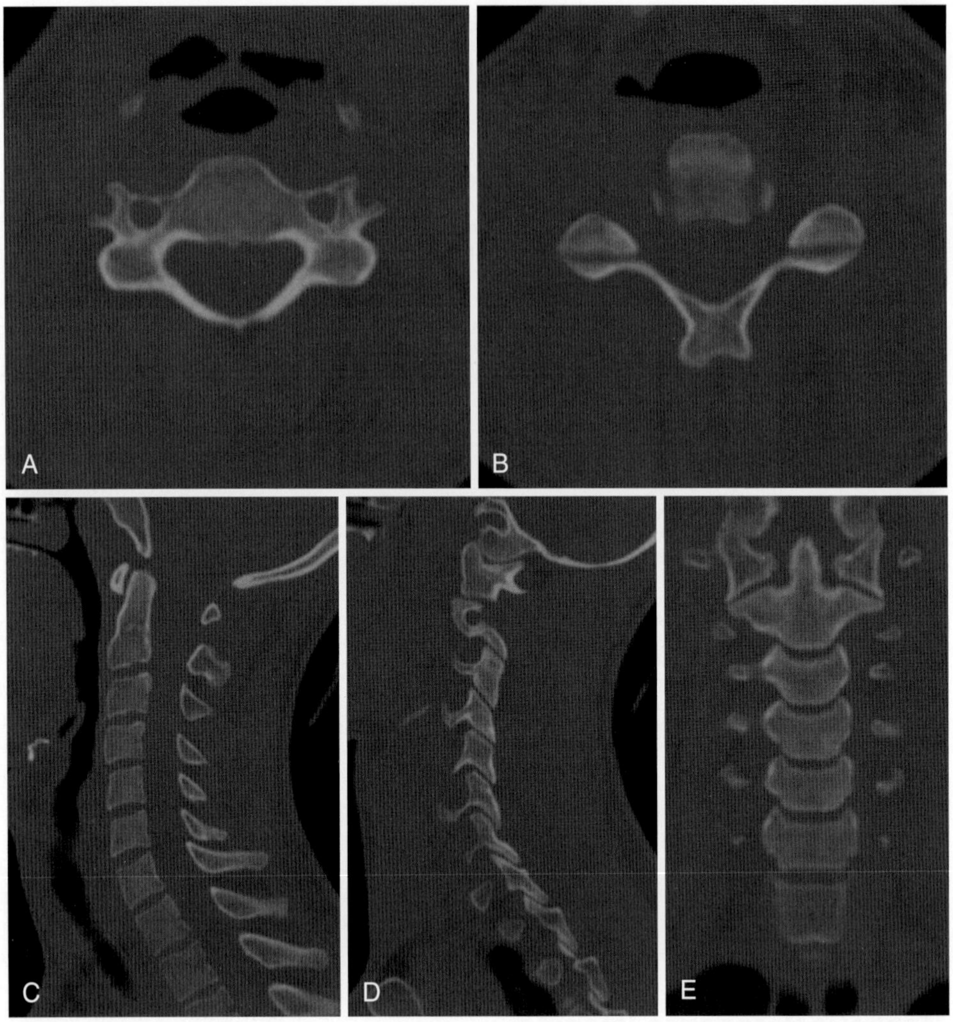

Figure 6-1 Normal cervical spine computed tomography (CT). A and B, Transaxial images shows complete intact bony ring surrounding the spinal canal. Normal facet articulations are present bilaterally in a "hamburger bun" configuration. Normal prevertebral soft tissues. C, Midsagittal CT reformation shows normal prevertebral soft tissues, as well as normal alignment of anterior and posterior vertebral body lines, and spinolaminar line. The basion-dens interval is less than 9.5 mm, and the atlantodental interval is less than 3 mm. D, Parasagittal CT reformation demonstrates normal relationship between occipital condyles and lateral mass of C1. Facet alignment is normal with an appearance of "shingles on a roof." E, Coronal CT reformation shows alignment between occipital condyles, C1, and C2, with centered dens.

ligamentum flavum, the facet joint capsules, and the interspinous and supraspinous ligaments. Injury of two or three columns is considered unstable, with the key contributing factor being disruption of the middle column.

■ INJURY PATTERNS—CRANIOCERVICAL SPINE

Atlantooccipital Dissociation

Atlantooccipital dissociation (AOD) results from high-energy trauma sufficient to separate the skull base from the upper cervical spine. It is invariably accompanied by severe neurologic dysfunction and concomitant injuries to the torso and extremities. The spectrum of AOD ranges from true dislocation, which is usually lethal, to subluxation, which is unstable but survivable. Most injuries in AOD are limited to soft tissue trauma (alar ligaments and tectorial membrane). Fractures are uncommon and when present are usually bilateral occipital condyle and clival avulsion fractures. Mixed bony and ligamentous injury patterns consist of bilateral occipital condyle fractures with associated tectorial membrane disruption.

Cross-sectional imaging, particularly CT, is most accurate in detecting AOD in the acute setting. Abnormal

findings in AOD include prevertebral soft tissue swelling at C2, a basion-dens interval greater than 9.5 mm measured in the midsagittal plane, and atlantooccipital condyle articulations greater than 1.4 mm in width (Fig. 6-3, A and B). Associated vascular injury can be evaluated with CTA, MR angiography, or catheter angiography.

Occipital Condyle Fractures

Several classification schemes for occipital condyle fractures have been proposed. However, in the absence of findings for AOD, description rather than classification of occipital condyle fractures seems warranted because no outcome differences by subtype have been demonstrated.

Atlantoaxial Rotatory Fixation

Atlantoaxial rotatory fixation (AARF) is a form of atlantoaxial dissociation characterized by rotational malalignment between the C1 and C2 vertebrae. AARF occurs within the physiologic range of motion at the C1/C2 joints and is thought to be secondary to muscle spasm and swelling or tearing of joint capsular soft tissues. In adults, AARF is invariably traumatic in cause and is associated with cervical pain and torticollis.

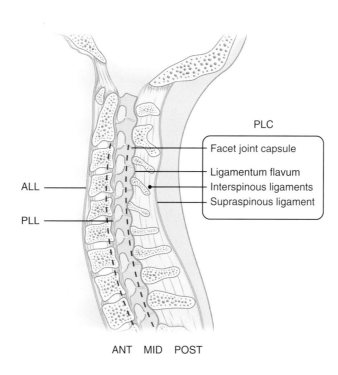

PLC
Facet joint capsule
Ligamentum flavum
Interspinous ligaments
Supraspinous ligament

ALL

PLL

ANT   MID   POST

Figure 6-2 Three-column theory of Denis. Denis's three-column theory has been applied to the subaxial cervical spine (C3-C7) for assessment of spinal stability. The anterior column includes the anterior longitudinal ligament (ALL), and anterior vertebral body and disk. The middle column includes the posterior longitudinal ligament (PLL), the posterior vertebral body cortex, and posterior disk anulus. The posterior column involves the posterior ligament complex (PLC), facets, and posterior vertebral bony arches. Injury involving two or three columns is considered unstable.

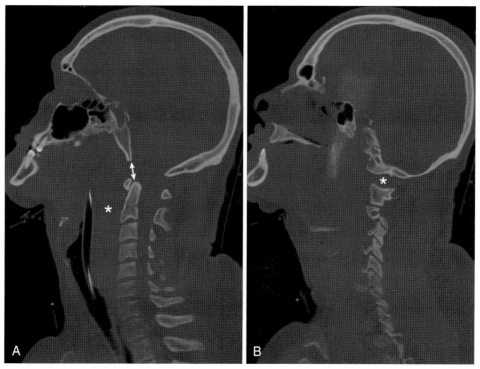

Figure 6-3 Atlantooccipital dissociation. A, Midsagittal computed tomography (CT) reformation shows marked prevertebral soft tissue swelling anterior to C2 (*) and increased basion-dens interval *(double headed arrow)*. **B,** Parasagittal CT reformation shows a noncongruent and wide atlantooccipital interval (*).

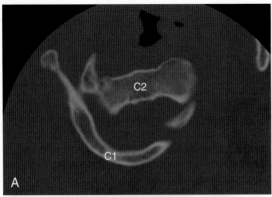
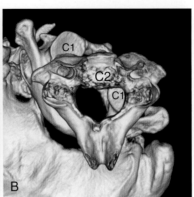
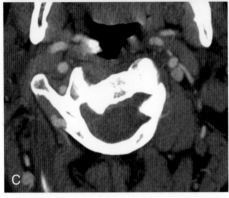

Figure 6-4 Atlantoaxial rotatory fixation (AARF). A, Transaxial computed tomography (CT) image shows rotational malalignment between C1 and C2. **B**, Three-dimensional (3-D) CT reconstruction viewed from inferiorly shows rotational malalignment with exposed portions of C1 lateral masses. **C**, CT angiogram fails to show filling of the left vertebral artery.

AARF is most commonly a pure rotational injury, with the odontoid as the pivot. In type I injuries, intact transverse and alar ligaments prevent excessive anterior displacement. In type II injuries, isolated disruption of the transverse ligament produces 3 to 5 mm anterior translation with rotation centered on one of the articular masses. Type III injuries have more than 5 mm translation with rotation because of a combination of transverse ligament and alar ligament disruption. Posterior displacement of C1 on C2 secondary to alar and transverse ligament injury combined with a deficient odontoid characterizes type IV injuries.

Computed tomography shows rotation or dislocation at the C1-C2 lateral masses, where the jaw and the neck appear pointed in different directions (Fig. 6-4, *A* and *B*). True fixation versus simple head turning can be confirmed clinically or by repeating CT with patient in maximal rotation to the opposite direction, though this is rarely necessary. Potential rotational injury to the stretched contralateral vertebral artery is best evaluated with CTA (see Fig. 6-4, *C*). Early diagnosis leads to improved outcome.

C1—Jefferson and Variant Jefferson Fractures

The first cervical vertebra (C1, atlas) supports the cranium through its articulations with the occipital condyles. Anatomically it is a simple bony ring with two lateral masses connected anteriorly and posteriorly by the neural arches. This unique shape allows for great range of motion. The odontoid process of C2 (axis) articulates with the anterior arch of C1 and is held in place by the transverse ligament, the integrity of which is the key determinant of atlantoaxial stability.

Transverse ligament disruptions are most commonly avulsions that heal with nonoperative management; however, a few purely ligamentous failures will remain truly unstable.

The classic Jefferson fracture results from axial loading on a straight cervical spine with forces transmitted from the vertex through the occipital condyles to the C1 lateral masses (Fig. 6-5, *A*). The result is a four-part fracture. Fractures occur at the weakest points of the ring, the anterior and posterior junctions of the arches and lateral masses (see Fig. 6-5, *B*). In the classic Jefferson fracture, the transverse ligament remains intact and there is no subluxation between C1 and C2. Thus, in the absence of concomitant fractures or ligamentous disruption, the classic Jefferson burst is both mechanically and neurologically stable.

Asymmetric axial loading produces the atypical Jefferson fracture, with two or three rather than four fractures of the C1 ring. In this fracture the transverse ligament is disrupted, and C1 fragments are laterally subluxed relative to C2 (see Fig. 6-5, *C*). Transverse separation of fracture fragments, greater than 5.4 mm on CT or 7 mm on radiographs (odontoid view), indicates transverse ligament injury and instability. This measurement, known as the *rule of Spence*, can be made on transverse or coronal CT. Other signs of instability include avulsion of the C1 tubercle (transverse ligament insertion), two anterior ring fractures with an intact posterior arch, and an atlantodental interval greater than 3 mm in adults or 5 mm in children. Magnetic resonance imaging is highly sensitive in directly identifying transverse ligament discontinuity. Pitfalls in the evaluation of C1 fractures include congenital fusion anomalies and aplasias that may simulate fractures. These are identified by their smooth, well-corticated margins.

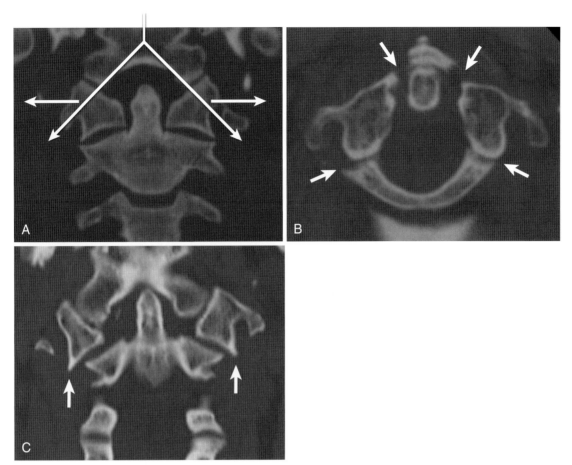

Figure 6-5 Jefferson fracture. A, Coronal computed tomography (CT) image shows mechanism of injury with axial load force on a straight cervical spine transmitted through the skull base *(vertical arrow)*, across the occipital condyles *(oblique arrows)*, and onto the C1 lateral masses *(horizontal arrows)*. **B,** Transaxial CT image of a classic Jefferson fracture shows two anterior *(arrows)* and two posterior *(arrows)* arch fractures with a normal atlantodental interval. **C,** Coronal CT reformation of a Jefferson variant shows lateral subluxation of C1 lateral masses, overhanging the lateral margins of C2 *(arrows)*. Widening of the spaces between the dens and lateral masses indicates transverse ligament rupture.

C2—Odontoid Fractures

C2 (axis) fractures represent approximately 15% to 20% of all cervical spine fractures, and the majority of these involve the odontoid process. Odontoid fractures are especially common in older adults and may occur following even minor trauma. In patients younger than 50 years, odontoid fractures often result from high-energy events and are commonly associated with other fractures and subluxations, frequently unstable in the aggregate.

A type I fracture is a small apical avulsion at the alar or apical ligament insertion (Fig. 6-6, *A*). Type II, the most common C2 fracture, is a simple transverse odontoid fracture (see Fig. 6-6, *B*). Type III fractures extend variably into the C2 body (see Fig. 6-6, *C*). In the absence of other indications of craniocervical instability (increased dens-basion distance, incongruous articular surfaces), type I fractures are considered stable. Type II fractures that show 4 mm or greater displacement or are comminuted have a high incidence of nonunion. Patients in this group are also more likely to have an associated neurologic injury or respiratory compromise. Type III odontoid fractures almost always heal with rigid collar immobilization.

C2—"Hanged-Man" Fractures

The hanged-man fracture, or traumatic C2 spondylolisthesis, classically results from hyperextension with fracture of both of the pars interarticularis or pedicles of C2 (Fig. 6-7, *A*). Although the eponym *hanged-man fracture* is derived from historic cases of judicial hanging, today most result from falls and motor vehicle crashes. They are often asymmetric and are considered *atypical* if the fracture propagates into the posterior vertebral body. Atypical fracture patterns are actually quite common and may involve the transverse foramen, placing the vertebral artery at risk for injury (see Fig. 6-7, *B*). The classification system devised by Effendi and modified by Levine and Edwards is the most widely used.

Type I fracture: Bilateral pars fractures without significant translation or angulation. These result from hyperextension or axial loading and are considered mechanically and neurologically stable.

Type II fractures: C2-3 disk disruption with anterior translation of the C2 body. These are the most common type of hanged-man fracture and result from hyperextension and axial loading with subsequent hyperflexion. Type II fractures are unstable.

Type IIA fractures: Unstable flexion-distraction injury resulting in C2 body angulation without translation.

Type III fractures: Anterior translation and angulation with facet subluxation or frank dislocation. These are highly unstable injuries that result from hyperflexion and compression.

Hanged-man fractures may be radiographically subtle and can be overlooked but should be easily identified on CT with multiplanar reformations. Atypical fractures, involving the transverse foramen, or those associated with neurologic deficit should be followed with angiographic imaging, usually CTA, to exclude vertebral artery injury. Types IIA and III fractures require internal fixation and therefore must be differentiated from Types I and II. Concurrent craniocervical fractures are common and should be excluded. These include odontoid

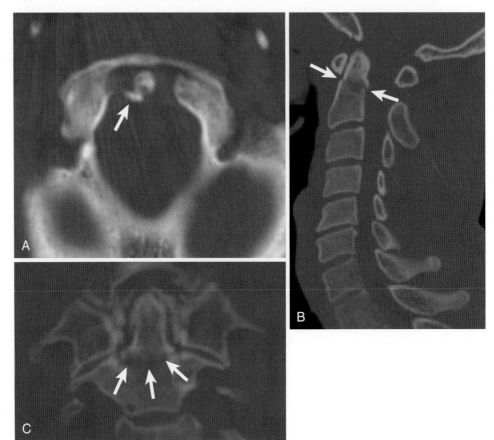

Figure 6-6 Odontoid (dens) fractures. A, Transaxial computed tomography (CT) image shows small avulsion fracture from the tip of the odontoid *(arrow)*, representing a type I fracture. **B,** Midsagittal CT reformation shows an undisplaced fracture through the odontoid (between *arrows*), representing a type II fracture. **C,** Coronal CT reformation shows an undisplaced fracture below the odontoid involving the C2 body *(arrows)*, representing a type III fracture.

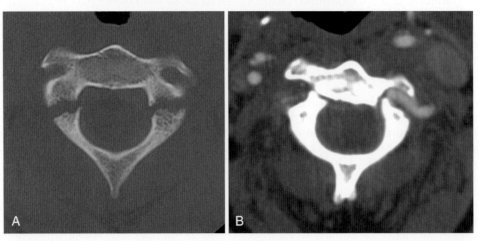

Figure 6-7 Hanged-man fracture. A, Transaxial computed tomography (CT) image demonstrates bilateral fractures through the pars interarticularis, or pedicles, of C2. (Reproduced with permission from Naderi S, Bernsyein M. Computed tomography. In: Legome E, Schockley LW, eds. *CT Trauma: A Comprehensive Emergency Medicine Approach.* Cambridge, UK: Cambridge University Press; 2011.) **B,** Transaxial CT angiogram image shows an atypical hanged-man fracture extending into the C2 body and involving the transverse foramina. There is occlusion of the right vertebral artery with normal flow on the left.

fractures, posterior C1 arch fractures, and hyperextension teardrop fractures.

■ INJURY PATTERNS—SUBAXIAL CERVICAL SPINE

Most subaxial cervical spine injuries occur in younger patients, involve high-energy mechanisms, and occur at or around the C5-C6 level. In older patients, injuries may follow lower-energy trauma (such as fall from standing height). Hyperextension injuries are more common than flexion injuries in older adults.

Hyperflexion Injuries

Hyperflexion injuries describe a spectrum of progressive ligamentous disruption from posterior to anterior, encompassing hyperflexion sprain, anterior subluxation, bilateral interfacetal dislocation (BID), and the flexion teardrop fracture (Fig. 6-8, *A* to *E*). Hyperflexion injuries are best evaluated on sagittal CT reformations. Specific findings include (from posterior to anterior; see Fig. 6-8, *F*):
1. Fanning of spinous processes/interspinous widening.
2. Uncovered or nonparallel facet articulations.

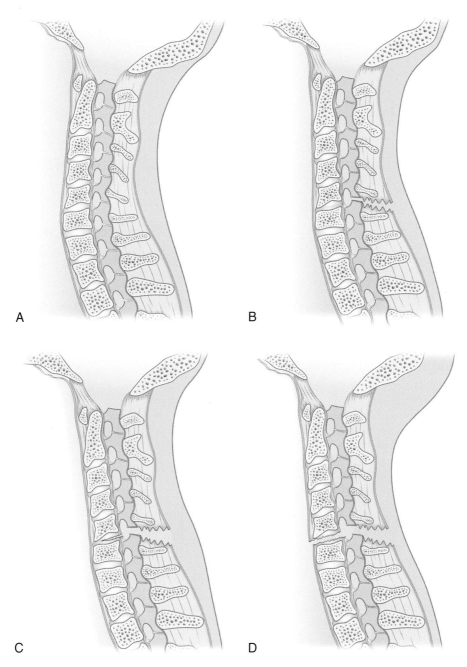

A   B

C   D

Figure 6-8 *Spectrum of hyperflexion injuries.* **A**, Normal cervical alignment. **B**, Hyperflexion sprain with disruption of posterior ligament complex (PLC), with intact posterior longitudinal ligament (PLL) and anterior longitudinal ligament (ALL). **C**, Anterior subluxation with PLC and PLL disruption, focal kyphosis, facet joint incongruity, and mild anterior subluxation. This injury is unstable. **D**, Bilateral interfacetal dislocation (BID) with perched facets. All ligaments are disrupted from posterior to anterior with kyphosis.

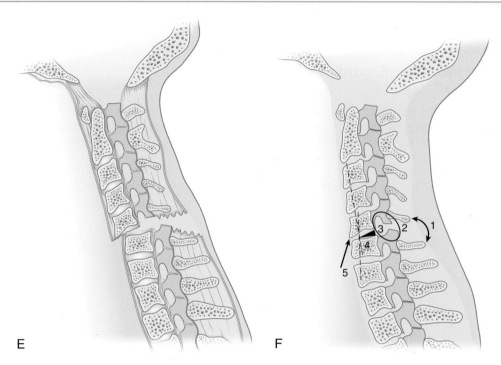

E   F

Figure 6-8, cont'd **E**, BID with jumped facets. **F**, Schematic showing the hallmarks of hyperflexion injuries: *1*, Interspinous widening; *2*, facet widening; *3*, wide posterior disk space; *4*, focal kyphosis; and *5*, anterior subluxation.

3. Widened posterior disk space.
4. Focal kyphosis.
5. Anterior subluxation.
6. Vertebral body compression and/or anterior-inferior teardrop fractures; these occur with severe hyperflexion and subsequent axial loading (e.g., sudden deceleration and striking head on the windshield).

Hyperflexion Sprain, Anterior Subluxation

Isolated PLC disruption defines the hyperflexion sprain and does not result in spinal instability. Anterior subluxation, in contrast, follows disruption of the posterior longitudinal ligament and posterior disk anulus (middle column of Denis), as well as PLC injury, and is always unstable (Fig. 6-9).

Evaluation of hyperflexion sprain and anterior subluxation can be challenging. Imaging findings on both radiographs and CT are subtle, and even when identified, their significance may be unappreciated. A missed injury can lead to significant morbidity, including pain, subluxation/dislocation, kyphosis, and neurologic deficit. Because of these dangers, if CT findings are equivocal, MRI should be performed to detect cervical ligament and soft tissue edema. Flexion and extension radiographs should not be performed in the presence of muscle spasm to avoid false-negative results.

Bilateral Interfacetal Dislocation

Bilateral interfacetal dislocation refers to either perched or jumped cervical facets (see Fig. 6-8, *D* and *E*). In both cases the inferior articulating facet no longer lies

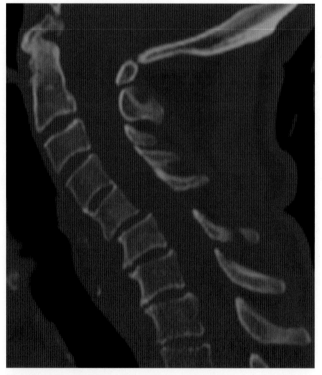

Figure 6-9 Anterior subluxation. Midsagittal computed tomography (CT) reformation reveals focal kyphosis at C5-C6, interspinous widening, and posterior disk space widening with mild anterior subluxation, hallmarks of hyperflexion injury. (Reproduced with permission from Naderi S, Bernsyein M. Computed tomography. In: Legome E, Schockley LW, eds. *CT Trauma: A Comprehensive Emergency Medicine Approach.* Cambridge, UK: Cambridge University Press; 2011.)

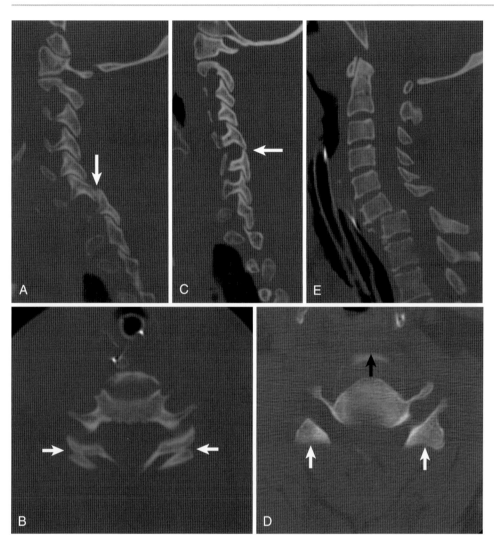

Figure 6-10 Bilateral interfacetal dislocation (BID). **A**, Parasagittal computed tomography (CT) reformation shows jumped facets at C6-C7 *(arrow)*. **B**, Transaxial CT image shows reversal of the normal "hamburger bun" bilaterally *(arrows)*. **C**, Parasagittal CT reformation of a patient with perched facets at C5-C6 *(arrow)*. **D**, Transaxial CT image in a case of perched BID shows bilateral "naked facets" *(white arrows)*. Subluxation between levels is evident *(black arrow)*. **E**, Midsagittal CT reformation in BID shows approximately 50% anterior translation of C6 on C7 with mild kyphosis.

posterior to the superior articular facet from the level below. When the facets of the upper vertebra are anterior to those of the lower vertebra, they are considered jumped (the term *locked* should be avoided because it falsely implies stability), and transaxial CT images reveal the "reverse hamburger bun" sign (Fig. 6-10, *A* and *B*). Alternatively, the facets may be perched upon one another, and transaxial CT shows "naked facets," in which no articulation is present (see Fig. 6-10, *C* and *D*). In BID the superior vertebra is anteriorly subluxed relative to the inferior vertebra by approximately 50% of the anteroposterior (AP) dimension of the vertebral body (see Fig. 6-10, *E*).

Hyperflexion combined with rotation can result in a unilateral interfacetal dislocation (UID), in which only one facet has jumped or become perched (Fig. 6-11, *A*). In contrast to BID, anterolisthesis of the superior vertebral body approximates 25% in UID (see Fig. 6-11, *B*). Bilateral interfacetal dislocation and UID are unstable, primarily ligamentous, injuries, though small impaction fractures (of no real significance) are often present at the facet tips. Magnetic resonance imaging is indicated in these injuries to assess the extent of injury to the spinal cord, the integrity of intervertebral disks and ligaments, and to detect any associated epidural hematoma.

Flexion Teardrop Fracture

The most severe hyperflexion injury is the flexion teardrop fracture, which results from marked hyperflexion followed by axial loading. Axial forces applied to an unstable flexed spine cause the upper vertebra to impact the vertebra below, shearing off its anterior-inferior corner (teardrop fragment) (Fig. 6-12, *A*). Significant interspinous and facet joint widening, as well as a sagittally oriented vertebral body fracture, are commonly seen in conjunction with the teardrop fragment (see Fig. 6-12, *B*). An anterior cord syndrome with quadriplegia and pain and temperature insensitivity, but often with preservation of vibration and position sense, is always associated with these severe injuries.

Hyperextension Injuries

Approximately 25% of cervical spine injuries result from hyperextension, either direct frontal impact or through a whiplash effect. Direct-impact injuries are often associated with facial or frontal head injuries. Conditions predisposing to injury include age greater than 65 years with increased fall risk, motor vehicle crashes, spinal canal stenosis, and osteopenia.

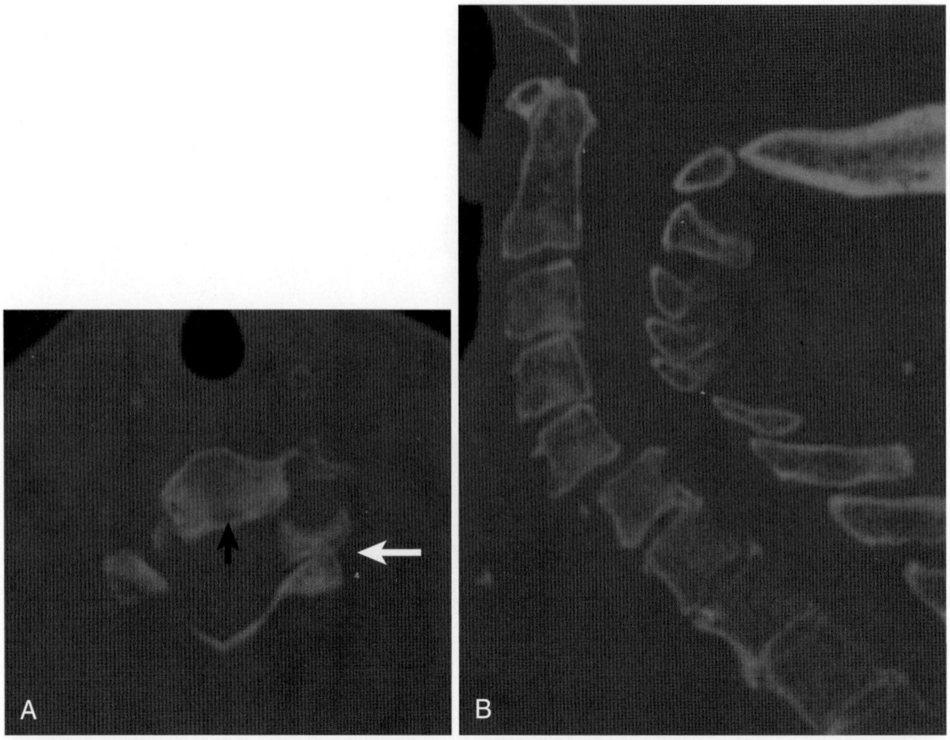

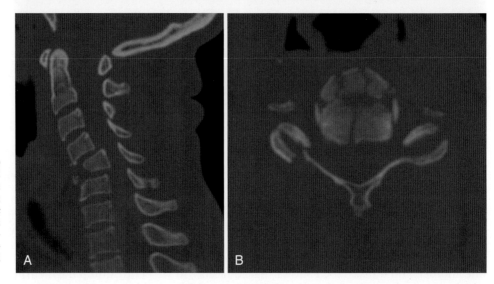

Figure 6-11 Unilateral interfacetal dislocation (UID). A, Transaxial computed tomography (CT) image shows reversed "hamburger bun" only on the left *(white arrow)* with mild anterior translation *(black arrow)*. B, Midsagittal CT reformation in UID injury shows approximately 25% anterior translation.

Figure 6-12 Flexion teardrop fracture. A, Midsagittal computed tomography (CT) reformation shows C4 teardrop fracture with kyphosis. B, Transaxial CT image shows wide facets bilaterally with C4 body teardrop fracture fragments anteriorly and sagittally oriented fracture posteriorly, typical of this injury.

Cervical spine hyperextension injuries are predominately ligamentous and range from the stable hyperextension teardrop fracture to the highly unstable hyperextension-dislocation. Ligamentous disruption progresses from anterior to posterior with increasing energy transfer sequentially involving the anterior longitudinal ligament, anterior anulus fibrosus, the posterior anulus, posterior longitudinal ligament, and ligamentum flavum. The hyperextension-dislocation injury often results in a central cord syndrome, characterized by quadriparesis with more severe upper extremity weakness and variable sensory deficits below the level of injury.

Extension Teardrop Fracture

The extension teardrop is an avulsion fracture of the anteroinferior process of C2 in which the anterior longitudinal ligament is disrupted above the fracture (Fig. 6-13). This common injury is limited to the anterior column and, unless associated with C2-C3 disk disruption, is stable.

Hyperextension-Dislocation

The hyperextension-dislocation is an unstable injury characterized by disruption of all three columns. Despite its pathophysiologic severity, imaging signs are often subtle, and subluxation can be masked by muscle spasm and cervical collar immobilization. Neurologic deficit, concurrent head trauma, or facial fracture should raise suspicion for this potentially unstable injury and lead to further investigation by MRI.

Hyperextension-dislocation injuries usually involve the lower cervical spine. Lateral radiographs and sagittal CT

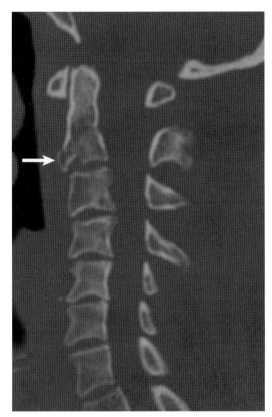

Figure 6-13 Extension teardrop fracture. Midsagittal computed tomography (CT) reformation shows teardrop fracture at C2. Alignment of middle and posterior columns is normal. As an isolated injury, this fracture is mechanically stable.

reformations show mild anterior disk space widening, facet widening, or malalignment and horizontally oriented anterior vertebral body avulsion fractures (Fig. 6-14, A to C). The latter should be distinguished from the vertically oriented hyperextension teardrop fracture, which involves the upper cervical spine, typically at C2. Magnetic resonance imaging reveals the full extent of discoligamentous injury. T2 and inversion recovery images show ligamentous disruption, soft tissue edema, disk protrusion, epidural hematoma, and associated spinal cord injury.

Fused Spine Hyperextension Injury

Ankylosing spondylitis and diffuse idiopathic skeletal hyperostosis produce both intervertebral bridging and fusion with poor bone quality. The rigid fused segment is susceptible to fracture with even mild hyperextension forces, and cord injury with profound neurologic deficit is common. In those patients with no neurologic deficit, failure to identify a fracture when present results in delayed neurologic deficit in at least 20%.

Fused spine hyperextension fractures may be occult on plain radiographs and CT (Fig. 6-15, A). This is due to both frequent spontaneous reduction and underlying osteoporosis, particularly in patients with advanced disease. Fractures may be horizontal or oblique and traverse the vertebral body, the fused disk space, or both (see Fig. 15, B and C). They typically involve the lower cervical spine, crossing all ossified ligaments from anterior to posterior and leading to marked instability. Because fractures are often horizontal, transaxial images are of limited utility, and careful review of sagittal or coronal CT reformations is necessary to exclude a nondisplaced or subtle fracture. Identification of one fracture mandates evaluation of the entire spine because there is a high incidence of noncontiguous concomitant fracture.

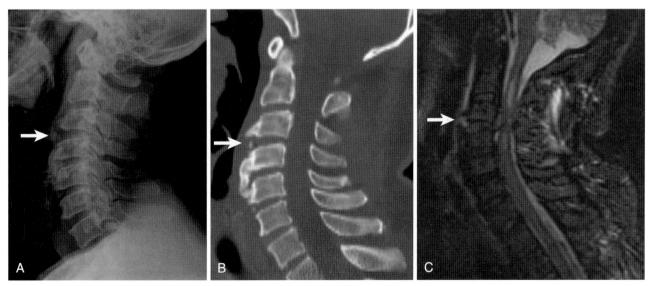

Figure 6-14 Hyperextension dislocation. **A,** Cross-table lateral cervical radiograph shows very subtle anterior widening at C3-C4 with fractured anterior osteophyte *(arrow)*. **B,** Midsagittal computed tomography (CT) reformation shows the same subtle findings *(arrow)*. **C,** T2-weighted midsagittal magnetic resonance imaging (MRI) shows prevertebral edema with anterior longitudinal ligament (ALL) disruption *(arrow)* at C3-C4. There is an associated traumatic disk herniation and buckling of the ligamentum flavum causing spinal cord edema and hemorrhage with central cord syndrome. (Reproduced with permission from Naderi S, Bernsyein M. Computed tomography. In: Legome E, Schockley LW, eds. *CT Trauma: A Comprehensive Emergency Medicine Approach.* Cambridge, UK: Cambridge University Press; 2011.)

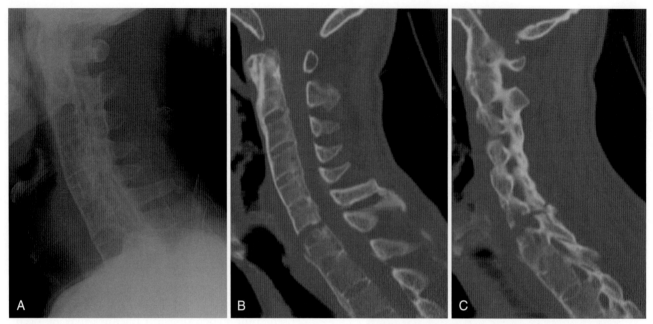

Figure 6-15 Fused spine hyperextension injury. A, Cross-table lateral cervical radiograph shows ankylosing spondylitis. No fracture seen. B, Midsagittal computed tomography (CT) reformation shows transverse fracture between C6 and C7 vertebral bodies. C, Parasagittal CT reformation shows fracture extending through the facets.

Thoracic and Lumbar Spine Emergencies
Mark Bernstein and Alexander B. Baxter

Thoracolumbar spine fractures occur in up to 18% of blunt trauma victims and can be difficult to diagnose. Many of these are associated with major extraspinal injuries and can be subtle on imaging, contributing to diagnostic delay or misdiagnosis. Because missed fractures are associated with neurologic injury and increased morbidity, careful and thorough workup of the multitrauma patient with dedicated spinal imaging is essential. This section reviews the major thoracolumbar spine fractures and imaging findings with attention drawn to subtle and easily overlooked features.

■ IMAGING GUIDELINES

The incidence of noncontiguous, multilevel vertebral injuries is as high as 20%. Consequently, the ACR advocates imaging the entire spine in multitrauma patients. In patients undergoing CT of the chest and abdomen, sagittal and coronal reformations of the spine should be produced from the thin-section thoracoabdominal data sets. Thoracic and lumbar spine radiographs may be reserved for patients whose other injuries do not mandate thoracoabdominal CT.

Dedicated overpenetrated coned-down AP and breathing lateral thoracic spine radiographs are superior to standard chest films for evaluation of the spinal injury. Fifty percent of portable trauma chest radiographic studies are nondiagnostic, and the radiographic findings of traumatic aortic injury overlap with those of significant thoracic spine injuries (Fig. 6-16). In patients with abnormal, incomplete, or inadequate radiographs, thoracolumbar spine CT with MPRs should be performed.

Multidetector CT is more accurate than spine radiographs for evaluation of bony injury and alignment. Multidetector CT with thin-section reconstruction and MPRs identifies the exact location of fractures and bone fragments, defines fracture morphologic characteristics, and shows the extent of any potential spinal canal, neuroforaminal, or vascular compromise.

Magnetic resonance imaging is indicated in patients with neurologic deficits and potentially unstable fracture patterns to assess injury to the spinal cord, nerve roots, intervertebral disks, and ligaments, and for the diagnosis of epidural hematoma.

■ DIRECTED SEARCH PATTERNS

Clinical history specifying injury mechanism, neurologic status, and location of pain is essential for accurately interpreting subtle findings, particularly in the setting of degenerative disk disease. To avoid search pattern errors, it is helpful to have a checklist in mind that will ensure all important structures are examined, as outlined in the following subsections.

Axial Images

Examine the integrity and rotational alignment of each vertebra, ensuring a complete bony ring surrounding the spinal canal (Fig. 6-17, A). Examine facet joint spacing and alignment, the adjacent soft tissues, spinal canal diameter, and neuroforaminal patency.

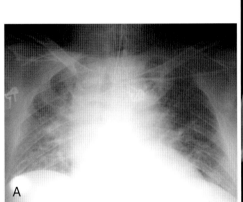

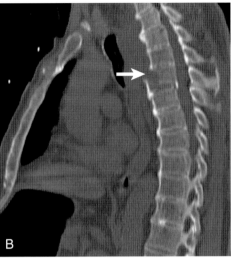

Figure 6-16 Hyperextension thoracic spine fracture. **A,** Supine anteroposterior (AP) portable chest radiograph with loss of normal aortic and mediastinal contours, widened right paratracheal stripe, and rightward deviation of the trachea. These signs are more commonly associated with traumatic aortic injury. **B,** Sagittal computed tomography (CT) reformation reveals thoracic spine hyperextension fracture *(arrow)*. No aortic injury was present.

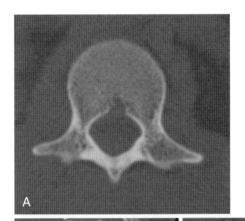

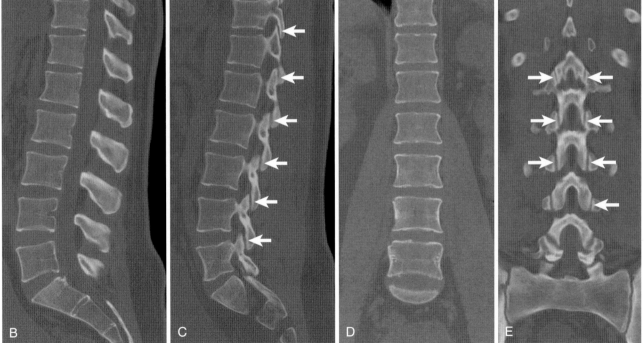

Figure 6-17 Normal thoracolumbar computed tomography (CT). **A,** Axial CT with complete bony ring forming the vertebral foramen. Midline defect in the posterior vertebral body represents the osseous entry of the basivertebral vein. **B,** Midsagittal CT reformation shows smooth anterior and posterior vertebral body and spinolaminar lines and normal interspinous spacing. **C,** Parasagittal CT image shows normal uniform facet joint alignment *(arrows)*. Anterior and posterior coronal images (**D** and **E**) show normal vertebral body alignment and lumbar facet relationships *(arrows)*, respectively.

Midline Sagittal Images

The anterior spinal line, posterior spinal line, and spinolaminar line should be continuous following the normal thoracic kyphosis and lumbar lordosis. The interspinous distances should be uniform. Spinal canal diameter is well evaluated on these images (see Fig. 6-17, *B*).

Parasagittal Images

The right and left facet joints should align normally with the inferior articulating facet of the upper vertebral body and posterior to the superior articulating facet of the adjacent lower vertebral body. Normal facet joints should be parallel and less than 2 mm wide (see Fig. 6-17, *C*).

Coronal Images

Vertebral bodies should be normally aligned and intact (see Fig. 6-17, *D*). Thoracic facets are coronally oriented and not well evaluated in this plane; however, lumbar facets are obliquely oriented and should be properly seated with inferior facets of the upper vertebral body medial to the superior facets from the lower vertebra (see Fig. 6-17, *E*).

■ CONCEPTS OF STABILITY

A stable spine is able to withstand physiologic loads without producing mechanical deformity or progressive neurologic injury or pain. These concepts may be difficult to translate to imaging, and therefore predicting posttraumatic thoracolumbar spine stability on an imaging study is challenging.

Both clinically and radiologically, the three-column concept of Denis is most widely applied for determining thoracolumbar spine stability (Fig. 6-18). The anterior column includes the anterior longitudinal ligament and the anterior vertebral body and disk. The middle column includes the posterior vertebral body cortex, posterior disk anulus, and the posterior longitudinal ligament. The posterior column includes the posterior bony arch, facets, and the PLC composed of the ligamentum flavum,

the facet joint capsules, and the interspinous and supraspinous ligaments. According to Denis, injury of two or three columns is considered unstable, with the key contributing factor being disruption of the middle column.

■ INJURY PATTERNS

The major thoracolumbar spine fracture patterns described by Denis are compression fractures, burst fractures, flexion-distraction injuries (or Chance fractures), and fracture dislocations. Two additional fracture types are described, pincer and hyperextension injuries, because these may be particularly subtle and warrant discussion. Table 6-2 outlines these major fracture patterns based on mechanism of injury and column involvement.

Compression Fractures

Compression fractures result from axial loading on a flexed spine with failure of the anterior column. Isolated anterior compression fractures are mechanically stable injuries, typically without neurologic deficit. It is crucial, however, to ensure that the posterior vertebral body cortex (middle column) and the posterior elements (posterior column) are intact.

Imaging

The hallmarks of a simple compression fracture are anterior vertebral body impaction with anterior cortical step-off and anterior superior end plate fracture (Fig. 6-19, *A* to *E*). Subtle linear density dorsal to the cortical step-off can sometimes be seen and reflects impacted trabeculae (see Fig. 6-19, *D* and *E*).

Unstable injuries that can mimic a compression fracture include pincer fractures, subtle burst fractures, and flexion-distraction injuries. On lateral radiographs, pay close attention to the posterior vertebral body cortex for signs of disruption or buckling. On AP radiographs, assess for interpedicular (transverse) and interspinous (vertical) widening. Radiographs of the thoracolumbar spine should be considered a screening study, and CT is indicated when potential abnormalities exist or when evaluation of the middle or posterior columns is limited by technique or overlying artifact.

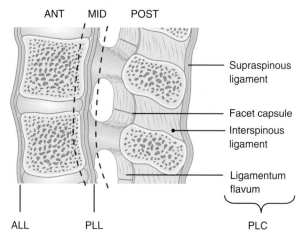

ANT   MID   POST

Supraspinous ligament

Facet capsule
Interspinous ligament

Ligamentum flavum

ALL   PLL   PLC

Figure 6-18 *Thoracolumbar spine anatomy and three-column concept of Denis.*

Table 6-2   Modes of Failure and Column Involvement of Major Thoracolumbar Fracture Types

	Anterior	Middle	Posterior
Compression	Compression	—	—
Pincer	Compression	—	—
Burst	Compression	Compression	None or compression
Flexion-distraction	None or compression	Distraction	Distraction
Fracture dislocation	Compression, rotation, shear	Distraction, rotation, shear	Distraction, rotation, shear
Hyperextension	Distraction	Distraction	None or compression

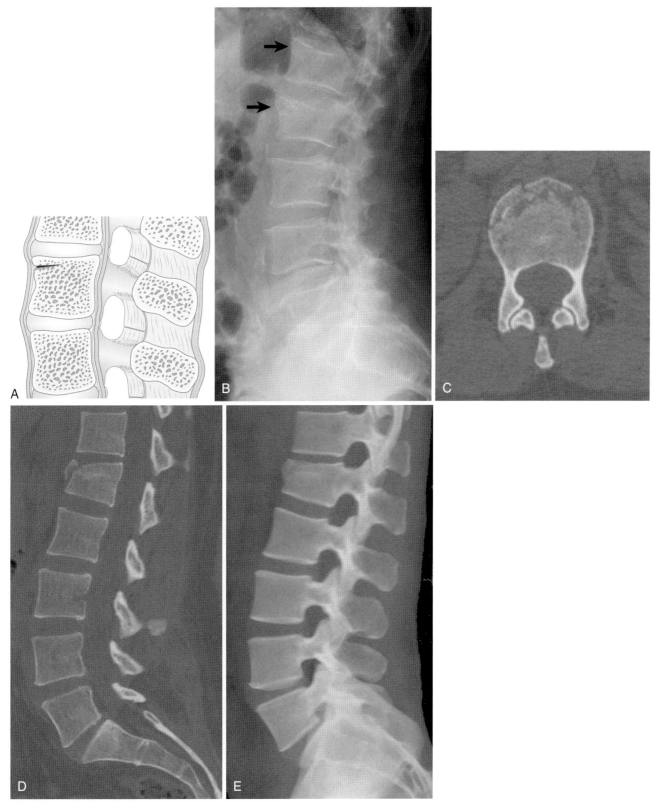

Figure 6-19 Compression fracture. **A**, Impacted anterior-superior aspect of the vertebral body with step-off deformity. The ligaments are intact, with the injury isolated to the anterior column. **B**, Lateral radiograph of L1 and L2 compression fractures *(arrows)*. **C**, Axial computed tomography (CT) image shows anterior comminution with intact posterior vertebral body cortex and normal facets. **D**, Midsagittal CT image confirms intact middle column. **E**, Three-dimensional (3-D) CT reconstruction in transparent bone algorithm ("virtual radiograph"); facets and spinous process spacing are normal.

Illustrative Case 1 (Fig. 6-20)

A 54-year-old intoxicated man presented to the emergency department after a fall on Halloween. Computed tomography of the head and cervical spine were negative. Lumbar spine x-ray examination was performed for back pain. The initial report described loss of anterior height of T12 vertebral body; suspicious for compression fracture. The next day CT of the abdomen and pelvis was performed for left flank pain, and the findings were preliminarily reported as negative. The attending review identified a fracture of T12. The patient returned 2 days later for a dedicated CT

of the thoracolumbar spine, where a burst fracture was diagnosed. No posterior column injury was seen, and nonoperative management was undertaken. Follow-up thoracolumbar radiographs revealed progressive collapse of the T12 vertebral body and increased kyphosis.

Pincer Fractures

The pincer fracture is a coronal split vertebral body fracture with central collapse and herniation of disk material into the fracture gap (Fig. 6-21, A). The fracture

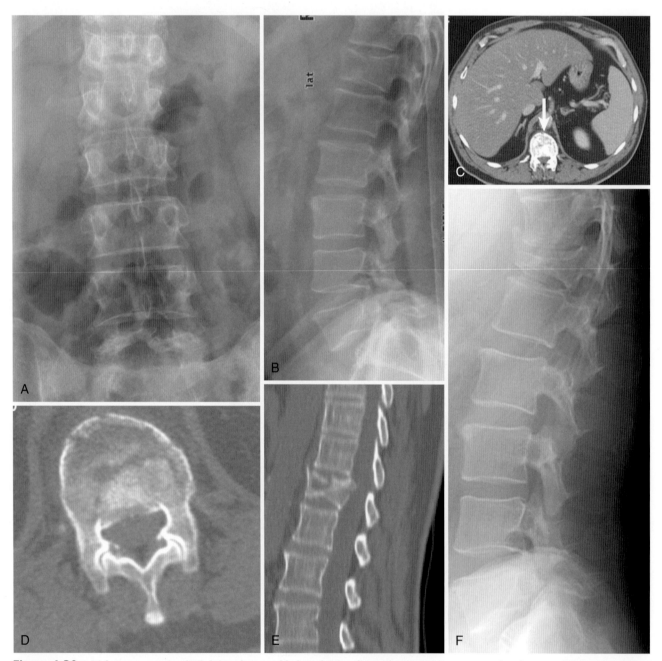

Figure 6-20 Initial anteroposterior (AP) (**A**) and cross-table lateral (**B**) radiographs reported as compression fracture of T12 with minimal loss of anterior vertebral height. Patient was discharged. **C**, Transaxial computed tomography (CT) image from abdominal and pelvic CT was performed the next day after the patient returned with complaints of abdominal pain. A burst fracture with posterior cortex retropulsion and mild paraspinal hemorrhage was missed on the initial study (*arrow*) and evident on the abdominal CT. Dedicated spine CT was obtained 2 days later. **D**, Transaxial CT image of T12 shows posterior cortical disruption with retropulsion. No posterior column injury is present. **E**, Midsagittal CT reformation better demonstrates the T12 burst fracture. **F**, Follow-up radiograph performed 9 days after initial presentation shows marked collapse of T12 with increased kyphosis consistent with an unstable burst fracture. (Reprinted with permission. Bernstein M. Easily missed thoracolumbar spine fractures. *Eur J Radiol.* 2010;74[1]:6-15.)

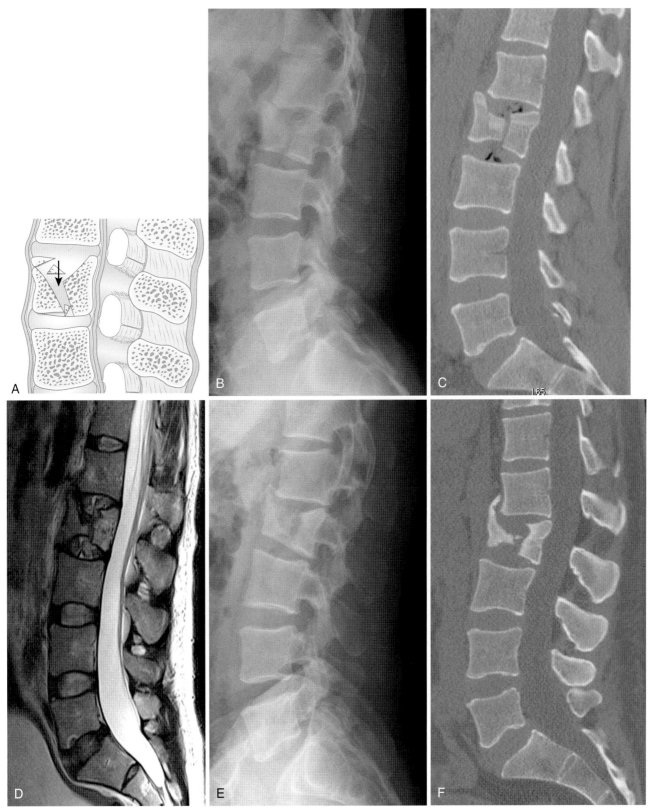

Figure 6-21 Pincer fracture. A, Diagram of coronal plane fracture and central comminution of the vertebral body with disk herniation into the fracture gap *(arrow)*. As in compression fractures, the middle and posterior columns are intact, but in this case instability is due to failure to support axial loads with delayed collapse and kyphosis. **B** and **C,** Initial lateral radiograph and midsagittal computed tomography (CT) image show the L2 coronal vertebral body fracture. **D,** Magnetic resonance imaging (MRI) reveals intact posterior longitudinal ligament (PLL) and posterior column. The patient was managed without surgery. Follow-up x-ray examination at 2 months **(E)** and midsagittal CT at 15 months **(F)** show progressive central collapse and increasing kyphosis.

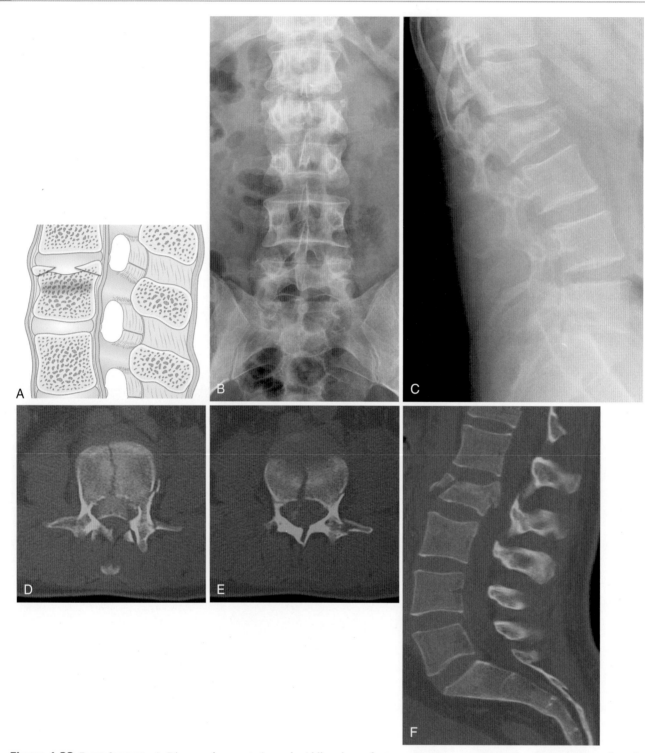

Figure 6-22 Burst fracture. A, Diagram shows anterior and middle column fractures. **B,** Anteroposterior (AP) radiograph shows flattening and slight widening of L2. **C,** Lateral radiograph demonstrates loss of vertebral body height, trabecular impaction, and kyphosis. **D & E,** Axial computed tomography (CT) images reveal middle column involvement with large retropulsed fragment (D), and posterior neural arch fracture (E). **F,** Sagittal CT reformation clearly depicts canal compromise secondary to the retropulsed bony fragment.

splits the vertebral body into anterior and posterior fragments running from the superior to inferior end plates. Though limited to the anterior column, the pincer fracture is mechanically unstable—the fractured vertebra is no longer able to support axial loads and, left untreated, may collapse (see Fig. 6-21, *B* to *F*).

Burst Fractures

Burst fractures result from axial loading on a neutral, nonflexed spine causing failure of at least the anterior and middle columns (Fig. 6-22, *A*). In many instances CT reveals posterior column failure as well. Disruption

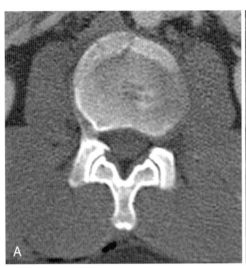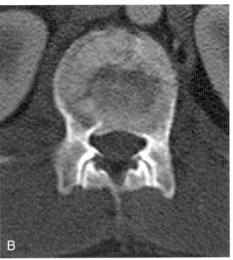

Figure 6-23 Compression versus subtle burst fracture. A, Axial computed tomography (CT) image of L2 compression fracture shows anterior vertebral body cortical fractures. Posterior cortex is intact. **B,** Axial CT image of L1 burst fracture in the same patient reveals a subtle posterior vertebral body cortical fracture in addition to anterior body fractures. Facet joints appear normal. (Reprinted with permission. Bernstein M. Easily missed thoracolumbar spine fractures. *Eur J Radiol.* 2010;74[1]: 6-15.)

of the posterior vertebral body cortex (middle column) is characteristic of burst fractures. A retropulsed posterior vertebral body fracture fragment into the spinal canal is primarily responsible for acute neurologic deficit, which is seen in one half to three quarters of such patients.

Imaging

Anteroposterior radiographs show flattening and sometimes widening of the vertebral body. Widening of the interpedicular distance indicates posterior column involvement (see Fig. 6-22, *B*). Lateral radiographs demonstrate loss of vertebral body height, trabecular condensation, and associated kyphosis. Disruption of the posterior vertebral body cortex and retropulsed fragment (see Fig. 6-22, *C*) is subtle or obscured in 30% of patients. Because unstable burst fractures can be confused with simple stable compression fractures, anterior compression deformities in the setting of acute trauma should be further evaluated by CT with MPRs.

Computed tomography characterizes the injury pattern and evaluates the integrity of each of the three columns. Axial images show superior end-plate comminution, distortion of the posterior vertebral body cortical contour, any retropulsion of fracture fragments into the spinal canal (see Fig. 6-22, *D*), and when present, posterior neural arch fractures (signifying a three-column injury) (see Fig. 6-22, *E*). Sagittal reconstructions provide the best measure of canal compromise (see Fig. 6-22, *F*). Burst fractures may be subtle, and middle column involvement can be limited to slight posterior vertebral body cortical buckling. Figure 6-23 compares a stable anterior compression fracture with a subtle burst fracture in the same patient.

Magnetic resonance imaging is indicated for patients with acute neurologic deficits and optimally evaluates spinal cord and nerve root injury, as well as integrity of the posterior ligamentous complex, traumatic disk herniation, and epidural hematoma.

Stability

The definition of a "stable" burst fracture is controversial. Some authors consider all burst fractures unstable. Others point to successful nonoperative management of burst fractures that involve only the anterior and middle

column. From an imaging standpoint, any posterior column injury, whether osseous or ligamentous, constitutes instability. In cases in which nonoperative management is pursued, close radiologic follow-up is recommended to identify early signs of failure (see Fig. 6-20).

Illustrative Case 2 (Fig. 6-24)

A 51-year-old man fell off a ladder, landing on his low back and buttocks. He presented to the emergency department with severe back pain. Initial lumbar spine radiographs showed compression deformities of L1 and L2 vertebral bodies anteriorly. Widening of the facet joints at this level were identified and described. Computed tomography of the thoracolumbar spine performed the next day confirmed these findings. The significance and inherent instability resulting from the facet distraction was unrecognized until 10-week follow-up radiographs showed further collapse of L1 and L2 anteriorly and increased distraction posteriorly.

Flexion-Distraction Injuries

Flexion-distraction injuries, or Chance fractures, predominately involve the thoracolumbar junction and result from forward flexion over a fixed object, such as a lap belt, where the axis of rotation lies at the anterior abdominal wall, subjecting the entire spine to distraction forces (Fig. 6-25, *A* and *B*). The posterior and middle columns are always involved, defining these fractures as unstable. Approximately 40% of patients with flexion-distraction injuries have associated intra-abdominal injuries, most commonly bowel and mesenteric, both of which may be very subtle on imaging. Delayed diagnosis of spinal or visceral injuries is common, occurring in up to 50% of patients.

Imaging

Radiographic diagnosis of flexion-distraction injuries is challenging because loss of posterior element integrity may be subtle or difficult to ascertain. When present, the most common radiographic finding is the "empty body" sign, visible on AP images, seen as a normal-appearing vertebral body without its corresponding spinous process. This is due to distraction and vertical separation

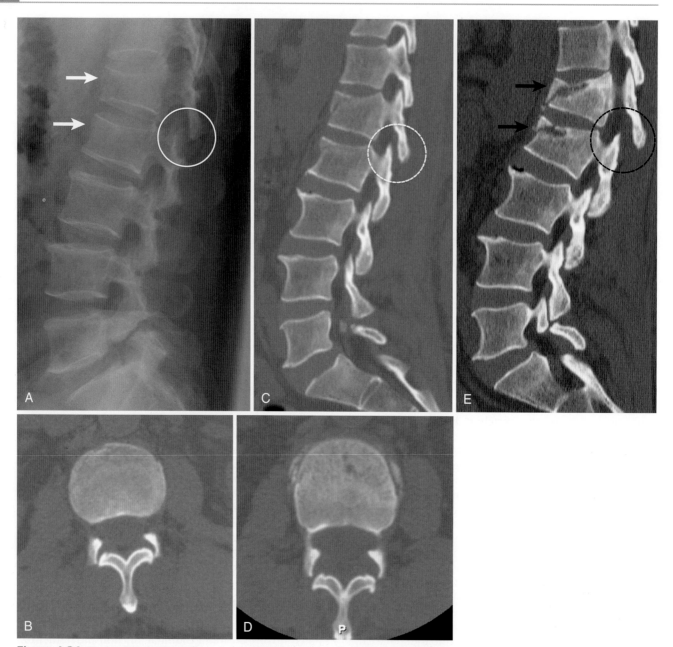

Figure 6-24 Flexion-Distraction Injury. A, Lateral lumbar spine radiograph shows subtle compression deformities of L1 and L2 vertebral superior end plates *(white arrows)*. The facets at L1 and L2 *(white circle)* are distracted. Computed tomography (CT) examination was performed the following day (**B** and **C**). **B,** Axial CT image at L2 shows subtle anterior vertebral body fractures and distraction of the facet joints. **C,** Parasagittal CT reformation through the left facet joints shows L1 and L2 widening *(white dashed circle)*. Follow-up CT examination 10 weeks later with axial (**D**) and parasagittal (**E**) reformations show failed nonoperative management with increased distraction of the facets *(black dashed circle)*, further collapse of the anterior vertebral bodies *(black arrows)*, and increased kyphosis. (Reprinted with permission. Bernstein M. Easily missed thoracolumbar spine fractures. *Eur J Radiol.* 2010;74[1]:6-15.)

of the posterior elements (see Fig. 6-25, *C*). Horizontal fractures through the pedicles or transverse processes may also be seen. A well-penetrated lateral view will usually show distraction of posterior elements and widening of the facet articulations (see Fig. 6-25, *D*).

The "dissolving pedicle" reflects the gradual loss of definition of the pedicle on serial axial CT images as the image plane crosses the transverse pedicle fracture (see Fig. 6-25, *E* to *G*). The "naked facet" sign reflects facet distraction in injuries involving the posterior ligaments (see Fig. 6-25, *F*). Both signs may be present on the same axial image, with a pedicle fracture on one side, and facet widening on the

other (see Fig. 6-25, *F*). Sagittal CT reconstructions demonstrate the distracted posterior elements and transverse pedicle fracture to advantage (see Fig. 6-25, *H* and *I*). A burst component may complicate the injury and when present, is best evaluated on sagittal images, which permit accurate measurement of any canal compromise.

Fracture Dislocations

Fracture dislocations result from complex forces that disrupt all three spinal columns. These are highly unstable injuries closely associated with severe neurologic deficits.

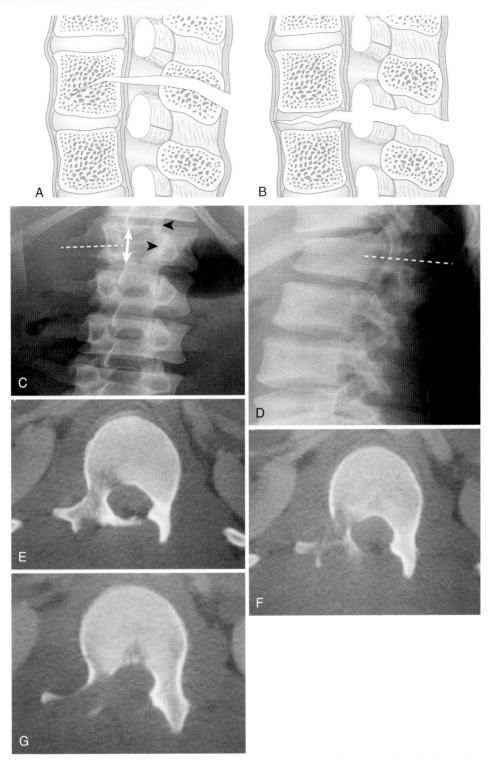

Figure 6-25 Diagrams of Chance fracture (**A**) and flexion-distraction injury (**B**). Both injuries result from flexion at the anterior abdominal wall with dorsal distraction. When the injury is osseous, a Chance fracture results; when it is ligamentous, a flexion-distraction injury results. **C**, Anteroposterior (AP) radiograph, though slightly oblique, shows vertical distraction and separation of the spinous processes *(double arrow)* leaving an L1 "empty body." Transverse right pedicle fracture *(dashed line)* and left T12/L1 facet distraction *(arrowheads)* are also seen. **D**, Lateral radiograph shows horizontal fracture line through the pedicle *(dashed line)*. Serial axial images (**E** to **G**) show an asymmetric injury with right "dissolving pedicle" and left "naked facet" signs. (**C** to **G** Reprinted with permission. Bernstein M. Easily missed thoracolumbar spine fractures. *Eur J Radiol.* 2010;74[1]:6-15.)

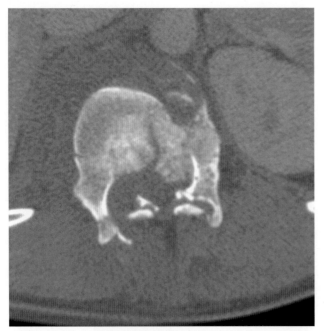

Figure 6-26 Fracture dislocation. Axial computed tomography (CT) image shows fracture fragments from two vertebral bodies on the same image with rotation and translation, diagnostic of fracture dislocation.

Imaging

Severe comminution, translation, and/or rotation are hallmarks of these grossly unstable injuries, and multiplanar reconstructions are essential in their analysis. Any horizontal translation, or visualization of two vertebral bodies on the same axial image, strongly suggests a fracture dislocation (Fig. 6-26).

Hyperextension Injuries

An important variant of spinal fracture dislocation, the hyperextension fracture constitutes less than 3% of all thoracolumbar spine fractures. Severe hyperextension forces cause distraction of the spine with subluxation and canal compromise. In the normal nonfused spine, such injuries are produced by severe forces, including motor vehicle ejection and "lumberjack paraplegia," in which the individual is struck in the back by a large heavy object, such as a falling tree.

Certain conditions, including ankylosing spondylitis and diffuse idiopathic skeletal hyperostosis, result in unusually brittle spines. In these patients, even minor trauma, such as a fall from standing, can result in devastating hyperextension injury.

Imaging

The hyperextension fracture dislocation may be quite subtle on plain radiographs and is often overlooked or misinterpreted (see Fig. 6-16). Osteoporosis and poorly defined disk spaces in the ankylosed spine contribute to diagnostic difficulty. Lateral radiographs can reveal anterior disk space widening or distraction of anterior vertebral body fracture fragments. When the mechanism of injury and patient risk factors suggest a hyperextension injury, CT is mandatory and MRI often very useful because it best identifies the disrupted anterior longitudinal ligament and anulus fibrosis.

Selected Reading

American College of Radiology. ACR Appropriateness Criteria—suspected cervical spine trauma. http://www.acr.org/~/media/ACR/Documents/AppCriteria/Diagnostic/SuspectedSpineTrauma. Published 1999. Accessed June 11, 2013.

Bernstein M. Easily missed thoracolumbar spine fractures. *Eur J Radiol.* 2010;74(1):6–15.

Bernstein MP, Baxter AB, Harris JH Jr. Imaging thoracolumbar spine trauma. In: Pope TL Jr, Harris JH Jr, eds. *Radiology of Emergency Medicine.* 5th ed Philadelphia, PA: Lippincott Williams & Wilkins; 2013:265–305.

Daffner RH. Daffner SD Vertebral injuries: detection and implications. *Eur J Radiol.* 2002;42:100–116.

Denis F. The three column spine and its significance in the classification of acute thoracolumbar spinal injuries. *Spine.* 1983;8(8):817–831.

Hoffman JR, Mower WR, Wolfson AB, et al. Validity of a set of clinical criteria to rule out injury to the cervical spine in patients with blunt trauma. National Emergency X-Radiography Utilization Study Group. *N Engl J Med.* 2000;343:94–99.

Magerl F, Aebi M, Gertzbein SD, et al. A comprehensive classification of thoracic and lumbar injuries. *Eur Spine J.* 1994;3(4):184–201.

Rao SK, Wasyliw C, Nunez DB Jr. Spectrum of imaging findings in hyperextension injuries of the neck. *Radiographics.* 2005;25:1239–1254.

Steill IG, Wells GA, Vandemheen KL, et al. The Canadian c-spine rule for radiography in alert and stable trauma patients. *JAMA.* 2001;286:1841–1848.

CHAPTER 7

Nontraumatic Spine Emergencies

Thomas Ptak

Infection of the vertebral column represents up to 20% of all osteomyelitis and is the most common infection of the axial skeleton. The presentation is often insidious. It is not uncommon for symptoms to be present for 6 to 8 weeks before being diagnosed. If ignored or misdiagnosed, infection of the spine can have a chronic, destructive, and significantly debilitating course. The general characteristics of spinal infections are summarized in Table 7-1.

Infection is commonly spread hematogenously, although direct extension from adjacent infection such as pneumonia or pyelonephritis is also possible. In 60% to 70% of patients the most common infectious agents encountered are gram-positive cocci, especially skin flora such as *Staphylococcus* (in about 60% of positive cultures), and less commonly *Streptococcus* with *Peptostreptococcus*, *Escherichia coli*, and *Proteus*. Although often implied by examination findings, a definitive infectious source is identified in less than 50% of patients with pyogenic spinal osteomyelitis. In unusual circumstances, such as immunodeficiency or patients from underdeveloped countries, one should consider atypical agents such as fungi or *Mycobacteria*.

Patients at risk include older adults, intravenous drug abusers, those with chronic illness, and those with a recent history of surgery, especially of the back or genitourinary system. Insidious onset of diffuse back pain (in 90%) and fever (in 50% to 70%) should suggest spinal infection. A history of recent back or genitourinary surgery, intravenous drug use, or infection of the soft tissue or respiratory or genitourinary system should increase the likelihood of spinal infection. Infection involves the vertebral body in 95% of cases, with the posterior elements being involved in less than 5%. Although neurologic symptoms such as radiculopathy may be present, they are uncommon and often present later in the course as the infection spreads from the disk and vertebra to the epidural, subarticular, and external foraminal spaces. Weight loss may also be present, but this constitutional symptom is less helpful in that it may also be associated with both inflammatory and neoplastic disease.

When thinking about where to look for infectious involvement of the vertebrae, it is helpful to consider the pathophysiologic manifestations. Blood-borne organisms seed from the vascular system. Intervertebral disks are the largest avascular organs in the body. The nucleus pulposus of the disk receives nutrients typically by diffusion from the subchondral vascular bed of the vertebral end plate. In addition, the outer annulus fibrosis has a direct capillary supply via spinal canal arteries, also contributing nutrients across the concentric fibrous layers of the annulus. The blood-borne organism is able to establish itself at the more vascular outer free margin of the disk and at the end plate in the capillaries of the subchondral vascular bed. From here the organism can spread contiguously into the more avascular central disk and into the adjacent bony vertebrae. Using this model, it is understandable that the earliest changes of infection should appear at the disk margin closest to the vascular source anteriorly and anterolaterally, as well as anywhere along the disk-margin interface. Advanced infection is characterized by an abnormal intervertebral disk and abnormal adjacent vertebral end plates.

■ DIAGNOSTIC IMAGING

Plain Film

Initial imaging in the emergency department (ED) may include plain film and/or nonenhanced computed tomography (CT). Both are directed at identifying bony changes that may indicate infection of the vertebral bodies. Plain film has limited sensitivity because of many overlying confluent shadows and other technical difficulties in obtaining an image. Gross findings such as vertebral sclerosis, vertebral collapse with acute angulation of the spine (e.g., Pott disease with gibbous deformity [Fig. 7-1]), or paraspinal soft tissue mass may be helpful, but the sensitivity is low and the images do not provide a complete evaluation of this potentially multifocal process.

Multidetector Computed Tomography

Sagittal reconstructions from CT provide greater diagnostic detail with respect to large-scale or multilevel osteomyelitis (Fig. 7-2). On CT the acute or active infection may show low-attenuation paraspinal swelling and edema, focal fluid collections, fat stranding, or gas (Fig. 7-3). Contrast administration may produce enhancement of the actively inflamed tissue with nonenhancing areas of central liquifactive debris in early abscess formation, if present. Attention should also be directed to adjacent organ systems such as the kidneys or lungs to provide clues to the origin of infection.

Typical findings suspicious for acute or active infectious involvement of the bone include focal or regional

Table 7-1   Common Locations and Characteristics of Spinal Infections

Infection	Characteristics	Common Location
Vertebral osteomyelitis	Elderly and debilitated Male predominance	Lumbar more common than thoracic
Spinal epidural abscess	Hematogenous gram-positive cocci	Thoracic more common than lumbar
Diskitis	Adult postdiscectomy most common Rare in pediatrics; often accompanies chronic infections (e.g., cystic fibrosis)	Lumbar more common than thoracic
Granulomatous disease	Rare in developed countries	Thoracic approximately equal to lumbar

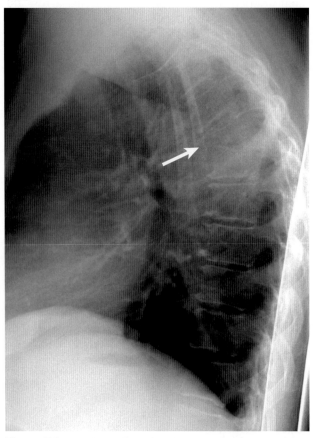

Figure 7-1 Lateral plain film of the thoracic spine showing collapse of the anterior-inferior T5 vertebral body *(white arrow)*, with acute angulation (gibbous deformity).

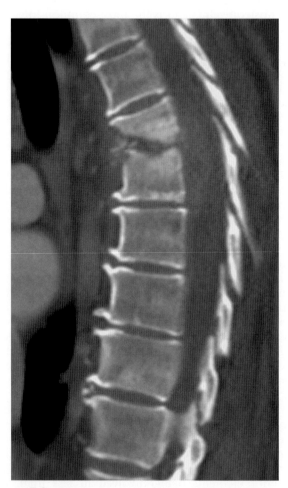

Figure 7-2 Sagittal reconstructions of the thoracic spine computed tomographic (CT) scan show the same angulation and destruction of the anterior-inferior end plate of T5 seen in Fig. 7-1 but reveal more detail of bony demineralization, resorption, and fragmentation. Also note involvement of the superior end plate of the T6 vertebra, not appreciated on the plain film.

demineralization, periosteal edema, and erosive or destructive changes in the cortex or end plates (Fig. 7-4). Contrast-enhanced CT (CECT) is useful for defining and characterizing areas of soft tissue infection and identifying any abscess formation or extension to the epidural or adjacent paravertebral spaces. Mature abscesses are readily recognizable by their nonenhancing, low-attenuation central area of liquifactive debris surrounded by a thick rim with ill-defined margins (Fig. 7-5).

Magnetic Resonance Imaging

Magnetic resonance imaging (MRI) is most sensitive for evaluating infections of the vertebral column. A contrast-enhanced MRI of the affected spinal segment should

include a precontrast T1- and T2-weighted sagittal series, with axial T1- and T2-weighted series performed through the level of interest. It is crucial to include fat suppression in the evaluation because abnormal signal indicating infection on T2-weighted and postcontrast T1-weighted sequences may be confused with hyperintense signal produced in the normal fat planes of the epidural space, marrow compartment, and in the interstitial spaces of spinal ligaments. This is especially true in the case of T1

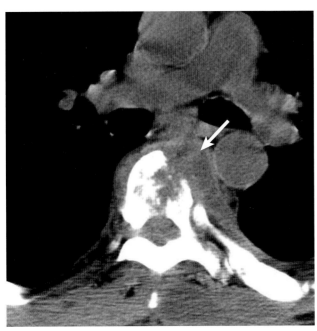

Figure 7-3 Nonenhanced computed tomographic (CT) image of T8 osteomyelitis with paraspinal abscess. Even without contrast, the 32-HU low-attenuation measurement of the collection *(white arrow)* suggests a proteinaceous liquifactive character.

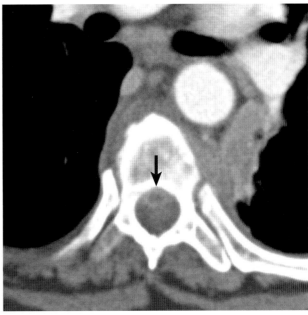

Figure 7-5 Contrast-enhanced computed tomographic (CECT) image shows a thick rimmed, enhancing abscess in the extradural space of the spinal canal *(black arrow)*.

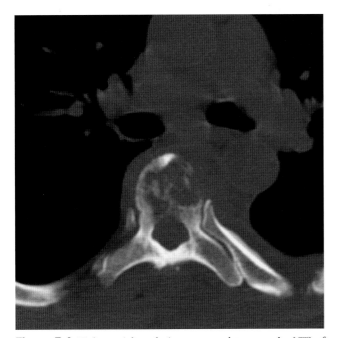

Figure 7-4 High–spatial resolution computed tomography (CT) of the patient in Fig. 7-3 using bone windows demonstrates demineralization, erosion, and fragmentation in the T8 vertebral body.

signal contamination on T2-weighted images obtained using fast-imaging protocols (e.g., multiecho, turbo spin echo). Precontrast T1-weighted images are customarily performed without fat suppression so that anatomic detail is preserved (and to save time), with T2-weighted sagittal and postcontrast T1-weighted images being fat suppressed in all planes. Fat suppression allows increased sensitivity in detecting infectious deposits by ensuring that hyperintense regions identified indicate areas of edema and enhancing inflammation and are not due to the normal soft tissue fat planes and interstitial fat encountered in the spine. Chemical fat suppression is typically employed but is prone to inhomogeneity due to off-resonance excitation resulting from local susceptibility effects and static field inhomogeneity. Some sites prefer to augment or replace the T2-weighted sagittal series with a sagittal short tau inversion recovery (STIR) sequence. The STIR technique results in fat suppression based on the intrinsic relaxation properties of the protons and does not rely on spectral excitation to diminish fat signal. More homogeneous suppression is attained, and the signal-to-noise ratio of water and edema with respect to the surrounding tissue is optimized.

When interpreting the spinal MRI, it is helpful to keep in mind that the infection may be multifocal or may extend some distance from the obvious lesion. Starting with a T2-weighted, fat-suppressed, large field-of-view image may be helpful and efficient for determining the extent and involvement of inflammation. The increased signal-to-noise characteristics and coverage in a sagittal STIR or fat-suppressed T2-weighted sequence may help to identify even small areas of hyperintensity indicating inflammation and will provide coverage over a large area (Figs. 7-6 and 7-7). Once inflammation is identified, further evaluation can be carried out with more focused T1-weighted precontrast and postcontrast imaging in additional planes optimized to best show the lesion(s) identified. Inflammation and/or enhancement identified adjacent to or within potential spaces should include additional orthogonal views (typically axial if sagittal was already used to survey the region) along the full length of the soft tissue space involved to ensure identification of the full extent of involvement. For example, inflammation in the psoas muscle

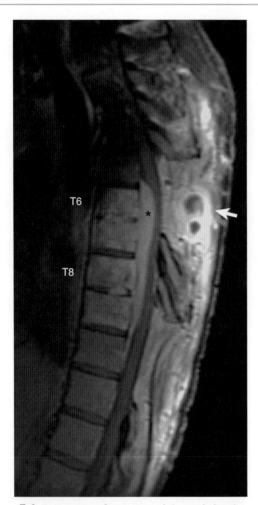

Figure 7-6 Postcontrast, fat-suppressed (note dark subcutaneous fat) T1-weighted sagittal image shows the extent of involvement of the osteomyelitis with extension to the extradural space *(black asterisk)* and surrounding soft tissues, including an abscess of the operative laminectomy bed *(white arrow)*.

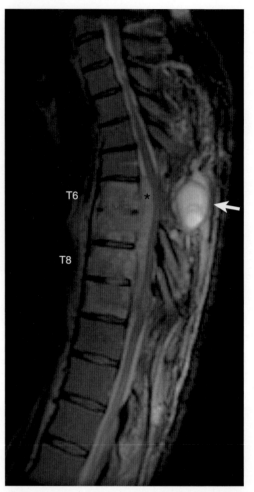

Figure 7-7 Fat-suppressed T2-weighted sagittal image shows the extent of involvement of the osteomyelitis with extension to the extradural space *(black asterisk)* and surrounding soft tissues, including an abscess of the operative laminectomy bed *(white arrow)*.

adjacent to a disk space should also include a full evaluation of the disk space. Enhancement adjacent to the central spinal canal should lead to a careful evaluation of the extradural space to identify any infection or abscess formation. This evaluation can be carried out using two orthogonal planes through the region of interest.

Evaluation of the bony structures is especially important, particularly in areas of adjacent soft tissue swelling or enhancement. Again, fat-suppressed T1-weighted imaging in the optimal plane for visualization is imperative. T2-weighted imaging may show hyperintensity in the marrow space adjacent to the soft tissue inflammation, and with the addition of fat suppression this will make certain that marrow edema from infection/inflammation is not confused with marrow space fat signal. Precontrast T1 weighting with fat-suppressed imaging should show the normally hypointense densely calcified bony cortex as very hypointense, but inflamed edematous cortical mantle may appear relatively hyperintense or nearly isointense to adjacent marrow signal, making it indistinguishable from adjacent marrow. On postcontrast T1-weighted imaging, areas of infectious involvement of the bony cortex will enhance, producing a hyperintense disruption in the normally sharply defined, thin hypointense signal of the normal bony cortical stripe.

As discussed earlier, one might expect diskitis to begin in the periphery at the outer annulus or along the disk–end plate margin; these are the regions of vascular supply and are the most likely points of origin for a blood-borne infection. Infection can then take hold in the avascular portion of the disk, where the immune response would be minimal. Infection, once established, can then spread to the adjacent bone. Fat-suppressed T2-weighted imaging may show hyperintensity in the thickened outer annular fibers, potentially extending to the disk-vertebrae margin. Evaluation of postcontrast images demonstrates enhancement in this same distribution (Fig. 7-8).

In most cases abscesses are readily recognizable on T1-weighted fat-suppressed postcontrast images as thick, rim-enhancing lesions, often with ill-defined margins owing to the infiltrative nature of the infectious process (Fig. 7-9). Do not be concerned if the central liquifactive debris appears slightly more or less intense

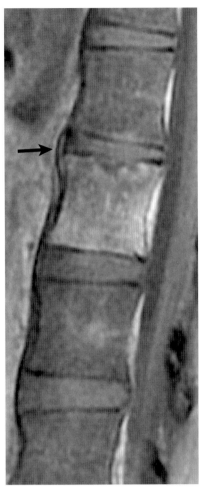

Figure 7-8 Postcontrast, fat-suppressed, T1-weighted sagittal image demonstrating enhancement in the affected ventral disk annulus extending to the anterior longitudinal ligament (ALL) and Sharpey fibers at the vertebral margin *(arrow)*, as well as vertebral body enhancement.

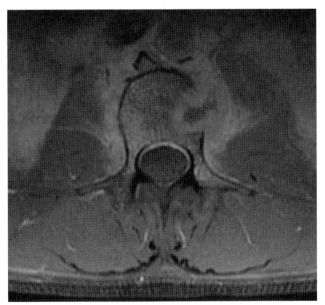

Figure 7-9 Postcontrast, fat-suppressed, T1-weighted axial image of well-formed abscess with central low-signal core of liquifactive necrosis and thick rim with hazy, ill-defined borders.

than expected. An infection begins from a central nidus of microorganism deposition. As the infection spreads centrifugally outward to involve contiguous adjacent tissues or along a potential space, the debris from metabolic waste and from the body's immune response is left behind. The central debris is typically highly concentrated with cellular elements and other lipoproteinaceous milieu, resulting in shortened T1 relaxation and causing the central debris to appear slightly more hyperintense than expected on nonenhanced T1-weighted images. Similarly, phase dispersion caused by the relatively proteinaceous material may cause increased T2 relaxation. As a result, the T2-weighted images may show this area to be more hypointense than expected. Abscesses that are more long-standing may produce a more pronounced effect on these signal changes because of desiccation or inspissation. Gas-forming organisms may produce small gas bubbles. Gas may be recognized not only by a lack of signal on any sequence, but also by air–soft tissue interface susceptibility introduced at the margin of the gas pocket. On spin echo images one may see a small crescent of hyperintensity in the phase-encoding direction paralleling the gas pocket margin. More consistently this effect may be seen as low signal on T^{2*}-weighted gradient refocused imaging sequences.

■ POSTPROCEDURE SPINE

Patients who have had back surgery, especially those with stabilization devices implanted, are relatively prone to infection at the surgical site and are likely to present to the ED. Although all of the principles of evaluation are the same, the presence of stabilization hardware makes evaluation difficult, especially near the interface with the device.

Computed tomography evaluation is fraught with beam-hardening artifact, obscuring image detail in the presence of metallic stabilization hardware and hence reducing sensitivity for detecting soft tissue infection. Evaluation of the central canal for epidural inflammation or abscess by CT may necessitate the introduction of contrast into the thecal sac and as such is less likely to occur in the ED.

Magnetic resonance imaging provides a better modality for evaluation of infection, although it remains hampered by physical constraints. Manufacturers try to incorporate low-magnetic-susceptibility materials into their devices to minimize magnetic interaction, making hardware devices safer for use in MRI. The materials used vary in degree of magnetic interaction and also vary with field strength. When possible, check the specific hardware device for safety and potential field interaction to help optimize imaging. An MRI-safe implant that is composed of metal and carbon composites will still cause field distortion. Even low-susceptibility metals such as titanium result in a big enough field disturbance to distort the local tissue signal and obscure images at the interface. Choosing an MRI pulse sequence designed to reduce metallic field effects (such as a short echo spacing multiecho sequence) may help minimize distortion.

Selected Reading

Butler JS, Shelly MJ, Timlin M, et al: Nontuberculous pyogenic spinal infection in adults: a 12-year experience from a tertiary referral center, *Spine* 31:2695–2700, 2006.

Colmenero JD, Jimenez-Mejias ME, Sanchez-Lora FJ: Pyogenic, tuberculous, and brucellar vertebral osteomyelitis: a descriptive and comparative study of 219 cases, *Ann Rheum Dis* 56(12):709–715, 1997.

Dagirmanjian A, Schils J, McHenry M, et al: MR imaging of vertebral osteomyelitis revisited, *AJR Am J Roentgenol* 167:1539–1543, 1996.

Dunbar JA, Sandoe JA, Rao AS, et al: The MRI appearances of early vertebral osteomyelitis and discitis, *Clin Radiol* 65(12):974–981, 2010.

Fernandez M, Carrol CL, Baker CJ: Discitis and vertebral osteomyelitis in children: an 18-year review, *Pediatrics* 105(6):1299–1304, 2000.

Gillams AR, Chaddha B, Carter AP: MR appearances of the temporal evolution and resolution of infectious spondylitis, *AJR Am J Roentgenol* 166:903–907, 1996.

Gold RH, Hawkins RA, Katz RD: Bacterial osteomyelitis: findings on plain radiography, CT, MR, and scintigraphy, *AJR Am J Roentgenol* 157:365–370, 1991.

Hadjipavlou AG, Mader JT, Necessary JT: Hematogenous pyogenic spinal infections and their surgical management, *Spine* 25(13):1668–1679, 2000.

Ledermann HP, Schweitzer ME, Morrison WB, et al: MR imaging findings in spinal infections: rules or myths? *Radiology* 228(2):506–514, 2003.

Murillo O, Roset A, Sobrino B, et al: Streptococcal vertebral osteomyelitis: multiple faces of the same disease. *Clin Microbiol Infect.* 20(1):033–8, 2014.

Resnik D: Osteomyelitis, septic arthritis and soft tissue infection: axial skeleton. In Resnick D, editor: *Diagnosis of Bone and Joint Disorders*, ed 4, Philadelphia, PA, 2002, Saunders, pp 2481–2509.

Ritchie DA: Commentary on the MRI appearances of early osteomyelitis and discitis, *Clin Radiol* 65(12):982–983, 2010.

Stäbler A, Reiser MF: Imaging of spinal infection, *Radiol Clin North Am* 39(1):115–135, 2001.

THORACIC EMERGENCY RADIOLOGY

CHAPTER 8

Blunt Chest Trauma

Lisa A. Miller and Stuart E. Mirvis

■ NONMEDIASTINAL INJURY

Chest trauma is directly responsible for 25% of all trauma deaths and is a major contributor in another 50% of all trauma mortality. Chest trauma may be blunt (90% of cases) or penetrating. Blunt thoracic injuries are the third most common injuries in polytrauma patients, following those of the head and extremity. Although 50% of blunt chest injuries are minor, 33% will require hospital admission. Rib fractures and pulmonary contusions are the most common injuries encountered. A chest radiograph is generally the first modality of radiologic evaluation of the chest trauma patient. It is essentially a screening examination and is used to identify life-threatening conditions such as a large hemothorax, tension pneumothorax, dangerously malpositioned lines and tubes, and mediastinal hematoma. Contrast-enhanced (CE) chest computed tomography (CT) is the gold standard for radiologic evaluation of the chest trauma patient. This chapter will review the spectrum of radiographic and CT imaging findings seen in patients sustaining major thoracic trauma, including the lungs, pleura, bones, and mediastinal structures.

■ LUNG INJURY

Pulmonary Contusion

Pulmonary contusions are the most common pulmonary injury and occur in 17% to 70% of blunt chest trauma patients, most commonly from motor vehicle collisions or falls from height. A pulmonary contusion results from injury to the alveolar wall and pulmonary vessels, allowing blood to leak into the alveolar and interstitial spaces of the lung. The causes are thought to include compression of the lung against the chest wall, shearing forces, rib fracture, or previously formed pleural adhesions tearing peripheral tissue as the lung separates from the chest wall at impact. Blast injuries also commonly cause pulmonary contusion.

The appearance of pulmonary contusion on the chest radiograph depends on its severity. Minimal contusion may not be visible or may appear as an ill-defined area of patchy air space opacity (Fig. 8-1). Severe contusion may appear as consolidation of a large area of lung (Fig. 8-2). Air bronchograms may be seen in contused lung if there has not been filling of the airways with blood. Pulmonary contusion is typically nonsegmental and geographic, and it readily crosses pleural fissures, unlike pneumonia or atelectasis.

Compared with radiography, CT is much more sensitive in detection of pulmonary contusion (Fig. 8-3). The appearance of pulmonary contusion may be delayed up to 6 hours on chest radiography but is seen immediately on chest CT. The CT appearance is similar to that of chest radiography. Minimal contusion may manifest as ground-glass density, often with subpleural sparing of 1 to 2 mm (especially in the pediatric population), often in the periphery of the lung or adjacent to bony structures such as the spine (see Fig. 8-3). On both radiography and CT, pulmonary contusion often "blossoms" in the first 24 to 48 hours after the injury as blood progressively accumulates in the lung parenchyma (Figs. 8-4 and 8-5).

Contusions are a risk factor for development of pneumonia or acute respiratory distress syndrome. Patients with contusions seen only on the CT image and not on the chest radiograph may have a prognosis similar to those that do not have pulmonary contusions at all on CT (i.e., "CT-only" contusion may have a better outcome than contusions that are visible on both CT and chest x-ray examination). Pulmonary contusion usually resolves in 1 to 14 days (Fig. 8-6). Generally, if the chest radiograph or CT has not cleared by day 14, alternate diagnoses such as development of pneumonia, acute respiratory distress syndrome, or aspiration should be considered.

Pulmonary Laceration

The mechanism of injury causing a pulmonary laceration is thought to be similar to that of pulmonary contusion: tearing of lung parenchyma due to compression, shearing forces, direct injury from rib fracture(s), or at the site of previously formed pleural adhesions. Pulmonary lacerations are round or oval in shape due to the elastic recoil of the lung (Fig. 8-7). There may be single or innumerable lacerations with size ranging from a few millimeters to several centimeters in diameter (Fig. 8-8). Air, blood, or both may fill in the laceration (see Fig. 8-5), and there will often be a thin pseudomembrane due to the compression of surrounding lung tissue. On the chest radiograph, pulmonary lacerations are often obscured for the first 48 to 72 hours because of surrounding pulmonary contusion (see Fig. 8-6). Computed tomography is much more sensitive in detection of pulmonary lacerations compared with radiography.

Active bleeding into a pulmonary laceration may occasionally be seen. On intravenous (IV) CECT active bleeding will appear as linear high density, with Hounsfield units (HU) similar to that of the aorta, within or

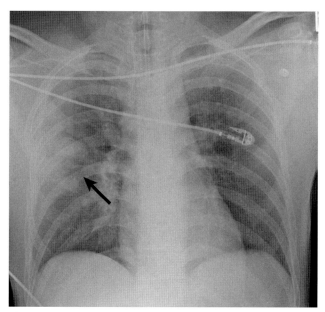

Figure 8-1 *Supine chest radiograph of a patient struck by a motor vehicle.* There is patchy, ill-defined opacity in the peripheral aspect of the right midlung *(arrow)*. Note adjacent right-sided rib fractures. Although commonly seen in association with pulmonary contusion, fractures need not be present, especially in the more compliant bones of the pediatric population.

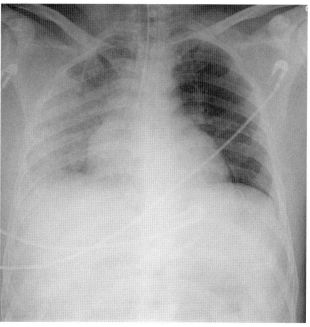

Figure 8-2 *Supine chest radiograph of a patient involved in motorcycle accident.* There is diffuse air-space opacification throughout the entire right lung, indicating severe, widespread pulmonary contusion. Note is made of right mainstem endotracheal tube intubation.

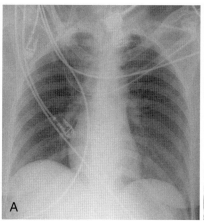
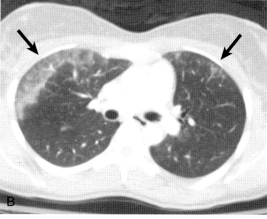

Figure 8-3 *Supine chest radiograph of a trauma patient.* **A,** Essentially clear lungs. **B,** Computed tomography (CT) of the same patient demonstrates a small to moderate amount of peripheral contusions in both lungs, right greater than left *(arrows)*. Note the 1 to 2 mm of subpleural sparing, a common finding in pulmonary contusion but not in other air-space processes such as pneumonia.

adjacent to the laceration (Fig. 8-9). A pulmonary laceration will typically take several weeks or months to resolve. During healing the laceration will gradually fill completely with blood and then gradually decrease in size (Fig. 8-10). A blood-filled rounded healing pulmonary laceration could be mistaken for a pulmonary neoplasm if the history of relatively recent chest trauma is not known.

An uncommon complication of a pulmonary laceration is formation of a bronchopleural fistula. This condition is more likely to occur if the laceration is in the periphery of the lung, with only the thin pseudomembrane between it and the pleural space. Bronchopleural fistula should be suspected if there is a persistent pneumothorax, unrelieved by appropriately positioned single or multiple chest tubes. Rarely, a pulmonary abscess may complicate a pulmonary laceration.

■ INJURIES INVOLVING THE PLEURAL SPACE

Pneumothorax

A pneumothorax is a collection of air in the pleural space. Air may enter the pleural space during trauma because of penetrating injury from a knife or gunshot, puncture from a fractured rib, rapid deceleration forces causing pulmonary laceration, or alveolar rupture from suddenly increased intrathoracic pressure at the time of impact.

The appearance of a pneumothorax on the chest radiograph will depend greatly on the patient position. The initial chest radiograph of the trauma patient is usually a supine film obtained in the emergency department or trauma bay. When the patient is in the supine position,

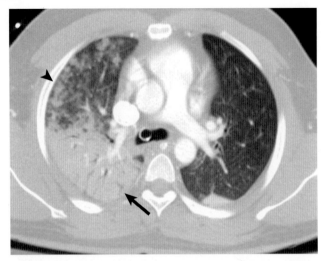

Figure 8-4 Chest computed tomography (CT) of a patient involved in motor vehicle collision. There is extensive pulmonary contusion throughout the entire visualized right lung. The pleural fissures are not respected in pulmonary contusion. Note air bronchograms *(arrow)* and subpleural sparing *(arrowhead)*.

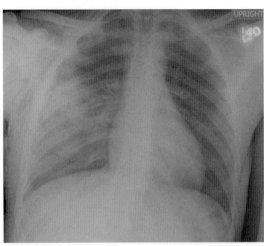

Figure 8-5 Chest radiograph of a patient who fell off a roof. Pulmonary contusion in the mid and lower portions of the right lung. Note a small right pneumothorax and subcutaneous air in the right chest wall.

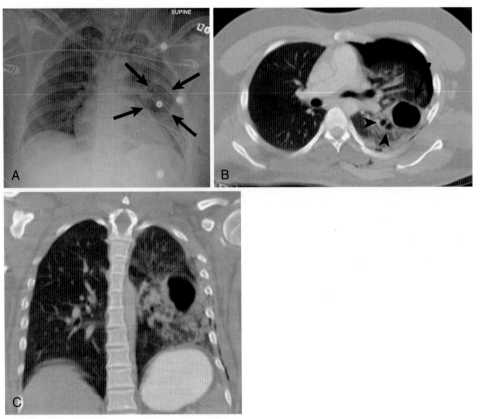

Figure 8-6 Chest radiograph of a patient involved in a jet-ski accident. A, Minimal patchy opacity and a large oval lucency *(arrows)* in the midportion of the left lung. Axial (**B**) and coronal (**C**) computed tomographic (CT) images better show the minimal pulmonary contusion in the left lung, a large pulmonary laceration *(arrow)*, and at least two smaller pulmonary lacerations *(arrowheads)*. A left pneumothorax is noted.

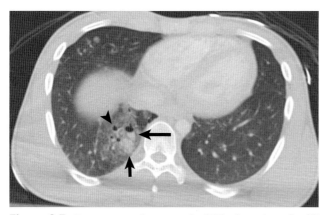

Figure 8-7 Chest computed tomography (CT) of a patient who fell out of a moving vehicle shows multiple pulmonary lacerations of various sizes in the right lower lobe. Note that pulmonary lacerations may be filled with blood *(short arrow)*, air *(arrowhead)*, or both *(long arrow)*, in which case a meniscus sign is seen. Patchy pulmonary contusion surrounds the lacerations.

air will collect in the anterior and medial aspects of the pleural space. On the chest radiograph this may manifest as increased lucency over the lower thorax/upper abdominal quadrant (Figs. 8-11 and 8-12), a deep costophrenic angle sign (Fig. 8-13), or a sharply defined border of the heart or diaphragm. The "double diaphragm" sign, seen when air in the pleural space outlines both the dome and the anterior insertion of the diaphragm, may also be identified. A thin lucency adjacent to the heart border may also be seen and represents air between the medial lung margin and the soft tissues of the mediastinum (Fig. 8-14). In the upright patient a pneumothorax is typically seen as a thin, sharply defined line of the visceral pleura with no lung markings beyond this border (Fig. 8-15).

There are numerous mimics of pneumothorax on chest radiography, including bullae, skin folds (Fig. 8-16), bedding or clothing, and overlying tubes or catheters. Computed tomography is much more sensitive for

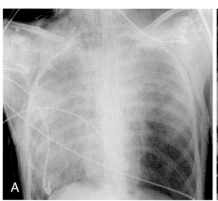
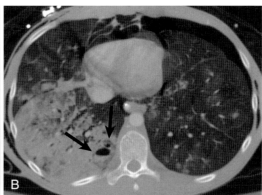

Figure 8-8 Chest radiograph of a patient who was hit by a train. A, Extensive pulmonary contusion throughout the right lung and upper medial aspect of the left lung. **B,** Computed tomography (CT) demonstrates presence of pulmonary lacerations in right lower lobe *(arrows)*, findings not seen on the chest radiograph.

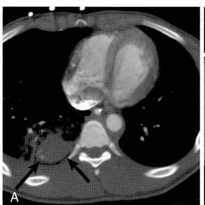
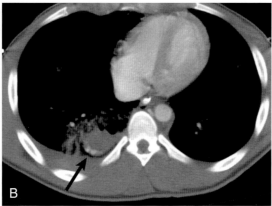

Figure 8-9 Arterial phase chest computed tomography (CT). A, A large oval pulmonary laceration in the right lower lobe *(arrows)* that is nearly completely filled with blood. **B,** There are several small foci of high density along the right lateral margin of the laceration *(arrow)* that increase in size and remain dense on the portal venous images. These findings indicate active bleeding within the laceration.

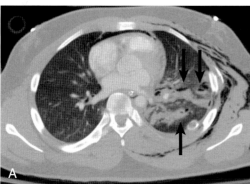
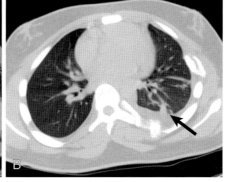

Figure 8-10 Admission chest computed tomography (CT) of a patient kicked by a horse. A, Multiple pulmonary lacerations in left lower lobe *(arrows)* with surrounding pulmonary contusion. **B,** Follow-up chest CT obtained 2 months later shows near complete resolution of multiple pulmonary lacerations. A single, blood-filled residual laceration is seen *(arrow)*. Small left hemothorax and healing left rib fractures are noted.

Figure 8-11 Supine chest radiograph of a patient struck by a moped. A, There is a thin rim of lucency above the right hemidiaphragm *(arrow)*, suspicious for inferior pneumothorax. Air in the soft tissues of the right lateral chest wall is another clue that pneumothorax may be present *(arrowheads)*. **B,** Coronal reformatted chest computed tomographic (CT) image confirms the presence of a small right inferior pneumothorax *(arrow)*.

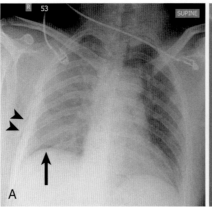
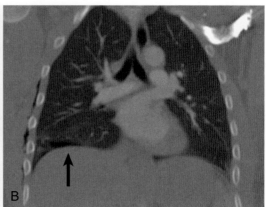

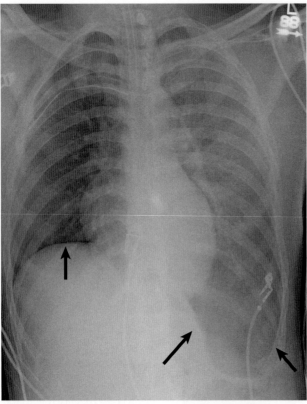

Figure 8-12 Supine chest radiograph of a patient involved in a motor vehicle collision. There is increased lucency of the left upper quadrant *(long arrows)*, indicating presence of a left pneumothorax. Also note a small residual right inferior pneumothorax after placement of right-sided chest tube *(short arrow)*.

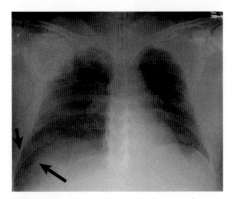

Figure 8-13 Supine chest radiograph of a trauma patient demonstrates increased lucency of the right lower hemothorax *(arrows)* producing deep costophrenic sulcus indicating pneumothorax.

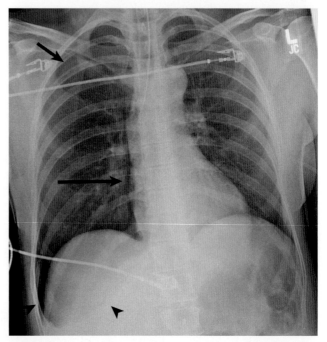

Figure 8-14 Supine chest radiograph of a patient involved in four-wheeler accident demonstrates several signs of pneumothorax: lucency between medial lung and heart border *(long arrow)*, deep costophrenic sulcus sign and hyperlucent right upper quadrant *(arrowheads)*, and the thin linear density over the right upper lung field with no lung marking distal to this line *(short arrow)*.

detection of pneumothorax. It is estimated that up to 78% of pneumothoraces are missed by chest radiography.

Generally a chest tube is placed for all pneumothoraces seen on the supine chest radiograph or in any unstable patient with a potential pneumothorax. Occult pneumothorax, defined as a pneumothorax seen only on chest CT and not on the supine chest radiograph, is thought to occur in up to 15% of blunt chest trauma patients (Fig. 8-17). Optimal management of the occult pneumothorax is currently debated. It was previously thought that an occult pneumothorax required a prophylactic chest tube because of risk for enlargement or development of tension pneumothorax, especially in patients on mechanical ventilation. There is growing evidence that a small occult pneumothorax can be safely managed in the majority of patients with close observation, without thoracostomy tube placement. About 10%

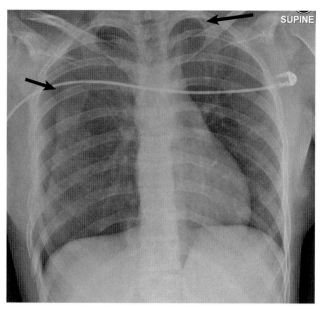

Figure 8-15 Supine chest radiograph of a patient who fell from a balcony demonstrates the typical signs of a pneumothorax: a thin dense line along the periphery of the right hemithorax with no lung markings beyond this line *(short arrow)*. There is also a tiny left apical pneumothorax *(long arrow)*. Note right rib fractures.

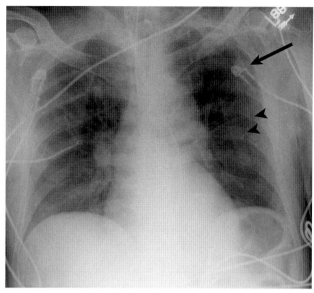

Figure 8-16 Semiupright chest radiograph of a trauma patient shows a linear density along the periphery of the left hemithorax *(arrow)*, which upon casual inspection would be suspicious for a pneumothorax. However, there are lung markings distal to this line and two additional linear densities medial to the first *(arrowheads)*. These findings are due to folds of skin or bedding, and not a pneumothorax.

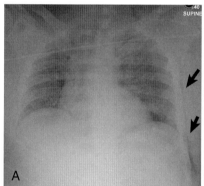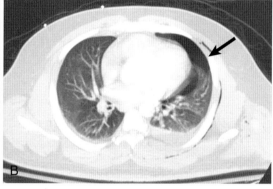

Figure 8-17 Supine chest radiograph of a patient involved in a farming accident. A, Only a small amount of subcutaneous air in the soft tissues of the left chest wall *(arrows)*. **B,** Axial chest computed tomographic (CT) image demonstrates a left pneumothorax *(arrow)* in addition to the soft tissue air. This would be considered an occult pneumothorax because there were no definite signs of pneumothorax on the supine radiograph.

of patients managed using this guideline will fail conservative management and ultimately require thoracostomy tube placement for symptomatic pneumothorax.

A tension pneumothorax occurs because of a one-way valve mechanism in which air can enter the pleural space but cannot get out. This results in rapid and progressive accumulation of air in the pleural space with increasing pressure causing contralateral shift of the mediastinum and compression of the vena cavae resulting in decreased cardiac output from impaired venous return (Fig. 8-18). Note that tension pneumothorax is a clinical diagnosis but can be suggested by radiologic signs of increased lucency of the affected hemithorax, contralateral shift of the mediastinum, widened ipsilateral rib interspaces, depression of the ipsilateral hemidiaphragm, and lung collapse toward the hilum. Treatment is immediate decompression with chest tube thoracostomy. Rapid reexpansion of the lung after treatment of tension pneumothorax can lead to pulmonary edema. This occurs immediately after treatment of the pneumothorax and may be unilateral or bilateral.

This condition occurs more commonly in patients 20 to 50 years of age. Although tension pneumothorax may be completely asymptomatic, there is a reported mortality rate of up to 20%. If there is persistent pneumothorax or air leak after chest tube placement, incorrect tube placement, bronchopleural fistula, or tracheobronchial injury should be suspected (Fig. 8-19).

Hemothorax

Hemothorax is seen in 50% cases of blunt chest trauma. Sources of bleeding can be the intercostal arteries, thoracic spine, lung, great vessels, or heart. Hemothorax can also occur with hemoperitoneum and concurrent ruptured diaphragm.

On chest radiography at least 150 to 200 mL of blood are needed to detect pleural fluid on an upright chest radiograph. A meniscus sign is often seen with pleural fluid of any type and appears as a concave sloping of fluid in the costophrenic angle toward the lateral chest

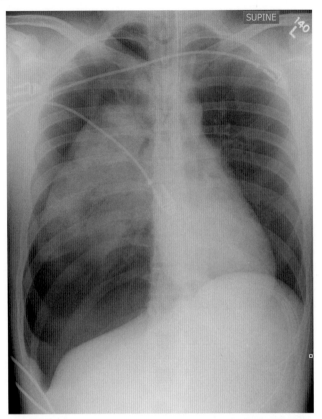

Figure 8-18 Chest radiograph shows signs suspicious for the clinical diagnosis of a tension pneumothorax: right lung collapsed toward the hilum with decreased density around the collapsed lung, deep costophrenic angle sign, depressed right hemidiaphragm, and shift of mediastinum to the left. Clinically the patient had severe dyspnea and hypotension that was relieved with chest tube placement.

wall. A straight air-fluid level indicates hemopneumothorax. Because most trauma chest radiographs are performed with the patient in the supine position, blood will collect in the dependent portion of the thorax. A hemothorax will be seen on the supine film as a diffuse increase in density over the entire hemithorax. A dense rim of blood may be seen along the lateral lung margin as blood progressively fills the dependent pleural space and compresses the lung medially (Fig. 8-20). A very large hemothorax can cause complete opacification of the affected hemithorax with contralateral shift of the mediastinum (Fig. 8-21).

On CT, acute hemothorax is seen as hyperdense fluid in the dependent portion of the pleural space. Hounsfield units of acute hemorrhage will be higher than 15, generally in the range of 20 to 45 HU. Slightly higher density in the dependent portion of the hemothorax may be seen because of settling of blood products. As blood clots, the density of the blood increases to 50 to 90 HU. If there is intermittent bleeding in the pleural space, layers of different densities may be seen, constituting the "hematocrit effect." Active bleeding within the pleural space will appear as a linear tract of high density (within 10 HU of the IV CE aorta) within the pleural space (Fig. 8-22). Angiography with selective embolization may be used for treatment of active bleeding or pseudoaneurysm (Fig. 8-23). The exact site of bleeding needs to be determined whether surgery or catheter embolization is the chosen treatment.

Simple or serous effusion, bile, chyle, and urine may also accumulate in the pleural space. A sympathetic serous effusion may be seen if there are injuries to the liver, spleen, or pancreas and will have HU density less

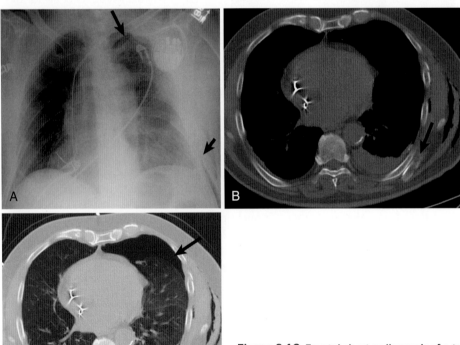

Figure 8-19 Frontal chest radiograph of a trauma patient. A, A pneumothorax persists *(long arrow)* despite the presence of a left chest tube. Note that the distal side hole of the chest tube projects outside of the bony thorax *(short arrow)* and could be responsible for the residual pneumothorax. **B,** Chest computed tomography (CT) on soft tissue windows shows the position of the chest tube to be in the subscapular space *(arrow)*. **C,** Lung window CT shows the residual left pneumothorax *(arrow)*.

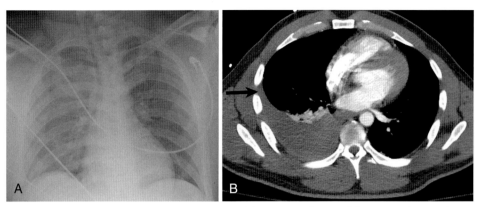

Figure 8-20 *Supine chest radiograph of a patient who fell.* **A,** Mild increase in density of the entire right hemithorax. **B,** Axial chest computed tomographic (CT) image shows blood accumulating in the dependent portion of the right pleural space. A meniscus sign is seen as blood slopes up toward the lateral chest wall *(arrow)*.

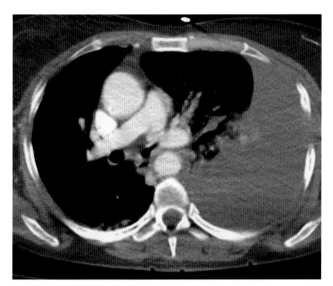

Figure 8-21 Tension hemothorax. Chest computed tomography (CT) of a trauma patient shows a large left hemothorax causing shift of the mediastinum to the right, findings concerning for the clinical diagnosis of tension hemothorax.

than 15. Chylous effusion is due to an injury to the thoracic lymphatic duct and may have negative HU density because of the presence of fat. An effusion composed of bile or urine is seen with injury to the biliary or urinary system and a concurrent full-thickness diaphragm tear. Differentiating between bile and urine on CT can be very difficult and may require thoracentesis and analysis of fluid to establish the correct diagnosis (Fig. 8-24). Delayed imaging of the renal collecting system may also be diagnostic if direct contrast leak is identified.

Extrapleural Hematoma

Extrapleural hematoma refers to blood that has collected between the parietal pleural and endothoracic fascia. The cause is usually a rib fracture that has lacerated an intercostal artery. On chest radiograph an extrapleural hematoma typically appears as a focal convex mass along the periphery of the lung. It may also be seen at the lung apex after subclavian vessel trauma or aortic

injury (Fig. 8-25). Unlike a pleural effusion or a hemothorax, an extrapleural hematoma will not change shape with a change in patient position. On CT an extrapleural hematoma appears as a fluid collection that causes inward displacement of the extrapleural fat (Fig. 8-26). Active bleeding within the hematoma may be seen and can be treated with angiographic embolization.

◼ BONY THORAX AND CHEST WALL

Soft Tissue Contusion

Soft tissue contusion or hematoma may be arterial or venous in origin. A hematoma from a high-pressure arterial injury may enlarge rapidly, whereas a hematoma from a low-pressure venous injury is usually self-limited. The trauma patient who is taking anticoagulants is at higher risk for developing a soft tissue contusion or hematoma from minor trauma.

On the chest radiograph a soft tissue contusion is not usually apparent unless there is a large amount of associated soft tissue hematoma. A large amount of hematoma may appear as increased density of the soft tissues or asymmetry of the soft tissues when compared to the uninjured side. Extensive soft tissue hematoma affecting one side of the chest wall can be hard to distinguish from a layering hemothorax on the supine chest radiograph. Excess soft tissues in an obese patient or a female patient with large breasts may mimic or obscure a chest wall hematoma.

The appearance of chest wall soft tissue trauma on CT will depend on the severity of the injury and can range from minimal fat stranding of the chest wall to a large hematoma with or without active bleeding (Fig. 8-27). A seatbelt mark, identified as soft tissue bruising on the lower neck and center chest, is often seen in patients injured in motor vehicle collisions. The presence of a seat belt bruise or hematoma in the neck may be a marker for underlying cervical vessel injury, and a neck CT angiography may be warranted for further evaluation.

Rib Fractures

Rib fractures are the most common thoracic skeletal injury in blunt chest trauma, with an incidence of 50%.

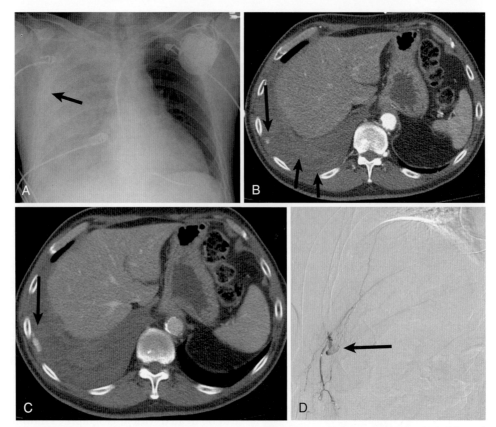

Figure 8-22 Supine chest radiograph of a patient involved in a motor vehicle collision. **A,** Opacification of the entire right hemithorax and a thin rim of density along the lateral margin of the right lung *(arrow),* indicating right hemothorax. **B,** Arterial phase chest computed tomography (CT) shows the "hematocrit effect" of layers of slightly different densities in the right pleural space *(short arrows),* indicating intermittent bleeding. A hyperdense focus is seen in the periphery of the hemothorax *(long arrow).* **C,** On the portal venous phase CT image this focus remains hyperdense and increases in size, indicating active bleeding *(arrow).* **D,** Selective intercostal angiography image shows active bleeding *(arrow)* from the right tenth intercostal artery. This was treated with angiographic embolization.

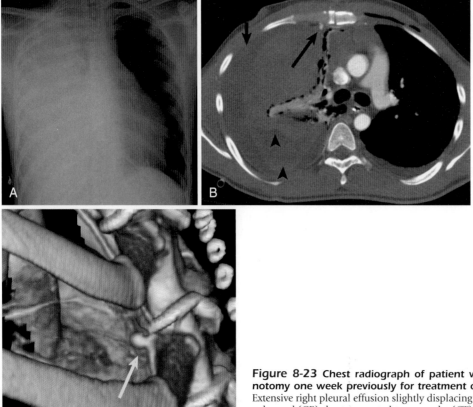

Figure 8-23 Chest radiograph of patient who had undergone median sternotomy one week previously for treatment of traumatic mediastinal injury. **A,** Extensive right pleural effusion slightly displacing the heart to the left. **B,** Axial contrast-enhanced (CE) chest computed tomography (CT) demonstrates fluid of different densities layering in the right thorax *(arrowheads)* with significant compression of the right lung. A more peripheral rim of lower density indicates more acute hemorrhage *(short arrow).* There is a lobular appearance of the right internal mammary artery *(long arrow).* **C,** Three-dimensional (3-D) reformatted CT image confirms the presence of a traumatic pseudoaneurysm of the right internal mammary artery *(arrow).*

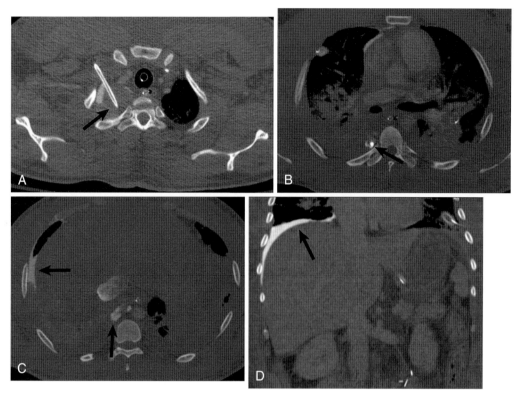

Figure 8-24 A more unusual cause of fluid in the pleural space. A, Contrast-enhanced (CE) chest computed tomography (CT) shows a malpositioned right central venous catheter (*arrow*). **B,** CT image of the lower hemithorax shows the very hyperdense tip of the central venous line in the posterior aspect of the hemithorax (*arrow*) surrounded by ill-defined, slightly less dense material. **C,** Another axial CT image slightly lower in the chest shows active bleeding. **D,** A coronal reformatted CT image show that the dense material is in the pleural space (*arrow*). These findings represent intravenous (IV) contrast material in the right pleural space secondary to malpositioned right subclavian central venous catheter.

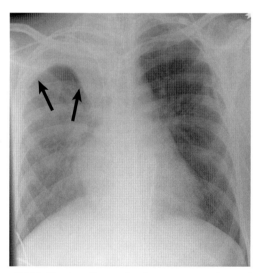

Figure 8-25 Chest radiograph of a trauma patient who just had a right subclavian central venous catheter placed. A rim of increased density along the apex of the right lung (*arrows*).

Rib fractures are most commonly the result of a motor vehicle collision in the adult patient. Rib fractures in older adults are most commonly due to falls. The lateral aspects of the ribs are the site most commonly fractured because of the chest wall architecture and decreased muscular support in this region. Chest radiography has sensitivity as low as 15% for detection of rib fractures. Computed tomography has a much higher sensitivity, especially when coronal reformatted images are reviewed.

Fractures of the eighth to eleventh ribs are associated with a higher incidence of injury to the spleen (left-sided fractures) or liver (right-sided fractures). When CT is obtained in the trauma patient with lower rib fractures, a routine search for injury involving these organs should be performed. Fractures of the first, second, and third ribs indicate high-velocity trauma and are associated with brachial plexus or subclavian vessel injury in 3% to 15% of blunt chest trauma patients. The rib number and site of each rib fracture should be specified in the radiology report because this provides prognostic information to the trauma surgeon. It has been shown that mortality increases 19% and pneumonia increases 27% in elderly patients with each additional rib fracture.

Flail chest, seen in 6% of blunt trauma patients, indicates the presence of at least two fractures in three or more consecutive ribs (Fig. 8-28). Flail chest is associated with a mortality of 33%. The chest wall instability, paradoxical motion of the fractured segment, and invariable presence of underlying pulmonary contusion cause altered pulmonary mechanics that lead to atelectasis, stasis of secretions, and pneumonia. Recent research shows that open reduction and internal fixation of flail chest may lead to improved outcomes.

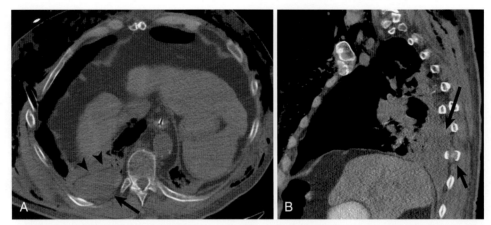

Figure 8-26 Computed tomography (CT) of a multitrauma patient. A, An oval high-density collection representing extrapleural hematoma adjacent to the posterior right ribs *(arrow)*. Note the thin rim of fat that separates it from the lung *(arrowheads)*. **B,** Sagittal reformatted CT again demonstrates the extrapleural hematoma *(long arrow)*, thin rim of extrapleural fat anterior to the hematoma and the probable cause of the hematoma: a right posterior rib fracture *(short arrow)*.

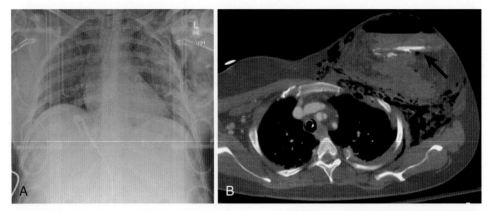

Figure 8-27 Chest radiograph of a female trauma patient. A, Extensive chest injuries, including scattered left pulmonary contusion, soft tissue air in left chest wall, and left clavicle and bilateral rib fractures. A right mainstem endotracheal tube intubation is also noted. **B,** Axial chest computed tomographic (CT) image shows a large hematoma in the left breast with central foci of linear high density *(arrow)*, indicating active bleeding.

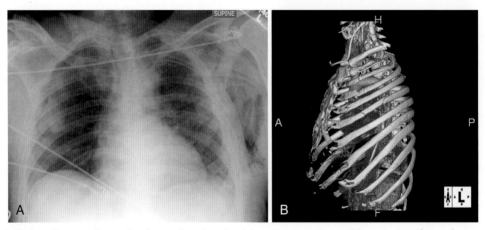

Figure 8-28 Admission chest radiograph of a patient involved in a motorcycle collision. A, Significant chest trauma, including a right pneumothorax, scattered bilateral pulmonary contusions, soft tissue air in the left chest wall, and multiple bilateral rib fractures. **B,** Three-dimensional (3-D) reformatted computed tomographic (CT) image of the chest better demonstrates the presence of multiple rib fractures. Analysis of the number and site of rib fractures indicates presence of a flail chest.

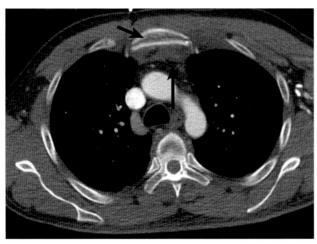

Figure 8-29 Axial computed tomographic (CT) image of patient involved in a motor vehicle collision shows a sagittal fracture of the sternum *(short arrow)*. There is a small amount of anterior mediastinal hemorrhage (MH) in association with the fracture *(long arrow)*. Note the preserved fat plane between the hemorrhage and the anterior aortic wall.

Sternal Fractures

Sternal fractures are seen in 3% to 8% of blunt chest trauma patients. Fractures of the sternum are high-impact injuries. Motor vehicle collision is the most common cause, and the injury is usually due to the chest striking the steering wheel or the airbag impacting the chest wall. Sternal fractures are associated with rib fractures, cardiac contusion (1.5% to 6%), pericardial effusion, and cervicothoracic spine injuries. Although commonly associated with additional injuries, a nondisplaced sternal fracture can be seen as an isolated injury.

The supine chest radiograph will rarely demonstrate the fractured sternum unless the sternum is significantly displaced laterally. A properly exposed lateral chest radiograph, though rarely obtained in the acute trauma setting, will usually permit identification of at least mildly displaced fractures. Axial CT images will demonstrate most but not all sternal fractures. A clue on the axial CT images that there may be a sternal fracture is the anterior mediastinal or retrosternal hemorrhage that accompanies nearly all of these fractures. There will be a preserved fat plane between the posterior aspect of the retrosternal blood and the aorta (Fig. 8-29). Traumatic aortic injury can also be a source of anterior mediastinal hemorrhage, but there will be no preserved fat plane and hemorrhage will be in direct contact with the aortic wall. Sagittal and coronal reformatted CT images are a significant aid in detection of a sternal fracture (Figs. 8-30 and 8-31). Treatment is conservative in the vast majority of cases. Rarely, nonunion, severe pain, or sternal instability may require open reduction and internal fixation.

■ MEDIASTINAL INJURY

Tracheobronchial Injury

Tracheal and bronchial injuries from blunt trauma are rare. Actual full-thickness tears are more common in the thoracic than cervical segment and are associated

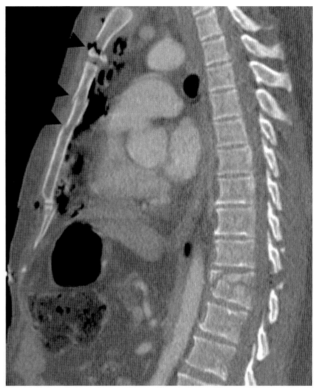

Figure 8-30 Sagittal reformatted computed tomographic (CT) image shows a severely comminuted but minimally displaced sternal fracture *(arrowheads)*. A Chance fracture of the lower thoracic spine is noted.

with higher mortality. Most transbronchial tears occur close to the carina and more frequently on the right (Fig. 8-32). Ruptures usually occur in the weaker posterior membranous portion. Mechanisms of the injury involve anterior-posterior compression of the chest forcing the lungs and mainstem bronchi laterally near the carina and exceeding the connective tissue strength of the airway, a sudden rise in intraluminal pressure when the glottis is closed, or by direct trachea crushing between the sternum and spine. The cervical portion can be sheared in rapid deceleration between the relatively immobile carina and cricoid and the more flexible trachea in between, by direct impact, or with sudden hyperextension and longitudinal traction. Tears typically occur across the weaker transverse plane. Injury can also result from a linear force applied across the cervical airway from a "clothesline" horizontal force when the neck impacts fixed linear obstacles like ropes, tree limbs, or wires (Fig. 8-33).

The injury may be suggested by clinical signs/symptoms, including hemoptysis, cough, respiratory distress, cyanosis, subcutaneous air, hoarseness, aphonia/dysphonia from recurrent laryngeal nerve injury, and the Hamman "crunch" sign, when cardiac motion impacts adjacent mediastinal air. These findings are neither sensitive nor specific and may not be present with small or incomplete tears. Because of their rarity and other more overt coincident injuries, airway injuries are not suspected based on bedside findings and may be recognized only by imaging or when overt clinical complications arise.

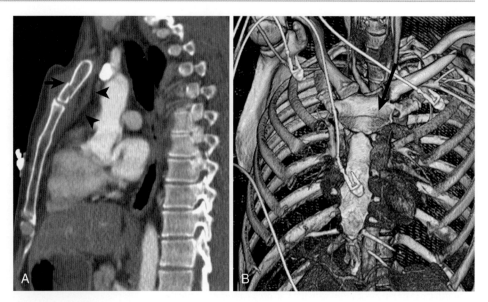

Figure 8-31 Sagittal reformatted computed tomographic (CT) image of a patient involved in a motor vehicle collision. A, An oblique fracture of the manubrium *(arrow)* and a small amount of retrosternal blood *(arrowheads).* **B,** Coronal three-dimensional (3-D) reformatted image shows the extent of the fracture across the manubrium *(arrow).*

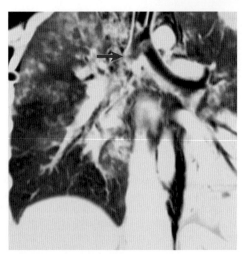

Figure 8-32 Mainstem bronchus injury. Coronal multidetector computed tomography (MDCT) reformation demonstrates complete cutoff across right mainstem bronchus *(arrow).* There is diffuse lung contusion, mainly in the right upper lobe and pneumomediastinum, well seen around the aorta and subcarinal region. The left lower lobe is collapsed.

Radiologic findings are more likely when there is positive pressure ventilator support. Air leaks into the mediastinum usually progress rapidly through tissue planes of the chest and beyond along fascial planes throughout the body. Pneumothorax can occur through dissection of air through the lung interstitium and visceral pleura, particularly from peripheral lung tears or through a direct tracheobronchial fistula (Fig. 8-34). A finding suggesting a major airway-pleural communication is failure of a properly placed thoracostomy tube to relieve a simple or tension pneumothorax. When a major airway is breached, air enters the pleural space at the same rate it is evacuated by suction, maintaining the pneumothorax at constant pressure (Fig. 8-35). Rarely an abrupt interruption or irregular tapering of the airway (bayonet sign) can be directly visualized radiographically. If there is a complete mainstem

bronchial disconnection, the entire distal lung may collapse and fall into a gravity-dependent position (fallen lung; see Fig. 8-35). Airway interruption from blood clot or lacerated tissue occlusion will lead to persistent distal atelectasis.

If the cervical trachea is disrupted, an inflated endotracheal tube cuff may overexpand into the weakened or torn wall, producing an overdistended or caudally displaced balloon (Fig. 8-36; see Fig. 8-32). A normally inflated balloon cuff is barely visualized radiographically. The course of the endotracheal tube may rarely deviate from the expected path of the trachea through a wall defect. Small portions of the balloon cuff may protrude/herniate through small tears.

The vast majority of blunt trauma patients with rapid onset and progressive mediastinal air leaks will NOT have injury to a major airway, but positive pressure respiratory support combined with lung laceration. Pneumomediastinum can be absent despite major airway injury when the adventitia remains intact or the tear is occluded by clot or an endotracheal tube balloon.

Computed tomography will display the same signs as chest radiographs with greater sensitivity and can detect airway tears directly (Figs. 8-36 to 8-38). Major airway injuries can occur in association with clavicular, sternal, upper rib, and vertebral body extension fractures, but these are nonspecific indicators of airway injury and principally indicate a high level of impacting force. Concurrent major vascular injuries should be sought as indicated by mediastinal blood given the same chest compression or a shearing force mechanism of injury responsible for some cases of major airway disruption.

A large amount of mediastinal air around the trachea and mainstem bronchi does not indicate adjacent airway injury, but direct visualization of an airway-mediastinal connection is diagnostic.

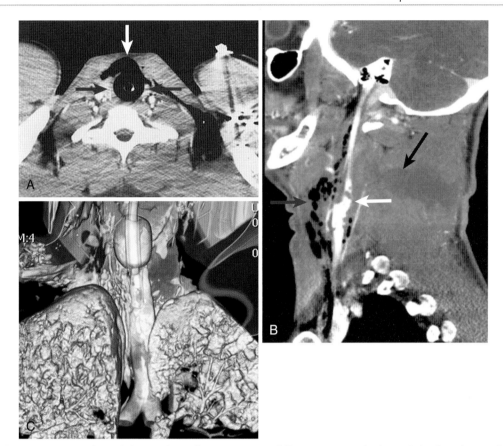

Figure 8-33 Transverse laceration of the trachea of a young man riding a motorcycle through backyards sustaining an actual "clothesline" laceration. **A,** Axial computed tomographic (CT) image across high cervical trachea shows overdistention of endotracheal balloon *(red arrows)* and extraluminal air anteriorly *(white arrow)*. **B,** Sagittal reformatted parasagittal image through the left side of the neck shows extraluminal air in anterior neck *(red arrow)*, thrombus, and dissection of distal common and left internal carotid artery *(white arrow)*, and linear soft tissue laceration through posterior cervical muscles *(black arrow)*. The patient survived the injury with restoration of airway and without cerebral injury. **C,** Three-dimensional (3-D) image better demonstrates overdistended balloon in ruptured trachea.

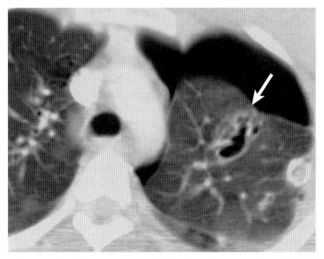

Figure 8-34 Bronchopleural fistula. Contrast-enhanced (CE) axial computed tomographic (CT) image in a blunt trauma patient reveals peripheral left upper lobe lung laceration with central hematoma creating trachea-to-pleural space connection *(arrow)*. There is a large pneumothorax despite a chest tube.

The diagnosis of complete airway disruption can be supported by volumetric rendering, including endoluminal views (virtual bronchoscopy; see Figs. 8-32, 8-34, 8-37) or verified with bronchoscopy. Earlier diagnosis of this injury improves the chances for successful surgical airway repair, preserving pulmonary function, and preventing long-term complications of chronic airway narrowing.

■ ESOPHAGEAL INJURY

Esophageal injury sustained from blunt chest trauma is extremely rare. The injuries occur in the cervical and upper thoracic portions below the cricopharyngeal muscle and at the gastroesophageal junction, where there are transition points between relatively fixed and mobile segments. Not surprisingly, given the central protected location of the esophagus, injury typically requires high-force impacts and thus is likely to be accompanied by other thoracic injuries (Fig. 8-39). Injury mechanisms include crushing between the impacted anterior chest wall and the spine, hyperextension of the spine mainly at the diaphragmatic hiatus, and laceration or entrapment related to fractures or dislocations of the thoracic spine (Fig. 8-40). A sudden increase in intraesophageal pressure by compressive forces may also cause rupture.

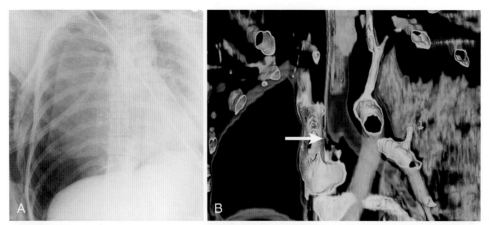

Figure 8-35 Completely torn right mainstem bronchus. **A,** Anteroposterior (AP) chest radiograph demonstrates a right tension pneumothorax with depression of right hemidiaphragm, displaced heart and mediastinum to the left, and spread right ribs. A chest tube that was appropriately placed overlies the right hemithorax, and the right lung is partially collapsed. **B,** Coronal slab three-dimensional (3-D) image highlights complete cutoff of right mainstem bronchus *(arrow)*.

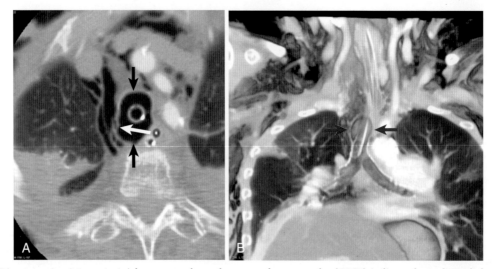

Figure 8-36 Direct tracheal tear. **A,** Axial contrast-enhanced computed tomography (CECT) indicates hyperdistended endotracheal tube balloon cuff *(black arrows)* and focal linear tear in right lateral wall of thoracic trachea *(white arrow)*. There is surrounding pneumomediastinum. **B,** Coronal slab three-dimensional (3-D) image verifies overdistended balloon cuff *(arrows)* and marked soft tissue air. (From Mirvis SE, Shanmuganathan K, Miller LA, et al. Case 89. *Emergency Radiology.* Case Review Series. Philadelphia, PA: Mosby Elsevier; 2009:181.)

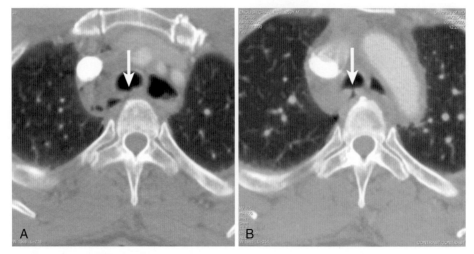

Figure 8-37 Direct tracheal tear. **A** and **B,** Axial contrast-enhanced computed tomographic (CECT) images through the carina shows a posterior defect in the membranous trachea *(arrows)* with adjacent mediastinal air and bilateral posterior mediastinal hematoma.

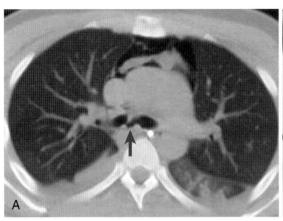

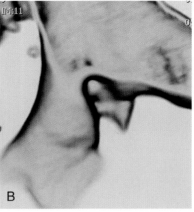

Figure 8-38 Airway injury at the carina. A, Axial computed tomographic (CT) image indicates an irregular lumen at level of the carina *(arrow)* in a blunt trauma patient. **B,** Coronal volumetric view through the carina verifies a tear and its proximity to the carina. Injury was verified bronchoscopically and successfully managed nonoperatively.

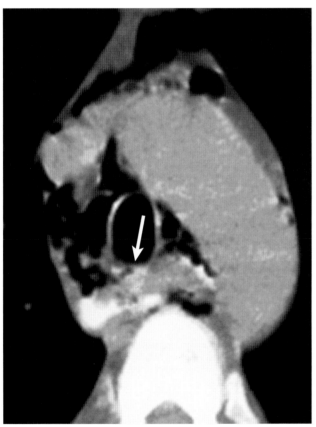

Figure 8-39 Tracheoesophageal injury. Axial computed tomographic (CT) image with oral contrast shows extravasation of contrast into the peritracheal mediastinum and mediastinal soft tissue air, most likely arising from a posterior defect *(arrow)* in the trachea wall. (From Mirvis SE. Diagnostic imaging of thoracic trauma. In: Mirvis SE, Shanmuganathan K, eds. *Imaging in Trauma and Critical Care.* Philadelphia, PA: Elsevier; 2003:297-389.)

Injuries are typically in the proximal right posterior and distal left posterior portions. Radiographic signs of full-thickness injury are often absent early but could include pneumomediastinum, left pleural effusion, and abnormal mediastinal contour related to leakage of esophageal content or associated mediastinal hemorrhage. An atypical course of a nasogastric tube traversing a tear is another rare indirect radiologic finding.

Computed tomography is more likely to provide signs of esophageal injury. Because air in the esophagus is not under positive pressure, there may be no or only small air bubbles adjacent to a tear (Fig. 8-41). Adjacent pneumomediastinum will obscure this finding. Fluid and air may leak from the esophagus and may track into the left pleura through torn parietal pleura adjacent to the distal esophagus. Delayed presentation of this finding may occur if a leak is initially blocked by hematoma or delayed breakdown of an injured ischemic esophageal wall segment. When this injury is suspected based on CT findings, further assessment of the esophagus by contrast opacification/esophagram (with dilute barium-based contrast) followed by CT and/or endoscopy can be definitive diagnostically, with both studies together achieving the highest accuracy.

Injuries, which include mucosal dissection, intramural hematoma, and complete tears, can be quite focal or extensive in length. Given high-energy central thoracic impact and proximity, injuries to the adjacent trachea, chest wall, and spine should always be sought.

Esophageal injury from blunt trauma is exceeding rare. There may be no direct imaging signs. A small quantity of mediastinal air adjacent to the esophagus or a low-attenuation left pleural effusion may be suggestive but quite nonspecific in the blunt trauma setting. Often the diagnosis is not suspected until mediastinal or pleural cavity infection develops.

■ CARDIOPERICARDIAL INJURY

Pneumopericardium

Pneumopericardium is an unusual consequence of blunt thoracic trauma that requires a tear in the tough pericardium and direct communication with an air-containing structure that is either under positive pressure or has a one-way valve–like connection with the pericardial space, allowing air to enter the pericardial space without possible egress. The trachea and pleural spaces are the most likely sources of air. Air typically completely surrounds the heart and is limited in rostral extent by the pericardial reflection at the root of the aorta (Fig. 8-42). Pneumopericardium can also occur as a consequence of dissection of gas along the pulmonary perivascular connective

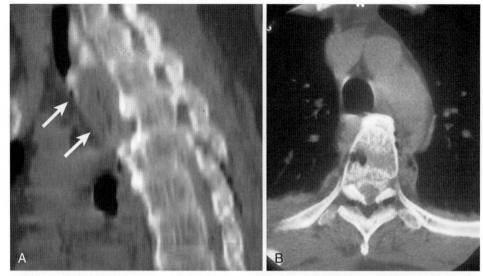

Figure 8-40 Esophageal entrapment. A, Sagittal multiplanar reformation (MPR) intravenous (IV) contrast–enhanced computed tomography (CECT) of the upper thoracic spine demonstrates retropulsion of T3 or T4. The proximal esophagus is distended and tracks into the subluxed level *(arrows)*. **B,** Axial slice across the level of subluxation shows air in the T3-T4 facet joints and intervertebral disk. The esophagus was not identified below this level. At surgery the esophagus was caught between the vertebrae and torn. (From Mirvis SE. Diagnostic imaging of thoracic trauma. In: Mirvis SE, Shanmuganathan K, eds. *Imaging in Trauma and Critical Care.* Philadelphia, PA: Elsevier; 2003:297-389.)

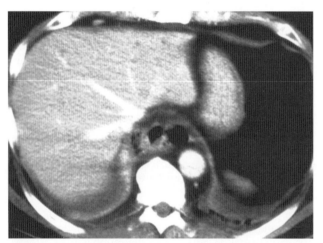

Figure 8-41 Ruptured esophagus. Axial image across the gastroesophageal junction shows two air bubbles adjacent to the distal esophagus, but no dissection of air beyond more distant air tracking. (From Mirvis SE. Diagnostic imaging of thoracic trauma. In: Mirvis SE, Shanmuganathan K, eds. *Imaging in Trauma and Critical Care.* Philadelphia, PA: Elsevier; 2003:297-389.)

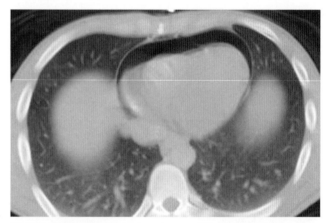

Figure 8-42 Pneumopericardium. Axial computed tomography (CT) demonstrates anterior pneumopericardium with compression of the right ventricle indicating tension component.

tissue or ostia of the pulmonary veins into the pericardium. This latter mechanism may occur acutely or days to weeks after initial trauma, particularly in the setting of concurrent major pulmonary parenchymal damage and high-pressure ventilator support.

Pneumopericardium needs to be distinguished from the much more common pneumomediastinum (see earlier discussion) given the potential for pericardial tamponade. The pericardium is thicker than the parietal pleura and completely surrounds the heart. Intrapericardial air shifts location with change in patient position, but this is difficult to demonstrate.

Pneumomediastinum pushes the parietal pleural laterally away from the mediastinum, is a thinner structure, and usually tracks roughly parallel to the mediastinal border descending below the midportion of the diaphragm, usually seen best on the left side (Fig. 8-43). There are typically concurrent findings of pneumomediastinum at multiple locations along soft tissue planes of the chest, including the "continuous diaphragm" sign, when air from the mediastinum extends between the parietal pleura and the central diaphragm, and the V sign of Naclerio, seen as air lucency outlining the medial portion of the left hemidiaphragm and the lower lateral mediastinal border (Figs. 8-43 and 8-44). Air surrounding the pulmonary artery or either of its main branches can result in the lucent "ring around the artery" sign, particularly when the air surrounds the mediastinal segment of the right pulmonary artery. When there is air adjacent to the major branches of the aorta, both sides of the vessel are depicted as mediastinal air outlines the medial side and the aerated lung is adjacent to the lateral

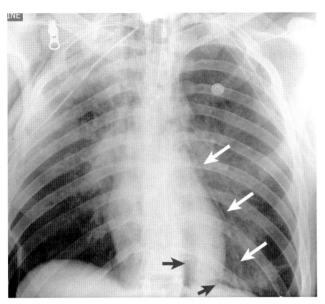

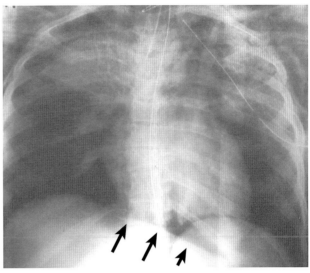

Figure 8-43 Pneumomediastinum. Anteroposterior (AP) supine chest radiograph of a blunt trauma patient shows the thin line of parietal pleura displaced away from the left mediastinum and continuing along the mediastinal border to descend below the left hemidiaphragm *(white arrows)*. There is superior mediastinal air. Naclerio's V sign *(red arrows)* is seen as an air lucency outlining the medial portion of the left hemidiaphragm and the lower lateral mediastinal border.

Figure 8-44 Pneumomediastinum. Anteroposterior (AP) chest radiograph shows a continuous collection of air between the central tendon of the diaphragm and the heart *(arrows)*, a sign of pneumomediastinum. There is soft tissue air in the upper chest walls, a large right pneumothorax, and partial collapse of the right upper lobe.

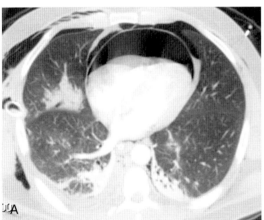

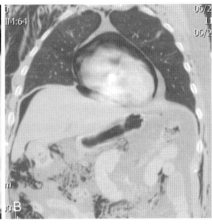

Figure 8-45 A, Axial and B, Coronal scans through mid-ventricular levels show a distended anterior pericardium and some flattening of the anterior heart, indicating tension. There are small bilateral pneumothoraces, soft tissue emphysema, and right middle lobe pulmonary contusion.

side, producing the "tubular artery" sign. Mediastinal air often extends along fascial planes throughout the body, particularly the chest wall and neck, and may rupture into the abdominal cavity. Of course pneumopericardium and pneumomediastinum may coexist.

Although pneumopericardium is generally innocuous, intrapericardial pressure can increase enough to produce tamponade physiological characteristics. This development may not be appreciated at all on imaging but may manifest as "ballooning" of the pericardium and/or global compression of cardiac size (Fig. 8-45). These findings can be appreciated radiographically with an appropriate comparison study but are more likely to be diagnosed by noting compression/flattening of the right ventricle on CT (see Figs. 8-41 and 8-44). The vena cavae and its more distal venous tributaries may be distended by elevated venous return pressure. Also,

elevated pressure in the draining hepatic and gallbladder lymphatics may produce CT findings of periportal and gallbladder wall (subserosal) edema (Figs. 8-45 and 8-46). The finding of pneumopericardium in the blunt trauma setting should promptly be communicated to the clinical service managing the patient to either follow or place a pericardial drain prophylactically.

Hemopericardium

Hemopericardium can develop as an acute consequence of blunt chest trauma from crush injuries or direct impact, usually over the anterior chest wall. Bleeding can arise from any cardiac chamber (clinically bleeding from the low-pressure atria is most commonly the source of cardiac rupture given the extremely high mortality associated with ventricular rupture), a coronary artery, retrograde bleeding into the pericardium from traumatic proximal aortic pseudoaneurysm, and myocardial or pericardial contusion. In the acute clinical setting, chest radiography is highly insensitive because a relatively small amount of blood can produce cardiac tamponade given the limited potential for acute distension of the pericardium. The small quantity of pericardial blood required to create tamponade is extremely unlikely to alter the usual cardio-pericardial radiographic contour acutely so as to suggest the diagnosis. However, the diagnosis should be very straightforward by IV CECT indicated by high-attenuation fluid (between liquid blood and clot attenuation) in the pericardial space and/or active bleeding (Figs. 8-46 to 8-48).

As with pneumopericardium the physiologic effects of tamponade may be best reflected in secondary signs of elevated venous return pressure such as distension of the vena cavae, hepatic and renal veins, periportal lymphatics, and subserosal gallbladder wall edema (see Figs. 8-46 and 8-47).

Atypical causes of pericardial tamponade include compression of the anterior heart (right ventricle) by an enlarging anterior mediastinal hematoma (Fig. 8-49), most likely from bleeding internal mammary arteries or, exceptionally uncommon, herniation of the stomach into the pericardium through a tear in the diaphragm and pericardium (Fig. 8-50).

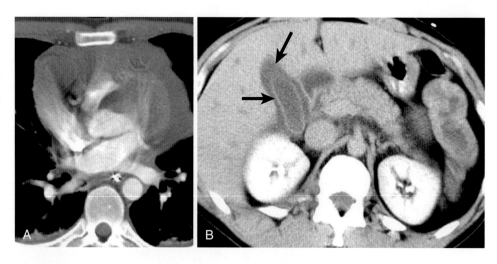

Figure 8-46 Hemopericardium. **A,** Pericardial blood collects mainly anteriorly and laterally. Note the small caliber of the aorta, indicating diminished blood pressure related to tamponade. **B,** Axial image through the upper abdomen with intravenous (IV) contrast illustrates subserosal edema *(arrows)* related to elevated lymphatic and venous pressure from cardiac tamponade. (From Mirvis SE. Diagnostic imaging of thoracic trauma. In: Mirvis SE, Shanmuganathan K, eds. *Imaging in Trauma and Critical Care.* Philadelphia, PA: Elsevier; 2003:297-389.)

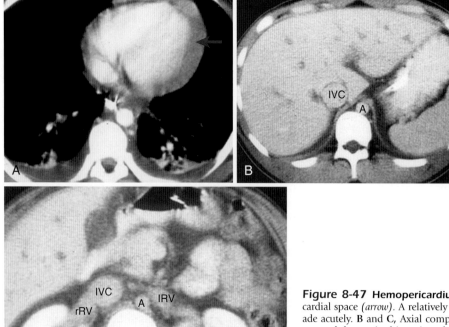

Figure 8-47 Hemopericardium. A, Blood collects in the left lateral pericardial space *(arrow).* A relatively small quantity of blood can create tamponade acutely. **B** and **C,** Axial computed tomographic (CT) images through the upper abdomen in this patient show distended inferior vena cava (IVC), small aortic lumen, and diffuse periportal low density from lymphatic distension. (From Mirvis SE. Diagnostic imaging of thoracic trauma. In: Mirvis SE, Shanmuganathan K, eds. *Imaging in Trauma and Critical Care.* Philadelphia, PA: Elsevier; 2003:297-389.) Right renal vein (rRV). Left renal vein (lRV). Aorta (A).

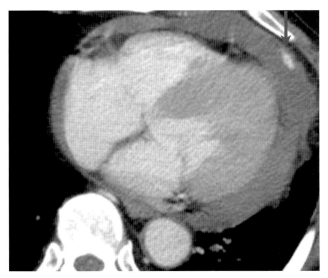

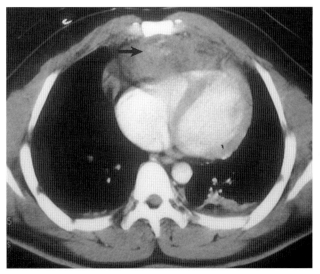

Figure 8-48 Hemopericardium and active bleeding. There is high-density contrast *(arrow)* indicating bleeding into pericardium, which is filled with blood.

Figure 8-49 Cardiac compression. Axial contrast-enhanced computed tomography (CECT) at the midventricular level reveals compression of the anterior heart and a large anterior mediastinal hematoma with active bleeding *(arrow)*. The blood does not surround the heart as expected with hemopericardium. (From Mirvis SE. Diagnostic imaging of thoracic trauma. In: Mirvis SE, Shanmuganathan K, eds. *Imaging in Trauma and Critical Care*. Philadelphia, PA: Elsevier; 2003:297-389.)

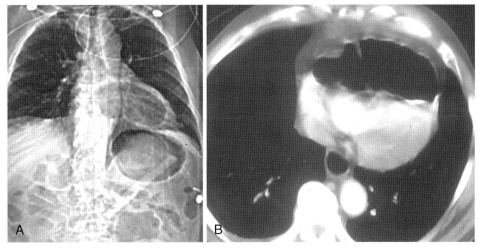

Figure 8-50 Intrapericardial herniation. A, Chest radiograph shows a "double bubble" with rostral air collection over the heart. The collection conforms to the shape of the pericardium and produces no mass effect on the heart or mediastinal, suggesting intrapericardial localization. There is a constriction between the bubbles. **B,** Axial computed tomography (CT) with intravenous (IV) contrast confirms rupture of the gastric fundus into the pericardium, compressing the cardiac chambers. The patient manifests tamponade physiological characteristics clinically. (From Glaser DL, Shanmuganathan K, Mirvis SE. General case of the day. Acute intrapericardial diaphragmatic hernia. *Radiographics*. 1998;18:799-801.)

Active pericardial hemorrhage may be directly evident on IV CECT, which would help guide surgical repair (see Fig. 8-48). Increasing use of bedside screening sonography can permit detection of pericardial fluid and can, given appropriate equipment and personnel, concurrently assess chamber size, valve integrity, and overall cardiac function, potentially allowing diagnosis in the acute setting.

■ CARDIAC INJURY—MULTIDETECTOR COMPUTED TOMOGRAPHY

Myocardial injury

Multidetector computed tomography (MDCT) is the most widely used imaging method to screen hemodynamically stable patients with blunt chest trauma for cardiac injury. Bedside sonography is typically used for stable patients with penetrating chest trauma to rapidly assess for the presence of pericardial fluid. Cardiac injury is far less common from blunt than penetrating trauma. Blunt injuries usually occur from direct crushing of the thorax when the heart is compressed between the sternum and spine in motor vehicle accidents or less commonly in direct crushing as may occur in industrial accidents. Injury may also result from abdominal compression via sudden increase in inferior vena cava pressure or upward movement of abdominal contents into the chest, thus increasing intrathoracic pressure. The anterior right ventricle is the region most prone to injury. Increases in transmural pressure are greatest in the left ventricle, increasing the risk for damage to the left-sided cardiac valves compared to the right.

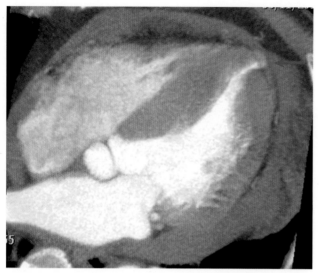

Figure 8-51 Cardiac rupture. Axial intravenous (IV) contrast–enhanced computed tomographic (CECT) image shows deep laceration of the left ventricle sustained in blunt trauma *(arrow)* with leak into the pericardial space.

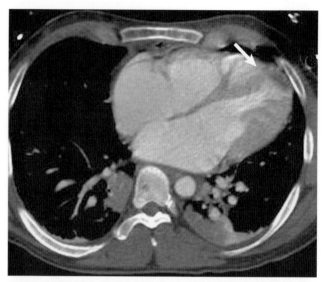

Figure 8-52 Traumatic ventricular septal defect. Axial intravenous (IV) contrast–enhanced computed tomographic (CECT) image shows linear defect in the inferior septum.

Figure 8-53 Cardiac herniation. A and B, Axial intravenous (IV) contrast–enhanced computed tomographic (CECT) images illustrate herniation of the heart into the left hemithorax. There is cardiac constriction at the free margin of the pericardial tear *(arrows)*. Portions of the torn pericardium *(curved arrows)* are shown. T=Tension pneumothorax.

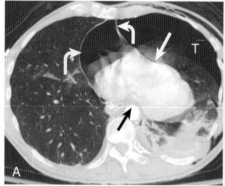

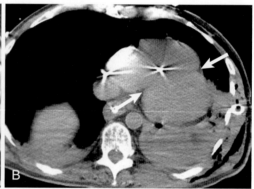

Blunt cardiac injury can produce myocardial "concussion" in which there are functional abnormalities of the heart, but no direct parenchymal damage, elevated levels of specific cardiac enzyme levels (troponin I is most accurate), or arrhythmias. Myocardial "contusion" includes parenchymal damage, elevated levels of cardiac-specific enzymes, and areas of necrosis and hemorrhage; this is an appearance similar to infarction. Rib, sternal, and clavicle fractures, as well as pneumothorax, are commonly associated with blunt cardiac injury, but none of these need be present. Abnormal findings on electrocardiogram, particularly showing more "malignant" arrhythmias, predict other complications that will require treatment.

Myocardial wall lacerations from blunt force are uncommon (Figs. 8-51 and 8-52) and usually lead to patient death. Disruption of the atria and right ventricular walls permits longer survival because of lower luminal pressure and rate of bleeding. Injuries to the valves, papillary muscles, and ventricular septum (see Fig. 8-52) usually lead to congestive failure as will severe contusion of the left ventricle. Bedside transthoracic sonographic screening most likely will identify pericardial fluid and perhaps tamponade-related findings but could also detect echogenic myocardial contusion and valve dysfunction. Complex injuries are diagnosed with greater accuracy using dedicated cardiac sonography with flow/volume measurements and color Doppler to identify abnormal flow direction. Transesophageal sonography is rarely used in the acute setting given the time required and relative invasiveness. Also this approach is contraindicated in patients who may have high spinal injury.

If cardiac injury is clinically suspected before CT, then prospective electrocardiographic gating may be helpful to see details of cardiac anatomy to assess cardiac valves, coronary arteries, wall-motion abnormalities, myocardial defects, and injuries of the proximal great vessels. Some of these injuries will not become clinically evident until the subacute period, perhaps several days from injury. Thorium single-photon emission computed tomography (SPECT) has not been shown to predict positive findings or the development of cardiac-related complications.

Cardiac Herniation

Pleuropericardial rupture with cardiac herniation is a rare injury from blunt chest trauma, but two thirds of pleuropericardial and diaphragmatic tears lead to subsequent cardiac herniation. The left pericardium paralleling the course of the left phrenic nerve is the most common site of tearing (Fig. 8-53) followed by the right and then superior pericardium. Displacement of the heart through the pericardium produces a number of MDCT signs, including a malpositioned heart, a discontinuous pericardium, an empty pericardial sac, a collar sign of cardiac constriction by the edges of the torn diaphragm, and a deformed ventricular silhouette (see Fig. 8-53). Cardiac torsion can also develop and produces strangulation of the inferior vena cava and great vessels, significantly impairing cardiac output and return.

■ INJURY TO THE AORTA AND PROXIMAL BRANCH VESSELS

Mediastinal Hemorrhage

The identification of blunt traumatic aortic injury (TAI) has been made considerably easier by the advent of MDCT. Before availability of MDCT the diagnosis was based on appreciation of abnormality of the mediastinal contour created by mediastinal hemorrhage (MH) and to some extent the aortic pseudoaneurysm itself as seen radiographically. A large number of signs of varying sensitivity and specificity were used in this assessment, including widening of the paraspinal stripes, increased opacity along the right paratracheal region, extrapleural blood extending from the mediastinum over the left lung apex (apical pleural cap), shift of the trachea and esophagus to the right, depression of the left mainstem bronchus, obliteration of the aortic-pulmonary window, or loss of the aortic arch or descending aortic walls due to adjacent hemorrhage (Fig. 8-54). Measurements of the absolute width of the mediastinum or the mediastinum-to-chest width ratio at the level of the aortic arch were, at various times in the past, believed to accurately select patients for aortography.

There are two major pitfalls with radiologic assessment of the mediastinum:

1. The limited capacity to perform a technically adequate chest radiograph for interpretation that ideally requires the patient to be able to sit for an upright AP chest view leaning slightly forward to more faithfully reproduce true mediastinal contours
2. The inability to rely on radiographic signs with sufficient predictive value to accurately diagnose or exclude MH as a potential sign of aortic injury

The concurrent absence of several radiologic signs of MH, on technically adequate chest radiographs, provides a negative predictive value of 98% for excluding major arterial injury. However, a very large number of blunt trauma patients did not fulfill these radiographic criteria and could not be "cleared" for potential aortic injury, generating a high volume of false-positive radiologic findings of abnormal mediastinal contours suggesting MH potentially associated with major thoracic arterial injury. For this reason a large number of thoracic arteriograms were required to exclude aortic and major branch vessel arterial injury with a very high negative-to-positive result.

Intravenous CECT, and particularly MDCT angiography, has allowed definitive assessment of the presence, quantity,

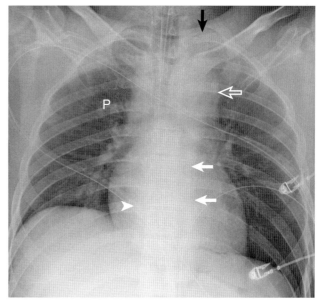

Figure 8-54 Hemomediastinum. Anteroposterior (AP) chest radiograph shows signs of mediastinal hemorrhage (MH), including mild displacement of the trachea and esophagus to the right, widened right paratracheal strip *(red arrow)*, widened left paraspinal line *(white arrows)*, widened right paraspinal line *(white arrowhead)*, abnormal, ill-defined aortic arch contour *(open arrow)*, and an apical extrapleural hematoma *(black arrow)*.

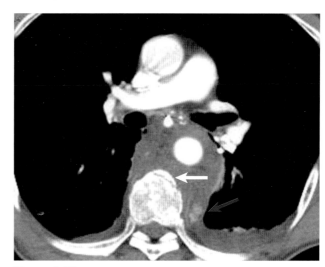

Figure 8-55 Computed tomography (CT) of mediastinal hemorrhage (MH). Intravenous (IV) contrast–enhanced (CE) axial CT image of a blunt trauma patient shows a mediastinal hematoma surrounding the descending thoracic aorta. Note the compression fracture of the adjacent vertebral body *(white arrow)* and active bleeding in the left paraspinal region *(red arrow)*. The thoracic aorta was intact on the study.

and localization of MH and identification or exclusion of major arterial injuries (aorta and its major branches) with near 100% sensitivity and specificity (Fig. 8-55).

The vast majority of patients with injury of major mediastinal arteries have blood directly in contact with or surrounding the aorta. Mediastinal hemorrhage limited to the anterior or posterior mediastinum, not in direct contact with the aorta, does not increase the likelihood of aortic or proximal branch injury. Of even

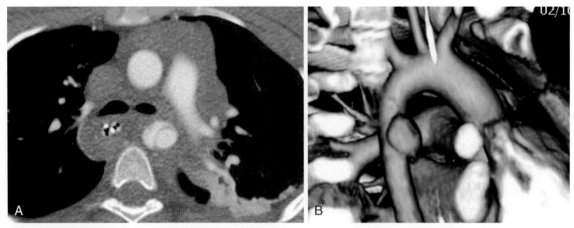

Figure 8-56 Aortic pseudoaneurysm. A, Axial intravenous (IV) contrast–enhanced computed tomographic (CECT) image shows a pseudoaneurysm surrounding the anteromedial aorta compressing the aortic lumen. A large mediastinal hematoma causes displacement of the carina and nasogastric tube to the right. The pseudoaneurysm itself generally contributes a minimal amount of mass effect relative to the hematoma. **B,** Volume-rendered three-dimensional (3-D) view shows the important relationship between the pseudoaneurysm and the left subclavian origin needed for stent-graft planning.

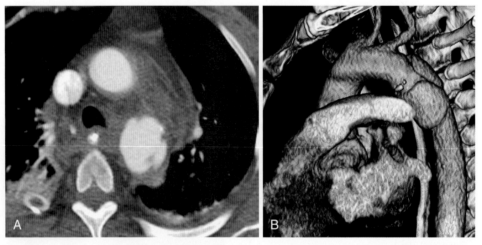

Figure 8-57 Aortic pseudoaneurysm. A, Axial intravenous (IV) contrast–enhanced computed tomographic (CECT) image reveals irregular pseudoaneurysms with adjacent intimal flaps. There is diffuse mediastinal hemorrhage (MH). **B,** Volumetric three-dimensional (3-D) view shows two distinct pseudoaneurysms draped over the aortic lumen.

greater import is the accuracy of MDCT angiography to directly assess the major arteries to diagnosis or exclude TAI with near 100% sensitivity and specificity. Despite the highly accurate technology available at the time of preparation of this chapter, a number of challenging cases still occur as are described later.

Intravenous CECT, and particularly MDCT angiography, allows definitive assessment of the presence, quantity, and location of MH to suggest a source and directly diagnosis or exclude major arterial injury with very high predictive value.

Typical Pseudoaneurysm

The typical aortic pseudoaneurysm is an oval to elliptical protrusion from the aortic lumen, usually projecting anteromedially at the level of the left mainstem bronchus and left pulmonary artery (isthmic region) (Figs. 8-55 to 8-58). A traumatic aortic tear traverses the intima and media with blood extending under the serosal layer creating the pseudoaneurysm. Rarely, injuries can transect

all layers of the aorta and result in immediate exsanguination or very temporary containment of bleeding by the surrounding tissue and parietal pleura. Typical pseudoaneurysms can progress to complete transection at any time, demanding expedient diagnosis.

The internal wall of a pseudoaneurysm can be smooth or irregular (see Figs. 8-55 to 8-58). The aneurysm can project outwardly from the aorta with a narrow base (see Fig.8-58) or drape over the intact wall of the adjacent aorta (see Figs. 8-56 and 8-57). Linear intima-media flaps at the base of the pseudoaneurysm (Figs. 8-56 to 8-59) are one of the most useful signs differentiating TAI from nontrauma aortic pathologic conditions and congenital or developmental anomaly (Figs. 8-60 to 8-63). Mediastinal hemorrhage is present in the vast majority of TAIs and is believed to arise from small adjacent arteries and/or the vasa vasorum of the aorta. The hematoma can focally surround the circumference of the aorta or extend into any portion(s) of the mediastinum (see Figs. 8-56 to 8-60). In our experience, minor injuries, subsequently discussed, can be seen without any or minimal hemorrhage, usually limited to the periaortic region

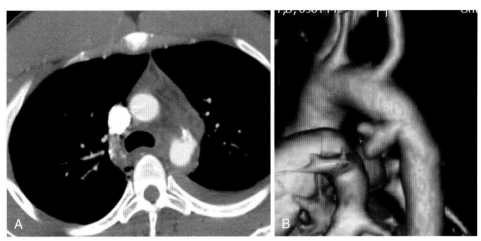

Figure 8-58 Aortic pseudoaneurysm. **A,** Axial intravenous (IV) contrast–enhanced computed tomographic (CECT) image demonstrates an irregular-shaped pseudoaneurysm projecting from the anterior aorta. Note calcification in the remnant of the ligamentum arteriosum. There is diffuse mediastinal blood. **B,** Volumetric three-dimensional (3-D) rendering shows an atypical branching appearance of pseudoaneurysm extending toward the left pulmonary artery.

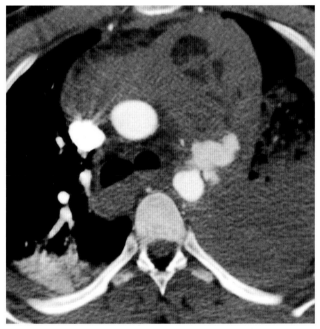

Figure 8-59 Ruptured aortic pseudoaneurysm. Axial intravenous (IV) contrast–enhanced computed tomographic (CECT) image demonstrates a complete tear of the anterior aortic wall with bleeding into the mediastinum, large mediastinal hematoma, and extension into the left pleural space. The patient did not survive this injury.

(Fig. 8.64; see Fig. 8-61). Very rarely a major injury occurs without hemorrhage (Fig. 8-65). Hemorrhage around the proximal descending aorta in the left superior mediastinum typically causes displacement of the trachea and esophagus anteriorly and to the right (see Figs. 8-55 to 8-59) and rarely depresses the left mainstem bronchus.

Traumatic aortic injury can be associated with traumatic pseudocoarctation in proximity to the wall injury. A large pseudoaneurysm can sufficiently narrow the aortic lumen to decrease distal blood flow and pressure (Figs. 8-66 and 8-67). A large luminal clot or intimal flap can also cause diminished distal flow. In up to 15% of patients with TAI, periaortic hematoma may extend caudally to the level of the diaphragmatic crura (see Fig. 8-66). Both pericrural hemorrhage and a diminished aortic caliber may be detected on abdominal MDCT (see Figs. 8-66 and 8-67), which would be evidence of potential TAI and of great import in the event that a chest CT was not performed. Clinically, traumatic pseudocoarctation would be expected to produce a weak femoral pulse because of diminished flow below the injury site and cause a noteworthy difference in blood pressure between the upper and lower extremities.

In the presence of otherwise unexplained MH, close inspection of the entire aorta and proximal major branches in a technically satisfactory study is required to search for atypical sites of injury. In our experience the aortic arch has been the second most common location of TAI (Fig. 8-68). Almost all patients who sustain ascending aortic injuries will die before a reaching medical care facility because of severe concurrent cardiac injury or bleeding into the pericardium leading to tamponade and thus are very rarely encountered clinically. Injury to the proximal ascending aorta is a site more commonly seen in autopsy series because of its high lethality. Paraspinal localization suggests spinal fracture as the cause, and an anterior mediastinal site suggests sternal fracture. Hemorrhage confined to these areas will not surround the aorta and may be clearly separated from it by intervening mediastinal fat. Rarely, major veins may be the bleeding source producing MH (see later discussion).

Intima-media flaps at the base of the pseudoaneurysm are one of the most useful signs differentiating traumatic aortic injury from a nontrauma aortic pathologic condition or congenital or developmental anomaly.

In the presence of any MH, close inspection of the entire aorta and major branches is required to exclude atypical sites of injury.

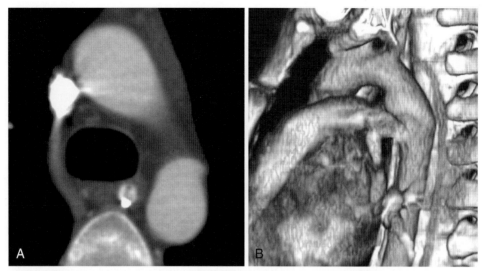

Figure 8-60 Ductus diverticulum. A, Axial intravenous (IV) contrast–enhanced computed tomographic (CECT) image displays smooth "bump" from the anterior aorta above the typical level of a pseudoaneurysm (above the carina). There is no mediastinal blood and no intimal flaps distinguishing this appearance from an injury. **B,** Volumetric three-dimensional (3-D) rendering shows completed smooth contour of the ductus with obtuse margins with the aortic wall.

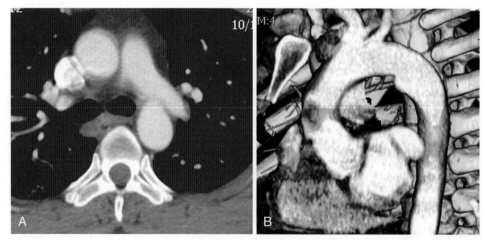

Figure 8-61 Ductus diverticulum. A, Axial intravenous (IV) contrast–enhanced computed tomography (CECT) image shows a smooth ductus arising from the isthmic portion of the aorta and extending toward the left pulmonary artery. The ductus has obtuse margins with the aortic lumen, no intimal flaps, and no mediastinal blood. **B.** Parasagittal three-dimensional (3-D) cut-away view through aorta verifies ductus.

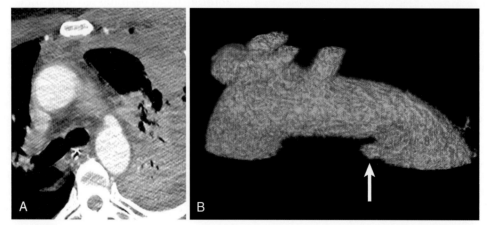

Figure 8-62 Atypical ductus. A, Axial intravenous (IV) contrast–enhanced computed tomographic (CECT) image illustrates smoothly contoured elliptical extension from the aorta pointing toward the left pulmonary artery. There is no intimal flap and actually no mediastinal blood. There is displacement of the mediastinum to the right, which is related to fluid in the left hemithorax. This contour abnormality was diagnosed as an atypical ductus, and no treatment was undertaken. **B,** Volumetric view of the aortic arch depicts a rectangular ductus with smooth contour and right-angle margins with the aortic lumen *(arrow)*.

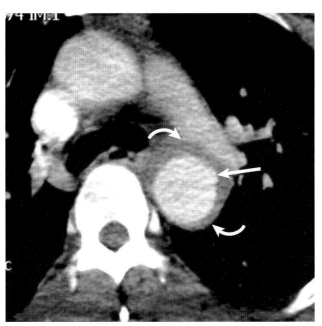

Figure 8-63 Shallow aortic pseudoaneurysm. Axial intravenous (IV) contrast–enhanced computed tomographic (CECT) image demonstrates a subtle outpouching *(arrow)* from the anterolateral aorta, which measured less than 10% of the normal adjacent aortic diameter and qualifies as a "minor" injury in our practice. There is a surrounding collar of periaortic blood *(curved arrows)*.

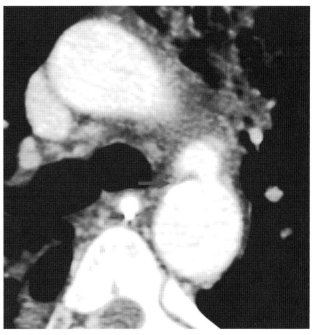

Figure 8-65 Aortic pseudoaneurysm. Axial intravenous (IV) contrast–enhanced computed tomographic (CECT) image reveals an irregular-shaped outpouching from the anterior the aorta at the level of the carina. Note intimal flap *(arrow)*. There is slight carinal displacement to the right but no clear mediastinal blood.

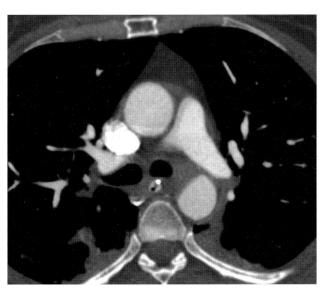

Figure 8-64 Aortic contour abnormality. Axial intravenous (IV) contrast–enhanced computed tomographic (CECT) images shows a flat contour of the anteromedial aorta most likely due to intramural blood. There is an associated periaortic hematoma. In our practice this would be considered a "minor" aortic injury.

Minor Traumatic Aortic Injury

The increase in temporal and spacial resolution of current MDCT allows for identification of more subtle aortic injuries than were generally observed in the era of conventional or low number–detector row CT. At the time of this writing a uniformly accepted definition of what constitutes a "minor" blunt TAI has not been established. In our center these injuries include intimal

irregularities with or without attached thrombus, contour irregularities (mainly flattening) of the aortic wall, and shallow pseudoaneurysms measuring 10% or less of the normal adjacent aortic lumen (Figs. 8-63 to 8-70). The definition of minor TAI varies among centers. These injuries typically have no or limited periaortic blood, although this is not always the case. Again, in our center's experience to date these injuries usually show some healing within a few days (see Figs. 8-69 and 8-70) after injury. An increase from initial injury size is distinctly uncommon. Also the exact treatment and follow-up regimen is not uniform even within an institution, nor is the best way to follow these injuries uniform, particularly given the high x-ray exposures required for multiple repeat CT scans. Generally we recommend performing MDCT limited to the region of the injury at 24 hours and 7 days to exclude progression or demonstrate healing. As noted later, the allowed diameter of aortic pseudoaneurysms considered minor is much less at the Maryland Shock Trauma Center, and the designation of "minor" is not influenced by the presence or absence of MH (Box 8-1). An earlier proposed classification from University of Tennessee at Memphis does include the extent of MH and sets a larger size limit for pseudoaneurysm to still be considered minor (Box 8-2).

Several anatomic variants and acquired aortic pathological conditions can potentially cause confusion with a diagnosis of TAI (Figs. 8-71 to 8-76; see Figs. 8-60 to 8-62). The most common variant is the ductus diverticulum, a smooth rounded bulge arising from the medial aspect of the proximal descending aorta, which has obtuse interfaces with the aortic lumen and no intimal flaps (see Fig. 8-61). Atypical features of the ductus

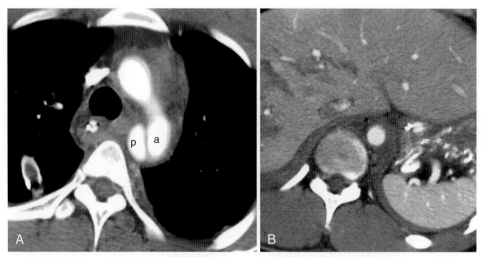

Figure 8-66 Traumatic aortic coarctation. **A,** Axial intravenous (IV) contrast–enhanced computed tomographic (CECT) image shows smooth pseudoaneurysm (p) arising from the medial aorta (a) at a typical level. Note compression of the aortic lumen. **B,** Axial image through the aortic hiatus demonstrates narrow aortic diameter due to decreased "downstream" flow and surrounding periaortic hematoma extending from upper mediastinum.

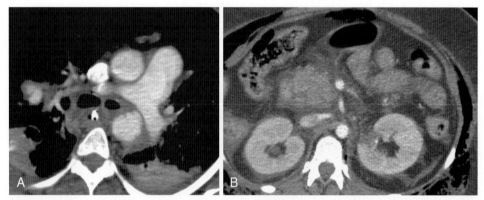

Figure 8-67 Traumatic aortic coarctation. **A,** Axial intravenous (IV) contrast–enhanced computed tomographic (CECT) image shows an irregular pseudoaneurysm projecting from the left anterior descending aorta with surrounding mediastinal hemorrhage (MH). **B,** Axial image at the level of the diaphragmatic crura demonstrates a small aorta, indicating traumatic aortic coarctation.

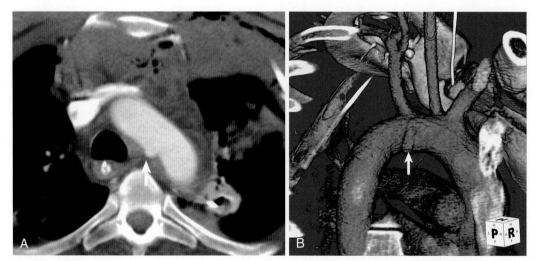

Figure 8-68 Atypical aortic injury. **A,** Axial intravenous (IV) contrast–enhanced computed tomographic (CECT) image shows a small pseudoaneurysm arising from the posterior aortic arch *(arrow)*. Also noted is a sternal fracture and substernal mediastinal hemorrhage (MH). **B,** Volume-rendered image shows aortic pseudoaneurysm *(arrow)* arising from the posterior arch and extending to the base of the left subclavian artery. This injury location has significant implications regarding stent-graft placement.

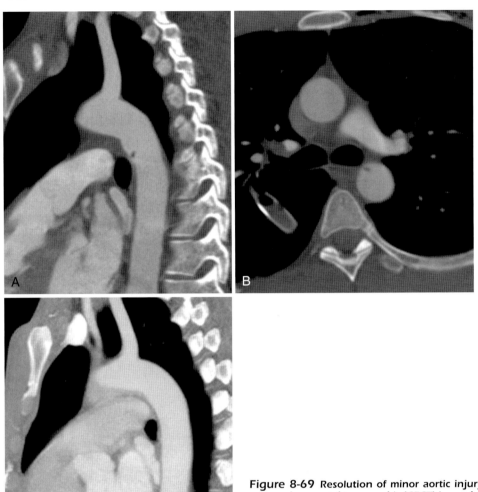

Figure 8-69 Resolution of minor aortic injury. A, Axial intravenous (IV) contrast–enhanced computed tomographic (CECT) image demonstrates an irregular anterior filling defect, most likely torn intima and clot, treated with low-dose aspirin. **B,** Two days after injury, follow-up CT shows a decrease in the size of the filling defect. **C,** At 8 days after injury, follow-up CT shows resolution of the filling defect, but residual contour abnormality of the anterior aortic wall. No further treatment was maintained.

include alteration of the usual shape, irregular inner walls, and nonobtuse interface with the aortic lumen (see Fig. 8-62). The absence of periaortic hemorrhage strongly supports the diagnosis of an anatomic variant rather than TAI. A diverticular origin of the bronchial arteries can simulate aortic wall injury but can be discriminated by following the diverticulum into the artery and toward the mainstem and lobar bronchi (see Fig. 8-71). A ductus remnant is another potential source of confusion with TAI. This is usually a linear, often partially calcified strand of tissue arising from the site of the ductus arteriosus (see Fig. 8-72). There is no associated MH, and the calcification marks this as a chronic finding.

Congenital anomalies of aortic branching can potentially cause confusion with the diagnosis of TAI (see Figs. 8-73 and 8-74), and recognition of these variants has significant impact regarding treatment selection, such as the feasibility of stent-graft placement. Also, ulcerations of the aortic wall due to atheroma or inflammatory ulceration seen in the setting of possible blunt chest trauma could also be mistaken for traumatic injury. However, accompanying aortic wall findings

should provide enough evidence to distinguish these conditions from TAI (see Fig. 8-75).

Sometimes the CT angiographic appearance of an aortic abnormality cannot be determined unequivocally to be an injury despite a technically adequate study. Several alternative imaging options exist, including creation of additional multiplanar, volume-rendered and endoluminal CT images, intravascular sonography, magnetic resonance imaging (MRI), transesophageal sonography, and follow-up CT to look for any changes in appearance of a "suspicious lesion." Maximal utilization of MDCT data is the most practical initial step; the second would be repeat CT in 3 to 5 days to look for evidence of evolution in the appearance of the potential injury. We have no significant experience with the other alternatives.

Atypical Traumatic Aortic Injuries

Atypical TAIs include dissection of the media arising in the isthmic region and extending caudally (Figs. 8-76 and 8-77). Clinically patients with this injury do not have underlying aortic pathologic conditions that may predispose to this mechanism. Such injuries are treated

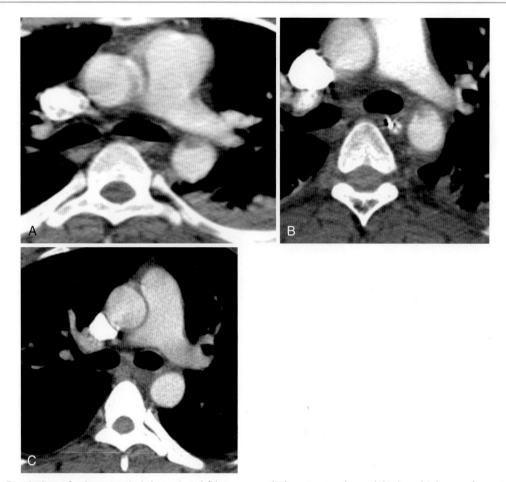

Figure 8-70 Resolution of minor aortic injury. A, Axial intravenous (IV) contrast–enhanced (CE) multiplanar reformation (MPR) computed tomographic (CT) image along the longitudinal aortic axis shows a small intimal flap and mild intimal irregularity in the anterior isthmic region. The patient received low-dose aspirin treatment. **B,** Intimal flap on axial view. **C,** Repeat CT 3 days later in equivalent projection as **A** shows resolution of the flap.

Box 8-1   University of Maryland Shock Trauma Center Traumatic Aortic Injury Grading System

Minor TAI: Contour irregularity, intimal flap with or without attached clot, intramural hematoma, pseudoaneurysm < 10% of "normal" aortic diameter at same level

Major TAI: Pseudoaneurysm > 10% of normal aortic diameter at same level, dissection

Catastrophic TAI: Aortic wall transection with bleeding into mediastinum

TAI, Traumatic aortic injury.

Forman MJ, Mirvis SE, Hollander DS. Blunt thoracic aortic injuries: CT characterisation and treatment outcomes of minor injury. *Eur Radiol.* 2013;23:2988-2995.

Box 8-2   Presley Trauma Center Grading System of Aortic Injury

  I. Normal aorta
    a. Nl thoracic aorta
    b. Nl aorta + MH
  II. Minimal aortic injury
    a. Flap, PsAn < 1 cm; no MH
    b. Flap, PsAn < 1 cm; + MH
  III. Confined TAI
    a. >1 cm well-defined PsAn with flap or thrombus; no great vessels injury + MH
    b. >1 cm well-defined PsAn with flap or thrombus; not isthmic aortic site, + MH
  IV. Total disruption with irregular poorly defined PsAn and MH

MH, Mediastinal hemorrhage; *PsAn,* pseudoaneurysm; *TAI,* traumatic aortic injury.

From Gavant ML. Helical CT grading of traumatic aortic injuries: impact on clinical guidelines for medical and surgical management. *Radiol Clin North Am.* 1999;37:553-574.

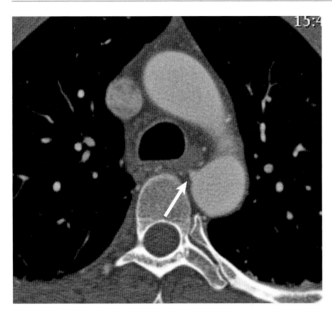

Figure 8-71 Diverticular origin of bronchial artery. Axial intravenous (IV) contrast–enhanced computed tomographic (CECT) image shows triangular outpouching from the lateral aortic arch *(arrow)*. The lumen narrows just beyond the origin. There is no periaortic blood, and the finding is in an atypical location for traumatic aortic injury (TAI).

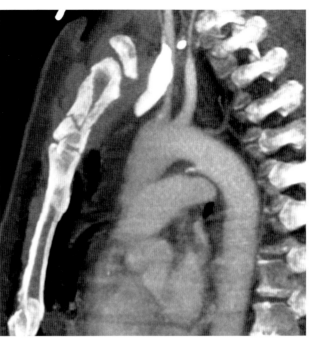

Figure 8-72 Remnant of ductus diverticulum. Axial intravenous (IV) contrast–enhanced computed tomographic (CECT) image depicts calcified linear remnant of ductus terminating near the left pulmonary artery. Note sternal fracture and substernal hematoma, which might raise concern that this finding was trauma related. (Mirvis SE. Thoracic vascular injury. In: Mirvis SE, Shanmuganathan K, eds. Emergency chest imaging. *Radiol Clin North Am.* 2006;44:189-192.)

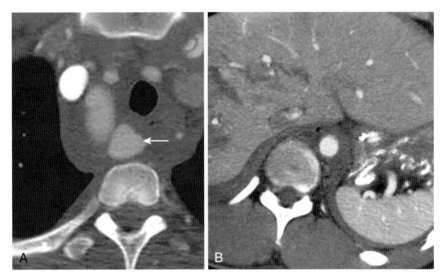

Figure 8-73 Aortic injury in a congenitally abnormal aorta. **A,** Axial intravenous (IV) contrast–enhanced computed tomographic (CECT) images indicate right aortic arch with diverticulum of Kommeral arising behind the trachea *(arrow)*. There is also mediastinal hematoma bilaterally. **B,** Anterior volume-rendered view of the proximal descending aorta demonstrates an irregular pseudoaneurysm *(arrow)* arising from the distal arch proximal to a diverticulum (D) feeding an atretic left subclavian artery.

in the same way as typical type B aortic dissections. Occasionally thrombi are present in proximity to aortic wall injury, particularly adherent to intimal flaps. Fragments of clot can embolize distally into major arterial branches, so this possibility should be clearly noted in reports and indicates treatment with platelet aggregation inhibitors or anticoagulants when there are no major contraindications (Fig. 8-78). Injuries to the descending aorta can occur with fracture and/or dislocations of the adjacent thoracic spine either from direct penetration of the posterior arterial wall by bone fragment(s) or overstretching of the aortic wall in hyperextension or rotation (Fig. 8-79). In the few examples encountered in our institution the injuries have been predominately minor and have occurred with major thoracic spine fracture-dislocations.

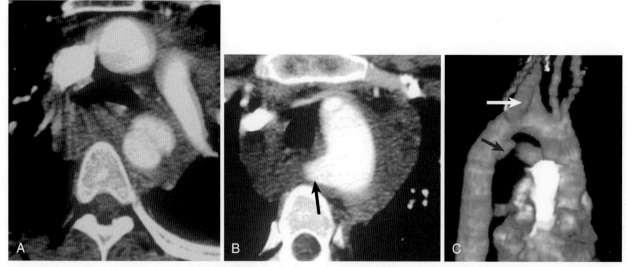

Figure 8-74 Aortic injury in a congenitally abnormal aorta. A, Axial intravenous (IV) contrast–enhanced computed tomographic (CECT) image documents an aortic pseudoaneurysm arising in a typical location. There is surrounding mediastinal blood. **B,** More rostral image shows aberrant origin of the right subclavian artery behind the trachea *(arrow).* **C,** Volume-rendered image shows close proximity of the pseudoaneurysm *(red arrow)* and left subclavian origin *(white arrow),* increasing the likelihood of at least partial occlusion of the aberrant branch vessel origin with stent-graft management of the pseudoaneurysm.

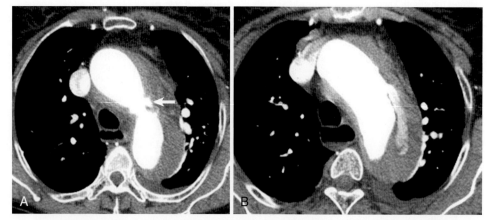

Figure 8-75 Aortic ulcer mimicking injury. A, Axial intravenous (IV) contrast–enhanced computed tomographic (CECT) image obtained in a 74-year-old woman shows irregularity of the lateral proximal descending aortic contour with a rectangular outpouching *(arrow).* There is blood surrounding the aorta, which appears to be intramural rather than mediastinal and is more likely associated with bleeding from ulceration. This location would be very atypical for traumatic aortic pseudoaneurysm. **B,** Active bleeding is noted arising from the ulcer.

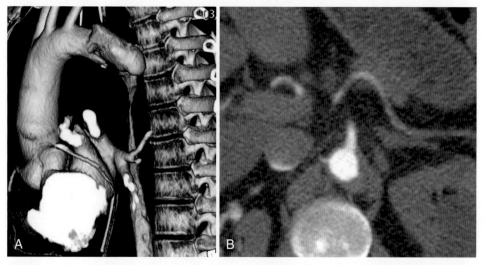

Figure 8-76 Traumatic aortic pseudoaneurysm and dissection. A, Contrast-enhanced (CE) volume-rendered three-dimensional (3-D) image shows a large irregular pseudoaneurysm arising from the proximal descending aorta with marked tapering of the opacified lumen of the more distal thoracic aorta. **B,** Axial image through the proximal abdominal aorta demonstrates a small lumen and pericrural hematoma.

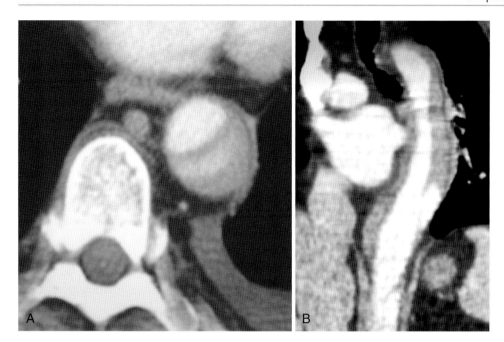

Figure 8-77 Traumatic dissection of aorta. Axial (**A**) and coronal (**B**) multiplanar reformation (MPR) intravenous (IV) contrast–enhanced (CE) images of a blunt trauma patient show aortic dissection beginning in the proximal descending aorta extending to the upper abdomen. The false lumen is partially thrombosed. The patient had no known underlying vasculopathy. (From Mirvis SE. Thoracic vascular injury. In: Mirvis SE, Shanmuganathan K, eds. Emergency chest imaging. *Radiol Clin North Am.* 2006;44:185-186.)

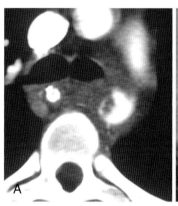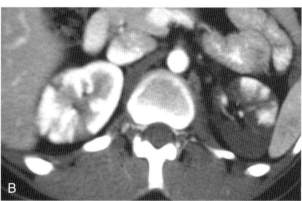

Figure 8-78 Clot embolization from injured thoracic aorta. A, Axial intravenous (IV) contrast–enhanced computed tomographic (CECT) image shows a large clot in the aortic lumen at level of the carina. There is surrounding mediastinal hematoma. **B,** Axial IV CECT image through the upper abdomen reveals a large infarct involving the majority of the left kidney, and smaller wedge-shaped infarcts on the right most likely as a result of emboli from a proximal aortic clot.

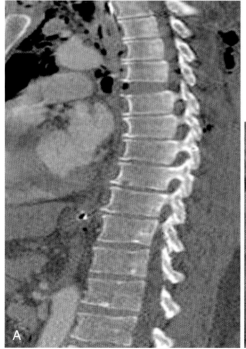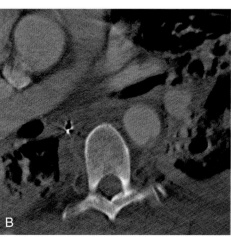

Figure 8-79 Concurrent spine and thoracic aortic injury. A, Coronal computed tomographic (CT) reformation shows a vertebral distraction fracture in the midthoracic spine. **B,** Axial intravenous (IV) contrast–enhanced (CE) image demonstrates an intimal flap *(arrow)* in the posterior descending thoracic aorta with surrounding mediastinal hematoma.

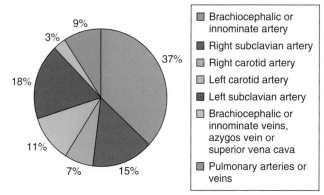

Figure 8-80 Incidence of blunt traumatic injury to major mediastinal vessels. (Wintermark M, Wick S, Bettex D, et al. Trauma of the mediastinum. In: Schnyder P, Wintermark M, eds. *Radiology of Blunt Trauma of the Chest.* Berlin-Heidelberg: Springer; 2000:71-127.)

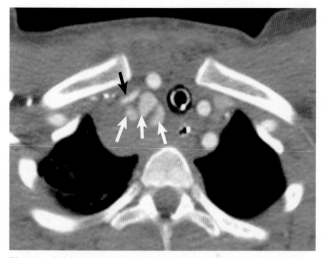

Figure 8-81 Proximal aortic branch injury. Axial intravenous (IV) contrast–enhanced computed tomographic (CECT) image shows proximal right subclavian pseudoaneurysms *(white arrows)*. The right subclavian artery is compressed *(black arrow)*. There is an extensive surrounding hemothorax and mass effect displacing the trachea and esophagus to the left because of prominent concentration of hematoma on the right.

Aortic Proximal Branch Vessel Injury

Blunt injuries to the proximal major aortic branch vessels are far less common than TAIs. The brachiocephalic artery is the most common major aortic branch injury (Fig. 8-80). Concurrent major branch vessel injury must always be excluded both with and without aortic injury. Usually branch vessel injuries occur with surrounding superior MH (Figs. 8-81 and 8-82). Injuries at the root of the major branch vessel may be difficult to appreciate in the area of insertion into the aortic lumen. Coronal reformations are helpful to better visualize such injuries and, along with sagittal views, should be routinely obtained. The lumen of the injured vessel may appear narrowed from spasm, direct injury to the segment, or injury to a more proximal portion decreasing rostral flow. Multiple branches may be injured given their close proximity to the shearing or traction strain from neck hyperextension and rotation (Fig. 8-83). It is vital to fully display the cerebral arterial vascular anatomy and flow for planning surgery or stenting. The patency of other major branches as a source of collateral flow must be established by MDCT angiography. Detection of intimal flaps and thrombi is vital to instituting therapy to minimize embolization.

Other Major Thoracic Vascular Injuries

Blunt force injuries to major mediastinal veins are rare and far less common than those caused by penetrating objects. Because these injuries are so rare, hemomediastinum is assumed to arise from an arterial origin and major venous structures are seldom considered. In patients with MH and no clear arterial origin, the major venous structures should be assessed using appropriate MDCT timing. The vena cavae are usually injured from shearing forces as they enter the pericardium. These may be associated with concurrent cardiac injuries, such as to the attached atria. Most major venous injuries are due to penetrating trauma. The azygos or hemiazygos veins can be torn at their insertion into the superior vena cava

Figure 8-82 Intraluminal thrombus of aortic branch. A, Axial intravenous (IV) contrast–enhanced computed tomographic (CECT) image shows thrombus in the proximal left common carotid artery *(arrow)* with some surrounding hematoma. **B,** Coronal reformation demonstrates proximal mural hematoma indenting lumen, segmental dilatation, and intimal flaps with attached thrombus distally.

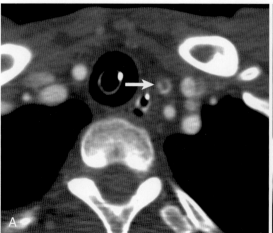
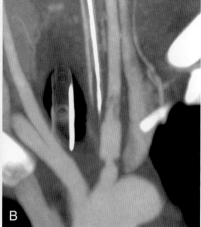

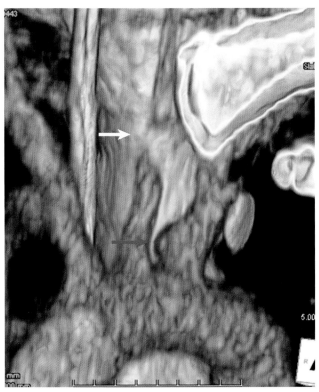

Figure 8-83 Multiple aortic branch vessel injury. Volume-rendered three-dimensional (3-D) view of the proximal aortic branches demonstrates a pseudoaneurysm arising from the base of the left subclavian artery *(red arrow)* and near complete occlusion of the left common carotid artery, probably from wall hematoma *(arrow)*.

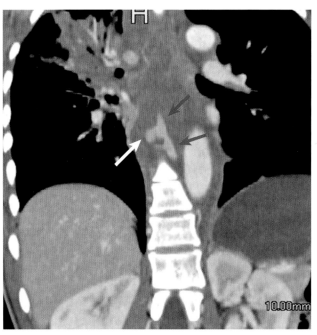

Figure 8-84 Azygos vein injury. Intravenous (IV) contrast–enhanced (CE) coronal reformation shows irregular contour of azygos vein *(red arrows)* and pseudoaneurysm *(white arrow)*. There is a large quantity of posterior mediastinal blood.

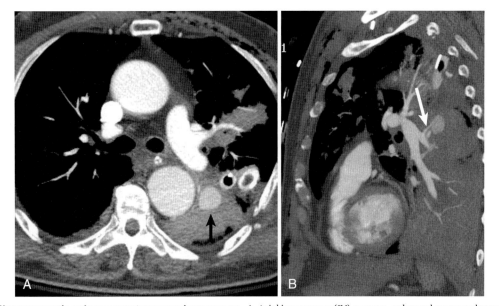

Figure 8-85 Blunt traumatic pulmonary artery pseudoaneurysm. **A,** Axial intravenous (IV) contrast–enhanced computed tomographic (CECT) image showing left main pulmonary artery. There is a round pseudoaneurysm *(black arrow)*, lateral to the aorta with surrounding consolidated lung. **B.** An oblique reformation shows the pseudoaneurysm supplied by a branch arising from the left upper lobe pulmonary artery *(white arrow)*.

or azygos vein, respectively (Fig. 8-84). Major thoracic venous injuries from blunt trauma are very rare. Injuries to the pulmonary arteries also rarely occur and may vary from intimal tears to pseudoaneurysms to massive hemorrhage (Fig. 8-85) and may be associated with cardiac and pulmonary parenchymal injury.

Planning and Imaging Aortic Stent-Grafts

Use of intravascular aortic stents has virtually replaced open repair of TAI given appropriate aortic anatomy. It is well established that this method of injury management has a lower mortality and complications, such as spinal cord ischemia (paraplegia), and decreased transfusion requirements, operative time, and length of stay. The procedure is minimally invasive and does not require a prolonged recovery period. Stent-graft placement has gained wide acceptance and has become the primary treatment of TAI. To facilitate stent placement, there are numerous factors that must be assessed by the initial CT angiogram as listed in Box 8-3.

There should be at least 1.5 to 2 cm of normal aorta as a "landing zone" for the proximal stent without covering a major arterial branch. The intact aorta should have a diameter between 18 and 20 mm and 36 and 40 mm in the region of the proximal and distal landing zones, respectively. The stent is oversized 10% to 20% to ensure complete exclusion of the lumen. In the

majority of patients occlusion of the left subclavian artery is tolerated, if necessary for acceptable graft positioning. Sharp aortic angulation can cause a decrease in aortic-stent opposition and increase the risk for type I endograft leaks. If a typical femoral artery approach is planned, then the diameter of the femoral artery (usually 6 to 9 mm) and the presence of tortuosity, severe atherosclerotic changes, or stenosis must be determined to assess the probability of successful access to the injury site.

An aortogram is performed immediately after graft deployment to assess placement. Optimally the stent should be centered over the injury site. A slight bulge in the stent at the level of the pseudoaneurysm may be seen (Fig. 8-86). There should be no appreciable space between the stent and aortic intima along the entire length and no site of focal narrowing or angulation of the stent. The region of injury should be completely covered. The amount of occlusion of any major branches and status of collateral flow should be assessed.

Complications of stent-graft placement have decreased with greater experience with the procedure. Potential early complications include endoleak, failure to adequately cover the injury (Fig. 8-87), kinking leading to loss of apposition to the aortic wall, stroke, paraplegia, upper extremity ischemia, and access site complications (thrombosis, hematoma, dissection, infection). Delayed complications include stent migration, endoleak, endograft collapse (Fig. 8-88), infection, and structural failure of the graft.

Box 8-3 Assessment of Aorta for Planning Stent-Graft Placement

- Total length of injury (measure in long axis of aorta perpendicular to central line—sagittal oblique)
- Distance from proximal site of injury to nearest adjacent major aortic branch (1.5 to 2.0 cm for landing zone)
- Aortic diameter of normal aortic lumen within 1 cm proximal and distal to the injury to size graft
- Presence of abnormal aortic and major branch anatomy
- Presence of acute angulation proximal or distal to injury that may lead to stent kinking
- Integrity of head and neck arterial flow must be assessed to verify adequate circulation if left subclavian artery must be occluded
- Vertebral artery dominance

■ BLUNT INJURY TO THE HEMIDIAPHRAGMS

Injury to the hemidiaphragms from blunt force trauma can be a difficult diagnosis, particularly when right sided

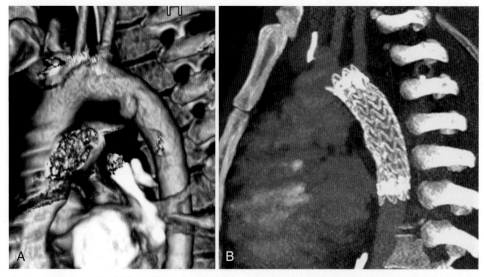

Figure 8-86 Aortic stent placement. A, Three-dimensional (3-D) volumetric image through the longitudinal aorta axis reveals a pseudoaneurysm arising from the medial proximal descending aorta. **B,** Maximum intensity projection (MIP) in sagittal orientation shows stent centered over injury with slight bulge at site of pseudoaneurysm. (From Mirvis SE, Shanmuganathan K, Miller LA, et al. Case 14. *Emergency Radiology. Case Review Series.* Philadelphia, PA: Mosby Elsevier; 2009:7.)

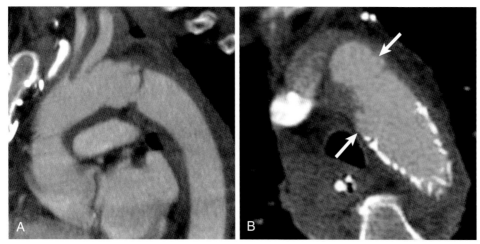

Figure 8-87 Failure to stent entire aortic injury. A, Oblique sagittal computed tomography (CT) with intravenous (IV) contrast demonstrates an irregular pseudoaneurysm extending from the aortic arch to the origin of the left subclavian. **B,** Axial IV contrast-enhanced CT shows length of injured aorta (between *arrows*) that was not covered by the stent.

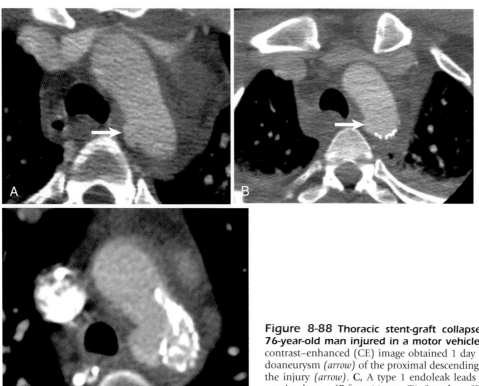

Figure 8-88 Thoracic stent-graft collapse; failure to exclude injury in a 76-year-old man injured in a motor vehicle collision. A, Axial intravenous (IV) contrast–enhanced (CE) image obtained 1 day after stent placement depicts a pseudoaneurysm *(arrow)* of the proximal descending aorta. **B,** The stent-graft fails to cover the injury *(arrow)*. **C,** A type 1 endoleak leads to displacement/compression of the proximal stent. (**B** from Morgan TA, Steenburg SD, Siegel EL, et al. Acute traumatic aortic injuries: posttherapy multidetector CT findings. *Radiographics.* 2010;30:851-867.)

or when herniation of abdominal contents fails to occur initially. On the other hand, there are other entities that can simulate the injury, leading to a false-positive interpretation. Proposed mechanisms of diaphragm tearing include a sudden increase in intra-abdominal pressure at the time of impact with release of energy at the weakest structure containing the abdominal viscera, avulsion of the peripheral diaphragm attachments to the chest wall, particularly from lateral impact, penetration by fracture fragments, primarily the ribs, and shearing forces that act across relative fixed and mobile portions of the muscle. Most injuries occur from sudden deceleration, as in motor vehicle collisions, and are about threefold more common from lateral than frontal impacts. Seat belts contribute to injury by creating further compression of the abdomen and increasing intraperitoneal pressure. Right-sided injuries require greater force to produce and are commonly associated with hepatic and other injuries causing higher mortality than that associated with left-sided rupture.

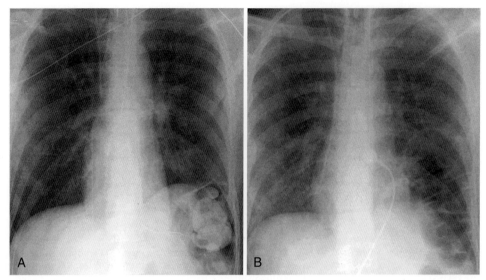

Figure 8-89 Effect of positive pressure ventilator support on transhemidiaphragm herniation. A, Anteroposterior (AP) chest radiograph obtained with a patient on positive ventilator support shows the left colon projecting slightly above the left hemidiaphragm. This is suspicious for transhemidiaphragm herniation but lacks other characteristic features. **B,** Follow-up radiograph after extubation now shows marked ascent of the colon into the left chest with negative pleural pressure reestablished. (From Mirvis SE. Diagnostic imaging of thoracic trauma. In: Mirvis SE, Shanmuganathan K, eds. *Imaging in Trauma and Critical Care.* Philadelphia, PA: Elsevier; 2003:297-389.)

Left Hemidiaphragm Injury

The left hemidiaphragm is weaker than the right because it is thinner and provides decreased support across the line of embryologic fusion between the costal and lumbar portions and because of the lack of energy absorption by an adjacent solid visceral structure like the liver. The esophageal hiatus also contributes to weakening of the left hemidiaphragm. Left hemidiaphragm injuries are detected at least three times more often than those on the right based on diagnostic imaging but predominate to a far lesser degree when operative findings, which identify a greater number of right-sided injuries, are considered. Left hemidiaphragm injuries are typically long, 10 cm or more, and usually begin in the posterior-lateral portion and extend radially toward the central tendon. The precise orientation of the tear is in part related to the vector and force of the impact. It is very common for left hemidiaphragm injuries to occur in association with rib fractures, spleen lacerations, and lung contusions. Less common but important associations include thoracic aortic tears and pelvic fractures, which should be sought.

Left-sided injuries are not suspected immediately in at least 50% of cases because the tear is too short, there is some protection by adjacent organs to block herniation, or there is positive ventilator support to reverse the usual pressure gradient between the chest and abdomen, preventing herniation (Fig. 8-89). Herniation may become evident days to weeks after injury (Fig. 8-90). In suspicious cases, oral contrast, a nasogastric tube, or air can outline the stomach, the most frequently herniated structure (Fig. 8-91), and may help solve difficult cases. Simple elevation of the left diaphragm is nonspecific, having many potential causes (Fig. 8-92).

The radiographic diagnosis of left hemidiaphragm injury depends on herniation of abdominal content because tears cannot be directly seen. A herniated stomach or air-containing bowel can mimic the air-containing gastric fundus beneath an intact diaphragm, but the wall of the herniated hollow viscus, "the apparent hemidiaphragm," alone is too thin to account for both the normal thickness of the gastric/bowel wall and apposed intact hemidiaphragm together (Fig. 8-93). Usually some hemothorax will occupy the left pleural space, but this is nonspecific after blunt chest trauma. The diaphragm may appear blurred or deformed, but these are insensitive and nonspecific findings. The presence of lower rib fractures and left lower lung contusion should increase suspicion for left hemidiaphragm injury. The presence of a transesophageal gastric tube elevated into the lower left chest also suggests the diagnosis (see Fig. 8-91). Left hemidiaphragm injury with herniation of abdominal content establishes the radiologic diagnosis with far higher specificity. Herniated structures are usually narrowed at the line of passage across the torn edges of the diaphragm (hourglass or collar sign) (Figs. 8-93 to 8-95; see Fig. 8-91).

When there is herniated air-filled stomach or bowel, the line of constriction is easier to appreciate. A herniated mass of sufficient size will displace the heart and mediastinum to the right (see Figs. 8-90 and 8-95). On radiography, even without a collar sign, significant elevation of abdominal content high into the thorax should, by itself, strongly suggest the diagnosis in the blunt trauma setting (see Figs. 8-90, 8-91, 8-93, 8-95). The herniated stomach is often dilated because of ileus or outlet obstruction.

Multidetector CT provides the capacity to directly identify edges of the torn diaphragm, establishing the diagnosis with or without minimal herniation, not likely to be diagnosed by radiography. Computed tomography slice thickness should be no more than 2 mm, perhaps

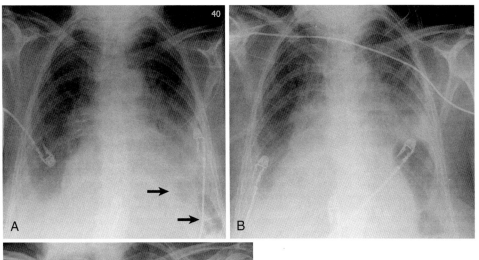

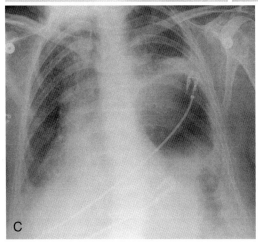

Figure 8-90 Delayed progression of herniation across left hemidiaphragm. A, Anteroposterior (AP) admission chest radiograph shows an enlarged cardiac contour and right pleural effusion. The left base is obscured, probably by pleural fluid and atelectasis. Gas shadows in left upper quadrant (*arrows*) may be mildly elevated. **B,** Repeat AP chest radiograph 2 days later shows the much more elevated gastric fundus with mass effect on the heart. The diagnosis of herniation was not made. **C,** Another chest radiograph 4 days after the first now shows marked elevation of the air-containing gastric fundus and a marked shift of the heart and mediastinum to the right. A delayed diagnosis was made.

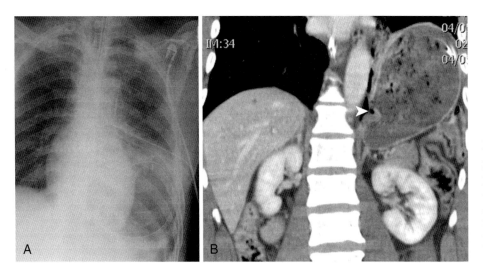

Figure 8-91 Nasogastric tube verifying gastric fundus. A, Anteroposterior (AP) chest radiograph at admission demonstrates a coiled gastric tube in the fundus conforming to an air bubble clearly above the normal level of the left hemidiaphragm. **B,** Intravenous (IV) contrast–enhanced (CE) coronal reformation shows the food-filled fundus with the collar sign at the level of the diaphragm *(arrowhead)*.

with 50% overlap whenever possible, easily obtained with current MDCT scanners. The diaphragm is abruptly interrupted in its course, and the free edge of the diaphragm may "dangle" within the abdominal fat, losing its normal orientation to the chest wall, and also appear thickened at its edge (Figs. 8-96 and 8-97). When the left hemidiaphragm is disrupted, the herniated content is

likely to fall directly against the dependent posterior thoracic wall (the "dependent viscera" sign; Figs. 8-98 and 8-99). More subtle constrictions of herniated structures are likely to be seen by CT. Hemorrhage is occasionally seen near the edges of a tear. Subtle or confusing cases may be resolved by use of coronal and sagittal reformations, which should be routinely performed. Axial views

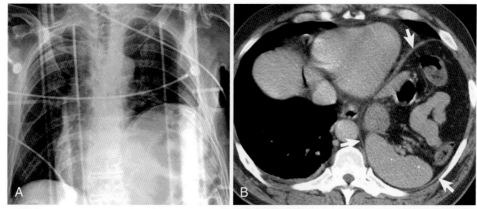

Figure 8-92 Elevated intact left hemidiaphragm. A, Anteroposterior (AP) supine chest radiograph on admission of a blunt trauma patient shows marked elevation of a normally contoured left hemidiaphragm with a normal left hemithorax. **B,** Axial intravenous (IV) contrast–enhanced computed tomographic (CECT) image verifies that the smooth, intact left diaphragm encloses the intraperitoneal structures. Again, the finding may be due to the eventration of the diaphragm or a phrenic nerve pathologic condition. (From Mirvis SE. Diagnostic imaging of thoracic trauma. In: Mirvis SE, Shanmuganathan K, eds. *Imaging in Trauma and Critical Care.* Philadelphia, PA: Elsevier; 2003:297-389.)

Figure 8-93 Variation in apparent diaphragm thickness with gastric herniation. A, Posteroanterior upright chest radiograph shows the thickness of the gastric fundic wall (outlined by air) combined with the thickness of the adjacent left hemidiaphragm. There are bilateral pneumothoraces. **B,** Anteroposterior (AP) supine chest radiograph of a different patient with gastric herniation into the chest shows diminished thickness without the adjacent intact diaphragm compared to the patient in **A.**

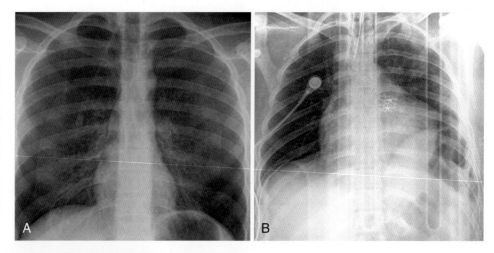

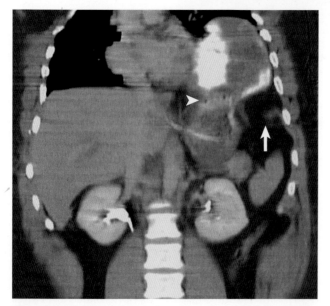

Figure 8-94 Gastric herniation through a torn left hemidiaphragm. Coronal reformatted computed tomography (CT) with intravenous (IV) contrast demonstrates an edge of the torn diaphragm *(arrow)*. The stomach and abdominal fat are constricted *(arrowhead)* crossing diaphragm rent.

should show the hemidiaphragm completely surrounding (external to) abdominal content (see Fig. 8-92), whereas herniated tissue will traverse a tear and project outside to the ring of the diaphragm on axial images (see Fig. 8-96).

A variety of anatomic and physiologic situations can mimic diaphragm injury on the left, including congenital eventration (noncontracting fibrous hemidiaphragm), phrenic nerve paresis or paralysis, acute gastric distention, adhesions that tether the diaphragm producing "pseudo" herniation (Fig. 8-100), left lower lobe atelectasis pulling up the diaphragm (Fig. 8-101), subpulmonic effusion creating apparent elevation of the diaphragm, cystic pulmonary lacerations mimicking the stomach or bowel, loculated hemopneumothorax, and Bochdalek (Fig. 8-102), Morgagni, or paraesophageal hernias. Most of these situations are more likely to be confusing radiographically. Discontinuity of the diaphragm between the crura and the lateral arcuate ligaments is a normal variation that tends to increase with age and should not be confused with diaphragmatic rupture. No hemorrhage will be present at the "apparent" tear. Traumatic diaphragm tears through the crura certainly can

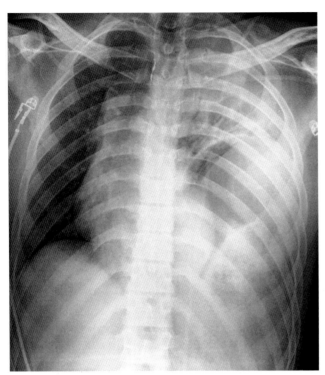

Figure 8-95 Gastric herniation radiograph. Anteroposterior (AP) supine chest radiograph shows marked elevation of the air-filled stomach with compression of the body at the level of the torn diaphragm. There is a large amount of left pleural fluid and cardiomediastinal shift to the right.

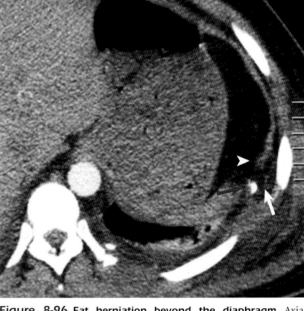

Figure 8-96 Fat herniation beyond the diaphragm. Axial intravenous (IV) contrast–enhanced computed tomography (CECT) shows discontinuity of the lateral left hemidiaphragm *(arrowhead)*. There is fat *(white arrow)* extending outside (external to) the diaphragm, indicating herniation. There is a small bone fragment *(red arrow)*, which probably arose from the adjacent broken rib that lacerated the diaphragm.

occur (Fig. 8-103); crural dehiscence can also mimic a tear. In most of these conditions an intact diaphragm, even thinned with eventration, should still completely surround the abdominal contents, excluding true herniation.

Right Hemidiaphragm Injury

Right hemidiaphragm injury is less common than on the left for the reasons described earlier. If there is a diaphragm tear but no herniation of abdominal contents, then the diagnosis is very challenging given the direct proximity of the liver and lack of the contrast provided by abdominal fat. An elevation of the apparent right diaphragm that is at least 4 cm above the left in a supine patient increases specificity of right diaphragm injury (Fig. 8-104). A lengthy tear of the right diaphragm and intra-abdominal ligament support is required for the bulk of the liver to dislocate into the right hemithorax and also requires higher energy than left-sided injury. There is also a higher likelihood of injury to the liver and other structures. The liver is by far the most common herniated visceral structure and tends to block other structures from herniating. However, extensive tears may also allow herniation of the hepatic flexure of colon. Radiographically the herniated mass of the liver mimics the right hemidiaphragm contour, making its identification as liver extremely difficult (Fig. 8-105). On MDCT there may be a collar sign where the liver crosses the diaphragm tear (Fig. 8-106). On reformatted coronal and sagittal images

the liver constriction creates a camel's hump appearance because of elongation of the herniated portion, and potentially a relatively lucent line (band sign) may appear where the liver is indented by the torn edges of the hemidiaphragm with uniformly dense liver parenchyma above and below the relatively lower density line (see Figs. 8-104 and 8-105). This low-attenuation band could also be caused by relative hypoperfusion of the compressed portion of the liver. Bilateral hemidiaphragm rupture rarely occurs, involving 1% to 2% of all cases (Fig. 8-107).

Magnetic Resonance Imaging

Rarely, in cases where CT is not diagnostic for presence or absence of diaphragm disruption, MRI can be used as an alternative study. Magnetic resonance imaging is particularly accurate for detection of left-sided injury because of fat occupying the subphrenic space that is easily detected on T1-weighted images when crossing a diaphragm tear (Fig. 8-108). Diagnosis of right-sided injury is more challenging because liver and diaphragm are similar in signal characteristics.

■ CONCLUSION

In most blunt trauma patients, chest radiographs are still obtained upon admission for the detection of immediately life-threatening injuries, such as major hemothorax, tension pneumothorax, diaphragm rupture with major compression of lung by herniated

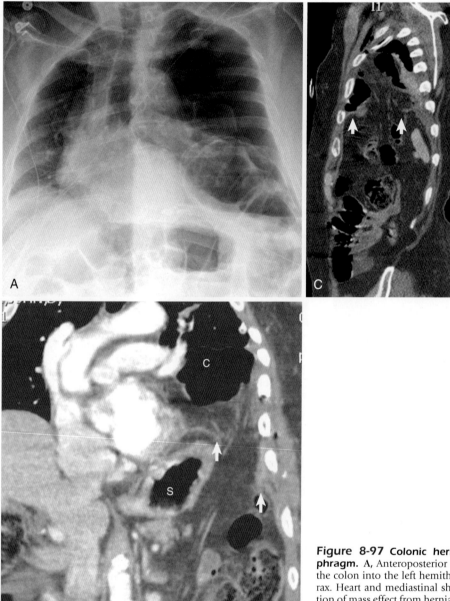

Figure 8-97 Colonic herniation through a torn left hemidiaphragm. A, Anteroposterior (AP) chest radiograph shows herniation of the colon into the left hemithorax. There is a complete left pneumothorax. Heart and mediastinal shift to the right is likely due to a combination of mass effect from herniated viscera and left tension pneumothorax. Rotation of the patient to the right also contributes to this appearance. Coronal (**B**) and sagittal (**C**) intravenous (IV) contrast–enhanced computed tomographic (CECT) images show markedly elevated colon (C), stomach (S), and torn edges of the diaphragm *(arrows).*

tissue, potential airway disruption, and major chest wall collapse, and for verification of positioning of initial monitoring and resuscitation devices. When patients are stabilized hemodynamically, full-body single-scan CT is performed in the majority of major trauma centers to assess all potentially significant injuries from the head through the pelvis. In the majority of challenging trauma patients, using today's high-detector-number ultrafast scanners, bolus IV CECT without need for oral contrast will rapidly acquire images of excellent quality with the ability to immediately generate multiplanar and volume reformations for optimal injury display. Computed tomography has proven the ideal general purpose technique for assessing blunt trauma patients, providing high accuracy for recognition of even subtle injuries that may ultimately affect patient course and management. Although most chest diagnoses are straightforward, the interpreting radiologist must be prepared to encounter findings that simulate or mask acute injury and injuries that can be recognized only by indirect findings and are subtle or atypical in their imaging presentation.

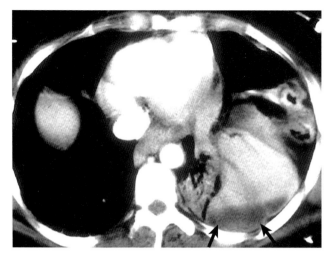

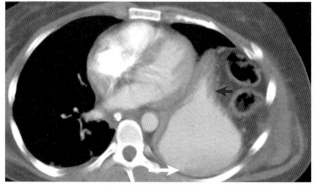

Figure 8-99 Dependent viscera sign. Axial computed tomography (CT) shows gastric fundus lying directly on posterior chest wall (*white arrow*). There is tapering of the stomach anteriorly as it crosses defect in diaphragm (*red arrow*).

Figure 8-98 Dependent viscera sign. Axial oral and intravenous (IV) contrast–enhanced computed tomographic (CECT) image demonstrates the gastric fundus in full contract with the posterior chest wall (*arrows*). Note the narrowing and swirl in the gastric body as it ascends through the diaphragm defect. The heart is displaced to the right.

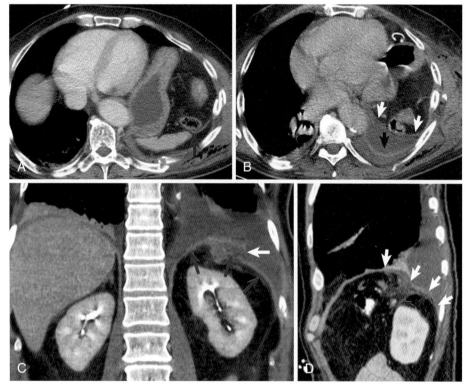

Figure 8-100 Left diaphragm pseudorupture. A, Axial intravenous (IV) contrast–enhanced computed tomographic (CECT) image demonstrates an apparent defect in the left hemidiaphragm *(red arrow)* with fat on either side. There are left posterior and lateral rib fractures and rightward displacement of the mediastinum. **B,** Another axial view shows apparent dangling torn left hemidiaphragm *(red arrow)*, dependent atelectatic lung *(black arrow)* with surrounding effusion and third curvilinear line *(white arrows)*, which is the actual intact hemidiaphragm. **C,** Coronal reformation shows an apparent tear in the left hemidiaphragm *(white arrow)*. The actual diaphragm *(red arrows)* has a thin central portion but is intact. **D,** Sagittal reformation shows the intact diaphragm *(white arrows)* and adhesion *(red arrow)*. There is pleural effusion and posterior left lower lobe atelectasis. At abdominal surgery an intact diaphragm was found with attached linear adhesions. An old healed injury was not ruled out.

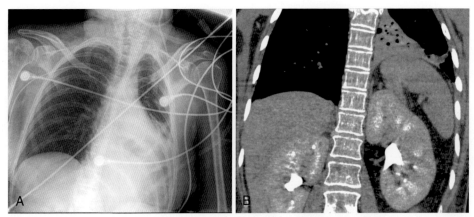

Figure 8-101 Atelectasis mimicking left hemidiaphragm injury. A, Anteroposterior (AP) chest radiograph shows elevation of the air-containing colon into the left lower chest. However, note the shift of the heart to the left, indicating left lower lobe volume loss. Surgery was initially planned. **B,** Coronal multiplanar reformation (MPR) intravenous (IV) contrast–enhanced computed tomography (CECT) indicates that the spleen and intact diaphragm are elevated by left lower lobe atelectasis.

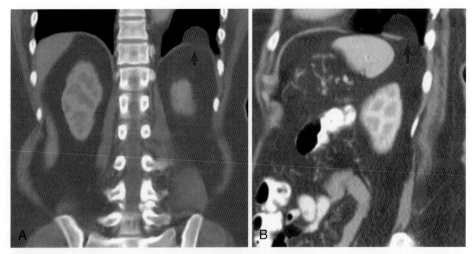

Figure 8-102 Foramen of Bochdalek hernia. Coronal (**A**) and sagittal (**B**) reformations from intravenous (IV) contrast–enhanced computed tomography (CECT) show a defect in the posterior left hemidiaphragm *(arrow)* with smoothly contoured fat herniation. The appearance is most consistent with Bochdalek hernia.

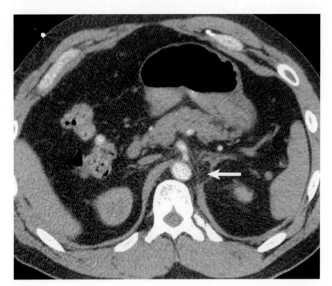

Figure 8-103 Traumatic crural tear. Axial intravenous (IV) contrast–enhanced computed tomography (CECT) demonstrates an irregular tear across the anterior left crus *(arrow)* with some surrounding fat infiltration.

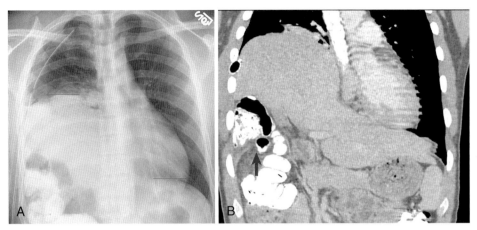

Figure 8-104 Elevation of the apparent right hemidiaphragm 4 cm or more above the left hemidiaphragm on supine radiograph increases specificity that the elevation is due to rupture of the right hemidiaphragm **A,** Anteroposterior (AP) supine chest radiograph shows marked elevation of the right hemidiaphragm compared to the left *(black lines).* **B,** Coronal multiplanar reformation (MPR) computed tomographic (CT) image obtained with oral and intravenous (IV) contrast shows a large hump of the liver displaced into the chest with currently colon herniation. Torn lateral edge of the right diaphragm is detected *(arrow)* and the heart and mediastinum are displaced to the left. (From Rees O, Mirvis SE, Shanmuganathan K. Multidetector-row CT of right hemidiaphragm caused by blunt trauma: a review of 12 cases. *Clin Radiol.* 2005;60:1280-1289.)

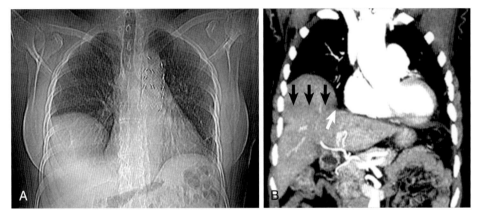

Figure 8-105 Rupture of the right hemidiaphragm with liver herniation. **A,** Anteroposterior (AP) chest radiograph illustrates elevation and abnormal medial contour of the apparent right hemidiaphragm. **B,** Coronal intravenous (IV) contrast–enhanced computed tomographic (CECT) image shows a well-defined hump of liver projecting above the diaphragm with a slight indentation of the medial border where the liver crosses the diaphragm *(white arrow).* Also note the low-attenuation "band" across the base of the herniated portion of the liver at the torn diaphragm *(black arrows),* also resulting from compression of the parenchyma and decreased density on that coronal slice.

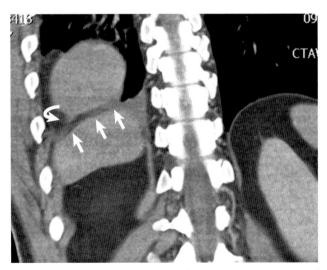

Figure 8-106 Liver herniation through a torn diaphragm. Coronal reformatted computed tomographic (CT) image through the lower chest shows a portion of the herniated liver above the hemidiaphragm with the collar sign *(curved arrow)* and the low-density-band sign *(straight arrows).*

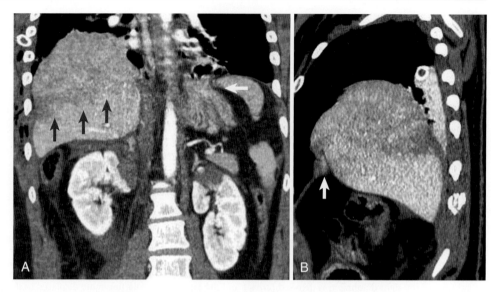

Figure 8-107 Liver herniation through a torn right diaphragm. Coronal (**A**) and sagittal (**B**) intravenous (IV) contrast–enhanced computed tomographic (CECT) images show the irregular band sign *(arrows)* at the level of the hemidiaphragm tear and the shallow collar sign at the level of the tear. The herniated portion of the liver is of lower attenuation, suggesting perfusion delay. The coronal image also shows the herniated gastric fundus though a tear in the medial left hemidiaphragm *(white arrow)*.

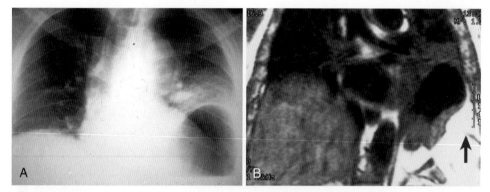

Figure 8-108 Magnetic resonance image (MRI) of a torn right hemidiaphragm and gastric herniation. A, Chest radiograph demonstrates an elevated apparent left hemidiaphragm. A large air-fluid level suggests gastric herniation. **B,** Coronal T1-weighted MRI shows a large tear in the left hemidiaphragm *(arrow)* with herniation of the stomach and left lower lobe atelectasis. (From Mirvis SE. Diagnostic imaging of thoracic trauma. In: Mirvis SE, Shanmuganathan K, eds. *Imaging in Trauma and Critical Care.* Philadelphia, PA: Elsevier; 2003:297-389.)

Selected Reading

Bean MJ, Johnson PT, Roseborough GS, et al. Thoracic aortic stent-grafts: utility of multidetector CT for pre and postprocedural evaluation. *Radiographics.* 2008;28:1835–1851.

Bernardin B, Troquet JM. Initial management and resuscitation of severe chest trauma. *Emerg Med Clin North Am.* 2012;30:377–400.

Beslic S, Beslic N, Sofic A, et al. Diagnostic imaging of traumatic pseudoaneurysm of the thoracic aorta. *Radiol Oncol.* 2010;44:158–163.

Chen JD, Shanmuganathan K, Mirvis SE, et al. Using CT to diagnose tracheal rupture. *AJR Am J Roentgenol.* 2001;176:1273–1280.

Cohn SM, DuBose JJ. Pulmonary contusion: an update on recent advances in clinical management. *World J Surg.* 2010;34:1959–1970.

Forman MJ, Mirvis SE, Hollander DS. Blunt thoracic aortic injuries: CT characterisation and treatment outcomes of minor injury. *Eur Radiol.* 2013 Nov;23(11):2988–2995. doi: 10.1007/s00330-013-2904-0.

Gavant ML. Helical CT grading of traumatic aortic injuries: impact on clinical guidelines for medical and surgical management. *Radiol Clin North Am.* 1999;37:553–574.

Glaser DL, Shanmuganathan K, Mirvis SE. General case of the day. Acute intrapericardial diaphragmatic hernia. *Radiographics.* 1998;18:799–801.

Kaewlai R, Avery LL, Asrani AV, et al. Multidetector CT of blunt thoracic trauma. *Radiographics.* 2008;28:1555–1570.

Linsenmaier U, Krötz M, Häuser H, et al. Whole-body computed tomography in polytrauma: techniques and management. *Eur Radiol.* 2002;12:1728–1740.

Miller LA. Chest wall, lung, and pleural space trauma. In: Mirvis SE, Shanmuganathan K, eds. Emergency chest imaging. *Radiol Clin North Am;* 2006;44:213–224.

Mirvis SE. Thoracic vascular injury. In: Mirvis SE, Shanmuganathan K, eds. Emergency chest imaging. *Radiol Clin North Am;* 2006;44:181–198.

Mirvis SE, Shanmuganathan K. Imaging hemidiaphragm injury. *Eur Radiol.* 2007;17:1411–1421.

Mirvis SE. Diagnostic imaging of thoracic trauma. In: Mirvis SE, Shanmuganathan K, eds. *Imaging in Trauma and Critical Care.* Philadelphia, PA: Elsevier; 2003:297–389.

Moore FO, Goslar PW, Coimbra R, et al. Blunt traumatic occult pneumothorax: is observation safe?—Results of a prospective, AAST multicenter study. *J Trauma.* 2011;70:1019–1025.

Morgan TA, Steenburg SD, Siegel EL, et al. Acute traumatic aortic injuries: posttherapy multidetector CT findings. *Radiographics.* 2010;30:851–867.

Rees O, Mirvis SE, Shanmuganathan K. Multidetector-row CT of right hemidiaphragm rupture caused by blunt trauma: a review of 12 cases. *Clin Radiol.* 2005;60:1280–1289.

Restrepo CS, Gutierrez FR, Marmol-Velez JA, et al. Imaging patients with cardiac trauma. *Radiographics.* 2012;32:633–649.

Scaglione M, Romano S, Pinto A, et al. Acute tracheobronchial injuries: impact of imaging on diagnosis and management implications. *Eur J Radiol.* 2006;59:336–343.

Sliker CW. Imaging of diaphragm injuries. In: Mirvis SE, Shanmuganathan K, eds. Emergency chest imaging. *Radiol Clin North Am;* 2006;44:199–212.

Steenburg SD, Ravenel JG, Ikonomidis JS, et al. Acute traumatic aortic injury: imaging evaluation and management. *Radiology.* 2008;248:748–762.

Symbas JD, Halkos ME, Symbas PN. Rupture of the innominate artery from blunt trauma: current options for management. *J Card Surg.* 2005;20:455–459.

Wintermark M, Wick S, Bettex D, et al. Trauma of the mediastinum. In: Schnyder P, Wintermark M, eds. *Radiology of Blunt Trauma of the Chest.* Berlin-Heidelberg: Springer; 2000:71–127.

Wong H, Gotway MB, Sasson AD. Periaortic hematoma at diaphragm crura at helical CT: sign of blunt aortic injury in patients with mediastinal hematoma. *Radiology.* 2004;231:185–189.

CHAPTER 9

Nontraumatic, Nonvascular Chest Emergencies

Anuj M. Tewari, Jamlik-Omari Johnson, and Waqas Shuaib

Use of imaging services in the emergency department (ED) continues to outpace the growth of actual ED patient visits. This imaging surge places the emergency radiologist at the forefront of acute care. Chest imaging constitutes a large percentage of examinations generated through the ED. In the time-sensitive acute care environment, efficiency is paramount; conventional radiographs are a common triage screening tool. It is not uncommon for the radiologist to "examine" the patient before the emergency physician does.

Navigating the multitude of acute and chronic diseases in the ED can be a daunting task for emergency radiologists. Applying a pattern-based approach and recognizing common disease states provides a road map for accurate and prompt diagnosis of chest emergencies. Understanding radiologic manifestations of these emergencies requires knowledge of the basic anatomy of the thoracic cavity.

◼ ANATOMIC CONSIDERATIONS

Anatomic clues facilitate a pattern-based approach to image interpretation. Distinguishing whether opacity lies in the alveolar space, airway, or pleural space seems basic but is requisite for accurate diagnosis. Basic anatomic landmarks such as the bronchi, fissures, vascular and nonvascular mediastinal structures, pleura, and soft tissues are important when navigating conventional radiography, especially if only a single view is obtained.

Not all opacities represent disease. Common anatomic variants such as pectus excavatum and benign masses can mimic acute disease. Recognition of these entities can help resolve diagnostic dilemmas. Displacement of fissures or mediastinal structures can be the first clue in recognizing lobar collapse or even pneumothorax. Left upper lobe collapse can be confounding and is often misinterpreted if secondary signs are not identified (Fig. 9-1). Secondary signs include tenting of the diaphragm, hilar retraction toward the collapsed lung, and the Luftsichel sign (due to compensatory hyperinflation of the superior segment of the left lower lobe). When opacities abut and silhouette the pleura, the presence of obtuse or acute interfaces can help localize the lesion to the pleural or subpleural compartments, respectively. Accurate localization is vital in the setting of aspirated foreign bodies or penetrating trauma for surgical planning. Infiltrative diseases such as a necrotizing pneumonia or neoplasm can be multispacial. Thin-section computed tomography (CT), through the use of 1- to 2-mm collimation, provides exquisite anatomic detail as compared to conventional radiography but requires a greater understanding of segmental and subsegmental pulmonary anatomy to interpret the multitude of patterns that can be encountered.

Beyond lobar and segmental anatomy (Fig. 9-2), the emergency radiologist should be familiar with the smallest unit visible on CT, which is the secondary pulmonary lobule. The walls of the secondary pulmonary lobule are composed of the interlobular septa. The interlobular septa are composed of connective tissue and house the pulmonary veins and lymphatic drainage to each lobule. Additional venolymphatic drainage is provided via the subpleural interstitium along the fissures and the periphery of the lung. At the center of each lobule is a bronchovascular bundle composed of a terminal bronchiole and pulmonary artery that supply oxygenated air and deoxygenated blood to the alveoli, where gas exchange occurs. They can be seen in disease states such as pulmonary interstitial edema when the septa become thickened due to vascular engorgement and increased hydrostatic pressure; radiographically these are manifested as Kerley B lines.

◼ PATTERN-BASED APPROACH

Common patterns can be seen across varying disease states. For example, hematogenous spread of disease will manifest as randomly distributed nodules throughout the lungs regardless of cause. Therefore metastatic disease can mimic septic emboli. Cavitation can be seen in both metastatic disease and infection. Recognizing these blood-borne disease patterns helps to guide clinical treatment. Nodules in a perilymphatic distribution with septal involvement are more commonly associated with insidious disease processes such as sarcoidosis or lymphangitic carcinomatosis. Similarly, alveolar opacities, often characterized as ground-glass opacities, can represent a variety of disease states, including infection, hemorrhage, edema, neoplasm, or inflammation.

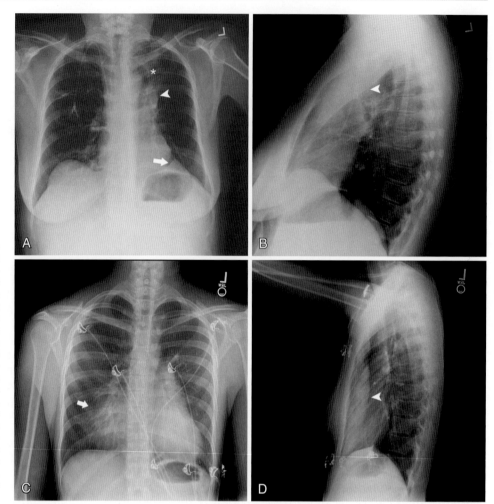

Figure 9-1 Left upper lobe collapse in a 60-year-old woman with B-cell lymphoma. **A,** Posteroanterior (PA) radiograph demonstrates secondary signs of left upper lobe collapse, including diaphragmatic tenting *(arrow)*, hilar retraction *(arrowhead)*, and Luftsichel sign *(asterisk)*. **B,** Lateral radiograph demonstrates the collapsed left upper lobe as an anterior density *(arrow)*. The collapse was due to a bronchial tumor, which represented recurrent disease. **C,** Right middle lobe opacity with ill-defined border *(arrow)* on PA radiograph. **D,** Lateral radiograph showing an anterior density *(arrow)* corresponding to pectus excavatum variant of the sternum. (Courtesy Media Services, Emory University.)

The commonly described tree-in-bud pattern seen on thin-section CT was first attributed to endobronchial spread of *Mycobacterium* tuberculosis (TB; Fig. 9-3). It described linear branching centrilobular opacities corresponding to impaction of distal airways. This finding is associated with other disease states where fluid, debris, pus, and mucus fill the distal bronchioles or if significant thickening of the distal bronchiolar walls is present. This pattern can indicate endobronchial spread of other bacterial, viral, or fungal infections such as cytomegalovirus and allergic bronchopulmonary aspergillosis (ABPA). The tree-in-bud pattern can also be seen in the setting of chronic airway disease states such as cystic fibrosis, after toxic inhalation or aspiration. Correlation with clinical and laboratory data is necessary when there is severe underlying chronic airways disease to exclude superimposed acute infection.

Several other common patterns of pulmonary disease can be seen in the acute setting. The "crazy-paving" pattern (Fig. 9-4) seen on thin-section CT is characterized by scattered or diffuse ground-glass attenuation with superimposed interlobular septal thickening. This was initially described in acute pulmonary alveolar proteinosis but subsequently has been reported in a wide range of infectious and inflammatory diseases such as *Pneumocystis jiroveci* pneumonia (Fig. 9-5), acute respiratory distress

syndrome (ARDS), organizing pneumonia, and even pulmonary edema. The presence of this pattern should prompt the radiologist to alert the clinician about possible underlying immunodeficiency disorders, most commonly acquired immunodeficiency syndrome (AIDS). Another commonly encountered pattern is "mosaic" perfusion of the lungs, which can be seen in chronic thromboembolic disease, small airways disease with air trapping, and hypersensitivity pneumonitis (HP).

Cavitary masses are commonly associated with fungal and tuberculous infections. Community-acquired pneumonias can also be complicated by necrosis and cavitation. In adults cavitary lesions typically contain mixed flora, including anaerobes such as *Klebsiella*. In children staphylococcal pneumonia is the most common cause of cavitary pneumonia. Primary lung neoplasm and metastatic disease may cavitate and are usually included as differential considerations particularly in smokers or patients with known primary malignancy. Computed tomography can be important for additional characterization to exclude bronchopulmonary abscess and empyema.

■ CLINICAL CONSIDERATIONS

For the emergency radiologist, acquiring accurate history can be a challenge because patients are often triaged

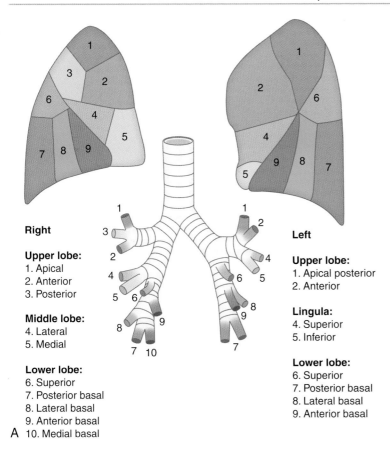

Right

Upper lobe:
1. Apical
2. Anterior
3. Posterior

Middle lobe:
4. Lateral
5. Medial

Lower lobe:
6. Superior
7. Posterior basal
8. Lateral basal
9. Anterior basal
A 10. Medial basal

Left

Upper lobe:
1. Apical posterior
2. Anterior

Lingula:
4. Superior
5. Inferior

Lower lobe:
6. Superior
7. Posterior basal
8. Lateral basal
9. Anterior basal

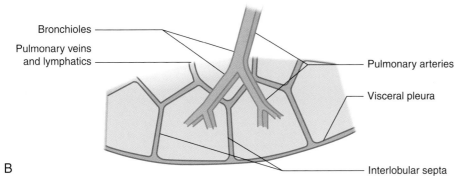

Bronchioles

Pulmonary veins
and lymphatics

Pulmonary arteries

Visceral pleura

B

Interlobular septa

Figure 9-2 A, Basic segmental lung anatomy. **B,** Anatomy of the secondary pulmonary lobule. (Courtesy Eric Jablonowski.)

quickly before relevant clinical information is obtained or available. Vague clinical indications such as "cough," "chest pain," or "shortness of breath" are commonplace. Direct communication with clinical providers can yield important data that can augment radiologic interpretation. The added history of chronic disease states such as chronic renal failure, sickle cell disease, or malignancy sheds light on imaging findings. Clinical data regarding acute exposure to inhalational toxins, thermal injury, or patient's immune status allow the radiologist to refine his or her interpretation. Reviewing basic laboratory data and patient medical records is frequently a worthwhile endeavor that can yield information unbeknownst even to the clinician.

Recognizing parenchymal lung disease patterns of susceptible populations can alert the radiologist to assess for associated potential complications. For example,

sickle cell anemia is a frequently encountered disease in the acute care setting. Patients are predisposed to infection, as well as bouts of acute vasoocclusive crises known as *acute chest syndrome*. Even without history, the recognizable radiographic stigmata of sickle cell disease such as osteonecrosis and cardiomegaly can alert the radiologist to assess for changes suggestive of acute chest syndrome—which is defined as the presence of a new consolidation on chest radiography (Fig. 9-6). Sickle cell patients are 100 times more susceptible to pneumonia than the general population, with a 30% recurrence rate. Pulmonary edema related to left ventricular failure can also be seen. Chronic findings of pulmonary hypertension related to microvascular occlusion and chronic hypoxia are manifested as scarring, architectural distortion, and enlargement of the pulmonary arteries.

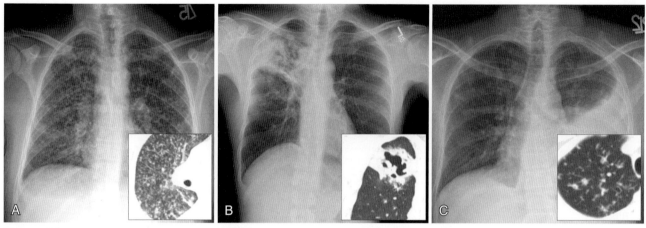

Figure 9-3 A, Miliary tuberculosis (TB) in a 46-year-old man. Radiograph shows randomly distributed pulmonary nodules confirmed on computed tomography (CT). Patient had disseminated infection with positive sputum, blood, and cerebrospinal fluid (CSF) cultures for acid-fast bacilli. **B,** Cavitary TB in a 40-year-old man with history of incarceration. Radiograph shows a right upper lobe mass with rounded central lucency confirmed to be cavitation on CT. **C,** Endobronchial spread of TB in a 45-year-old man who presented with worsening shortness of breath and fever. Large left effusion and reticulonodular opacities were seen on the radiograph, which had tree-in-bud pattern on the accompanying CT. (Courtesy Media Services, Emory University.)

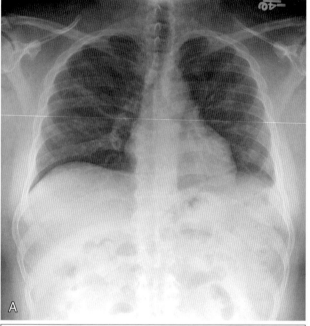

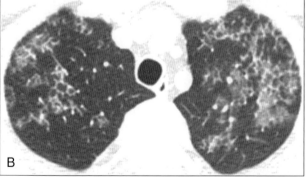

Figure 9-4 Pulmonary alveolar proteinosis (PAP) in a 41-year-old man who presented initially to the emergency department (ED) with shortness of breath. **A,** Chest radiograph was ordered to rule out pneumonia, which showed streaky bronchocentric opacities. **B,** Axial computed tomography (CT) demonstrated classic "crazy-paving" pattern with ground-glass attenuation superimposed with interlobular septal interstitial thickening. Alveolar proteinosis was eventually confirmed after biopsy. (Courtesy Media Services, Emory University.)

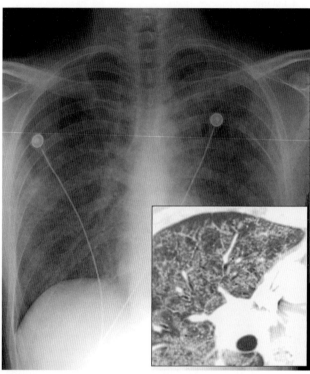

Figure 9-5 Pneumocystis pneumonia in a 28-year-old man with progressive shortness of breath, fever, and thrush. The patient was newly diagnosed with human immunodeficiency virus (HIV) with CD4 count of 62. Radiograph and computed tomographic (CT) scan show diffuse bilateral reticulonodular prominence and air-space opacities. (Courtesy Media Services, Emory University.)

Patients with obstructive lung physiological findings, most commonly long-time smokers, appear to have hyperinflated lungs because of pulmonary emphysema and are predisposed to infection and neoplasm. Parenchymal damage due to cystic or bullous changes can predispose this population to secondary spontaneous pneumothorax. Another commonly encountered entity is cystic fibrosis. Patients present with frequent respiratory tract complaints, including cough, dyspnea, and fever. The radiographic findings

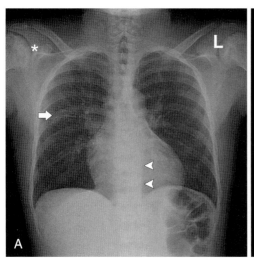 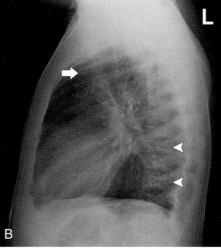

Figure 9-6 Acute chest syndrome in a 29-year-old man who presented with chest pain. Posteroanterior (PA), **A,** and lateral, **B,** radiographs demonstrate a new right upper lobe opacity *(arrow)* and stigmata of sickle cell disease, including osteonecrosis of the proximal humerus *(asterisk)* and "fish-mouth" or H-shaped vertebral bodies *(arrowheads)* and enlarged pulmonary arteries. (Courtesy Media Services, Emory University.)

of cystic fibrosis include bronchiectasis and parenchymal scarring. Computed tomography findings include bronchial wall thickening, progressive bronchiectasis, and mucoid plugging within the bronchi with upper lobe predominance. Hyperinflation and secondary spontaneous pneumothorax can also be seen. Consideration should also be given to the wide range of disease states that result in immunosuppression. In addition to human immunodeficiency virus (HIV)/AIDS, patients undergoing chemotherapy, long-term corticosteroid use, or recent organ transplantation are susceptible to opportunistic infections.

■ INFECTION

Infectious disease processes of the thoracic cavity are diverse in clinical and radiologic presentation depending on the pathophysiological characteristics of the offending organism. Lobar and interstitial pneumonias, cavitary pneumonias, endobronchial infection, pleural-based infections, and hematogenous spread of infection are all encountered in the acute care setting, and the emergency radiologist should be alert to the radiographic findings and common associations of these disease states.

Community-Acquired Pneumonia

Community-acquired pneumonia is a common cause of significant morbidity and mortality, especially in older adults. *Mycoplasma, Streptococcus,* and viral respiratory pathogens account for the majority of community-acquired pneumonias encountered. Radiographic findings vary from normal to patchy, or confluent air-space opacities with air bronchograms to occasional progression to cavitation. Opacities within the lingula and right middle lobe may silhouette the cardiac margins. Lower lobe opacities may obscure the diaphragm or appear as a retrocardiac density. Differentiating viral from bacterial pneumonias on radiography is rarely possible; however, interstitial patterns with lymphadenopathy tend to typify viral pneumonias, whereas bacterial pneumonias are more likely to be lobar in distribution with occasional effusions and cavitation. Radiographic follow-up

is beneficial to exclude underlying lung pathologic conditions after treatment.

Although CT is more sensitive than radiography in detecting community-acquired pneumonia, practical issues of radiation, time, and cost argue against routine use unless complication such as abscess formation is suspected. Computed tomography imaging findings vary greatly depending on route of spread. The most common finding on CT is air-space consolidation with or without bronchograms. Other common findings include centrilobular nodules in viral and *Mycoplasma* pneumonias. Lymphadenopathy and effusions can also be seen. Airway-predominant disease may show bronchial wall thickening, bronchocentric ground-glass opacities, and tree-in-bud type opacities.

Atypical Infections

Atypical pneumonia is a nonspecific term that includes rare and opportunistic infections caused by fungal, viral, and bacterial pathogens typically encountered in patients with comorbidities such as AIDS or immunosuppression related to transplant or chemotherapy and in longtime smokers. Chronic debilitating diseases such as renal failure, diabetes, sickle cell disease, and cystic fibrosis may also render patients prone to atypical infections. The emergency radiologist should be familiar with common radiographic manifestations of these infections because prompt and accurate diagnosis can greatly affect the clinical course.

Pulmonary Tuberculosis

Risk factors for pulmonary TB include acquired, innate, or iatrogenic immunodeficiency and exposure to infected individuals. Prisoners and recent immigrants from countries where TB is endemic have higher risks for infection. Primary TB may manifest as lymphadenopathy, parenchymal disease, miliary disease, or pleural effusion. Multiple patterns can be seen concomitantly. Classic findings of reactivation TB include a predilection for the upper lobes, cavitation, and relative absence of lymphadenopathy; however, recent studies report overlapping radiographic findings in primary and postprimary TB.

Miliary TB is found mainly in immunocompromised patients with disseminated disease affecting multiple organ systems (see Fig. 9-3). Distinct radiographic findings consist of innumerable, 1- to 3-mm diameter nodules uniformly distributed throughout both lungs with slight lower lobe predominance. High-resolution CT depicts nodules in a random distribution. These nodules resolve with treatment, but they may coalesce to form focal areas of consolidation. Thickening of interlobular septal networks is frequently present. Diffuse or localized ground-glass opacity may indicate superimposed ARDS.

Cavitary TB is a hallmark of reactivation TB (see Fig. 9-3). Typical cavities are irregular and thick walled and can occur within surrounding areas of consolidation. Cavitary neoplasms or fungal infections should also be considered in the differential diagnosis depending on the clinical scenario. Complications of cavitary lesions include rupture into pleural space and bronchopleural fistula. A small percentage of cavities showing air-fluid levels may indicate the presence of superinfection.

Computed tomography findings of bronchocentric TB are circumferential mural thickening and luminal narrowing, which may cause lobar collapse or hyperinflation, obstructive pneumonia, and mucoid impaction. In active disease the airway lumens are irregularly narrowed and have thick walls, whereas in fibrotic disease the airways are smoothly narrowed and have thin walls. Tree-in-bud opacities and traction bronchiectasis of the upper lobes may be evident (see Fig. 9-3). Radiographic evidence of lymphadenopathy is seen in up to 90% of children and 50% of adults. Adenopathy is more often unilateral and tends to be right-sided, involving the paratracheal and hilar regions, but may be bilateral in 30% of cases. Nodes larger than 2 cm tend to have low-attenuation centers because of necrosis and are highly suggestive of active disease. Nontuberculous mycobacterial species such as *Mycobacterium avium-intracellulare* complex can manifest as chronic right middle lobe and lingular bronchiectasis and tree-in-bud opacities.

Fungal Infections

Fungi are uncommon pathogens in otherwise healthy populations. Fungal infections occur more frequently in susceptible populations. Fungal infections can manifest with unique radiologic findings. Pulmonary aspergillosis is an opportunistic infection that has four distinct forms: ABPA, aspergilloma, and invasive and semi-invasive aspergillosis. ABPA can be seen in long-standing asthmatic patients typically under the age of 40 years. Eosinophilia and elevated serum immunoglobulin E levels are features of ABPA. During the initial stages of ABPA, chest radiographs may appear normal or depict asthmatic changes. If mucoid impaction within the dilated central bronchi is present, the classic "finger-in-glove" appearance may be seen (Fig. 9-7). Computed tomography findings include fleeting alveolar opacities, central upper lobe bronchiectasis, bronchial wall thickening, and mucoid impaction. Lung distal to the impacted region may become hyperinflated or atelectatic.

Aspergilloma or fungus ball can appear as an air crescent sign, a round focal intracavitary mass surrounded by crescent of air (Fig. 9-8). Early signs include increasing

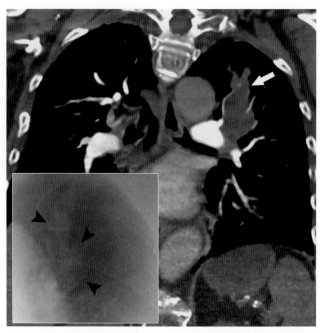

Figure 9-7 Allergic bronchopulmonary aspergillosis (ABPA) in a 63-year-old woman. Radiograph inset demonstrates "finger-in-glove" left suprahilar opacity *(black arrowheads)*. On coronal computed tomography (CT) a left upper lobe soft tissue mass was identified within dilated bronchi *(white arrow)*. (Courtesy Media Services, Emory University.)

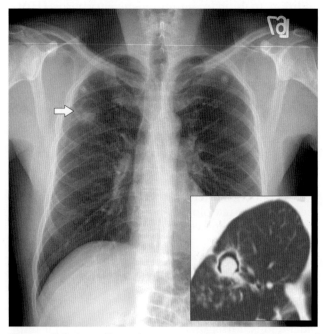

Figure 9-8 Aspergilloma in a 50-year-old man with history of incarceration and tuberculosis (TB) 10 years earlier. Radiograph demonstrates a thin-walled cavitary mass *(arrow)* with increased density within the cavity. On coronal computed tomography (CT) inset, a mobile fungus ball within the cavity creates classic air crescent sign of the aspergilloma. (Courtesy Media Services, Emory University.)

wall thickness of a preexisting cavity or cyst, most commonly prior cavitary TB. The mass may shift with patient position. Invasive aspergillosis appears mainly in severely immunocompromised patients, and it may demonstrate patchy nodular opacities or lobar type of air-space disease in cases with vascular invasion. Computed tomography

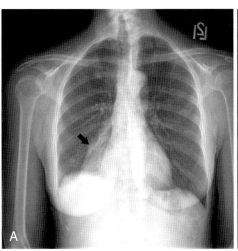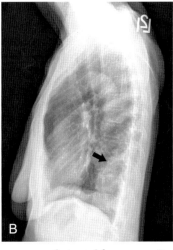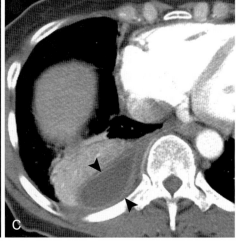

Figure 9-9 Empyema in a 48-year-old woman who was recently treated for community-acquired pneumonia. She returned to the emergency department (ED) because of worsening shortness of breath and fever. **A** and **B,** Posteroanterior (PA) and lateral radiographs demonstrate a right lower lobe pleural-based opacity *(black arrows)* with obtuse margins to the chest wall. **C,** The split pleura sign *(black arrowheads)* was evident on axial computed tomography (CT). (Courtesy Media Services, Emory University.)

may disclose a halo or ground-glass attenuation and is more accurate in the detection of early disease. Cavitation frequently develops with time and typically results in the air crescent sign. Semi-invasive aspergillosis has an indolent course of onset. Radiologic features of semi-invasive pulmonary aspergillosis include areas of focal consolidation or masslike lesions with upper lobe predilection and pleural thickening.

Pneumocystis pneumonia is an opportunistic infection caused by the yeastlike fungus *P. jiroveci.* It is seen most commonly in HIV patients with a CD4 count of less than 200 cells/mm. Patients present with worsening dyspnea and a nonproductive cough. Plain radiographic features vary and may include a fine reticular interstitial pattern or patchy ground-glass peribronchial opacities (see Fig. 9-5). Computed tomography is more sensitive than radiography and may identify diffuse ground-glass opacities, septal thickening, and pneumatoceles (30% of cases). The crazy-paving pattern seen in pneumocystis pneumonia is characterized by scattered or diffuse ground-glass attenuation with superimposed interlobular septal thickening. Atypical radiologic features in those treated prophylactically include cavitating nodules, lymphadenopathy, consolidation, and pleural effusion. The upper lobe–predominant, cystic form poses an increased risk for pneumothorax.

Blastomycosis is an airborne fungal disease endemic in the southern and central United States. Imaging manifestations are nonspecific but most commonly include air-space disease, nodular masses, interstitial disease, and cavitation. Histoplasmosis is a systemic fungal infection caused by breathing the spores of *Histoplasma capsulatum,* mostly found in the Mississippi and Ohio River valley regions. Although immunocompetent hosts may be asymptomatic with no abnormal radiographic findings, disseminated histoplasmosis mostly occurs among the immunocompromised and those with chronic, debilitating diseases. Nearly 50% of these patients will initially have normal radiographic findings. In others radiographic findings may include diffuse, interstitial, reticulonodular or miliary opacities. Smaller nodules may coalesce and produce air-space disease and ARDS.

Hematogenous Spread of Disease

The diagnosis of a septic emboli or disseminated fungal infection is typified by randomly distributed pulmonary nodules, often with cavitation. Hematogenous nodules can extend to the periphery and involve upper and lower lung zones (see Fig. 9-3). Prompt recognition of this miliary pattern plays a pivotal role in early diagnosis and patient prognosis. Septic pulmonary emboli may result as a complication of bacterial endocarditis, septic thrombophlebitis, osteomyelitis, infected venous catheters, or odontogenic infections. Chest radiography may show randomly distributed nodular opacities extending to the lung periphery. Early in the course of septic pulmonary emboli, CT can detect the tiny nodules. Computed tomography can detect wedge-shaped nodules adjacent to the pleura or located at the end of vessels (feeding vessel sign). Empyema, adenopathy, cavity formation, or pneumothorax may be associated with septic emboli.

■ PLEURAL AND CHEST DISEASE

Pleural effusions are common and can accompany infection, pulmonary edema, renal failure, or malignancy. Simple pleural effusions have thin, imperceptible pleural surfaces. Hepatic hydrothorax refers to the frequent build-up of pleural fluid due to chronic liver failure and a presumed diaphragmatic defect. Calcified pleural plaques can be seen in the setting of asbestos exposure.

Empyema, a collection of pus in the pleural space, can result as a complication of pneumonia, trauma, chest tube placement, or esophageal rupture. Common pathogens include *Staphylococcus aureus* and *Pseudomonas aeruginosa.* Radiographically empyema can mimic pleural effusion or peripheral pulmonary abscess. However, abscesses form acute angles with the chest wall. Empyemas are usually lentiform or triangular and form obtuse angles with the chest wall (Fig. 9-9). On CT, abscesses have thick, irregular walls and interrupt bronchovascular structures. Empyemas typically have smoothly enhancing walls with separation of the visceral and parietal pleura (split pleura sign) and compression of the adjacent lung. Empyema treatment typically requires more aggressive measures, including chest tube placement with or without intrapleural fibrinolytic therapy, video-assisted thoracic surgery, or traditional open thoracotomy

Chest wall involvement is a rare complication of TB and can occur because of contiguous or hematogenous spread of pulmonary disease. Abscess or sinus tract can occur in 25% of cases. Pleural effusion can occur with primary infection and is sometimes the initial radiologic manifestation (see Fig. 9-3). Bone destruction and soft tissue mass can be seen in pyogenic osteomyelitis of the ribs or sternum. Computed tomography can be helpful for treatment planning when percutaneous drainage is required. Poststernotomy complications such as dehiscence and mediastinitis occur rarely but are important to recognize due to high mortality (>50%). Other atypical causes of chest wall infection include actinomycosis, which can present with rib destruction and sinus tract formation and aspergillosis, more often seen in immunocompromised hosts. Primary tumors of the chest wall, including soft tissue sarcomas, lymphoma, and metastatic disease, can present as chest wall masses with obtuse angles, mimicking pleural-based infections. Chest wall variants and deformities such as pectus excavatum and benign masses such as lipomas, neurogenic tumors, and fibrous dysplasia can mimic acute disease. Overall, pleural and chest wall diseases are rare. Identifying and localizing these diseases radiographically can be challenging. Computed tomography provides greater anatomic detail.

Pulmonary Abscess

Pulmonary abscess can arise as a complication of aspiration of anaerobic bacteria, necrotizing pneumonia, or hematogenously spread disease. Abscesses are more commonly found in dependent lung on the right side (Fig. 9-10). Patients present with subacute signs of infection or may have recent diagnosis of pneumonia. Patients may complain of pleuritic chest pain, productive cough with bloody sputum and/or fetid odor, and night sweats. Lung abscesses typically respond well to long-term antibiotic therapy but can require percutaneous drainage or surgical resection when therapy is unsuccessful.

Airways

Small Airways and Obstructive Lung Disease
Small airways disease encompasses a variety of disease states. In the acute setting, asthma is most commonly encountered. Radiographically the most common finding of asthma is hyperinflation with flattened diaphragms due to air trapping. Air trapping in asthma occurs as a result of architectural changes of the lung parenchyma. Inflamed or stenotic distal airways bronchoconstrict and cause a ball-valve effect leading to hyperaeration. The end result is typically a mosaic pattern of normal and hyperaerated lung. Diffuse air trapping can be harder to recognize due to lack of contrast with surrounding normal lung. Additional findings related to small airway

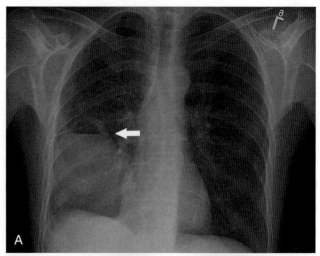
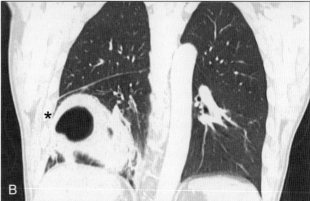

Figure 9-10 Pulmonary abscess in a 39-year-old man with fever and cough. **A,** Posteroanterior (PA) radiograph demonstrates a right lower lobe mass with air-fluid level *(white arrow)*. **B,** Coronal computed tomography (CT) confirms diagnosis of a pulmonary abscess forming acute angles *(black asterisk)* with pleural surface. (Courtesy Media Services, Emory University.)

disease on CT are subsegmental atelectasis, mild bronchial wall thickening, and bronchiectasis.

Chronic disease states like bronchiolitis obliterans or smoking-related bronchiolitis also affect the small airways. Thin-section CT can provide more detailed assessment of the small airways. Common findings include thickened airway walls, mucus plugging within small and large airways, centrilobular nodules, subsegmental atelectasis, and mosaic perfusion due to air-trapping and superimposed infection. Normal, small airways are typically invisible but become more prominent when filled with mucus, pus, or debris. Dilated, thick-walled airways can result in the tree-in-bud pattern seen on thin-section CT.

Small airways disease among pediatric patients is usually viral, commonly respiratory syncytial virus. Hyperinflation may be the only radiologic clue of lower respiratory infection. Identifying hyperinflation in infants can be challenging. Many radiologists use the anterior sixth rib to identify the normal diaphragm position and consider deviation from this landmark as criteria for hyperinflation or hypoinflation. Reactive airways disease is considered a distinct clinical entity from asthma. Reactive airways disease can accompany viral pneumonia and presents as episodic airflow obstruction, wheezing, and airway hyperreactivity. Anatomic considerations that predispose younger patients to bouts of respiratory compromise include diminished airway size, poor collateral ventilation, decreased elastic recoil, and a less developed diaphragmatic muscle.

Cigarette smoking is a significant cause of morbidity, and patients are often seen in the ED for exacerbations of underlying chronic obstructive pulmonary disease. Emphysema is characterized by permanent enlargement of air spaces due to parenchymal destruction. Airway collapse occurs on expiration because of increased elasticity and results in abnormal pulmonary function test results. Findings on radiographs include hyperinflation, flattening of diaphragms, increased retrosternal air space (>4.4 cm), and the presence of bullas. Paraseptal, centrilobular, and panlobular emphysema can be distinguished on CT.

Bronchial Disease

A basic understanding of airway anatomy and physiology can be useful to the emergency radiologist. There are over 300,000 branch points between the trachea and respiratory bronchioles through which air is transported to the alveoli, where gas exchange occurs. The mucus-producing respiratory epithelium lines the tract to the level of the bronchioles. Any impairment in the production or movement of mucus via cilia along the respiratory tract, from primary cilia dyskinesia to smoking, can give rise to a variety of disease states.

Bronchiectasis, permanent bronchial dilatation and wall thickening, is typically the sequela of previous inflammation or infection. Forms of bronchiectasis include cylindric, varicose, and cystic. Computed tomography more readily distinguishes these patterns. Causes of bronchiectasis include cystic fibrosis, childhood viral infection, ABPA, pulmonary fibrosis, and chronic aspiration. Patients with bronchiectasis are prone to infections and may present with clinical signs of pneumonia. Mucus impaction, bronchial wall thickening, and peribronchial opacities are indicators of superimposed infection but may be hard to distinguish from baseline scarring. Cystic fibrosis patients may have upper lobe–predominant mucus impaction.

Airway Obstruction and Aspiration

Bronchial obstruction is an important cause of respiratory distress in the acute setting, and therefore the emergency radiologist must always assess airway patency. Causes include aspiration of foreign bodies; gastrointestinal (GI) or oral secretions; infected material such as pus, food, or water; and toxic substances. Subglottic obstruction can result from tracheal edema related to infection, giving rise to the steeple sign, where the air column assumes the configuration of an inverted V. Risk factors for acute obstruction include chronic physical and/or neurologic debilitation, anatomic abnormalities of the GI tract such as strictures or achalasia, sedation, and intoxication. Radiographic findings are nonspecific and can mimic those of other conditions, but suspicion should be raised when there are known risk factors. Dependent pulmonary opacities can be seen. When

there is high-grade bronchial obstruction, lobar collapse can occur.

Massive gastric acid aspiration can be seen in the setting of trauma, alcoholic stupor, cerebrovascular accident or other neurologic impairment, seizure, or cardiac arrest. The low pH of gastric secretions can result in severe alveolar damage and hemorrhage. In severe cases, bilateral, symmetric heterogeneous opacities progressing to diffuse ARDS pattern occur. The aspiration of partially digested food typically is less severe. It may result in a more focal pulmonary abnormality such as focal opacity or atelectasis. Resolution commonly occurs within 24 to 48 hours. Persistent opacities suggest superimposed infection. Aspiration of secretions in patients with poor oral hygiene and advanced periodontal disease can manifest as cough and fever initially and progress to pneumonia and lung abscess, particularly when anaerobic bacterial species are present. Aspiration of anaerobic bacteria can also result in empyema or bronchopleural fistula. Recurrent aspiration can manifest as recurrent bouts of coughing, wheezing, or dyspnea and tends to occur in patients with anatomic predispositions such as hiatal hernias or esophageal stricture, as well in patients with gastroesophageal reflux and chronic neurologic impairment.

Near-drowning events can result in severe pulmonary complications. The radiologic features of fresh or salt water aspiration are similar and include scattered pulmonary opacities and atelectasis that can progress to diffuse lung opacification over several days. Patients are typically dyspneic at presentation and may require intubation. Chemical and organic contaminants in the water can contribute to the acute lung injury and subsequent permeability edema.

Foreign body aspiration is more common in pediatric patients but can be seen occasionally in adults. The clinical manifestations are dependent on the size and location of the aspirated material. Large objects can become lodged in the trachea and result in immediate asphyxiation and death. Small foreign bodies such as nuts can lodge distally, causing bronchial obstruction. Resultant postobstructive atelectasis or pneumonia may be the only radiologic manifestation if the object is not radiopaque. Aspirated teeth or bridgework is a common cause of bronchial obstruction after trauma or emergent intubation (Fig. 9-11). The aspiration of mineral oil, leading to exogenous lipoid pneumonia, is not encountered frequently but can be seen in patients who ingest mineral oil to treat chronic constipation. A variety of findings have been described, including the crazy-paving pattern, but the presence of fat-attenuation foci amidst pulmonary opacities is a reliable indicator.

Inflammatory Disease

Hypersensitivity Pneumonitis

Hypersensitivity pneumonitis is an immune-mediated inflammation of the alveoli caused by hypersensitivity to inhalation of an antigen. Sufferers are commonly exposed to organic dusts related to occupational or recreational exposure. In 40% of cases the offending agent is never found. This exposure mediates an exaggerated immune response that leads to HP. Hypersensitivity pneumonitis is categorized into acute, subacute, and chronic forms based on the duration of the illness.

Acute symptoms develop following heavy exposure to the inciting antigen, usually in 4 to 6 hours. Patients may present with dyspnea, chest tightness, cough, chills, fever, and headache. Symptoms may resolve within 12 hours to several days upon removal of the irritant. Histologically, acute HP is characterized by noncaseating interstitial granulomas and mononuclear cell infiltration in a peribronchial distribution with prominent giant cells. Chest radiographs often demonstrate a diffuse micronodular interstitial pattern in the middle and lower lung zones with or without ground-glass density that can mimic pulmonary edema. Findings are normal in approximately 10% of patients. High-resolution CT demonstrates ground-glass or reticular opacities. Patients demonstrate reduced diffusion capacity of lungs for carbon monoxide on pulmonary function tests, have hypoxemia at rest, and desaturate with exercise.

Subacute phase symptoms include progression to anorexia, weight loss, fatigue, productive cough, dyspnea, and pleurisy. Symptoms may overlap acute disease but tend to be more insidious. The subacute form produces bronchiolitis with or without organizing pneumonia and interstitial fibrosis. Classic findings include centrilobular nodules and mosaic attenuation on inspiratory images (Fig. 9-12).

Chronic forms reveal additional findings of chronic interstitial inflammation and alveolar destruction (honeycombing) associated with dense fibrosis. On chest radiographs, progressive fibrotic changes with loss of

lung volume particularly affect the upper lobes. Nodular or ground-glass opacities are usually not present. Chronic HP can be difficult to diagnose because the functional and clinical presentations are nonspecific. Hypersensitivity pneumonitis may be distinguished from occupational asthma in that it is not restricted to only occupational exposure. Unlike asthma, HP targets lung alveoli rather than bronchi. HP frequently mimics chronic interstitial pneumonias such as idiopathic pulmonary fibrosis and nonspecific interstitial pneumonia. Each disease is managed differently, thus distinguishing HP from idiopathic pulmonary fibrosis and nonspecific interstitial pneumonia is important. In chronic HP, removing the patient from the inciting antigen remains a key factor in successful management.

Acute Respiratory Distress Syndrome

Acute respiratory distress syndrome, also known as *respiratory distress syndrome* or *adult respiratory distress syndrome* (in contrast with infant respiratory distress syndrome) is a life-threatening reaction to injuries or acute infection to the lung. ARDS is not a specific disease; rather it is a syndrome with direct and indirect causes. Inflammation of the lung parenchyma leads to impaired gas exchange with systemic release of inflammatory mediators. Inflammation, hypoxemia, and multiple organ failure follow. Untreated patients survive only 10% of the time. With treatment, including supportive care and mechanical ventilation in an intensive care unit, the mortality rate is 50%.

The majority of ARDS cases can be traced to three settings: sepsis, trauma, and aspiration. Sepsis syndrome is most common (Fig. 9-13). Some cases of ARDS are

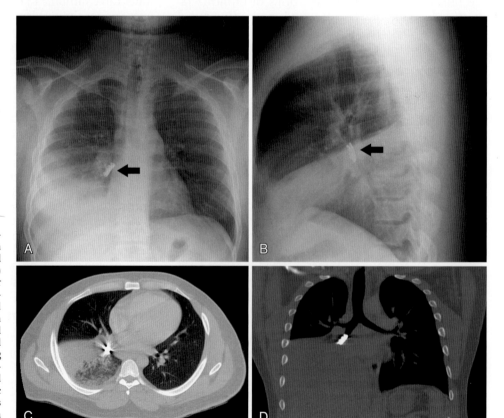

Figure 9-11 Foreign body aspiration in a 30-year-old man with chronic renal failure who presented to the emergency department (ED) in sepsis. **A** and **B**, Posteroanterior (PA) and lateral radiographs demonstrate the patient's gold dental bridgework *(black arrows)* within the bronchus intermedius. **C** and **D**, Axial and coronal computed tomography (CT) images showing the bridgework lodged in the bronchus intermedius with associated postobstructive pneumonia. The patient "swallowed" his gold caps 6 months earlier. (Courtesy Media Services, Emory University.)

linked to aggressive fluid resuscitation after trauma. Other causes include shock, near-drowning, multiple transfusions, and inhalation of irritants or toxic fumes that damage the alveolar epithelium. Patients usually present with shortness of breath, tachypnea, and hypoxia. ARDS usually occurs within 72 hours after the trigger such as an acute illness—sepsis or infectious pneumonia, trauma, burns, aspiration, or massive blood transfusion. Chest imaging demonstrates bilateral air-space opacities or consolidation sparing the costophrenic angles.

Alveolar Proteinosis

Pulmonary alveolar proteinosis (PAP) is characterized by impaired gas exchange due to an abnormal accumulation of surfactant within the alveoli. The majority of cases are idiopathic, but PAP can occur secondarily in the setting of neoplasm such as myeloid leukemia, pulmonary infection, or environmental exposure. The disease is more common in males and in tobacco smokers between the ages of 20 and 50 years. The symptoms of PAP are insidious, such as low-grade fever, dyspnea, nonproductive cough, malaise, and weight loss. Classic features on radiographs include bilateral symmetric alveolar opacities in a perihilar distribution that can resemble pulmonary edema. Typical features on thin-section CT include diffuse ground-glass attenuation with superimposed interlobular and intralobular septal thickening in the crazy-paving pattern (see Fig. 9-4). Histopathologic diagnosis is confirmed when alveolar specimens demonstrate lipid-rich PAS-positive proteinaceous material. The clinical course of PAP widely varies, ranging from spontaneous remission to stable disease to death. The standard treatment for PAP is whole-lung lavage, in which sterile fluid is instilled into the lungs and then aspirated. Lung transplantation is a last-line treatment.

■ MISCELLANEOUS ACUTE CHEST EMERGENCIES

Thermal Injury

Inhalational injury related to burns includes direct thermal effects as well as chemical effects. Pulmonary complications are a major cause of morbidity and mortality despite advances in burn care. The presence of inhalational injury in patients with cutaneous burns increases the mortality rate by 20% to 40%. The total mortality rate for burn victims with pulmonary complications is as high as 80% to 90%. Patients with facial and perioral burns, singed nasal hairs, soot within the oral or nasal cavity, and stridor should alert the clinician to the possibility of inhalational injury. The extent of respiratory tract injury from inhalational stress depends on the temperature, duration of exposure, and smoke particle size. When direct pulmonary parenchymal damage is

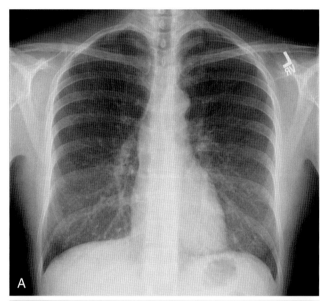

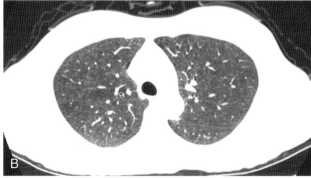

Figure 9-12 Hypersensitivity pneumonitis (HP) in a 43-year-old woman due to drug reaction. **A,** Posteroanterior (PA) radiograph showing essentially clear lungs. **B,** Axial computed tomography (CT) demonstrating subtle centrilobular nodules with ground-glass attenuation consistent with likely subacute HP. (Courtesy Media Services, Emory University.)

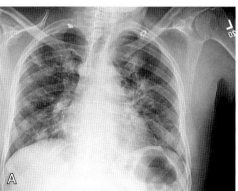

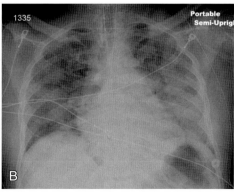

Figure 9-13 *Legionella* pneumonia in a 66-year-old male smoker with recent travel to Florida. **A,** Initial portable radiograph showing multifocal pneumonia. **B,** Progression to more confluent air-space disease representing acute respiratory distress syndrome (ARDS) on the follow-up study after patient deteriorated and required intubation. (Courtesy Media Services, Emory University.)

present, patients develop acute respiratory insufficiency. Respiratory tract injury can be complicated by intubation and ventilation, fluid overload from aggressive resuscitation, and infection. Pulmonary complications related to burn injuries can be subdivided into three categories based on time of development: early phase, subacute or delayed phase, and late phase.

Early radiographic manifestations of thermal injury occur within the first 24 hours and represent direct inhalational damage to the lungs and respiratory epithelium. Injury to small airways and tracheobronchial mucosa is due to toxic products of combustion and smoke. Changes include air-space opacities related to chemical injury, atelectasis, and tracheobronchial wall thickening related to edema (Fig. 9-14). Atelectasis may occur because of airway collapse from direct respiratory epithelial injury and impairment of ciliary clearance or from bronchoconstriction. Upper respiratory tract injury is often concomitant but beyond the scope of this chapter. Pulmonary edema, including pulmonary vascular engorgement and effusions, can be seen after aggressive resuscitation in older patients.

In the subacute phase of burn injury between 2 and 5 days, lung abnormalities include pulmonary edema, atelectasis, microembolism, and ARDS. Radiographic findings of microembolism are varied and can range from normal to rapidly changing patchy infiltrates, which represent hemorrhage. Radiographic changes of ARDS can mimic edema, which further clouds the clinical picture. In the late phase (beyond 5 days), pulmonary thromboembolism, pneumonia, septicemia, and ARDS are the primary complications seen. Again, the clinical picture is often clouded by superimposition of multiple complications.

Toxic Gas Exposure

Though infrequently encountered, toxic gas exposure can cause significant pulmonary complications, including airway and alveolar damage through direct chemical injury. Potential toxic agents span a large variety of substances that are used for commercial, scientific, and recreational purposes. Chlorine inhalation is a more frequently encountered toxic agent due to its common commercial use, though it was also used in World War I as an agent of chemical warfare. Symptoms can vary from mild to serious, but most patients do not experience long-term complications. Organophosphates exert their effects on muscarinic and nicotinic receptors, causing a wide range of symptoms, but mortality from organophosphate exposure results from pulmonary complications. Organophosphates have been used in chemical warfare and terrorist acts, but accidental exposure has also been reported from pesticides. Pulmonary complications, including bronchorrhea with mucus plugging and hypoxia, severe bronchospasm, and diaphragmatic paralysis, can result in asphyxiation and death. Welding is associated with inhalational exposure to ozone, phosgene, and nitrogen dioxide gases. Crowd control agents such as chloroacetophenone (Mace) are respiratory irritants with transient effects. However, prolonged exposure in enclosed spaces may result in more severe damage to the respiratory tract, resulting in delayed ARDS. There are a variety of recreational inhalants abused for their euphoric effects, including nitrous oxide, adhesives, aerosols, cleaning agents, and solvents. Known by many terms, including *huffing* or *bagging*, these types of exposures rarely result in direct inhalational injury but can potentially result in central nervous system toxicity, which can lead to seizures and aspiration.

Spontaneous Pneumothorax

Pleural air collections should always be included in the emergency radiologist's search pattern, even in the absence of trauma. Primary spontaneous pneumothorax refers to pneumothorax that occurs without any known lung disease; risk factors include male sex, smoking, and family history of pneumothorax. Secondary spontaneous pneumothorax denotes the presence of an underlying lung pathologic condition, most commonly bullous emphysema. Secondary spontaneous pneumothorax has also been reported in the setting of cystic lung disease such as lymphangiomyomatosis (Fig. 9-15) and pulmonary Langerhans cell histiocytosis, connective tissue diseases such as Marfan syndrome, and cavitary disease such as TB. Architectural damage to lung parenchyma with involvement of the pleura is the underlying mechanism that predisposes to bouts of pneumothorax. Computed tomography can be useful for identifying underlying parenchymal disease in cases of spontaneous pneumothorax.

Pericardial Disease

Pericardial effusions are abnormal accumulations of fluid in the pericardial space that can result from an imbalance of production and/or reabsorption. A small effusion may remain asymptomatic, but large-volume collections that accumulate rapidly can cause increased intrapericardial pressure leading to cardiac tamponade. Normal levels of pericardial fluid range from 15 to 50 mL. Like pleural effusions, pericardial effusions can be tran-

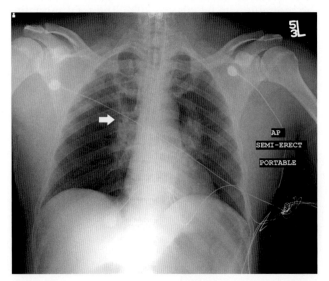

Figure 9-14 Early thermal inhalational injury in a 52-year-old man with flash burns involving 20% of total body surface area. Marked central bronchial wall thickening *(white arrow)* reflects edema related to respiratory epithelium injury. (Courtesy Media Services, Emory University.)

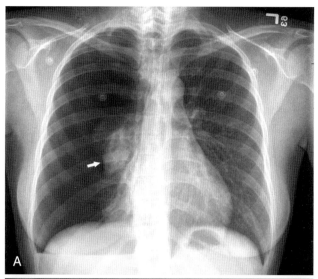

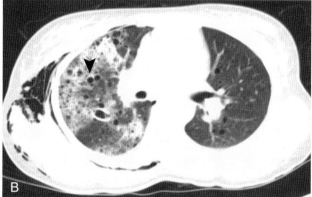

Figure 9-15 Spontaneous pneumothorax in a 26-year-old woman who presented to the emergency department (ED) with shortness of breath. **A,** Posteroanterior (PA) radiograph shows complete collapse of the right lung with a large pleural air collection. **B,** Axial computed tomography (CT) demonstrates multiple bilateral thin-walled cysts *(black arrowhead)* throughout the lung parenchyma after chest tube placement. Diffuse ground-glass opacification of the right lung is consistent with reexpansion pulmonary edema. (Courtesy Media Services, Emory University.)

sudative, exudative, hemorrhagic, or malignant. Transudative effusions are associated with congestive heart failure, myxedema, or nephrotic syndrome. Exudative effusions are associated with infections such as TB. Hemorrhagic effusions may be seen in the setting of trauma or rupture of aneurysms. Malignant effusions are associated with metastasis and may be accompanied by smooth or nodular thickening of the pericardium, also seen with TB. Chest radiography demonstrates an enlarged cardiac silhouette; the classic water bottle–shaped heart may be noted (Fig. 9-16). Computed tomography signs of cardiac tamponade include engorgement of the superior and inferior vena cava, reflux of contrast into the azygous and hepatic veins, and bowing of the interventricular septum. Treatment depends on the underlying cause and the severity of cardiac impairment. Pericardial effusions due to a viral infection are usually self-limited and resolve after a few weeks. In the setting of cardiac tamponade or large effusions with unknown cause, pericardiocentesis is warranted.

Noncardiogenic Pulmonary Edema

Pulmonary edema is most commonly associated with chronic cardiac dysfunction but can also arise from noncardiogenic sources in the setting of diffuse alveolar damage or increased permeability. Reexpansion pulmonary edema is an occasional complication of thoracentesis or chest tube placement in which the pleural space is rapidly evacuated (see Fig. 9-15) causing rapid reexpansion of the collapsed lung. The development of edema is multifactorial, but hypoxia, rapid restoration of blood flow, and increase in negative pressure within the pleural space are the primary contributing factors. Early identification of reexpansion edema is vital because the process proves fatal in 20% of patients. Neurogenic pulmonary edema is multifactorial but can be seen in up to 50% of patients with a major neurologic insult such as stroke, subarachnoid hemorrhage, or status epilepticus.

High-altitude pulmonary edema occurs in otherwise healthy individuals exposed to lower partial oxygen

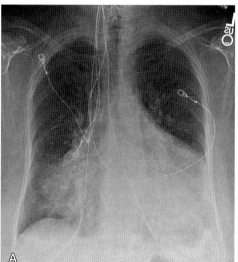

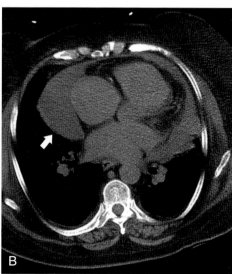

Figure 9-16 Large pericardial effusion in an 80-year-old woman who presented with symptoms of congestive heart failure. **A,** Posteroanterior (PA) radiograph shows the classic water bottle–shaped cardiac contour. **B,** Axial computed tomography (CT) confirms the presence of a large pericardial effusion, which required drainage because of the patient's symptoms. (Courtesy Media Services, Emory University.)

pressures. The condition most commonly affects younger males 24 to 48 hours following rapid ascent to higher altitudes (>3000 m) and can be preceded by acute mountain sickness. The proposed mechanisms are multifactorial, including endothelial leakage and diffuse alveolar damage. Recognized radiographic patterns include central interstitial edema with peribronchial cuffing and patchy alveolar opacities.

Other types of noncardiogenic pulmonary edema that can be seen in the acute setting include cocaine- or heroin-induced pulmonary edema, the mechanism of which is poorly understood but is thought to be related to permeability edema. Acute pancreatitis and acute asthma can also cause pulmonary edema. Mimics of edema include multifocal pneumonia or ARDS and are often only distinguished by response to therapy.

Selected Reading

Boitsios G, Bankier AA, Eisenberg RL: Diffuse pulmonary nodules, *AJR Am J Roentgenol* 194:W354–W366, 2010.

Chen TM, Malli H, Maslove DM, et al: Toxic inhalational exposures, *J Intensive Care Med*, 28:323–333, 2012.

De Wever W, Meersschaert J, Coolen J, et al: The crazy-paving pattern: a radiological-pathological correlation, *Insights Imaging* 2:117–132, 2011.

Friedman PJ, Harwood IR, Ellenbogen PH: Pulmonary cystic fibrosis in the adult: early and late radiologic findings with pathologic correlations, *AJR Am J Roentgenol* 136:1131–1144, 1981.

George A, Gupta R, Bang RL, et al: Radiological manifestation of pulmonary complications in deceased intensive care burn patients, *Burns* 29:73–78, 2007.

Gluecker T, Capasso P, Schnyder P, et al: Clinical and radiologic features of pulmonary edema, *Radiographics* 19:1507–1531, 1999.

Guan Y, Zeng Q, Yang H, et al: Pulmonary alveolar proteinosis: quantitative CT and pulmonary functional correlations, *Eur J Radiol* 81:2430–2435, 2012.

Halvorsen RA, Duncan JD, Merten DF, et al: Pulmonary blastomycosis: radiologic manifestations, *Radiology* 150:1–5, 1984.

Hartman TE, Primack SL, Lee KS, et al: CT of bronchial and bronchiolar diseases, *Radiographics* 14:991–1003, 1994.

Hoffman CK, Goodman PC: Pulmonary edema in cocaine smokers, *Radiology* 172:463–465, 1989.

Iwasaki Y, Nagata K, Nakanishi M, et al: Spiral CT findings in septic pulmonary emboli, *Eur J Radiol* 37:190–194, 2001.

Jeong YJ, Lee KS: Pulmonary tuberculosis: up-to-date imaging and management, *AJR Am J Roentgenol* 191:834–844, 2008.

Jeung MY, Gangi A, Gasser B, et al: Imaging of chest wall disorders, *Radiographics* 19:617–637, 1999.

Kangarloo H, Beachley MC, Ghahremani GG: The radiographic spectrum of pulmonary complications in burn victims, *AJR Am J Roentgenol* 128:441–445, 1977.

Katabathina VS, Restrepo CS, Martinez-Jimenez S, et al: Nonvascular, nontraumatic mediastinal emergencies in adults: a comprehensive review of imaging findings, *Radiographics* 31:1141–1160, 2011.

Kim YK, Kim Y, Shim SS: Thoracic complications of liver cirrhosis: radiologic findings, *Radiographics* 29:825–837, 2009.

Marom EM, McAdams HP, Erasmus JJ, et al: The many faces of pulmonary aspiration, *AJR Am J Roentgenol* 172:121–128, 1999.

Panselinas E, Judson MA: Acute pulmonary exacerbations of sarcoidosis, *Chest* 142:827–836, 2012.

Restrepo CS, Lemos DF, Lemos JA, et al: Imaging findings in cardiac tamponade with emphasis on CT, *Radiographics* 27:1595–1610, 2007.

Rossi SE, Erasmus JJ, Volpacchio M, et al: "Crazy-paving" pattern at thin-section CT of the lungs: radiologic-pathologic overview, *Radiographics* 23:1509–1519, 2003.

Rossi SE, Franquet T, Volpacchio M, et al: Tree-in-bud pattern at thin-section CT of the lungs: radiologic-pathologic overview, *Radiographics* 25:789–801, 2005.

Rovner AJ, Westcott JL: Pulmonary edema and respiratory insufficiency in acute pancreatitis, *Radiology* 118:513–520, 1976.

Rubin SA, Winer-Muram HT: Thoracic histoplasmosis, *J Thorac Imaging* 7:39–50, 1992.

Silva CI, Churg A, Müller NL: Hypersensitivity pneumonitis: spectrum of high-resolution CT and pathologic findings, *AJR Am J Roentgenol* 188:334–344, 2007.

Sun JS, Park KJ, Kang DK: CT findings in patients with pericardial effusion: differentiation of malignant and benign disease, *AJR Am J Roentgenol* 194:489–494, 2010.

Teel GS, Engeler CE, Tashijian JH, et al: Imaging of small airways disease, *Radiographics* 16:27–41, 1996.

Traber DL, Maybauer MO, Maybauer DM, et al: Inhalational and acute lung injury, *Shock* 24:82–87, 2005.

Wang ZJ, Reddy GP, Gotway MB, et al: CT and MR imaging of pericardial disease, *Radiographics* 23:167–180, 2003.

Webb WR: Radiology of obstructive pulmonary disease, *AJR Am J Roentgenol* 169:637–647, 1997.

Wong KS, Lin TY, Huang YC, et al: Clinical and radiographic spectrum of septic pulmonary embolism, *Arch Dis Child* 87:312–315, 2002.

CHAPTER **10**

Vascular Chest Emergencies

Sanjeev Bhalla and Constantine A. Raptis

With chest pain representing one of the most common presenting symptoms in the emergency department (ED), radiologists are frequently called upon for the noninvasive evaluation of aortic and pulmonary vascular diseases. Adequate assessment relies on the ability to understand the spectrum of the pathologic conditions and the significance of each of these entities.

■ THORACIC AORTA

Anatomy

The thoracic aorta begins at the level of the aortic valve and extends to the level of the diaphragmatic hiatus (Fig. 10-1). The aortic root is said to be made of three outpouchings or sinuses of Valsalva and the aortic valve with its annulus. The tubular ascending aorta begins just above the sinuses at a waist known as the *sinotubular junction*. At the level of the innominate or brachiocephalic artery the ascending artery gives way to the arch. Just distal to the left subclavian artery the descending aorta begins. The most proximal portion of the descending aorta is referred to as the *aortic isthmus*. A majority of the thoracic aorta is extrapericardial in its location. Only the first 2 to 3 cm of the ascending aorta resides within the pericardial sac.

The aortic wall has three layers. Although not distinguishable by computed tomography (CT) or magnetic resonance imaging (MRI), these layers include the intima, media, and adventitia. The media is the muscular layer in which many of the acute aortic syndromes may propagate. The inner two thirds of the media has concentric fibers that are orthogonal to the outer one third consisting of longitudinal muscle fibers. The net effect is a natural cleavage plane. If blood can access the space within the media, it can easily travel along the course of the media as either a false lumen or intramural hematoma (IMH).

Imaging

Computed tomography has remained the workhorse for aortic imaging in the ED. Its ubiquitous use comes from the proximity of many scanners to the ED, often with 24-hour technologist staffing and high speed of image acquisition. In addition, many of our surgical colleagues are quite comfortable with CT image review. The advent of multidetector computed tomography (MDCT) has only strengthened the role of CT in the evaluation of acute aortic pathologic conditions. With increased detector rows, thinner section images can be obtained at faster speeds. These thinner sections allow for higher quality multiplanar and three-dimensional reconstructions. In the modern era CT has close to 100% accuracy in depicting acute aortic pathologic conditions. Neither echocardiography nor MRI is more accurate.

Our nontraumatic aortic CT protocol begins with a noncontrast acquisition. The noncontrast images are helpful for looking for high attenuation within the wall, indicative of IMH. The IMH should be higher in attenuation than the blood pool, but not as high as calcium. It usually involves only a portion of the wall, not 360 degrees. The images are acquired as 3-mm thick images with a 3-mm reconstruction interval to avoid any gap. The noncontrast images are followed by a CT angiogram using bolus tracking software and a rapid injection rate of 4 to 5 mL/sec. These images are reconstructed as 1- to 2-mm thick images with 1- to 2-mm reconstruction intervals. A noncontrast study should not be used to exclude acute aortic pathologic conditions. If the patient cannot receive intravenous contrast, a noncontrast study can be performed to exclude aortic rupture, but it should be followed by another test, either echocardiography or MRI.

Although MDCT allows for electrocardiogram (ECG) gating, it is not routinely used in our ED for assessment of the aorta. With fewer than 4% of these studies being positive for aortic pathologic conditions, the potential for increased radiation and the added technical prowess of ECG gating have not been justified in our practice. Instead, we have relied on ECG gating as a problem-solving tool once an aortic pathologic condition is encountered. If a question arises as to whether the ascending aorta is truly involved by a process, the patient may be rebolused and rescanned using ECG gating (Fig. 10-2). With the advent of dual-source CT, we have also begun to rely on ultrahigh-pitch imaging (pitch of 3.2) for the evaluation of the ascending aorta. With its lower radiation dose profile, this technique has shown greater promise in evaluating the ascending aorta on a more regular basis.

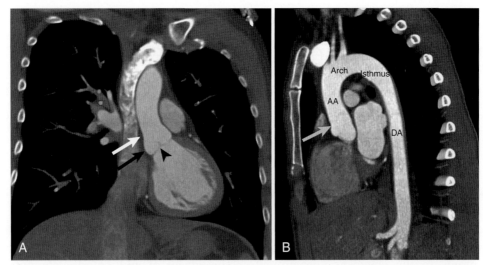

Figure 10-1 Volume-rendered images from an electrocardiogram (ECG)-gated computed tomographic angiogram (CTA) showing normal aortic anatomy in a 28-year-old man. **A,** The normal aortic root. *Arrowhead,* Aortic valve; *black arrow,* sinus of Valsalva; *white arrow,* sinotubular junction. **B,** The ascending aorta (AA), aortic arch, and descending aorta (DA). The portion of the aorta just distal to the arch and left subclavian artery is known as the *isthmus.* In this case the isthmus is slightly dilated, a variant sometimes called the *aortic spindle. White arrow,* Sinotubular junction.

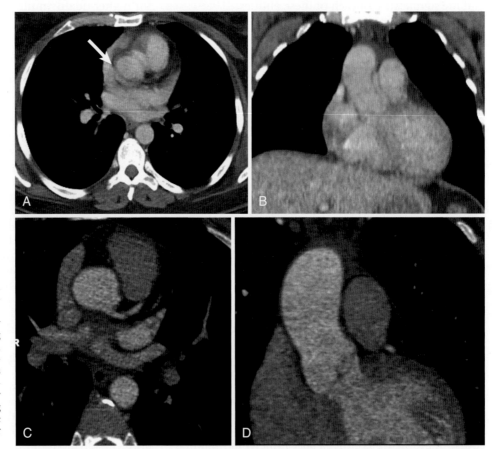

Figure 10-2 A 44-year-old woman with chest pain and concern for ascending aortic dissection. Original computed tomography (CT) scan (**A**) had a linear filling defect *(arrow)*, which persisted on coronal image (**B**). Pulsation artifact was favored, but the patient was brought back for a low-dose electrocardiogram (ECG)-gated study (**C**), which cleared the ascending aorta. Coronal image (**D**) from the gated study has no potential for confusion.

Oblique sagittal reconstructions are created directly at the scanner for all aortic CTs. The candy cane reconstruction allows for a close approximation of an angiogram view and allows for clear delineation in the z-axis of any aortic process. Volume-rendered and shaded surface images are rarely performed in real time. Although the images can be very artistic, they rarely add to the diagnosis.

Magnetic resonance imaging is increasingly being used as a secondary study when the patient is unable to receive iodinated contrast material or if a question arises from the CT. With technologic improvements and improved MR angiography techniques, MRI offers a nonradiation alternative. Unfortunately, distance from the ED and longer examination times have kept MRI as a second-line test at

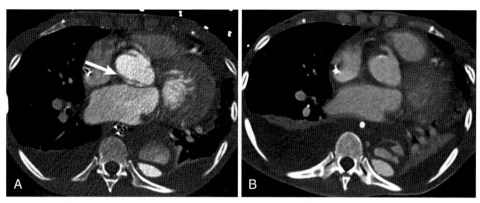

Figure 10-3 Pulsation artifact in the ascending aorta in a 47-year-old woman with a known type B aortic dissection. Arrow in **A** delineates an apparent filling defect, representing pulsation artifact. Note how the anterior wall also has motion. Pulsation artifact usually involves at least two sides of the aorta. Follow-up study (**B**) performed 5 days later shows that the apparent flap (pulsation) is no longer seen.

many institutions. Although gadolinium may allow for images that appear more similar to CT, contrast material is not required for diagnosis of acute aortic conditions. This allows for the potential of noncontrast MRI in the evaluation of the aorta in patients in renal failure. An added benefit of MRI is the use of black-blood sequences and fat-suppressed T2-weighted or short tau inversion recovery (STIR) images. These sequences can be useful for the evaluation of increased signal within the aortic wall, which may be indicative of an IMH and may help clarify a subtle CT finding.

No discussion of aortic imaging in the ED would be complete without discussing conventional radiography and angiography. Conventional radiography is useful when findings are positive because it allows the team to mobilize while support lines are being placed before CT. Radiography findings include widening of the mediastinum, effacement of mediastinal lines, and mass effect on the trachea and the left mainstem bronchus. A majority of the time the radiography signs can be subtle. The most useful finding is change in the mediastinal contour compared to a prior radiograph. A negative radiograph should not be used to exclude acute aortic pathologic conditions.

Angiography was once considered the gold standard for the evaluation of the acute nontraumatic aorta. In the current era, angiography is mainly used in the deployment of endovascular stents.

Mimics and Pitfalls on Computed Tomography

Artifacts and mimics of aortic disease are more commonly encountered than real aortic pathologic conditions. To avoid sending a patient for needless surgery, one must be comfortable with some of the more common mimics of acute disease. The most commonly encountered artifact is pulsation of the aorta at the root (Fig. 10-3). This pulsation artifact can simulate a dissection flap at the root. Despite advances in CT technology, pulsation is still encountered. Clues to pulsation artifact include visualization of a flap in the pulmonary artery at the same level, lack of pericardial effusion or aortic wall thickening, and an ill-defined craniocaudal extension on

multiplanar imaging. Although pulsation can usually be excluded, sometimes an echocardiogram or a repeat CT with ECG gating or ultrahigh-pitch imaging is required.

Other artifacts may stem from other diseases, such as a vasculitis or an adjacent neoplasm that may simulate aortic wall thickening or hematoma. The presence of lymphadenopathy can be helpful in suggesting these other entities.

Aortic Aneurysms

An aneurysm can be defined as failure of tapering of the aorta or even dilatation of the distal aorta. In the ascending aorta 4 cm is often used as the minimal size of an ascending aortic aneurysm; in the descending aorta, 3 cm is the minimal size. Measurements must be performed orthogonal to the long axis of the aorta. Occasionally this can be performed on transverse images, but usually these measurements require multiplanar reconstructions. Although patients with known aneurysms are often followed to determine a rate of change (if any) over time, in the ED the radiologist is not often afforded the luxury of a prior study for comparison. It becomes imperative then that certain imaging signs are used to determine when a thoracic aneurysm is unstable.

One of the most important findings is the shape of the aneurysm. Most aneurysms can be described as fusiform (diffuse concentric enlargement) or saccular (eccentric outpouching). Although fusiform aneurysms can become unstable, saccular outpouchings are more often indicative of a pseudoaneurysm that has the potential of being unstable. Most saccular aortic aneurysms are indicative of infection, traumatic injury, or a postoperative complication, such as dehiscence of a suture line. The one major exception is the pseudoaneurysm from a penetrating atherosclerotic ulcer (PAU; see later discussion).

Other imaging findings of an unstable aneurysm include high attenuation within the wall (sometimes referred to as the *impending rupture sign*) (Fig. 10-4), irregular shape, calcium that is somewhat tangential to the arc of the aorta, and periaortic stranding. All of these signs require careful attention. Usually more than one of these are present. The impending rupture sign and tangential calcium may be easier to see on noncontrast images.

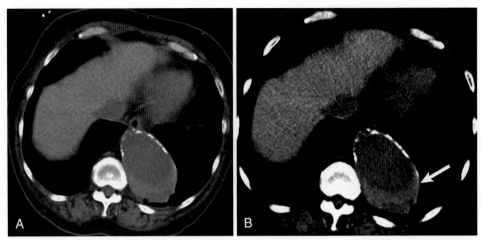

Figure 10-4 Unstable descending thoracic aortic aneurysm in a 77-year-old woman presenting with chest pain. Noncontrast image shows high attenuation in the left and posterior wall of the aorta (**A**). A narrow window width (150 HU width; 30 HU center) can make this high attenuation more apparent (*arrow* in **B**). When combined with an aneurysm, this high attenuation (akin to an intramural hematoma [IMH]) suggests that the aneurysm is unstable. The patient went for emergent endoluminal repair.

Rarely, high attenuation indicative of blood may be seen in the mediastinum and in the pleural space (hemothorax). More commonly, mild fat stranding is seen with a low-attenuating pleural effusion. This transudate is felt to represent a sympathetic effusion. In fact, it is very unusual to see an unstable aorta without a left pleural effusion. Care must be taken to not mistake the concomitant left-sided atelectasis, which often briskly enhances, for contrast extravasation. In the past the visualization of blood would result in termination of the scan and immediate contact with the surgeon. In the era of endoluminal therapy the presence of blood in the mediastinum or pleura results in immediate contact with the surgeon, but often the postcontrast images are continued because they are key in planning appropriate therapy. Even more rarely, extravasation of intravenous contrast may be seen. Of all the signs, this one has the gravest prognosis.

Acute Aortic Syndromes

Over the past decade the term *acute aortic syndrome* has come into use as an aortic equivalent of the *acute coronary syndrome* as an explanation for an aortic cause of chest pain. Although some authors include unstable aneurysms in this grouping, most reserve the term for the spectrum of aortic medial pathologic conditions, namely, aortic dissection, IMH, and PAU. These entities are rare but can be lethal and require a high index of suspicion. Because CT is critical in the diagnoses of these entities, every radiologist working in the ED must be familiar with their imaging appearances.

Aortic Dissection

Aortic dissection represents the most common of the acute aortic syndromes to present to the ED and the most common to result in premature death. Simply put, an aortic dissection represents a breach of the aortic intima with access of blood to the media. As described earlier, the inner two thirds of the media travel circumferentially within the wall, whereas the outer one third

of the media travels longitudinally parallel to the long axis of the aorta. If flowing blood can gain access to the plane between the two orthogonally directed fibers, a false passage can easily be created. Entities that either weaken the medial wall or exaggerate the space between the planes of the media can predispose to dissection as can those conditions that increase aortic luminal pressures. These include conditions associated with cystic medial necrosis (such as Marfan syndrome or bicuspid aortic valve), aortic hypertension, and conditions that transiently elevate aortic pressures, such as pregnancy, cocaine use, and weight lifting. Atherosclerotic disease may increase the risk for dissection by way of a PAU but does not usually directly result in dissection.

Once flowing blood gains access to the media, two lumens are created (a true lumen corresponding to the actual aortic lumen and a false lumen) (Fig. 10-5). The wall that separates the two channels is often referred to as an *intimal flap*, though technically it is an intimomedial flap (because it contains the intima and the inner two thirds of the media).

Accurate delineation of the true from the false lumen is key on cross-sectional imaging in case surgical treatment is required. In the ascending aorta the true lumen is usually contiguous with the aortic valve orifice and is the smaller of the two lumens. The true lumen tends to be on the left of the false lumen (closer to the pulmonary artery). When a fenestration is present in the ascending aorta, the flaps on both sides of the defect point away from the true lumen, a finding sometimes referred to as the *intimomedial rupture sign*. In the arch and descending aorta the most reliable way to distinguish the true from the false aortic lumen is the ability to directly trace the suspected true lumen to the intact "normal" lumen of the proximal aorta. Other findings include the size, because the true lumen is usually smaller than the false lumen, and the presence of calcifications, which are usually in the intima surrounding the true lumen. Care must be used in chronic dissections because the false lumen can occasionally calcify. In the descending aorta the true lumen is usually anterior and

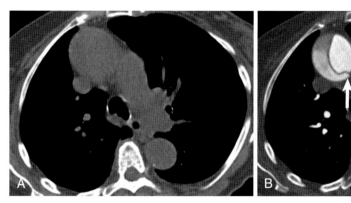

Figure 10-5 Acute Stanford type A aortic dissection in an 84-year-old woman presenting with acute chest pain. Noncontrast image (**A**) shows the dilated aorta but not the intimomedial flap. Postcontrast image (**B**) clearly shows the flap within the ascending aorta. The arrow denotes a region where the false lumen creates an acute angle with the flap, known as the *beak sign*. Unfortunately, the patient died before surgery.

to the right of the false lumen. Although variable, classically the celiac artery, superior mesenteric artery, and inferior mesenteric artery arise from the true lumen, and the left renal artery tends to arise from the false lumen. As a result, left renal ischemia with resultant left flank pain may be the presenting symptom of an acute aortic dissection. Another helpful finding in the false lumen is the presence of thin strands, representing fibers of the media that remain as blood has dissected in this false space. These are occasionally referred to as *aortic cobwebs* and are indicative of the false lumen. The angle created by the flap and the outer aortic wall can also be used for separating the true from the false lumen. Generally, the angle is more acute in the false lumen, a finding sometimes known as an *aortic beak* or *beak sign* (see Fig. 10-5).

A mainstay of aortic dissection treatment is blood pressure control, but clearly some patients require surgical intervention. The location of the dissection flap is the main determinant. Classification of a dissection is usually based on the location of the flap. Two main categorization schemes include the Stanford and DeBakey classifications. At our institution, we use the Stanford classification, in which involvement of the ascending aorta is considered a Stanford type A dissection, requiring surgery. Arch and descending aortic involvement alone are considered Stanford type B dissections and may be amenable to medical therapy alone. Of note, although some authors have previously described the left subclavian artery as the landmark for delineation between Stanford A and Stanford B, increasingly ascending aortic involvement is used. In other words, only when the ascending aorta is involved is the dissection considered type A. In the DeBakey scheme, ascending aortic and descending aortic involvement is considered type I, ascending involvement alone is considered type II, and descending aortic involvement alone is considered type III.

Ascending aortic involvement prompts surgical intervention because of the risk for acute aortic valve regurgitation, coronary artery involvement, or tamponade from hemopericardium. The risk for death from the dissection exceeds the potential risk from surgery (including paralysis). Although most isolated descending aortic dissections are considered medical lesions, occasionally these dissections can become surgical. Potential rupture

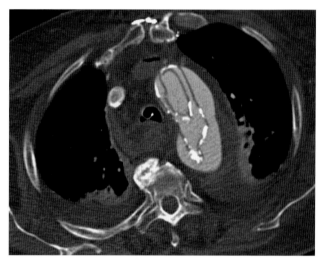

Figure 10-6 Intimal intussusception in an 86-year-old man with a type A aortic dissection. In this case the intima and inner media have completely separated from the remainder of the aorta. The dissection flap can then telescope akin to an enteric intussusception.

of the false lumen and end-organ ischemia may prompt either surgical or endoluminal therapy. A concise report therefore must include signs of unstable false lumen. These are exactly the same as those for the unstable aneurysm described earlier. The report should also include information about end-organ ischemia and the nature of the ischemia. If the ischemia is from propagation of the flap into the vessel for that organ, the patient may be stented. If the flap occludes the orifice of the feeding artery without directly involving it, the patient may undergo fenestration at that level.

Most aortic dissections will present with a linear filling defect in the aortic lumen that corresponds to the intimomedial flap. Occasionally the aortic dissection can take on an unusual appearance. Rarely the dissection will involve 360 degrees of the aorta so that the false lumen completely surrounds the true lumen. In this instance the intimomedial flap may become free of the remainder of the aorta and form an irregular filling defect. Occasionally this circumferential flap will begin to infold or intussuscept similar to bowel intussusception. This unusual dissection is referred to as an *intimointimal intussusception* (Fig. 10-6).

In another variation a dissection involving the ascending aorta may rupture just above the valve plane into a shared sheath with the pulmonary artery. The blood in the wall of the pulmonary artery will compress the pulmonary artery and may occlude it. Sometimes the blood will dissect around the pulmonary artery to the segmental arterial level. A third unusual manifestation of aortic dissection is a focal dissection at the level of the aortic root near the sinotubular junction. This localized process has been referred to as an *incomplete aortic dissection* and is almost always associated with cystic medial necrosis and aortic root enlargement. This incomplete dissection can mimic pulsation artifact. As a general guideline, one should have a low threshold for reimaging the aortic root when a linear defect is encountered in the setting of annuloaortic ectasia or in a patient with known Marfan syndrome or bicuspid valve.

Focal dissections of the abdominal aorta are rare in the absence of prior trauma or aortic catheterization. However, imaging of an aortic dissection should include the abdominal aorta and the iliac vessels to the level of the common femoral arteries. Inclusion of the abdomen and pelvis is performed to look for any end-organ ischemia and to delineate the extension of the dissection. Increasingly surgeons are relying on peripheral cannulation for initial bypass in aortic repair. The role of imaging is to help distinguish true from false lumen so that any peripheral cannulation for bypass avoids cannulating the false lumen, which would preclude adequate bypass and could potentially be lethal.

Intramural Hematoma

Intramural hematoma refers to blood within the aortic media that does not have a communication with the aortic lumen. In other words, no fenestration is noted within the intima. The effect on imaging is that the aortic wall will be eccentrically thickened with blood, but the thickening will not enhance with intravenous contrast. The blood will result in high attenuation on CT (usually better seen on noncontrast images) or high signal on black-blood MRI (Fig. 10-7). In an idiopathic IMH the blood is believed to arise from rupture of the vasa vasorum into the media. An IMH may also be secondary to a PAU (see next section).

As with dissections, IMH is associated with hypertension and cystic medial necrosis. Patients tend to be older than dissection patients. An IMH may resolve with medical therapy, but it may also progress into a true aortic dissection. If the pressure in the media exceeds luminal pressure, the media may create a fenestration with the true lumen. This process has been sometimes referred to as a *reverse dissection*, although the imaging will mimic a true aortic dissection that begins on the luminal side. Rarely the IMH will rupture. As with the other entities, signs of impending rupture include irregular shape of the IMH and adjacent fat stranding. As with dissection, an IMH may rupture into the shared sheath with the pulmonary artery. This event can result in a very unusual appearance of the pulmonary arteries and can be quite confusing to the unaware reader.

Because of the potential for progression of an IMH to dissection or rupture, an IMH is often treated similarly to aortic dissection. Many centers will classify an IMH with the Stanford or DeBakey classifications described in the prior section. Intramural hematoma involving the ascending aorta is usually treated surgically, whereas descending aortic IMH is often treated medically. Literature mostly coming from Asia has suggested that in certain patients there may be a role for close observation of a patient with an ascending aorta IMH instead of surgery. These patients may do as well (if not better) than patients undergoing median sternotomy. Other literature has suggested that thickness of the IMH in the ascending aorta or presence of an ulcer may predict which patients are at increased risk for rupture. These features of IMH are currently under investigation. For now the ED radiologist should be aware that most patients with ascending aortic involvement will undergo surgical repair, but that a minority fitting certain criteria may be closely observed instead.

Occasionally a contrast blush may be seen within an IMH (see Fig. 10-7). This may arise from the lumen and a tiny ulcerlike projection or from retrograde flow from an intercostal artery. These blushes can lead to confusion in the categorization of which entity of acute aortic syndrome is present. The key is to clearly report whether the ascending aorta is involved and if possible, why the blush is present. Some of the literature has shown that a blush from an ulcerlike projection is at increased risk for progressing to a true aortic dissection. These patients may be more closely followed with subsequent imaging.

Penetrating Atherosclerotic Ulcer

The PAU is the newest entity to have been described, with many of the early papers appearing in the late 1980s.

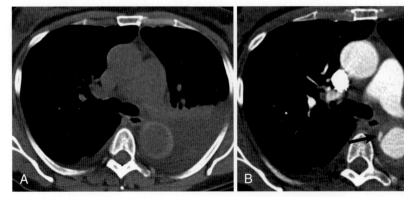

Figure 10-7 Intramural hematoma (IMH) in a 63-year-old woman presenting with chest pain. Note the high attenuation on the noncontrast image (**A**). The small focal blush (*arrow* in **B**) can be seen with an IMH and is not indicative of an aortic dissection.

The PAU represents ulceration of an atherosclerotic plaque so that blood from the lumen now has access to the aortic media. The belief is that the macrophages within the plaque weaken the intima and allow for this focal ulceration. The key from an imaging perspective is to make sure that the ulceration truly penetrates through the intima and does not simply represent an ulcerated plaque without an intimal breach. From an imaging perspective, most PAUs will have an eccentric outpouching of the outer wall (saccular aneurysm; Fig. 10-8).

Unlike aortic dissection and IMH, PAUs have a high association with aortic atherosclerosis. Patients with PAUs tend to be older and tend to have a greater atherosclerotic burden. PAUs may spontaneously resolve, but they may also present with an IMH. Because of the intimal breach, flowing blood in a PAU will occasionally create an aortic dissection. Rarely a PAU may go on to rupture. Signs of rupture are similar to those of the unstable aneurysm. The treatment goal in a patient with PAU is to make the patient free of chest pain. If the patient has persistent pain, there is increased risk for IMH, dissection, or rupture. These patients will be closely followed and if possible, may undergo endoluminal treatment. Location of the PAU and the size of the neck will play a role in determining which patients will receive endoluminal repair.

Aortic Thrombus

Occasionally a patient with chest pain will undergo CT and a large filling defect will be seen within the aorta (Fig. 10-9). This acute aortic thrombus is increasingly being recognized as an embolic source. The thrombus is believed to arise from an area of intimal irregularity. Some authors have postulated that a scar from the ductus arteriosus may serve as a nidus for thrombus formation. Others have suggested that differential flow may promote an area of relative stasis along the lesser curve of the aorta at the level of the isthmus.

The thrombus itself should not present with chest pain, but emboli from the clot may result in symptoms of abdominal or extremity pain. These filling defects are usually encountered within the aorta at the level of the isthmus and within the descending thoracic aorta. They should not enhance with intravenous contrast, but when they are chronic, areas of recanalization may create pseudoenhancement if they are included in measurements of attenuation on CT or signal on MRI. Radiologists should be aware of the acute aortic thrombus to avoid confusion with an aortic tumor. The latter almost always has soft tissue that extends beyond the aortic wall. Treatment for an acute aortic thrombus begins with anticoagulation but may include a thrombectomy and rarely endoluminal stent placement to trap the thrombus.

Aortic Fistula

Another rare manifestation of aortic disease in the ED is an aortic fistula. Unfortunately, the imaging of an aortic fistula can be quite subtle despite the high lethality of this entity. Clinically the course of a patient with a fistula may be tricky as well. These patients usually report a large episode of hematemesis or rectal bleeding (the herald bleed). Because the fistula is only intermittently patent, the bleeding subsides, so the patient is hemodynamically stable enough to present to the ED and undergo cross-sectional imaging.

Aortic fistulas can be primary, usually from rupture of an aortic aneurysm or in the setting of an infection, such as mediastinitis. When findings of mediastinitis are encountered (such as gas or diffuse mediastinal fat infiltration), careful inspection of the aortic contour is required. Any subtle outpouching of the aorta may be

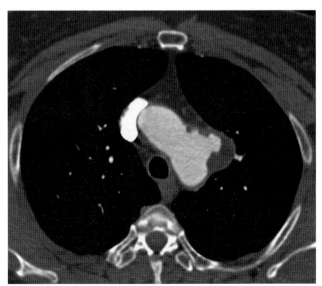

Figure 10-8 Penetrating atherosclerotic ulcer (PAU) in an 84-year-old woman. Note the extension beyond the confines of the aorta (saccular pseudoaneurysm) and associated intramural hematoma. These features allow distinction from an ulcerated atherosclerotic plaque.

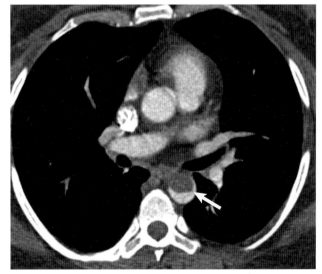

Figure 10-9 Aortic thrombus in a 40-year-old woman who presented with abdominal pain and a superior mesenteric artery embolism. Computed tomography (CT) was performed to evaluate for an embolic source in the descending aorta. This filling defect *(arrow)* was found to represent a bland thrombus at surgery.

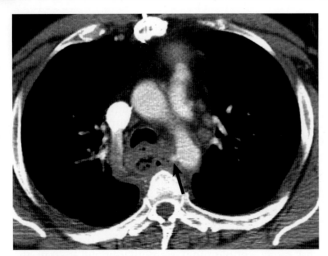

Figure 10-10 Aortoesophageal fistula in a 62-year-old man who presented with hematemesis after an episode of mediastinitis. The fistula *(arrow)* required emergent surgical correction.

indicative of the development of a fistula (Fig. 10-10). Patients with aortic fistulas from mediastinitis tend to have less of an atherosclerotic burden than those with PAUs. Rarely an aortic aneurysm may rupture and fistulize to an adjacent organ. This phenomenon is more common in the abdomen and has been reported with adjacent bowel and the inferior vena cava.

An aortic fistula is more likely to result as a complication from prior surgery. In the thorax the fistula may be to the esophagus or an adjacent bronchus (usually the left main bronchus). Fistulas may follow either open or endoluminal surgery. Clues to the diagnosis rest on seeing gas next to the repair site, irregular contour of the aorta, and clinical history. Sometimes endoscopy is used to confirm a suspected fistula.

■ PULMONARY EMBOLISM

The pulmonary arteries serve as the main conduit of blood from the right ventricle to the lungs and serve as the main path of oxygenation of the circulatory system. They begin as a main pulmonary artery that bifurcates into a right pulmonary artery, which travels slightly posterior and inferior to the right main bronchus, and a left pulmonary artery, which travels superior to the left main bronchus. The arteries continue to divide into lobar, segmental, subsegmental arteries, eventually reaching a microscopic capillary level. The result is that these smallest of vessels serve as a net to stop any emboli from gaining access to the left heart and the systemic (aortic) circulation. In other words, the pulmonary arteries should be the final recipient of emboli from the venous system to prevent systemic complication. Many types of embolic disease can manifest within the lungs. In thromboembolic disease the thrombi form in peripheral veins from an antecedent condition (e.g., long period of sitting still, hypercoagulability) and then dislodge to the lungs.

When acute, the embolism may result in right heart failure and even death. Usually the acute emboli go unnoticed clinically. In fact up to 3% to 5% of outpatients may have asymptomatic embolic disease. If the emboli result in a cascade of cytokine-mediated scarring in the pulmonary arteries, pulmonary pressures may elevate, and the result is chronic pulmonary emboli (PEs) or chronic thromboembolic pulmonary hypertension. This is occurs in about 1% to 3% of patients with acute embolic disease. Sometimes the embolized thrombus is infected. These septic emboli are unlikely to result in right heart failure (because the burden is small), but they tend to be markers of a bacteremic patient.

Not all emboli arise from embolized thrombi. In trauma, bone marrow may be embolized, as can amniotic fluid in the setting of a difficult delivery. These latter two entities result in a microvascular disease with characteristic CT appearance. Other emboli include tumor and iatrogenic material. As imaging for suspected emboli increases, radiologists must be familiar with the entire spectrum of embolic disease.

Acute Pulmonary Embolism

Acute PE represents the third most common cause of cardiovascular death in the United States, following stroke and myocardial infarction. As with the acute aortic syndromes and the other entities previously described, clinical history is only modestly helpful. Patients with PE range from being asymptomatic to asystolic. The nonspecific clinical presentation has resulted in the proliferation of imaging that any radiologist with even one night in the ED can appreciate.

Computed tomography has become the main imaging technique for acute PE. Since its introduction in the 1990s, CT has risen to become the dominant modality for imaging of acute PE, especially in the ED. The popularity of CT for PE, as with acute aortic syndromes, rests on its availability in most EDs and its rapid turnaround times. In the emergency setting, ventilation-perfusion ($\dot{V}/\dot{Q}$) scintigraphy has taken a backseat to CT, owing largely to the limited availability of technologists and the longer examination times. Another explanation for the dominance of CT is its ability to diagnose alternative conditions. In many centers only 5% to 10% of CT scans for PE will be positive for PE. Up to one third may reveal another explanation for the patient's presentation. Often these alternative diagnoses are not possible by $\dot{V}/\dot{Q}$ scan.

Computed tomography findings of PE rely mostly on direct visualization of the PE (Fig. 10-11). These include a central filling defect that usually expands the vessel. Contrast may be seen between the embolism and the wall. When the vessel with embolism is cut in cross-section, it is referred to as the *rim sign*, and when the vessel is in plane, the surrounding contrast is sometimes called a *tram-track sign*. Key in diagnosing an acute PE is to remember that every bronchus should have a corresponding artery. This point is key in preventing confusion of a vein for an artery and key in detecting an occluded artery. Another potential pitfall in the diagnosis of an acute PE is the confusion of a mucoid impacted bronchus for PE. Again, if the radiologist remembers that a bronchus should accompany an artery, he or she will realize that the enhancing structure is the artery and the apparent adjoining filling defect is actually in the bronchus.

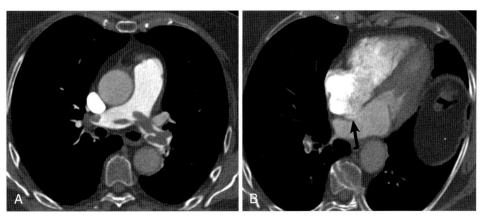

Figure 10-11 Acute pulmonary embolism (PE) in a 78-year-old woman with a history of hypercoagulable state. The filling defects in **A** are central with contrast outlining them, in keeping with acute PE. The right heart was noted to be enlarged in **B** with bowing of the interventricular and interatrial septa leftward. The finding of right heart enlargement without right ventricular hypertrophy is in keeping with right heart strain. Note the patent foramen of ovale (*arrow* in **B**) from the elevated pressures.

A true PE should withstand two tests. The first is that the apparent filling defect should be within the artery. Often the filling defect is detected on the soft tissue windows. Previous authors have written on a variety of techniques to calculate the ideal viewing window. In our practice we try to choose a window that allows for adequate visualization of the cardiac valves, figuring that if the valve can be seen so should any PE. The lung windows are used to confirm the PE and to ensure that the finding resides within the artery and not a vein or bronchus. The second test is to verify that the PE can be seen in at least one other plane. If the suspected embolism cannot be seen in the other planes, it is likely artifactual.

Although a variety of scoring systems have been published, we have not found any of these to be useful in the clinical setting. Instead, one should look for any signs of right heart strain (see Fig. 10-11). These include right ventricular enlargement and bowing of the interventricular and interatrial septa leftward. When these signs are encountered, the patient may be more closely observed. Usually the CT findings will prompt an echocardiogram for confirmation.

Ventilation-Perfusion Scintigraphy or Computed Tomography

One of the big questions that often arise in an ED setting is which modality should be used for the diagnosis of PE: $\dot{V}/\dot{Q}$ scintigraphy or CT. Of course the major determinant resides in the availability of each modality. If both are readily available, the issue becomes more complicated. Computed tomography is inherently faster and potentially offers alternative diagnoses, but $\dot{V}/\dot{Q}$ has about 20% the effective dose of a standard CT scan. We tend to use the patient's age and the chest radiograph to help triage. If the chest radiograph findings are normal, we have found that the $\dot{V}/\dot{Q}$ scan results will tend to be normal or have a high likelihood ratio in most young patients. As a result, in younger patients (less than 40 years) we tend to consider $\dot{V}/\dot{Q}$ scan a lower-radiation option when the chest radiograph findings are normal.

In our ED practice the most common cause of a nondiagnostic or indeterminate CT is bolus related, either transient interruption of the contrast column or a poor bolus in the setting of an obese patient. In both young patients and obese patients the $\dot{V}/\dot{Q}$ scan tends to offer a diagnosis (either normal or high likelihood).

Recently the Society of Thoracic Radiology, working in conjunction with the American Thoracic Society, has issued an approach to the pregnant patient, which is similar to our own experience. In their consensus statement they recommend that the chest radiograph be used as a decision point. When findings are normal, a $\dot{V}/\dot{Q}$ scan is recommended. If the chest radiograph findings are abnormal, then a CT is recommended. In our practice we have adopted this approach. We also find that the use of a $\dot{V}/\dot{Q}$ scan avoids any concern about iodinated contrast, which crosses the placenta.

Chronic Pulmonary Embolism

Chronic PE is rarely an issue in the ED. Chronic PE refers to cytokine-mediated scarring that may occur even after only one episode of PE. The net effect of the scarring is that the pulmonary artery volume decreases, and as a result, pulmonary pressures increase. The resultant pulmonary hypertension may be debilitating but is potentially curable with a thromboendarterectomy.

Computed tomography features of chronic PE include eccentric filling defects within the arteries, beading of the vessels, thread vessels, and vascular cutoffs (Fig. 10-12). Other findings include enlarged main pulmonary artery, mosaic attenuation, bronchiectasis, and enlarged bronchial arteries. The goal in making the diagnosis of chronic PE is to direct treatment toward the pulmonary hypertension. Rarely an acute PE can present with an eccentric embolism. Care should be taken to look for the other findings before diagnosing chronic PE so that the clinical approach will be appropriate for an acute PE, namely, anticoagulation and search for an underlying explanation.

Septic Emboli

Occasionally a patient will present to the ED and the clinical question will focus on septic emboli as a potential diagnosis. Either the chest radiograph will point the

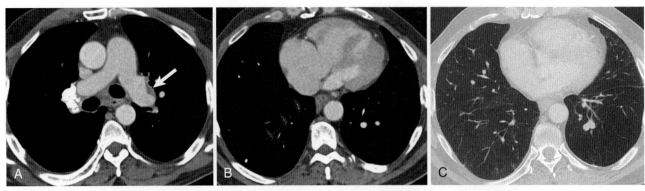

Figure 10-12 A 53-year-old man with a history of pulmonary hypertension found to be secondary to chronic pulmonary embolism (PE). The eccentric, flat filling defect (*arrow* in **A**) is typical of this condition along with the right ventricular hypertrophy in **B** and mosaic attenuation in **C**. Bronchiectasis also seen in **C** is another feature of chronic PE.

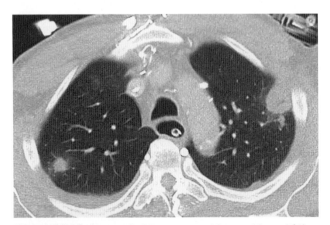

Figure 10-13 Septic emboli in a 64-year-old man with renal failure on dialysis who presents with fever and dyspnea. Although no filling defects were seen in the pulmonary arteries, multiple peripheral nodules were seen, in keeping with septic emboli. Some of the nodules (as in the left upper lobe) were cavitary. Blood cultures were positive for *Staphylococcus aureus*.

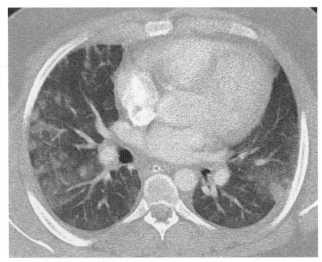

Figure 10-14 Fat emboli in a 19-year-old man who sustained a femur fracture 2 days before undergoing a pulmonary embolism (PE) computed tomographic (CT) scan. No filling defects were seen in the arteries, but multiple ground-glass opacities, mostly in the upper lobes and middle lobe, were in keeping with fat emboli.

way with cavitary nodules, or the patient will be febrile. Septic emboli represent a unique subset of PE in which the emboli are infected and the main sequelae are cavitary infections within the lung (Fig. 10-13). The key is to remember that the embolic burden is low. Although the pathologic condition is called *septic emboli*, emboli are rarely seen. The key to the radiologic diagnosis is peripheral cavitary nodules. In other words, the lung windows combined with the clinical history are more likely to make the diagnosis than the detailed analysis of the CT angiographic images.

Fat and Amniotic Emboli

Fat and amniotic emboli represent another class of embolic disease in which the lung windows are more likely to make the diagnosis than the soft tissue windows. Both entities represent a form of microembolic disease in which the breakdown products of the emboli result in a chemical pneumonitis. The effect is that the pneumonitis results in dyspnea and hypoxia. As the pathophysiology would suggest, the key in diagnosis is the visualization of the breakdown products. On CT these usually manifest as ground-glass opacities associated with terminal arte-

rioles (Fig. 10-14). The appearance can look very much akin to the tree-in-bud pattern usually seen with bronchiolar dilatation (bronchiectasis). This vascular tree-in-bud pattern (which is most pronounced in the apices) is usually associated with more confluent ground-glass opacities and consolidation in the lower lungs. Pleural effusions, lymphadenopathy, and cavitation are rare.

Tumor Emboli

Rarely, intra-arterial emboli may force a patient to seek care in the ED. Tumor emboli usually present in one of two ways: macroscopic emboli and microscopic emboli. The macroscopic tumor emboli tend to present with filling defects seen on the CT angiographic windows. The key in distinguishing these from routine PE is to realize that these filling defects enhance similarly to the primary tumor (Fig. 10-15). Although reported with any tumor, tumor emboli are most commonly seen with adenocarcinomas, most notably renal cell cancer, hepatocellular cancer, and adrenal cortical carcinomas, owing to their propensity for vena caval extension.

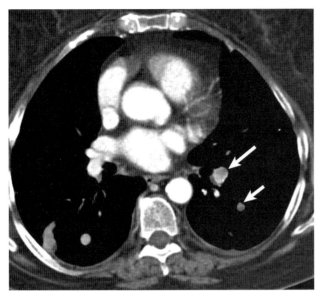

Figure 10-15 A 60-year-old woman with adrenal cortical carcinoma and macroscopic tumor emboli. Note how the intra-arterial filling defect *(anterior arrow)* is similar in attenuation to one of the pulmonary metastases *(posterior arrow)*.

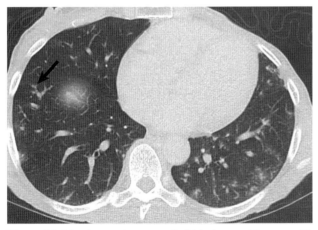

Figure 10-16 Microscopic tumor emboli in a 58-year-old woman with diffusely metastatic pancreatic cancer. Note the beaded artery *(arrow)* and multiple ground-glass nodules. As with the fat and septic emboli, no filling defects were seen in the arteries. The patient died 3 months later.

Another variation of tumor emboli is the microscopic variant. These tend to be much harder to diagnose. The emboli are usually not seen on the CT angiographic window. The key is to see beading of the small arteries and arterioles, usually better detected on the lung windows (Fig. 10-16). The small emboli are believed to initiate a cascade of thrombosis and remodeling that only exacerbate the patient's dyspnea. This cycle is sometimes referred to as *pulmonary tumor thrombotic microangiopathy* (PTTM). Findings of lymphangitic carcinomatosis may be present with nodular septal line thickening, lymphadenopathy, and pleural effusions. Although PTTM may also be seen with any primary tumor, it is also most commonly seen with adenocarcinomas, most often gastric and other gastrointestinal primary tumors. PTTM has been reported to be the initial clinical manifestation of neoplasm and may be seen in younger adults.

Iatrogenic Emboli and Foreign Material

Although any device that gains access to the venous system has the potential to embolize, these emboli rarely tend to be symptomatic. It is hard to imagine a radiology resident who has not seen an embolized catheter fragment, guidewire, or even inferior vena cava filter. These are often removed because of fear of serving as a nidus for thrombus formation or infection.

Liquid and semisolid medications serve as another variant of iatrogenic emboli. Probably the most commonly currently is methylmethacrylate, which is often impregnated with barium and used for bone fixation, as in vertebroplasty (Fig. 10-17). If the material gains access to the spinal veins, it can embolize via the azygous system. To avoid this potential complication, many radiologists will perform a preprocedural venogram to make sure that the needle for injection is not in a major vein. If the methylmethacrylate is embolized, usually the dose is small and the patient will experience transient chest pain and dyspnea. Rarely, the embolized dose is large enough to result in an infarct. If the infarct is large enough, it may cavitate. This necrotic lung may need resection in extreme cases. On CT the methylmethacrylate will be very high in attenuation. Emboli may be masked by a dense contrast bolus. When a wide

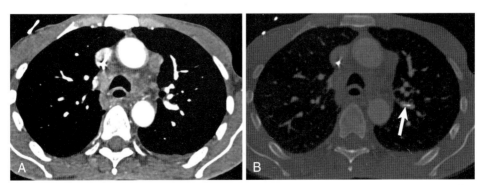

Figure 10-17 Embolized methylmethacrylate (MMA) in a 53-year-old man with metastatic lung cancer requiring vertebroplasty. The MMA is difficult to see on a standard window (**A**; 400 HU width, center 30 HU) but is much more apparent on the bone window (*arrow* in **B**; 2000 HU width, center 500 HU).

window width is used for viewing, such as a bone window, emboli are much easier to detect. Occasionally one may see ground-glass opacities in a tree-in-bud distribution. These represent fat emboli from the vertebral marrow that has also embolized.

Mercury and talc represent two medications that may embolize to the lungs and result in symptoms prompting an ED admission. Both are usually seen in patient self-inflicted conditions. Mercury will present with very dense linear filling defects with a propensity for very peripheral arterioles. Although less common than a few years back, mercury is usually used by patients with depression who seek the wasting and debilitation that mercury poisoning is well known to cause.

Talc, conversely, is usually used by patients with Munchausen syndrome who inject their pills. Many of the capsules and pills use talc and their derivatives to stabilize the oral preparation. The talc particles are not dense, but they are inert and lodge in small arterioles. The net effect is visualization of small arterioles on CT in a centrilobular pattern. Because of the increased vascular resistance, right heart enlargement may be seen.

■ CONCLUSION

The acute aorta and PE represent two ends of the spectrum in the ED presentation of chest pain. The former is rare, but the potential lethality of the acute aorta requires a high index of suspicion. Pulmonary embolism, conversely, is common and may be lethal, although usually it is not. Because of the nonspecificity of symptoms of both entities, imaging has become a first line for both. The radiologist therefore must become familiar with the usual cross-sectional appearance of both and also the uncommon manifestations. Commonly encountered artifacts (motion, bolus-related, pulsation) must also be mastered to avoid needless treatment or additional imaging. Finally, less common variants may render a patient symptomatic and should be learned; these include aortic fistulas, thrombi, fat emboli, tumor emboli, and foreign substance emboli.

Selected Reading

Attia R, Young C, Fallouh HB, et al: In patients with acute aortic intramural haematoma is open surgical repair superior to conservative management? *Interact Cardiovasc Thorac Surg* 9:868–871, 2009.

Bhalla S, West OC: CT of nontraumatic thoracic aortic emergencies, *Semin Ultrasound CT MR* 26:281–304, 2005.

British Thoracic Society Standards of Care Committee Pulmonary Embolism Guideline Development Group: British Thoracic Society guidelines for the management of suspected acute pulmonary embolism, *Thorax* 58:470–483, 2003.

Erbel R, Alfonso F, Boileau C, et al: Diagnosis and management of aortic dissection, *Eur Heart J* 22:1642–1681, 2001.

Evangelista A, Mukherjee D, Mehta RH, et al: Acute intramural hematoma of the aorta: a mystery in evolution, *Circulation* 111:1063–1070, 2005.

Fleischmann D, Mitchell RS, Miller DC: Acute aortic syndromes: new insights from electrocardiographically gated computed tomography, *Semin Thorac Cardiovasc Surg* 20:340–347, 2008.

Harris JA, Bis KG, Glover JL, et al: Penetrating atherosclerotic ulcers of the aorta, *J Vasc Surg* 19:90–98, 1994.

Hayter RG, Rhea JT, Small A, et al: Suspected aortic dissection and other aortic disorders: multi-detector row CT in 373 cases in the emergency setting, *Radiology* 238:841–852, 2006.

Hiratzka LF, Bakris GL, Beckman JA, et al: 2010 ACCF/AHA/AATS/ACR/ASA/ SCA/SCAI/SIR/STS/SVM guidelines for the diagnosis and management of patients with thoracic aortic disease: a report of the American College of Cardiology Foundation/American Heart Association Task Force on Practice Guidelines, American Association for Thoracic Surgery, American College of Radiology, American Stroke Association, Society of Cardiovascular Anesthesiologists, Society for Cardiovascular Angiography and Interventions, Society of Interventional Radiology, Society of Thoracic Surgeons, and Society for Vascular Medicine, *Circulation* 121:e266–e369, 2010.

Kitai T, Kaji S, Yamamuro A, et al: Impact of new development of ulcer-like projection on clinical outcomes in patients with type B aortic dissection with closed and thrombosed false lumen, *Circulation* 122:574–580, 2010.

Meszaros I, Morocz J, Szlavi J, et al: Epidemiology and clinicopathology of aortic dissection, *Chest* 117:1271–1278, 2000.

Moizumi Y, Komatsu T, Motoyoshi N, et al: Clinical features and longterm outcome of type A and type B intramural hematoma of the aorta, *J Thorac Cardiovasc Surg* 127:421–427, 2004.

Remy-Jardin M, Pistolesi M, Goodman LR, et al: Management of suspected acute pulmonary embolism in the era of CT angiography: a statement from the Fleischner Society, *Radiology* 245:315–329, 2007.

Ridge CA, McDermott S, Freyne BJ, et al: Pulmonary embolism in pregnancy: comparison of pulmonary CT angiography and lung scintigraphy, *AJR Am J Roentgenol* 193:1223–1227, 2009.

Song JK, Kim HS, Kang DH, et al: Different clinical features of aortic intramural hematoma versus dissection involving the ascending aorta, *J Am Coll Cardiol* 37:1604–1610, 2001.

Song JK, Yim JH, Ahn JM, et al: Outcomes of patients with acute type A aortic intramural hematoma, *Circulation* 120:2046–2054, 2009.

Sostman HD, Stein PD, Gottschalk A, et al: Acute pulmonary embolism: sensitivity and specificity of ventilation-perfusion scintigraphy in PIOPED II study, *Radiology* 246:941–946, 2008.

Stanson AW, Kazmier FJ, Hollier LH, et al: Penetrating atherosclerotic ulcers of the thoracic aorta: natural history and clinicopathologic correlations, *Ann Vasc Surg* 1:15–23, 1986.

Stein PD, Fowler SE, Goodman LR, et al: Multidetector computed tomography for acute pulmonary embolism, *N Engl J Med* 354:2317–2327, 2006.

Torbicki A, Perrier A, Konstantinides S, et al: Guidelines on the diagnosis and management of acute pulmonary embolism: the Task Force for the Diagnosis and Management of Acute Pulmonary Embolism of the European Society of Cardiology (ESC), *Eur Heart J* 29:2276–2315, 2008.

Tsai TT, Nienaber CA, Eagle KA: Acute aortic syndromes, *Circulation* 112:3802–3813, 2005.

Vilacosta I, Román JA: Acute aortic syndrome, *Heart* 85:365–368, 2001.

von Kodolitsch Y, Csösz SK, Koschyk DH, et al: Intramural hematoma of the aorta: predictors of progression to dissection and rupture, *Circulation* 107:1158–1163, 2003.

Wittram C, Waltman AC, Shepard JA, et al: Discordance between CT and angiography in the PIOPED II study, *Radiology* 244:883–889, 2007.

Yoo SM, Lee HY, White CS: MDCT evaluation of acute aortic syndrome, *Radiol Clin North Am* 48:67–83, 2010.

ABDOMINAL EMERGENCIES

Blunt Abdominal and Retroperitoneal Trauma

Computed Tomography Protocols and Scan Optimization

Thorsten R. Fleiter and Krystal Archer-Arroyo

Trauma is one of the leading causes of mortality in the United States, responsible for approximately 100,000 deaths per year. The majority of the trauma cases are due to blunt force, with more than two thirds of these caused by motor vehicle collisions. Additional causes of blunt trauma include falls and assaults. Penetrating trauma, including stab and gunshot wounds, is also a leading cause of death in the United States. The Centers for Disease Control and Prevention (CDC) reported 31,224 firearm-related deaths in 2007. Moreover, it is estimated that there are 200,000 nonfatal gun-related injuries in the United States annually. Given the potential severity of the injuries, the majority of these patients are evaluated in emergency departments (EDs) and trauma centers.

■ WHOLE-BODY MULTIDETECTOR COMPUTED TOMOGRAPHY

Computed tomography (CT), with its continually advancing technology, allows rapid scanning of critically injured patients detailing internal injuries from head to toe, assessing traumatic brain, cervical spine, chest, abdomen, and pelvic injuries—a one-stop shop for traumatic injury diagnosis. Computed tomography angiograms can reveal vascular injuries and active bleeding requiring acute intervention. Performing whole-body multidetector computed tomography (WBMDCT) early in the initial care of polytrauma patients with multisystem injury (injury severity score ≥ 16) significantly increases the probability of survival. This result is achieved because WBMDCT is a comprehensive diagnostic test that quickly identifies all major injuries so that the trauma team can optimize treatment and reduce missed injuries.

At our institution, 40- and 64-slice CT scanners are used for WBMDCT examinations (Tables 11-1 and 11-2). The examination begins with a non–contrast-enhanced head CT scan to assess for intracranial injuries, including hemorrhage or herniation. After the head CT scan, if there is no clear clinical indication of shoulder girdle injury, the patient's arms are then raised above the head, placed alongside the neck. This positioning provides the best overall image quality for the single scanning run through the head, neck, chest, and abdomen/pelvis with the least total radiation. Other arm positions that can be used in patients with shoulder girdle injury include placing the arms alongside the torso or ventrally over the chest. In both these positions, lifting the arms on pillows can reduce artifact arising from the arms and decrease total exposure.

The patient is initially scanned from the vertex of the head through the inferior pubic rami in the arterial phase to assess for nonbleeding vascular injuries and acute bleeding usually best seen in this phase; this also contributes to detection of nonvascular injury (Fig. 11-1). A portal venous phase is obtained about 60 seconds after the contrast injection from the diaphragm to the iliac crest to facilitate the diagnosis of nonvascular parenchymal injuries in the solid organs, especially given the often heterogeneous parenchymal enhancement seen in the arterial phase, particularly the spleen (Fig. 11-2). This dual-phase imaging approach optimizes detection of both vascular and nonvascular injury (see Solid Intraperitoneal Organ Injury).

Axial images of the head CT are immediately sent to the picture archiving and communication system (PACS) for rapid interpretation of traumatic brain injuries. The axial cervical spine images are reconstructed with a smaller field of view from the same data set to provide detail of bony and vascular structures. A bone filter is also used to provide detailed high-resolution images of the osseous structures. Sagittal and coronal multiplanar reformats are routinely performed to provide orthogonal axes that improve visualization of some injures based on their orientation. Imaging the cervical spine with intravenous contrast material as part of the WBMDCT serves as a screening technique to identify carotid or vertebral artery injuries not infrequently seen in patients with no risk factors for these injuries. This technique does not limit the diagnosis of cervical spine fractures.

Axial images of the chest, abdomen, and pelvis are reconstructed as single continuous coronal and sagittal images to facilitate "seamless" assessment of the thoracoabdominal region, given the continuity of

Table 11-1   64-Slice Whole-Body Multidetector Computed Tomography Protocol*

Parameter	Dry Head	Arterial Phase	Portal Venous Phase
Patient positioning	Arms fully extended adducted	Affected arm fully abducted	Affected arm fully abducted
Detector collimation and configuration (mm)	16 × 0.625	64 × 0.625	32 × 1.25
Pitch		0.625	0.656
Rotation time (sec)	1.5	0.5	0.5
kV	120	120	120
Current (mA)	350	250	250
Area scanned	Skull base through the vertex	Circle of Willis through the lesser trochanters	Diaphragms to the iliac crests
Contrast volume (mL)	—	100	—
Contrast injection rate	—	60 mL at 6 mL/sec 40 mL at 4 mL/sec	—
Scan delay (sec)	—	18*	60
Source axial images (mm)[†,‡]	1.25	2 × 1	2 × 1
Reconstruction filter	Brain	Soft tissue	Soft tissue
Diagnostic axial images to PACS[‡] (mm)	5 × 10	3 × 3	3 × 3
Sagittal MPR[‡] (mm) for chest, abdomen and pelvis		4 × 3	4 × 3
Coronal MPR[‡] (mm) for chest, abdomen and pelvis		4 × 3	4 × 3
Thin-section axial images to independent workstation (mm)		2 × 1	2 × 1

*For patients less than 50 years old.
[†]Source axial images used to construct all routine diagnostic images.
[‡]Thickness × interval.
MPR, Multiplanar reformats; PACS, picture archiving and communication system.

Table 11-2   Reconstructions for 64-Slice Whole-Body Multidetector Computed Tomography

Parameter	Face	Cervical Spine	Thoracic/Lumbar Spine
Source axial images (mm)[†,‡]	1 × 0.5	1 × 0.5	1.5 × 0.75
Reconstruction filter	Bone	Bone	Bone
Diagnostic axial images to PACS[‡] (mm)	1 × 0.5	1 × 0.5	2 × 1
Sagittal MPR[‡] (mm)	2 × 2	1 × 0.5	2 × 1
Coronal MPR[‡] (mm)	1 × 0.5	1 × 0.5	2 × 1
Thin-section axial images to independent workstation (mm)	1 × 0.5	1 × 0.5	1.5 × 0.75

[†]Source axial images used to construct all routine diagnostic images.
[‡]Thickness × interval.
MPR, Coronal multiplanar reformats; PACS, picture archiving and communication system.

these body regions, and to decrease radiation exposure compared to scanning these body regions separately with overlapping fields of coverage (Fig. 11-3). Sagittal and coronal multiplanar reformatted images of the chest, abdomen, and pelvis are routinely generated for both the arterial and portal venous phase scans, and dedicated targeted studies of the thoracic and lumbar spines, often requested, are created from the original data set.

■ COMPUTED TOMOGRAPHY PROTOCOLS

Protocol for Assessing Extremity Vascular Injuries

Vascular injuries constitute 3% of trauma cases with the potential for significant morbidity. Penetrating injuries from gunshot or stab wounds are the most common source of vascular injury producing disruption of the vessel wall via direct impact injury or blast effect (Fig. 11-4). The most

Figure 11-1 Post motor vehicle accident. A, Non–contrast-enhanced computed tomography (CT) of the head demonstrates diffuse edema in the right hemicerebrum with mild mass effect and loss of the gray-white matter differentiation, suggesting ischemia. B, Axial image of the subaxial cervical spine from whole-body multidetector computed tomography (WBMDCT) demonstrates an intraluminal filling defect *(red arrows)* in the distal right internal carotid artery causing 80% stenosis. C, Coronal image of the subaxial cervical spine better delineates the location, size, and extent of the intraluminal filling defect *(white arrow)* in the distal right internal carotid artery causing 80% stenosis. D, Sagittal image of the subaxial cervical spine best demonstrates an intraluminal filling defect *(white arrow)* in the distal right internal carotid artery causing 80% stenosis (grade 2b blunt cerebrovascular injury [BCVI]) in relation to the carotid bifurcation.

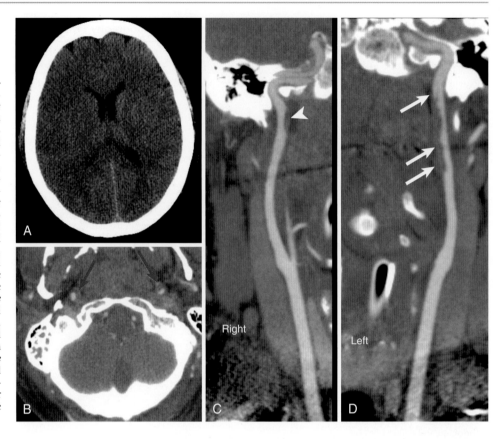

Figure 11-2 Solid organ injury: arterial versus portal venous phase. A, Arterial phase of whole-body multidetector computed tomography (WBMDCT) demonstrates a laceration in the posterior right hepatic lobe *(black arrow)* and devascularization of the right kidney *(red arrow)*. Normal heterogeneous enhancement of the spleen in the arterial phase *(white arrow)*. B, Portal venous phase of the abdomen from WBMDCT best demonstrates the laceration in the posterior right hepatic lobe *(black arrows)*. The homogeneous appearance of the spleen facilitates the evaluation for lacerations *(white arrow)*. C, Coronal reformat of the portal venous phase of the abdomen from WBMDCT best demonstrates the viable tissue *(curved arrows)* and areas of devascularization in the shattered right kidney.

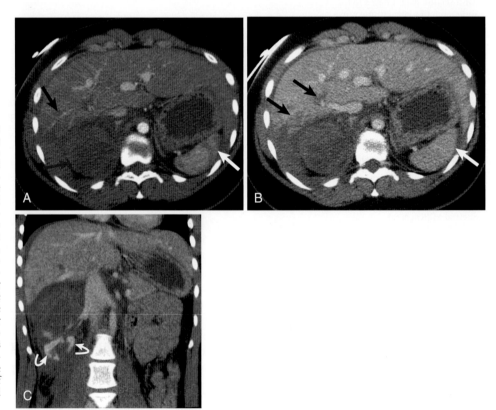

common cause of blunt vascular injury is crushing that can produce intimal flaps with secondary thrombosis or complete disruption of the vessel and thrombosis. Box 11-1 shows indications for extremity CT angiography (CTA).

Typically the affected upper extremity can be raised above the patient's head to reduce beam-hardening artifact in the absence of shoulder girdle injury (see earlier discussion). The lower extremities may also be evaluated at the same time given adequate table length. When studying the lower extremities, a larger than typical intravenous contrast bolus will be required to ensure adequate vascular opacification (Table 11-3). Intravenous contrast

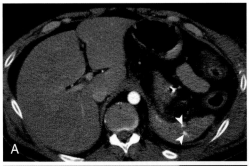

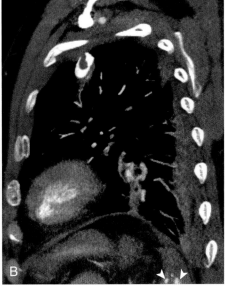

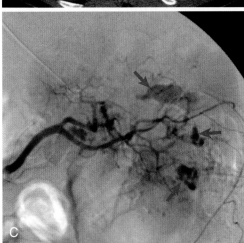

Figure 11-3 Patient transferred from an outside hospital post motor vehicle accident. A, The last axial image from a computed tomographic angiogram (CTA) of the chest to reevaluate an aortic injury demonstrates multiple foci of arterial enhancement in the superior pole of the spleen *(arrowheads)* suspicious for pseudoaneurysms or active bleeding. **B**, Sagittal image from a CTA of the chest to reevaluate an aortic injury demonstrates multiple foci of arterial enhancement in the superior pole of the spleen *(arrowheads)* suspicious for pseudoaneurysms or active bleeding. **C**, Subsequent angiogram of the splenic artery confirms the presence of multiple pseudoaneurysms within the spleen *(red arrows)*.

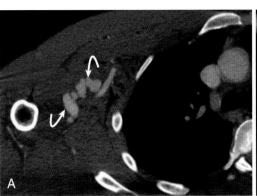

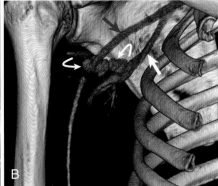

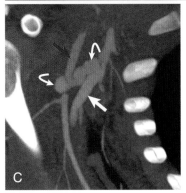

Figure 11-4 Post gunshot wound to the right anterior chest wall. A, Axial image from a computed tomographic angiogram (CTA) of the upper extremity reconstructed from whole-body multidetector computed tomography (WBMDCT) demonstrates the axillary artery *(red arrow)*. Extraluminal contrast is seen in the axilla *(curved arrows)*. **B**, Volume rendered image demonstrates an abnormal connection *(curved arrows)* between the right axillary artery *(red arrow)* and vein *(white arrow)* consistent with a traumatic arteriovenous fistula. **C**, Maximum intensity projection (MIP) image of the right axilla demonstrates abnormal connection *(curved arrows)* between axillary artery *(red arrow)* and vein *(white arrow)* consistent with a traumatic arteriovenous fistula. (Courtesy Uttam Bodanapally, MD.)

should be injected on the contralateral side of a suspected upper extremity injury. This technique helps avoid artifact arising from the contrast bolus that can obscure injuries in the adjacent arteries or soft tissues.

Protocol for Follow-up of Solid Organ Injury

Controversy persists regarding the merits of routine CT follow-up of solid organ injuries before discharge to document healing and exclude injury progression or

---

Box 11-1 Indications for Upper/Lower Extremity Computed Tomographic Angiogram

Asymmetric pulses
Nonexpanding hematoma
Proximity of the wound to major vessels
Peripheral neurologic deficit
History of arterial bleeding at the scene
Abnormal ankle-brachial index

---

complications. Indications in our practice for follow-up CT include clinical deterioration and initial diagnosis of high-grade injury. A follow-up CT typically is obtained between 48 to 72 hours after admission. The protocol will vary if angiographic intervention has been previously performed to treat the injury. Contrast material used during the angiographic procedure can extravasate into or around the injured organ and mimic active hemorrhage on a follow-up contrast-enhanced CT. Therefore it is important to document the presence of any previously extravasated angiographic contrast material by performing a non–contrast-enhanced CT in patients who have had recent angiography before performing a follow-up CTA. This will optimize distinction of previously extravasated contrast from continuing bleeding. The protocol used is shown in Table 11-4.

Protocol for Bladder Injury

Bladder injuries are seen in approximately 2% of blunt trauma patients involving the abdomen and pelvis and often involve concurrent pelvic fractures. Injury to the

---

Table 11-3 Multidetector Computed Tomography Upper/Lower Extremity Computed Tomographic Angiogram Protocols

Parameter	Upper Extremity	Lower Extremity
Patient positioning	Affected arm fully abducted	—
Detector collimation and configuration (mm)	40 × 0.625	64 × 0.625
Pitch	1.076	1.076
Rotation time (sec)	0.5	0.5
kV	120	120
Current (mA)	200	230
Area scanned	Mid thorax through fingertips	Mid abdomen to the toes
Contrast volume (mL)	100	125
Contrast injection rate	4 mL/sec	4 mL/sec
Scan trigger threshold (HU)[†]	120	120
Source axial images (mm)[‡,§]	1 × 0.5	1.5 × 0.75
Reconstruction filter	B (soft tissue)	B (soft tissue)
Diagnostic axial images to PACS[§] (mm)	2 × 1	2 × 1
Sagittal MPR[§] (mm)	5 × 2 MIP	5 × 2 MIP
Coronal MPR[§] (mm)	5 × 2 MIP	5 × 2 MIP
Thin-section axial images to independent workstation (mm)	1 × 0.5	1.5 × 0.75

*Do not inject the injured extremity.
[†]Bolus Pro Triggering System (Philips Medical Systems) with region of interest at distal ascending aorta.
[‡]Source axial images used to construct all routine diagnostic images.
[§]Thickness × interval.
MIP, Maximum intensity projection; MPR, coronal multiplanar reformats; PACS, picture archiving and communication system.

Table 11-4 Multidetector Computed Tomography Solid Organ Injury Protocol

Parameter	Arterial Phase	Portal Venous Phase
Patient positioning	Affected arm fully abducted	Affected arm fully abducted
Detector collimation and configuration (mm)	40 × 0.625	64 × 0.625
Pitch	0.671	1.093
Rotation time (sec)	0.5	0.5
kV	120	120
Current (mA)	250	300
Area scanned	Diaphragm to the lesser trochanters	Diaphragm to the iliac crests
Contrast volume (mL)	100	—
Contrast injection rate	4 mL/sec	—
Scan trigger threshold (HU)*	120	—
Scan delay (sec)	—	70 sec
Source axial images (mm)[†,‡]	0.9 × 0.45	1.5 × 0.75
Reconstruction filter	B (soft tissue)	B (soft tissue)
Diagnostic axial images to PACS[‡] (mm)	3 × 3	3 × 3
Sagittal MPR[‡] (mm)	5 × 3 MIP	4 × 3
Coronal MPR[‡] (mm)	5 × 3 MIP	4 × 3
Thin-section axial images to independent workstation (mm)	0.9 × 0.45	0.9 × 0.45

*Bolus Pro Triggering System (Philips Medical Systems, Cleveland, Ohio) with region of interest at distal ascending aorta.
[†]Source axial images used to construct all routine diagnostic images.
[‡]Thickness × interval.
MIP, Maximum intensity projection; MPR, coronal multiplanar reformats; PACS, picture archiving and communication system.

bladder is often related to how distended the bladder is at the time of injury. Gross hematuria is the most common clinical finding. Bladder ruptures are intraperitoneal in 25%, extraperitoneal in 62%, and combined in 12% of cases. Dedicated evaluation of the bladder can be conducted at the conclusion of the WBMDCT examination and is advised in the setting of pelvic fractures with or without gross hematuria.

If CT cystography is being performed, the bladder should be emptied and continually drained by an indwelling Foley catheter before the scan is started. After the portal venous phase is obtained, the bladder should be filled with a water-soluble iso-osmolar radiopaque contrast (35 mL of Omnipaque 350 diluted in 450 mL of sterile water). The contrast is instilled under gravity through the Foley catheter from a bag of contrast 1 m above the CT table. The pelvis is then imaged when the bladder is full (approximately 300 mL) or the column of contrast stops flowing. Axial views are obtained at a slice thickness of 0.9 mm for high resolution with sagittal and coronal reformations (Table 11-5). Postvoid images are routinely obtained in an attempt to see possible injuries posterior to the bladder. Given the superior ability of multidetector computed tomography (MDCT) to assess the soft tissues surrounding the bladder, there is no need to image the pelvis with CT after emptying the bladder unless there is the rare question of contrast retained in the bladder versus extravasated contrast.

Renal injuries, such as lacerations, extending to the renal collecting system may cause hematuria. Lacerations disrupting the collecting system may lead to complications associated with urine leaks, which can

be easily managed with nephroureteral stents. These injuries may be easily missed on the arterial and portal venous phases of the whole-body CT given the lack of radiopaque contrast within the renal collecting system. It is advised that patients with renal injuries extending to the renal collecting system have additional imaging through the kidneys at least 5 minutes after the injection of contrast if the study is being actively monitored or return to the CT scanner for delayed imaging if a question of collecting system injury is raised by review of the initial whole-body scan.

ORAL AND RECTAL CONTRAST MATERIAL

Protocol for Blunt Trauma

Intravenous contrast is routinely administered to patients undergoing CT after trauma to improve recognition of both vascular and parenchymal injury. However, the use of oral contrast for admission CT examinations has decreased significantly over the past few years. The routine availability of high spatial resolution axial and reformatted images, increased familiarity with CT signs of bowel and mesenteric injury, and the low sensitivity of spilled gastrointestinal contrast with full-thickness bowel injury are some reasons for this development. Although oral contrast aspiration is also mentioned as a contraindication for its use, this is in fact an extremely rare event. Computed tomography without oral contrast can typically show subtle bowel wall thickening, minimal pneumoperitoneum, direct defects in the bowel wall, a small quantity of intraperitoneal free fluid, and small mesenteric contusion or hematomas.

At our institution, patients needing a repeat CT of the abdomen and pelvis for indeterminate initial CT findings of bowel or mesenteric injury, isolated free intraperitoneal fluid beyond a trace amount without a clear source, or clinical deterioration possibly related to an abdominal source following a negative admission CT are reimaged with inclusion of oral contrast material (Fig. 11-5). A total volume of 600 mL of oral contrast material (50 mL Omnipaque 300 diluted in 950 mL of water) is given in two equal doses orally or per orogastric tube, the first about 30 to 45 minutes before and the second immediately before performing the scan.

Protocol for Penetrating Trauma

In the setting of penetrating trauma to the torso (entry site between nipple line and upper third of thigh), a triple-contrast MDCT examination of the chest, abdomen, and pelvis should be performed. The triple-contrast technique includes the use of iodinated intravenous contrast and water-soluble oral and rectal contrast material. The patient is scanned using the solid organ injury protocol (see Table 11-4) following administration of both oral (600 mL in two divided doses) and 1 to 1.5 L of rectal contrast (50 mL Omnipaque 300 diluted in 950 mL of water) through a rectal tube as an enema. The enema is administered under gravity (the enema bag is 1 m above the CT table) before performing the scan in the CT suite. Patients

Table 11-5   64-Slice Multidetector Computed Tomographic Cystogram* Protocol

Parameter	
Detector collimation and configuration (mm)	64×0.625
Pitch	0.984
Rotation time (sec)	0.75
kV	120
Current (mA)	250
Area scanned	Iliac crests to the ischial tuberosities
Source axial images (mm)[†,‡]	0.9×0.45
Reconstruction filter	B (soft tissue)
Diagnostic axial images to PACS[‡] (mm)	4×3
Sagittal MPR[‡] (mm)	4×3
Coronal MPR[‡] (mm)	4×3
Thin-section axial images to independent workstation[‡] (mm)	0.9×0.45

*Parameters are used for the initial non-filled and full bladder.
[†]Source axial images used to construct all routine diagnostic images.
[‡]Thickness × interval.
MPR, Coronal multiplanar reformats; *PACS*, picture archiving and communication system.

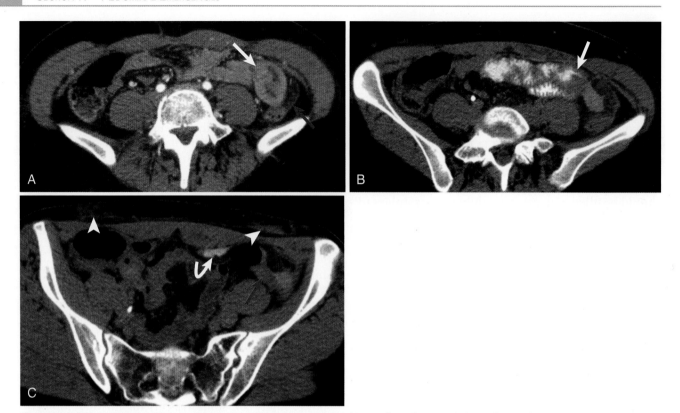

Figure 11-5 Post motor vehicle accident with seat belt sign. A, Axial image from the arterial phase of whole-body multidetector computed tomography (WBMDCT) demonstrates thickened and hyperemic loops of small bowel in the left lower quadrant *(white arrow)*. Small amount of fluid and mesenteric stranding adjacent to abnormal-appearing loop of small bowel *(red arrow)*. **B,** Image of the same area 6 hours later with oral contrast demonstrates thickened loops of small bowel *(white arrow)* in the left lower quadrant. Small amount of hemorrhage *(red arrow)* is now seen in the adjacent mesentery. **C,** Axial image demonstrates extravasation of oral contrast *(curved arrow)* into the peritoneal cavity consistent with a full-thickness bowel injury. Small amount of hemorrhage *(red arrow)* present in the adjacent mesentery. A seat belt mark *(arrowheads)* is seen over the anterior abdominal wall.

requiring urgent CT on admission may be scanned with a single dose of oral and rectal contrast material.

■ SPECIAL CONSIDERATIONS

Protocol for Pregnant Patients

Blunt trauma may complicate up to 7% of pregnancies and is a leading cause of maternal death, with the majority of injuries sustained in motor vehicle collisions. Penetrating trauma as a result of domestic violence or accidental gunshot wounds account for as many as 36% of maternal deaths. Although there is always concern for radiation exposure to the fetus, this should not impede the performance of radiographic or CT examinations to evaluate life-threatening injuries sustained by the mother (Fig. 11-6). In hemodynamically stable pregnant patients following major blunt trauma, WBMDCT should be used to screen for injuries. Automatic exposure control (AEC) should be used to reduce radiation dose. A formal obstetric ultrasound (US) examination is also performed in hemodynamically stable patients by an experienced physician or ultrasonographer to document the age of the fetus and to assess viability and placental integrity.

Protocol for Obese Patients

The CDC, National Institutes of Health, and World Health Organization define obesity as a body mass index

of 30 or more, which is calculated by dividing the weight (in kilograms) by the square of the height (in meters). The prevalence of obesity among adults in the United States has increased steadily since 1985, when the CDC conducted its first Behavioral Risk Factor Surveillance System survey. In 2006 more than 72 million Americans 20 years or older were obese with a slightly higher prevalence among women (35.5%) than men (33.2%).

The most common technical difficulties experienced with obese patients are the bore size of the CT scanner and the weight limit of the scanner table. This has been accommodated by CT manufacturers now offering CT tables with weight limits approaching 700 pounds and selected vendors increasing bore size with the largest aperture of 90 cm and a 70-cm acquired field of view.

The most common artifact encountered in the CT images of obese patients is photon starvation. Increased body fat raises photon attenuation, resulting in insufficient photon transmission to the detectors. This in turn results in excessive quantum mottle, reduced contrast-to-noise ratio, and streak artifact. Increasing the milliamperes and decreasing the pitch increases the number of photons transmitted to the detectors, decreasing the photon starvation artifact. The peak kilovoltage (kVp) can also be increased to raise the energy of the photons to better penetrate the soft tissues. The use of 140 kVp is advised for morbidly obese patients (body mass index ≥ 40) to improve the contrast-to-noise ratio in soft tissues. The use of 120 kVp is advised for CTA in most

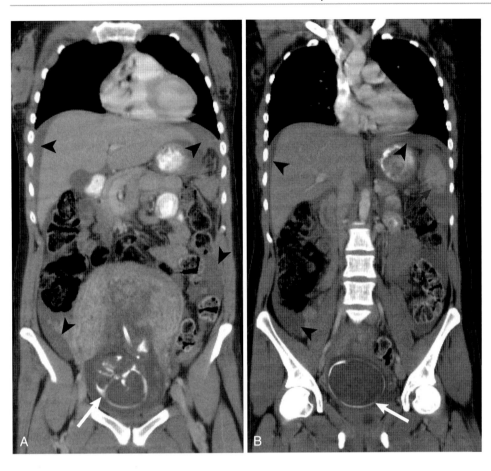

Figure 11-6 Splenic injury with hemoperitoneum. A, Coronal reformat of the arterial phase of the whole-body multidetector computed tomography (WBMDCT) demonstrates hemoperitoneum throughout the abdomen *(arrowheads).* Gravid uterus contains a single fetus in a vertex position *(white arrow).* **B,** Coronal reformat of the arterial phase of the WBMDCT demonstrates hemoperitoneum *(arrowheads)* throughout the abdomen and a laceration through the inferior pole of the spleen *(red arrow).*

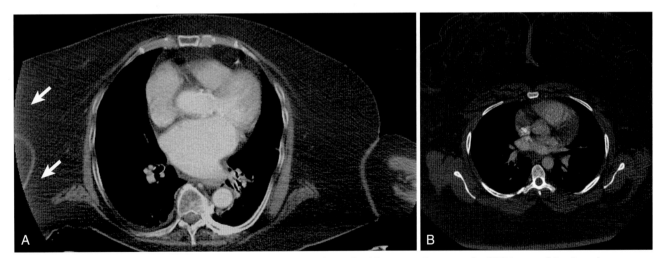

Figure 11-7 Beam hardening in obese patient. A, Contrast-enhanced axial computed tomography (CT) image of the chest demonstrates artifact commonly seen in obese patients. *White arrows* indicate beam hardening. Photon starvation artifact is seen throughout the image because of the attenuation of the photons by the thick subcutaneous soft tissues. **B,** Contrast-enhanced axial CT image of the chest demonstrates the lack of beam hardening in this obese patient given the symmetry of the breasts by bundling them with the CT table restraint.

obese patients to optimize iodine-induced attenuation. Slice thickness can be widened to increase the number of photons used to produce each image. Iterative reconstruction algorithms also reduce noise created by diminished detector exposure. Beam-hardening artifact may also be encountered when obese patients lay flat and large breasts or subcutaneous fat falls to the side, creating an asymmetric profile and leading to beam hardening and photon starvation artifacts in lateral CT projection, which is exacerbated by the bowtie filter effect (see Chapter 1). This may be overcome by bundling or wrapping the patient in sheets or CT restraint devices to reduce artifact by providing a symmetric profile of excess soft tissues (Fig. 11-7).

With the increase in milliamperes and kVp to obtain diagnostic images, obese patients receive higher radiation doses than nonobese patients. Automatic exposure control may be used to help reduce radiation dose to the obese patient. However, special attention needs to be given to specific protocols that include AEC. The maximum milliamperes must be restricted, otherwise AEC will automatically increase tube output to compensate and may result in very large radiation doses, the opposite of what is desired when trying to reduce the patient's overall radiation exposure.

Sonography

Alexandra Platon and Pierre-Alexandre Poletti

Imaging plays a key role in the screening of blunt abdominal trauma patients because clinical examination is insufficient to rule out a major intra-abdominal traumatic injury. The imaging method to be used for the screening of traumatic intra-abdominal injuries should be adapted to the available institutional imaging facilities and to the hemodynamic status of the patient. Imaging a polytrauma patient should take into consideration the balance between the quality of the examination and the time required to obtain these images to fit with the concept of "the golden hour": the shorter the time elapsed between trauma and treatment, the higher the chances of survival. Thus, because time constraint is a major issue in hemodynamically unstable patients, the imaging management must be performed as fast as possible, for immediate depiction of the life-threatening condition. The situation is different in a hemodynamically stable patient, with sufficient time to obtain a more detailed examination. In this case the main concern is to select the most appropriate imaging algorithm and to avoid missing subtle or potentially life-threatening injuries, which may become apparent only in a delayed fashion.

In this section we will present several aspects of the current imaging methods used for the initial triage and diagnostic work-up of blunt abdominal trauma patients.

■ ULTRASONOGRAPHY

Focused Assessment Sonography for Trauma

In clinical practice, focused assessment sonography for trauma (FAST) consists of regarding and using US as a rapid diagnostic test for depiction of free fluid only. This technique can be performed by emergency medical staff with a relatively limited level of training in US, including nonradiologist physicians or surgeons.

FAST examination is realized by using a sector probe with a frequency in the range of 2.5 to 5 MHz, according to the patient's morphologic characteristics.

To check for the presence of free peritoneal fluid, the technique of FAST examination consists of assessing at least three abdominal regions:
1. The right upper quadrant, for visualization of the hepatorenal recess (Morison pouch), where free fluid may freely accumulate from the upper abdomen and from the right pericolic gutter because there is no ligament to hinder fluid movement. The detectability of fluid in the Morison pouch may be improved, when feasible, by the Trendelenburg position.
2. The left upper quadrant, to assess the presence of perisplenic fluid. Both the splenorenal and subphrenic areas should be carefully examined.
3. The rectovesical recess in males and the Douglas pouch in females, which are the most dependant areas of the pelvis. A full bladder is required to optimize the depiction of free fluid in this region.

Views of the right and left paracolic gutters are also considered as part of the FAST examination by some authors, but their added value has not been demonstrated yet.

The presence of pleural fluid will be sought during the examination of the right and left upper quadrants.

It is also classically recommended that a subxiphoid view be obtained to assess for the presence of pericardial fluid. However, the actual benefit of doing so is not well established, and it may also be a source of overdiagnosis.

Focused Assessment Sonography for Trauma Findings
ASPECT

Intraperitoneal blood may have a different appearance at US. It may vary according to the quantity of blood and to the delay elapsed between the onset of bleeding and the examination (Fig. 11-8). Blood may appear completely anechoic, anechoic with some internal echoes, or as an echogenic mass, corresponding to a clotted hematoma. These various forms may also coexist.

Where as a large quantity of free fluid is easily detected as a hypoechoic area in all peritoneal recesses, with floating bowel loops, a small quantity of blood is more difficult to assess and may be detected as a sliver of anechoic fluid in the Morison pouch, in the left subphrenic space, and/or in the pelvis.

MINIMUM BLOOD VOLUME TO BE DETECTED
The minimum amount of blood to be detected by US is impossible to assess because it will depend not only on the volume of blood, but also on its echogenicity (free fluid or clotted blood) and on the skill of the operator. It has been reported that the minimum quantity of free peritoneal fluid that can be detected by US in the Morison pouch is 250 mL, although a minimum of 620 mL would be required to be depicted by the majority of the operators.

QUANTIFICATION OF FREE FLUID
The estimation of the quantity of free intraperitoneal fluid as small, moderate, or large is important and is subject to interpersonal variability. However, such

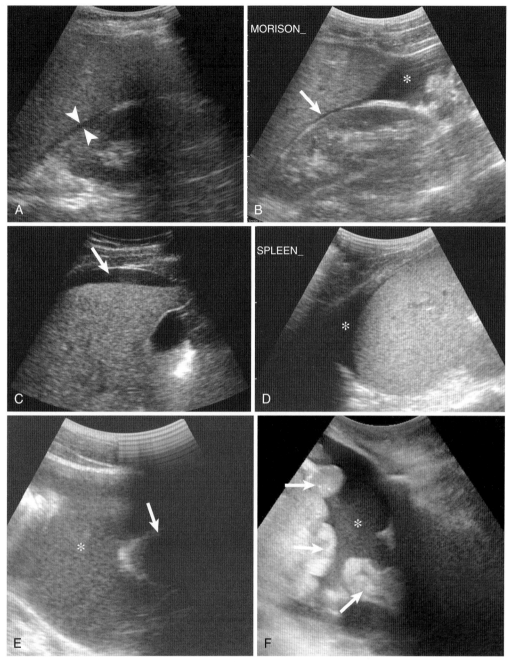

Figure 11-8 *Various presentations of peritoneal blood at focused assessment sonography for trauma (FAST) examination in different trauma patients.* **A,** Small quantity of free peritoneal fluid *(arrowheads)* in the Morison pouch. **B,** Sliver of free fluid in the Morison pouch *(arrow)* and at the tip of the liver *(asterisk).* **C,** Large quantity of perihepatic fluid *(arrow).* **D,** Large quantity of perisplenic fluid *(asterisk).* **E,** Large quantity of hyperechoic pelvic free fluid *(asterisk);* the bladder is empty, drained by a urinary catheter *(arrow).* **F,** Small bowel loops *(arrows)* floating in a large quantity of free hyperechoic fluid *(asterisk).*

quantification may be useful for the triage of patients when correlated to the hemodynamic status. The detection of a large quantity of free peritoneal fluid in a patient who is hemodynamically unstable will certainly justify an immediate laparotomy, whereas a small quantity of peritoneal fluid in the same patient will alert the clinician to look for another source of bleeding. Some authors proposed various scoring systems to more precisely estimate the quantity of free peritoneal fluid, according to its depth and location. However, these

scores have not been validated by large series and are currently not used in most trauma centers.

TRAINING OF THE OPERATOR FOR FOCUSED ASSESSMENT SONOGRAPHY FOR TRAUMA

The wide majority of FAST examinations in the United States are now performed by nonradiologists in both university and community hospitals.

The minimum training required for a nonradiologist to become proficient in FAST is one of the more controversial topics in trauma US. There is no consensus or standard guidelines for the minimum number of FAST examinations that should be performed under supervision before a surgeon or emergency physician can be considered trained in this technique. This number fluctuates from 10 to 200 according to the various authors, institutions, or medical associations. This variability is easy to understand when considering the fact that the skill to depict a large quantity of free fluid will be lower than that necessary to depict a sliver of free fluid. Many authors consider that a minimum of 30 proctored examinations is necessary to become proficient in FAST, taking into consideration that the trainee must be confronted with a sufficient number of positive cases.

VALUE OF A FOCUSED ASSESSMENT SONOGRAPHY FOR TRAUMA EXAMINATION

The practical value of a FAST examination depends on the hemodynamic status of the patient. In a hemodynamically unstable patient, positive FAST results mandate laparotomy, following the recommendations of the 1997 International Consensus Conference in Baltimore. When the FAST results are negative, the clinician will look for a nonabdominal source of bleeding.

In a hemodynamically stable patient the value of the FAST examination will be more dependent on the existing resources of a given institution, and the guideline should be adapted in consequence. No general rules can be enacted. Thus it is even questionable whether a FAST examination should be performed in a stable patient who will undergo a CT examination anyway. In this situation, performing FAST may be helpful for choosing the priority order for CT, when many patients are managed simultaneously. Positive FAST results are usually considered an indication for performing an abdominal CT.

Although negative CT results are sufficient to rule out an intra-abdominal injury, negative FAST examination results alone cannot do so and must therefore be integrated in the clinical situation to be correctly interpreted. Thus, in alert patients who underwent minor blunt abdominal trauma, without any other reason to perform a CT, negative FAST examination results may be useful, in addition to normal clinical examination results and normal biologic parameters, to decide whether the patient can be discharged without performing a CT scan. Depending on the clinical scenario, serial negative FAST examination results along with 12 hours of clinical observation have been advocated before discharging a patient without performing CT.

PITFALLS

The subphrenic space may be difficult to screen due to the accumulation of bowel gas in the splenic flexure. However, this area should be carefully scrutinized because a small quantity of fluid will preferentially accumulate in this space rather than in the splenorenal interface.

A small quantity of free fluid may only be depicted in the Douglas pouch (rectovesical space in males), which corresponds to the most dependent space of the abdomen. A proper analysis of this requires a distended bladder. If the bladder is empty, FAST may miss a small amount of free fluid.

Clotted blood may appear hyperechoic and thus be overlooked or misinterpreted as normal abdominal content.

False-positive FAST results are much less common than false-negative ones. Fat may sometimes appear hypoechoic and mimic fluid, especially between the kidney and the liver. Similarly, normal pericardial fat may often be considered as pericardial effusion. Intraintestinal fluid content may also be falsely interpreted as free fluid when the operator does not pay attention to the bowel movements. The detection of normal fluid in the Douglas pouch in a woman in the middle of her menstrual period may be source of diagnostic dilemma and should be integrated in the clinical setting. Similarly, a preexisting ascites in a trauma patient may be misinterpreted as hemoperitoneum.

A large percentage of intra-abdominal organ injuries (up to 34%) are not associated with free peritoneal fluid and therefore remain undetectable by FAST. Up to 16.5% of these lesions have been considered life threatening because they required surgery or embolization. Besides, the limitation of FAST for detecting free fluid originating from bowel and mesenteric injuries has also been documented, with a sensitivity not exceeding 44%.

Blood associated with retroperitoneal injuries (kidney, pancreas, vessels) is classically missed by FAST because it does not appear hypoechoic and therefore remains undistinguishable from retroperitoneal fat.

Parenchymal Analysis

Parenchymal injuries may have various presentations at direct US examination (Fig. 11-9). An acute liver injury classically appears as a hyperechoic area when compared to the normal parenchyma; it may also be detected as a heterogenous or hypoechoic structure, depending on the time elapsed from the trauma and the severity of the injury. In the spleen and kidney, injuries are usually hypoechoic or heterogenous, with possible foci of cysticlike lesions and disorganization of the normal parenchyma.

The capsule of the organ must be scrupulously scrutinized for the presence of hypoechoic or hyperechoic layers, corresponding to hematoma. Doppler examination does not clearly improve the detection of parenchymal injuries when compared to B mode alone and is therefore not recommended in this setting. However, a Doppler examination may be useful to detect an occlusion of a renal artery.

To improve the sensitivity of US to suggesting an intra-abdominal injury, it is recommended, in addition to the search for free peritoneal fluid, to systematically analyze the parenchyma of solid intra-abdominal organs. Doing so requires a higher level of prior training in abdominal US, which should be achieved in a radiologic ward, when compared to limiting the screening to a sole FAST examination. However, the added value of complete US examination to confirming the suspicion of organ injury with regard to free-fluid analysis only is subject to controversy. About 50% of CT-proven organ injuries remain undetectable at parenchymal examination by US. When abdominal free fluid is detected in an unstable patient, it is probably of no clinical benefit to spend additional time searching for the source of bleeding by US.

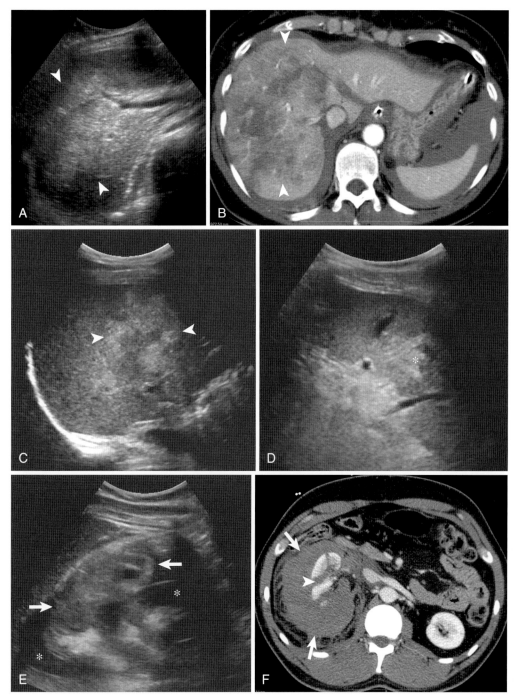

Figure 11-9 **Various presentations of intraparenchymal traumatic injuries at ultrasonography (US) in different trauma patients.** **A,** The center of the right liver lobe appears hyperechoic *(arrowheads).* **B,** The corresponding axial computed tomography (CT) image confirms the presence of a large liver laceration *(arrowheads).* **C,** Mixed aspect of a liver laceration *(arrowheads):* the periphery of the injury appears hyperechoic, whereas the center is hypoechoic. **D,** Mixed aspect of a splenic laceration *(asterisk):* the periphery of the injury appears hyperechoic, whereas the center is hypo-echoic. **E,** Disruption of the normal renal cortex *(asterisks)* by a large heterogenous mass, protruding in the perirenal space *(arrows).* **F,** The corresponding axial CT image confirms the rupture of the renal cortex *(arrowhead)* surrounded by a large hematoma *(arrows).*

Contrast-Enhanced Ultrasonography in Abdominal Trauma

Value and Limitations of a Contrast Ultrasonographic Examination

Contrast-enhanced US has been reported to be much more efficient than B-mode US only for the depiction of liver, spleen, and kidney injuries (Fig. 11-10). The sensitivity for depiction of traumatic organ injuries is classically between 50% and 80% at US, and between 90% and 94% after administration of ultrasound contrast media. Contrast US examination requires specific training in this technique and can therefore be performed only by a skilled operator. Contrast-enhanced US should be performed in optimal conditions and is completed in approximately 10 to 15 minutes. These constraints prevent this technique from being used at

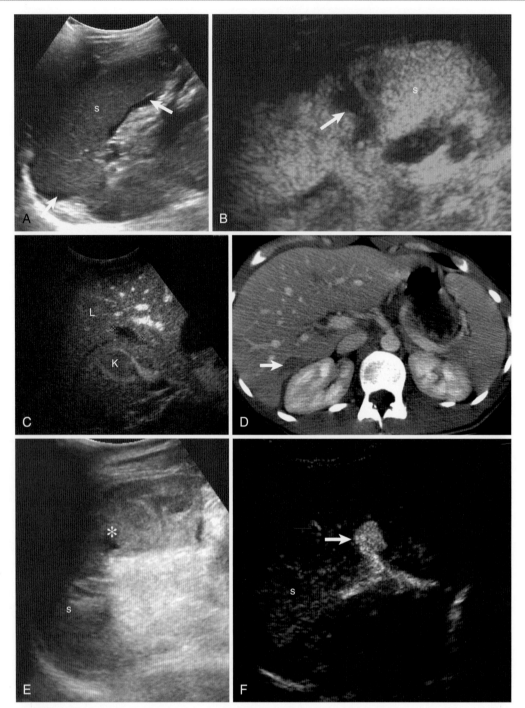

Figure 11-10 Contrast-enhanced ultrasonographic examinations in different trauma patients. **A,** The splenic parenchyma (S) appears homogenous before administration of contrast media. The spleen is surrounded by free fluid *(arrows)*. **B,** After injection of ultrasonographic contrast media, a splenic laceration appears as a hypoechoic rent *(arrow)* within the normally enhancing parenchyma (S). **C,** A hypoechoic rent (between *calipers*) is depicted in the lateral aspect of the liver (L), at the level of the kidney (K). **D,** Subsequent enhanced computed tomography (CT) confirms the presence of a laceration *(arrow)*. **E,** Unenhanced ultrasonographic examination: a splenic hematoma *(asterisk)* appears as a heterogenous mass in the central aspect of the spleen (S). **F,** Twenty seconds after injection of ultrasonographic contrast media, a large hyperechoic blush *(arrow)* is depicted in the central aspect of the spleen (S), consistent with a pseudoaneurysm.

a patient's admission. However, it can play an interesting role in ruling out a solid organ injury in the follow-up of a patient who underwent minor abdominal trauma, with no clinical indication for undergoing a CT scan. Contrast-enhanced US has also been reported useful for follow-up of solid organ injuries detected by CT. However, this technique is still limited by its inability to depict bowel injuries and by the cost

of US contrast agent, which is similar to that of CT contrast media.

Contrast-enhanced US has been reported useful for the depiction of traumatic vascular injuries. Thus it can play an interesting role in the screening of delayed splenic pseudoaneurysms, which may appear some days after trauma and are considered a cause of failure of nonoperative management. A contrast-enhanced US

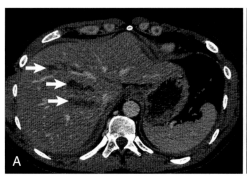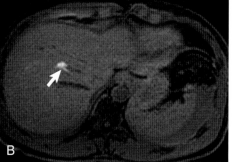

Figure 11-11 Biliary leak in a patient with liver trauma. **A,** Contrast-enhanced computed tomography (CT) performed 5 days after trauma, for abdominal pain and elevated serum bilirubin level. Multiple well-delineated hypodense lacerations are depicted in the right liver lobe *(arrows)*. **B,** Magnetic resonance imaging (MRI) after intravenous injection of a hepatobiliary-specific contrast agent (gadoxetic acid) shows an extravasation of the contrast agent *(arrow)*, corresponding to the site of the bile leak.

examination that is positive for the presence of a pseudoaneurysm mandates an angiographic embolization.

Technique

Second-generation US contrast agents consist of stabilized microbubbles filled with an inert innocuous gas and are characterized by both stability and resistance to pressure. Unlike the first generation of contrast agents, the bubbles are not massively destroyed during their first pass into the pulmonary vascular microcirculation. Thus they can be used during several minutes after a single intravenous bolus. The US contrast agent is eventually eliminated through the pulmonary route and is thus innocuous for the kidney.

An initial analysis of parenchyma is first performed on standard B-mode imaging. Then the operator switches on a specific mode for contrast media (such as a pulse inversion harmonic mode) with a reduced mechanical index. The contrast agent is then injected intravenously, using a 20-gauge catheter placed into an antecubital vein, followed by a 10-mL flush of saline water. The maximal parenchymal enhancement is obtained about 1 minute after injection for the liver and spleen and earlier (20 to 30 seconds) for the renal cortex. Solid organ injuries appear as deep hypoechoic (nonenhancing) areas, when compared to the hyperechoic enhancement of the normal surrounding parenchyma. A focal pooling of contrast medium within the splenic parenchyma during the arterial phase, with enhancement similar to the splenic artery, surrounded by a normally enhancing or nonenhancing (injured) parenchyma, is highly suggestive of a pseudoaneurysm (Fig. 11-10F).

Multidetector Computed Tomography Imaging

Multidetector CT has become a key diagnostic tool for the management of polytrauma patients and is now equipping most emergency centers. It allows a rapid and accurate assessment of the whole body. Computed tomography is not only valuable to get a thorough assessment of soft and bony structures, but also plays a key role in determining the need for surgery or nonoperative management of intra-abdominal injuries. In a polytrauma patient CT is useful for obtaining a detailed analysis of multiple lesions. In patients who underwent minor trauma, CT is necessary to rule out an injury.

Indeed, normal abdominal CT results have been considered sufficient to safely discharge a patient with no other reason to be hospitalized. Performing a systematic CT scan in every abdominal trauma patient will expedite the work flow in the ED and has been reported to be cost-effective by saving the institution's resources. On the other hand, doing so raises the problem of exposing to radiation doses and contrast media some patients who could otherwise have been managed by US and clinical observation only. This dilemma between overuse of CT in mild trauma patients and improving the work flow in a busy emergency center is unresolved; specific guidelines should therefore be tailored to every institution.

A follow-up CT scan is usually indicated for the monitoring of nonoperative management in patients with major abdominal organ injuries and for the depiction of complications after abdominal surgery.

Magnetic Resonance Imaging

Magnetic resonance imaging (MRI) plays a limited role in abdominal trauma patients because it is technically difficult to perform in an acute setting. Magnetic resonance imaging is sometimes used as a complement to CT in a limited number of well-targeted indications. Thus MRI has been reported useful for showing the integrity of hemidiaphragms and to demonstrate the herniation or entrapment of abdominal contents when CT images are ambiguous.

In a liver trauma patient with suspicion of bile leak in the peritoneum (Fig. 11-11), MRI may be useful for confirming a lesion of the biliary ducts and to depict the exact site of the injury, allowing optimal management (drainage or surgical repair). In this setting, MRI must be used with injection of hepatobiliary-specific contrast agents.

In pancreatic injuries the diagnosis of pancreatic transection is often difficult to ascertain on CT images. Information about the presence and location of a pancreatic duct rupture is of paramount importance to determining the proper treatment (i.e., surgery in proximal disruptions, drainage in distal injuries) and to preventing complications. Magnetic resonance imaging is now used as a noninvasive alternative to endoscopic retrograde cholangiopancreatography (ERCP) to assess the integrity or the disruption of the pancreatic duct. Unlike ECRP, MR pancreatography (Fig. 11-12) allows visualization of the pancreatic duct beyond the injury site.

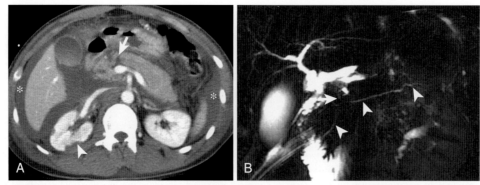

Figure 11-12 Pancreatic injury. A, Admission axial computed tomography (CT) image shows a large amount of free fluid (*asterisk*), a hypodense rent within the pancreatic neck (*arrow*), and a right renal injury (*arrowhead*). **B,** Magnetic resonance pancreatography shows a leak of pancreatic fluid (*arrow*) arising from the main pancreatic duct (*arrowheads*), consistent with a partial ductal disruption.

Solid Intraperitoneal Organ Injury

Alexis Boscak and Kathirkamanathan Shanmuganathan

The spleen and liver are the two most frequently injured organs after blunt trauma to the abdomen, most commonly caused by motor vehicle collision, fall, assault, or sports or workplace accident. Exsanguinating hemorrhage may result from disruption of either of these highly vascular organs; if there is hemoperitoneum after blunt abdominal trauma, spleen and liver injuries should sought initially. Imaging protocols for investigation of spleen and liver injuries are almost identical. Both organs are best evaluated in the acute setting by contrast-enhanced CT with arterial, portal venous, and, in some cases, delayed phase imaging, which play similar roles in the assessment of both organs. Blunt splenic and hepatic injuries may require emergent laparotomy for surgical therapy, generally in the setting of hemodynamic instability, or may be amenable to nonoperative management with or without angiographic intervention. Splenectomy provides definitive control of life-threatening splenic hemorrhage, although with a lifetime risk for overwhelming postsplenectomy sepsis, whereas surgical management of severe liver injury is necessarily more complex. Liver trauma is also complicated by the possibility of coexistent biliary injury. Treatment of both splenic and hepatic blunt trauma has evolved over the past several decades toward conservative nonoperative management for a majority of cases, even with high-grade injuries. This trend is concurrent with increased use of CT as the primary diagnostic imaging modality after blunt abdominal trauma, allowing improved diagnosis and injury characterization, which not only facilitates appropriate selection of patients for initial operative versus nonoperative therapy, but also allows patients undergoing conservative management who show signs of deterioration to be readily and accurately reevaluated without requiring immediate recourse to laparotomy. There are many similarities between the imaging findings after blunt splenic and hepatic injury and some important differences. The posttrauma imaging evaluation of each of these organs is addressed in separate sections to follow.

■ BLUNT SPLENIC INJURY

Splenic Anatomy and Traumatology

Although relatively small and sheltered within the left upper quadrant, the spleen is a delicate organ consisting of soft, friable, and extremely vascular parenchyma constrained by a thin capsule. The spleen receives as much as 5% (200 mL/min) of the cardiac output and may contain as much as 500 mL of blood at a time. The spleen is primarily perfused by the splenic artery, which also gives rise to pancreatic branches, several short gastric arteries, and, in some cases, a posterior gastric artery, as well as having an anastomosis with the left gastroepiploic (left gastro-omental) artery near the splenic hilum. The intrasplenic arterioles, which are surrounded by lymphoid tissue constituting the splenic white pulp, are end vessels that may feed into the intrasplenic red pulp or directly into venous sinuses. Venous outflow is through the main splenic vein to the portal vein. Although primarily intraperitoneal, the spleen has limited extraperitoneal bare areas at its vascular hilum and along the confluence of its peritoneal attachments. The spleen is suspended within the left upper quadrant by the partially continuous phrenicosplenic, gastrosplenic, and splenorenal ligaments and rests upon the phrenicocolic ligament below. Unless unusually long, the splenic vascular pedicle affords the organ only limited mobility. The nonenlarged spleen does not generally protrude below the costal margin, but a pathologically enlarged spleen may be significantly exposed, in addition to being abnormally fragile. Displaced fracture of the overlying ribs may result in splenic laceration. Direct compression and acceleration/deceleration shear forces are the other major mechanisms of splenic disruption in blunt trauma. The spleen is the only injured abdominal organ in approximately 60% to 75% of cases, although extra-abdominal injuries may be present in up to 80% of patients with blunt splenic injury.

■ SPLENIC TRAUMA IMAGING MODALITIES AND PROTOCOLS

Computed Tomography

Computed tomography is the primary modality for definitive evaluation of the spleen after blunt trauma. Contrast enhancement is necessary for optimal diagnostic performance, rendering splenic parenchymal injuries, which can be inconspicuous on noncontrast CT, visible as defects within the otherwise enhancing organ. Such injuries are best depicted in the portal venous phase during which splenic parenchymal enhancement is most homogeneous; the heterogeneity of the arterial phase spleen and decreased parenchymal attenuation in delayed phases (3 to 5 minutes post injection of intravenous contrast material) make these unsuitable for primary diagnosis of splenic parenchymal injury. Arterial phase imaging, however, can demonstrate contained splenic vascular injuries (pseudoaneurysms and arteriovenous fistulas) that may become imperceptible in later phases. Active bleeding can appear in any phase but may be indistinguishable from contained vascular injury unless CT images are acquired in more than one phase. For this reason, delayed imaging may be of value if a contrast "blush" is seen on a portal venous phase image, although late-phase CT is otherwise of limited utility for splenic evaluation. Some trauma centers routinely acquire portal venous phase images and perform immediate image review to determine whether or not delayed-phase images should be acquired; if necessary, dedicated arterial phase imaging would then require additional contrast agent injection. Other trauma centers use a primary dual-phase protocol including both arterial and portal venous phase CT imaging to optimize diagnosis of both vascular and parenchymal injuries on the admission study.

Other Modalities

Conventional radiography has limited value for evaluation of the abdomen after blunt trauma, although left lower rib fractures and displacement of the gastric air bubble from the left upper quadrant by a perisplenic hematoma can raise suspicion for splenic injury. FAST protocol US examination is limited to interrogation for perisplenic hemorrhage. Dedicated ultrasonographic imaging can certainly identify splenic parenchymal injuries but is highly operator dependent and can be time consuming. Magnetic resonance imaging is not routinely used in the setting of splenic trauma because of limited availability, increased imaging time, and restrictions on patient access and instrumentation imposed by safety considerations in the magnetic field. Because of increased use of CTA for diagnosis, catheter angiography after splenic injury is now primarily performed for therapeutic or prophylactic embolization.

Computed Tomography Findings in Acute Splenic Trauma

Computed tomography evaluation after acute blunt splenic trauma may identify various injuries, including splenic lacerations, parenchymal devascularization and infarction,

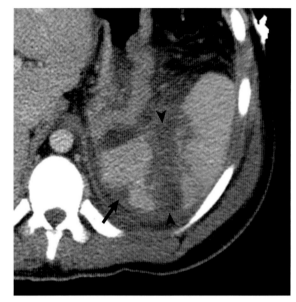

Figure 11-13 Splenic laceration and fracture. Axial computed tomography (CT) in portal venous phase shows through-and-through fracture *(black arrowheads)*, as well as a shallow laceration *(black arrow)* of the spleen.

hematomas, and vascular injuries, including uncontained active bleeding, as well as contained pseudoaneurysms and arteriovenous fistulas. These various lesions can all be diagnosed by contrast-enhanced CT, but their appearance and conspicuity vary in different phases; in some cases comparison between phases at the exact same anatomic location is necessary for accurate characterization.

■ SPLENIC INJURIES

Lacerations

Lacerations are the most common traumatic injury of the spleen. On postcontrast CT, lacerations typically appear as linear or branching areas of abnormal low attenuation within the otherwise enhancing spleen. Lacerations are most conspicuous in the portal venous phase, when intact splenic parenchymal enhancement is most homogeneous and intense. Splenic lacerations may be partial or full thickness; through-and-through lacerations may be termed *fractures* (Fig. 11-13). Lacerations may or may not violate the splenic capsule; perisplenic hematoma suggests capsular disruption unless there is another likely source of hemorrhage. Laceration depth should be measured perpendicular to the splenic surface, although length can be assessed in any plane.

Infarctions

Sharply marginated geographic areas of splenic parenchymal nonenhancement typically extending to the capsule indicate devascularization resulting in infarction (Fig. 11-14). Acute infarctions are edematous and may appear slightly bulky compared to intact portions of the spleen, whereas chronic infarctions become atrophic. Posttraumatic splenic infarctions can be of any size and number; it is useful to estimate the approximate percentage of

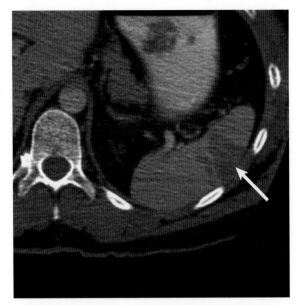

Figure 11-14 Splenic segmental infarction. Axial computed tomography (CT) in portal venous phase demonstrates a well-defined triangular area of low attenuation extending to the splenic periphery *(white arrow)*, consistent with segmental infarction.

splenic involvement by sizable infarctions. Hilar vascular injury or avulsion can result in total splenic infarction (Fig. 11-15).

Hematomas

Acute hematomas from blunt trauma in and around the spleen show intermediate attenuation (40 to 70 HU). Hematomas are therefore slightly higher in attenuation than intact splenic parenchyma on noncontrast CT but are lower in attenuation than perfused splenic tissue on portal venous phase postcontrast CT. Splenic intraparenchymal hematomas may be distinguished from lacerations and infarcts by their typically rounded or ovoid shape with associated mass effect (Fig. 11-16). Their maximum diameter should be reported. Splenic subcapsular hematomas accumulate at the splenic periphery but are constrained by an intact overlying capsule. They exert mass effect on the underlying splenic parenchyma, resulting in a characteristic crescentic or lenticular form (Fig. 11-17). Maximal hematoma thickness should be reported. Perisplenic hematoma suggests underlying splenic injury with capsular disruption, but it must be kept in mind that hemoperitoneum from a remote source can also pool around the spleen. The term *sentinel clot* refers to the finding of the highest-attenuation

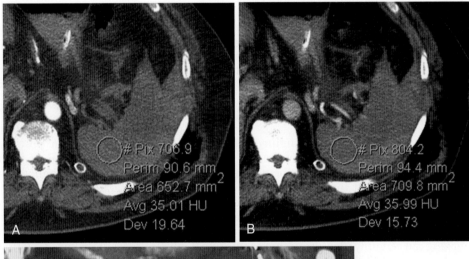

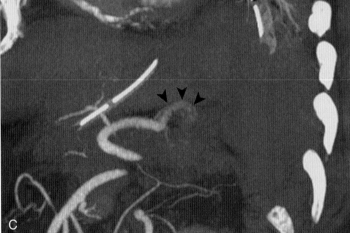

Figure 11-15 Splenic hilar arterial injury with splenic devascularization. Axial computed tomography (CT) in arterial (**A**) and portal venous (**B**) phases demonstrates complete absence of splenic parenchymal enhancement; a coronal arterial phase maximum intensity projection (MIP) image (**C**) shows loss of enhancement within the distal splenic artery *(black arrowheads)*.

hematoma near the site of bleeding in the setting of hemoperitoneum after blunt abdominal trauma. Perisplenic sentinel clot is therefore highly suspicious for underlying splenic injury (Fig. 11-18).

Splenic Vascular Injuries

Blunt traumatic disruption of intrasplenic arteries can result in contained or uncontained arterial hemorrhage. Contained splenic arterial injuries include pseudoaneurysms and arteriovenous fistulas, whereas uncontained splenic arterial injury is manifest as frank active bleeding. Both types of injury are visible on postcontrast CT as extravasation of contrast-enhanced blood resulting in focal accumulation of contrast agent outside of intact vessel contours. The term *contrast blush* is commonly used for such lesions but is not specific for contained versus uncontained extravasation.

Uncontained active bleeding can be confidently diagnosed by single-phase CT when the extravasated blood tracks beyond the confines of the spleen, spilling into the peritoneal cavity (Fig. 11-19). Uncontained intrasplenic active bleeding, however, can have the same appearance as contained intrasplenic arterial injury in a single phase, both appearing as foci of intrasplenic contrast extravasation, requiring multiphase CT for distinction.

Uncontained intrasplenic arterial bleeding (Fig. 11-20) typically increases in volume and changes in form on sequentially obtained CT images, reflecting the ongoing active extravasation. The shape of the extravascular collection is often linear or irregular. Intrasplenic active bleeding may progress to extrasplenic (intraperitoneal) hemorrhage on subsequent phases during a single CT study. The extravasated enhanced blood is no longer in continuity with the vascular system, and so its attenuation does not wash out with time, although it may decrease by dilution into an accompanying hematoma.

Contained intrasplenic arterial injuries (Fig. 11-21), which may include intrasplenic pseudoaneurysms as well as arteriovenous fistulas, appear as rounded or ovoid foci of contrast enhancement with attenuation matching (not less than 10 HU) that of intra-arterial blood, regardless of the acquisition phase, because these lesions remain in communication with the vascular system. Therefore sequential CT imaging of a

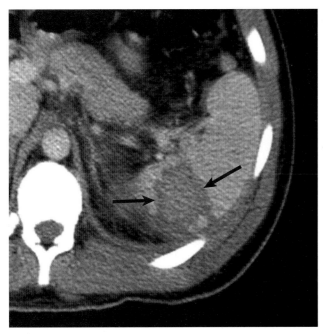

Figure 11-16 Intrasplenic hematoma. Axial computed tomography (CT) in portal venous phase shows a bulky collection of nonenhancing material expanding a splenic laceration *(black arrows)*, consistent with intrasplenic hematoma.

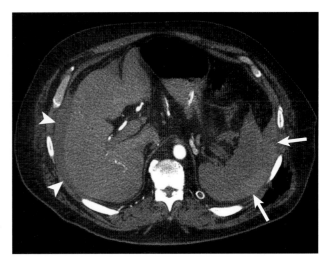

Figure 11-18 Perisplenic sentinel clot. Axial computed tomography (CT) in arterial phase demonstrates perihepatic hemoperitoneum *(arrowheads)*, as well as more hyperattenuating perisplenic sentinel clot *(white arrows)*.

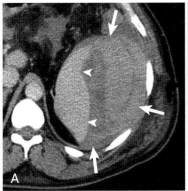

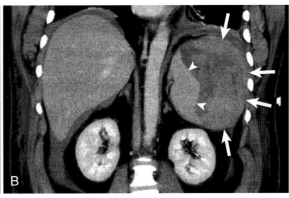

Figure 11-17 Subcapsular splenic hematoma. Axial **(A)** and coronal **(B)** portal venous phase computed tomography (CT) images demonstrate compressive deformation of splenic parenchyma *(white arrowheads)* by an acute subcapsular hematoma *(white arrows)*.

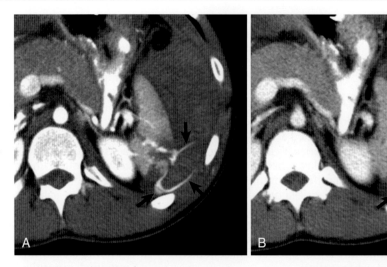

Figure 11-19 Splenic active bleeding with extravasation into the peritoneal compartment. Axial computed tomography (CT) in arterial phase (A) demonstrates extravasation of contrast material into a perisplenic hematoma *(black arrows)*, constituting uncontained active bleeding into the peritoneal compartment. Portal venous phase (B) demonstrates persistent, increased extravasation *(black arrows)* without washout of hyperattenuation.

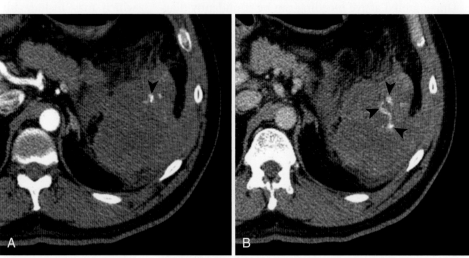

Figure 11-20 Intrasplenic active bleeding. Axial computed tomography (CT) in arterial phase (A) shows a tiny intrasplenic focus of contrast extravasation *(black arrowhead)* within the spleen, which could represent active bleeding or a contained injury such as a pseudoaneurysm. Portal venous phase (B) shows increase in volume of extravasated blood *(black arrowheads)* without washout of hyperattenuation.

contained intrasplenic arterial injury will demonstrate arterial phase enhancement followed by washout of contrast material synchronous with decreasing arterial attenuation. The lesion may become indistinguishable from surrounding parenchyma in the portal venous or delayed phases, depending on lesion size (which affects contrast transit). Early splenic venous enhancement in association with such a lesion is specific for arteriovenous fistula (Fig. 11-22), but this finding is infrequently observed on CT and so these cannot usually be distinguished from pseudoaneurysms. The distinction is of limited clinical significance because catheter angiography is indicated in either case.

Splenic Injury Scoring

Numerous clinical, surgical, and radiologic systems exist for grading the severity of injury after trauma. Splenic injury grading scales allow the summarization of multiple features of injury as a single score. Such simplification facilitates rapid communication and is of value to subsequent research investigations but can also obscure clinically important detail. Although no currently available system can be relied upon as the sole determinant of patient management, splenic injury grading based

on CT does factor into clinical decision making and is a component of many institutional trauma management protocols. Two different splenic injury grading scales are discussed in the following sections (Table 11-6).

American Association for the Surgery of Trauma Scale

The most widely used system for grading the severity of blunt splenic trauma is the American Association for the Surgery of Trauma (AAST) Spleen Injury Scale, which was developed to facilitate clinical investigation and outcomes research but is frequently used as a factor in determining clinical management in the acute setting. This is a surgical grading system but can (with some limitations) be applied based on CT findings after blunt splenic injury. The AAST splenic injury grade is determined by the depth of splenic lacerations, the surface area occupied by subcapsular hematomas, the maximum diameter of intraparenchymal hematomas, and the extent of devascularization (infarction), as well as the presence of expanding or ruptured hematoma; splenic fragmentation ("shattered spleen") or complete devascularization constitutes the highest grade of injury. Multiple lacerations and hematomas advance the injury grade by one, up to grade III. Computed tomography

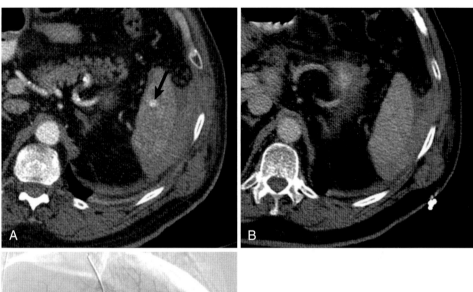

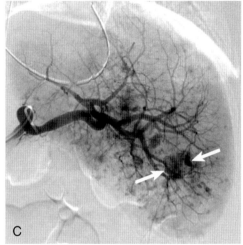

Figure 11-21 Intrasplenic pseudoaneurysm. Axial computed tomography (CT) in arterial phase (**A**) demonstrates a small rounded collection of contrast *(black arrow)* within the spleen, which could represent active bleeding or a contained injury such as a pseudoaneurysm. Portal venous phase (**B**) shows decreased lesion attenuation (washout) without increase in size or change in shape, consistent with a contained vascular injury. Catheter angiography (**C**) demonstrates intrasplenic pseudoaneurysm *(white arrows)*.

findings of contained vascular injury or uncontained active bleeding do not directly affect the AAST grade. The primary advantage of using the AAST scale to grade splenic injury identified on CT is the near-universal familiarity of trauma surgeons with the AAST system, facilitating the goal of clear communication between the radiologist and the treating physician.

Modified Computed Tomography Classification

Despite its wide use by radiologists, the AAST scale was not designed as an imaging-based system, which limits its application to CT findings after blunt splenic trauma. Most importantly, the CT findings of contained vascular injury and uncontained active bleeding, which have clinical and prognostic significance, are not accounted for by AAST scoring. To address these shortcomings, alternative CT-based grading systems have been developed as CT has gained dominance as the primary modality for trauma imaging. A recently proposed system closely mirrors the AAST scale for grades 1 through 3 to maintain legibility but assigns the finding of intrasplenic vascular injury the new grade of 4a, and the finding of active bleeding into the peritoneal compartment the new grade of 4b. Splenic fragmentation ("shattered spleen") is considered a grade 4a injury by this particular scale, which does not include

a grade 5 and does not explicitly address the finding of parenchymal devascularization.

Fine Points of Splenic Injury Grading

Splenic injury grade is frequently used as one of the many factors determining clinical management after trauma, but it has limited predictive value regarding the need for specific interventions and the potential for failure of nonoperative management in any given case. The CT diagnoses of contained and uncontained arterial injury, which are included in the CT scale but not in the AAST scale, are proven risk factors for ongoing splenic hemorrhage requiring intervention and should be clearly described in the radiologist's report, as well as being emergently communicated directly to the trauma team. Reporting a grade for splenic injury may improve the clarity of communication between the radiologist and the surgeon; however, because AAST and CT scale grades for a given splenic injury may not be concordant because of differences between the two systems, the radiologist should indicate not only the numeric grade but also which system has been used, as well as providing a full detailed description of the injuries themselves.

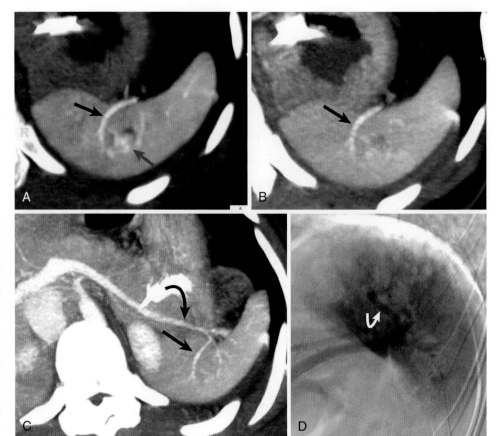

Figure 11-22 Splenic arteriovenous fistula. Axial computed tomography (CT) in arterial phase (**A**) demonstrates a focus of intrasplenic contrast extravasation *(red arrow)* and a prominent adjacent vessel *(black arrow)*. I portal venous phase (**B**) the vessel persists *(black arrow)* while the extravasation is no longer apparent, indicating that it is a contained vascular injury. A maximum intensity projection (MIP) CT image (**C**) reveals that the prominent vessel *(black arrow)* is a draining vein leading to the main splenic vein *(curved black arrow)*. Catheter angiogram (**D**) confirms early appearance of the intrasplenic draining vein *(curved white arrow)*, indicating arteriovenous fistula.

Table 11-6   Splenic Injury Grading by Type of Splenic Injury: Criteria of the AAST Scale* Compared to a Modified Computed Tomography–Based System†

AAST Grade	Laceration	Hematoma	Vascular Injury	CT Grade
I	<1 cm depth	Subcapsular < 10% surface area (AAST) or < 1 cm thick (CT)	—	1
N/A	—	Intraparenchymal < 1 cm diameter	—	1
II	1-3 cm depth	Subcapsular 10%-50% surface area (AAST) or 1-3 cm thick (CT)	—	2
II	—	Intraparenchymal < 5 cm (AAST) or 1-3 cm (CT) diameter	—	2
III	>3 cm depth	Subcapsular > 50% surface area (AAST) or > 3 cm thick (CT)	—	3
III	—	Intraparenchymal > 5 cm (AAST) or > 3 cm diameter (CT)	—	3
III	—	Expanding or ruptured hematoma (AAST) or splenic capsular disruption (CT)	—	3
IV	laceration involving hilar or segmental vessel	—	>25% devascularization	N/A
V	—	—	Total devascularization	N/A
V	"Shattered spleen"	—	—	4a
N/A	—	—	Contained or uncontained intrasplenic arterial injury (pseudoaneurysm, arteriovenous fistula, intrasplenic or subcapsular active bleeding)	4a
N/A	—	—	Active intraperitoneal bleeding	4b

†Data from TraumaSource, The American Association for the Surgery of Trauma, http://www.aast.org/library/traumatools/injuryscoringscales.aspx#spleen.

‡Data from Marmery H, Shanmuganathan K, Alexander M, et al. Optimization of selection for nonoperative management of blunt splenic injury: comparison of MDCT grading systems. *AJR Am J Roentgenol.* 2007;189:1421-1427.

AAST, American Association for the Surgery of Trauma; *CT,* computed tomography; *N/A,* not applicable.

■ IMAGING PEARLS AND PITFALLS IN BLUNT SPLENIC TRAUMA

Overdiagnosis and Underdiagnosis of the Arterial Phase Spleen

Peculiarities of splenic perfusion result in marked heterogeneity of parenchymal enhancement in the arterial phase (Fig. 11-23). The resulting interspersed areas of hypoattenuation and hyperattenuation can convincingly mimic the appearance of an injured spleen and can as readily obscure real parenchymal disruptions. If only arterial phase CT images have been obtained, interpretation should be cautious, and repeat study for acquisition of portal venous phase images may be necessary.

Underdiagnosis of Injury in Delayed Phase (3 to 5 Minutes Post Injection of Intravenous Contrast)

Normal splenic parenchymal enhancement becomes and remains homogeneous by the portal venous phase; subsequently, decreasing parenchymal attenuation diminishes the conspicuity of nonenhancing splenic injuries in later phases. Even perisplenic hematoma may become difficult to distinguish on delayed CT (Fig. 11-24). If only delayed-phase CT images have been obtained, interpretation should be cautious, and repeat study for acquisition of portal venous phase images may be necessary.

Preserved Splenic Parenchymal Islands

Small areas of parenchyma can remain intact within an otherwise devascularized portion of the spleen. These perfused splenic islands appear as relatively high attenuation areas and can be misinterpreted as foci of vascular contrast extravasation (Fig. 11-25). The distinction can be made by discerning that such islands follow the enhancement pattern of other intact portions of the spleen; evaluation of multiple phases is helpful in such cases. Diagnosis of contrast extravasation should be confirmed by checking that the attenuation of the contrast blush is close to or higher than that of intravascular contrast in the same phase.

Other Artifacts and Normal Structures Mimicking Splenic Injury

Developmental lobulations may persist in the mature spleen as visible clefts, which can be confused with

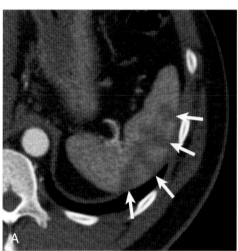
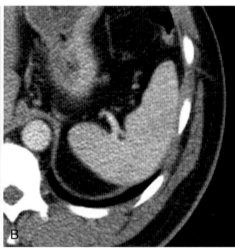

Figure 11-23 Splenic parenchymal heterogeneity in arterial phase. Axial computed tomography (CT) in arterial phase (**A**) shows multiple linear areas of low attenuation *(white arrows)* that cannot be distinguished from lacerations. Portal venous phase (**B**) demonstrates normal parenchymal enhancement with no residual defect to indicate injury.

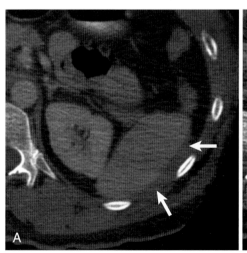
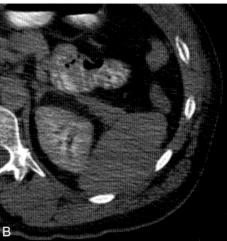

Figure 11-24 Perisplenic blood obscured on delayed imaging. Axial computed tomography (CT) in portal venous phase (**A**) demonstrates perisplenic hematoma *(white arrows)*, which is lower in attenuation than the enhancing spleen. On delayed phase imaging (**B**), splenic attenuation has decreased such that the perisplenic blood is much less conspicuous and could be overlooked.

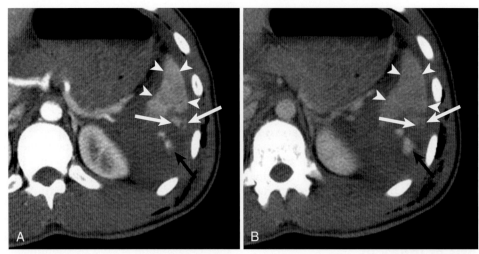

Figure 11-25 Splenic parenchymal island. Axial computed tomography (CT) in arterial phase (**A**) shows intact anterior pole splenic paren-chyma *(white arrowheads)* with an adjacent isolated perfused parenchymal island *(white arrows)*, which could be mistaken for extravasation; note, however, that its attenuation matches that of adjacent parenchyma, in contradistinction to a true focus of contrast extravasation *(black arrow)* within the devascularized area of the spleen. In portal venous phase (**B**) the isolated fragment *(white arrows)* is unchanged in size and shape and continues to match the attenuation of intact spleen *(white arrowheads)*, while the extravasated contrast remains hyperdense but has increased in volume *(black arrow)*, consistent with active bleeding.

splenic lacerations. Splenic clefts appear as smoothly marginated indentations of the splenic surface with nor-mal parenchymal enhancement and an intact overlying capsule clearly defined by adjacent extrasplenic fat (Fig. 11-26). Multiplanar and volume-rendered reformatted images should be used in problematic cases.

Artifact resulting from dense structures, including overlying ribs and devices, can produce linear bands of low attenuation through the spleen that can be mistaken for lacerations (Fig. 11-27). Such artifacts can best be identified by confirming their correlation with the over-lying structure and in some cases their extension outside the spleen. Respiratory motion can result in blurring or duplication of the splenic outline, which can mimic perisplenic hematoma; the presence of similar artifacts elsewhere on the same scan and the altered appearance in other respiratory phases are clarifying features.

Nontraumatic Splenic Lesions

Nontraumatic low-attenuation lesions in the spleen, including cysts and other masses, can be mistaken for injuries. The typically round or ovoid shape and often distinct margins of such lesions may aid in their distinc-tion from lacerations or contusions. Enhancing lesions are less common but may prompt erroneous diagnosis of contrast blush, as can intrasplenic calcification. Evalu-ation of lesion appearance in multiple phases is helpful. In all cases, comparison to prior imaging, if available, may allow the most confident diagnosis.

■ FOLLOW-UP AND COMPLICATIONS OF SPLENIC TRAUMA

The goals of therapy for blunt splenic injury are control of hemorrhage and preservation of splenic function. As in the immediate posttrauma setting, CT is the mainstay of follow-up imaging, regardless of the treatment strat-

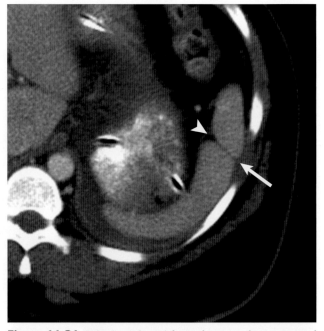

Figure 11-26 Splenic cleft. Axial portal venous phase computed tomography (CT) shows a splenic cleft contacted laterally by unrelated perisplenic blood *(white arrow)*, which could result in misdiagnosis of laceration, but demarcated medially by perisplenic fat *(white arrow-head)*, which delineates the typical smooth rounded margins.

egy employed. Ultrasound examination may be used in some cases, depending upon institutional expertise. Repeat imaging after splenic trauma is most frequently requested for suspected ongoing or recurrent bleeding, which can occur after splenic embolization, splenor-rhaphy, or even splenectomy, as well as in the nonop-eratively managed patient. Computed tomography performed for this reason can use the same trauma pro-tocol (using both arterial and portal venous phase imag-ing through the solid organs) as the initial examination.

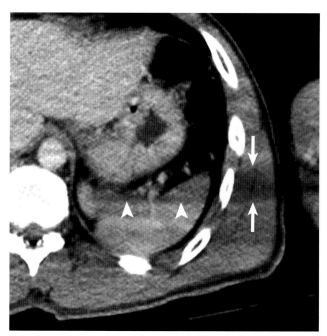

Figure 11-27 Splenic beam-hardening artifact. Axial portal venous phase computed tomography (CT) demonstrates bands of linear low attenuation within the spleen *(white arrowheads)*, which could be mistaken for lacerations but can be identified as artifactual by their uniformity and more conclusively by their extension beyond the spleen *(white arrows)*. In this case the patient's arm accounts for the beam-hardening effect.

The study is interpreted in the same fashion, with evaluation for splenic parenchymal disruption, contained vascular injuries, and active bleeding. Assessment must also include determination of whether or not there appears to have been interval recurrent intraabdominal hemorrhage based on comparison of hemoperitoneum volume versus the initial scan. Initially missed injuries to structures other than the spleen should be searched for on any such study. Repeat CT may also be indicated to investigate other developments, including splenic infarction, infection, and surgical complications. There are no absolute indications for follow-up imaging in the asymptomatic patient recovering from splenic injury; practice patterns vary depending on patient age, severity of injury, and local preference.

■ IMAGING STATUS POST MANAGEMENT

Nonoperative

Nonoperative management is the reference standard of care for hemodynamically stable patients with splenic injury after blunt trauma. The primary feared complication is delayed splenic hemorrhage (rupture). Failure of conservative management can present catastrophically with life-threatening hemorrhage requiring emergent laparotomy. Any evidence of ongoing hemorrhage or worsening pain in an otherwise stable patient being observed after blunt splenic trauma should trigger prompt repeat CT imaging using a trauma protocol. In the subacute phase, delayed hemorrhage becomes less likely, but other complications, including infarction and infection,

should be sought if repeat imaging is performed for persistent or new symptoms after splenic injury.

Angioembolization

Transcatheter splenic embolization may be performed as a therapeutic intervention for treatment of splenic vascular injury diagnosed by CT or as a prophylactic adjunct to nonsurgical management due to the very high clinical failure rate in high-grade splenic injury (grades IV and V) even without visible vascular injury on initial CT. Selective intrasplenic arterial embolization may be required to gain control of specific injuries, but occlusion of end arteries with partial splenic infarction may result. Proximal main splenic artery embolization effectively reduces intrasplenic arterial pressure and so has utility as both a therapeutic and a prophylactic measure, with reduced incidence of infarction because of preserved collateral perfusion. Computed tomography after successful embolization, regardless of the technique used, should ideally demonstrate no new or persistent contrast extravasation. Both arterial and portal venous phase imaging should be performed in these cases to optimize evaluation of vasculature and parenchyma. If contained intrasplenic vascular injuries persist on postembolization CT, and, depending on clinical factors, small persistent lesions can be followed by short-interval CT and typically resolve subsequently without need for repeat angiography or surgery. The distal main splenic artery typically appears occluded after proximal embolization, but splenic parenchymal perfusion will be preserved (Fig. 11-28). Areas of infarction may be observed after either proximal or selective splenic arterial embolization. Less commonly, total infarction can occur. Partial or complete splenic atrophy may ultimately result. Infection is a relatively uncommon complication of embolization. Small amounts of gas within the spleen can be a normal finding shortly after embolization (Fig. 11-29). Increasing gas or fluid collection, however, should raise suspicion for necrosis or abscess formation.

Splenorrhaphy

Although nonsurgical management has supplanted spleen-conserving surgery as the most common approach to splenic conservation after injury, splenorrhaphy is still an option in appropriate cases. Splenorrhaphic techniques range from suturing to cautery or application of other topical hemostatic agents, to subtotal splenectomy. Regardless of the surgical technique employed, ongoing or recurrent bleeding is the primary early complication of splenorrhaphy. Clinical evidence of hemodynamic compromise may warrant repeat laparotomy rather than CT, but if repeat imaging is performed for suspected hemorrhage, a trauma protocol CT should be performed. An important consideration after splenorrhaphy is that some hemostatic materials, including suture pledgets and surgical mesh, may be radiopaque (Fig. 11-30) and can be mistaken for contrast extravasation on postsurgical CT. When in doubt, direct discussion with the surgical team is recommended. Gas may be seen in and around the spleen after splenorrhaphy but

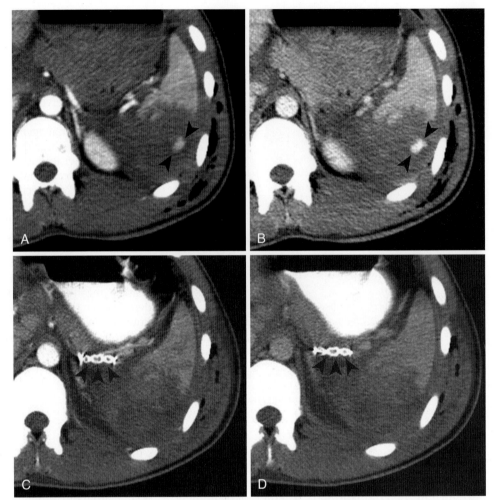

Figure 11-28 Proximal main splenic artery embolization with preserved distal perfusion. Preembolization axial computed tomography (CT) in arterial (**A**) and portal venous (**B**) phases demonstrates an enlarging focus of contrast extravasation *(black arrowheads)* within a devascularized area of the spleen. Postembolization axial CT in arterial (**C**) and portal venous (**D**) phases demonstrates metal-density embolization material in the main splenic artery *(red arrowheads)* with preservation of anterior pole splenic parenchymal perfusion but no residual contrast extravasation.

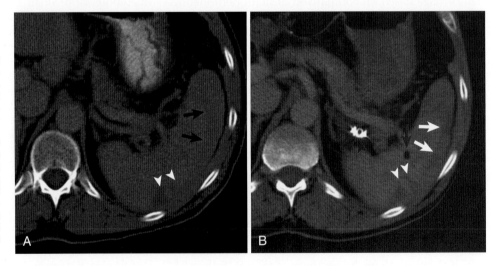

Figure 11-29 Intrasplenic gas after embolization. Axial portal venous phase computed tomography (CT) obtained at admission after blunt abdominal trauma (**A**) shows splenic parenchymal injuries *(white arrowheads)* and perisplenic hematoma *(black arrows)*. Axial portal venous phase CT obtained 3 days after proximal main splenic artery embolization (**B**) demonstrates metal coils *(red arrowheads)* with a bubble of residual intrasplenic gas *(red arrow)*; the perisplenic hematoma *(white arrows)* and parenchymal injuries *(white arrowheads)* are unchanged.

should resolve within several days. Traumatic or superimposed iatrogenic injury to the spleen may result in partial or complete splenic infarction after splenorrhaphy, which may or may not be symptomatic. Iatrogenic injury to other structures, particularly the pancreas and stomach, has also been reported after splenorrhaphy.

Splenectomy

Imaging evaluation after splenectomy may be indicated if there is clinical concern for postoperative hemorrhage or infection. Small amounts of blood and trace gas within the splenectomy bed are normal findings in the first several days after surgery. A large or increasing hematoma

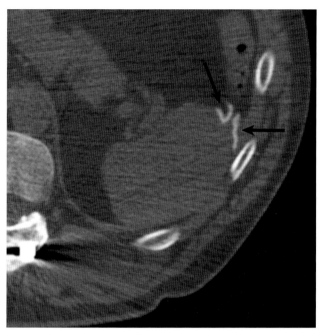

Figure 11-30 High-attenuation hemostatic material after splenorrhaphy. Noncontrast axial computed tomography (CT) image demonstrates linear high-attenuation material adjacent to the anterior pole of the spleen *(black arrows)*, representing radiopaque hemostatic mesh applied during splenorrhaphy performed for splenic injury after blunt trauma.

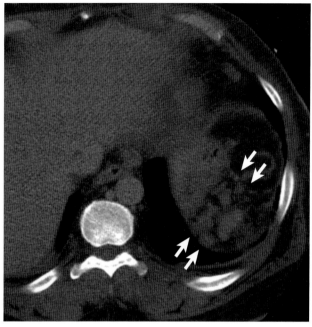

Figure 11-31 Posttraumatic splenosis. Noncontrast axial computed tomography (CT) image obtained 7 years after splenectomy for blunt trauma shows multiple ovoid nodules within the left upper quadrant, representing hypertrophic residual splenic tissue consistent with splenosis *(white arrows)*.

in the splenic fossa or worsening hemoperitoneum (not otherwise explained), however, should raise suspicion for abnormal postoperative bleeding. Other initially missed posttraumatic injuries, as well as iatrogenic injuries (particularly of the pancreas and stomach), may also present after splenectomy and should be searched for if imaging is requested for postsplenectomy pain, bleeding, or sepsis. Postsurgical infection can result in a splenic fossa abscess, which may contain complex fluid and/or gas. It is not always possible to definitively distinguish abscess from hematoma by imaging; although a perceptible wall and intralesional gas are more suggestive of abscess, an evolving subacute hematoma may develop a wall, and gas can be seen within an acute hematoma after recent surgery.

Following surgical removal of a shattered spleen, it is not unusual for small residual fragments of detached splenic parenchyma to remain vital and enlarge to form visible posttraumatic splenules, appearing as soft tissue nodules usually within the left upper quadrant (Fig. 11-31) although occasionally more distant, a condition termed *splenosis*. Preexisting accessory spleens may also increase in size after splenectomy. The splenic origin of either can be demonstrated by radiolabeled sulfur colloid imaging or by superparamagnetic iron oxide colloid–enhanced MRI.

Routine Follow-up

Routine follow-up imaging for the asymptomatic patient after splenic injury is controversial and not mandatory for any injury grade. Low-grade injuries (AAST grades I and II or CT grades 1 and 2) are rarely reimaged without

clinical indication, but higher-grade injuries are sometimes reevaluated by CT before hospital discharge. Follow-up CT may also be requested for the asymptomatic patient after splenorrhaphy or embolization, although standard guidelines are lacking. Postsplenectomy imaging is not commonly performed in the absence of specific clinical concerns.

Computed tomography is sometimes performed after splenic trauma to document resolution of visible splenic injury before a patient is given medical clearance to return to work or sport. Most splenic injuries appear healed by 2 months, but the healing time varies and can exceed 3 months for higher-grade lesions.

■ BLUNT HEPATIC TRAUMA

Hepatic Anatomy and Traumatology

The liver's large size, limited mobility, partially exposed position, firm but brittle parenchyma, and relatively thin capsule contribute to its susceptibility to blunt injury. This primarily intraperitoneal organ, which has extraperitoneal bare areas at its dome against the right hemidiaphragm and at the porta hepatis, is suspended by the coronary (including the hepatorenal) and left triangular ligaments superiorly and posteriorly and by the falciform ligament extending inferiorly along the ventral aspect of the liver to the ligamentum teres. The lesser omentum extends between the stomach and the liver from the porta hepatis to the dome. The liver receives approximately 25% of the cardiac output via a dual vascular inflow with 75% of incoming blood arriving through the portal venous system and 25% supplied by the hepatic artery. Portal vein and hepatic artery branches travel together with bile ducts accompanying the portal triads, which are surrounded by invaginations of the liver capsule, whereas the hepatic veins run separately. The large-caliber, thin-walled intrahepatic portal and systemic veins are readily torn and held open by disruption of the surrounding nonpliable liver parenchyma and can therefore contribute substantially to hemorrhage after liver injury. In blunt abdominal trauma the liver may be subject to direct impact, secondary compression, and shear forces. The right lobe is more frequently injured than the left, predisposed by its greater bulk and proximity to the relatively inflexible retroperitoneal body wall. Isolated liver injury is relatively uncommon, with associated injuries to other structures in 75% to 90% of cases. The spleen is injured in up to 45% of cases of blunt hepatic trauma. Other extrahepatic injuries associated with right lobe liver injury include right lower rib fractures, right lung base contusions, right hemidiaphragmatic disruption, and right adrenal gland and renal injuries. Injuries associated with left lobe liver disruption include pancreatic, duodenal, colonic, and myocardial.

■ HEPATIC TRAUMA IMAGING MODALITIES AND PROTOCOLS

Computed Tomography

Computed tomography is the primary imaging modality for evaluation of liver trauma. Contrast enhancement is required for optimal diagnostic performance. As is the case with the spleen, arterial phase CT imaging is limited for evaluation of parenchymal integrity because of incomplete enhancement but is of value for detection and characterization of arterial injury. Portal venous phase images are relied upon for diagnosis of liver parenchymal and portal venous injuries. Delayed (excretory) phases may be useful for characterization of vascular injuries, particularly those involving the systemic venous system, but are not suitable for primary diagnosis because of decreased conspicuity of many posttraumatic findings.

Other Modalities

Conventional radiography has limited value in the setting of suspected blunt hepatic trauma, although right lower rib fractures may be seen in cases of direct impact or crush mechanisms. FAST protocol US is used to assess for perihepatic hematoma and intrahepatic injuries, including lacerations and some vascular injuries that can be discerned by US given an experienced operator, but may require prolonged scan time. Magnetic resonance imaging is not typically used in the immediate posttrauma setting but may be of value for follow-up imaging of specific injuries. Catheter angiography after liver injury is primarily performed for therapeutic or prophylactic embolization but retains diagnostic utility for characterization of complex posttraumatic intrahepatic intervascular or biliary fistulas.

■ COMPUTED TOMOGRAPHY FINDINGS IN ACUTE HEPATIC TRAUMA

Computed tomography evaluation after acute blunt liver trauma may identify various injuries, including hepatic lacerations, parenchymal devascularization and infarction, vascular injuries including contained pseudoaneurysms and intervascular fistulas, as well as uncontained active bleeding and juxtahepatic venous injury. These various lesions can all be assessed by contrast-enhanced CT but are optimally depicted in different phases; in some cases comparison of lesion appearance between phases is necessary for accurate characterization.

Lacerations

Lacerations are the most common traumatic lesion of the liver, appearing on postcontrast CT as typically linear or stellate areas of abnormal low attenuation delineated by surrounding enhancing liver parenchyma (Fig. 11-32). Hepatic lacerations are most conspicuous in the portal venous phase, during which the attenuation difference between injured and intact liver parenchyma is greatest. Laceration depth should be measured perpendicular to the liver surface, whereas length may be measured in any plane. Preservation or disruption of the overlying capsule should be assessed; perihepatic hematoma adjacent to a laceration is good evidence for capsular tear. Laceration proximity to or intersection of structures, including the hepatic veins, portal triads, porta hepatis, and gallbladder, suggests the likelihood of their associated injury, and these structures should be carefully evaluated and specifically reported.

Devascularization and Infarction

The dual (arterial and portal venous) vascular inflow of the liver makes it relatively resistant to ischemic injury, although total interruption of both arterial and portal supply can result in frank infarction. Subtotal traumatic disruption of blood supply and/or drainage can result in altered parenchymal perfusion visible on CT as areas of geographic attenuation differences (Figs. 11-33 and 11-34), which may vary in appearance depending upon scan phase. Multiphase CT imaging is usually required to characterize such injuries, and catheter angiographic correlation may be necessary.

Hematomas

Acute hematomas in and around the liver appear as intermediate-attenuation (40 to 70 HU) nonenhancing fluid collections. Intraparenchymal hematomas lie within liver lacerations and may diffusely or focally expand the parenchymal defect (see Fig. 11-35); their maximum diameter should be reported. Hepatic subcapsular hematomas appear as crescentic or lenticular collections deep to the liver capsule, with mass effect upon the underlying liver parenchyma (Fig. 11-36). The maximal dimensions and surface area of hematoma involvement should be reported. Perihepatic hematoma

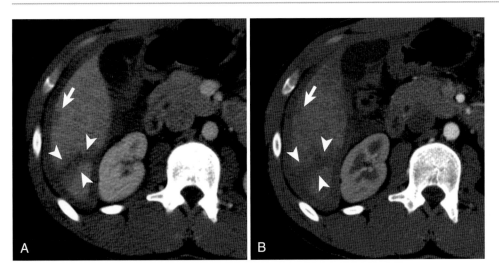

Figure 11-32 Hepatic lacerations. Axial computed tomography (CT) in arterial (**A**) and portal venous (**B**) phases demonstrates through-and-through liver laceration *(white arrowheads)* as well as a shallow laceration *(white arrow)*.

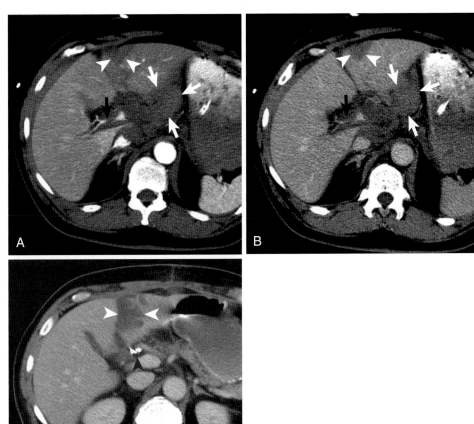

Figure 11-33 Hepatic ischemic injury from arterial disruption. Axial computed tomography (CT) in arterial (**A**) and portal venous (**B**) phases demonstrates a small triangular subsegmental infarction in the left lobe of the liver *(white arrowheads)*, surrounded by an area of arterial phase hypoattenuation that resolves in portal venous phase; the attenuated right hepatic artery *(black arrow)* is visualized with surrounding hematoma *(white arrows)*. At laparotomy an injury to the common hepatic artery adjacent to the porta hepatis was repaired. Follow-up CT (**C**) obtained 2 weeks later demonstrates metal surgical clips in the left hepatic artery *(red arrowhead)* with a residual left lobe parenchymal defect *(white arrowheads)*.

implies underlying liver injury with capsular tear, unless the blood around the liver represents hemoperitoneum from a nonhepatic source. Injury involving the bare area of the liver can result in retroperitoneal hematoma, rather than hemoperitoneum. The presence of the highest-density hematoma around the liver compared to other sites supports hepatic origin of bleeding, the sentinel clot sign (Fig. 11-37).

Hepatic Vascular Injuries

Blunt trauma to the liver can injure any of the hepatic vascular structures. Bleeding resulting from arterial, portal venous, or hepatic venous injury may be specifically diagnosed if extravasation is seen and the source vessel is identified. Both contained and uncontained vascular injuries with extravasation of blood result in a focal blush on postcontrast CT, appearing as a collection of

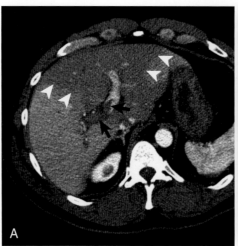

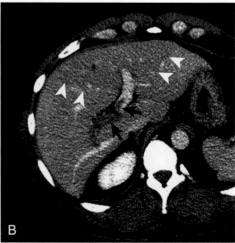

Figure 11-34 Intrahepatic portal vein injury with thrombosis. Axial computed tomography (CT) in arterial (**A**) and portal venous (**B**) phases demonstrates thrombosis of the right portal vein (*black arrows*) and an associated transient hepatic parenchymal attenuation difference manifest as a geographic area of lower attenuation (*white arrowheads*) most prominent in arterial phase.

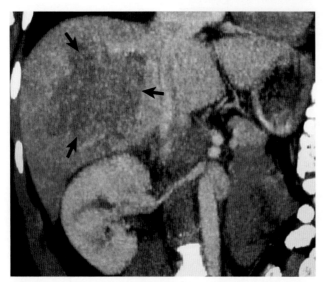

Figure 11-35 Intrahepatic hematoma. Coronal portal venous phase computed tomography (CT) image demonstrates a large intrahepatic hematoma (*black arrows*).

contrast-enhanced blood accumulating outside normal intact vessel contours. Extravasated enhanced blood extending beyond the confines of the liver, into either the peritoneum or retroperitoneum, can be confidently diagnosed as uncontained active bleeding even based on a single CT image (Fig. 11-38). Extravasation of vascular contrast within the liver can represent either intrahepatic active bleeding or a contained vascular injury. Accurate distinction between contained and uncontained intrahepatic vascular injury generally requires comparison between two CT phases acquired as part of a multiphase scan. Active bleeding results in an extravascular collection of contrast, which usually increases in size and changes in shape on sequential imaging while remaining relatively high in attenuation, even as the source vessel undergoes contrast washout (Fig. 11-39). A contained vascular injury (e.g., a pseudoaneurysm) is constrained by surrounding tissue and retains communication with the vascular system, such that extravasated blood subsequently reenters a vessel and is carried away. Pseudoaneurysms therefore exhibit attenuation values

that typically measure not less than 10 HU of their source vessel regardless of the imaging phase. For this reason, although uncontained active bleeding persists and may increase in conspicuity on sequentially obtained CT phases, contained vascular injuries will become less visible with time elapsed since contrast injection and may become imperceptible in phases performed beyond their initial appearance (Fig. 11-40).

Contained vascular injuries of the liver include intervascular fistulas and pseudoaneurysms. Arteriovenous, arterioportal, and portal venous fistulas may occur after liver trauma. Although fistulas may be less likely to enlarge and rupture than pseudoaneurysms, high-flow fistulas can cause intrahepatic systemic or portal venous hypertension and associated complications, including varix formation and variceal bleeding as well as hemobilia, and can result in high-output cardiomyopathy. Differentiation of fistulas from pseudoaneurysms is not always possible, but arterial phase CT imaging may allow identification of early enhancement of the draining vein adjacent to an enhancing artery in which a transient hepatic parenchymal attenuation difference may also be observed. Catheter angiography is usually required for accurate diagnosis and treatment.

Central hepatic venous injury or vena caval disruption may result in exsanguinating hemorrhage, even if the patient receives prompt surgical intervention. Whereas both hepatic arterial and portal venous bleeding can be brought under rapid, if temporary, intraoperative control by the Pringle maneuver (clamping at the porta hepatis), juxtahepatic venous hemorrhage cannot be easily controlled, requiring more extensive manipulation for total venous vascular exclusion, including both infrahepatic and suprahepatic caval clamping. These injuries have persistently high mortality rates ranging from 65% to 100%, although improved survival has been achieved at major transplant centers with involvement of experienced liver surgeons. Hepatic parenchymal lacerations extending to the region of the intrahepatic venous confluence and inferior vena cava should raise suspicion for injury to these structures. Perivascular hematoma, which may compress the

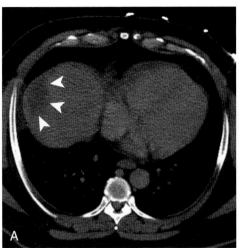
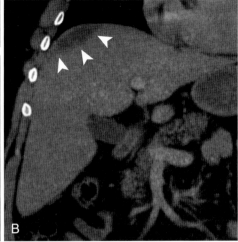

Figure 11-36 Subcapsular hepatic hematoma. Axial (**A**) and coronal (**B**) portal venous phase computed tomography (CT) images demonstrate a small lenticular hepatic subcapsular hematoma with mild mass effect compressing the underlying liver parenchyma (*white arrowheads*).

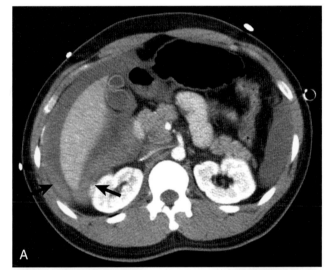
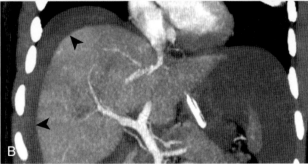

Figure 11-37 Perihepatic sentinel clot. Portal venous phase computed tomography (CT) images demonstrate higher attenuation of hematoma around the liver in axial (**A**; *arrows*) and coronal (**B**; *arrowheads*) images than elsewhere, indicating a hepatic source of bleeding.

underlying vessel, is particularly worrisome. Thrombosis may be observed, in addition to extravasation.

■ HEPATIC INJURY SCORING

Organ-specific injury grading systems attempt to synthesize and rank the key features of organ injury to facilitate communication, clinical research, and patient care. Ideally, organ injury grades would reliably correlate with clinical

outcome and predict need for specific interventions. Although the literature results are inconsistent, in practice, injury grades are used to guide clinical decision making and are incorporated into many institutional trauma management protocols. As for the spleen, both surgical and CT-specific liver injury grading systems have been developed, with different strengths and weaknesses (Table 11-7).

American Association for the Surgery of Trauma Scale

The AAST Liver Injury Scale is familiar to most trauma surgeons worldwide. Although developed as a surgical grading scale, it can be readily applied to CT findings after blunt liver injury and is the most commonly used such system. The AAST liver injury grade is determined by the depth of hepatic lacerations, the surface area occupied by subcapsular hematoma, the maximum diameter of intraparenchymal hematomas, and the extent of parenchymal disruption (maceration or devascularization) based on hepatic segmental and lobar anatomy; juxtahepatic venous injury is a separate consideration, and complete hepatic avulsion constitutes the highest injury grade. Multiple lacerations and hematomas advance the injury grade by one, up to grade III. Direct CT evidence of vascular injury, including identification of contained or uncontained extravasation, is not accounted for by this scale and does not affect the AAST grade.

Modified Computed Tomography Classification

The first CT-specific system for grading blunt liver injury was adapted directly from the AAST scale with little modification and can be used almost interchangeably. The only significant deviations from the surgical system are the inclusion of focal periportal blood tracking in the region of hepatic injury as a grade 1 lesion and the omission of juxtahepatic venous injury. This early system, however, like the AAST scale, does not account for direct CT evidence of vascular injury. A recently published report supports the incorporation of contrast extravasation, as well as other potentially salient imaging findings, such as the presence

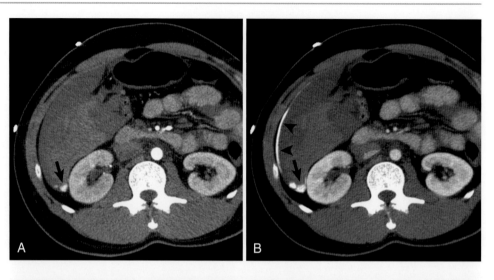

Figure 11-38 Hepatic active bleeding into the peritoneal compartment. Axial arterial phase computed tomography (CT) (**A**) demonstrates a focus of contrast extravasation at the periphery of the right hepatic lobe *(black arrow)*. Axial portal venous phase CT (**B**) demonstrates increased extravasation *(black arrow)* also tracking outside the liver *(black arrowheads)*, consistent with uncontained active bleeding into the peritoneum.

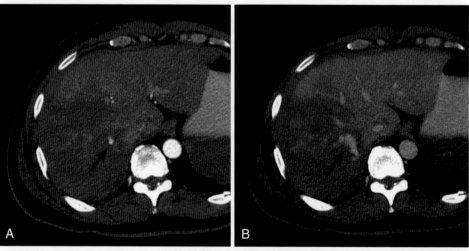

Figure 11-39 Intrahepatic active bleeding. Axial arterial phase computed tomography (CT) image (**A**) shows a tiny focus of extravascular contrast extravasation within the right lobe of the liver *(black arrow)*. Axial portal venous phase CT (**B**) shows increase in volume of extravasated blood *(black arrow)* without washout, consistent with active bleeding.

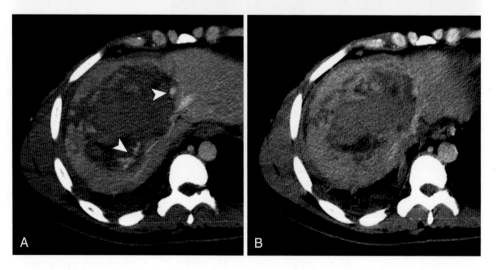

Figure 11-40 Intrahepatic pseudoaneurysms. Axial portal venous phase computed tomography (CT) (**A**) shows a large intrahepatic hematoma with tiny nodular foci of peripheral contrast extravasation *(white arrowheads)*. Delayed-phase CT at the same level (**B**) demonstrates decreased conspicuity of the lesions, which have not increased in size or changed in shape, typical of pseudoaneurysms.

of sentinel clot, into the structure of a proposed novel CT liver injury grading system that has yet to be finalized and validated.

Fine Points of Liver Injury Grading

Contradictory reports have been published regarding the value of the AAST and correlating CT-based liver injury grades for predicting patient outcome, need for specific interventions, and risk for failure of nonoperative management. Despite the apparent limitations, liver injury grade is commonly incorporated into trauma management protocols and considered in decision making in individual cases. A numeric grade may be included in the CT report but must be accompanied by a complete description of the discrete lesions

Table 11-7 Liver Injury Grading by Type Of Liver Injury: Criteria of the AAST Scale* Compared to a Modified Computed Tomography–Based System†

AAST Grade	Laceration	Hematoma	Vascular Injury	CT Grade
I	<1 cm depth	Subcapsular < 10% surface area (AAST) or < 1 cm thick (CT)	—	1
N/A	—	Periportal blood tracking (*not* diffuse periportal edema)	—	1
II	1-3 cm depth, <10 cm length	Subcapsular 10%-50% surface area (AAST) or 1-3 cm thick (CT)	—	2
II	—	Intraparenchymal < 10 cm (AAST) or < 3 cm (CT) diameter	—	2
III	>3 cm depth	Subcapsular > 50% surface area (AAST) or > 3 cm thick (CT)	—	3
III	—	Intraparenchymal > 10 cm (AAST) or > 3 cm (CT) diameter	—	3
III	—	Expanding or ruptured hematoma (AAST)	—	N/A
IV	Disruption of 1-3 segments or 25%-75% of a lobe (AAST); lobar maceration (CT)	—	Lobar devascularization (CT)	4
V	Disruption of > 3 segments or > 75% of a lobe (AAST); bilobar maceration (CT)	—	Bilobar devascularization (CT)	5
V	—	—	Juxtahepatic venous injuries (retrohepatic vena cava/central major hepatic veins)	N/A
VI	—	—	Hepatic avulsion	N/A

*Data from TraumaSource, The American Association for the Surgery of Trauma, http://www.aast.org/library/traumatools/injuryscoringscales.aspx#liver.
†Data from Mirvis SE, Whitley NO, Vainwright JR, et al. Blunt hepatic trauma in adults: CT-based classification and correlation with prognosis and treatment. *Radiology.* 1989;171:27-32.
AAST, American Association for the Surgery of Trauma; *CT,* computed tomography; *N/A,* not applicable.

identified, with specific mention made of any evidence for juxtahepatic venous injury. Separate attention should be drawn to observation of contained or uncontained contrast extravasation.

■ IMAGING PEARLS AND PITFALLS IN BLUNT HEPATIC TRAUMA

Unenhanced intrahepatic vessels can mimic lacerations. The hepatic veins enhance later than the portal veins and will be nonopacified on arterial and even early portal venous phase CT, appearing as linear low-attenuation structures that can be mistaken for hepatic lacerations. Intrahepatic bile ducts, particularly if dilated, can similarly be confused with lacerations in any phase. Conversely, liver lacerations adjacent to unenhanced intrahepatic vessels can be overlooked. The intrahepatic vessels should be specifically identified and evaluated during image interpretation, which should prevent such misdiagnosis. The hepatic veins should be traced to the caval confluence, and the portal veins and bile ducts should be traced to the porta hepatis.

Periportal low attenuation can represent injury or edema. Linear areas of low attenuation paralleling the portal tracts may be observed on CT after abdominal trauma. Hematoma can accumulate along the portal tracts after liver injury and produce this appearance focally. This finding has been considered to represent

a low-grade (grade 1) liver injury. The more commonly observed phenomenon of diffuse periportal hypoattenuation, however, is more likely to reflect edema resulting from fluid resuscitation (Fig. 11-41), or in rare cases may be a manifestation of elevated central venous pressure from intrathoracic processes, including tension pneumothorax and pericardial tamponade. Generalized periportal hypoattenuation within an otherwise intact liver is not suggestive of significant hepatic injury.

Intact tissue in an area of devascularization can mimic extravasation. Isolated islands of perfused tissue and skeletonized intact vessels within an area of non-enhancing parenchymal injury both appear as foci of contrast enhancement that can be mistaken for extravasation, leading to false-positive diagnosis of pseudoaneurysms, fistulas, or active bleeding (Fig. 11-42). Intact vessels retain continuity with the rest of the vascular tree and can be contiguously traced to other vessels. Parenchymal islands follow the enhancement pattern of other intact portions of the liver on multiphase imaging, whereas the attenuation of contrast blush is close to or higher than that of intravascular contrast in the same phase.

Artifacts Mimicking Hepatic Injury

Streak artifact emanating from overlying ribs or devices can produce linear bands of low attenuation through the liver that can be mistaken for lacerations (Fig. 11-43) but can be correctly identified by their correlation with the overlying structure and in many cases their extension beyond the liver. Respiratory motion can result in blurring or duplication of the hepatic outline, which can sometimes mimic perihepatic hematoma. The presence of similar artifact elsewhere on the same scan and inconsistent appearance in other phases are clarifying features.

Normal Structures Mimicking Hepatic Injury

Normal hepatic fissures, including those for the ligamentum teres and the ligamentum venosum and particularly unexpected normal variant accessory fissures, have the potential to be mistaken for lacerations. Diaphragmatic indentations of the liver surface can also produce apparent peripheral linear parenchymal defects. These lesions are smoothly marginated by an intact overlying capsule delineated by perihepatic fat. Alternatively, small lac-

erations lying adjacent to any of these structures could be overlooked, requiring careful review of all obtained images, including multiplanar and volume-rendered reformats in problematic cases.

Nontraumatic Hepatic Lesions

Preexisting low-attenuation liver lesions, including cysts, can usually be distinguished from injuries by their more distinct margins and typically round or ovoid shape. High-attenuation lesions such as intrahepatic calcification and enhancing lesions such as hemangiomas can be mistaken for vascular extravasation on single-phase imaging but can be accurately diagnosed by multiphase CT. Comparison to prior imaging, if available, may be most definitive.

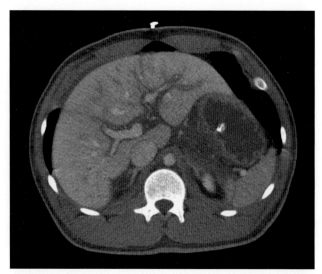

Figure 11-41 Periportal edema. Axial portal venous phase computed tomography (CT) demonstrates diffuse hypoattenuation along the intrahepatic portal tracts, consistent with edema secondary to fluid overload in this patient who had received crystalloid resuscitation after trauma but had no evidence of abdominal injury.

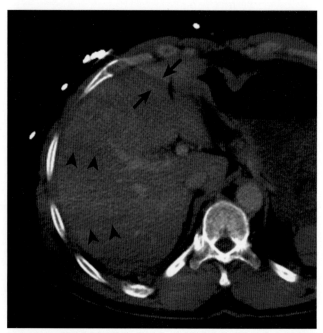

Figure 11-43 Device and rib artifacts. Axial portal venous phase computed tomography (CT) demonstrates linear streak artifact through the liver emanating from an overlying metal lead (black arrows), and more ill-defined bands of hypoattenuation representing rib shadows (black arrowheads).

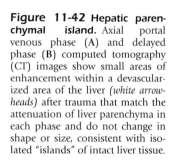

Figure 11-42 Hepatic parenchymal island. Axial portal venous phase (**A**) and delayed phase (**B**) computed tomography (CT) images show small areas of enhancement within a devascularized area of the liver (white arrowheads) after trauma that match the attenuation of liver parenchyma in each phase and do not change in shape or size, consistent with isolated "islands" of intact liver tissue.

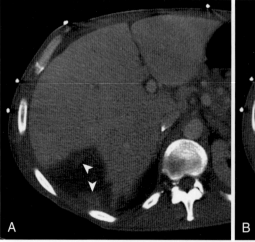

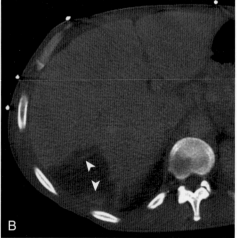

■ FOLLOW-UP AND COMPLICATIONS AFTER HEPATIC INJURY

Nonoperative management is increasingly applied to blunt liver trauma, even for high-grade and complex injury. The development and improvement of adjunctive therapeutic techniques, including angiographic embolization, biliary endostent placement, and imaging-based percutaneous drainage of sterile and infected collections, have been fundamental to the decreased requirement for surgery in such cases. The primary complications of liver injury, whether operatively or nonoperatively managed, are hemorrhage, infarction (which can result in necrosis and delayed bleeding), infection, and liver failure, as well as biliary injuries, which are discussed in a separate section. In most cases, follow-up CT performed in the first few days after injury should use a trauma protocol, and image interpretation should include a search for newly visible or previously overlooked hepatic and extrahepatic injuries, as well as for developing secondary lesions.

Noninterventional Management

The hemodynamically stable patient with liver injury clearly defined by CT and with no evidence of concomitant injury requiring surgery (particularly hollow viscus injury) can be considered for nonoperative management. Free air or free fluid not otherwise explained on CT should be considered suspicious for hollow viscus injury, but the incidence is only 1% when the liver is the only other injured organ. Computed tomography findings of hemoperitoneum and contrast extravasation from liver injury portend early failure of nonoperative management, as in the case of the spleen, although liver injuries appear more amenable to spontaneous hemostasis. Nevertheless, when high-grade liver injuries are managed conservatively, the risk for complication remains higher than for lower-grade injuries. Although early surgery will usually be prompted by bleeding, failure of nonoperative management of liver injury most often results from biliary complications.

Angioembolization

The success of angioembolic or endostent therapy for hepatic vascular injury is often reevaluated by follow-up CT after 24 to 72 hours and/or clinical findings become suspicious for failure. Computed tomography in this setting should include noncontrast, arterial, and portal venous phase acquisitions, and image evaluation should include assessment for recurrent bleeding and persistent or new vascular injuries, as well as for other complications, including parenchymal infarction, necrosis, infection, and abscess formation. Liver parenchymal infarction is uncommon after hepatic arterial embolization because of parallel portal venous perfusion, but arterial compromise alone can result in biliary necrosis. Some embolic materials, including glue agents, are high in attenuation and could be mistaken for foci of contrast extravasation. Images obtained at completion of angiography should be reviewed, if available. Small amounts of gas may be seen within the liver for a short time after embolization, but increasing gas or progressive fluid accumulation after embolization should raise suspicion for necrosis or infection (Fig. 11-44).

Surgery

Because nonoperative management has become the dominant paradigm for treatment after blunt hepatic injury, surgical intervention is now generally reserved for the most severe liver injuries. For this reason, many of the cases taken to surgery will be managed with a damage-control approach, consisting of early laparotomy with rapid systematic exploration and temporizing control of hemorrhage and contamination with expedited temporary closure of the abdomen. Prolonged surgery for definitive resection or repair is deferred until after a 48- to 72-hour period of resuscitation and stabilization. Techniques for management of hepatic hemorrhage during damage-control surgery may include application of topical hemostatic agents, electrocautery, parenchymal suturing, balloon tamponade, and perihepatic packing. Resectional débridement may be required during the initial operation or be reserved for the second-look

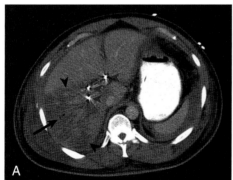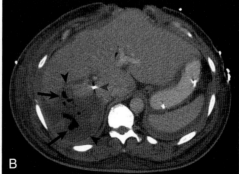

Figure 11-44 Progressive necrosis after hepatic embolization. Axial portal venous phase computed tomography (CT) (**A**) obtained 3 days after embolization of a high-grade right lobe liver injury demonstrates metal embolization coils *(red arrowheads)* and punctate gas *(black arrow)* within a geographic area of parenchymal disruption *(black arrowheads)*, all normal findings. Follow-up CT (**B**) obtained 3 weeks after embolization demonstrates an increased volume of gas *(black arrows)* within the injured area, which is liquifying *(black arrowheads)*, consistent with necrosis and raising the possibility of infection.

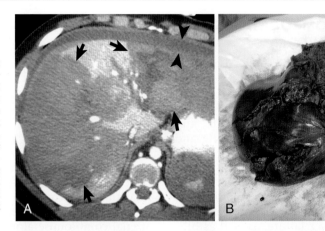

Figure 11-45 Devastating liver injury requiring transplantation. Axial portal venous phase computed tomography (CT) (**A**) demonstrates complete destruction of the majority of right and left lobe parenchyma *(black arrows)*, with perihepatic hematoma *(black arrowheads)*, caused by an industrial wrecking ball striking the patient's abdomen. The macerated liver was entirely resected (**B**), and the patient received an emergent liver transplant.

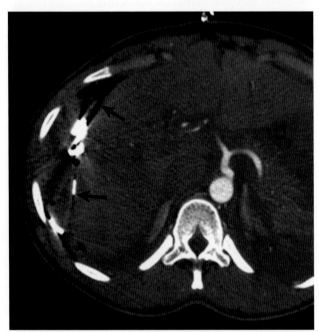

Figure 11-46 Damage-control surgery with hepatic packing. Axial arterial phase computed tomography (CT) demonstrates a perihepatic collection of gas, fluid, and high-attenuation surgical materials *(black arrows)*, reflecting perihepatic packing placed during "damage-control" laparotomy.

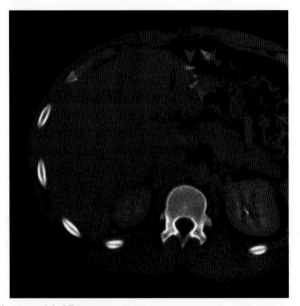

Figure 11-47 Hepatorrhaphy. Axial unenhanced computed tomography (CT) demonstrates high-attenuation pledgets along the left liver margin *(red arrowheads)* after partial resection for injury.

procedure. Rarely, catastrophic liver injury may necessitate removal of the entire organ and liver transplantation for survival (Fig. 11-45).

Early complications after liver trauma surgery include rebleeding, abdominal compartment syndrome, and hepatic necrosis from traumatic, postembolic, or ligature devascularization. Clinical decompensation in the early phase may prompt immediate return to surgery rather than repeat imaging, depending on the urgency of the clinical situation. Repeat CT may be ordered before second-look surgery for complex cases, to aid in surgical planning. After definitive surgery, repeat CT may be requested for the patient with evidence of ongoing bleeding, persistent or worsening pain, signs of infection, or jaundice.

Postsurgical CT interpretation requires reassessment for all the possible types of liver injury, with critical evaluation for evidence of interval recurrent or ongoing active bleeding and special attention to the possibilities of new pseudoaneurysm, progressive necrosis, or developing fluid collection (biloma or abscess). The radiologist must be familiar with the expected appearance of surgical interventions, including packing materials, which commonly entrain gas and can be mistaken for abscess collections (Fig. 11-46), and high-attenuation hemostatic materials such as suture pledgets and repair mesh, which can mimic foci of contrast extravasation (Fig. 11-47). Incomplete abdominal closure, often with a "Bogota bag" or negative-pressure (vacuum) dressing placement, is standard after damage-control laparotomy to reduce the risk for abdominal compartment syndrome, to allow removal of packing material, and to perform definitive repair or resection. Review of the operative notes, if available, or direct consultation with the surgeon can improve the accuracy of postsurgical image interpretation.

Routine Follow-up

If patient recovery from liver injury appears clinically uneventful, routine follow-up CT is not mandated. How-

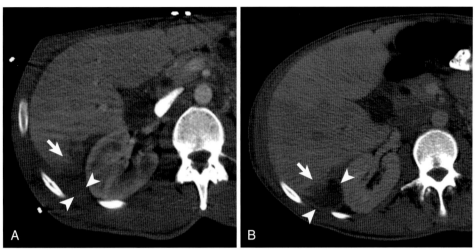

Figure 11-48 Maturing liver injuries. Axial portal venous phase computed tomography (CT) (**A**) obtained at admission after blunt abdominal trauma shows right lobe liver laceration *(white arrow)* with perihepatic hematoma *(white arrowheads)*. Follow-up axial portal venous phase CT (**B**) obtained 2 weeks later demonstrates decreased conspicuity of parenchymal laceration *(white arrow)*, with organization and liquefaction of the perihepatic hematoma *(white arrowheads)*, which has decreased in attenuation and is surrounded by a thin enhancing rim.

ever, repeat CT at 7 to 10 days after high-grade or complex liver injury may be requested in hopes of early identification of complications, either after surgical intervention or in the course of nonoperative management. In either case, reassessment of liver parenchymal and vascular integrity should be performed with attention to the development of infarction or necrosis. Abnormal intrahepatic or perihepatic collections developing on follow-up CT should raise suspicion for biloma or abscess formation.

Computed tomography may be requested before a patient is cleared to return to significant physical activity such as a contact sport, which may be considered at 3 to 6 months. Healing liver lacerations may become more clearly defined on short-interval follow-up imaging but should decrease in size over time. Maturing hematomas will decrease in attenuation and may develop a perceptible thin rim, but not thick irregular walls (Fig. 11-48). There is no validated reference indicating what extent of improvement on CT may be considered safe for such activity, so complete absence of any residual abnormality is, by default, generally the conservative end point.

Gallbladder and Biliary System Injury

Uttam K. Bodanapally and
kathirkamanathan Shanmuganathan

■ BILIARY TRACT TRAUMA

Biliary tract injury is rare, occurring in 0.1% of trauma admissions. Injuries to the extrahepatic bile ducts are difficult to detect and are associated with high morbidity and mortality, especially if diagnosis is delayed. Diagnosis of extrahepatic bile duct injury may be difficult, even at surgery, with up to 20% of injuries missed at surgery.

Biliary injuries are highly associated with liver, splenic, and duodenal injuries. Biliary injury may occur because of torsion, shearing, or compression forces.

■ GALLBLADDER INJURIES

The most common location of biliary injury involves the gallbladder, which occurs in up to 2% to 3% of blunt trauma patients undergoing laparotomy. The low prevalence may be due to protective effect of the liver. Gallbladder injuries may be classified into three main categories: contusion, laceration/perforation, or complete avulsion. Contusions are considered to be the mildest of injuries with intramural hematomas and are treated conservatively. Lacerations and perforations are full-thickness wall injuries. Distention of the bladder in a preprandial state increases the risk for rupture. Lacerations and perforations requires cholecystectomy. Avulsion injuries may involve variable portions of the gallbladder, cystic duct, and artery. Injuries associated with cystic artery transection may result in major blood loss. Cholecystectomy remains a gold standard for management of this form of gallbladder injury.

■ BILE DUCT INJURY

The spectrum of severity ranges from severe injuries such as transection or lacerations to contusion and mural hematomas. Bile duct injury is usually associated with other intra-abdominal organ injuries, most commonly blunt hepatic trauma.

Intrahepatic Bile Duct Injury

Injuries to the intrahepatic bile ducts are usually seen in patients with severe liver injuries. Intrahepatic biliary injury most commonly affects small subsegmental ducts; however, major ducts may also be injured, usually adjacent to the hilum. Biliary leakage after hepatic trauma is usually self-limiting; however, percutaneous, endoscopic,

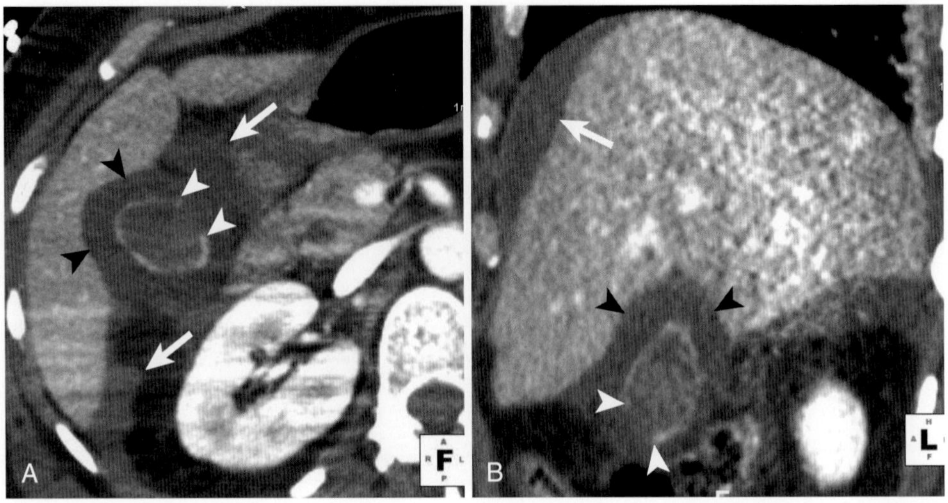

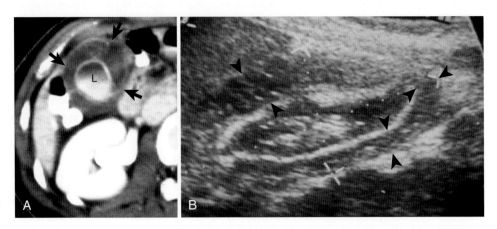

Figure 11-49 Discontinuous mucosal enhancement of gallbladder due to traumatic gangrene. Axial contrast-enhanced computed tomography (CT) (**A**) and coronal multiplanar reformat image (**B**) of the abdomen demonstrates focal nonenhancement of the mucosa *(white arrowheads)* with diffuse wall thickening *(black arrowheads)* and pericystic and right subphrenic fluid *(arrows).*

Figure 11-50 Diffuse thickening of the gallbladder wall due to contusion. A, Axial contrast-enhanced computed tomography (CT) of the abdomen demonstrates diffuse wall thickening *(arrows)* with vicarious excretion of contrast into the lumen (L). **B**, Ultrasonogram of the gallbladder demonstrated a similar finding of diffuse wall thickening *(arrowheads).*

or operative interventions may be required. Simple percutaneous drainage with additional endoscopic sphincterotomy and stenting for prolonged or high-volume biliary fistula is recommended for intrahepatic bile duct injuries.

Extrahepatic Bile Duct Injury

Extrahepatic duct injuries may occur at anatomic fixation, such as the intrapancreatic portion of the common bile duct, because of blunt impact or deceleration. Injury to the extrahepatic biliary tree is much less frequent and is very unlikely to resolve without percutaneous, endoscopic, or operative interventions. The majority of trauma-related injuries are distant to the hepatic confluence, in contrast to biliary duct injury after laparoscopic cholecystectomy. Roux-en-Y hepaticojejunostomy remains the gold standard for extrahepatic injuries. Injury within the pancreatic head is always associated with pancreatic or duodenal trauma. Treatment is predominantly related to management of pancreatic injuries.

Complications

Delayed complications due to biliary injury results from bile leak and superinfection. Sterile bile undergoes continuous peritoneal reabsorption and may lead to very few symptoms. Bile usually does not cause symptoms until infected, but when symptomatic they are nonspecific and include vague abdominal pain, nausea, vomiting and occasionally jaundice. Occasionally, bile leak can result in biloma formation both in the intrahepatic and extrahepatic locations. Extrahepatic biloma are most likely caused due to bile leak from intrahepatic bile duct injury. Injury to the gallbladder and extrahepatic ducts is uncommon sources for extrahepatic bilomas.

■ IMAGING

Gallbladder injuries and bile duct injury can be suggested with CT. Confirmation of bile duct injury can be done with hepatobiliary iminodiacetic acid (HIDA) or ERCP. Magnetic resonance imaging or magnetic resonance cholangiopancreatography (MRCP) may have a limited role because of peritoneal fluid and tissue edema due to injury, causing artifacts. But normal MRCP results essentially exclude biliary injury.

Computed Tomography

Computed tomography findings helpful in diagnosing gallbladder trauma are thickened wall (Figs. 11-49 and 11-50) with or without pericystic fluid (see Fig. 11-49).

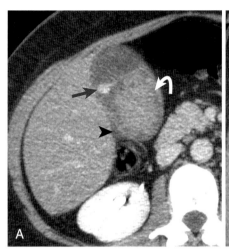
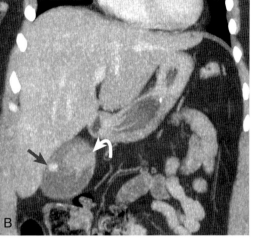

Figure 11-51 Layering blood in the gallbladder with mural active bleeding. Axial contrast-enhanced computed tomography (CT) (**A**) and coronal maximum intensity projection (MIP) image (**B**) of the abdomen demonstrate layering intraluminal blood *(curved arrows)* with focus of mural active bleeding *(red arrows)* and trace pericystic fluid *(arrowhead)*.

Thickened wall may be a highly suggestive sign of gallbladder injury but not specific for any particular type of injury. Intramural hematoma with a well-distended gallbladder may indicate contusion without perforation. Collapsed gallbladder with thickened and indistinct wall or discontinuous mucosal enhancement (see Fig. 11-49) with pericystic fluid is suggestive of perforation. Layering blood within the gallbladder lumen (Fig. 11-51) also indicates an injury but can be mimicked by milk of calcium and vicarious excretion of contrast (see Fig. 11-50). Cystic artery injuries may manifest as active bleeding or transection. Cystic artery active bleeding may result in major blood loss.

Extrahepatic bile duct injuries can be suggested with CT, which shows fluid in the subhepatic or perihepatic spaces (Fig. 11-52). Distal common bile duct injury is almost always associated with pancreatic or duodenal trauma (see Fig. 11-52).

Computed tomography of intrahepatic and extrahepatic biloma includes a low-attenuation collection in and around the liver (Figs. 11-53 and 11-54). Percutaneous imaging–guided aspiration or radiotracer accumulation during hepatobiliary scintigraphy within the collection (see Fig. 11-53) confirms the diagnosis.

Hepatobiliary Iminodiacetic Acid

HIDA is sensitive in detecting biliary leak and useful in detecting gallbladder perforation or ruptured biliary ductal system. Delayed imaging at 4 hours is essential because slow leaks may not be detected with early termination of the study.

Magnetic Resonance Imaging/ Magnetic Resonance Cholangiopancreatography

MRI/MRCP with contrast may demonstrate the same findings as those of CT with collapsed gallbladder, intramural and intraluminal hemorrhage, pericystic fluid, or thickened and indistinct wall, or discontinuous mucosal enhancement. Intraluminal hemorrhage can be mimicked by biliary stasis and sludge. Evaluating bile duct perforation with MRCP may be limited because of adjacent bilomas, hematomas, ascites, and organ injuries, all limiting the quality of MRCP. Nonperforating injuries like intramural hematomas can be evaluated with T1-weighted MRI/MRCP. Gadoxetic acid is the new hepatobiliary contrast agent that is specifically taken up by hepatocytes using the same molecular mechanism as bile acids and has 50% biliary excretion. Biliary excretion causes T1 shortening of bile and can be used for contrast-enhanced T1-weighted MRCP. This in combination with conventional T2-weighted MRCP can help in biliary anatomy and leak.

ERCP

ERCP continues to be the reference standard in diagnosis and therapy of biliary tract injuries. It may demonstrate the exact site of a leak (see Fig. 11-52) or narrowing from intramural hematoma or stricture and may allow placement of a stent across the segment.

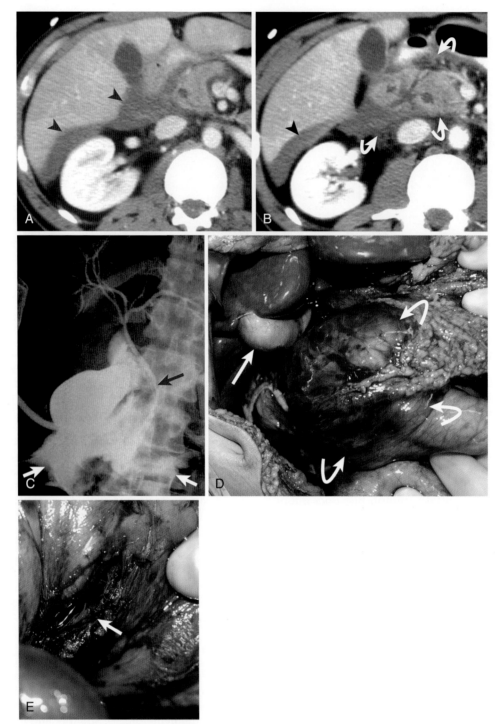

Figure 11-52 Extrahepatic bile duct injury. A, Axial contrast-enhanced computed tomography (CT) of the abdomen demonstrates fluid in the right subhepatic space *(arrowheads).* **B,** A caudal axial image demonstrates contusion and hematoma around the duodenopancreatic complex *(curved arrows)* with perihepatic fluid *(arrowhead).* **C,** Intraoperative cholangiogram demonstrates contrast leak *(white arrows)* and distal common bile duct injury *(red arrow).* Surgery confirmed avulsion injury of the distal common bile duct. **D,** Bile staining in the lesser sac *(curved arrows)* and intact gallbladder *(straight arrow).* **E,** Disconnected distal common bile duct *(arrow).*

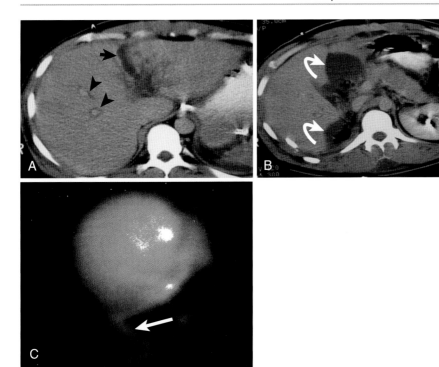

Figure 11-53 Intrahepatic and extrahepatic biloma. A, Axial contrast-enhanced computed tomography (CT) of the abdomen demonstrates intrahepatic biloma as a linear low-attenuation collection *(arrow)* with mild intrahepatic biliary duct dilatation *(arrowheads)*. **B,** A caudal axial image demonstrates extrahepatic fluid collections *(curved arrows)*. **C,** Hepatobiliary iminodiacetic acid scan demonstrated bile leak from the liver (arrow).

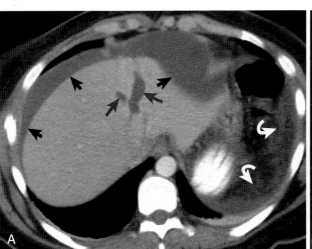 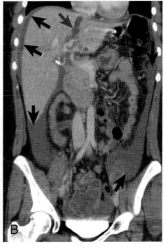

Figure 11-54 Intrahepatic and extrahepatic biloma. Axial contrast-enhanced computed tomography (CT) **(A)** and coronal multiplanar reformat image **(B)** of the abdomen demonstrate intrahepatic biloma as a linear low-attenuation collection *(red arrows)* and extrahepatic biloma with fluid in the right subphrenic and bilateral pericolic spaces *(black arrows)* and left subphrenic space *(curved arrows)*.

Pancreatic Injury

Uttam K. Bodanapally and
Kathirkamanathan Shanmuganathan

Multidetector CT is the first-line imaging tool in pancreatic trauma and has a major role in early diagnosis. Computed tomography can demonstrate pancreatic parenchymal injuries, which include lacerations and contusions; it also demonstrates additional abdominal injuries that are commonly associated with pancreatic trauma. The improved z-axis resolution of MDCT has made it possible to reconstruct multiplanar or maximum-intensity projection images, which have enhanced the sensitivity and specificity in detecting pancreatic trauma. This

section reviews the relevant imaging techniques in the evaluation of pancreatic trauma, with emphasis on MDCT as the primary imaging modality. Other modalities of imaging such as MRI, MRCP, and ERCP typically used to confirm the CT findings and demonstrate the exact anatomic site of the pancreatic ductal injuries are also discussed. Knowledge of the mechanism of injury, types of associated injuries, and the roles of various imaging modalities is essential for prompt and accurate diagnosis.

■ INCIDENCE

The pancreas is situated in the anterior pararenal space of the upper retroperitoneum, in a relatively protected zone. This location in a protected zone is the cause of the uncommon nature of pancreatic injury, with an incidence of 1% to 2% after severe blunt abdominal trauma. Only a third of pancreatic injuries occur as a result of blunt trauma; the rest are associated with penetrating trauma. Pancreatic injuries caused by blunt trauma are difficult to detect and are associated with high morbidity and mortality, especially if diagnosis is delayed. The reported morbidity and mortality rates range from 30% to 60% and 9% to 34%, respectively. Delayed complications occur in up to 20% of cases if initial injury is unrecognized. Most of the acute deaths in pancreatic trauma are due to associated injuries. In contrast, death due to delayed complications is from multiorgan failure and sepsis.

■ MECHANISM OF INJURY

The injuries usually result from severe anteroposterior compression trauma against the spinal column, deceleration trauma, and handlebar compression. Less common mechanisms include sports injuries, falls, and blows to the upper abdomen. Children are more prone to injury due to less protection by a thinner layer of peripancreatic fat and more intense transmission of energy to the pancreas. Two thirds of injuries occur in the pancreatic body, the remainder with equal distribution in the head, neck, and tail. In adults the majority of injuries are due to high-energy motor vehicle collision. In children, bicycle handlebar injuries are common, and child abuse may result in pancreatic injuries in infants.

■ LABORATORY VALUES

Elevation of serum amylase and lipase levels can be seen in up to 70% and 80% of cases, respectively. The presence of hyperamylasemia is time dependent. The results can remain normal in early stages after injury, and serial determination increases the sensitivity. The values do not correspond to the severity of injury, and an increasing enzyme level is more reliable than a single value. Hyperamylasemia was as likely to occur after pancreatic contusion as after ductal injury and hence cannot be used to determine the grade of injury. Because hyperamylasemia has been observed in the majority of pancreatic injury patients, it should be considered as a sign of probable pancreatic injury. Abnormal amylase levels associated with trauma to the salivary gland, bowel injury, cerebral trauma, alcoholism, and liver disease can cause difficulty in interpretation of the test results.

■ GRADING OF PANCREATIC INJURY

The pancreatic injury scale is based on the extent of hematoma, laceration, and the presence and location of pancreatic duct injury. Identification of a ductal injury is the single most significant predictor of morbidity following pancreatic trauma. Pancreatic injuries are classified into five categories on the basis of location and severity (Table 11-8). Determining ductal integrity is crucial to the management of pancreatic injuries. Pancreatic duct injury determines the success of endoscopic, interventional radiologic, and surgical intervention. Ductal injuries can be divided into major and minor injuries. Major injuries include complete disruption, also called *disconnected*

Table 11-8   Pancreatic Injury Scale

AAST Grade	Modified CT Grade	Type	Description
I	1, 2	Contusion Laceration	Minor contusion without duct injury Superficial laceration without duct injury
II		Contusion Laceration	Major contusion without duct injury Major laceration without duct injury
III	3	Laceration	Distal transection or parenchymal injury with duct injury to the left of SMV
IV	4	Laceration	Proximal transection or parenchymal injury with duct injury to the right of SMV
V	5	Laceration	Massive disruption of pancreatic head and duodenum

AAST, American Association for the Surgery of Trauma; *CT,* computed tomography; *SMV,* superior mesenteric vein.

pancreatic duct syndrome, in which access to the upstream duct by the ERCP guidewire will not be possible (Fig. 11-55). Minor injuries include partial disruption of the main duct or side branch disruption, in which a guidewire can be passed into the upstream duct (Fig. 11-56). Pancreatic duct injury is more common to the left of the superior mesenteric vessels and occurs when there is compression over the spine. Identifying the location and severity of pancreatic duct injury has major surgical implications. In patients with disconnected pancreatic duct, injury to the left of the mesenteric vessels is usually managed by distal pancreatectomy, and injury to the right of the superior mesenteric vessels usually requires subtotal pancreatectomy and Roux-en-Y pancreaticojejunostomy. An associated injury to the ampulla requires pancreatoduodenectomy. In patients with partial duct disruption, a conservative approach of ERCP-guided stent placement across the injury site should be attempted, and surgery should be considered after failure of conservative treatments.

Grades I and II (Minor Injuries)

Minor pancreatic injuries are parenchymal contusions or lacerations without pancreatic duct injuries. Minor superficial contusions and lacerations are frequently managed conservatively and sometimes may require drainage procedures. Extensive contusions may require débridement and drainage.

Grade III

Grade III injury involves pancreatic ductal injury in the neck or body and usually requires ERCP-guided stent placement or surgical intervention. Management of partial duct disruption can be attempted with a drainage procedure or stent placement. Disconnected duct syndrome warrants distal pancreatectomy or Roux-en-Y pancreaticojejunostomy. Distal pancreatectomy is a safe, reliable procedure with a 15% incidence of pancreatic

9

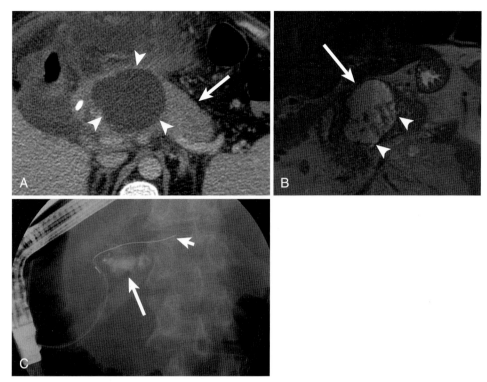

Figure 11-55 Pancreatic duct disconnection in a patient with prior episode of acute pancreatitis. A, Axial contrast-enhanced computed tomography (CT) of the abdomen demonstrates fluid collection in the pancreatic head and neck *(arrowheads)* with viable upstream segment of pancreas *(arrow)*. B, Coronal T2-weighted turbo spin echo magnetic resonance image (MRI) demonstrates the complex fluid collection in the head and neck *(arrow)* with main pancreatic duct entering and exiting the collection *(arrowheads)*. C, Endoscopic retrograde cholangiopancreatography (ERCP) image demonstrates extravasation of contrast material from the region of the neck *(arrow)*. A guidewire *(arrowhead)* could not be passed into the upstream duct of the body, hence it was not opacified.

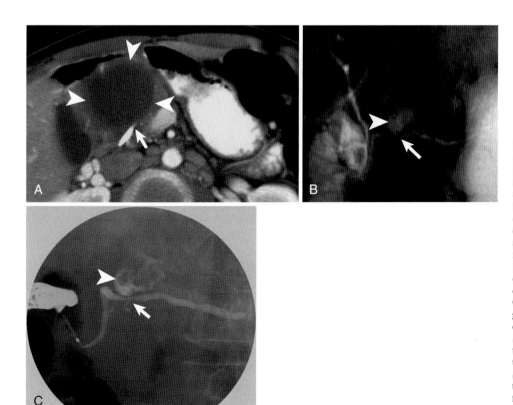

Figure 11-56 Pancreatic duct disruption in a patient with prior episode of acute pancreatitis. A, Axial contrast-enhanced computed tomography (CT) of the abdomen demonstrates fluid collection *(arrowheads)* in the pancreatic head with a pancreatic duct stent *(arrow)*. B, Magnetic resonance cholangiopancreatogram (MRCP) demonstrates a narrowed duct in the neck *(arrow)* with adjacent fluid collection *(arrowhead)*. C, Endoscopic retrograde cholangiopancreatography (ERCP) image demonstrates ductal narrowing *(arrow)* without duct disconnection. There is extravasation of contrast material into the collection *(arrowhead)* with opacification of the upstream pancreatic duct, a finding indicative of disruption of the main duct or side branch.

fistula and resultant pseudocyst (Fig. 11-57), which almost always resolves spontaneously.

Grade IV

Pancreatic duct injury is usually to the right of the superior mesenteric vessels. Similar to grade III injuries, partial duct disruptions can be managed by pancreatic duct stent

placement. Duct disconnection usually requires subtotal pancreatectomy but, unlike grade III injuries, requires pancreas preservation such as Roux-en-Y pancreaticojejunostomy to prevent the complication of diabetes.

Grade V

Grade V injury involves major destruction and devascularization of the pancreatic head. This exceptional injury requires pancreatoduodenectomy. Because these injuries are associated with other life-threatening trauma, damage control with débridement and drainage is performed in the initial stage, followed by a second-stage operation that usually involves reconstruction procedures such as Roux-en-Y pancreaticojejunostomy.

■ COMPUTED TOMOGRAPHY

Pancreatic contusions appear as focal areas of hypoattenuation in the background of normally enhancing parenchyma (Fig. 11-58). Lacerations appear typically as linear or branching hypoattenuations perpendicular to the long axis of the pancreas (Figs. 11-59 and 11-60). Direct signs of pancreatic injury include parenchymal laceration or contusion. Pancreatic injuries are also manifested on

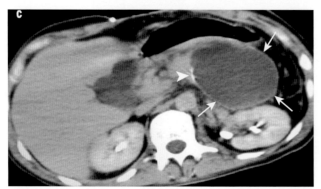

Figure 11-57 Pseudocyst formation after distal pancreatectomy. Axial contrast-enhanced computed tomography (CT) of the abdomen demonstrates pseudocyst *(arrows)* at the pancreatectomy site. Surgical sutures *(arrowhead)* are seen at the pancreatectomy site.

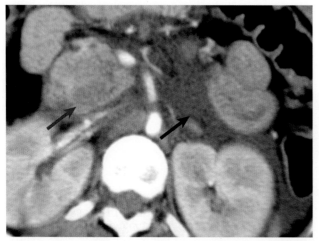

Figure 11-58 Pancreatic contusion. Axial contrast-enhanced computed tomography (CT) of the abdomen demonstrates a contusion as an ill-defined area of hypoattenuation *(red arrow)* within normally enhancing pancreatic parenchyma. Low-attenuation fluid *(black arrow)* is seen in the left anterior pararenal space.

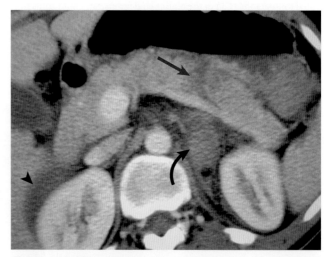

Figure 11-60 Pancreatic laceration. Axial contrast-enhanced computed tomography (CT) of the abdomen demonstrates laceration at the junction of the body and tail of the pancreas *(red arrow)* with adjacent hematoma in the retroperitoneum *(curved arrow)* and right free intraperitoneal fluid *(arrowhead)*.

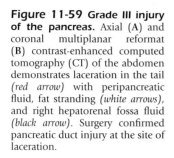

Figure 11-59 Grade III injury of the pancreas. Axial (A) and coronal multiplanar reformat (B) contrast-enhanced computed tomography (CT) of the abdomen demonstrates laceration in the tail *(red arrow)* with peripancreatic fluid, fat stranding *(white arrows)*, and right hepatorenal fossa fluid *(black arrow)*. Surgery confirmed pancreatic duct injury at the site of laceration.

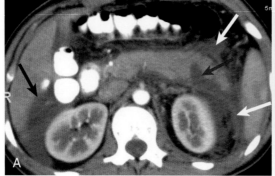
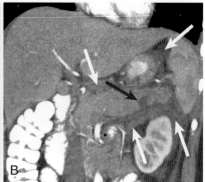

CT as focal enlargement and edema, pancreatic hematoma, and rarely active bleeding from the parenchyma. Secondary signs of injury include peripancreatic hemorrhage (Fig. 11-61) or fluid (Fig. 11-62), fat stranding (see Fig. 11-59), sentinel clot, fluid in the anterior pararenal space (see Fig. 11-58), and fluid between the splenic vein and pancreas (see Fig. 11-62). Other CT findings include thickening of the anterior renal fascia and fluid or blood in the lesser sac or along the transverse mesocolon. Isolated injuries are rare, and associated injuries, especially to the liver, stomach, duodenum, spleen (see Fig. 11-62), kidneys (see Fig. 11-61), and peripancreatic vascular structures (see Fig. 11-61), occur in over 90% of cases.

The accuracy of CT in detecting pancreatic injuries increases with time after the initial trauma because various findings are slow to develop. Computed tomography within the first 12 hours of injury may have normal findings, and repeat evaluation at 24 to 48 hours may be recommended in the presence of high clinical suspicion or abnormal serum amylase or lipase values, which may well demonstrate features of pancreatic injury that initially were barely apparent.

Computed tomography is not a reliable method for grading pancreatic injury or identifying pancreatic duct injury. False-negative and false-positive predictions of ductal injury are very common with CT. Hence CT prediction of ductal injury cannot be relied on. Pancreatic duct injury can also occur in the face of an intact pancreatic surface, which makes it all the more difficult to identify ductal injury. The degree of parenchymal injury may indicate the probability of ductal injury, with deep lacerations and full-thickness lacerations increasing the chances of ductal injury (see Fig. 11-60). Presence of full-thickness laceration should not be considered a sign of ductal injury because the pancreatic duct itself is more resistant to injury when compared to the parenchyma due to its higher tensile strength. Though there is a limited utility of CT in identification of pancreatic duct injuries in acute stages, it can suggest duct injuries after development of posttraumatic complications such as pancreatic parenchymal necrotic collections or pseudocyst formation.

■ MAGNETIC RESONANCE IMAGING/ MAGNETIC RESONANCE CHOLANGIOPANCREATOGRAPHY

Because the integrity of the pancreatic duct is the main factor determining the outcome and guiding therapy, evaluating the ductal anatomy is essential. MRCP allows direct imaging of the pancreatic duct and can help in identification of the site of duct injury. MRCP has the advantage of being noninvasive, faster, and more readily available than ERCP. MRCP with secretin stimulation (SecreFlo) has been suggested to increase the sensitivity in assessing ductal injury. Secretin induces pancreatic secretion of water and bicarbonate, resulting in temporary distension and better visualization of the pancreatic ducts. It may be preferable to scan trauma patients with suspected pancreaticobiliary injury on a 1.5 T scanner due to the limitations from magnetic field heterogeneity and standing wave artifacts caused on a 3.0 T scanner. Pancreaticobiliary injuries are rarely isolated and usually

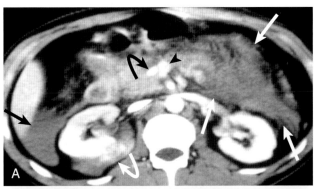

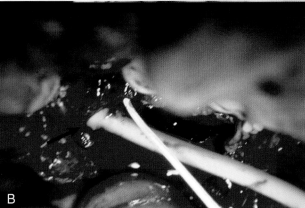

Figure 11-61 Pancreatic injury with active bleeding in a patient involved in a motor vehicle collision. A, Conventional computed tomography (CT) images show active bleeding *(arrowhead)* adjacent to superior mesenteric vein *(black curved arrow)*. Peripancreatic hematoma *(white arrows)* is seen around body and tail of pancreas. Free intraperitoneal blood in right paracolic gutter *(black arrows)* and actively bleeding right perinephric hematoma *(white curved arrow)* are also seen. **B,** Intraoperative photograph shows a Foley balloon used to tamponade hemorrhage from an injured superior mesenteric vein *(arrow)*.

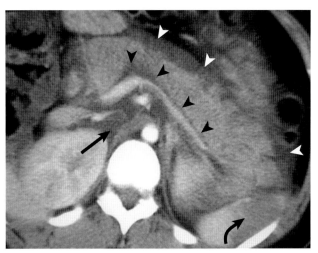

Figure 11-62 Secondary signs of pancreatic injury. Axial contrast-enhanced computed tomography (CT) of the abdomen demonstrates fluid between the splenic vein and pancreas *(black arrowheads)* with peripancreatic fluid anterior to the body and tail *(white arrowheads)* and right perinephric space *(arrow)*. Associated splenic contusion *(curved arrow)* was also demonstrated.

are associated with fluid in various peritoneal spaces, including subhepatic spaces, subphrenic spaces, anterior pararenal spaces, and the lesser sac and fluid along the transverse mesocolon. Apart from the free peritoneal fluid, these patients have significant peritoneal and retroperitoneal edema from third spacing of fluid, resulting in anasarca. The increase in field strength at 3.0 T translates into a decrease in radio frequency (RF) wavelength. The decreased RF wavelength may approximate the size of the field of view, resulting in a standing wave effect, seen more often in patients with anasarca and patients with ascites. In patients with ascites, peritoneal and retroperitoneal edema, a rapidly changing magnetic field like that in RF transmission induces a circulating electric field, and in a highly conductive medium (fluid), a circulating electric current is established. This current acts as an electromagnet that opposes the changing magnetic field, reducing the amplitude and dissipating the energy of the RF field, resulting in local regions of signal loss. Various techniques are being developed to meet such challenges.

Technique

To evaluate the pancreaticobiliary system the following sequences are used: T1-weighted gradient echo, T2-weighted axial and coronal turbo spin echo, two-dimensional (2-D) and three-dimensional (3-D) MRCP, and T1-weighted 3-D gradient echo before and after gadolinium. Secretin-enhanced MRCP is used for optimal assessment of the pancreatic ducts. Table 11-9 gives the MRI parameters for these sequences on a 1.5-T scanner.

Patient Preparation

Negative oral contrast is given to reduce the signal from the stomach and duodenal fluid. Silicone-coated superparamagnetic iron oxide particle suspension (ferumoxil) is a commonly used oral contrast. Pineapple and blueberry juice can also be used as oral contrast because of their manganese content, which results in increased signal on T1-weighted images and decreased signal on T2-weighted images. If possible, patients should be scanned in the fasting state (4 hours) to improve the exocrine response of the pancreas to secretin so that the pancreatic duct is optimally distended and visualized.

Magnetic Resonance Cholangiopancreatography Findings

MRCP can be a sensitive test for evaluating main pancreatic duct injuries but can be nonspecific for the injury and type of injury due to various factors. An MRCP image that shows a normal pancreatic duct usually excludes a main duct injury. Acute injuries are usually manifested as focal obstruction or irregular narrowing of the main duct. The low specificity can be due to the peripancreatic fluid collections that often obliterate the view of the main duct; respiratory motion artifacts, especially in trauma patients, that compromise the quality of the study, limiting duct visualization; and the technical limitations of MRCP, sometimes resulting in poor visualization of the duct in the tail. ERCP has no similar limitations. The nonspecific nature of the test warrants an ERCP in such cases. MRCP also has the advantage of providing a road map to ERCP and ERCP-guided therapy when either congenital or acquired pancreatic or ductal anomalies are present. Though MRCP with secretin has been suggested to increase the sensitivity in assessing ductal injury, its sensitivity is lower than that of ERCP.

Table 11-9   Magnetic Resonance Imaging Protocol for Pancreas on 1.5-T Magnetic Resonance Imaging Scanner

Parameters	3-D SPGR Dixon	T2 2-D SSFSE	T2 2-D STIR	T2 2-D SSFSE	MRCP 2-D Slab	MRCP 3-D	MRCP Secretin	3-D SPGRFS
FOV	400	360	360	360	290	350	290	360
TR/TE (msec)	7.47/4.76 (in), 2.38 (out)	1100/90	2900/132 (TI 150)	1100/90	2000/755	2500/691	2000/756	5.17/2.52
ST/SG (mm)	3.4/—	4/4	7	4/4	40	1/—	40	3/—
NEX	1	1	1	1	1	2	1	1
RBW (Hz/pixel)	290	475	250	476	300	372	300	300
Echo-train length	1	160	33	192	320	189	256	1
Matrix	256 × 120	256 × 192	256 × 180	256 × 192	256 × 256	384 × 346	256 × 256	256 × 144
Fat saturation	No	No	Inversion recovery	No	Fat sat	Fat sat	Fat sat	Fat sat
Respiration	Breath-hold	Breath-hold	Breath-hold	Breath-hold	Breath-hold	Navigator	Breath-hold	Breath-hold

The parameters are on Magnetom Avanto 1.5-T MRI scanner (Siemens Healthcare).
2-D, Two-dimensional; *3-D,* three-dimensional; *3-D SPGR Dixon,* 3-D nonfat-saturated spoiled gradient-echo sequence for chemical shift imaging; *3-D SPGRFS,* fat-saturated 3-D spoiled gradient-echo T1-weighted sequence for contrast-enhanced imaging; *FOV,* field of view; *MRCP,* magnetic resonance cholangiopancreatography; *NEX,* number of excitations; *RBW,* receiver bandwidth; *SSFSE,* half single-shot fast spin-echo sequence; *STIR,* short tau inversion recovery; *ST/SG,* slice thickness and slice gap.

ENDOSCOPIC RETROGRADE CHOLANGIOPANCREATOGRAPHY

Although MRCP has become the noninvasive-imaging method of choice in evaluating pancreatic duct injury, ERCP remains the reference standard diagnostic test and also the choice for guiding therapy. ERCP is indicated when there is a high suspicion of ductal injury. The ERCP findings of pancreatic duct injury include contrast extravasation (see Figs. 11-55 and 11-56), ductal stenosis or obstruction with or without contrast extravasation (see Fig. 11-56), and inability to access the upstream pancreatic duct seen in disconnected pancreatic duct syndrome (see Fig. 11-55).

A hemodynamically unstable patient usually is taken directly to surgery. A pancreatic ductogram can be performed in the operating room during laparotomy. This can be obtained either by on-table ERCP or by direct cannulation, in the presence of obvious duct disconnection or disruption.

COMPLICATIONS

Computed tomography can demonstrate acute complications such as parenchymal necrosis, peripancreatic fat necrosis, pancreatitis, and subacute complications like fistula or pseudocyst. Late complications like chronic pancreatitis or ductal strictures can also occur and can be identified by CT. A patient with posttraumatic pseudocyst is considered to have ductal injury with pancreatic leak until proven otherwise. The minor ductal injuries may be complicated with stricture formation with or without endoscopic-guided treatments, resulting in upstream duct dilatation and changes of chronic pancreatitis with parenchymal atrophy. Undetected pancreatic duct injuries invariably lead to complications. After the complications have developed, MDCT and MRI can detect duct injury more accurately by demonstrating viable pancreatic tissue upstream to the area of necrosis and persistent pancreatic fistula or fluid collection along the expected course of the pancreatic duct (see Figs. 11-55 and 11-56), despite a course of conservative medical management. When the pancreatic duct is visible, it enters the pancreatic fluid collection at an angle of approximately 90 degrees in patients with disconnected duct (see Fig. 11-55). In patients with partial main duct disruption or side branch disruption, the pancreatic duct usually makes an oblique angle with the wall of the collection (see Fig. 11-56).

Bowel and Mesenteric Injury

Uttam K. Bodanapally and
Kathirkamanathan Shanmuganathan

BOWEL AND MESENTERIC TRAUMA

Bowel and mesenteric injuries occur in 1% to 5% of major blunt abdominal trauma patients. Common modes of injury are falls, motor vehicle collisions, and automobile-pedestrian collisions. The basic mechanisms involved in bowel and mesenteric injuries in blunt trauma are shearing caused by deceleration, crushing from direct impact, and burst injuries from sudden increase in intraluminal pressure. Half of bowel injuries involve the small bowel, with colonic, duodenal, and gastric injuries occurring in decreasing order of frequency. Unrecognized bowel injuries are associated with significant morbidity, including fatal peritonitis from perforation, sepsis, and life-threatening hemorrhage. Mesenteric injuries may produce significant blood loss or may result in bowel ischemia and necrosis with resultant delayed rupture or ischemic strictures. Delayed diagnosis of bowel or mesenteric injuries, by as few as 8 hours, may result in severe complications and high mortality rates.

This section reviews the relevant diagnostic techniques in the evaluation of bowel and mesenteric trauma, with emphasis on MDCT as the primary imaging modality. Noninvasive methods of evaluation such as FAST and MDCT have led to a significant paradigm shift in the management of bowel injuries, minimizing the role of diagnostic peritoneal lavage (DPL) and laparotomy.

Physical Assessment

Physical examination is notoriously inaccurate in the diagnosis of bowel injury. There is an association between bowel and mesenteric injuries with abdominal wall injuries (wall hematoma, seat belt sign [Fig. 11-63], abdominal wall tear [Fig. 11-64], traumatic lumbar hernias [see Fig. 11-63] and traumatic abdominal wall hernias [see Fig. 11-64)]); however, the accuracy of these findings is relatively low. Seat belt sign is a transverse abdominal wall ecchymosis and may be associated with seat belt syndrome, which is a complex of injuries resulting from sudden deceleration and flexion of the upper body around the fixed lap belt. Such injuries most commonly include abdominal viscera such as the small bowel, mesentery, duodenum, and pancreas with concomitant fracture and distraction or subluxation of the thoracic or lumbar spine. Spilled blood products and intestinal contents into the peritoneal cavity may cause peritonitis, and clear clinical signs may not appear for several hours. In addition, associated neurologic injuries, intra-abdominal solid organ injuries, or altered mental status makes clinical examination difficult and inaccurate.

Diagnostic Peritoneal Lavage

In the past, to increase diagnostic accuracy in hemodynamically stable patients, four-quadrant paracentesis of the peritoneal cavity was used as an adjunct to physical examination. Although sensitive to the presence of free intraperitoneal hemorrhage, DPL is not specific regarding the quantity of blood, its site(s) of origin, or the extent of injury. Thus even relatively minor injuries that could be treated nonsurgically may produce a positive DPL result. Celiotomy on the basis of a positive DPL aspiration of 10 mL of blood from the peritoneal cavity will result in a nontherapeutic celiotomy rate of

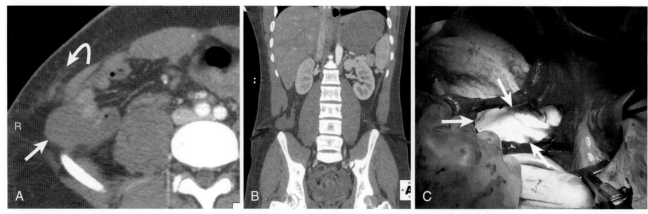

Figure 11-63 Bowel injury associated with traumatic lumbar hernia. A, Axial contrast-enhanced computed tomography (CT) of the abdomen demonstrates a right traumatic lumbar hernia associated with free fluid *(arrow)* adjacent to the distal ileum. Seat belt sign appears as subcutaneous fat stranding *(curved arrow)*. B, Coronal contrast-enhanced CT of the abdomen in the same patient indicates bilateral traumatic lumbar hernias *(red arrows)*. C, Photograph at surgery confirms segmental avulsion of the distal ileum with a large mesenteric tear *(arrows)*.

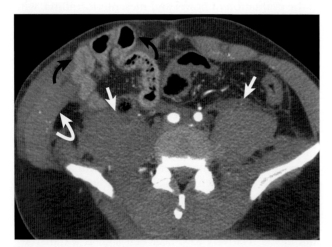

Figure 11-64 Traumatic abdominal wall tear with small bowel hernia. Axial contrast-enhanced computed tomography (CT) of the abdomen shows a segmental herniation of small bowel *(curved black arrows)* through the disrupted anterior abdominal wall musculature *(curved white arrow)* and fascia. A retroperitoneal hematoma *(arrows)* is also present. Surgery confirmed infarcted bowel due to associated mesenteric avulsion.

3% to 6%. Nontherapeutic laparotomies performed for positive DPL results have been associated with 12% morbidity and 3.5% mortality. This may have been appropriate before the era of nonoperative management of solid organ injuries, when the belief was held that every injured spleen or liver required hemostasis and repair. The availability of US, MDCT, and transcatheter angiographic embolization techniques have relegated the role of DPL to diagnosis of peritoneal hemorrhage in a small number of unstable blunt trauma patients or in patients requiring immediate surgical intervention for severe head injuries.

Bowel injuries may be missed if DPL is performed early in the hospital course (4 to 6 hours) because these injuries bleed minimally and the degree of inflammation is insufficient to generate the peritoneal leukosequestration required to produce a positive DPL finding of over 500 white blood cells/mm^3. Diagnostic peritoneal lavage also cannot assess retroperitoneal bowel segment injuries. Elevated amylase and alkaline phosphatase levels in the peritoneal lavage are also suggestive of bowel injury.

■ COMPUTED TOMOGRAPHY FEATURES OF BOWEL AND MESENTERIC INJURY

Multidetector CT is the imaging modality of choice in evaluating blunt trauma to the bowel and mesentery in hemodynamically stable patients. Computed tomography can demonstrate direct and indirect signs of bowel injury along with additional associated sold organ injuries. The results from various recent studies have shown MDCT to have sensitivity of 84% to 95% and specificity from 84% to 99% in detecting bowel injuries.

The diagnostic performance of various specific and nonspecific CT signs to demonstrate bowel and mesenteric injuries has been well described. The significance of each individual sign varies. Typically the presence of a single sign or a combination of direct and specific signs indicates a bowel injury that requires surgery. However, the presence of a combination of the signs increases the likelihood of injury.

Small Bowel and Colonic Injuries

The common sites of blunt trauma in the small bowel are the proximal jejunum, near the ligament of Treitz, and the distal ileum, near the ileocecal valve. In these regions, mobile and fixed portions of the gut are continuous and therefore are susceptible to shearing force. Colonic injuries are rare, with the transverse colon being the most frequently injured segment due to its anterior location.

Specific CT signs in bowel injury:
1. *Discontinuity of the bowel wall* occurs due to perforation (Figs. 11-65 to 11-67), and direct visualization of the defect on CT is uncommon, likely due to the small size of the defects. Such small defects are seen only at surgery with careful inspection. This particular sign has high specificity but has low sensitivity. The advances in CT technology, enabling image

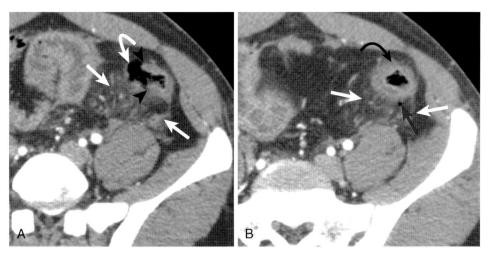

Figure 11-65 Discontinuity of bowel wall. A, Axial contrast-enhanced computed tomography (CT) of the abdomen reveals a focal wall defect *(arrowheads)* and pericolonic fat stranding *(arrows)* due to mesenteric contusion involving the descending colon. Intestinal content *(curved arrow)* is seen outside the lumen of bowel. **B,** Caudal axial image demonstrates focus of extraluminal air *(red arrow)*, colonic wall thickening *(curved arrow)*, and pericolonic fat stranding *(white arrows).*

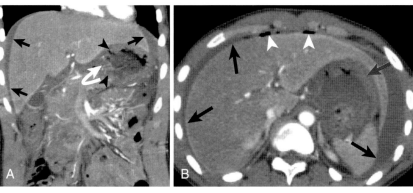

Figure 11-66 Traumatic gastric perforation. A, Coronal multiplanar reformatted image from contrast-enhanced computed tomography (CT) of the abdomen demonstrates focal wall defect *(arrowheads)* involving the gastric body with leakage of intraluminal content *(curved arrow)* from the site of injury. Large amount of free intraperitoneal fluid *(arrows)* is also seen. **B,** Axial image of the upper abdomen shows thickened gastric wall *(red arrow)*, free air *(arrowheads)* anterior to the liver, perisplenic and perihepatic free fluid *(black arrows).*

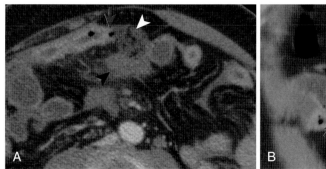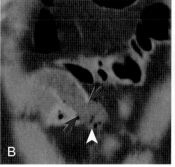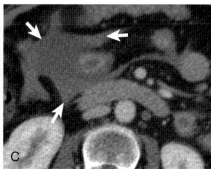

Figure 11-67 Ileal transection with bowel wall defect and leakage of enteric contents. A, Axial image of the upper abdomen reveals segmental thickening of the mid ileum with discontinuity of the wall *(red arrow)*, mesenteric hematoma *(black arrowhead)*, and extraluminal enteric contents *(white arrowhead)*. **B,** Coronal multiplanar reformat image from contrast-enhanced computed tomography (CT) of the abdomen establishes focal wall defect *(red arrows)* involving the mid ileum with leakage of enteric content *(arrowhead)* from the site of injury. **C,** Cephalad axial image verifies interloop fluid (triangular collections between the mesenteric leaves) *(white arrows).*

acquisition in thin sections, has improved the accuracy of this sign.

2. *Pneumoperitoneum and pneumoretroperitoneum* are highly specific signs of bowel perforation when certain additional criteria are met (see Figs. 11-65 and 11-66). Retroperitoneal air is usually seen in conjunction with intraperitoneal air and is seen because of the retroperitoneal course of the ascending and descending colon. The high specificity is associated with modest sensitivity (20% to 55%). The low sensitivity may be due to a lack of bowel distension at the time of trauma, limiting the transmural pressure gradient for the air to be forced out of the lumen. It may also be caused by a small quantity of intraperitoneal air, which can certainly be missed unless it is searched for using wide window settings. At times, pneumoperitoneum can be seen in blunt trauma patients without bowel perforation because of a pneumothorax or pneumomediastinum from thoracic injuries decompressing into the peritoneum or retroperitoneum, iatrogenic introduction of air into the peritoneum, or air within the bladder following placement of a Foley catheter entering the peritoneum via an intraperitoneal urinary bladder rupture (Fig. 11-68). When pneumoperitoneum is an isolated finding, it would be prudent to exclude free air from these other causes.

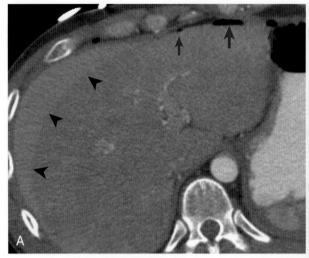
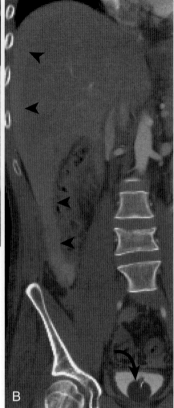

Figure 11-68 Pneumoperitoneum from intraperitoneal urinary bladder rupture. **A,** Axial contrast-enhanced computed tomography (CT) of the upper abdomen demonstrates free peritoneal air anterior to the liver *(red arrows)* and a large amount of high-attenuation urinary contrast in the right subphrenic space *(arrowheads)*. **B,** Coronal multiplanar reformat image demonstrates a Foley catheter within a minimally distended urinary bladder *(curved arrow)* and an intraperitoneal urinoma *(arrowheads)*.

3. *Extravasation of oral contrast material into the peritoneum or retroperitoneum,* if CT is performed following administration of oral contrast material, is a highly specific sign of bowel perforation, but it has a very low sensitivity (Fig. 11-69). Extravasated oral contrast material can be confused with active bleeding and contrast-opacified urine in patients with urinoma (see Fig. 11-68). Reviewing delayed images at the same anatomic location and measuring the attenuation values of extravasated contrast material and comparing the attenuation values of contrast material within the adjacent vascular, urinary, or gastrointestinal system can help to determine the exact source of contrast leak.

4. *Abnormal bowel wall enhancement, segmental lack of enhancement* (Figs. 11-70 and 11-71), *or decreased enhancement* (Fig. 11-72) of bowel is highly suggestive of devascularization of a segment, resulting in ischemia and infarction. Unlike diminished or complete lack of enhancement, hyperenhancement of the bowel wall is a nonspecific finding. Focal nonenhancement or hypoenhancement of the wall can be seen following perforation (Fig. 11-73). Focal hyperenhancement can be seen within areas of bowel wall contusion. In contrast, diffuse hyperenhancement of the entire small bowel is a nonspecific sign and is usually seen in shock bowel and is associated with other signs of hypovolemic shock. Typically administration of positive contrast material to opacify the bowel will *decrease* the sensitivity of this sign.

Nonspecific signs of bowel injury:

1. *Bowel wall thickening* can be either circumferential (Figs. 11-74 and 11-75; see Figs. 11-65, 11-69, and 11-73) or eccentric and may be focal or diffuse. The thickening could be due to edema or hematoma (see Fig. 11-74). Bowel wall thickening is defined as greater than 3 mm (small bowel) and 5 mm (large bowel) in the presence of adequate distention of the lumen. Focal thickening of the wall is a more specific sign of injury (Fig. 11-76; see Fig. 11-69), than diffuse thickening. In general, large bowel wall thickening is more specific for bowel injury than small bowel wall thickening is (see Figs. 11-65 and 11-76). Lack of bowel distention is a common cause for false-positive diagnosis of bowel wall thickening. In the absence of other CT signs of bowel injury, this sign in isolation should raise the possibility of underdistention.

Diffuse bowel wall thickening is less specific for bowel injury and is typically seen in systemic volume overload or shock bowel syndrome. These two entities typically involve the entire small bowel and spare the colon. However, with prolonged periods of volume overload or shock, colonic wall thickening can be observed. Other CT findings of hypoperfusion complex and fluid overresuscitation accompanied by bowel wall thickening may help in distinguishing small bowel injury from these two mimicking entities. Moreover, there should be careful scrutiny in patients with hypoperfusion complex and fluid overload to identify concurrent bowel or mesenteric injuries, where the CT signs for bowel and mesenteric injury can easily be masked. Small bowel injury usually appears as a focal rather than diffuse

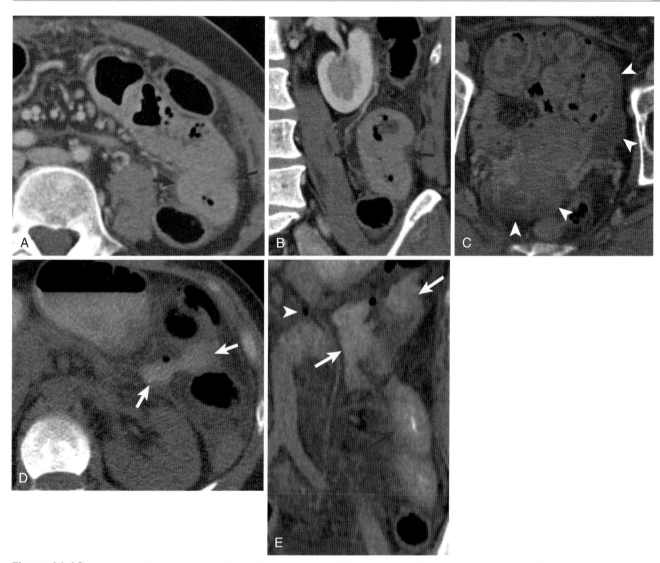

Figure 11-69 Jejunal perforation with oral contrast leak. Axial (A) and coronal (B) multiplanar reformatted images display circumferential wall thickening *(red arrows)* of the jejunum. **C,** Axial image in the pelvis reveals a small amount of free fluid in the pelvis *(arrowheads).* **D,** Follow-up computed tomography (CT) obtained following administration of oral contrast shows intraperitoneal leak of oral contrast material *(white arrowheads).* **E,** Coronal multiplanar image confirms extraluminal contrast *(white arrows)* with small focus of pneumoperitoneum *(arrowhead)* and wall thickening of the jejunum *(red arrow).*

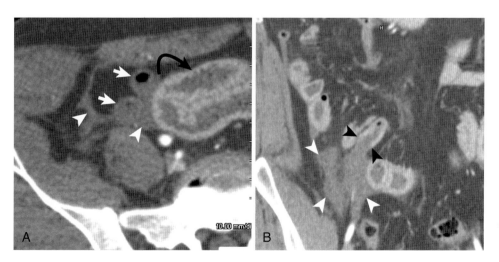

Figure 11-70 Segmental devascularization of the bowel manifested as absence of wall enhancement. A, Axial contrast-enhanced computed tomography (CT) of the abdomen demonstrates absent wall enhancement of distal ileum *(arrows)* secondary to devascularization with small amount of free fluid *(arrowheads).* Compare with normal enhancing ileum *(curved arrow).* **B,** Coronal multiplanar reformatted image exhibits abrupt termination in the enhancement of distal ileum *(black arrowheads)* with extravasation of intestinal content *(white arrowheads)* into peritoneum.

abnormality on CT. When any of the specific findings are present, it could indicate concurrent bowel injury. All patients with CT findings of shock bowel or volume overload and high index of suspicion for small bowel injury should be followed up with repeat CT.

2. *Free intraperitoneal fluid* is the most sensitive but nonspecific sign of bowel or mesenteric injury (Fig. 11-77; see Figs. 11-66 and 11-67). Free intraperitoneal fluid as the sole finding on CT in blunt abdominal trauma may indicate an occult bowel or mesenteric injury. Other causes of free fluid include previous

intraperitoneal fluid not associated with trauma (ascites), occult surface lacerations to solid organs, intraperitoneal bladder injury, and decompression or diapedesis of red blood cells from pelvic hematoma into the peritoneal cavity. Women of reproductive age may have a small amount of "physiologic" free fluid in the cul-de-sac. Interloop or intermesenteric fluid (triangular collections between the mesenteric leaves) (see Fig. 11-67) and high-attenuation fluid (greater than 15 HU) (see Fig. 11-70) are more likely to be associated with a bowel or mesenteric injury.

There is no clear consensus on how these patients with isolated free intraperitoneal fluid should be managed to identify occult bowel or mesenteric injury. The important factors that should be taken into consideration in planning management of patients with isolated free intraperitoneal fluid on CT include the quantity and location of the free intraperitoneal fluid, the sex of the patient, the result of physical examination, and the presence of leukocytosis. With the advancement of CT technology, small amounts of free fluid in the deep lower pelvis or fluid attenuation can be seen in male patients without a bowel or mesenteric injury. However, presence of moderate to large amounts of isolated free fluid, a small amount of fluid in multiple locations, or intermesenteric fluid require aggressive follow-up with CT, DPL, or laparotomy.

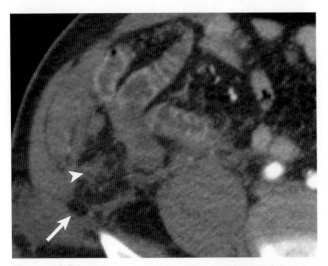

Figure 11-71 Mesenteric tear resulting in segmental devascularization of the bowel. Axial image displays no wall enhancement of distal ileum *(red arrow)* secondary to devascularization. There is also mesenteric fat stranding *(arrowhead)* and a small traumatic lumbar hernia *(white arrow)*.

■ DUODENAL INJURIES

The prevalence of duodenal injuries is 0.2%, with only a small minority of these patients sustaining full-thickness injury. It is essential to distinguish duodenal wall contusion, wall hematoma, perforation, and devascularization because of the varied treatment implications.

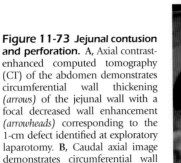

Figure 11-72 Mesenteric hematoma associated with mesenteric tear. A, Coronal contrast-enhanced computed tomography (CT) of the abdomen demonstrates mesenteric hematoma *(curved arrow)* with decreased wall enhancement of the attached small bowel loop. B, Surgery confirmed a long mesenteric tear.

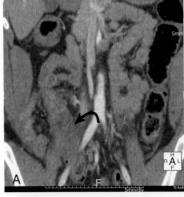
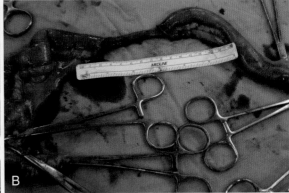

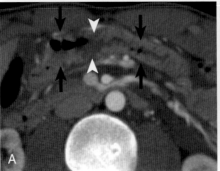

Figure 11-73 Jejunal contusion and perforation. A, Axial contrast-enhanced computed tomography (CT) of the abdomen demonstrates circumferential wall thickening *(arrows)* of the jejunal wall with a focal decreased wall enhancement *(arrowheads)* corresponding to the 1-cm defect identified at exploratory laparotomy. B, Caudal axial image demonstrates circumferential wall thickening of jejunal wall *(arrows)*.

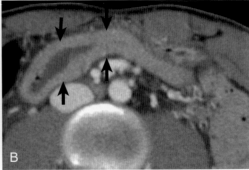

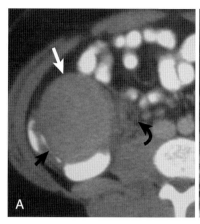
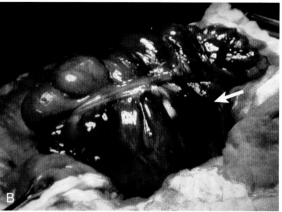

Figure 11-74 Large eccentric intramural hematoma. A, Axial computed tomography (CT) image demonstrates a large eccentric hematoma within the ascending colonic wall *(white arrow)* with luminal narrowing *(black arrow)* and pericolonic fat stranding *(curved black arrow).* **B,** Photograph at surgery shows the mural hematoma *(arrow).* A hemicolectomy was performed.

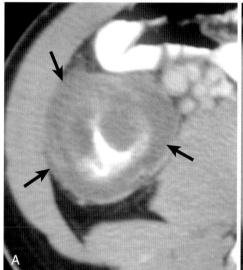
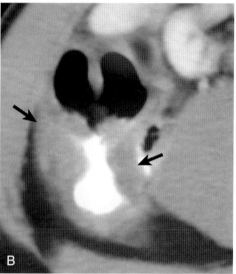

Figure 11-75 Bowel contusion manifested as circumferential wall thickening. A, Axial contrast-enhanced computed tomography (CT) of the abdomen demonstrates concentric thickening of the ascending colonic wall *(arrows)* with mild pericolonic fat stranding. **B,** Follow-up axial contrast-enhanced CT 8 hours after the first study demonstrates persistent but improved colonic wall thickening *(arrows),* suggesting a nonsurgical injury.

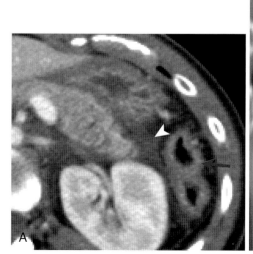
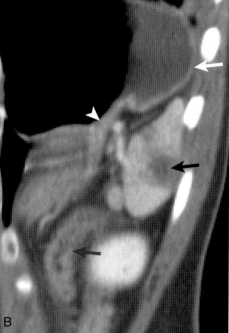

Figure 11-76 Colonic contusion with circumferential wall thickening. A, Axial contrast-enhanced computed tomography (CT) of the abdomen demonstrates distal transverse colonic wall thickening *(red arrow)* with pericolonic fat stranding and fluid in the left anterior pararenal space *(arrowhead)* due to associated pancreatic laceration (not shown in the image). **B,** Sagittal multiplanar reformat image demonstrates colonic wall thickening *(red arrow),* associated diaphragmatic rupture with gastric herniation into the thoracic cavity with "dependent viscera sign" *(white arrow),* and "waist sign" *(arrowhead).* Also demonstrated is a splenic contusion *(black arrow).*

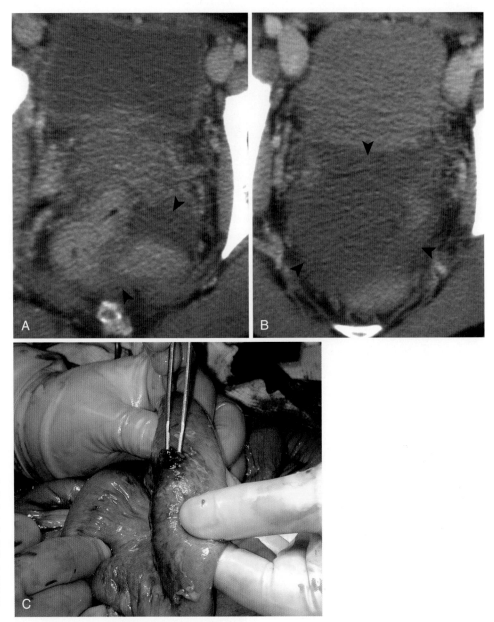

Figure 11-77 Jejunal injury manifested as increasing free fluid in the pelvic peritoneum. A, Admission axial contrast-enhanced computed tomography (CT) of the pelvis demonstrates a small amount of free fluid in the pelvic peritoneum *(arrowheads)*. B, Seven-hour follow-up CT demonstrates an increase in the fluid *(arrowheads)*. C, Surgery confirmed a small jejunal perforation.

Full-thickness perforations or devascularized duodenum are surgical injuries, whereas wall contusions, hematomas, or partial-thickness wall lacerations can often be managed conservatively. Delays in diagnosis and treatment and failure to identify perforation or devascularization can considerably increase morbidity and mortality. The high complication rate associated with duodenal injuries is due to diagnostic delays and missed injuries because surgical repair becomes more difficult the later the injury is recognized. When the diagnosis is delayed by more than 8 hours, the complication rate increases significantly.

Anatomic Consideration

The duodenum is divided into the bulb, descending part, transverse part, and ascending part. The bulb is predominantly intraperitoneal. The descending, transverse, and ascending parts are retroperitoneal. Within the ret-

roperitoneum the duodenum is located in the anterior pararenal space.

Mechanism of Injury

The deep, central, retroperitoneal location usually protects the duodenum from many instances of trauma. The injuries usually result from severe anteroposterior compression force against the spinal column, deceleration trauma, and handlebar compression. Less common mechanisms include sports injuries, falls, and a blow to the upper abdomen.

Computed Tomography Findings

Computed tomography is an essential means of diagnosing traumatic lesions of the duodenum. Duodenal injuries range from minor wall hematomas and partial-thickness lacerations and wall contusions to

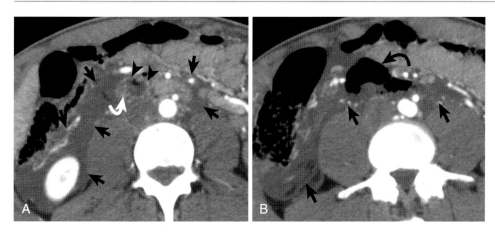

Figure 11-78 Duodenal perforation. **A,** Axial contrast-enhanced computed tomography (CT) of the abdomen demonstrates duodenal perforation involving the horizontal portion *(arrowheads)* with wall thickening *(curved arrow)* and paraduodenal fluid *(arrows)*. **B,** A caudal axial image demonstrates extraluminal air *(curved arrow)* and paraduodenal fluid *(arrows)*.

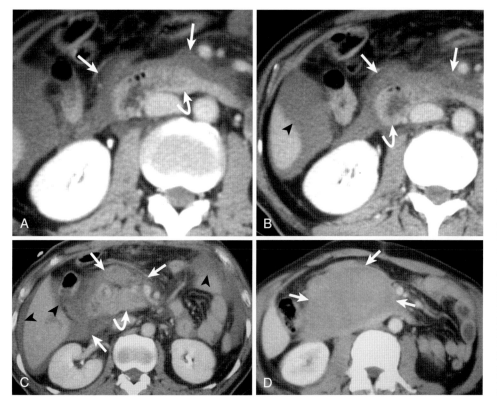

Figure 11-79 Duodenal wall contusion. **A,** Axial contrast-enhanced computed tomography (CT) of the abdomen demonstrates duodenal wall thickening involving the horizontal portion *(curved arrow)* with paraduodenal blood *(arrows)*. **B,** A caudal axial image demonstrates paraduodenal sentinel clot *(arrows)* with wall thickening *(curved arrow)* and blood along the right anterior pararenal space and right subhepatic space *(arrowhead)*. **C** and **D,** Follow-up axial contrast-enhanced image demonstrates increased duodenal wall thickness *(curved arrow)* and paraduodenal hematoma *(arrows)*. Free intraperitoneal fluid persists *(arrowheads)*.

complex or full-thickness lacerations and massive disruption of the duodenopancreatic complex. Duodenal injury is suspected with wall thickening (Figs. 11-78 and 11-79), edema, paraduodenal fluid (see Fig. 11-78), and intramural hematoma. Free air (see Fig. 11-78) and oral contrast extravasation are the specific signs of duodenal perforation but are insensitive. Perforation is most likely to occur in the descending and horizontal portions (see Fig. 11-78). Lack of continuity of the wall also indicates perforation. Devascularization is manifested as lack of focal or segmental mucosal enhancement. The latter two conditions mandate surgical treatment. Fluid in the anterior pararenal space (see Fig. 11-79), sentinel clot (see Fig. 11-79), and thickening of the wall are useful secondary signs for both perforation (see Fig. 11-78) and contusion (see Fig. 11-79).

■ ANORECTAL INJURY

Anorectal injuries are associated with high morbidity and mortality due to their propensity to be associated with pelvic fractures (Fig. 11-80) and urinary bladder, urethral, and pelvic vascular injuries. Pubic symphysis diastasis and anteroposterior compression type of fractures of the pelvis have been shown be independent predictors of rectal injuries. Distinction between intraperitoneal and extraperitoneal rectal injuries is important for treatment implications. The intraperitoneal segment consists of the anterolateral sidewalls of the upper one third and anterior wall of the middle third of the rectum. The extraperitoneal segment consists of the posterior wall of the upper two thirds, sidewalls of the middle third, and circumference of the lower one third of the rectum. Extraperitoneal injury occurs because of shearing at the anorectal junction, where the bowel is relatively fixed. Management of intraperitoneal rectal injuries is similar to that of colonic injury. Extraperitoneal injuries are difficult to access and manage, but the mainstay of treatment includes four main components: fecal diversion with colostomy, presacral drainage, distal rectal washout, and repair of the injury when possible. Specific and nonspecific CT findings for intraperitoneal rectal injuries are similar to those described for the remainder of bowel injuries. Primary CT findings for extraperitoneal anorectal injuries with high specificity include extraperitoneal air, contrast leak, and bowel wall defects. These specific signs are, however, insensitive. The nonspecific signs include wall thickening, perirectal fat stranding, and hematomas, including the involvement of the ischiorectal fossa (see Fig. 11-80). Unrecognized extraperitoneal anorectal injuries may result in local infectious complications ranging from abscess formation (see Fig. 11-80) to necrotizing fasciitis.

SPECIFIC COMPUTED TOMOGRAPHY SIGNS OF MESENTERIC INJURY

1. *Extravasation of contrast from mesenteric vessels* (active bleeding) manifests as contrast extravasation from the mesenteric blood vessels (Fig. 11-81) and usually is a very specific sign of injury that requires surgery. It is also associated with a high incidence of bowel ischemia or infarction due to devascularization of the attached bowel segment.
2. *Abrupt termination of mesenteric vessel or vascular beading* (Fig. 11-82) is a less severe form of vascular injury when compared to active bleeding. As with active bleeding, the radiologist should pay special

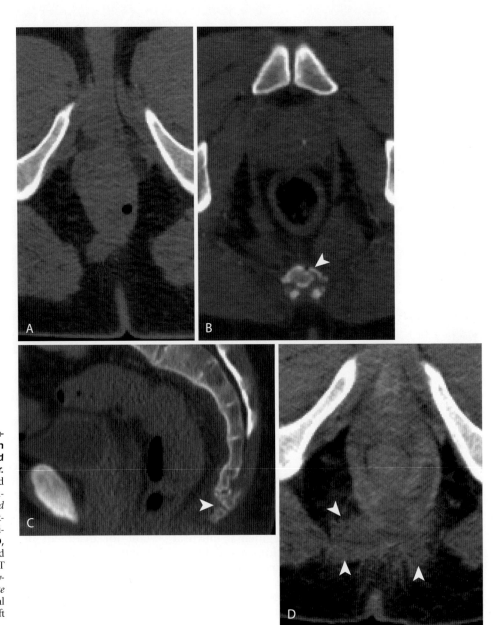

Figure 11-80 Missed extraperitoneal rectal perforation in a 35-year-old man who jumped from a bridge into the water. **A,** Axial contrast-enhanced computed tomography (CT) of the pelvis demonstrates perirectal hematoma *(red arrow)*. Cephalad axial **(B)** and sagittal **(C)** images demonstrate an associated coccyx fracture *(arrowheads)*. **D,** Follow-up axial contrast-enhanced study after 12 days from initial CT demonstrates a large rectal *(red arrowheads)* and perirectal abscess *(white arrowheads)*, which required local incision, drainage, and a diverting left colostomy.

attention to the attached bowel loop for ischemia or infarction.

■ NONSPECIFIC COMPUTED TOMOGRAPHY SIGNS OF MESENTERIC INJURY

Mesenteric fat stranding with free fluid or hematoma (Fig. 11-83; see Figs. 11-81 and 11-82) is a sensitive sign of mesenteric contusion. Contusion associated with hemorrhage may result in mesenteric hematoma (see Figs. 11-81 to 11-83) or high-density interloop fluid (see Fig. 11-67). The presence of mesenteric contusion or hematoma should alert the radiologist to look for associated bowel injuries (see Figs. 11-65 and 11-67) or ischemia (see Figs. 11-71 and 11-72). Bowel wall thickening associated with adjacent hematoma indicates a higher likelihood of a surgical bowel or mesenteric injury.

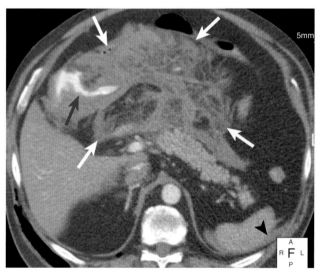

Figure 11-81 Active bleeding from mesenteric vessel. Axial contrast-enhanced computed tomography (CT) demonstrates active bleeding *(red arrow)* with a large mesenteric hematoma, fat stranding, adjacent small bowel loop *(white arrows)*, and a small amount of free fluid in the posterior left subphrenic space *(arrowhead)*.

■ MIMICS OF BOWEL CONTUSION

The radiologist should be familiar with abnormalities observed in the bowel in patients with hypovolemia or hypoperfusion complex (shock bowel) and fluid overload. These two entities can mimic bowel injury on CT. The CT findings of shock bowel include diffuse thickening of the small bowel wall, fluid-filled dilated loops, increased contrast enhancement of the wall from slow perfusion and interstitial leak of intravenous contrast material, and a flattened inferior vena cava (Fig. 11-84). The large bowel is usually spared. Follow-up CT obtained after correction of hypovolemia usually shows complete resolution of small bowel changes.

The bowel wall changes seen following vigorous fluid resuscitation may result in diffuse bowel wall edema, particularly the entire small bowel (Fig. 11-85, *A*). Other CT findings of intravenous volume expansion include periportal edema (see Fig. 11-85), distention of the inferior vena cava (see Fig. 11-85), retroperitoneal fluid, and occasionally ascites.

■ FOLLOW-UP COMPUTED TOMOGRAPHY IN BOWEL AND MESENTERIC INJURIES

There is no clear consensus in the radiologic or surgical literature regarding the ideal management of patients with nonspecific CT findings of bowel or mesenteric injuries. These CT findings include bowel wall thickening (see Figs. 11-69, 11-74, and 11-75), diffuse hyperenhancement of the wall, focal mesenteric infiltration, and a small amount of free intraperitoneal fluid (see Figs. 11-69 and 11-77). Follow-up of these patients can vary, based on initial CT findings, mechanism of injury, clinical examination, neurologic status (Glasgow Coma Scale score, presence of a spinal cord injury), time from injury to CT examination, and local surgical practices. Table 11-10 lists the various techniques that can be used to carefully evaluate these patients and prevent delays in diagnosis of surgical bowel or mesenteric injuries. It is important to have a discussion between the radiologist and surgeon to formulate an optimal management plan on an individual basis, combining

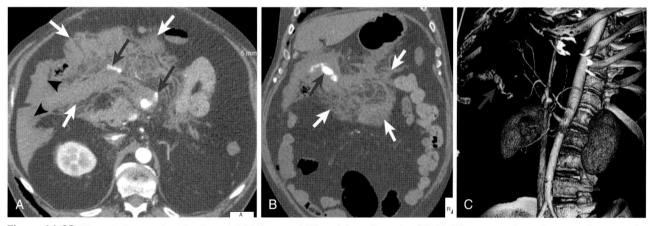

Figure 11-82 Mesenteric vascular bleeding. Axial (**A**), coronal (**B**), and three-dimensional (3-D) (**C**) contrast-enhanced computed tomography (CT) images of the abdomen demonstrate vascular beading *(red arrows)* and a large mesenteric hematoma with fat stranding *(white arrows)*. A moderate amount of free intraperitoneal blood *(arrowheads)* is also seen.

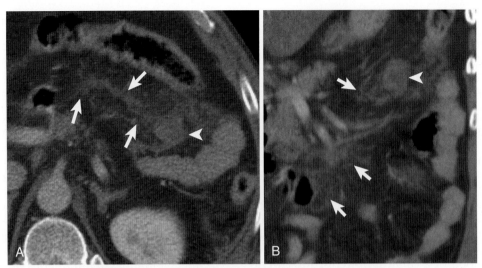

Figure 11-83 Mesenteric contusion. Axial contrast-enhanced computed tomography (CT) (**A**) and coronal multiplanar reformat image (**B**) of the abdomen demonstrate small mesenteric hematoma *(arrowheads)* and fat stranding *(white arrows)* along the transverse mesocolon and mesenteric root.

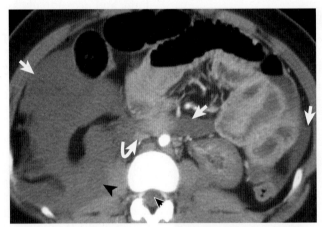

Figure 11-84 Shock bowel. Axial contrast-enhanced computed tomography (CT) of the abdomen demonstrates loops of small bowel with pronounced mucosal enhancement with flattened inferior vena cava *(curved arrow)* and delayed left nephrogram. The findings are consistent with shock bowel caused by hypotension secondary to large retroperitoneal hematoma *(arrows)* arising from the pelvis due to pelvic fractures (not shown).

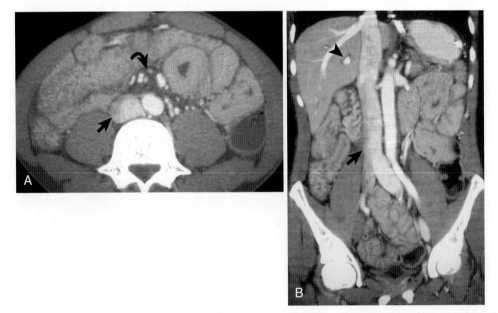

Figure 11-85 Volume overload due to vigorous fluid resuscitation. **A,** Axial contrast-enhanced computed tomography (CT) of the abdomen demonstrates diffuse bowel wall thickening and at the mesenteric root *(curved arrow)* with a distended inferior vena cava *(arrow)*. **B,** Coronal multiplanar reformat image demonstrates periportal edema *(arrowhead)*, distended inferior vena cava *(arrow)*, and diffuse bowel wall thickening.

Table 11-10   Follow-up Strategies for Nonspecific Computed Tomography Findings of Bowel or Mesenteric Injury

Technique	Positive Test	Advantages	Disadvantages
Serial physical examination	Development of peritonitis, fever, or tachycardia Development of hemodynamic instability Development or persistent pain and tenderness	Good sensitivity and negative predictive value	Hospital admission Frequent hemodynamic and physical examinations requires the same surgeon to perform serial evaluations
Serial US examination	Increase in peritoneal fluid	No radiation Easy to perform and repeat Available in all trauma centers	Operator dependant Cannot discriminate the source of fluid False-negative rate due to potential to miss small volumes of fluid
Follow-up CT (4 to 6 hours) with oral contrast	Development of peritonitis Development of new specific CT signs of bowel and mesenteric injuries	Accurate in demonstrating surgical lesion in bowel or mesentery Best assessment of retroperitoneal bowel segments Available in most trauma centers	Cumulative radiation dose
DPL	White blood cell count > 500 Lavage amylase level > 20 units/L Alkaline phosphatase level > 10 units/L	Performed immediately Easy to perform	Invasive Lack of good criteria for positive DPL for bowel injury Low sensitivity for retroperitoneal bowel injury High false-positive rate
Laparoscopy	Direct visualization of injury	Direct visualization of peritoneum Easy to convert to laparotomy	User dependent Not available in all centers Invasive Low sensitivity Limited evaluation of retroperitoneal bowel
Laparotomy	Direct visualization of injury	Reference standard technique	Invasive Associated with complications Extended hospital stays

CT, Computed tomography; *DPL,* diagnostic peritoneal lavage; *US,* ultrasound.

radiologic and clinical findings. Usually, most stable patients with nonspecific CT findings of bowel or mesenteric injuries are evaluated with a follow-up CT performed at 4 to 6 hours following administration of intravenous and oral contrast material. In specific cases, rectal contrast is used for colonic injuries. This usually allows time for the surgically important bowel and mesenteric injuries to evolve and manifest overt primary signs of injury or secondary signs due to complications such as peritonitis or bowel ischemia.

Genitourinary Tract Trauma

Lisa A. Miller

Multidetector CT has rapidly become the test of choice for prompt evaluation of acute injuries of the kidneys, ureters, and bladder. Reconstructed multiplanar, maximum intensity projection, and volumetric images can be readily created and enhance visualization and comprehension of select genitourinary system injuries. This section describes imaging findings seen with injury to the urinary system and male genitalia from both blunt and penetrating force. The emphasis is on the CT findings of acute genitourinary system injury, but the use of

other modalities such as intravenous pyelography, US, nuclear scintigraphy, and retrograde urography are also discussed. The use of angiographic and interventional radiology procedures in the diagnosis of acute vascular injury and management of complications associated with genitourinary system trauma are also discussed.

■ RENAL INJURY

Incidence

Approximately 10% of patients presenting with abdominal trauma will sustain a renal injury. Blunt force trauma such as motor vehicle collision or fall from height is responsible for about 90% of renal injuries, and 10% of cases are due to penetrating trauma. Penetrating trauma is most commonly due to gunshot or stab wounds; iatrogenic penetrating injuries sustained during renal biopsy or laparotomy are less frequent. Patients with congenital renal anomalies such as horseshoe kidney or ectopic kidney or those with an acquired renal abnormality such as hydronephrosis, neoplasm, or cyst are more vulnerable to traumatic renal injury from minor trauma. An underlying renal abnormality should be suspected in the patient who presents with CT findings of significant renal injury out of proportion to the mechanism of injury (Figs. 11-86 and 11-87).

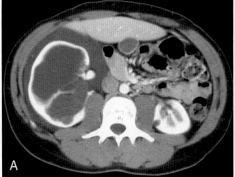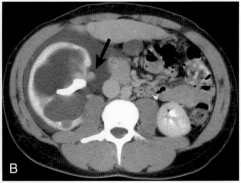

Figure 11-86 Computed tomography (CT) of trauma patient who fell down five steps. A, Axial image shows right hydronephrosis with hypodense fluid similar in density to urine surrounding the kidney. **B,** Delayed image obtained at 5 minutes shows contrast extravasation *(arrow)* from the ruptured right collecting system.

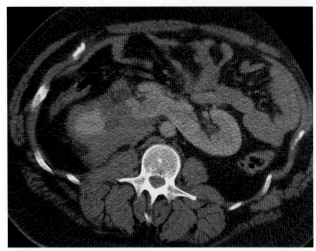

Figure 11-87 Forty-five-year-old patient who fell off a bike. Computed tomography (CT) shows laceration through right side of horseshoe kidney with moderate amount of perinephric hemorrhage.

Indications for Imaging

The indications for imaging evaluation of the genitourinary system depend foremost on the hemodynamic stability of the trauma patient. A patient who is unstable is usually taken directly to surgery. A rapid intravenous urogram can be performed in the operating room once hemodynamic stability is achieved. The intravenous urogram will give information regarding excretion from both kidneys and will detect major renal parenchymal injuries.

The adult trauma patient who is hemodynamically stable and is suspected of having a renal injury upon presentation should be evaluated with contrast-enhanced CT. Clinical indications for imaging include direct blunt trauma, pain, bruising, hematuria, or suspicion for renal injury based on the mechanism of injury (Table 11-11). The presence, absence, or degree of hematuria as an indicator of renal injury has been the subject of debate, but general guidelines for imaging include gross hematuria following blunt trauma. Although microscopic hematuria without signs of shock following abdominal trauma has a very low association with major renal trauma in adult patients, the absence of hematuria in the adult patient does not exclude a renal injury. Hematuria may be absent in patients with severe renal injury, particularly those with vascular pedicle

Table 11-11   Indications for Renal Imaging in Acute Trauma

Indication	Imaging Study
Blunt trauma + Gross hematuria	Chest, abdominal-pelvic CT with IV contrast medium Abdominal-pelvic CT with IV contrast medium if hemodynamically stable or resuscitated
Hemodynamically unstable requiring emergency surgery	Intraoperative IVU when stabilized
Hemodynamically stable with microscopic hematuria, but no other indication for abdominal-pelvic CT	Observation until resolution of hematuria
Hemodynamically stable with microscopic hematuria but other indications for abdominal-pelvic CT (positive abdominal examination, decreasing hematocrit, indeterminate result of peritoneal lavage or abdominal US, unreliable physical examination)	Abdominal-pelvic CT with IV contrast medium
Hemodynamically stable with or without microscopic hematuria with evidence of major flank impact (e.g., lower posterior rib or lumbar transverse process fracture, major contusion of flank soft tissues)	Abdominal-pelvic CT with and IV contrast medium

CT, Computed tomography; *IV,* intravenous; *IVU,* intravenous urogram; *US,* ultrasonography.

injury, ureteral transection, ureteropelvic disruption or penetrating urinary system injury. In the pediatric trauma patient, microscopic hematuria without hypotension can be associated with significant injury, and CT is recommended for both gross and microscopic hematuria. Overall, the decision to image a patient suspected of having a renal injury should not depend only on the presence or absence of hematuria, but also on the age of the patient, mechanism of injury, and hemodynamic stability of the patient.

Although US examination is often used in the diagnosis of medical renal disease and for rapid assessment of the peritoneal cavity for free fluid using the FAST examination, it cannot assess renal function and is relatively insensitive for detection of renal lacerations, extravasation of blood or urine, collecting system disruption, and parenchymal hematoma. Because of these limitations, negative findings from US examination cannot reliably exclude a renal injury, and the examination is not recommended for assessment of acute renal injury.

Computed Tomography Technique for Renal Injury

In general, the kidneys and proximal collecting systems are evaluated as part of the abdominal-pelvic CT study without special protocols. In our center the abdomen and pelvis are examined using 40- or 64-channel MDCT with nonionic intravenous contrast material as part of a whole-body trauma scan (for technique see Computed Tomography Protocols and Scan Optimization). Both the axial arterial phase and portal venous phase images are fused at 3 to 5 mm for review and storage on a PACS workstation. The original images are used for all 2-D or 3-D reformatted imaging and are also saved to a TeraRecon server (TeraRecon Inc., San Mateo, California) for reference, if required. Because MDCT covers the abdomen and pelvis very quickly, there is no opportunity for opacification of the renal pelvis and ureters, resulting in inability to diagnose potential proximal collecting system injury. If there is radiologic suspicion for collecting system injury on the initial CT image set, additional 3- to 20-minute delayed images may be obtained as necessary to evaluate for extravasation of urinary contrast material from the collecting system or ureters. Reduced radiation dose is adequate for additional delayed images because these images are used primarily for detection of high-attenuation contrast material rather than parenchymal injury.

The arterial phase images are most useful in demonstrating presence and symmetry of intravenous contrast by the kidneys and potential active bleeding or traumatic pseudoaneurysm, whereas the portal venous images provide more information about the extent of parenchymal damage and help differentiate active bleeding from traumatic pseudoaneurysm.

Grading of Renal Injury

A grading system for renal injuries based on surgical observations was developed in 1989 by the AAST. The grading system described renal injuries *as seen at surgery* on a scale of I to V, ranging from minor injuries such as renal contusion (grade I injury) to major renal injuries such as shattered kidney (grade V injury). This grading system correctly predicts that increasing grade of renal injury correlates with the following: need for renorrhaphy or nephrectomy after blunt or penetrating trauma, the need for hemodialysis, inpatient mortality, and decreased renal function after major renal injury. Although useful for guiding surgical management, grades IV and V were somewhat confusing, and not all types of renal injuries were included in the grading scale. In 2011 the original AAST renal grading system was revised to take into account CT findings as well

Table 11-12 *Revised AAST Renal Injury Grading System*

Grade	Location	Injury Definition
I	Parenchyma	Subcapsular hematoma and/or contusion
	Collecting system	No injury
II	Parenchyma	Laceration < 1 cm in depth and into cortex, small hematoma contained within the Gerota fascia
	Collecting system	No injury
III	Parenchyma	Laceration > 1 cm in depth and into medulla, hematoma contained within the Gerota fascia
	Collecting system	No injury
IV	Parenchyma	Laceration through the parenchyma into the urinary collecting system Vascular segmental vein or artery injury
	Collecting system	Laceration, one or more into the collecting system with urinary extravasation Renal pelvis laceration and/or complete ureteral pelvic disruption
V	Vascular	Main renal artery or vein laceration, avulsion, or thrombosis

*A renal unit can sustain more than one grade of injury and should be classified by the higher grade of renal injury.
AAST, American Association for the Surgery of Trauma.

as surgical findings and to include all types of renal injury (Table 11-12). Although most hospitals use the AAST renal grading system, it is wise to confirm before assigning a grade to a renal injury in the radiologic report.

Generally, patients with grades I to III renal injuries are managed nonoperatively. Grades IV and V renal injuries have historically required surgical management. Currently there is a shift in management to a more conservative approach, and some of these injuries will likely be managed with interventional angiography and aggressive monitoring of vital signs in a facility that has expertise to manage multitrauma patients rather than surgery. Some grade IV injuries, such as complete ureteral-pelvic junction avulsion, and many grade V injuries will still require surgical management.

Computed Tomography of Grades I to III Renal Injury

The vast majority (75% to 98%) of renal injuries are minor, represented by grades I to III, and will heal spontaneously. Renal contusions are seen on CT as low-attenuation, ill-defined areas with irregular margins (Fig. 11-88). A striated nephrogram pattern is occasionally seen in the region of contusion (Fig. 11-89). No follow-up imaging is required for renal contusions. Subcapsular hematomas are uncommon because the renal capsule does not readily separate from the underlying cortex. On contrast-enhanced CT a subcapsular hematoma typically appears as a

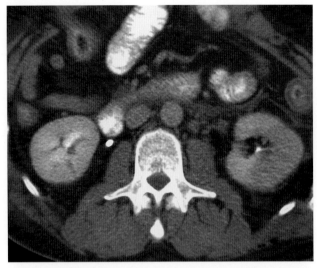

Figure 11-88 Computed tomography (CT) of multitrauma patient shows vague low attenuation area in the lateral aspect of the left kidney representing renal contusion.

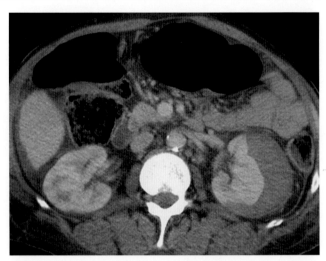

Figure 11-90 Left renal subcapsular hematoma in patient who was struck by a car. Note the typical crescentic shape of the hematoma with compression and deformity of the underlying renal parenchyma.

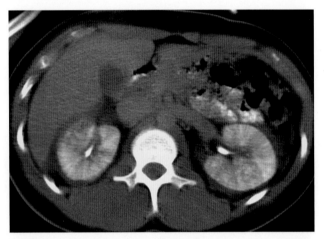

Figure 11-89 Twenty-six-year-old trauma patient with small bilateral perinephric hemorrhage and bilateral renal contusions demonstrating striated appearance. This appearance is due to a slight lag in blood flow through the contused parenchyma.

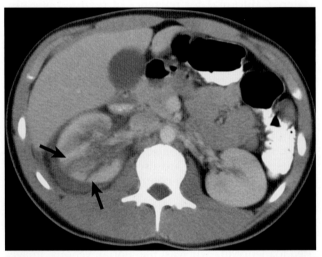

Figure 11-91 Computed tomography (CT) of patient who fell off a horse shows linear low attenuation right renal lacerations (*arrows*) with small amount of perinephric blood.

low-attenuation, convex-shaped collection of blood indenting the underlying renal parenchyma (Fig. 11-90). Delayed renal perfusion may be seen in the affected kidney because of increased resistance to arterial perfusion. Most cases of subcapsular hematoma will resolve completely. Acute or delayed onset of hypertension from renal parenchymal compression (Page kidney) may rarely be seen with a large subcapsular hematoma and may require surgical release of the renal tamponade.

Minor renal lacerations either can be superficial, involving only the renal cortex, or may extend deeper into the renal medulla. A minor renal laceration by definition does not involve the collecting system. On CT a laceration is seen as a linear or branching low-attenuation defect on a background of otherwise normally enhancing renal parenchyma (Fig. 11-91). There is often a small amount of accompanying perinephric hemorrhage seen as poorly defined isoattenuation or hyperattenuation fluid around

the kidney, contained by the Gerota fascia (Fig. 11-92). Minor renal lacerations are self-limited injuries and typically require no follow-up imaging.

Segmental renal infarctions are a common minor renal injury and result from stretching and occlusion of an accessory renal artery, extrarenal or intrarenal branches of the renal artery, or a capsular artery. A segmental infarction will appear as a sharply demarcated, wedge-shaped region of low attenuation with the base of the wedge at the renal capsule (Fig. 11-93). Segmental infarctions most commonly occur at the renal poles.

Computed Tomography of Grade IV Renal Injury

Grade IV injuries include deep renal lacerations that extend into the renal collecting system (with or without urinary extravasation), segmental vascular injury

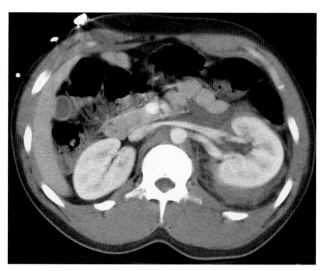

Figure 11-92 Moderate amount of left perinephric hemorrhage in a trauma patient involved in a motor vehicle collision. Unlike a subcapsular hematoma, perinephric hemorrhage will not indent the renal contour.

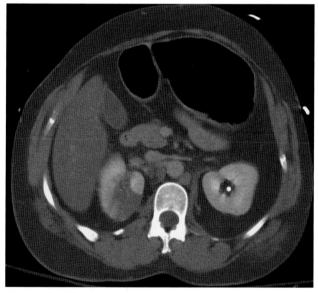

Figure 11-93 Trauma patient who fell off roof. Contrast-enhanced computed tomography (CT) shows a well-defined, wedge-shaped region of hypoattenuation in the posterior and medial aspect of the right kidney, a typical appearance of a segmental infarction.

within the kidney, and renal pelvis laceration or ureteropelvic junction (UPJ) disruption. On CT, findings such as a renal laceration that appears to extend into the collecting system or the presence of fluid near the renal pelvis may signal a potential collecting system injury. Typically CT portal venous images are obtained before intravenous contrast has reached the collecting system. If there is suspicion of a collecting system injury, additional 5- to 20-minute delayed CT images through the kidneys will be needed for complete evaluation. Delayed images of a collecting system injury will show high-attenuation, contrast-enhanced urine adjacent to the site of injury (Fig. 11-94). A missed collecting system may manifest as development of unexplained sepsis

or rising serum creatinine and urea levels. The vast majority of urine leaks from collecting system injury will resolve without treatment. Placement of a nephrostomy tube or double-J ureteral catheter or surgical repair may be required if the urine leak persists. Some urinoma may only be seen on follow-up CT because the mass effect from the contusion or hematoma can prevent urinary contrast leak on the admission CT. With healing, decrease in mass effect allows visualization of the urinoma on follow-up CT. Rarely, infection of the urinoma may develop if there is any impedance to antegrade flow of urine such as with an obstructing stone or blood clot in the ureter or bacterial contamination of the collection from penetrating renal injury. Infected urinomas can often be treated with percutaneous drainage.

Segmental vascular injuries include active bleeding and traumatic pseudoaneurysm. Active bleeding into the kidney or surrounding tissue appears as patchy or linear high-attenuation contrast material surrounded by hematoma, which may not be visualized on arterial phase images. If visualized on arterial phase images on portal venous imaging the area of extravasated contrast material will increase in size and remain hyperattenuated (Figs. 11-95 and 11-96). Hemorrhage can be differentiated from urine extravasation, when arterial extravasation appears before opacification of the renal collecting system. Typically the attenuation of extravasated arterial contrast medium is greater than 80 HU and is within 15 HU of an adjacent artery. A traumatic renal pseudoaneurysm will appear as a rounded or oval area of high attenuation on arterial phase imaging that becomes isodense on portal venous images (Fig. 11-97) compared to the adjacent normal parenchyma. If the patient is hemodynamically stable, traumatic pseudoaneurysm and active bleeding can be confirmed by selective renal angiography and treated by angioembolization.

A renal pelvis injury is seen on CT as gross contrast-opacified urine extravasation near the UPJ, often with no or minimal renal parenchymal injury (Fig. 11-98). The injury is thought to be the result of hyperextension with overstretching of the renal pelvis. As with intrarenal collecting system injuries, a renal pelvis injury can be missed if the images are obtained before intravenous contrast has reached the renal pelvis. This emphasizes the need for a high index of suspicion of injury when fluid is seen the near the UPJ with subsequent acquisition of additional delayed CT images. A right-sided UPJ injury may mimic duodenal rupture with leakage of oral contrast. A dilated renal pelvis due to congenital or acquired outflow obstruction is at increased risk for traumatic rupture (Fig. 11-86).

Computed Tomography of Grade V Injury

AAST grade V injuries are the most severe and often require angiographic or surgical intervention. A grade V renal injury indicates main renal artery or vein laceration, avulsion, or thrombosis. Main renal artery injury from blunt trauma is uncommon and is thought to be due to lateral displacement of the kidney with stretching of the intima, leading to clot formation and artery occlusion or

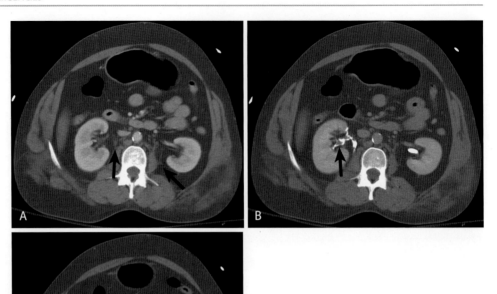

Figure 11-94 Portal venous phase computed tomography (CT) image of a patient involved in a high-speed motor vehicle collision. A, Image shows minimal fat stranding *(arrows)* near the renal pelvis. Note the left flank soft tissue contusion. **B and C,** Delayed images obtained at 5 minutes after injection of contrast show extravasation of contrast material from the right collecting system. A small amount of hypoattenuated clotted blood *(black arrow)* is seen in the right renal pelvis. A large traumatic left lumbar hernia *(red arrow)* is also seen.

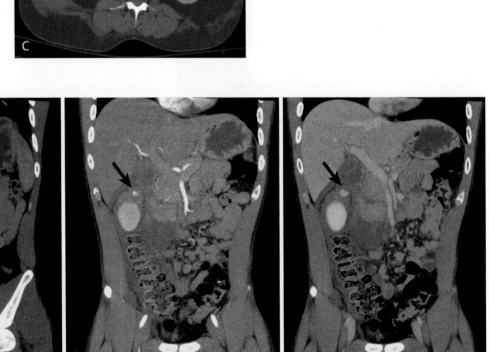

Figure 11-95 Renal active bleeding in a patient involved in a motorcycle accident. A, Coronal reformatted arterial phase computed tomography (CT) image shows a laceration extending from the renal hilum to the lower pole. There is a moderate amount of perinephric hemorrhage. **B,** Coronal reformatted arterial phase CT image shows a focus of hyperattenuation in the perinephric hemorrhage superior to the kidney *(arrow).* **C,** Coronal portal venous phase image shows the focus has remained hyperdense and is slightly bigger in size *(arrow),* indicating active bleeding.

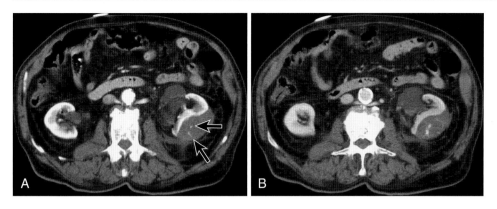

Figure 11-96 Arterial phase computed tomography (CT) image (**A**) of a patient involved in a motor vehicle collision shows a large left renal subcapsular hematoma containing two small foci of hyperattenuation *(arrows)*. A left extrarenal pelvis is noted. On portal venous phase imaging (**B**), the foci of hyperattenuation increases in size and remains hyperattenuated, diagnostic of active bleeding.

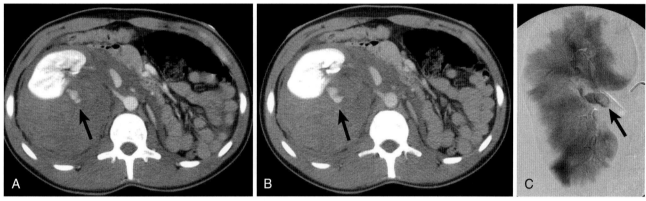

Figure 11-97 Arterial (**A**) and portal venous phase (**B**) computed tomography (CT) images of a patient who fell from a horse show a large right perinephric hemorrhage displacing the kidney anterolaterally and stretching the right renal artery. A lobular hyperattenuation along the posterior margin of the kidney *(arrows)* remains hyperdense and is unchanged in size on the portal venous image, findings consistent with a traumatic pseudoaneurysm. A renal angiogram (**C**) confirms the presence of a pseudoaneurysm *(arrow)*. This injury was treated successfully with angiographic embolization.

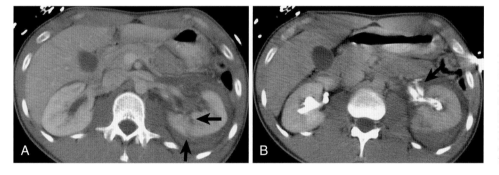

Figure 11-98 Portal venous phase computed tomography (CT) image (**A**) of patient involved in motor vehicle collision shows a small amount of perinephric hemorrhage and small lacerations *(arrows)* in the posterior aspect of the left kidney. Delayed images (**B**) show contrast extravasation *(arrow)* from the injured left renal pelvis.

dissection. The affected kidney will appear slightly small with decreased to no perfusion on contrast-enhanced CT but is often otherwise intact (Fig. 11-99). The rim sign may be seen in renal arterial occlusion and refers to a thin rim of preserved peripheral enhancement due to intact collateral blood flow (Fig. 11-100) from ureteric and perinephric soft tissues. Multiplanar images are often quite useful in determining the exact site of renal artery occlusion (Fig. 11-101).

Optimal management of main renal artery occlusion remains controversial. Treatment options include immediate nephrectomy, endovascular or surgical revascularization, or, most commonly, nonoperative management. Surgical revascularization preserves renal function in fewer than 25% of patients. There are only

scattered case reports of treatment of main renal artery occlusion with endovascular stent placement, and long-term results are mixed.

Major renal vein injury can produce extensive perinephric bleeding, but because the venous pressure is low, this is usually limited to the retroperitoneum and is not usually a clinically significant source of ongoing hemorrhage. Computed tomography findings include an enlarged renal vein containing thrombus (Fig. 11-102), increased renal size, a delayed and progressively dense nephrogram due to high venous outflow resistance, and delayed excretion of intravenous contrast into the collecting system (Fig. 11-103).

Severe fragmentation of the kidney is also considered a major renal injury (Fig. 11-104). Although it has historically been treated with nephrectomy, there have

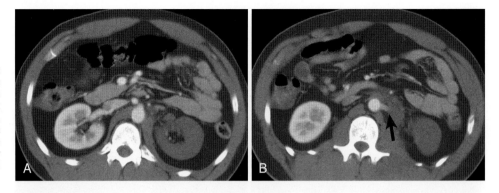

Figure 11-99 Arterial phase computed tomography (CT) image of a patient who fell (**A**) shows global hypoattenuation of the left kidney, indicating nonperfusion. There is no significant perinephric hemorrhage. Image at level of the left renal artery origin (**B**) clearly depicts the site of left main renal artery injury *(arrow)*.

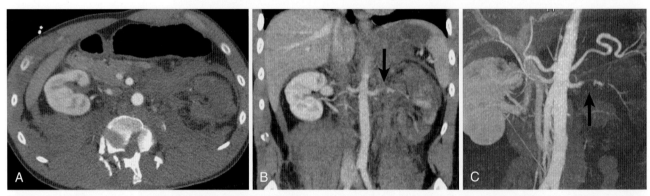

Figure 11-100 A, Axial arterial phase computed tomography (CT) of trauma patient demonstrates a nonperfused left kidney. There is minimal perinephric hemorrhage but a large amount of retroperitoneal hemorrhage in association with a lumbar spine burst fracture. **B,** Coronal reformatted image shows a filling defect in the mid left renal artery *(arrow)*, indicating a traumatic vascular injury. There is patchy perfusion of the left kidney. **C,** Coronal maximum intensity projection (MIP) image confirms the focal filling defect *(arrow)* in the left renal artery.

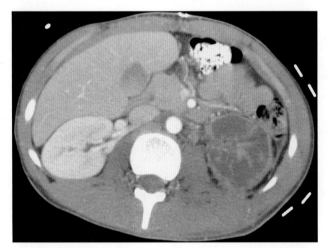

Figure 11-101 Arterial phase computed tomography (CT) image of a patient with traumatic left renal artery injury and "rim" sign. Note minimal patchy perfusion of the parenchyma of the left kidney.

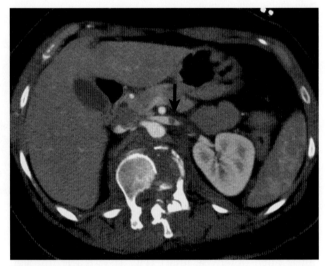

Figure 11-102 Computed tomography (CT) image of patient who fell out of a deer stand shows a comminuted spinal fracture and a small filling defect in the left renal vein *(arrow)*, thought to represent a traumatic intimal injury. The filling defect resolved on repeat CT done 4 days later.

been recent cases of successful nonoperative management using renal angiography and, if needed, percutaneous drainage.

Intervention in Renal Injury

Trauma patients who undergo surgical exploration of an injured kidney have a 64% chance of nephrectomy, regardless of operative intent. Interventional radiology procedures such as angiographic embolization and percutaneously placed nephrostomy catheters have become increasingly valuable in permitting nonoperative management of major renal injuries. Currently surgery is required in less than 10% of major renal injuries.

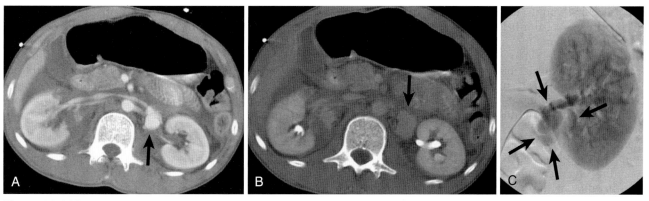

Figure 11-103 Patient with renal vein pseudoaneurysm following blunt trauma. A, Portal venous phase computed tomography (CT) shows multiple right renal lacerations and a small amount of bilateral perinephric hematoma. There is a rounded focus of high attenuation in the region of the mid left renal artery and vein *(arrow)*. **B,** On delayed images the rounded focus has become less dense with no change in size *(arrow)*. **C,** Selective left renal arteriogram in the venous phase shows the lobular density filling with contrast *(arrows)*, diagnostic of a traumatic left renal vein pseudoaneurysm. The left renal artery was normal. This patient underwent left nephrectomy.

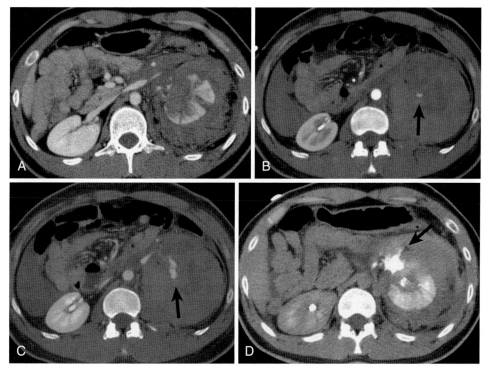

Figure 11-104 A, Axial computed tomography (CT) of patient involved in motor vehicle collision shows traumatic fragmentation of the left kidney and a large perinephric hematoma. **B,** There is a small focus of hyperattenuation *(arrow)* in the inferior portion of the shattered kidney on the arterial phase image. **C,** Portal venous phase image shows enlargement of high attenuation *(arrow)*, indicating active bleeding. **D,** A 10-minute delayed image shows extravasation of very high attenuation contrast from the left renal collecting system *(arrow)*, indicating concurrent collecting system injury.

The use of angiographic embolization for treatment of active bleeding or segmental traumatic renal artery pseudoaneurysm has become increasingly common. Currently there is no firm consensus on exactly what CT findings can predict or exclude the need for angiographic embolization. Criteria such as the AAST grade of injury, the complexity and site of laceration, the presence of active bleeding, and the size of perirenal hematoma have been studied. Renal injury, AAST grade III or higher treated with conservative management, CT findings of presence of active bleeding, and a perinephric hematoma greater than 25 in width had the best prediction for AE. None of the other findings, including AAST grade, complexity of laceration, and laceration site were useful in predicting the need for AE.

■ URETERAL INJURY

Blunt traumatic ureteral injuries are rare and account for less than 1% of all genitourinary injuries from blunt trauma. The ureters are protected by the vertebral column, psoas muscles, and pelvis, and significant force is needed to produce injury. Injuries to multiple organs are almost always present. There may be delay in diagnosis of ureteral injury due to emergent treatment of other injuries.

Types of ureteral injury include contusion, partial tear, or complete disruption. In the setting of blunt trauma, injuries typically occur at or near the UPJ. The mechanism of injury is thought to be due to hyperextension with ureteral stretching or compression of the ureter against the lumbar transverse processes. Computed tomography findings of blunt ureteral injury on arterial or portal venous phase imaging can be subtle; mild periureteral fat stranding or fluid around the ureter or kidney may be the only findings. Hematuria is absent in up to one third of patients with ureteral injury. Three- to 20-minute delayed, excretory phase images are usually needed to definitively make the diagnosis. High-attenuation urine from the injured ureter will collect in the periureteral soft tissues (Fig. 11-105). The integrity of the ureter (i.e., partial or complete ureteral tear) can be determined by demonstration of intraureteral contrast distal to the level of the injury (Figs. 11-105 and 11-106). If CT findings are inconclusive, intravenous pyelogram, retrograde pyelography, or radionuclide scintigraphy can be used to detect urine extravasation.

■ BLADDER INJURY

Incidence

Between 2% and 11% of patients with pelvic fractures will have a bladder injury. Up to 90% of patients with traumatic bladder rupture will have concurrent fractures of the pelvis. The severity of the pelvic injury correlates positively with the risk for bladder or urethral injury. Gross hematuria almost always is seen with significant bladder injury. Suprapubic pain or tenderness, difficulty or inability to void, guarding, rebound tenderness, shock, ileus, and ascites are additional signs and symptoms of a bladder injury.

Diagnostic Technique

Cystography, either by radiography or CT, must be performed in all patients suspected of having a bladder injury. Cystography is performed after urethral injury has been excluded and retrograde catheterization of the urethra is deemed safe. To reliably diagnose bladder injury, at least 250 to 300 mL of iodinated contrast material must be instilled into the bladder. Less than this amount can cause false-negative study results because of inadequate distention. A scout anteroposterior radiograph

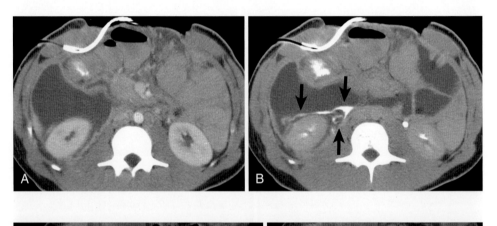

Figure 11-105 Postoperative computed tomography (CT) of multitrauma patient without known urinary system injury (**A**) shows large low-attenuation fluid collection surrounding the right kidney. Because a urinoma was suspected, 10-minute delayed images (**B**) were obtained and show contrast extravasation (*arrows*) from an injury to the proximal right ureter.

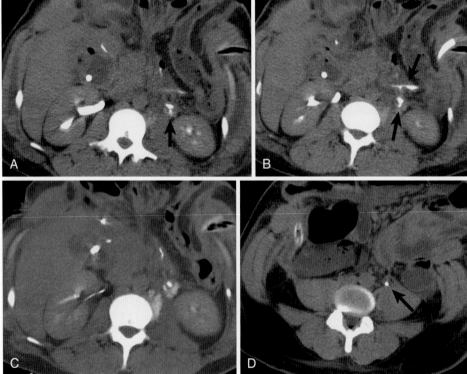

Figure 11-106 Delayed axial computed tomography (CT) images of multitrauma patient. A and **B,** Axial images show a small amount of extravasated contrast (*arrows*) from the proximal left ureter. There is progressive accumulation of periureteral contrast on the 10-minute delayed image (**C**). CT image distal to the site of ureteral injury (**D**) shows contrast opacification of the left ureter (*arrow*), indicating a partial rather than complete ureteral tear.

of the pelvis is initially obtained, 30% contrast medium is instilled into the bladder, and then full and postvoid radiographs of the pelvis are acquired. If the patient requires immediate pelvic angiography and embolization because of significant ongoing pelvic hemorrhage, cystography should be performed after pelvic angiography is complete. If performed before angiography, extravasated contrast material from the injured bladder could potentially obscure sites of pelvic bleeding. An on-table cystogram can be conveniently performed in the angiographic suite upon completion of the arteriogram.

Because most trauma patients will ultimately undergo abdominal-pelvic CT for evaluation of injuries, CT cystography is rapidly becoming the preferred study for suspected bladder trauma. In addition to gross hematuria, a cystogram should be performed when the abdominal-pelvic CT shows pelvic fractures (excluding isolated acetabular fractures) with free pelvic fluid or pelvic hematoma of unknown source (for technique see Computed Tomography Protocols and Scan Optimization). Multidetector CT cystography has proven to be as accurate as conventional cystography, with 95% sensitivity and

99% specificity in detecting bladder rupture. Although bladder injuries may be seen on standard CT with intravenous contrast bolus and a clamped bladder catheter, this antegrade approach to bladder distension cannot reliably exclude bladder injury.

Classification

Urinary bladder rupture is classified as intraperitoneal, extraperitoneal, or mixed. Intraperitoneal bladder rupture typically occurs at the anatomically weak bladder dome (Fig. 11-107) and most commonly results from blunt impact to a full bladder. Intraperitoneal bladder rupture accounts for up to 20% of all bladder ruptures in adults. Intraperitoneal bladder ruptures are thought to occur more frequently in small children involved in motor vehicle accidents than in adults; in the pediatric patient the seat belt fits over the anterior lower abdomen rather than the superior iliac spines, and the bladder is positioned in the lower abdomen rather than deep in the pelvis, thus putting the bladder in a more vulnerable position. An intraperitoneal bladder rupture will require surgical repair to avoid urinary peritonitis. Standard cystography or CT cystography will show high-attenuation urinary contrast medium extravasated from the bladder to the peritoneal cavity, outlining the peritoneal recesses and bowel loops (Figs. 11-107 and 11-108). High-attenuation contrast material from the ruptured bladder within the peritoneum can mimic bowel injury with extravasation of oral or rectal contrast. In addition, high-attenuation urinary contrast medium can obscure intraperitoneal blood or intestinal contents, diminishing overall diagnostic accuracy of abdominal-pelvic CT. Cystography can be falsely negative for bladder rupture when contrast is blocked from leaking by detrusor contraction, a small tear, a blood clot, or a balloon of the Foley catheter.

Extraperitoneal bladder rupture is caused either by bone spicules from a pelvic bone fracture perforating the bladder wall or by pulling of fascial connections between the bladder and pelvis during pelvic trauma. The most common site for extraperitoneal rupture is in the anterolateral bladder wall near the base (Fig. 11-109). On cystography or CT cystography the typical appearance is streaky or flame-shaped contrast extravasation into the extraperitoneal tissues surrounding the bladder. Contrast material may dissect through the fascial planes into the prevesical space of Retzius, the lateral

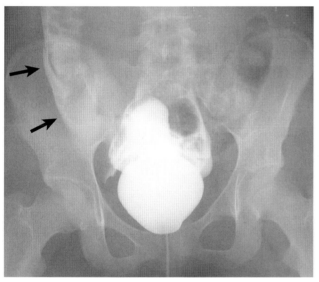

Figure 11-107 Cystogram of patient involved in a motorcycle accident demonstrates extensive contrast extravasation from the urinary bladder. The contrast appears to be coming from the bladder dome and also is seen outlining bowel loops *(arrows)*. These findings are diagnostic of intraperitoneal bladder rupture.

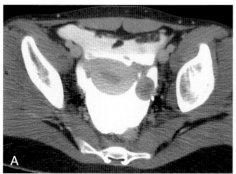
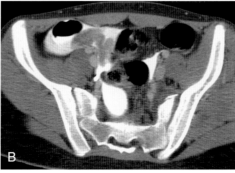

Figure 11-108 A, Computed tomography (CT) images of trauma patient with intraperitoneal bladder rupture show contrast from bladder pooling in the pelvis and outlining the uterus and adnexal structures. **B,** Contrast is also seen outlining bowel loops in the lower abdomen.

paravesical space, the anterior abdominal wall, or the retroperitoneum. If there is concurrent disruption of the urogenital diaphragm and bladder base, contrast may extend into the inguinal region or scrotum (Fig. 11-110). Most cases of extraperitoneal bladder rupture can be treated successfully with transurethral or suprapubic bladder catheterization. Ninety percent of extraperitoneal bladder ruptures will heal within 10 days. Combined intraperitoneal and extraperitoneal ruptures are seen in approximately 5% to 10% of all ruptures, and cystography will demonstrate features typical of both injuries.

Lacerations of the bladder mucosa and bladder wall contusions may produce hematuria or intravesicular hematoma. Clots arising in the region of the ureteral orifices may be due to renal or ureteral trauma rather than bladder injury. Intravesicular clots can rarely mask a full-thickness bladder injury by blocking urine leakage (see Fig. 11-111). In a patient with pelvic fractures and pubic symphysis diastasis, the bladder may herniate through the widened pubic symphysis (Fig. 11-112). Complications of a missed bladder injury include urinary tract infection, pelvic abscess, bladder fistula formation, and incontinence.

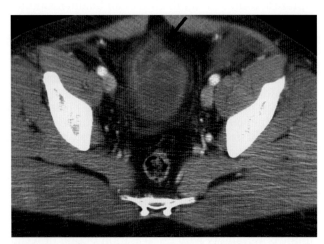

Figure 11-109 Computed tomography (CT) image of patient who fell from tree shows small amount of fluid surrounding the bladder and a focal wall defect *(arrow)* at the anterior bladder base. This is the most common site of extraperitoneal bladder rupture.

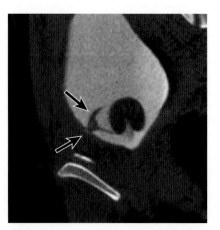

Figure 11-111 Reformatted sagittal computed tomographic cystogram image demonstrates contrast extravasation from a small tear in the bladder *(large arrow)*. An intravesicular filling defect *(small arrow)*, likely representing blood clot, lies adjacent to the site of bladder injury and may be partially blocking contrast egress.

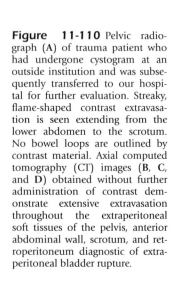

Figure 11-110 Pelvic radiograph (**A**) of trauma patient who had undergone cystogram at an outside institution and was subsequently transferred to our hospital for further evaluation. Streaky, flame-shaped contrast extravasation is seen extending from the lower abdomen to the scrotum. No bowel loops are outlined by contrast material. Axial computed tomography (CT) images (**B**, **C**, and **D**) obtained without further administration of contrast demonstrate extensive extravasation throughout the extraperitoneal soft tissues of the pelvis, anterior abdominal wall, scrotum, and retroperitoneum diagnostic of extraperitoneal bladder rupture.

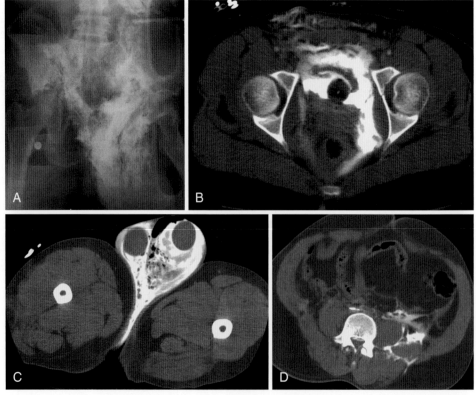

■ URETHRAL INJURY

Most urethral injuries occur in young males injured by high-velocity trauma who have pelvic fractures, especially unstable pelvic ring disruption or lateral compression type of injuries. Urethral injuries are uncommon in women due to the protective configuration of the female pelvic floor and shorter urethral length. Approximately 10% of patients with major pelvic fractures will sustain a urethral injury, typically involving the posterior (proximal) portion. In males, blood at the urethral meatus, inability to void, elevation of the prostate gland on rectal examination, or perineal swelling or hematoma should raise the suspicion for this injury. In women with urethral injury, pelvic fractures, the presence of vaginal bleeding, labial edema, dysuria, blood at the urethral orifice, hematuria, or urine leak through the rectum have all been described.

Anteroposterior pelvic radiography will almost always demonstrate pubic symphysis diastasis in a patient with a urethral injury. Imaging assessment of the urethra should precede cystography but should be delayed until after pelvic arteriography. A retrograde urethrogram is performed using 30 mL of 60% contrast medium via a Foley balloon catheter positioned in the distal urethra and inflated with 2 mL of saline. Ideally the study should be conducted using fluoroscopy, but it is often performed in the acute setting using oblique radiographs obtained with the shaft of the penis perpendicular to the femur to visualize the full extent of the urethra. Contrast extravasation into the periurethral soft tissues is usually readily apparent (Fig. 11-113). Posterior urethral injuries may be occasionally diagnosed with CT. Associated CT findings include regional hematoma and distortion of the urogenital diaphragm fat plane or prostatic contour. Computed tomography retrograde urethrography has recently been described. Urethrography results can be used to classify the injury using the Goldman system (Table 11-13), which helps in treatment planning.

Anterior (distal) urethral injury is more commonly caused by iatrogenic or penetrating rather than blunt trauma. The bulbous urethra may be injured in crush-type trauma. The injury may be limited to the corporal bodies if the Buck fascia remains intact or, if disrupted, may spread throughout the scrotum, perineum, and anterior abdominal wall.

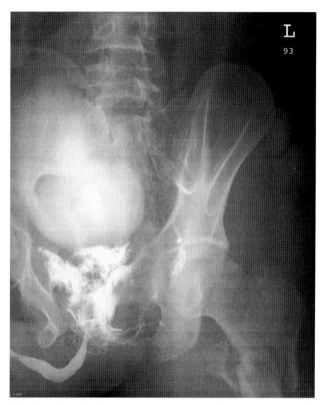

Figure 11-113 Retrograde urethrogram of patient involved in motor vehicle collision shows massive extravasation of contrast material from the posterior urethra. Note fractures of the left superior pubic ramus and femur.

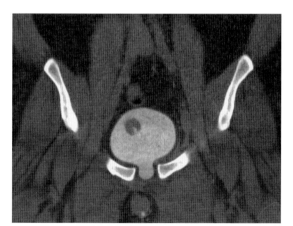

Figure 11-112 Coronal computed tomography (CT) image of a trauma patient shows diastasis of the pubic symphysis with traumatic herniation of the bladder, a finding critical for the orthopedic surgeon to know before surgical fixation of the pelvis.

Table 11-13   Classification of Urethral Injuries

	Colapinto and McCallum	Goldman and Sandler
Grade I	Posterior urethra stretched but intact	Posterior urethra stretched but intact
Grade II	Posterior urethral tear above intact UGD	Partial or complete posterior urethral tear above intact UGD
Grade III	Posterior urethral tear with extravasation through torn UGD	Partial or complete tear of combined anterior and posterior urethra with torn UGD
Grade IV	—	Bladder neck injury with extension to the urethra
Grade IVa	—	Injury to bladder base with extravasation simulating type IV (pseudo–grade IV)
Grade V	—	Isolated anterior urethral injury

UGD, Urogenital diaphragm.

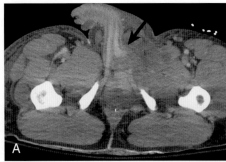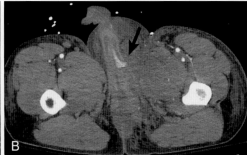

Figure 11-114 Axial contrast-enhanced images of a patient involved in a motorcycle collision (**A**) show diffuse swelling of the left hemiscrotum, left perineal hematoma, and a disruption of the left corpora cavernosa of the penis *(arrow)*. Due to increased size of the perineal hematoma, repeat computed tomography (CT) was performed 1 day later (**B**) and shows a focus of high attenuation within the left corpora cavernosa *(arrow)*, representing active bleeding.

■ SCROTAL INJURY

Testicular injury may be due to direct impact, penetrating wounds, or compression of the testis between the pubic arch and impacting object. About 50% of testicular injuries are seen in association with sports injuries. Differentiating testicular hematoma, rupture, or torsion is exceeding difficult by clinical examination. Rapid and accurate assessment is vital because a ruptured testis can be salvaged in 90% of patients if repaired within 72 hours, but salvage drops to 55% with increasing time since injury.

Ultrasound is the imaging technique of choice in acute scrotal trauma. A 5- or 7.5-MHz transducer is used. Both gray-scale and color Doppler US are required for complete examination. Ultrasound examination has 100% sensitivity and 65% specificity in detecting testicular rupture. Testicular rupture indicates tearing of the tunica albuginea with extrusion of the testis into the scrotal sac. On US the margins of the testicle are poorly defined and the testicle is diffusely heterogeneous. Color Doppler will show loss of vascularity to a portion or the entire testicle. Testicular laceration, hematoma, and fragmentation are also often seen.

Intratesticular hematomas are common after direct blunt trauma. The ultrasonographic appearance varies with the time of injury. Acute hematomas are typically isoechoic to normal testicular parenchyma and can be difficult to identify. A repeat US examination in 12 to 24 hours is indicated if initial results are equivocal. Although a hematoma will usually be managed conservatively, follow-up to resolution is recommended because of the risk for infection and necrosis, which may require orchiectomy.

Additional injuries seen with testicular trauma include dislocation and torsion. Traumatic torsion is uncommon and is seen in only 5% of all cases of torsion. Dislocation is most commonly seen in a patient involved in a motorcycle collision with impaction of the scrotum against the fuel tank. Dislocation is typically into the inguinal canal and can be diagnosed with US or CT. Prompt diagnosis is essential because a missed dislocation puts the patient at risk for development of intratesticular cellular changes that may predispose to malignant degeneration.

■ PENILE INJURIES

A penile fracture refers to fracture of the corpus cavernosum, typically due to vigorous sexual intercourse or masturbation. The "fracture" is actual rupture of the tunica albuginea, usually accompanied by a cracking sound from the erect penis, with pain and detumescence. Corporal laceration may be seen with direct trauma such as a kick to the flaccid penis. Physical examination is often quite limited due to painful swelling. Penile US examination can identify the site of the tear, seen as an interruption of the thin echogenic line of the tunica albuginea, with adjacent hematoma. Color Doppler may show blood flush through the tunica defect upon squeezing of the penile shaft. Magnetic resonance imaging or CT can demonstrates the discontinuity of the hypointense tunica albuginea (Fig. 11-114).

Selected Reading

http://www.aast.org/library/traumatools/injuryscoringscales.aspx#liver.

http://www.aast.org/library/traumatools/injuryscoringscales.aspx#spleen.

Albayram F, Hamper UM. Ovarian and adnexal torsion: spectrum of sonographic findings with pathologic correlation. *J Ultrasound Med.* 2001;20(10):1083–1089.

Anderson SW, Varghese JC, Lucey BC. Blunt splenic trauma: delayed-phase CT for differentiation of active hemorrhage from contained vascular injury in patients. *Radiology.* 2007;243:88–95.

Atri M, Hanson JM, Grinblat L, et al. Surgically important bowel and/or mesenteric injury in blunt trauma: accuracy of multidetector CT for evaluation. *Radiology.* 2008;249:524–533.

Ball CG, Dixon E, Kirkpatrick AW, et al. A decade of experience with injuries to the gallbladder. *J Trauma Manag Outcomes.* 2010;4:3.

Baron KT, Babagbemi KT, Arleo EK, et al. Emergent complications of assisted reproduction: expecting the unexpected. *Radiographics.* 2013;33(1):229–244.

Blaivas M, DeBehnke D, Phelan MB. Potential errors in the diagnosis of pericardial effusion on trauma ultrasound for penetrating injuries. *Acad Emerg Med.* 2000;7:1261–1266.

Bode PJ, Edwards MJ, Kruit MC, et al. Sonography in a clinical algorithm for early evaluation of 1671 patients with blunt abdominal trauma. *AJR Am J Roentgenol.* 1999;172:905–911.

Bradley EL 3rd, Young PR Jr, Chang MC, et al. Diagnosis and initial management of blunt pancreatic trauma: guidelines from a multinstitutional review. *Ann Surg.* 1998;227(6):861–869.

Branney SW, Wolfe RE, Moore EE, et al. Quantitative sensitivity of ultrasound in detecting free intraperitoneal fluid. *J Trauma.* 1995;39:375–380.

Brody JM, Leighton DB, Murphy BL, et al. CT of blunt trauma bowel and mesenteric injury: typical findings and pitfalls in diagnosis. *Radiographics.* 2000;20:1525–1536. discussion 1536–1537.

Brofman N, Atri M, Hanson JM, et al. Evaluation of bowel and mesenteric blunt trauma with multidetector CT. *Radiographics.* 2006;26:1119–1131.

Brown MA, Casola G, Sirlin CB, et al. Importance of evaluating organ parenchyma during screening abdominal ultrasonography after blunt trauma. *J Ultrasound Med.* 2001;20:577–583. quiz 585.

Buckley JC, McAninch JW. Revision of current American Association for the Surgery of Trauma renal injury grading system. *J Trauma.* 2011;70:35–37.

Catalano O, Aiani L, Barozzi L, et al. CEUS in abdominal trauma: multi-center study. *Abdom Imaging*. 2009;34:225–234.

Centers for Disease Control and Prevention. Sexually transmitted diseases treatment guidelines, 2010: pelvic inflammatory disease. http://www.cdc.gov/std/treatment/2010/pid.htm. Published 2013.

Charbit J, Manzanera J, Millet I, et al. What are the specific computed tomography scan criteria that can predict or exclude the need for renal angioembolization after high-grade renal trauma in a conservative management strategy? *J Trauma*. 2011;70(5):1219–1227.

Cohn SM, Arango JI, Myers JG, et al. Computed tomography grading systems poorly predict the need for intervention after spleen and liver injuries. *Am Surg*. 2009;75:133–139.

Daly KP, Ho CP, Persson DL, et al. Traumatic retroperitoneal injuries: review of multidetector CT findings. *Radiographics*. 2008;28:1571–1590.

Dreizin D, Munera F. Blunt polytrauma: evaluation with 64-section whole-body CT angiography. *Radiographics*. 2012;32:609–631.

Fang JF, Chen RJ, Wong YC, et al. Classification and treatment of pooling of contrast material on computed tomographic scan of blunt hepatic trauma. *J Trauma*. 2000;49:1083–1088.

Freitas ML, Frangos SG, Frankel HL. The status of ultrasonography training and use in general surgery residency programs. *J Am Coll Surg*. 2006;202:453–458.

Friese RS, Malekzadeh S, Shafi S, et al. Abdominal ultrasound is an unreliable modality for the detection of hemoperitoneum in patients with pelvic fracture. *J Trauma*. 2007;63:97–102.

Fulcher AS, Turner MA, Yelon JA, et al. Magnetic resonance cholangiopancreatography (MRCP) in the assessment of pancreatic duct trauma and its sequelae: preliminary findings. *J Trauma*. 2000;48(6):1001–1007.

Gupta A, Stuhlfaut JW, Fleming KW, et al. Blunt trauma of the pancreas and biliary tract: a multimodality imaging approach to diagnosis. *Radiographics*. 2004;24:1381–1395.

Huber-Wagner S, Lefering R, Qvick LM, et al. Effect of whole-body CT during trauma resuscitation on survival: a retrospective, multicentre study. *Lancet*. 2009;373:1455–1461.

Ingram MD, Watson SG, Skippage PL, et al. Urethral injuries after pelvic trauma: evaluation with urethrography. *Radiographics*. 2008;28:1631–1643.

Ishak C, Kanth N. Bladder trauma: multidetector computed tomography cystography. *Emerg Radiol*. 2011;18:321–327.

Jang T, Sineff S, Naunheim R, et al. Residents should not independently perform focused abdominal sonography for trauma after 10 training examinations. *J Ultrasound Med*. 2004;23:793–797.

Killeen KL, Shanmuganathan K, Boyd-Kranis R, et al. CT findings after embolization for blunt splenic trauma. *J Vasc Interv Radiol*. 2001;12:209–214.

Korner M, Krotz MM, Degenhart C, et al. Current role of emergency US in patients with major trauma. *Radiographics*. 2008;28:225–242.

Lingawi SS, Buckley AR. Focused abdominal US in patients with trauma. *Radiology*. 2000;217:426–429.

Linsenmaier U, Wirth S, Reiser M, et al. Diagnosis and classification of pancreatic and duodenal injuries in emergency radiology. *Radiographics*. 2008;28(6):1591–1602.

Lochan R, Sen G, Barrett AM, et al. Management strategies in isolated pancreatic trauma. *J Hepatobiliary Pancreat Surg*. 2009;16(2):189–196.

Lowdermilk C, Gavant ML. Screening helical CT for the evaluation of blunt traumatic injury in the pregnant patient. *Radiographics*. 1999;19:S243–S255.

Lozano JD, Munera F, Anderson SW, et al. Penetrating wounds to the torso: evaluation with triple-contrast multidetector CT. *Radiographics*. 2013;33:341–359.

MacLean AA, Durso D, Cohn SM, et al. A clinically relevant liver injury grading system by CT, preliminary report. *Emerg Radiol*. 2005;12:34–37.

Marmery H, Shanmuganathan K, Alexander M, et al. Optimization of selection for nonoperative management of blunt splenic injury: comparison of MDCT grading systems. *AJR Am J Roentgenol*. 2007;189:1421–1427.

Marmery H, Shanmuganathan K, Mirvis SE, et al. Correlation of multidetector CT findings with splenic arteriography and surgery: prospective study in 392 patients. *J Am Coll Surg*. 2008;206:685–693.

McCarter FD, Luchette FA, Molloy M, et al. Institutional and individual learning curves for focused abdominal ultrasound for trauma: cumulative sum analysis. *Ann Surg*. 2000;231:689–700.

McGahan JP, Horton S, Gerscovich EO, et al. Appearance of solid organ injury with contrast-enhanced sonography in blunt abdominal trauma: preliminary experience. *AJR Am J Roentgenol*. 2006;187:658–666.

McGahan JP, Richards J, Gillen M. The focused abdominal sonography for trauma scan: pearls and pitfalls. *J Ultrasound Med*. 2002;21:789–800.

McGahan JP, Wang L, Richards JR. From the RSNA refresher courses: focused abdominal US for trauma. *Radiographics*. 2001;21(spec No.):S191–S199.

Miller LA, Mirvis SE, Shanmuganathan K, et al. CT diagnosis of splenic infarction in blunt splenic trauma: imaging features, clinical significance and complications. *Clin Radiol*. 2004;59:342–348.

Miller MT, Pasquale MD, Bromberg WJ, et al. Not so FAST. *J Trauma*. 2003;54:52–59. discussion 59–60.

Mirvis SE, Dunham CM. Abdominal-pelvic trauma. In: Mirvis SE, Young JWR, eds. *Imaging in Trauma and Critical Care*. Baltimore, MD: Williams & Wilkins; 1992:145–242.

Mirvis SE, Whitley NO, Vainwright JR, et al. Blunt hepatic trauma in adults: CT-based classification and correlation with prognosis and treatment. *Radiology*. 1989;171:27–32.

Modica MJ, Kanal KM, Gunn ML, et al. The obese emergency patient: imaging challenges and solutions. *Radiographics*. 2011;31:811–823.

Natarajan B, Gupta PK, Cemaj S, et al. FAST scan: is it worth doing in hemodynamically stable blunt trauma patients?. *Surgery*. 2010;148:695–700. discussion 700-691.

Nuss GR, Morey AF, Jenkins AC, et al. Radiographic predictors of need for angiographic embolization after traumatic renal injury. *J Trauma*. 2009;67:578–582.

Park DH, Kim MH, Kim TN, et al. Endoscopic treatment for suprapancreatic biliary stricture following blunt abdominal trauma. *Am J Gastroenterol*. 2007;102(3):544–549.

Patel NY, Riherd JM. Focused assessment with sonography for trauma: methods, accuracy, and indications. *Surg Clin North Am*. 2011;91:195–207.

Patel SV, Spencer JA, el-Hasani S, et al. Imaging of pancreatic trauma. *Br J Radiol*. 1998;71(849):985–990.

Pieroni S, Foster BR, Anderson SW, et al. Use of 64-row multidetector CT angiography in blunt and penetrating trauma of the upper and lower extremities. *Radiographics*. 2009;29:863–876.

Poletti PA, Kinkel K, Vermeulen B, et al. Blunt abdominal trauma: should US be used to detect both free fluid and organ injuries? *Radiology*. 2003;227:95–103.

Poletti PA, Mirvis SE, Shanmuganathan K, et al. Blunt abdominal trauma patients: can organ injury be excluded without performing computed tomography? *J Trauma*. 2004;57:1072–1081.

Poletti PA, Mirvis SE, Shanmuganathan K, et al. CT criteria for management of blunt liver trauma: correlation with angiographic and surgical findings. *Radiology*. 2000;216:418–427.

Poletti PA, Platon A, Becker CD, et al. Blunt abdominal trauma: does the use of a second-generation sonographic contrast agent help to detect solid organ injuries? *AJR Am J Roentgenol*. 2004;183:1293–1301.

Rose JS. Ultrasound in abdominal trauma. *Emerg Med Clin North Am*. 2004;22:581–599. vii.

Rothlin MA, Naf R, Amgwerd M, et al. Ultrasound in blunt abdominal and thoracic trauma. *J Trauma*. 1993;34:488–495.

Saladyga A, Benjamin R. An evidence-based approach to spleen trauma: management and outcomes. In: Cohn SM, ed. *Acute Care Surgery and Trauma: Evidence Based Practice*. London, England: Informa UK; 2009:131–137.

Sandrasegaran K, Lin C, Akisik FM, et al. State-of-art pancreatic MRI. *AJR Am J Roentgenol*. 2010;195(1):42–53.

Sandrasegaran K, Tann M, Jennings SG, et al. Disconnection of the pancreatic duct: an important but overlooked complication of severe pancreatitis. *Radiographics*. 2007;27(5):1389–1400.

Sato M, Yoshii H. Reevaluation of ultrasonography for solid-organ injury in blunt abdominal trauma. *J Ultrasound Med*. 2004;23:1583–1596.

Scalea TM, Rodriguez A, Chiu WC, et al. Focused assessment with sonography for trauma (FAST): results from an international consensus conference. *J Trauma*. 1999;46:466–472.

Shackford SR, Rogers FB, Osler TM, et al. Focused abdominal sonogram for trauma: the learning curve of nonradiologist clinicians in detecting hemoperitoneum. *J Trauma*. 1999;46:553–562. discussion 553-562.

Shanmuganathan K. Multi-detector row CT imaging of blunt abdominal trauma. *Semin Ultrasound CT MR*. 2004;25:180–204.

Shanmuganathan K, Mirvis SE. CT scan evaluation of blunt hepatic trauma. *Radiol Clin North Am*. 1998;36:399–411.

Shanmuganathan K, Mirvis SE, Boyd-Kranis R, et al. Nonsurgical management of blunt splenic injury: use of CT criteria to select patients for splenic arteriography and potential endovascular therapy. *Radiology*. 2000;217:75–82.

Shanmuganathan K, Mirvis SE, Sherbourne CD, et al. Hemoperitoneum as the sole indicator of abdominal visceral injuries: a potential limitation of screening abdominal US for trauma. *Radiology*. 1999;212:423–430.

Shanmuganathan K, Mirvis SE, White CS, et al. MR imaging evaluation of hemidiaphragms in acute blunt trauma: experience with 16 patients. *AJR Am J Roentgenol*. 1996;167:397–402.

Sharpe JP, Magnotti LJ, Weinberg JA, et al. Impact of a defined management algorithm on outcome after traumatic pancreatic injury. *J Trauma Acute Care Surg*. 2012;72(1):100–105.

Soto JA, Alvarez O, Munera F, et al. Traumatic disruption of the pancreatic duct: diagnosis with MR pancreatography. *AJR Am J Roentgenol*. 2001;176:175–178.

Stassen NA, Bhullar I, Cheng JD, et al. Eastern Association for the Surgery of Trauma. Nonoperative management of blunt hepatic injury: an Eastern Association for the Surgery of Trauma practice management guideline. *J Trauma Acute Care Surg*. 2012;73:S288–S293.

Stassen NA, Bhullar I, Cheng JD, et al. Selective nonoperative management of blunt splenic injury: an Eastern Association for the Surgery of Trauma practice management guideline. *J Trauma Acute Care Surg*. 2012;73:S294–S300.

Stuhlfaut JW, Soto JA, Lucey BC, et al. Blunt abdominal trauma: performance of CT without oral contrast material. *Radiology*. 2004;233:689–994.

Thomson BN, Nardino B, Gumm K, et al. Management of blunt and penetrating biliary tract trauma. *J Trauma Acute Care Surg*. 2012;72(6):1620–1625.

Tkacz JN, Anderson SA, Soto J. MR imaging in gastrointestinal emergencies. *Radiographics*. 2009;29(6):1767–1680.

Vaccaro JP, Brody JM. CT cystography in the evaluation of major bladder trauma. *Radiographics*. 2000;20:1373–1381.

Valentino M, Serra C, Pavlica P, et al. Blunt abdominal trauma: diagnostic performance of contrast-enhanced US in children—initial experience. *Radiology*. 2008;246:903–909.

Valentino M, Serra C, Zironi G, et al. Blunt abdominal trauma: emergency contrast-enhanced sonography for detection of solid organ injuries. *AJR Am J Roentgenol.* 2006;186:1361–1367.

Whelan JG 3rd, Vlahos NF. The ovarian hyperstimulation syndrome: fertility and sterility. 2000;73(5):883-896

Williamson JM, Williamson RC. Managing pancreatoduodenal trauma. *Br J Hosp Med (Lond).* 2012;73(6):335–340.

Yu J, Fulcher AS, Turner MA, et al. Blunt bowel and mesenteric injury: MDCT diagnosis. *Abdom Imaging.* 2011;36:50–61.

Yu J, Fulcher AS, Turner MA, et al. Frequency and importance of small amount of isolated pelvic free fluid detected with multidetector CT in male patients with blunt trauma. *Radiology.* 2010;256:799–805.

CHAPTER 12

Imaging of Penetrating Trauma to the Torso and Chest

Kathirkamanathan Shanmuganathan and Thomas M. Scalea

Firearm-related injury is the second leading cause of death following motor vehicle collision. For every firearm death it is estimated that there are three to five other nonfatal firearm injuries. These injuries have become a major public health problem, creating a devastating impact on U.S. society with substantial emotional and financial cost. This chapter will describe the role of imaging in evaluating patients admitted with penetrating injuries to the abdomen and chest and the influence of imaging findings on management.

■ BALLISTICS

A missile exits the barrel of a weapon with significant kinetic energy. Military weapons and hunting rifles are high-energy weapons and have a muzzle velocity greater than 1000 ft/sec. Most civilian gunshot wounds (GSWs) result from medium-energy handguns, with a muzzle velocity less than 1000 ft/sec.

The extent of tissue damage caused by a projectile is more severe if the missile has high energy; yaws early in its path through tissue; is large in mass; hits bone, forming secondary missiles; or expands, deforms, or fragments when it strikes tissue. A permanent cavity results from the missile crushing the tissues it transits. The temporary cavity may enlarge from 20 to 25 times the diameter of the bullet fired from high-energy weapons. Severe damage results from the temporary cavity formation in fluid-filled organs (bladder or heart) and organs that have a dense parenchyma (Fig. 12-1) (liver, kidney, brain). The temporary cavity formed from a medium-energy weapon (handgun) is insignificant and does not contribute significantly to the amount of tissue damage in far- or intermediate-range civilian GSWs.

■ PENETRATING INJURIES TO THE TORSO

Mechanism of Injury

Most stab wounds are caused by knives, but they may also result from sharp objects or instruments. Unlike missiles, hand-driven low-energy weapons, such as a knife or ice pick, cause tissue damage only by their sharp cutting edge or point. Only 50% to 75% of victims of stabbing injuries to the anterior abdominal wall will have peritoneal penetration. Only 50% to 75% of these patients will have an injury that requires operative repair.

Unlike stab wounds, GSWs result in peritoneal penetration in 85% of abdominal gunshot wounds, and 80% of these patients will have significant organ injury. Surgeons use a penetrating abdominal trauma index (PATI) score to predict the severity of injury and risk for complications that occur following penetrating injuries. It takes into consideration the severity of the injury (1 minimal to 5 severe) to 14 organs and assigns a risk factor (1 to 5) for each organ. The PATI is obtained by multiplying the severity grade by the risk factor of all the injured organs and summing the individual organ scores. A high PATI score (>25) is typical of gunshot wounding and is associated with a higher likelihood of overtly positive peritoneal signs. Few, if any, further investigations are needed to confirm peritoneal violation.

Anatomic Regions

The torso (defined by the area between the internipple line and upper third of the thigh) is divided into five anatomic regions (Fig. 12-2) to categorize the site of injury, as follows:

1. The *thoracoabdominal* area defined by the internipple line superiorly, costal margins extended posteriorly, to the inferior tip of the scapula inferiorly.
2. The *anterior abdomen* defined by the costal margins superiorly, anterior axillary lines laterally, inguinal ligaments and symphysis pubis inferiorly.
3. The *flank* defined by the anterior and posterior axillary line (tip of the scapula superiorly and iliac crests inferiorly) and from the costal margin to the iliac crest.
4. The *back* defined by the tips of the scapula superiorly and iliac crests inferiorly.
5. The *pelvis* defined by the iliac crests and inguinal ligaments superiorly and upper thirds of the thighs inferiorly.

Mandatory Laparotomy

Before the mid-1960s it was believed that routine exploration for penetrating torso injuries would reduce mortality by 12% to 27% compared to expectant management. This concept arose from military experience since World War I. However, if such an approach were

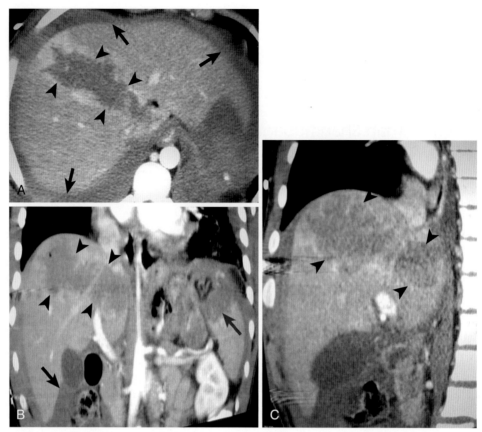

Figure 12-1 Severe liver injury from temporary cavity formation. Axial (**A**), coronal (**B**), and sagittal (**C**) multidetector computed tomography (MDCT) images show parenchymal contusion and hematoma *(arrowheads)* in the liver and spleen *(red arrow)* along temporary cavity formation outlining the bullet tract. Large amount of hemoperitoneum *(black arrows)* is seen around the liver.

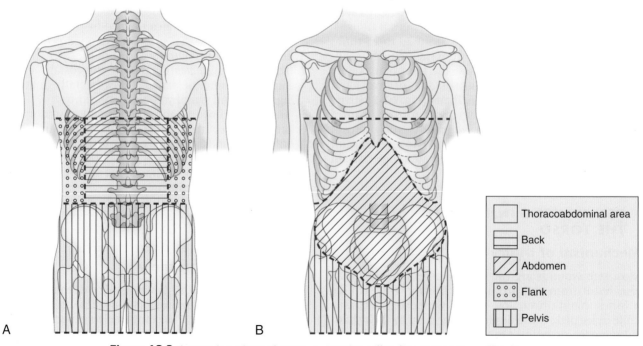

Figure 12-2 Anatomic regions of torso. **A,** Anterior axillary line. **B,** Posterior axillary line.

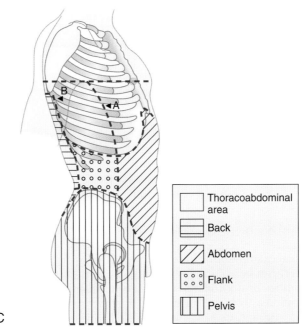

C

Figure 12-2, cont'd C, Blank, thoracoabdominal area. Horizontal lines, back. (From Shanmuganathan K, Mirvis SE, Chiu W, et al. Value of triple-contrast spiral CT in penetrating torso trauma: a prospective study to determine peritoneal violation and the need for laparotomy. *AJR Am J Roentgenol.* 2001;177:1247-1256.)

Box 12-1   Indications for Urgent Laparotomy

Hemodynamic instability
Peritonitis
Bleeding from rectum
Aspiration of frank blood via nasogastric tube
Evisceration of bowel
Positive FAST findings

FAST, Focused assessment sonography for trauma.

applied to all *civilian* penetrating injuries, 15% to 20% of GSWs and 35% to 53% of stab wounds to the torso would lead to an unnecessary (nontherapeutic) laparotomy.

Proponents of mandatory laparotomy based their belief on unproven assertions that intra-abdominal injury cannot be diagnosed short of exploration. They also believed that clinical examination was often unreliable in patients with serious injuries, that delay in diagnosis of these penetrating injuries would result in unacceptably high morbidity and mortality, and that nontherapeutic laparotomies were rarely associated with morbidity.

Indications for urgent laparotomy following penetrating trauma to the torso are shown in Box 12-1. The standard of care in the United States for patients who are hemodynamically unstable or have overt clinical signs of peritonitis after sustaining gunshot or stab wounds is laparotomy. Other clear indications for immediate laparotomy include aspiration of frank blood via a nasogastric tube, evisceration of bowel, and bleeding from rectum on clinical examination, proctoscopy, or sigmoidoscopy. The availability of new surgical concepts and techniques and sophisticated new radiologic technology, the use of antibiotics, and recognition of the potential morbidity

and increased hospital costs associated with laparotomy have challenged the dictum of mandatory exploration of the abdomen in the civilian setting.

Selective Conservative Management

The decision process of deciding which patient can be managed nonoperatively when there are no clear indications for surgery is termed *selective conservative management.* Over the past 4 decades, evidence of visceral injury has replaced simple peritoneal violation as the main indication for abdominal exploration. In the United States this policy is applied more often to stab wounds than GSWs in stable patients. Ideally a selective conservative approach should reduce the number of negative and nontherapeutic laparotomies without increasing the number, morbidity, or mortality of missed or delayed diagnoses of serious injuries.

The optimal method of ruling out peritoneal violation or significant visceral injury in hemodynamically stable patients with equivocal peritoneal signs following penetrating injury varies among institutions. The basic conservative management strategies, their strengths, and their weaknesses are listed in Table 12-1. The anatomic location of the entry wound and the local practice at any given trauma center may dictate the management approach selected.

■ MANAGEMENT STRATEGIES

Observation

Thirty-four percent to 72% of all patients with penetrating injury to the anterior abdomen or back are hemodynamically stable without overt signs of peritonitis and may be candidates for observation. The practice

Table 12-1   Selected Management Strategies

Technique	Strength	Weakness
Serial clinical examination	Low NTLR, noninvasive	Physician, bed, and time intensive
Local wound exploration and DPL	Easy to perform; if negative, discharge patient; sensitive for intraperitoneal injury	Invasive; if positive, DPL has to be performed; cannot evaluate entry site to retroperitoneum and thoracoabdominal region; does not evaluate the retroperitoneum; no uniform agreement on the criteria for a positive lavage; high NTLR
Computed tomography	High sensitivity for peritoneal violation and organ injury, evaluates retroperitoneum	No uniform agreement for specificity for surgical intestinal injury, radiation
Ultrasonography (FAST)	High specificity for injury, easy to perform, noninvasive, no radiation	Low sensitivity for injury
Laparoscopy	High sensitivity for peritoneal violation and diaphragm injury	Requires a skilled operator, known to miss intestinal injury

DPL, Diagnostic peritoneal lavage; FAST, focused assessment sonography for trauma; NTLR, non-therapeutic laparotomy rate.

of observation with serial physical examination (ideally performed by the same examiner) can be accomplished safely, thereby reducing the number of nontherapeutic laparotomies. This technique could easily be performed on abdominal stab wounds. In the appropriate clinical setting this practice may also be applied to GSWs. The majority of patients with a reliable clinical examination who have minimal or no abdominal tenderness can be discharged after 24 hours of observation. Missed injuries requiring subsequent surgical exploration may occur in 4% to 6% of patients in the observation group, with an average delay in treatment ranging from 3 hours to 5 days. Compared to mandatory laparotomy, this management approach reduces the nontherapeutic laparotomy rate from 53% to 3% to 8%.

One disadvantage of observation with serial examination is the need for admission to the hospital for up to 72 hours because a significant amount of time may be needed for clinical signs of peritonitis to develop after perforation, especially if the injury involves the retroperitoneal colon or duodenum. In a busy trauma center or in a small community hospital, staff may not be available to perform frequent examinations. This limits the number of patients that can be regularly observed. Physical examination may be unreliable, and it may be difficult to elucidate signs of peritonitis in patients with associated severe head or spinal cord injuries, intoxication with alcohol or drugs, or other distracting injury.

Local Wound Exploration and Diagnostic Peritoneal Lavage

Local wound exploration and diagnostic peritoneal lavage (DPL) have been used to evaluate hemodynamically stable patients without peritonitis who are at risk for penetration of the peritoneum. A positive tap in blunt trauma is aspiration of 10 mL of blood. In penetrating trauma the definition of a positive tap is less clear. A tap is considered positive if feces, bile, or food material is aspirated through a catheter placed in the peritoneal cavity. A negative peritoneal tap is followed by a peritoneal lavage performed through the same catheter using 1 L of normal saline. The lavage effluent is sent for analysis. Local wound exploration is generally performed in the admission area under local anesthesia and sterile conditions. Local wound

Table 12-2   Sensitivity and Specificity of Peritoneal Lavage Red Blood Cell Count for Detection of Peritoneal Injury

Mechanism of Injury	RBC Count (RBCs/mm³)	Sensitivity	Specificity
SW	5000	100%	0%
SW	50,000	94%-96%	75%-88%
SW	100,000	76%	75%
GSW	100,000	100%	71%

GSW, Gunshot wound; RBC, red blood cell; SW, stab wound.

exploration is appropriate only for anterior abdominal stab wounds. It should not be used for gunshot wounds or stab wounds to the back or flank. If the peritoneum has not been violated, the exploration site is closed and the patient can be discharged following wound care. If there is penetration of the peritoneum or if wound exploration is equivocal for peritoneal violation, DPL may then be performed to assess for intraperitoneal injuries.

There is no uniform agreement among surgeons on the peritoneal lavage red blood cell (RBC) count that is an appropriate trigger for exploration. Currently the number of RBCs per cubic millimeter sufficient to perform surgical exploration ranges from 1000 to 100,000/mm³; it varies among trauma centers and is based on the injury mechanism (Table 12-2). The lavage technique is highly sensitive when based on low RBC counts and highly specific using high RBC counts.

Significant injuries to the diaphragm and small bowel may occur with minimal hemorrhage and can be associated with false-negative DPL results. The inability to define the anatomic source of hemorrhage or severity of injury by DPL may increase the rate of nontherapeutic laparotomies in nonbleeding solid visceral injuries. Because DPL does not survey the retroperitoneum, it is unreliable in evaluating retroperitoneal organ injury and should not be used as the sole technique in the evaluation of patients with penetrating injuries to the flank and back. Local wound exploration may be difficult in obese patients, patients with thick back muscles, penetration in the thoracoabdominal region, or the presence of a large actively bleeding abdominal wall hematoma.

To improve patient flow, busy trauma centers prefer local wound exploration and DPL to observation with serial physical examination in order to triage asymptomatic patients with penetrating torso injury. Patients that have a DPL should be admitted for 24 hours to screen for any DPL complication and/or missed gastrointestinal injury. Unlike serial physical examination that warrants admission of a large number of patients for up to 3 days, these techniques can immediately eliminate patients who need not be observed. Intraperitoneal injuries in asymptomatic patients are also more likely to be detected acutely. This approach eliminates the risk for potential morbidity and mortality associated with a delay in injury diagnosis.

Multidetector Computed Tomography

Currently, triple-contrast multidetector computed tomography (MDCT) has become a valuable imaging modality to evaluate penetrating trauma to the torso considered for nonoperative management immaterial of the entry site or the number of gunshot or stab wounds. In this group of patients, MDCT can be very helpful and accurate in facilitating management decisions. Oral and intravenous contrast is also used routinely to optimize the detection of injuries to the intraperitoneal bowel, solid organs, mesentery, retroperitoneal genitourinary system, and duodenum. Penetrating trauma to the flank and back in asymptomatic patients is rarely associated with injury to critical retroperitoneal viscera because these organs are well protected by ribs, the spine, and the large back and paraspinal muscles. Patients with isolated retroperitoneal injuries resulting from these two anatomic locations may not present with overt clinical signs or symptoms and are not evaluated by DPL. It is important to routinely use rectal contrast material to opacify the entire colon to demonstrate contrast extravasation or focal colonic wall thickening, which enhances the ability to diagnose subtle colonic injuries that require surgical repair. Fifty-eight percent of patients with penetrating trauma to the back or flank incur intraperitoneal injuries. Combined intraperitoneal and retroperitoneal injuries may occur in about 16% of these patients.

Triple-contrast MDCT is highly sensitive and accurate in excluding peritoneal violation in patients with penetrating torso trauma. Among patients with peritoneal violation, MDCT has a high specificity, positive predictive value, and accuracy in predicting the need for laparotomy. It also helps to diagnose isolated liver injury, allowing nonoperative management for patients with penetration limited to the right upper quadrant.

Typically triple-contrast MDCT results are classified into negative, minor, or low risk for injuries and major or high risk for injuries. Patients with minor or low-risk injuries (small retroperitoneal hematoma or minor renal injury) are generally managed conservatively. Patients with major injuries are managed with surgery or angiography. In a busy trauma center, triple-contrast spiral MDCT is a safe and reliable technique to triage stable patients with penetrating injuries to the torso with no clinical or radiographic signs of peritoneal violation.

Diagnostic Laparoscopy

Laparoscopy enables direct visualization of the peritoneum and the intraperitoneal viscera to diagnose peritoneal violation and evaluate potential organ injury. Typically the diagnostic laparoscopy is converted to a laparotomy in the presence of peritoneal violation, major organ injury, or significant hematoma. Patients with no peritoneal penetration or with nonbleeding solid organ injuries may be observed or discharged. Laparoscopy still carries a 17% to 20% rate of nontherapeutic laparotomy and 17% negative laparotomy rate. Laparoscopy can prevent unnecessary laparotomies in 34% to 60% of patients with a concurrent reduction in hospitalization duration and costs.

The strength of diagnostic laparoscopy appears to be in the evaluation of patients with penetrating injuries to the left thoracoabdominal area with potential for small diaphragmatic rents. Local wound exploration is unreliable and associated with the risk for creating a pneumothorax. Laparoscopy reduces the number of nontherapeutic laparotomies, as compared to DPL, that may be performed among the subset of patients with minor splenic and liver injuries that have stopped bleeding by the time of surgery. Laparoscopy has also been shown to be optimally suited to evaluate the diaphragm for injuries in asymptomatic patients with less than 10,000 RBCs/mm^3 in the DPL effluent.

The limitations of laparoscopy include the need for general anesthesia and inadequate visualization of the retroperitoneum. Laparoscopy may also miss gastrointestinal injuries. The sensitivity can be as low as 18% for diagnosing bowel injury following penetrating trauma to the abdomen.

Tension pneumothorax may develop during laparoscopy in patients with diaphragm injury, and special precautions should be taken to avoid this complication. One major contraindication for laparoscopy includes prior history of multiple adhesions and patients with elevated intracranial pressure, who may suffer adverse effects from the insufflation of carbon dioxide. A significant cost savings will be gained only if laparoscopy is performed under local anesthesia.

Ultrasonography

There has been little enthusiasm to embrace ultrasonography as an initial screening study to evaluate patients with penetrating trauma to the torso. Though ultrasound can demonstrate free intraperitoneal fluid in blunt trauma patients, these results have not been reproduced in patients suffering penetrating injuries to the abdomen. The overall sensitivity of focused assessment sonography for trauma (FAST) to detect free fluid in the peritoneal cavity (in the perisplenic, perihepatic, pelvic, and pericardial spaces) is 47%. Ultrasonography is typically used only to detect free fluid. A significant number of patients with negative FAST study results have serious abdominal injuries requiring surgical repair. Positive FAST results are a strong predictor of intra-abdominal injury (specificity of 94%, positive predictive value of 90%). Thus positive FAST results should prompt immediate exploration.

■ IMAGING OF PENETRATING TORSO TRAUMA

Radiography

Radiographs are the initial imaging modality performed to localize a bullet and to evaluate for peritoneal violation. To determine the missile caliber from radiographs, the bullets should be seen on two views with no deformity, and the degree of magnification should be taken into account. Localization of a bullet or penetrating foreign body needs two radiographs obtained at 90 degrees or tomographic images (Fig. 12-3). Occasionally these two views may not be able accurately localize the exact site of the penetrating object (Figs. 12-4 to 12-6). It would be extremely risky to determine the course of a penetrating object using radiographs, by extrapolating a straight line between the entry and exit wounds or between the bullet and the entry site (see Fig. 12-3). Missiles do not take the shortest path between two points because the assailant may have been in motion when the injury occurred and

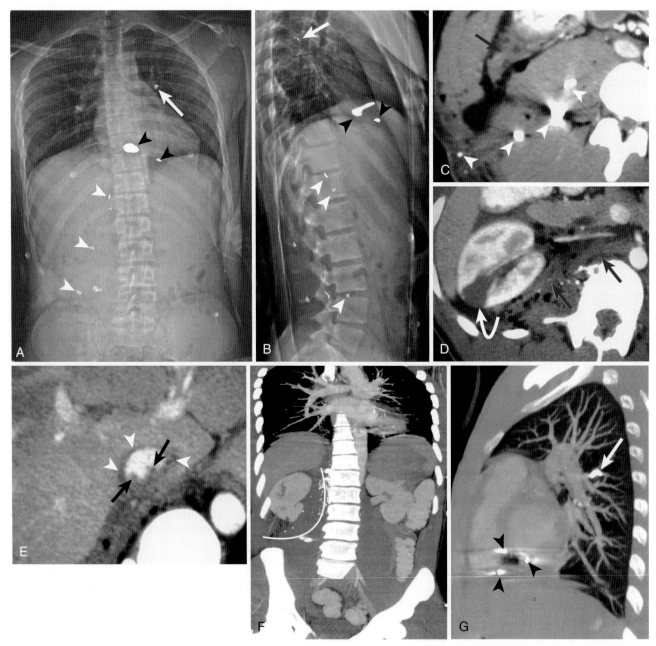

Figure 12-3 Unpredictable ballistic track with retroperitoneal, intracardiac, and left thoracic bullet fragments in a 26-year-old man shot in the right flank. Anteroposterior (AP) (**A**) and cross-table lateral (**B**) whole body digital radiographs show bullet fragments within retroperitoneum *(white arrowheads)*, heart *(black arrowheads)*, and left hemithorax *(white arrow)*. **C** and **D**, Axial computed tomography (CT) images obtained in mid and lower abdomen confirm wounding, gas bubbles, and bullet fragments in the retroperitoneum *(white arrowheads)* along the wound tract. A small retroperitoneal hematoma *(red arrows)* and a right renal contusion *(curved arrow)* are also seen. **E**, Axial image at the level of the intrahepatic vena cava shows fluid around the cava *(arrowheads)* and filling defects *(arrows)* within the lumen. Coronal (**F**) and sagittal (**G**) maximum intensity projection (MIP) images demonstrate bullet fragments outlining a curved path of the wound tract *(white line)* and the embolized bullet fragments through the vena caval injury into the heart *(arrowheads)* and branch of left pulmonary artery *(arrow)*.

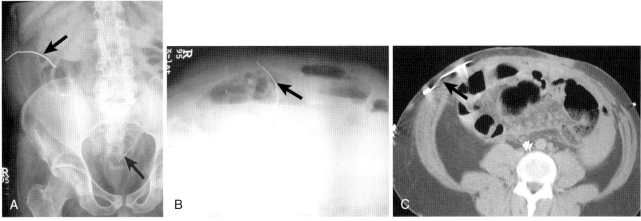

Figure 12-4 Attempted impalement with a metallic wire by a patient from a mental institution. Anteroposterior (AP) (**A**) and lateral (**B**) radiographs of abdomen show a metallic wire *(arrows)* with its tip in the peritoneal cavity. **C,** Axial computed tomography (CT) image at the level of the wire shows the wire *(arrow)* to be superficial to the abdominal wall muscles. Note a needle within the pelvis *(red arrow)* from a prior attempted impalement. (From Shanmuganathan K, Mirvis SE, Chiu W, et al. Value of triple-contrast spiral CT in penetrating torso trauma: a prospective study to determine peritoneal violation and the need for laparotomy. *AJR Am J Roentgenol.* 2001;177:1247-1256.)

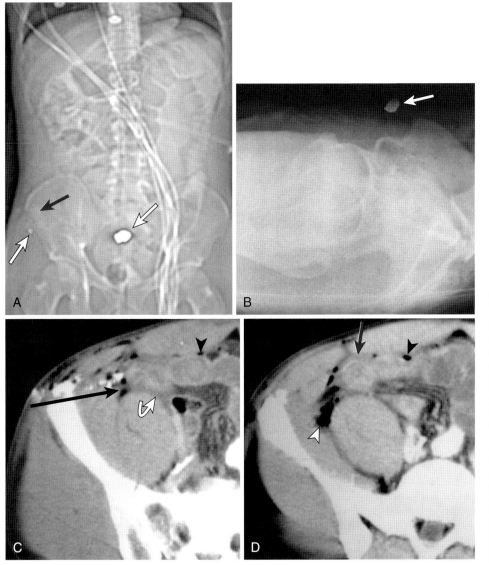

Figure 12-5 Gunshot wound to right side of pelvis. Anteroposterior (AP) computed tomography (CT) scan (**A**) and lateral radiograph (**B**) of the abdomen show a bullet *(white arrows)* in the anterior abdominal wall. The precise location of the bullet cannot be determined by the two views. A fracture *(red arrow)* of lateral right iliac wing and an adjacent bullet fragment *(white arrow)*. **C** and **D,** Axial images show the bullet tract outlined by bullet and bone fragments *(black arrow)*. Bubbles of gas are seen within the peritoneum *(black arrowheads)* and retroperitoneum *(white arrowhead)*. Small amount of free intraperitoneal fluid *(curved arrow)* and a loop of distal ileal wall thickening *(red arrow)* is seen. At surgery a full-thickness injury to ileum was repaired.

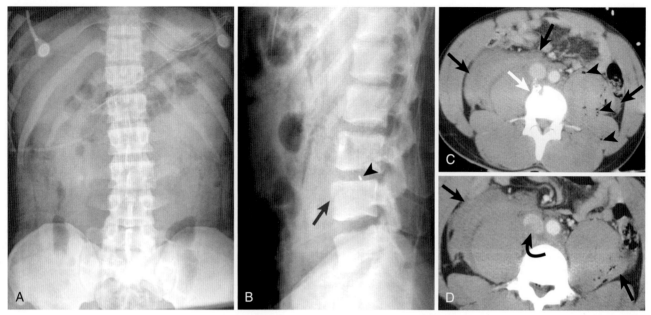

Figure 12-6 Gunshot wound to left lower back. Anteroposterior (AP) (**A**) and lateral (**B**) radiographs of the abdomen show a small bullet fragment *(arrowhead)* and an anterior L4 vertebral body fracture *(red arrow)*. **C** and **D**, Axial image confirms air bubbles *(arrowheads)* are seen within the left paraspinal and psoas muscle. A large retroperitoneal hematoma *(black arrows)* as a result of an injury to the posterior wall *(curved arrow)* of the inferior vena cava (IVC) is seen. Lumbar vertebral body fracture *(white arrow)* is also seen. At surgery the vena cava was ligated to control hemorrhage, and no intraperitoneal bowel injuries were seen.

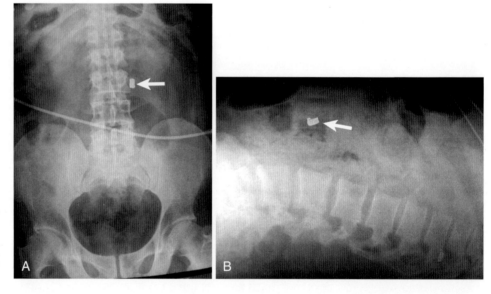

Figure 12-7 Gunshot wound to the left pelvis. Anteroposterior (AP) (**A**) and lateral (**B**) radiographs of the abdomen show an intraperitoneal bullet *(arrows)*. No free intraperitoneal air is seen.

missiles traveling through tissue with different density can change course.

Typically, trauma centers routinely obtain a chest radiograph and two views (anteroposterior [AP] and lateral projections) of the abdomen, usually performed without moving the patient (Fig. 12-7). Chest radiographs can be obtained in patients with penetrating trauma to the torso because penetrating injuries of the upper abdominal and thoracoabdominal regions are associated with thoracic pathologic conditions and need to be assessed for pneumoperitoneum. If feasible, chest radiographs should be obtained in the erect position to increase sensitivity for the detection of pneumoperitoneum. These three views help to evaluate for peritoneal penetration and localize

the penetrating object. Localized views may be required in obese patients or in regions of dense structure such as the pelvis (Figs. 12-8 and 12-9) to localize the penetrating object or evaluate for fractures. Radiographic findings of peritoneal violation include an intraperitoneal bullet (see Figs. 12-7 and 12-8) or a penetrating object and pneumoperitoneum (Figs. 12-10 and 12-11). Displacement of intraperitoneal organs by hematomas may help to localize the site and extent of injury. Abdominal and chest radiographs have a low sensitivity and lack specificity for intra-abdominal injuries (see Figs. 12-3, 12-8, and 12-11). The erect chest radiograph is positive for pneumoperitoneum in only approximately 18% of patients with surgically proven intestinal perforation.

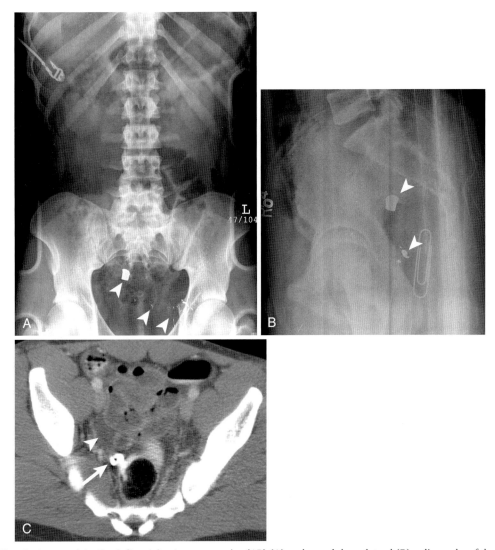

Figure 12-8 Gunshot wound to the left pelvis. Anteroposterior (AP) **(A)** and coned-down lateral **(B)** radiographs of the pelvis show bullet fragments *(arrowheads)* along the bullet tract. No free intraperitoneal air is seen. The largest bullet fragment is intraperitoneal in location. **C,** Computed tomography (CT) image shows small amount of free intraperitoneal fluid *(arrowhead)*, indicating peritoneal violation. The largest bullet fragment *(arrow)* is within the peritoneum and adjacent to the right lateral wall of sigmoid colon. At laparotomy a full-thickness injury to the ileum was repaired. No injury was seen to the sigmoid colon.

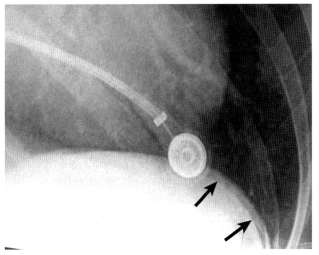

Figure 12-9 Small amount of pneumoperitoneum *(arrows)* seen beneath the hemidiaphragm of a patient with penetrating torso injury.

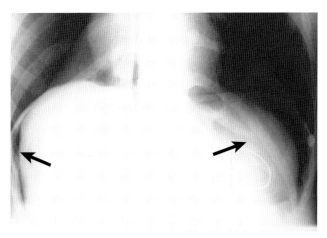

Figure 12-10 Large amount of pneumoperitoneum *(arrows)* is seen bilaterally in the upper abdomen.

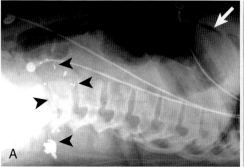
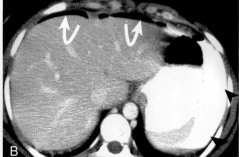
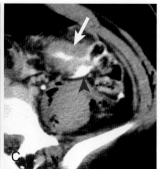

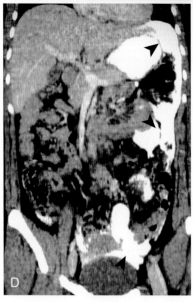

Figure 12-11 Subtle amount of pneumoperitoneum following a gunshot wound to the left flank. A, A cross-table lateral radiograph shows a small amount of pneumoperitoneum anterior to the liver *(arrow)* with multiple bullet fragments seen projected over the lower lumbar spine *(arrowheads)*. Axial computed tomography (CT) images (**B** and **C**) and multiplanar coronal reformatted CT images (**D**) confirm the pneumoperitoneum *(curved arrows)* anterior to the liver. Large amount of rectal contrast material extravasation *(arrowheads)* is also seen. Descending colonic wall thickening *(arrow)* represents the site of injury, which was confirmed at surgery.

Box 12-2   Contraindications for Multidetector Computed Tomography in Penetrating Torso Injury

Hemodynamic instability
Peritonitis
Bleeding from rectum
Aspiration of frank blood via nasogastric tube
Evisceration of bowel
Positive FAST findings

FAST, Focused assessment sonography for trauma.

Computed Tomography

Multidetector CT is the imaging modality of choice to evaluate patients who are hemodynamically stable following blunt trauma and has been shown during the last 2 decades to be accurate in diagnosing solid organ and hollow viscus injury. In the setting of penetrating trauma, MDCT is both far more sensitive and specific than radiography for identifying injuries to organs along a wound track. Multidetector CT is currently a popular diagnostic modality in hemodynamically stable patients with penetrating injuries to the torso without radiographic or clinical signs of peritonitis to detect peritoneal violation and intraperitoneal and retroperitoneal injuries. Contraindications for MDCT are listed in Box 12-2.

Technique

Triple-contrast MDCT scans are obtained from the internipple line to the symphysis pubis following administration of intravenous, rectal, and oral contrast material. The computed tomography (CT) parameters used at our institution for multislice spiral CT and for administration of intravenous contrast material are discussed in Chapter 11. A total volume of 600 mL of 2 % sodium diatrizoate (Hypaque) oral contrast material is administered 30 minutes before and immediately before initiation of the scan. An enema of 1 to 1.5 L of 2 % sodium diatrizoate is also administered on the CT table to opacify the colon before scanning. Delayed images are obtained routinely in the portal venous phase or at about 3 minutes following injection of intravenous contrast material to evaluate the renal collecting system.

Active Bleeding, Hemoperitoneum, and Free Fluid

Multidetector CT is extremely sensitive in detecting even small quantities of free intraperitoneal fluid or hemoperitoneum. Using attenuation measurements of free intraperitoneal fluid seen within the peritoneal cavity, CT is able to distinguish between free fluid, blood, hematoma, bile, and active bleeding (Figs. 12-12 and 12-13). On contrast-enhanced CT scans, free intraperitoneal fluid measures between 0 and 15 HU, free blood between 20 and 40 HU, clotted blood or hematoma between 40 and

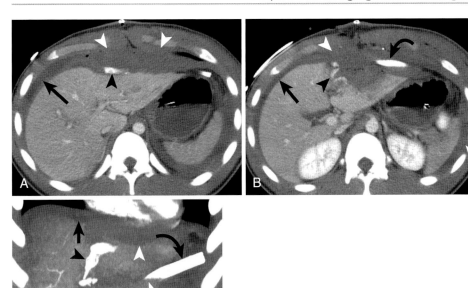

Figure 12-12 Multidetector computed tomography (MDCT) appearance of intraperitoneal blood. CT obtained following damage-control surgery for a thoracoabdominal gunshot wound. Axial (**A** and **B**) and coronal (**C**) maximum intensity projection (MIP) images show active bleeding *(black arrowheads)* from a liver injury. Large amount of clotted blood *(white arrowheads)* and small amount of nonclotted blood *(arrows)* seen in the upper abdomen. A surgical drain *(curved arrow)* is also placed adjacent to liver.

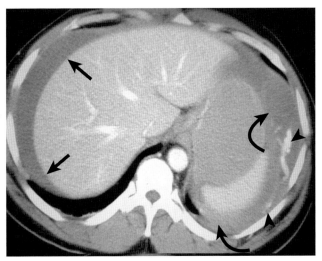

Figure 12-13 Multidetector computed tomography (MDCT) appearance of intraperitoneal blood. CT obtained following a stab wound to the left thoracoabdominal region. Axial image shows active bleeding *(arrowheads)* with perisplenic clot *(curved arrows)*. Lower-attenuation free intraperitoneal blood *(arrows)* is also seen adjacent to the liver.

70 HU, and active bleeding not less than 10 HU of the attenuation of intravenous contrast material seen within an adjacent major artery.

The significant difference in the attenuation value of extravasated contrast material (range, 85 to 350 HU; mean, 132 HU) and hematoma (range, 40 to 70 HU; mean, 51 HU) is helpful in differentiating active bleeding from clotted blood (see Figs. 12-12 and 12-13). This attenuation difference between clotted blood and active bleeding may often be appreciated on inspection and without need for measuring attenuation values using a region of interest.

The extended areas that can be scanned to obtain high-resolution imaging by MDCT during various phases (arterial, portal venous, and excretory) of intravenous contrast material administration help to better demonstrate active bleeding compared to conventional or spiral CT. On MDCT, ongoing hemorrhage may be seen as an increase in the amount of intravenous contrast material extravasated on images obtained in the identical anatomic region during dual-phase imaging (Fig. 12-14). Using MDCT scanners with greater than 40 slices with dual-phase imaging (arterial and portal venous phase), active bleeding may be seen only on the portal venous phase (see Fig. 12-14). This typically occurs when faster scanners outrun the vascular contrast bolus, especially when there is slow bleeding, bleeding from peripheral small arterial branches, venous hemorrhage, or vascular spasm. Blood and fluid show lower attenuation compared to the contrast-enhanced parenchyma of solid organs (see Figs. 12-12 to 12-14). Blood appears hyperattenuating compared to the parenchyma on unenhanced CT (Fig. 12-15). Blood or hematoma may appear isodense to suboptimally enhancing parenchyma, making it difficult to visualize by CT (see Fig. 12-14). To avoid this pitfall it is important to scan during peak parenchymal enhancement (portal venous phase) and to administer an adequate volume and concentration of intravenous contrast material based on patient body habitus. Bolus-tracking techniques and using a saline flush to use all the contrast material injected can be helpful to achieving peak arterial parenchymal enhancement without use of an excessive amount of contrast material. Oral and rectal contrast material to opacify the small bowel and the entire colon should also be administered routinely. This contrast helps demonstrate subtle bowel wall thickening (Fig. 12-16) and distinguish small quantities of intramesenteric blood, fluid, or hematoma from aggregated nonopacified bowel loops that can mimic these findings. Extravasation of a subtle amount of enteric contrast material may be the only specific finding of a surgical bowel injury (Fig. 12-17; see Fig. 12-16).

Small amounts of blood or free fluid are typically seen in the most gravity-dependent regions of the peritoneal cavity. In the supine position the most dependent region of the peritoneal cavity is the hepatorenal fossa (Morison pouch) (Fig. 20-18). Other areas where free fluid or blood is often seen in trauma patients are the pelvis between the sigmoid colon and the bladder, the paracolic gutters, and the perihepatic and perisplenic spaces (see Figs. 12-1, 12-5, and 12-11). Careful inspection of these areas is necessary to identify small quantities of fluid or blood

that may be the only CT sign of peritoneal violation, a subtle or occult intraperitoneal visceral injury (see Figs. 12-5, 12-8, and 12-18). Measuring the attenuation value of the free intraperitoneal blood in the various anatomic locations in the peritoneal cavity is important because the highest-attenuation blood will be seen adjacent to the injured organ and this is referred to as the *sentinel clot* (Fig. 12-19). This CT sign is reliable and helpful in localizing the source of hemorrhage when evaluating MDCT in patients with hemoperitoneum in multiple compartments or with multiple visceral injuries.

Performance of DPL can decrease the attenuation value of hemoperitoneum by dilution. Whenever DPL is performed before CT, this knowledge is required for

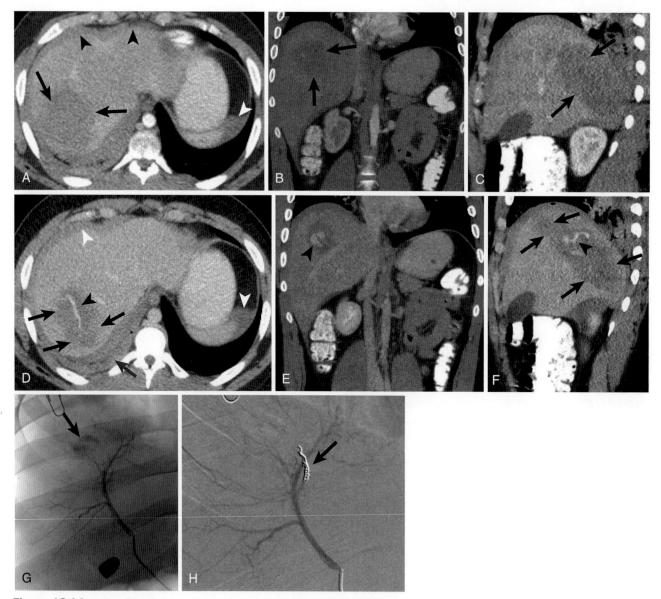

Figure 12-14 Active bleeding seen only on portal venous images in a patient with a gunshot wound to the right thoracoabdominal region. Axial (**A**), coronal (**B**), and sagittal (**C**) late arterial phase images show a contusion *(arrows)* along the bullet tract. Hemoperitoneum *(white arrowhead)* is seen adjacent to spleen. Perihepatic blood *(black arrowheads)* is also seen. Axial (**D**), coronal (**E**), and sagittal (**F**) portal venous phase images obtained at the same anatomic location show active bleeding *(black arrowheads)* within the contusion *(arrows)* with hemoperitoneum *(white arrowheads)* in the perihepatic and adjacent to spleen. A small right hemothorax *(red arrow)* is also present. **G,** Selective hepatic arteriogram shows active bleeding *(arrow)* from a right branch vessel. **H,** Postembolization image with multiple coils *(arrow)* shows arrest of hemorrhage.

accurate interpretation. Any fluid that measures more than 10 HU after a pre-MDCT DPL is performed is considered to contain either admixed blood or oral/rectal contrast material. Attenuation measurements should be obtained for all fluid collections identified by MDCT to help characterize their origin. Care should be taken to avoid volume averaging in assigning the region of interest within the fluid.

The CT attenuation value of bile is usually below 0 HU due to its high cholesterol content. Intraperitoneal or combined intraperitoneal and extraperitoneal bladder

injuries could result in urine leaking into the peritoneal cavity. Unopacified urine is usually similar in density to fluid and measures between 0 and 15 HU and thus can mimic free intraperitoneal fluid from other sources. However, on delayed images obtained during the excretory phase the attenuation of intraperitoneal urine will increase in value and may be similar in attenuation to urine in the bladder as a result of admixing extravasated urinary contrast material and unopacified urine within the peritoneal cavity.

Wound Tract and Peritoneal Violation

The presence of air, hemorrhage, or bullet fragments along a wound tract allows identification of the bullet or knife trajectory using CT. The greater amount of hemorrhage (Fig. 12-21; see Figs. 12-1 and 12-3), air, and metal fragments (see Figs. 12-3 and 12-5) usually seen along GSW tracts enables those tracts to be more clearly seen on CT compared to a low-energy stab wound tract (Fig. 12-20). Knife wound tracts may be subtle, and it is important to identify the wound tract, its extension into the peritoneal cavity, and its relationship to abdominal viscera (Fig. 12-22). Prior knowledge of the entry wound, use of a radiopaque marker to demonstrate the entry wound, and use of optimum CT windows and level (window, 550; level, 75) aid in identifying subtle wound tracts. Computed tomography findings should be considered positive for peritoneal violation in the presence of a wound tract outlined by air, hemorrhage, or bullet fragments due to a missile or knife with a missile or knife trajectory toward the peritoneal cavity. (It is important to review images on bone and lung window settings to determine the precise location of air bubbles seen along the wound tract that are located adjacent to the peritoneum. Intraperitoneal free air or fluid, bullet fragments, and visceral, mesenteric, or vascular injury are diagnostic findings of peritoneal violation (Figs. 12-5 to 12-8, 12-11 to 12-14, 12-19, and 12-20).

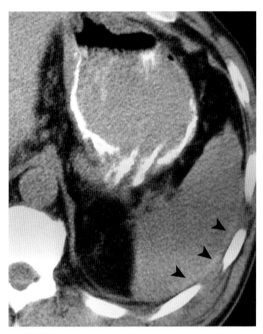

Figure 12-15 Appearance of blood on unenhanced computed tomography (CT). Unenhanced CT image in the region of the spleen in a trauma patient shows a small amount of subcapsular blood *(arrowheads)*. Blood appears hyperattenuated compared to the normal splenic parenchyma.

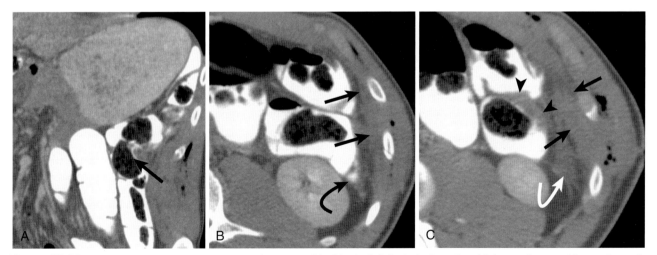

Figure 12-16 Subtle colonic wall thickening. Patient was stabbed in the left flank. **A,** Curved multiplanar reformatted image shows the wound tract outlined by hematoma and gas bubble extending from the skin to descending colon *(arrow)*. **B** and **C,** Axial images show subtle amount of colonic contrast material outside the lumen *(curved black arrow)* and colonic wall thickening *(arrowheads)*. An adjacent mesenteric hematoma *(white curved arrow)* and contiguous injury on either side of the diaphragm with thickening of the diaphragm *(arrows)* are also seen. Both the colonic and diaphragm injury were repaired at surgery.

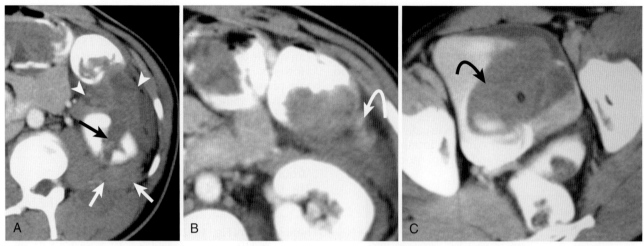

Figure 12-17 Subtle colonic contrast extravasation following stab wound to left back. A to C, Axial images show a laceration to the lower pole of the left kidney *(black arrow)* and large amount of clotted blood *(black curved arrow)* within the bladder as a result of bleeding from the renal injury. Posterior pararenal *(white arrows)* and perinephric *(arrowheads)* hematomas are seen. Subtle amount of rectal contrast extravasation *(curved white arrow)* is seen from the descending colon. This could be easily missed because of the obvious predominant renal injury. Colonic injury was repaired at surgery.

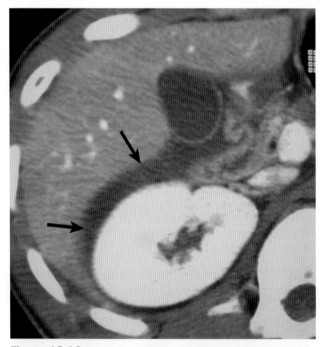

Figure 12-18 Free intraperitoneal fluid in a 35-year-old man admitted following a gunshot wound and small bowel injury (not shown). Axial computed tomography (CT) image shows low-attenuation free intraperitoneal fluid *(arrows)* in the Morison pouch. This was the only sign of peritoneal violation.

The most common MDCT finding seen in patients with peritoneal violation following entry site to the torso is intraperitoneal free fluid, and this may be the only finding in up to 11% of patients with peritoneal violation. This sign is more often associated with GSWs than stab wounds. Other CT signs useful for diagnosing peritoneal violation include direct visualization of the wound tract extending through the peritoneum (see Fig.12-22), intraperitoneal visceral injury (see Figs. 12-5, 12-8, and 12-12), seen in about 60% of patients, and free intraperitoneal air (see Figs. 12-5 and

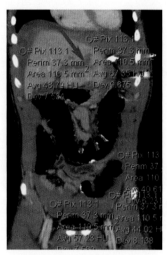

Figure 12-19 Sentinel clot sign. Patient was shot in the thoracoabdominal region. Coronal multiplanar reformatted image shows a left lobe liver laceration *(arrow)*. Hemoperitoneum is seen in multiple compartments of the peritoneum. Measurements of attenuation values in the various compartments show the highest attenuation value is seen adjacent to liver.

12-11), seen in 43% of patients. Multidetector CT is highly accurate and has a very high negative predictive value (97% to 100%) in determining peritoneal violation. Based on this performance of MDCT, the majority of the patients selected for nonoperative management without other injuries that require in hospital treatment can be discharged from the hospital with 24 hours of observation (see Fig.12-22). Information derived from triple-contrast MDCT helps triage patients with penetrating torso trauma and facilitates optimal use of medical resources.

Solid Organ Injury
The liver is the most commonly injured solid organ seen following penetrating torso trauma (Fig. 12-23). Injuries to the liver and spleen are seen more frequently following penetrating injuries to the thoracoabdominal

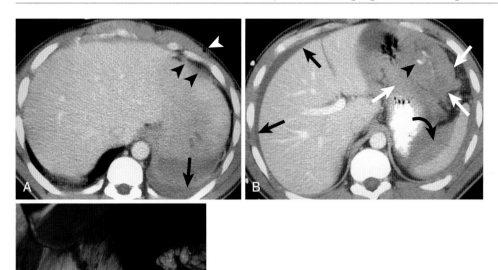

Figure 12-20 Subtle wound tract due to a stab wound to left thoracoabdominal region. A, Admission axial computed tomography (CT) image of the upper abdomen shows thickening of the left diaphragm *(black arrowheads)* and a single gas bubble *(white arrowhead)* at the overlying entry site. A small hemothorax *(arrow)* is also seen. **B,** Follow-up CT obtained 18 hours post admission for abdominal pain and distention now shows free intraperitoneal blood around the liver *(black arrows)* with a large mesenteric hematoma *(white arrows)* and active bleeding *(arrowhead)* in the center of the mesenteric hematoma. Perisplenic clot *(curved arrow)* is also seen. **C,** At surgery a mesenteric hematoma and left hemidiaphragm injury *(arrow)* were identified.

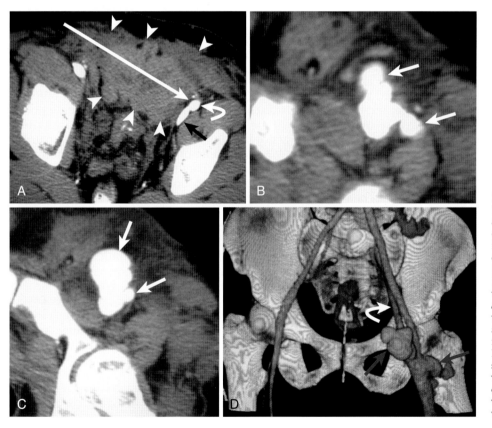

Figure 12-21 Wound tract outlined by hematoma in a patient admitted following a transpelvic gunshot wound. A, Axial image in the lower pelvis shows a large extraperitoneal pelvic hematoma *(arrowheads)* along the bullet tract *(white arrow)*. Both the left iliac vein *(black arrow)* and artery *(curved arrow)* are seen because of an arteriovenous fistula. **B** and **C,** Axial image at the level of the fistula shows multiple pseudoaneurysms *(arrows)*. **D,** Three-dimensional (3-D) image shows early filling of the left iliac vein *(curved arrow)*, multiple pseudoaneurysms *(arrows)*, and arteriovenous fistula. The vascular injury was repaired surgically.

region, upper abdomen, and flank. The principal types of parenchymal injury that may be seen on CT include contusions, hematoma, laceration, and active bleeding. Hematomas may be subcapsular (Fig. 12-24) or intraparenchymal (Figs. 12-25 and 12-26). Parenchymal hematomas typically occur along the wound tract and are isoattenuating or slightly hyperattenuating compared to normal liver parenchyma. Subcapsular hematomas are less frequently seen and are usually smaller in size with penetrating than blunt trauma. The penetrating object typically tears the Glisson capsule and allows decompression of the hematoma

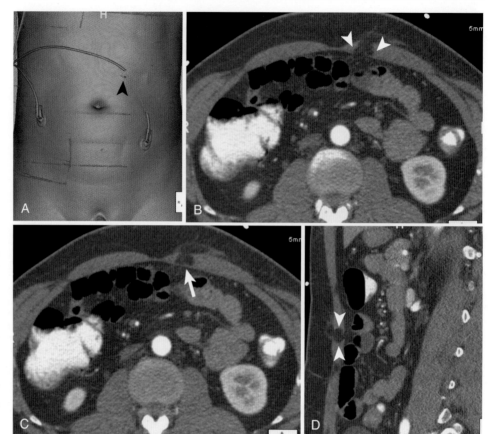

Figure 12-22 Stab wound to anterior abdomen in a 37-year-old man with peritoneal violation. A, Three-dimensional (3-D) image shows the entry site *(arrowhead)* in the left anterior abdomen. axial (**B** and **C**) and sagittal (**D**) reformatted images show wound tract extending through the anterior abdominal wall muscles *(arrowheads)* and peritoneum *(arrow)*. Because no wound tract, free intraperitoneal fluid, or air was seen, patient was observed for 10 hours post injury for development of peritonitis before discharge from the hospital.

into the peritoneal cavity rather than into the subcapsular space. Subcapsular hematomas are seen as low-attenuation collections between the parenchyma and the Glisson capsule. Subcapsular hematomas cause direct compression of the underlying liver parenchyma (see Fig. 12-24). This CT sign is helpful for differentiating a subcapsular hematoma from free intraperitoneal blood. Subcapsular or parenchymal hematomas may also occur some distance away from the wound tract without penetration of the solid organ. This is particularly true with high-energy injuries such as GSWs. These hematomas usually result from the temporary cavity formation transmitted via high-energy missiles into organs with dense parenchyma like the liver and spleen.

On contrast-enhanced CT, intraparenchymal contusions are seen along the wound tract as low-attenuation areas when compared to the normally enhancing parenchyma of the liver or spleen (Fig. 12-27). Intraparenchymal contusions and hematomas seen with the same wound tract are usually more extensive following a high-energy GSW, which generally causes more tissue damage than stab wounds (Fig. 12-28; see Figs.12-1, 12-12, 12-23, 12-25 to 12-27).

Lacerations also occur along the wound tract, resulting from crushing of parenchyma. On contrast-enhanced CT acute lacerations are seen as linear low-attenuation areas compared to the normal-enhancing parenchyma (see Figs. 12-23, 12-27, and 12-28). Computed tomography helps identify the relationship between lacerations and major vascular structures as hepatic veins, the porta hepatis, intrahepatic inferior vena cava (IVC), and splenic hilum

(Fig. 12-29; see Figs. 12-1 and 12-12). These CT findings may help plan management and predict outcome because extension of liver lacerations adjacent to one or more of the hepatic veins has a significant association with active bleeding and failed nonoperative management. Whereas lacerations resulting from blunt trauma typically display a parallel irregular linear or stellate pattern, such patterns do not occur from penetrating trauma. As a liver laceration heals, it typically enlarges, develops smooth margins, and assumes a round or oval shape (see Fig. 12-29).

Active hemorrhage (see Figs. 12-12, 12-14 and 12-28) resulting from penetrating injury is seen as an irregular or linear high-attenuation area of contrast extravasation surrounded by less dense hematoma that usually increases in amount on delayed images using MDCT (see Fig.12-28). With faster MDCT scanners (≥40 detector rows) a slow rate of bleeding may be visualized only on delayed images. Posttraumatic vascular injuries include pseudoaneurysms (Fig. 12-25), arteriovenous fistulas (Fig. 12-30; see Fig. 12-29), and porto-venous fistulas. Pseudoaneurysms are seen as well-defined high-attenuation areas, similar in attenuation to adjacent arteries. Posttraumatic vascular injuries typically become less dense or "wash out" on equilibrium phase images. It is important to review both the initial and delayed phase images obtained through the same anatomic location to diagnose small amounts of bleeding and differentiate ongoing bleeding from various other posttraumatic vascular injuries (see Fig. 12-14 and Figs. 12-28 to 12-30).

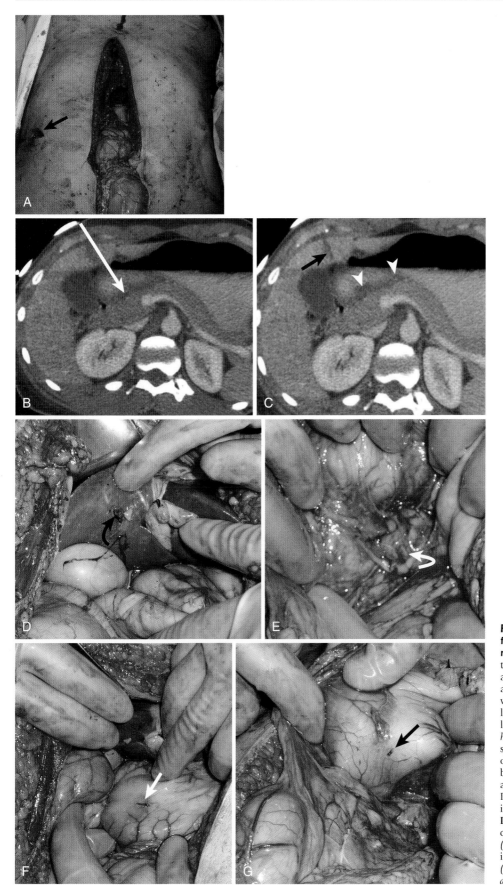

Figure 12-23 Liver laceration following stab wound to abdomen. A The stab wound (*arrow*) to the right anterior abdomen. **B,** and **C,** Axial images in the upper abdomen show the apparent knife wound tract (*white arrow*), a linear liver laceration (*black arrow*), and low-attenuation fluid (*white arrowheads*) in the anterior pararenal space. Though no direct evidence of an injury to the stomach is seen, based on the wound track the stomach is highly likely to be injured. Presence of anterior pararenal fluid indicates an injury to the pancreas. **D** to **G,** Intraoperative photographs confirm the injuries to the liver (*black curved arrow*) and pancreatic injury (*curved white arrow*) anterior (*white arrow*) and posterior (*black arrow*) wall of the stomach.

On dual-phase MDCT (arterial phase and portal venous phase), patients with posttraumatic arterio-portal fistula of the liver may demonstrate transient hepatic parenchymal attenuation differences (see Figs. 12-29 and 12-30), early increased attenuation of the peripheral portal vein

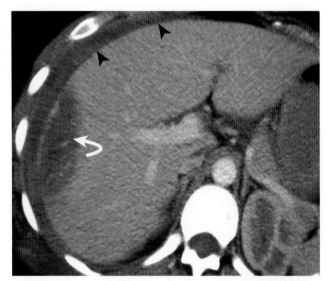

Figure 12-24 Subcapsular hematoma following gunshot wound to right thoracoabdominal region. Axial image shows a small mixed-attenuation subcapsular hematoma *(curved arrow)* causing mass effect on underlying liver parenchyma. Hemoperitoneum *(arrowheads)* is seen because of the subcapsular hematoma decompressing into the peritoneum through a tear in the Glisson capsule.

compared to the central portal vein, increased attenuation of the central and peripheral hepatic portal veins compared to the main portal vein, and simultaneous local enhancement of the hepatic artery and accompanying adjacent portal vein branch, the "double barrel" (see Figs. 12-29 and 12-30) or "rail track" (see Fig. 12-30) sign. The most sensitive MDCT finding to diagnose a hepatic arterio-portal fistula is transient hepatic parenchymal attenuation differences. Patients with active hemorrhage or posttraumatic vascular injuries usually require angiographic embolization (see Figs. 12-14 and 12-25), surgical repair (see Fig. 12-24), or a combined therapeutic approach (see Figs. 12-21 and 12-30).

Retrohepatic Vena Caval and Major Hepatic Vein Injury

Injuries to the major hepatic veins or retrohepatic IVC (juxtahepatic venous injuries) are fortunately rarely seen following abdominal trauma. However, up to 87% of all retrohepatic vena caval injuries result from penetrating trauma (Fig. 12-31; see Fig.12-3). Unlike the 11% mortality rate reported in surgically managed penetrating hepatic injuries without involvement of the intrahepatic IVC, retrohepatic caval injuries are typically associated with very high mortality (30% to 90%). In most series this mortality has been attributed to excessive blood loss, coagulopathy resulting in delayed recognition of the injury, and difficulty in obtaining surgical exposure for repair. A majority of these patients will proceed

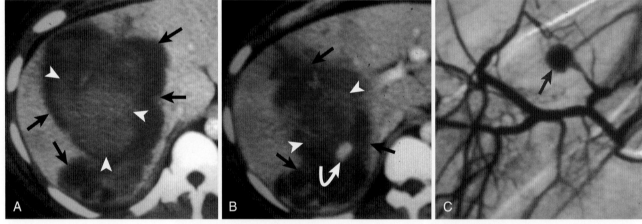

Figure 12-25 Gunshot wound to right thoracoabdominal region. **A** and **B,** Axial computed tomography (CT) image shows a large area of liver hematoma *(arrowheads)* and contusion *(arrows)* along the wound tract. A pseudoaneurysm *(curved arrow)* is also seen within the injury. **C,** Selective right hepatic arteriogram shows the pseudoaneurysm *(arrow)*, which was treated successfully with embolization.

Figure 12-26 Gunshot wound to right thoracoabdominal region. **A** and **B,** Axial images show a large mixed-attenuation *(arrowheads)* right lobe liver contusions and hematoma. There is moderate amount of hemoperitoneum *(arrows)* and a gas bubble *(curved arrow)* within the liver parenchyma brought in by the bullet.

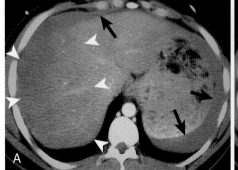
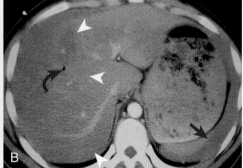

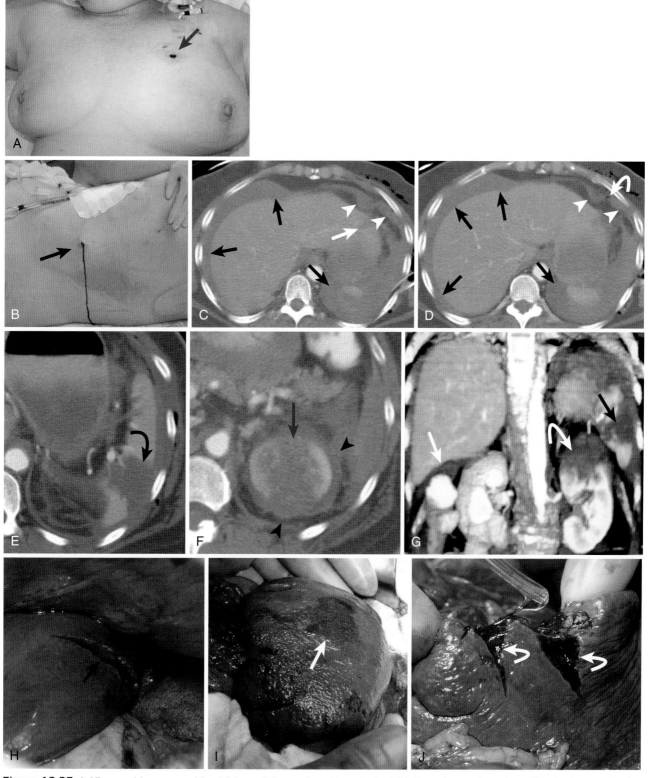

Figure 12-27 A 65-year-old woman with a history of depression attempted suicide by trying to shoot herself in the heart. A and B, Photographs show the entry site *(red arrow)* in the left "cardiac box" and exit wound *(black arrow)* in upper back. C to F, Axial images in the upper abdomen show thickening of the left hemidiaphragm due to a hematoma *(white arrowheads)* and a small rent *(curved white arrow)*. A surface liver laceration *(white arrow)* and hemoperitoneum *(black arrows)* are seen in the upper abdomen. There is also a splenic *(black curved arrow)* and left upper pole renal *(red arrow)* contusion. A small perinephric hematoma *(black arrowheads)* is seen. G Three-dimensional (3-D) image shows the mid-splenic contusion (black arrow). H to J, Intraoperative photographs show the surface liver laceration *(black arrow)*, splenic contusion *(white arrow)*, and left upper pole renal injuries *(curved arrows)*. The diaphragm injury was also repaired at surgery.

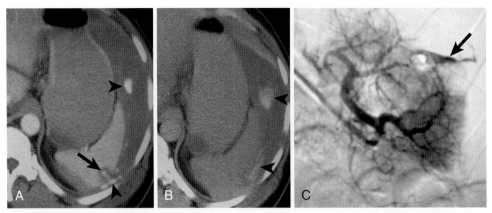

Figure 12-28 Stab wound to left thoracoabdominal region. Portal venous (**A**) and excretory phase (**B**) axial images obtained at the same anatomic location show active bleeding *(arrowheads)* arising from a splenic laceration *(arrow)*. The active bleeding increases in amount on delayed imaging. Moderate amount of perisplenic clot and hemoperitoneum are seen adjacent to the spleen and stomach. **C,** Splenic arteriogram confirms active bleeding *(arrow)* from the spleen. Embolization arrested the bleeding (not shown).

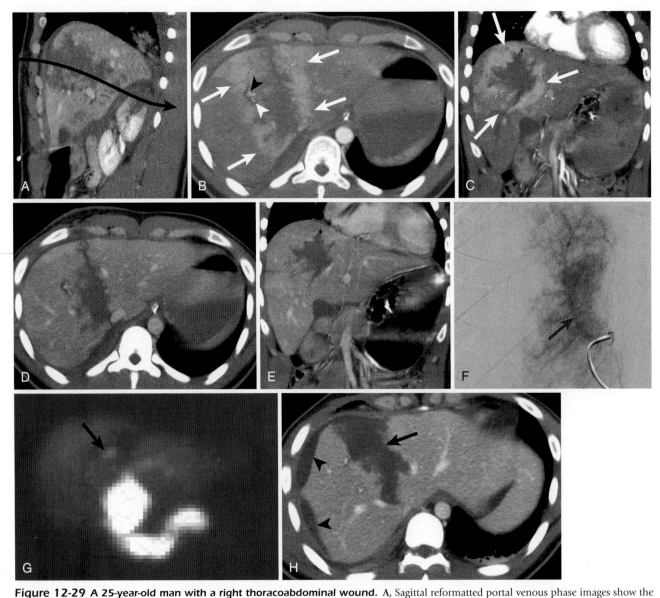

Figure 12-29 A 25-year-old man with a right thoracoabdominal wound. **A,** Sagittal reformatted portal venous phase images show the wound tract *(arrow)* extending adjacent to proximal branches of the right portal vein, hepatic artery, and bile duct. Axial (**B**) and coronal reformatted (**C**) late arterial phase and axial (**D**) and coronal reformatted (**E**) portal venous phase images at same anatomic location show an area of transient hepatic parenchymal enhancement *(arrows)* seen along the wound tract. Enhancement of both the right hepatic artery *(white arrowhead)* and portal vein *(black arrowhead)* are seen within the injured area. **F,** Selective right hepatic artery angiogram shows early enhancement of portal vein branches *(arrow)* because of arterioportal fistula. The fistula was embolized (not shown). **G,** Hepatobiliary iminodiacetic acid scan obtained 24 hours post injury shows a small biloma *(arrow)* within the injury. **H,** Follow-up axial portal venous phase image obtained 5 days post injury shows the injury has enlarged *(arrow)* and has smooth margins. Two new subcapsular *(arrowheads)* seromas or bilomas are also seen.

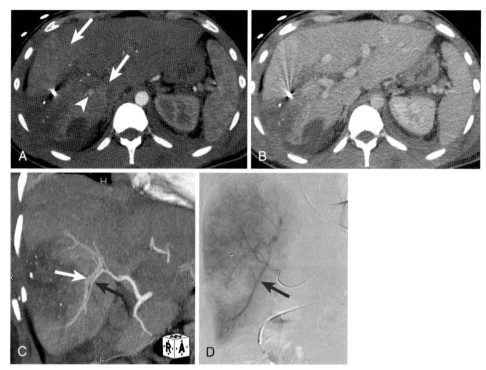

Figure 12-30 Arterioportal fistula of liver seen on follow-up multidetector computed tomography (MDCT) obtained 5 days post gunshot wound to right thoracoabdominal region. Late arterial phase (**A**) and portal venous phase (**B**) images at the same anatomic location show transient hepatic parenchymal enhancement *(arrows)* within the injured segments with the "double barrel" sign *(arrowhead)*. **C,** Coronal maximum intensity projection (MIP) image shows simultaneous enhancement of the branches of right hepatic artery *(red arrow)* and portal vein *(white arrow)*, the "rail track" sign. **D,** Selective right hepatic arteriogram confirms an arterioportal fistula *(arrow)*. This lesion was embolized.

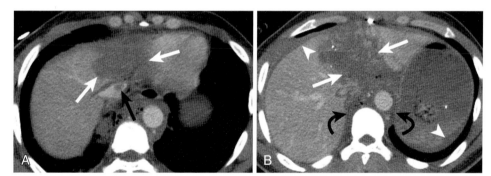

Figure 12-31 Retrohepatic vena caval injury following gunshot wound to right thoracoabdominal region. **A** and **B,** Axial images in the upper abdomen show a filling defect in the intrahepatic vena cava *(black arrow)*. A large liver injury is seen along the wound tract *(white arrows)* with hemoperitoneum *(arrowheads)* seen in the upper abdomen. A retroperitoneal hematoma *(curved arrows)* is also seen around the aorta.

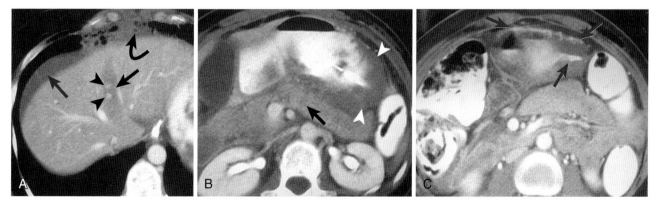

Figure 12-32 A 37-year-old woman stabbed multiple times in the lower chest and abdomen. **A,** Axial images show a large liver laceration *(straight black arrow)* with active bleeding *(arrowheads)*. Free intraperitoneal fluid *(red arrow)* is seen anterior to the liver. Anterior mediastinal hematoma *(curved arrow)* and gas bubbles are seen along the knife track. **B** and **C,** A linear laceration *(black arrow)* in the pancreatic body, and gastric contrast material extravasation *(red arrows)* is seen into the thickened wall of the stomach *(arrowheads)* and along outer surface of the anterior wall of the stomach. Injuries to the liver, stomach, and pancreas were confirmed surgically.

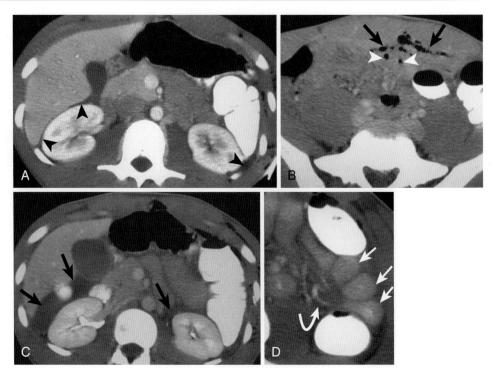

Figure 12-33 Subtle findings of intestinal injury on admission computed tomography (CT). A and B, Admission CT images show tiny amount of free intraperitoneal fluid *(black arrowheads)* in the upper abdomen and extraperitoneal gas *(arrows)* in the lower abdomen. Two additional gas bubbles *(white arrowheads)* are seen. It is difficult to know if they are within the bowel or in the peritoneal cavity. C and D, Follow-up CT obtained 4 hours post admission shows significant increase in the upper abdominal free intraperitoneal fluid *(black arrows)* and new small bowel wall thickening *(white arrows)* with adjacent intermesenteric fluid *(curved arrow).*

urgently to the operating room because of hemodynamic instability.

Retrohepatic IVC injuries should be suspected on CT on the basis of liver wound tracts extending into the major hepatic veins or IVC and/or profuse hemorrhage behind the right lobe of the liver into the lesser sac or near the posterior diaphragm (see Fig. 12-31). A combined therapeutic approach for high-grade liver lacerations with injury to the retrohepatic IVC may involve both the trauma surgeon and the interventional radiologist. Initially the trauma surgeon controls the massive hemorrhage with temporary perihepatic packing called *damage-control surgery*. Recurrent hepatic parenchymal hemorrhage following liver packing may be successfully managed by using transcatheter embolization of the venous and arterial sources of blood loss. Even bleeding from major hepatic veins can potentially be controlled by balloon occlusion, hepatic vein embolization, or intravenous stent placement.

Isolated Hepatic Injuries

The widespread availability of MDCT, its capacity to image both intraperitoneal and retroperitoneal viscera, to identify injury morphologic characteristics, and to relate the injury to adjacent major vascular structures has been the basis for nonoperative management of isolated hepatic injuries in hemodynamically stable patients without signs of peritonitis. This concept has become the standard of care for isolated penetrating injuries to the right upper quadrant (see Fig. 12-14). The associated high incidence of bowel injury seen following penetrating trauma with peritoneal violation makes it difficult for many surgeons to observe these patients (Fig. 12-32; see Fig. 12-23). However, the large number of nontherapeutic laparotomies performed on patients with nonbleeding hepatic injuries following penetrating

---

Box 12-3   Multidetector Computed Tomography Findings Representing a Bowel Injury Requiring Surgery

Gastrointestinal contrast extravasation outside the lumen of bowel
Bowel wall thickening
Wound tract extending up to bowel
Mesenteric hematoma adjacent to bowel
Discontinuity of bowel wall
Bleeding within bowel lumen or mesentery

---

injuries to the right lower chest and thoracoabdominal region has led to the adoption of this nonsurgical approach in some centers.

Multidetector CT can facilitate the selection of patients with isolated liver injury for nonoperative management after right thoracoabdominal penetrating trauma. Hepatic angiography and embolization can be used to treat hepatic active hemorrhage shown by MDCT (see Fig. 12-14). Triple-contrast MDCT provides the information required to attempt nonoperative management, including the ballistic trajectory, extent of liver injury, and, perhaps most importantly, exclusion of other injuries that would mandate celiotomy.

Bowel and Mesenteric Injuries

Hollow viscous injuries are the most common injury seen following all penetrating trauma. These injuries may remain clinically occult for several hours, especially injuries to the duodenum and retroperitoneal colon (Fig. 12-33). Concerns about the true sensitivity and specificity of CT in diagnosing bowel injury have limited the use of CT to evaluation of penetrating trauma to the

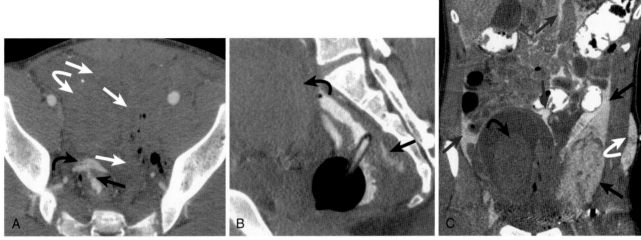

Figure 12-34 Rectal contrast material extravasation following a pelvic gunshot wound. **A,** Axial computed tomography (CT) image shows a defect *(black arrow)* in the thickened anterior wall of lower sigmoid colon with rectal contrast material extravasation *(curved black arrow)* into the perirectal soft tissues. A large left pelvic wall hematoma *(white arrows)* displaces a distended bladder with large amount of clot *(curved white arrow)*. Sagittal **(B)** and coronal **(C)** multiplanar reformatted images show extravasation of rectal contrast material through the wound tract into peritoneum *(red arrows)*, extrapelvic hematoma *(black arrows)*, and subcutaneous fat *(curved white arrow)*. Large amount of blood clot *(curved black arrows)* is seen within the bladder from an injury to the bladder wall.

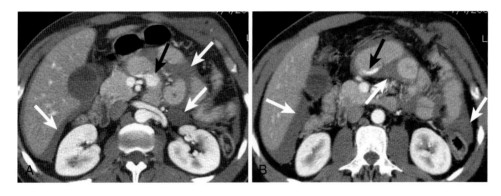

Figure 12-35 Active bleeding into jejunum following stab wound to left abdomen. **A** and **B,** Axial images show active bleeding *(black arrow)* into the lumen with moderate amount of free intraperitoneal fluid *(white arrows)* seen throughout the abdomen. The entry wound *(red arrow)* is seen in the left mid abdomen.

torso. In the recent past, MDCT has been shown to be safe and reliable in detecting penetrating injuries of the entire torso. Routine administration of oral and rectal contrast material is used to help opacify the bowel and increase CT sensitivity for detection of small amounts of intramesenteric fluid, mesenteric contusions, or infiltration of the mesenteric fat that may be the only evidence of a bowel injury (see Fig. 12-33). Also, adequate bowel distension by gastrointestinal contrast material enhances the ability of CT to directly demonstrate bowel wall pathologic changes. Specific CT findings of bowel or mesenteric injury in patients with penetrating trauma are listed in Box 12-3 and include extravasation of oral or colonic contrast material (Fig. 12-34; see Figs. 12-11, 12-16, and 12-32), bowel wall thickening (see Figs.12-5, 12-11, 12-16, and 12-32 to 12-34), mesenteric bleeding, bleeding within the bowel lumen (only seen if there is no oral contrast material within lumen of the bleeding bowel segment) (Fig. 12-35), discontinuity or defect in the bowel wall or focal mesenteric hematoma (Fig. 12-36; see Figs. 12-3 and 12-16), and infiltration

(Fig.12-37). A wound tract extending up to the wall of a hollow viscus (see Figs. 12-5 and 12-37) is also considered a CT sign of bowel injury. Table 12-3 shows the differences in diagnostic performance, sensitivity, and specificity of the various CT findings used to diagnose penetrating and blunt bowel injury.

The presence of pneumoperitoneum without evidence of a pneumothorax, pneumomediastinum, or retroperitoneal air decompressing into the peritoneal cavity is a specific CT finding of bowel injury and mandates surgery in *blunt* trauma. However, free air may be introduced into the intraperitoneal cavity by a bullet or knife during violation of the peritoneum (Fig.12-38). Therefore in penetrating trauma pneumoperitoneum is a sign of peritoneal violation and should not be considered a specific CT finding of bowel injury. In penetrating trauma, free intraperitoneal blood may be the result of bleeding from an injury to the abdominal wall, from the peritoneal lining itself, or from extraperitoneal blood extending through a defect caused by a wound tract into the peritoneal cavity (Fig. 12-39). Free intraperitoneal

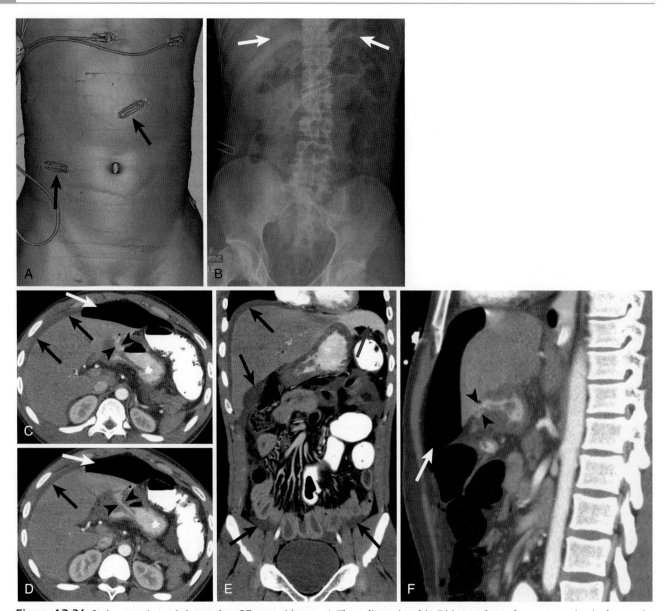

Figure 12-36 Stab wounds to abdomen in a 27-year-old man. A, Three-dimensional (3-D) image shows the two entry sites in the anterior abdomen marked with paper clips *(arrows)*. **B,** Abdominal radiograph shows a large lucency *(arrows)* in the epigastrium representing pneumoperitoneum. Axial (**C** and **D**), coronal (**E**), and sagittal (**F**) reformatted multiplanar images confirm the large amount of pneumoperitoneum *(white arrows)* in the anterior upper abdomen. A defect *(arrowheads)* is seen in the lesser curve of stomach wall. Oral contrast material is extravasating through the defect into the lesser sac and peritoneum *(red arrow)*. Free intraperitoneal fluid *(black arrows)* is seen throughout the peritoneum.

fluid in the absence of solid organ injury should be considered a CT finding of peritoneal violation and not a specific finding of bowel injury. For these reasons, the inability to use the presence of isolated free intraperitoneal air or fluid as a diagnostic CT sign of bowel injury makes diagnosis of bowel injury far more challenging for the radiologist in the setting of penetrating trauma compared to blunt trauma.

A wound tract extending adjacent to the injured bowel is the most common MDCT finding (sensitivity 67% to 77%) seen with penetrating bowel injury (Fig. 12-40; see Figs. 12-5 and 12-23). The most specific (100%) MDCT finding of bowel injury, oral or rectal contrast extravasation, has a low sensitivity (15% to 19%). Focal or diffuse bowel wall thickening has a high specificity (about 85% to 95%) and a moderate sensitivity (47% to 54%).

The majority of the patients with bowel wall thickening will require surgical intervention (see Figs. 12-5, 12-11, 12-16, 12-32, 12-33, and 12-40). Suboptimal accuracy of MDCT in demonstrating bowel wall thickening can result from blood tracking along the external surface of the bowel wall from adjacent injuries (Fig. 12-41) or apparent wall thickening from underdistention or mattering of bowel loops.

Commonly, active bleeding in the mesentery (Figs. 12-42 and 12-43) or mesenteric contusion occurs adjacent to injured bowel (see Figs. 12-3, 12-37, and 12-42). Isolated mesenteric injuries rarely occur following penetrating trauma. Given the frequent concurrence of mesenteric and bowel injury, it is important to carefully evaluate the bowel loops adjacent to a mesenteric contusion for subtle injury.

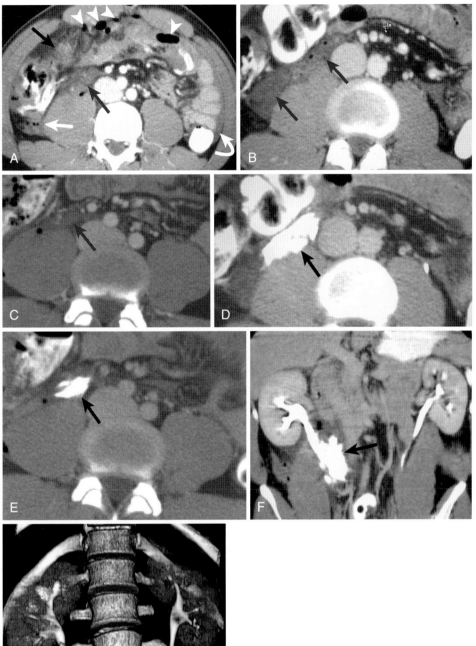

Figure 12-37 Combine intraperitoneal and retroperitoneal injuries following a gunshot wound to the abdomen. A to C, Axial portal venous phase images show mesenteric stranding *(black arrow)*, free intraperitoneal gas bubbles *(white arrowheads)*, free intraperitoneal fluid *(curved arrow)*, low-attenuation fluid along right psoas muscle *(red arrows)*, and retrocecal hematoma *(white arrow)* within which rectal contrast material is extravasating from a right colon injury. C and D, Excretory phase images obtained at the same anatomic location show urinary contrast material *(black arrow)* extravasation into the low-attenuation fluid. Coronal multiplanar (E and F) and three-dimensional (3-D) (G) reformatted images confirm complete transection of right ureter with extravasation of urinary contrast material *(arrows)* into the retroperitoneum. The lower right ureter is not visualized because of a complete transection.

Urinary Tract Injuries

The management of genitourinary injuries has evolved over time based on improvements in CT technology, validated grading scales for various injuries, new surgical techniques, and accumulating experience with operative and nonoperative management. Only a minority of urinary tract injuries occur from a penetrating mechanism.

However, up to half of the patients with hematuria will have high-grade renal injuries and require a complete imaging workup or exploration.

Contrast-enhanced MDCT has been clearly shown to be the imaging modality of choice to assess blunt trauma patients for urinary tract injuries. Often it is used for penetrating trauma as well. Computed tomography has been compared with excretory urography in patients with stab wounds to the flank and back. However, in many cases excretory urography findings of renal parenchymal injuries were indeterminate, underestimated, or overestimated. Excretory urography was not helpful in providing information pertinent to plan management. The role of excretory urography has been relegated to situations in which CT is not available or to obtaining a single image in the operating room to determine if excretion is seen from both kidneys.

Because there is no correlation between the magnitude of hematuria and extent of urinary tract injury, radiographic staging plays a major role in triaging patients for surgical or conservative management. Conservative management of stable penetrating renal injuries has become the preferred therapeutic option. Studies report

that more than half of the patients with renal parenchymal injuries can be treated nonoperatively based on radiologic, laboratory, and clinical criteria. Triple-contrast MDCT provides important information, including extent of renal parenchymal injury, amount of retroperitoneal hematoma, and injuries to the renal vascular pedicle and collecting system to plan management (Figs. 12-44 and 12-45).

"One Shot" Intravenous Pyelography

One-shot intravenous pyelography (IVP) is a quick method of examining renal integrity in unstable patients with hematuria who require urgent surgical intervention. The main role of IVP is to identify a contralateral normal kidney before impending

Table 12-3 Performance of Multidetector Computed Tomography Finding in Diagnosing Penetrating and Blunt Bowel Injury

MDCT Findings	Penetrating Trauma		Blunt Trauma	
	Sensitivity	Specificity	Sensitivity	Specificity
Free intraperitoneal air	N/A	N/A	15%-30%	80%–99%
Free intraperitoneal fluid	N/A	N/A	60%-70%	30%-55%
Oral contrast extravasation	15%-25%	100%	1%-10%	100%
Bowel wall thickening	45%-55%	85%-95%	50%-70%	25%-40%

MDCT, Multidetector computed tomography; *N/A,* not applicable because these are findings representing peritoneal violation.

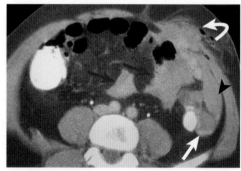

Figure 12-39 Hemorrhage within peritoneum from an extraperitoneal injury. Axial image in the lower abdomen shows a subcutaneous hematoma *(curved arrow)* and gas bubbles at the entry site. Large amount of high-attenuation blood and clot are seen in the mesentery *(red arrows)* and left paracolic gutter *(arrowheads).* Active bleeding *(white arrow)* is also seen. At laparotomy no mesenteric or bowel injury was seen. The inferior epigastric artery was lacerated and bleeding into the peritoneum.

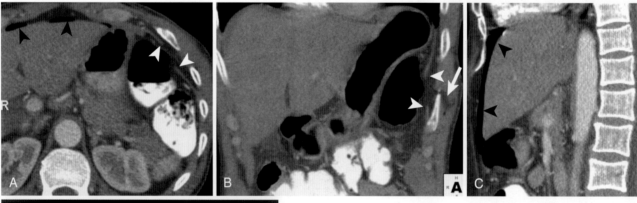

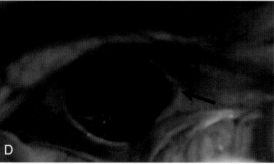

Figure 12-38 Pneumoperitoneum without bowel injury following a stab wound to left thoracoabdominal region. Axial (**A**), coronal (**B**), and sagittal (**C**) multiplanar images show moderate amount pneumoperitoneum *(black arrowheads)* in the upper abdomen. A 3-cm diaphragmatic defect *(white arrowheads)* is also seen with abdominal fat herniation *(white arrow)* through the rent. Wound tract *(arrow)* is seen extending up to the diaphragm injury. **D,** Intraoperative photographs show the diaphragm injury *(arrows).* No hollow viscus injury was identified at surgery.

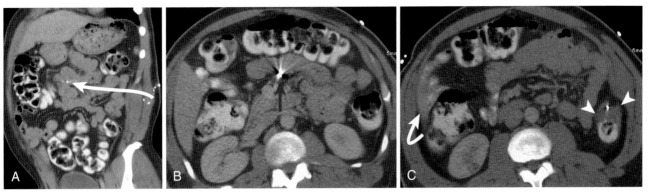

Figure 12-40 Wound tract extending up to bowel in a 50-year-old man shot in the left mid flank. Curved multiplanar (A) and axial (B and C) images show the wound tract *(white arrow)* extending from mid left flank to the proximal jejunum. A bullet fragment is within the jejunal wall *(red arrow)* and thickening *(arrowheads)* of the descending colon wall. Small amount of hemoperitoneum *(curved arrow)* is seen at the tip of the liver. Both the jejunum and descending colon injuries were repaired at surgery.

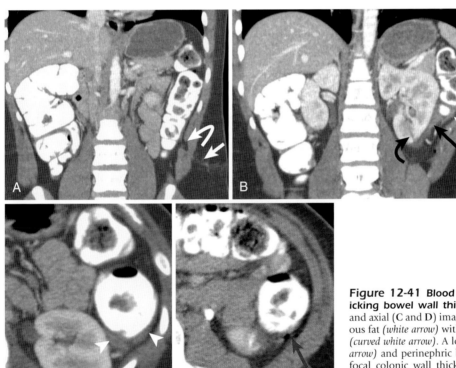

Figure 12-41 Blood tracking on outer wall of colon mimicking bowel wall thickening. Coronal multiplanar (A and B) and axial (C and D) images show the wound tract in the subcutaneous fat *(white arrow)* with a rent in the left abdominal wall muscles *(curved white arrow)*. A lower pole left renal laceration *(curved black arrow)* and perinephric blood *(black arrow)* are also seen. There is focal colonic wall thickening *(arrowheads)* and gas bubbles *(red arrow)* adjacent to colon. At surgery no injury to the left colon was seen.

renal exploration. A single abdominal radiograph is obtained approximately 5 to 10 minutes after administration of 100 mL of 300 mg iodine per milliliter of intravenous contrast material. The study quality may be limited, but it can potentially provide information that may influence operative decisions. The one-shot IVP can identify major structural abnormalities of the renal parenchyma, as well as establish the presence of bilateral kidneys and their anatomic location. Other findings may include displacement of the kidneys or ureters by retroperitoneal hematoma, bilateral excretion of contrast material from the kidneys, and urinary contrast material extravasation into the intraperitoneal or retroperitoneal spaces. Normal study results may obviate the need for renal exploration in 30% to 60% of patients.

Renal Injuries

Blunt trauma is the most common mechanism accounting for the majority of renal injuries, but there has been a steady increase in the incidence of penetrating renal injury with the rise in urban violence. Stab wounds are the most common mechanism of penetrating trauma to the kidney. Common entry sites associated with renal injury are the flank (see Fig. 12-41), abdomen (see Fig. 12-45), and back (see Figs. 12-17 and 12-44). Major renal injuries (grade II to V) are diagnosed more commonly with penetrating mechanisms (67%) compared to blunt trauma (4%). The amount of hematuria typically does not predict the injury severity in 30% of renal stab wounds, 13% of renal gunshot wounds, and 21% of penetrating renal vascular injuries that are not associated with hematuria on admission (see Fig. 12-45).

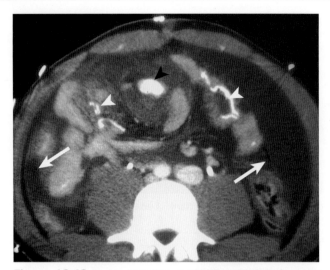

Figure 12-42 Active bleeding mesentery. Computed tomography (CT) image obtained for hypotension following surgery for abdominal gunshot wound shows active bleeding *(black arrowhead)* in the center of a large mesenteric hematoma. Surgical staples *(white arrowheads)* are seen related to recent surgery. Large amount of hemoperitoneum *(arrows)* is also seen. Repeat celiotomy revealed bleeding in mesentery.

Associated injuries are seen in 61% to 81% of patients (see Figs. 12-17, 12-27, and 12-45), including the liver (21%), bowel (25%), spleen (10%), and hemothorax or pneumothorax (19%).

The optimum radiologic evaluation of stable patients with grades II to grade V renal injuries is essential for the trauma surgeons and urologist to plan appropriate management (see Figs. 12-44 and 12-45). Indications for renal exploration in penetrating trauma include persistent renal hemorrhage, pulsatile or expanding retroperitoneal hematoma (see Fig. 12-45), large devitalized renal parenchyma seen by imaging or at surgery, and incomplete clinical or radiographic staging. Patients with no major blood loss, absence of a large amount of devitalized renal parenchyma, without injury to hilar renal vessels or pelvis, and absence of associate intraperitoneal injuries are ideal candidates for nonoperative management. Trauma centers attempting to manage penetrating renal injury patients nonoperatively should have facilities for bed rest, intensive monitoring, serial hematocrits, and transfusions as indicated for hypotension or decrease in hematocrit.

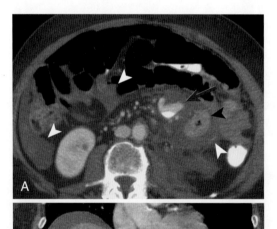

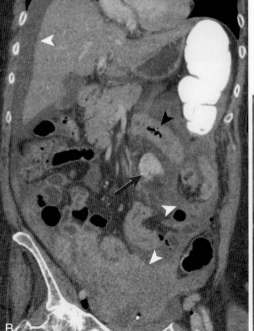

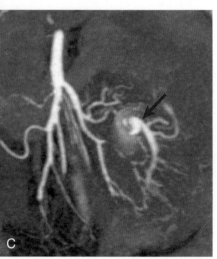

Figure 12-43 Active bleeding in the mesentery following a self-inflicted gunshot wound to abdomen in a 74-year-old woman. Axial (**A**), coronal multiplanar (**B**), and coronal maximum intensity projection (MIP) (**C**) images show an area of active bleeding *(arrows)* in the mesentery arising from a branch of the superior mesenteric artery with an adjacent loop of thick wall small bowel *(black arrowheads)*. Large amount of hemoperitoneum *(white arrowheads)* is also seen. At surgery the bleeding superior mesenteric artery branch was legated. About 30 cm of ischemic nonviable small bowel was resected.

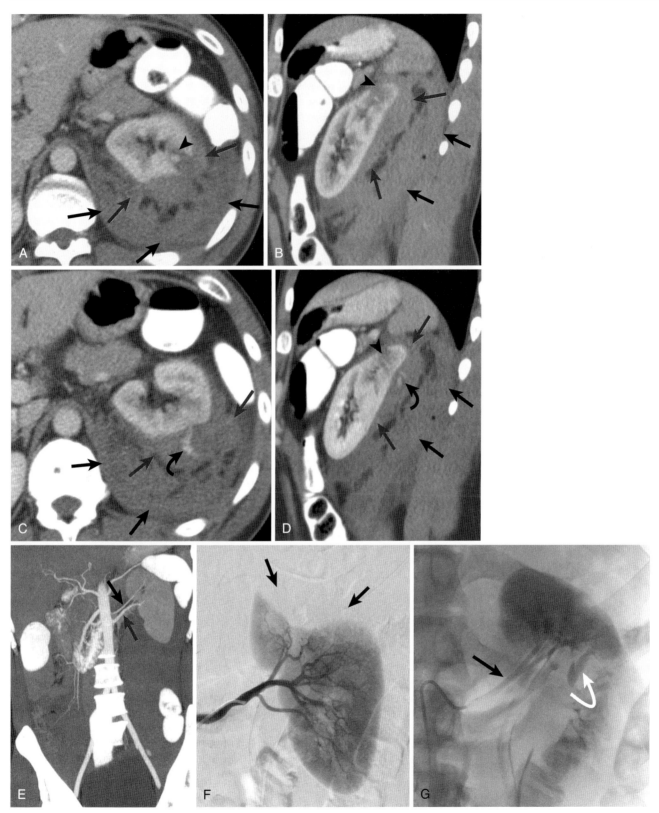

Figure 12-44 Renal laceration from stab wound to back. Axial (A) and sagittal (B) late arterial phase and axial (C) and sagittal (D) portal venous phase images obtained at the same anatomic location show a left upper pole renal laceration *(arrowheads)* with a large perinephric *(red arrows)* and posterior pararenal *(black arrows)* hematomas. Active bleeding *(curved arrows)* is seen only on the portal venous phase images. **E,** Coronal maximum intensity projection (MIP) image shows an accessory renal artery *(black arrow)* entering the injured upper pole of the left kidney. A large main renal artery *(red arrow)* is also visualized. **F,** Left main renal artery angiogram shows no active bleeding. No parenchymal enhancement is seen in upper pole *(arrows)*. **G,** Left accessory renal artery *(arrow)* arteriogram shows active bleeding *(curved arrow)* from a peripheral branch.

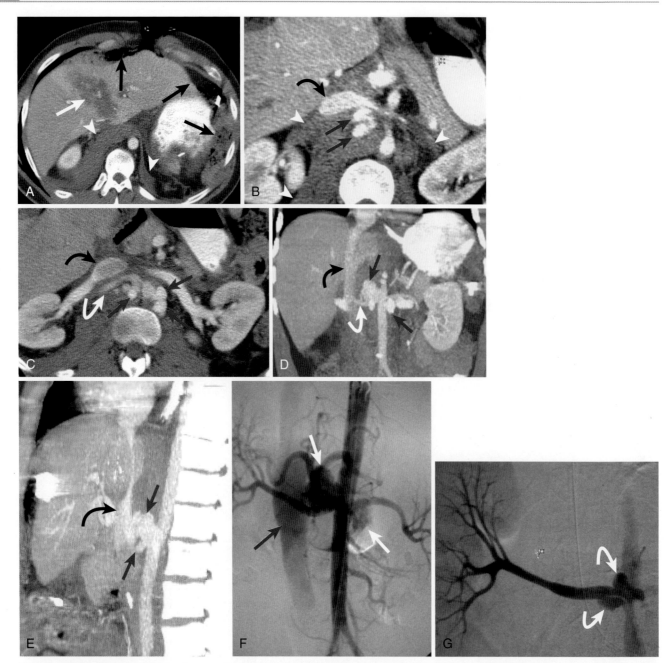

Figure 12-45 Renal artery, aortic pseudoaneurysms, and aortocaval fistula following a gunshot wound to thoracoabdominal region. Computed tomography (CT) was obtained for ongoing hemorrhage following damage-control surgery for liver injury. Axial (**A** to **C**), coronal (**D**), and sagittal (**E**) maximum intensity projection (MIP) images show surgical packing in the upper abdomen *(black arrows)* from damage-control surgery for a large liver injury *(white arrow)*. A moderate-sized retroperitoneal hematoma *(arrowheads)* with multiple pseudoaneurysms *(red arrows)* arising from the aorta and right renal artery *(white curved arrows)* is seen. Early filling of the upper inferior vena cava (IVC) *(black curved arrows)* is seen because of an aortocaval fistula. Aortogram (**F**) and right renal arteriograms (**G**) confirm the aortocaval fistula *(red arrow)* and renal *(curved arrows)* and aortic *(white arrows)* pseudoaneurysms. Both the pseudoaneurysms and aortocaval fistula were surgically repaired.

Common injuries seen on MDCT following penetrating torso trauma include renal contusions (see Figs. 12-3 and 12-27), perinephric hematomas (see Figs. 12-41 and 12-44), retroperitoneal hematoma (see Fig. 12-45), and renal lacerations (see Figs. 12-17, 12-41, and 12-44). The majority of these injuries can be safely managed without surgery (Fig. 12-46; see Figs. 12-3 and 12-41). Renal injuries that result from entry sites posterior to the anterior axillary line are more likely to involve the periphery and less vital parenchyma, resulting in less

severe injuries (see Figs. 12-41 and 12-46). Injuries that occur with entry sites to the anterior abdomen or medial aspect of the back are more likely to involve the renal hilum, resulting in more severe injuries to vital structures such as the renal pelvis or main renal artery or vein (see Figs. 12-17, 12-44, and 12-45).

Renal contusions are the most common parenchymal injury seen following penetrating trauma and are seen as focal or global low-attenuation areas compared to normal parenchyma (Fig. 12-47; see Figs. 12-3 and

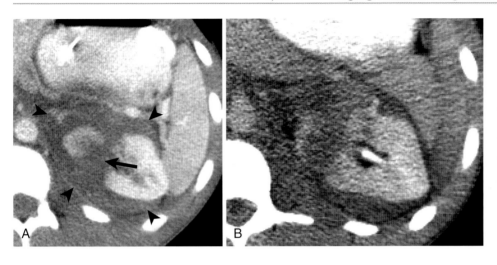

Figure 12-46 Minor renal injury following multiple stab wounds to left chest and back. Portal venous (**A**) and excretory phase (**B**) axial images obtained 5 minutes post injection of contrast material show a moderate-sized perinephric hematoma *(arrowheads)* and an upper pole renal laceration *(arrow)*. No extravasation of urinary contrast material is seen on delayed images to indicate involvement of the renal collecting system.

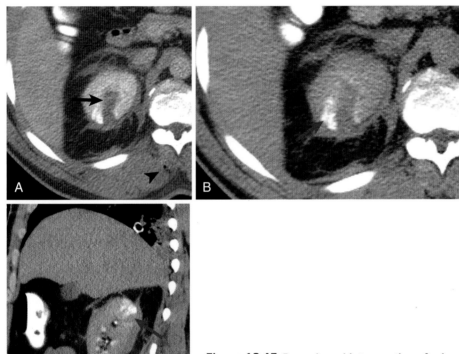

Figure 12-47 Parenchymal intravasation of urinary contrast material into a renal contusion. Axial portal venous (**A**), axial excretory phase (**B**), and sagittal multiplanar (**C**) images show a right upper pole renal contusion *(black arrow)* and a gas bubble *(arrowhead)* in the stab wound tract. Excretory phase images show urinary contrast material *(red arrows)* intravasation into the contusion.

12-27). On delayed images these areas may be seen as hyperattenuation compared to normal parenchyma, resulting from retained contrast within injured renal tubules or parenchymal intravasation of contrast from injured renal tubules (see Fig. 12-47). Renal contusions may result from the blast wave due to a high-energy proximity gunshot wound without direct penetration of the renal parenchyma.

Perinephric hematomas are seen as hyperattenuating areas in the perinephric fat with no mass effect on the renal parenchyma (see Figs. 12-41, 12-44, and 12-46). Compared to blunt trauma, subcapsular hematomas are less often seen following penetrating renal injuries. Subcapsular hematomas result from hemorrhage between the renal capsule and parenchyma and cause mass effect on the underlying normal parenchyma. This CT

finding helps to distinguish a subcapsular hematoma from perinephric hematomas. Renal lacerations are seen as linear low-attenuation areas with normal adjacent parenchyma (Figs. 12-17, 12-41, and 12-46). Compared to lacerations seen following blunt trauma, lacerations resulting from stab wounds tend to have well-defined margins and are more often associated with a perinephric hematoma (Figs. 12-17 and 12-46).

Pseudoaneurysms or arteriovenous fistulas result from injuries to medium and large renal artery branches or main renal arteries (see Fig. 12-45). The injury typically involves the media, leading to weakening of the wall and enlargement of the arterial diameter. Laceration of the wall of the adjacent vein can allow arterial hemorrhage to decompress into the venous lumen, resulting in an arteriovenous fistula. Both pseudoaneurysms and

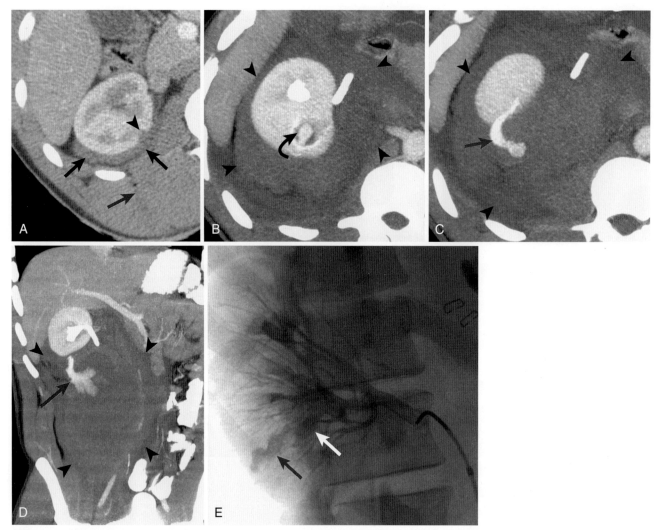

Figure 12-48 Delayed hemorrhage from renal pseudoaneurysm following a stab wound to the back. A, Admission computed tomography (CT) image shows a minor renal injury *(arrowhead)* and a small perinephric hematoma *(black arrows)*. The wound tract *(red arrow)* is seen in the right upper back. Axial (**B** and **C**) and coronal (**D**) reformatted maximum intensity projection (MIP) images obtained 10 days post injury for hypotension shows a pseudoaneurysm *(curved arrow)* with active bleeding *(red arrows)*. A larger retroperitoneal hematoma *(arrowheads)* is seen extending from the upper abdomen to the pelvis. **E,** Renal arteriogram confirms both the pseudoaneurysm *(white arrow)* and active bleeding (active bleeding). Transcatheter embolization was successful in arresting the hemorrhage.

arteriovenous fistulas are common causes for delayed hemorrhage, a well-recognized complication seen especially following stab wounds (Fig. 12-48).

Contrast-enhanced MDCT is much more sensitive than IVP in demonstrating urinary extravasation (see Fig. 12-47). Both the surgical and MDCT-based injury grading scales upgrade renal laceration from grade III to grade IV and from grade II to grade III, respectively, when associated with urinary extravasation. Delayed CT images should be *routinely* obtained during the excretory phase (5 to 10 minutes post administration of intravenous contrast material) after penetrating renal injuries when urinary contrast material is present within the collecting system (Fig. 12-49; see Figs. 12-37 and 12-47). This helps to avoid missing important injuries to the unopacified collecting system if only images are obtained during the arterial and portal venous phases. Computed tomography can distinguish active hemorrhage from extravasated oral contrast and

urinary contrast material. Contrast-opacified urine typically extravasates into the perinephric and anterior or posterior pararenal spaces and adjacent to the renal hilum, depending on the location of collecting system disruption. Extravasated urine arising from the renal collecting system should be contiguous with the collecting system and similar in attenuation to contrast within the collecting system (see Fig. 12-49). Bleeding from renal penetrating injuries is typically surrounded by high-attenuation clotted blood and is seen before opacification of the renal collecting system. Typically the attenuation of extravasated urine is higher than clotted blood and liquid blood.

Angiography with transcatheter embolization can manage active bleeding from penetrating renal injuries without need for surgical exploration among patients with CT evidence of persistent renal bleeding or expanding retroperitoneal hematoma. Angiography and transcatheter embolization is a safe and therapeutic technique

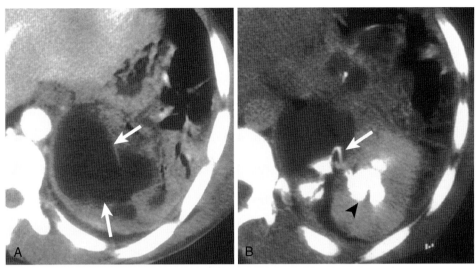

Figure 12-49 *Calyceal injury in a 23-year-old man who was shot in the back with injuries to the spleen and pancreas requiring admission splenectomy.* **A,** Axial portal venous phase image shows a low-attenuation collection *(arrows)* medial and superior to the upper pole of the left kidney. These computed tomography (CT) findings may represent a urinoma, pancreatic pseudocyst, or a resolving hematoma. **B,** Images obtained at 10 minutes post injection of intravenous contrast material at the same anatomic location shows urinary contrast material *(arrow)* leaking from an injured medial upper pole calyx *(arrowhead)* into urinoma.

for renal branch vessel injuries, including pseudoaneurysms, arteriovenous fistulas, and active bleeding. Because surgical intervention for penetrating renal injuries often results in partial or occasionally total nephrectomy, there is an advantage to use of superselective angiographic techniques to identify the precise origin of bleeding and control hemorrhage by transcatheter embolization with minimal loss of renal parenchyma. The rapid availability and expertise for selective angiographic treatment is paramount in considering this option.

Renal Pelvic and Ureteral Injuries

Renal pelvic and ureteral injuries are relatively rare following penetrating trauma and account for less than 1% of all urologic traumas. The anatomic location and narrow caliber makes the ureter less likely to be injured by external trauma. Penetrating trauma accounts for 84% of ureteral injuries (Fig. 12-50; see Fig. 12-37). Often these patients have multiple associated injuries, shock, and a high penetrating trauma index score. Ideal management for penetrating ureteral injury is primary surgical repair. Delayed diagnosis of ureteral injuries can result in nephrectomies in up one third of these patients.

Findings of ureteral injury as demonstrated on IVP include deviation, dilatation, or nonvisualization of the ureter. Up to 45% of patients with ureteral injury have no hematuria. High-dose IVP with nephrotomography (see Fig. 12-50) cannot be performed routinely in all patients and is often limited or incomplete.

Contusion of the ureter may result from blast effect of high-energy bullets passing in proximity to the ureter. The contusion may either resolve or progress to necrosis with potential for delayed urine extravasation. Patients with ureteral contusion typically have hematuria, but a normal ureter on both IVP and MDCT.

The sensitivity and specificity of contrast-enhanced MDCT in demonstrating ureteral injuries is not known. Computed tomography is more sensitive than IVP in

demonstrating urinary contrast extravasation. Delayed images, during the excretory phase (5 to 10 minutes post injection of contrast material), are mandatory to demonstrate urinary contrast extravasation from a site of ureteral injury (see Figs. 12-37, 12-47, and 12-49). Direct CT signs of ureteral injury include extravasation of urinary contrast material from the ureter, normal excretion of contrast material from the ipsilateral kidney, and an intact calyceal system and renal pelvis. Filling of the ureter distal to the injury is an important sign and indicates a partial tear (Fig. 12-51). Computed tomography signs suspicious for ureteral injury include periureteral fluid or hematoma (see Figs.12-37 and 12-51), a wound track seen extending into the region of the ureter, ureteral dilatation proximal to the site of the wound tract, and periureteral hematoma and ureteral wall thickening.

Bladder Injuries

From 25% to 43% of bladder injury results from penetrating trauma. The most frequent clinical findings include gross hematuria, abdominal tenderness, and shock. The lateral bladder wall is the most common location of rupture seen at surgery following penetrating trauma (see Fig. 12-34). Conventional cystography with postdrainage radiographs or MDCT cystography are imaging modalities of choice to evaluate patients with clinical findings suggestive of bladder injury or wound proximity to the bladder as determined by radiographs or CT.

Urinoma

Urinomas result from persistent extravasation of urine from a high-grade renal injury (grade IV surgical or grade 3 CT-based renal injuries) or full-thickness injury to the wall of the renal pelvis, ureter, or bladder (see Figs. 12-37 and 12-49 to 12-51). A majority (80% to 90%) of urinomas following major renal injuries will resolve spontaneously and only require expectant management.

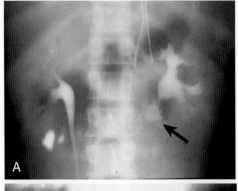

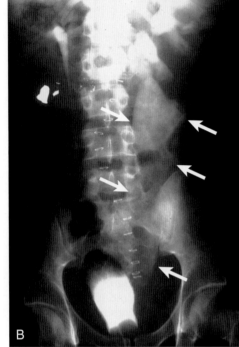

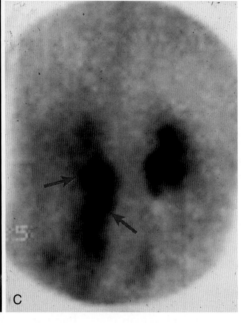

Figure 12-50 Missed left ureteral injury in a 25-year-old man who was shot in the back. A, Tomogram obtained during an intravenous pyeloureterogram shows extravasation of urinary contrast material *(arrow)* from site of injury to the proximal left ureter. **B,** Delayed image in the excretory phase shows extravasation of urine *(arrows)* into a large retroperitoneal urinoma extending from the left kidney to left pelvis. **C,** Posterior view of a technetium Tc 99m diethylenetriamine pentaacetic acid renogram also shows activity *(arrows)* within a left retroperitoneal urinoma.

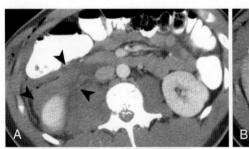

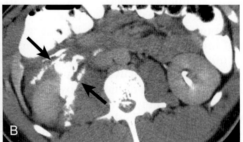

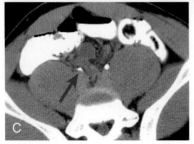

Figure 12-51 Partially transected right ureter following gunshot wound to right thoracoabdominal region. Axial **(A)** and portal venous **(B** and **C)** excretory phase images show a mixed-attenuation right retroperitoneal collection *(arrowheads)*. Excretory phase images show urinary contrast extravasation *(black arrows)* due to a right ureteric injury. Contrast material *(red arrow)* in the distal right ureter indicates partial transection of the ureter. These findings were confirmed at surgery.

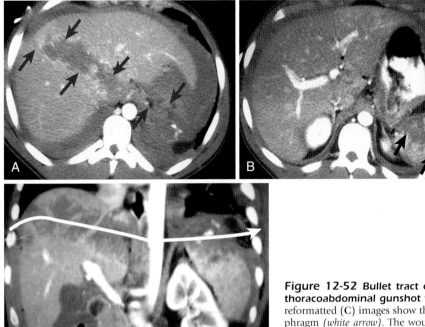

Figure 12-52 Bullet tract extending up to the diaphragm following a thoracoabdominal gunshot wound. Axial (**A** and **B**) and curved multiplanar reformatted (**C**) images show the bullet tract extending from the right to left diaphragm *(white arrow)*. The wound tract is also seen within the liver *(red arrows)* and splenic *(black arrows)* parenchyma. Thickening of the left hemidiaphragm *(arrowheads)* is also seen. Bilateral diaphragm injuries were confirmed at surgery. The left diaphragm injury was only repaired.

Though most urinomas are asymptomatic, they may present with low-grade fever, a palpable mass, adynamic ileus, electrolyte imbalance, and flank or abdominal pain. They develop insidiously and become symptomatic usually within a few weeks following the trauma incident (see Figs. 12-37, 12-49, and 12-50). Typical CT findings are a perinephric low-attenuation collection into which urinary contrast material will extravasate on excretory phase images (see Figs. 12-37, 12-49, and 12-50). It is mandatory to obtain delayed images at 5 to 10 minutes post injection of intravenous contrast material to demonstrate the urinoma and the exact anatomic site of the leak from the collecting system. Image-guided drainage of the urinoma and endourologic techniques are the preferred methods of treatment for infected, large, or persistent urinomas. Follow-up imaging should be obtained at routine intervals to demonstrate resolution.

Diaphragm Injury

Patients with any penetrating injury to the lower chest, thoracoabdominal area, or radiographic or CT evidence of a wound trajectory in close proximity to the diaphragm are likely to have a diaphragmatic injury. Most penetrating diaphragmatic injuries occur because of the bullet or knife tearing through the diaphragm and typically vary between 1 and 4 cm in length (Fig.12-52; see Figs. 12-20, 12-27, and 12-38). It is difficult to directly visualize these injuries on radiographs and conventional CT; they are diagnosed at surgical exploration, laparoscopy, or thoracoscopy via direct inspection. Unlike patients with blunt trauma, the CT signs of the short diaphragm tears typically produced with penetrating injury may be extremely subtle. The majority of stable patients (up to 68%) with penetrating injuries to

the thoracoabdominal region will have normal chest radiograph findings and no clinical indication for celiotomy. Chest radiographs demonstrate a slightly higher incidence of pneumothorax or hemothorax (in 35% of patients) with a diaphragm injury than without (in 24% of patients). Typically no abdominal viscera herniation into the thoracic cavity is seen at the time of definitive treatment. Small isolated diaphragm injuries are asymptomatic and often remain silent from hours to years after injury.

Currently MDCT is used to diagnose intraperitoneal and retroperitoneal injuries in hemodynamically stable patients with penetrating trauma to the torso. It is important for the radiologist to be familiar with the CT signs of short tears in the diaphragm generally seen with penetrating injury. All patients with a penetrating injury tract extending adjacent to the diaphragm should be considered to potentially have diaphragm injury (see Figs. 12-16, 12-23, 12-29, and 12-52). Specific CT signs of a full-thickness (injury requiring surgical repair) diaphragm injury include the CT "collar sign"(waistlike constriction of a herniating viscus at the diaphragmatic rent) (Figs. 12-53 and 12-54), herniation of abdominal content into the thoracic cavity through a diaphragmatic rent (Fig. 12-55; see Figs. 12-53 and 12-54), discontinuity of the diaphragm visualized along the wound tract (see Figs. 12-20 and 12-38), and the presence of injury on either side of the diaphragm in patients with single gunshot or stab wound (Fig. 12-56). Among the accurate signs for diagnosis of a diaphragm injury is a single entry wound contiguous on either side of the diaphragm (sensitivity 88%, specificity 82%). This sign is observed when there is injury on either side of the diaphragm along the wound tract as outlined by hematoma, gas bubbles, and bullet or bone fragments.

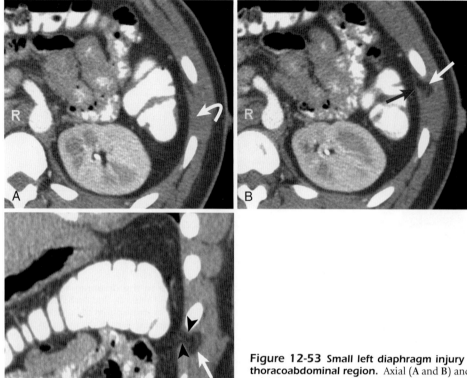

Figure 12-53 Small left diaphragm injury following a stab wound to the left thoracoabdominal region. Axial (**A** and **B**) and coronal oblique multiplanar reformatted (**C**) images show abdominal fat *(white arrows)* herniating through a small diaphragmatic tear *(red arrow)*. Thickening *(curved arrow)* of the diaphragm adjacent to the tear with constriction of the fat at the tear *(arrowheads)*, the "collar" sign, is seen. Injury was repaired surgically.

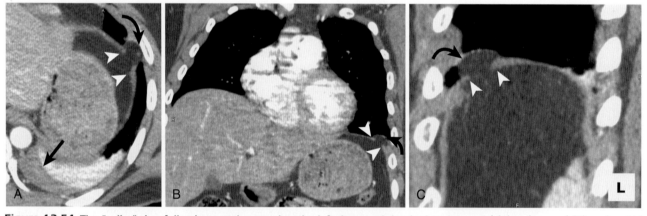

Figure 12-54 The "collar" sign following a stab wound to the left thoracoabdominal region. Axial (**A**) and coronal (**B**), and sagittal (**C**) multiplanar reformatted images show peritoneal fat *(curved arrows)* herniating into the thoracic cavity. The collar sign *(arrowheads)* is seen at the diaphragmatic rent with a small hemothorax *(arrow)*. The isolated diaphragm injury was repaired at surgery.

Some caution must be exercised for the identification of this sign because ballistic injuries occurring on one side of the diaphragm could conceivably injure the organ or structure on the other side through blast effect without direct penetration. The other signs discussed have higher specificity but are rarely seen on axial or reformatted MDCT because of the small length of diaphragmatic rents that occur with penetrating injury.

Multidetector CT findings suspicious for a diaphragm injury include a wound tract adjacent to the diaphragm, focal or diffuse thickening of the diaphragm as a result of hematoma or edema (see Figs. 12-16, 12-20, 12-52, and 12-53), and a defect in the continuity of the normal

diaphragm or crus without adjacent hematoma or stranding of the adjacent fat. Diaphragmatic thickening is considered as a nonspecific CT finding because hematomas may also result from injuries to adjacent organs like the spleen, adrenal glands, liver, bowel, or kidneys and track along the adjacent diaphragm.

■ IMAGING OF PENETRATING CHEST TRAUMA

Approximately 4% to 15% of all trauma admissions to major trauma centers are attributed to penetrating thoracic injuries. Most penetrating injuries to the chest

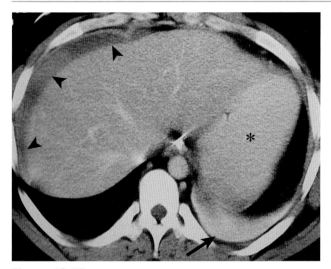

Figure 12-55 Oral contrast extravasation into the thoracic cavity through a left diaphragm injury in a 27-year-old man stabbed in the left lower thoracoabdominal region. Computed tomography (CT) image obtained through the upper abdomen shows free intraperitoneal fluid *(arrowheads)* and a high-density left pleural effusion *(arrow)*. Pleural effusion is similar in attenuation to contrast *(asterisk)* seen within the stomach.

are caused by knives or bullets from handguns. The prehospital mortality from transmediastinal penetrating injuries may be as high as 86% for cardiac, 92% for thoracic vascular, and 11% for pulmonary vascular injuries. Patients admitted to an emergency center with potential transmediastinal wounds or injury to the chest wall, pleura, and lungs that are symptomatic but physiologically stable require imaging studies to determine the location and extent of injury. Chest radiographs are the most common imaging study performed to quickly evaluate these patients (Figs. 12-57 to 12-59).

Injury to Chest Wall, Pleura, and Lung

From 88% to 97% of patients admitted with penetrating injuries to the chest have noncardiac thoracic injuries to the chest wall, pleura, or lung (Fig. 12-60). About 83% of patients with hemopneumothorax will require immediate intercostal tube drainage, and in 21% the initial hemopneumothorax worsens on follow-up. Patients with isolated small pneumothorax or hemothorax on admission chest radiographs are less likely to need a

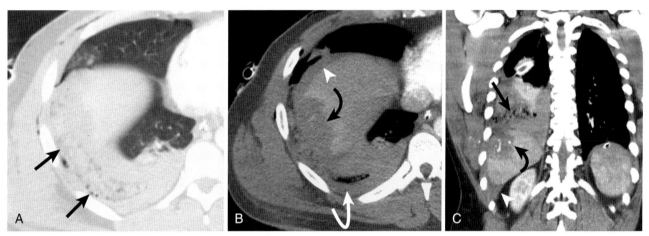

Figure 12-56 Contiguous organ injury on either side of hemidiaphragm following a single gunshot wound to the right thoracoabdominal region. Axial (**A** and **B**) and coronal multiplanar reformatted (**C**) images show pulmonary contusion in the right lower lung *(arrows)*, a small hemothorax *(white curved arrow)*, contusion *(black curved arrow)* at the dome of the right lobe of the liver, and perihepatic intraperitoneal fluid *(arrowhead)*. Presence of contiguous injuries on either side of hemidiaphragm indicates an injury to the right hemidiaphragm.

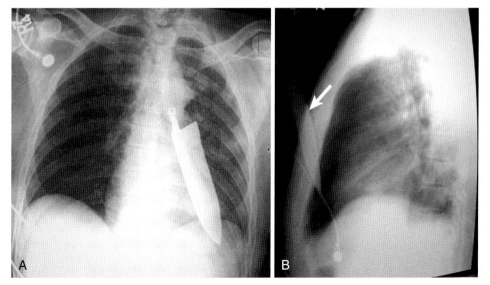

Figure 12-57 Stab wound to the left chest. Anteroposterior (AP) (**A**) and lateral (**B**) radiographs show a knife penetrating the left chest wall with the tip of the knife in the left pleural space *(arrow)*.

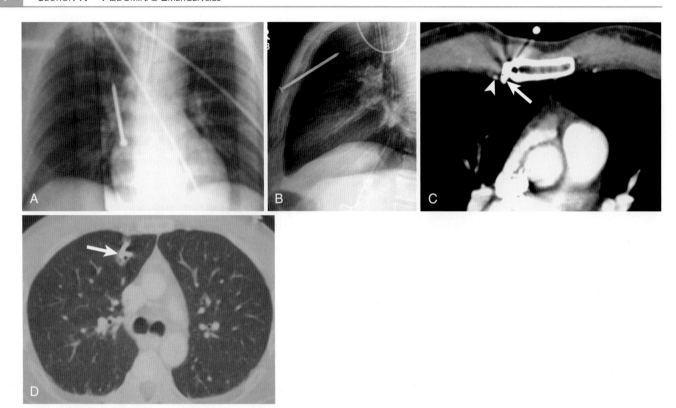

Figure 12-58 Nail gun injury to the chest. Anteroposterior (AP) (**A**) and lateral (**B**) radiographs show a nail in the right pleural space. Computed tomography (CT) images (**C** and **D**) show a nail *(arrows)* entering the right lung just medial to the right internal mammary artery *(arrowhead)*. No pneumothorax is seen.

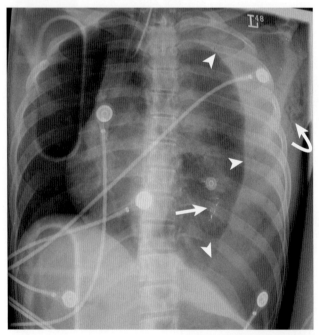

Figure 12-59 Tension hemothorax in an 18-year-old man shot in the left chest. Admission radiograph shows a large left hemothorax *(arrowheads)* with shift of mediastinum to contralateral side and depression of left diaphragm, indicating a tension hemothorax. Some bullet fragments *(arrow)* in lower left chest and soft tissue air *(curved arrow)* in the left axilla at the entry site are seen.

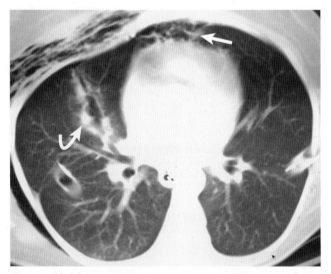

Figure 12-60 Lung laceration along wound tract following a stab wound to the chest. Axial computed tomography (CT) image shows a lung laceration *(curved arrow)* along the wound tract. Anterior mediastinal emphysema *(arrow)* is also seen from pneumothorax decompressing into the mediastinum.

thoracostomy tube. They are also less likely deteriorate on follow-up imaging compared to patients with hemopneumothorax.

Pneumothorax is common following penetrating thoracic trauma. Prompt diagnosis, even of a small pneumothorax, is important because significant respiratory and cardiovascular embarrassment may develop, especially for patients with impaired pulmonary

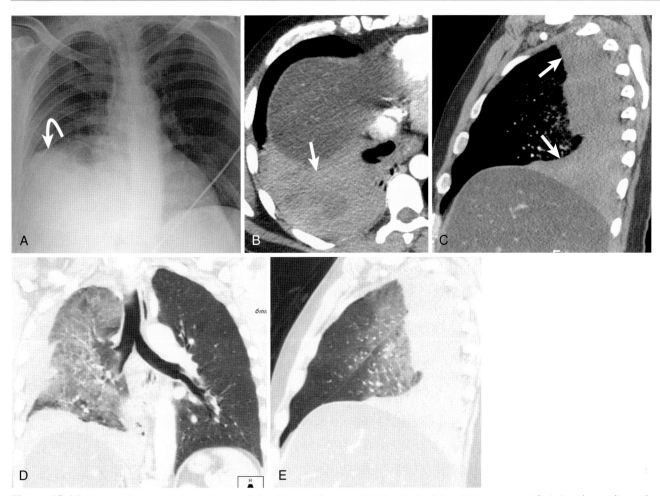

Figure 12-61 *Large subpulmonic hemothorax following a stab wound to the back of the right chest.* **A,** Admission chest radiograph shows elevation of the lateral aspect of the right diaphragm *(curved arrow)* with a large increase in density in the lower right hemithorax. Axial **(B)** and sagittal **(C)** soft tissue and coronal **(D)** and sagittal **(E)** multiplanar lung window images show a large subpulmonic hemothorax *(arrows)* tracking from the apex to the base of the right thorax with passive atelectasis of the lung. No lung injury is seen.

function or if mechanical ventilation is instituted for patients with normal lung function. Review of the literature indicates that small pneumothoraces are not initially recognized by clinical examination or by admission chest radiography in 30% to 50% of patients and are only diagnosed after thoracic CT. The location of pneumothorax depends on patient position, the amount of air in the pleural space, and the presence of pleural adhesions and regions of atelectasis. Typically air in the pleural space collects in the apicolateral aspect of the hemithorax in the erect or semierect patient. Air within the pleural space is diagnosed by visualizing the visceral pleura as a thin sharp white line with absence of lung markings beyond this line. In the supine position the most nondependent part of the hemithorax is the anterior costophrenic sulcus extending from the 7th costal cartilage laterally to the 11th rib in the midaxillary line.

Asymptomatic stab wounds with normal admission chest radiograph findings may occur in up to 62% of patients admitted following civilian penetrating thoracic injuries. Delayed complications are well recognized and occur in 8% to 12% of these patients as late as 48 hours to 5 days after injury. Overall, mortality in

asymptomatic patients is 0.1% and results from cardiac or major vascular injuries.

The appropriate length of time to observe these patients in a busy facility to identify those who will develop delayed complications is an ongoing controversy. By performing an admission and follow-up chest radiograph at 6 hours the negative predictive value for a thoracic injury could be increased from 87% to 99% and allow subsequent outpatient management.

Hemothorax and Pleural Effusions

Pleural effusions that present after acute thoracic trauma are usually due to hemorrhage (see Figs. 12-14, 12-20, and 12-59), and the majority of hemothoraces are managed by tube thoracostomy. Hemothorax in penetrating trauma may be the result of injury to the visceral pleura, a laceration/contusion of lung parenchyma, or injury to the internal mammary, intercostal arteries, heart, or great vessels. When more than 1500 mL of blood accumulates in the pleural space, it is called a *massive hemothorax* (Fig. 12-61; see Fig. 12-59). Indications for thoracotomy include immediate removal of 1500 mL of blood from the pleural space, continuing hemorrhage resulting in a

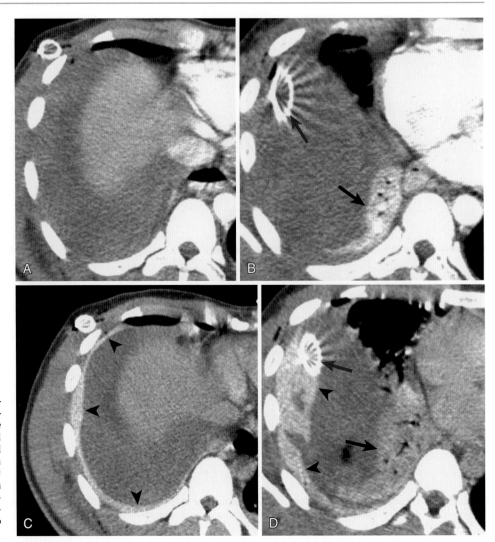

Figure 12-62 Active bleeding into the hemothorax following a stab wound to the chest. Axial arterial (**A** and **B**) and delayed (**C** and **D**) images obtained at the same anatomic location show active bleeding *(arrowheads)* seen only on delayed images into a retained large hemothorax. Thoracostomy tube *(red arrows)* and collapsed lung *(black arrows)* are also seen.

thoracostomy tube output of 200 mL/hr for 4 hours, or completely evacuating large amounts of clotted blood from the pleural space. However, it is vital to take into consideration the patient's physiologic characteristics as an important indication for intervention rather than absolute numbers of volume of the hemothorax or rate of chest tube output.

Chest radiographs should be routinely obtained without any delay in all patients to evaluate for pneumothorax and lung parenchymal, potential mediastinal, and osseous injuries. Multidetector CT is the reference standard imaging modality to demonstrate a hemothorax. Computed tomography attenuation values may help diagnose serous effusion (low attenuation, usually 0 to less than 20 HU) from hemothorax, which has a CT attenuation of 35 to 70 HU depending upon the degree of clot formation. Also, active hemorrhage (Figs. 12-62 and 12-63) into the pleural space can be demonstrated by MDCT using power-injected intravenous contrast.

Bedside ultrasonography has been reliably used in the acute setting to demonstrate pleural effusion. Smaller quantities of pleural fluid may be detected on ultrasonography compared to an erect chest radiograph. Pleural fluid or free blood in the pleural space is seen as an anechoic area above the hyperechoic band represent-

ing the diaphragm. Blood or complex fluid collections reveal echogenic foci within the anechoic area. Clotted blood is more difficult to detect by ultrasonography because it may be isoechoic with lung parenchyma, chest wall, and the mediastinum.

Retained hemothorax in the pleural space may trap significant amounts of normal lung with potential loss of function from compressive atelectasis, the ensuing fibrothorax, and adhesions. Clotted blood is an ideal nidus for secondary infection and development of pneumonia and empyema. To prevent or minimize these complications, surgeons have started using minimally invasive surgical techniques, including video-assisted thoracoscopy (VATS), to evacuate retained hemothorax. The optimum time for VATS is unknown. Though chest radiographs are the most frequently obtained imaging study to initially assess chest trauma and follow hemothoraces, they are not accurate in precisely measuring the volume of retained blood in the thoracic cavity to plan the need for thoracoscopic intervention. The chest radiograph can be normal in; 50% of the patients with a hemothorax of more than 300 mL. Multidetector CT is essential for accurately measuring the volume of retained hemothorax to select patients for thoracoscopy (see Figs. 12-20, 12-61, and 12-62). Very small retained

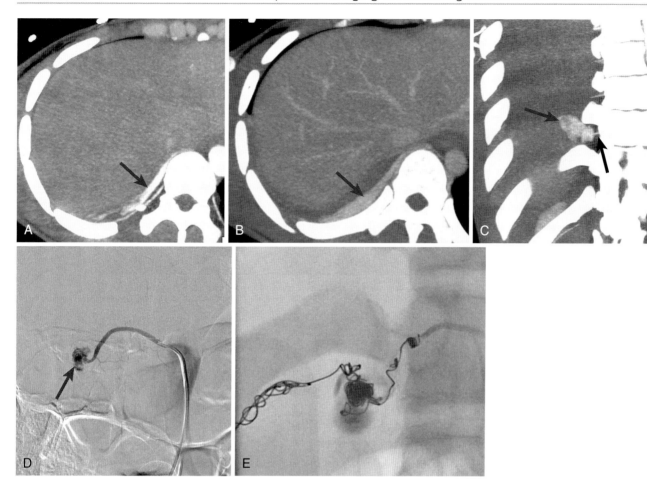

Figure 12-63 Active bleeding from intercostal artery injury. Patient was stabbed in the right back. Axial (**A** and **B**) and coronal (**C**) maximum intensity projection (MIP) images show active bleeding *(red arrows)* from the right 10th intercostal artery *(black arrow).* **D,** Intercostal arteriogram confirms the bleeding *(arrow)* from the intercostal artery. **E,** Embolization with multiple coils used distal and proximal to bleeding site to arrest the bleeding.

hemothoraces generally reabsorb and can be successfully managed with observation (see Figs. 12-14 and 12-20). A majority of the retained hemothoraces greater than 900 mL will require VATS or thoracostomy for definitive treatment.

Chylothorax is another cause of pleural fluid that should be considered in the setting of penetrating trauma and results from interruption of the thoracic duct. The injury is suggested by low or negative pleural fluid attenuation values. Most thoracic duct injuries (88%) occur within the superior mediastinum at the junction on the thoracic duct and left subclavian vein in the Poirier triangle and should be treated by early surgical intervention. A bilious effusion is very rare and results from concomitant laceration of the right hemidiaphragm and liver with formation of a biliary-pleural fistula (Fig. 12-64).

Transmediastinal Wounds

Unlike injury to the chest wall, pleura, and lung, penetrating transmediastinal wounds (Figs. 12-65 and 12-66) are associated with potential for injury to vital structures, including the heart, great vessels (Fig. 12-67), esophagus, and trachea. Most civilian transmediastinal

penetrating wounds warrant admission to a major emergency center. A majority of hemodynamically unstable patients with a GSW are likely to have a major cardiac or vascular injury and will proceed directly to the operating room for immediate surgery. The hemodynamically stable patients may have no injuries or have occult vascular, cardiac, pericardial, tracheal, bronchial, or esophageal injuries. A significant increase in morbidity and mortality is associated with delayed recognition of these injuries.

Traditionally radiography, angiography, esophagoscopy, bronchoscopy, contrast barium swallow, pericardial window, and echocardiography are considered the appropriate studies to diagnose mediastinal vascular and aerodigestive injury in hemodynamically stable patients. This aggressive workup often removes the patient from an environment of ideal clinical support and monitoring. Multidetector CT is readily available in most institutions in the United States, and it is a safe, cost-effective, and rapid imaging modality to triage patients. In this group of patients the goal of contrast-enhanced MDCT is to demonstrate the trajectory of the penetrating object. This can help to select patients for further invasive investigations like angiography, endoscopy, or surgery (see Figs. 12-65 and 12-66).

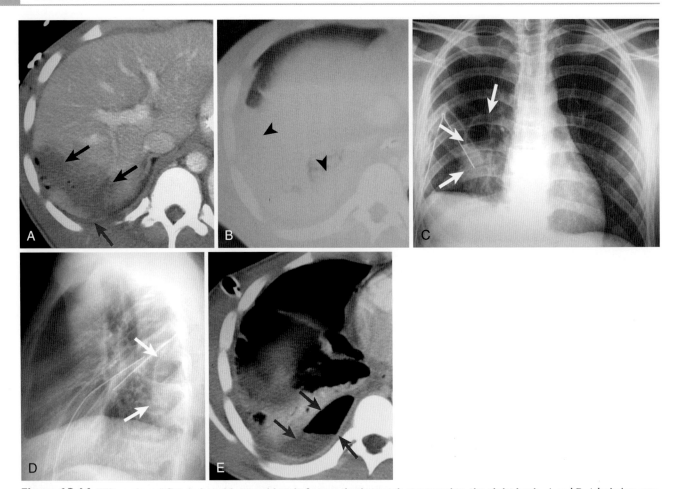

Figure 12-64 Biliary-pleural fistula in a 16-year-old male from a single gunshot wound to the right back. A and B, Admission computed tomography (CT) images show mixed-attenuation injury *(black arrows)* to the posterior segment of the right hepatic lobe. Right lower lobe parenchymal contusion *(arrowheads)* and a small hemothorax *(red arrow)* are also seen. Contiguous injuries to the liver and right lower lobe of the lung indicate injury to the right hemidiaphragm. Anteroposterior (AP) (C) and lateral (D) chest radiographs performed 3 weeks post admission show a fluid-containing cavity *(arrows)* in the posterior right lower lobe. E, CT image of the lower chest shows a cavity *(arrows)* with an air-fluid level. Bile was aspirated under CT guidance from the cavity in the pleural space.

Multidetector CT is optimally suited to visualize individual mediastinal structures and can often demonstrate the trajectory of the objects penetrating the thorax. The mediastinal structures can be assessed at the peak of contrast enhancement, with minimal misregistration and motion artifact and with the possibility of excellent quality two- and three-dimensional (3-D) image reconstruction (Fig. 12-68; see Figs. 12-65 to 12-67). When a thoracic wound tract is clearly shown by CT not to be in close proximity to vital mediastinal structures, the traditional workup of these patients can be deferred.

Tracheobronchial Injuries

Tracheobronchial injury (TBI) has been reported in 0.8% to 3% of autopsy series of trauma victims and in 0.4% to 1.5% of clinical series of patients sustaining major trauma. These injuries are relatively uncommon and often go unrecognized as a result of lack of visible external signs of injury. Early symptoms may be nonspecific and minimal, resulting in diagnosis only when late symptoms of TBI develop. Isolated tracheal injuries account for 25% of all TBI. Tracheobronchial injury should be suspected in all patients with penetrating transmediastinal or neck wounds that extend deep to the platysma muscle. Penetrating trauma is less likely to injure the trachea (incidence of blunt trauma:penetrating trauma, 8:5) and generally involves the cervical trachea. Penetrating injuries most commonly involve the anterior aspect of the cervical trachea with injuries to the rings and the ligaments between the tracheal cartilages. There is a high incidence of associated esophageal and major vascular injuries (31%) occurring with penetrating TBI.

The most common radiologic finding in TBI is a persistent air leak into the mediastinum and deep cervical soft tissue planes. Up to 10% of patients with major airway injury have no radiologic findings in the immediate postinjury period. Soft tissue and mediastinal emphysema is usually extensive, progressive, and not relieved by chest tube placement. Soft tissue air can dissect into the superficial and deep tissues of the neck and chest wall and through the foramen of Bochdalek and Morgagni into the retroperitoneal and intraperitoneal spaces, potentially mimicking primary bowel injury. The resolution of the extrapulmonary air does not exclude this injury.

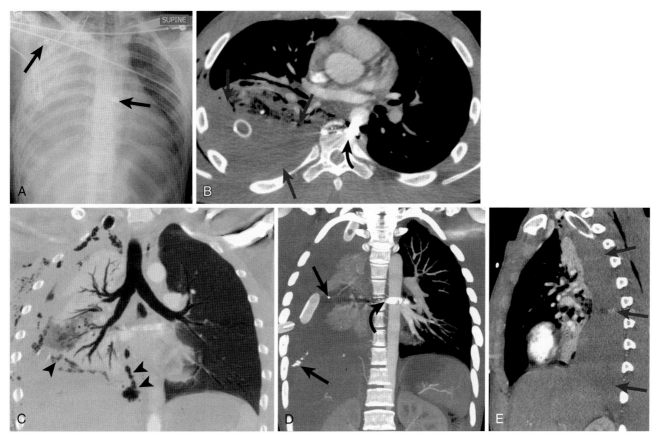

Figure 12-65 Transmediastinal gunshot wound in a 16-year-old boy. A, Anteroposterior (AP) radiograph shows a large right pleural effusion following placement of a right chest tube. Bullet fragments *(arrows)* are seen projected over the right axilla and middle mediastinum. Axial (**B**), coronal (**C**) minimum intensity, and coronal (**D**) and sagittal (**E**) maximum intensity images show a large residual hemothorax *(red arrows)* and extensive consolidation due to contusion and lacerations *(arrowheads)* in the right lung. Bullet fragments are seen in the pleural space *(black arrows)* and adjacent to the aorta and esophagus *(curved arrows)* in the posterior mediastinum. At right anterolateral thoracotomy, bleeding was seen from the posterior right lung. No aerodigestive injury was seen at endoscopy or surgery.

Pneumothorax is seldom seen following tracheal injuries and is more likely to be associated with distal bronchial tears. Persistent pneumothorax and distal atelectasis from obstruction of a ruptured bronchus may occur. Rarely, the proximal end of the ruptured bronchus can be visualized on chest radiographs as a tapering air-filled structure referred to as the *bayonet sign.* Highly diagnostic but rarely seen is the fallen lung sign, in which the lung is detached from its mainstem bronchus and falls by gravity into the most dependent part of the thoracic cavity. In such cases the hilum of the collapsed lung appears abnormally dependent in position. An extraluminal position of the endotracheal tube or balloon or overexpansion of the balloon may be the earliest radiologic finding of tracheal injury.

Computed tomography has an overall sensitivity of, 85% in detecting tracheal injury. With MDCT's ability to obtain volumetric data with less partial volume averaging and motion artifact improves reformatted coronal and sagittal images of the major airways. This capacity could potentially help delineate an airway injury site in cases with a subacute or chronic presentation of airway injury. Compared to chest radiographs, MDCT detects smaller quantities of mediastinal air, which may be the only sign of TBI. Visualization of extrapulmonary air in direct contact with the trachea (paratracheal air) by CT among patients with pneumomediastinum is not pathognomonic for TBI. Direct CT signs of airway injury include an overdistended endotracheal tube balloon (maximum transverse diameter measuring more than 2.8 cm) (Fig.12-69), herniation of the endotracheal balloon outside the airway (Fig. 12-70), the endotracheal tube projecting outside the airway, fracture or deformity of the cartilaginous rings of the airway (Fig. 12-71), and discontinuity of the airway wall.

Bronchoscopy is the diagnostic modality of choice to confirm TBI, and early diagnosis is essential to obtain successful primary reanastomosis and optimal long-term results. Though complete transection of the trachea is usually diagnosed soon after admission, partial tears of the trachea and complete or partial tears of the bronchi may be detected only as late sequelae of TBI, including tracheal stenosis, tracheoesophageal fistula, empyema, mediastinitis, or bronchiectasis.

Esophageal Injury

All forms of trauma accounted for only 10% to 19% of esophageal perforations. Isolated rupture of the esophagus is very uncommon, and most busy Level I trauma centers may see two to nine patients with penetrating esophageal injuries annually. In any case of

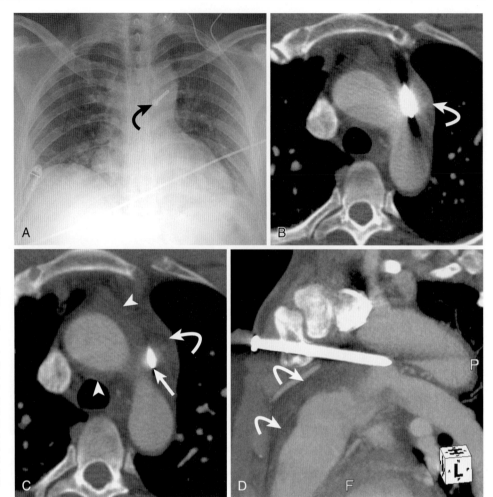

Figure 12-66 Transmediastinal nail gun injury in a 35-year-old man shot by his coworker. A, Anteroposterior (AP) chest radiograph shows a nail *(curved arrow)* projected over the aortopulmonary window. No pneumothorax or pleural effusion is seen. Axial (**B** and **C**) and maximum intensity coronal (**D**) reformatted images show the tip of the nail *(arrow)* is adjacent to the mid aortic arch and left pulmonary artery. Some mediastinal blood *(curved arrows)* and a subtle small pericardial effusion *(arrowheads)* are seen. At surgery both left pulmonary artery and pericardial injuries were repaired.

transmediastinal penetrating trauma with a wound tract in proximity to the esophagus, it is necessary to exclude esophageal injury (Fig. 12-72; see Figs. 12-65, 12-67, 12-70, and 12-71). Most penetrating injuries involve the cervical esophagus and are associated with injuries to the respiratory tract (81%), central nervous system (23%), and vascular system (21%).

Typically physical findings are present in only a third of patients with esophageal injury. The most common presenting symptom is pain, followed by fever, dyspnea, and crepitus. Other signs and symptoms include dysphagia, odynophagia, hematemesis, stridor, abdominal tenderness, and a mediastinal "crunching" sound from cardiac pulsation (the Hamman sign). The uncommon nature of this injury, lack of specific clinical signs or chest radiographic findings, and necessity for early diagnosis to avoid complications warrants a high index of clinical suspicion.

The most frequent chest radiographic signs are cervical and mediastinal emphysema (60%) and left pleural effusion (66%). Another radiologic sign of esophageal disruption is alteration of the mediastinal contour due to fluid leakage from the esophagus, associated mediastinal hemorrhage (see Figs. 12-67 and 12-72), or inflammatory reaction in the mediastinal fat.

Multidetector CT of the chest is currently used in trauma centers to verify the presence or absence of mediastinal involvement. Demonstration of gas bubbles, bone,

or bullet fragments (see Figs. 12-65, 12-67, and 12-70 to 12-72) in the mediastinum in close proximity to the esophagus indicates potential perforation. Direct MDCT findings of esophageal injury include wall thickening (see Fig. 12-72), a defect in the wall of the esophagus adjacent to the wound tract, and extravasation of oral contrast into the mediastinum. Demonstration of a ballistic penetrating tract that unequivocally misses the mediastinum avoids the need for evaluation of the esophagus, aorta, and mainstem bronchi. Knife wounds to the chest tend to have a less predictable course because of limited hemorrhage or air along the wound tract and are more likely to require further mediastinal imaging. If any doubt regarding the course of penetrating trauma exists, the mediastinal structures must be evaluated in a dedicated fashion.

Endoscopy or esophagography should be used to evaluate suspected cervical or transmediastinal penetrating injury with a wound tract adjacent to the esophagus on MDCT. Contrast esophagogram is performed first with water-soluble contrast (Fig. 12-73) and if findings are negative, with barium sulfate contrast. Fluoroscopic guidance is ideal, but if not possible due to the patient's overall condition, contrast can be instilled into the upper esophagus with chest radiographs performed during injection of water-soluble contrast once proper nasogastric tube position is verified. Contrast studies of the esophagus are approximately 57% to 100% sensitive in establishing a diagnosis of injury, with higher accuracy reported for

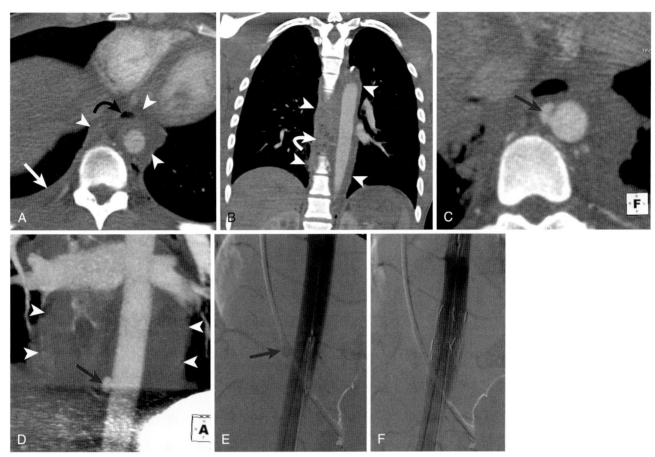

Figure 12-67 Posterior transmediastinal gunshot wound in a 19-year-old man. Axial (**A**) and coronal multiplanar (**B**) admission images show diffuse posterior mediastinal blood *(arrowheads)* abutting the lower thoracic aorta and esophagus *(black curved arrow)*. A small right hemothorax *(arrow)* and gas bubbles *(white curved arrow)* are also seen. Follow-up axial (**C**) and coronal (**D**) maximum intensity projection (MIP) images obtained 4 hours post admission show a new aortic pseudoaneurysm *(arrows)*; posterior mediastinal hemorrhage *(arrowheads)* is unchanged. **E**, Aortogram confirms the pseudoaneurysm *(arrow)*. **F**, A covered stent graft was used to treat the pseudoaneurysm.

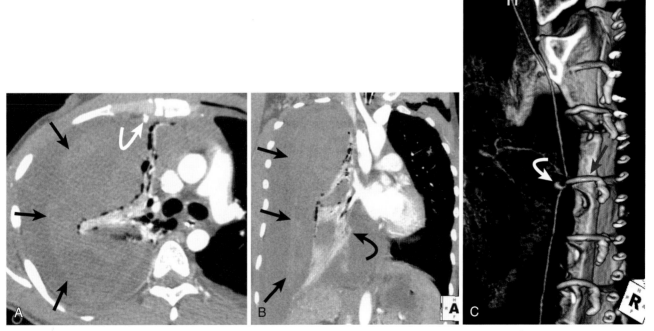

Figure 12-68 Iatrogenic injury to internal mammary artery. Multidetector computed tomography (MDCT) was obtained for hypotension following sternotomy 10 days ago for a transmediastinal gunshot wound. Axial (**A**), coronal (**B**), and three-dimensional (3-D) (**C**) images show a large tension hemothorax with clotted *(black arrows)* and nonclotted blood causing collapse of the entire right lung *(curved black arrow)*. A small right internal mammary artery pseudoaneurysm *(curved white arrow)* is seen because of an injury from the sternotomy wire *(red arrow)*. The pseudoaneurysm was resected at surgery.

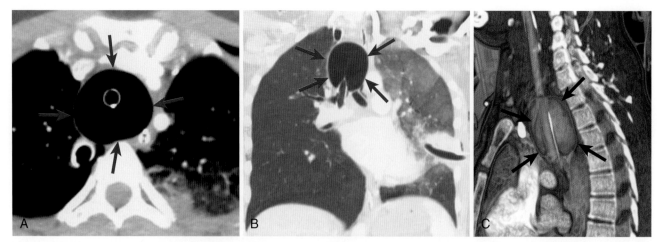

Figure 12-69 Overdistention of endotracheal tube balloon following emergent intubation. Axial (**A**), coronal multiplanar (**B**), and three-dimensional (3-D) (**C**) images show an overdistended endotracheal tube balloon *(arrows)*. Bronchoscopy showed a 14-cm longitudinal tear in the membranous trachea.

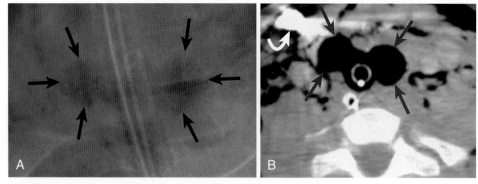

Figure 12-70 Bilateral herniation of endotracheal tube balloon through defects in tracheal wall in a 15- year-old boy who sustained a gunshot wound to the thoracic inlet region. Supine chest radiograph (**A**) and computed tomography (CT) image (**B**) show herniation of endotracheal balloon *(arrows)* through bilateral injury sites in trachea wall. A bullet *(curved arrow)* is seen in right thoracic inlet region. (From Chen J, Shanmuganathan K, Mirvis SE, et al. Using CT to diagnose tracheal rupture. *AJR Am J Roentgenol.* 2001;176:1273-1280.)

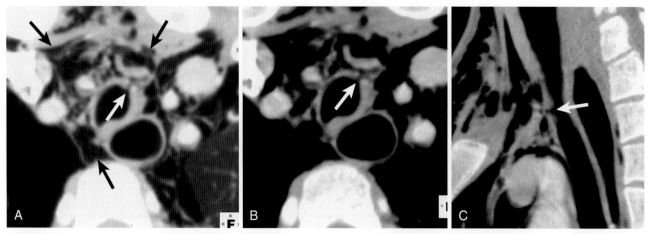

Figure 12-71 Fracture of tracheal ring following gunshot wound to thoracic inlet. Axial lung window (**A**), soft tissue window (**B**), and sagittal multiplanar reformatted (**C**) images show extensive soft tissue emphysema *(black arrows)* at the thoracic inlet. A subtle fracture *(white arrows)* of the left anterolateral ring of tracheal cartilage is seen. Bronchoscopy confirmed injury at the same anatomic location.

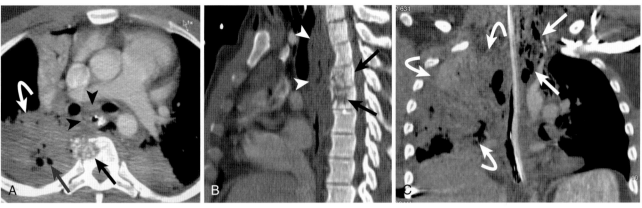

Figure 12-72 Esophageal injury following transmediastinal gunshot wound. Axial (A), sagittal (B), and coronal multiplanar (C) images show diffuse esophageal wall thickening *(arrowheads)*, T7 and T8 vertebral body fractures *(black arrows)*, and posterior mediastinal emphysema *(white arrows)*. There are extensive right lung contusions *(curved arrows)* and lacerations *(red arrow)*. At thoracotomy an injury to both anterior and posterior walls of mid esophagus was repaired.

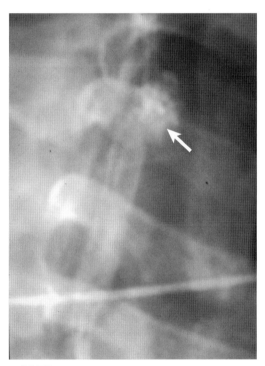

Figure 12-73 Esophageal injury in a patient with a stab wound to the lower neck and upper mediastinum. Contrast swallow shows oral contrast extravasation *(arrow)* from upper thoracic esophagus.

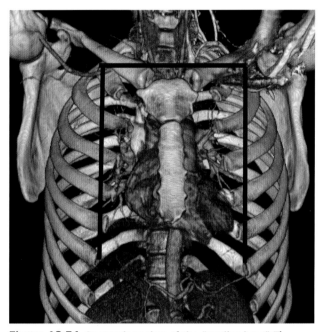

Figure 12-74 Anatomic region of the "cardiac box." The areas within the *black lines* form the cardiac box.

thoracic than cervical esophageal injuries. The high average false-negative rate (21%) reported in the literature may be related to inability to obtain multiple projections to evaluate all walls of the esophagus with barium sulfate.

Cardiac and Pericardial Injuries

Penetrating injuries to the heart and pericardium have a prehospital mortality of approximately 60% to 80%. Among the patients who reach a hospital with stable vital signs mortality can also be high (48% to 71%). Patients with entrance wounds in a juxtacardiac location, the "cardiac box" (Fig. 12-74), defined by the area between the midclavicular lines laterally, the clavicles superiorly, and

costal margins inferiorly, are at high risk for intrapericardial, aortic, pulmonary arteries (Figs. 12-75 and 12-76), or vein injury. The most frequently injured chambers are the ventricles (right, 35%, and left, 25%) with the atria (right, 33%, and left, 14%) and aorta (14%) less common.

The clinical presentation of patients with penetrating cardiac wounds is determined by the anatomic location of the cardiac injury, the rate of bleeding from the wound, and the size of the pericardial rent. The majority of patients who have penetrating injuries to the heart will present with unstable or absent vital signs. Up to 80% of patients with cardiac/pericardial stab wounds will present with cardiac tamponade (Fig.12-77). However, a small group of patients will be relatively asymptomatic with stable vital signs.

The preferred method of diagnosing cardiac injuries in stable patients with proximity injuries to the heart is echocardiography. At most trauma centers surgeons perform

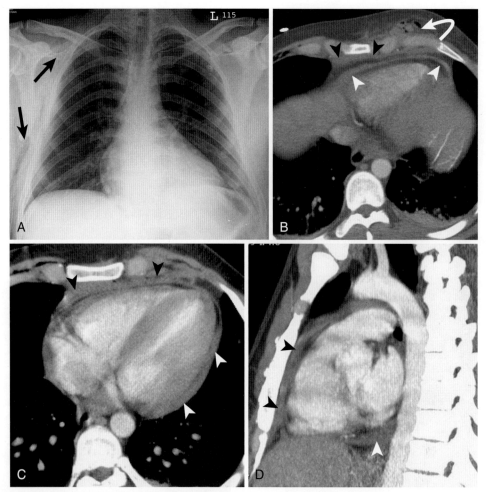

Figure 12-75 **Stab wound to the heart in a 25-year-old man.** **A,** Admission chest radiograph shows right chest wall emphysema *(arrows)*. Axial (**B** and **C**) and sagittal (**D**) maximum intensity projection (MIP) images show an entry site *(curved arrow)* in the cardiac box, anterior mediastinal blood *(black arrowheads)*, and a hemopericardium *(white arrowheads)*. Pericardial window was performed to confirm the hemopericardium. At surgery a 2-cm interventricular laceration to the heart was repaired.

ultrasound examination (extended-focus abdominal sonography for trauma), which has replaced echocardiography for demonstrating or excluding pericardial fluid. A subcostal window is typically used. If there is no evidence of pericardial fluid by CT, the likelihood of a cardiac injury is quite low. Typically this group of patients can be observed in hospital for a minimum of 24 hours. In patients with pericardial fluid a subxiphoid pericardial window or echocardiography can be performed, and if findings are positive, surgical exploration is required.

Multidetector CT findings of cardiac and pericardial injury include a wound tract extending to the pericardium, a defect in the pericardium or myocardium, hemopericardium (see Figs. 12-75 and 12-77), pneumopericardium, herniation of the heart through a pericardial rent, and an intrapericardial or intracardiac bullet. Still faster MDCT with the capability of obtaining 40 or 64-plus slices per subsecond rotation and use of cardiac gating will essentially eliminate cardiac and respiration motion, producing high-resolution images of the heart and coronary vessels. This technique is likely to be robust enough to reliable exclude or verify any injury to the cardiac structures, abolishing the need for sonography, pericardial window, and coronary arteriography.

■ CONCLUSION

Multidetector CT is the imaging modality of choice to evaluate hemodynamically stable patients admitted following penetrating injuries to the torso (Fig. 12-78) and chest. Triple-contrast spiral CT is highly accurate in excluding peritoneal violation in patients with penetrating torso trauma with no other indication for laparotomy. Patients with isolated liver injury can be selected for nonoperative management based on benign CT findings. Chest CT has been used to attempt to verify the presence or absence of mediastinal involvement from penetrating thoracic trauma. Demonstration of a ballistic tract that unequivocally *avoids* the mediastinum eliminates the need for dedicated imaging evaluation of the esophagus, aorta, and mainstem bronchi. Knife wounds to the chest tend to have a less predictable course and are more likely to require mediastinal imaging assessment. If any doubt regarding the course of penetrating wound tract exists, the mediastinal structures must be individually evaluated. Future studies will reveal what role advanced multislice CT scanning may play in replacing the current imaging regimen for penetrating torso and mediastinal trauma.

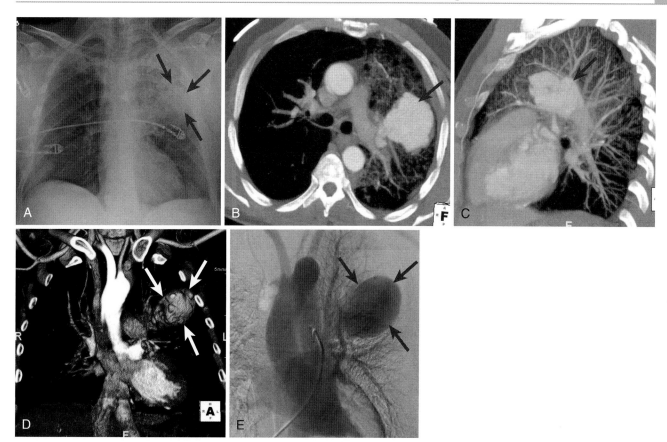

Figure 12-76 Pulmonary artery pseudoaneurysm in a 56-year-old man stabbed in the left chest with a screwdriver. A, Admission chest radiograph shows left upper lobe lung contusion. A large rounded dense region *(arrows)* within the contusion could represent posttraumatic pneumatocele or vascular lesion. Axial **(B)** sagittal **(C)**, and coronal **(D)** images show that a large pseudoaneurysm *(arrows)* appears to arise from the left main pulmonary artery. Lung contusion surrounds the pseudoaneurysm. **E,** Pulmonary angiogram confirms a large left main pulmonary artery pseudoaneurysm. At surgery the pseudoaneurysm was arising from a 2-cm diameter injury to the proximal left main pulmonary artery, which was repaired.

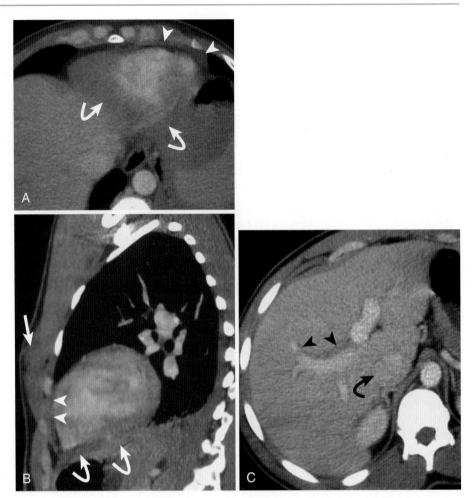

Figure 12-77 Cardiac tampon-ade following a stab wound to the chest. Axial (**A**) and coronal refor-matted (**B**) images show the entry site *(arrow)* in the "cardiac box." There is a small hemopericardium *(curved arrows)* and anterior mediastinal blood *(arrow-heads)*. **C,** Axial image obtained in the upper abdomen shows a distended intrahepatic vena cava *(curved arrow)* and diffuse periportal edema *(arrow-heads)* due to raised venous hydrostatic pressure from tamponade.

ALGORHYTHM TO TRIAGE PENETRATING TORSO TRAUMA PATIENTS

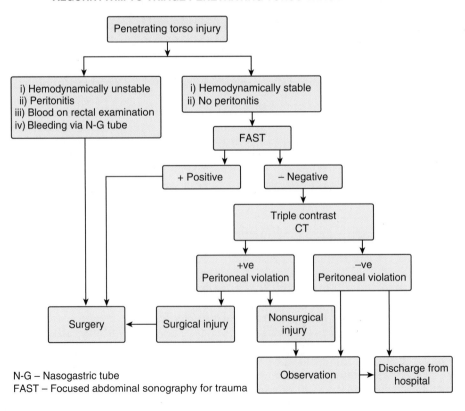

Figure 12-78 The algorithm used at our Shock Trauma Center at University of Maryland Medical Center.

N-G – Nasogastric tube
FAST – Focused abdominal sonography for trauma

Selected Reading

Asensio JA, Chahwan S, Forno W, et al. Penetrating esophageal injuries: multicenter study of the American Association for the Surgery of Trauma. *J Trauma*. 2001;50:289–296.

Biffl WL, Kaups KL, Cothren CC, et al. Management of patients with anterior abdominal stab wounds: a Western Trauma Association multicenter trial. *J Trauma*. 2009;66:1294–1301.

Biffl WL, Kaups KL, Pham TN, et al. Validating the Western Trauma Association algorithm for managing patients with anterior abdominal stab wounds: a Western Trauma Association multicenter trial. *J Trauma*. 2011;71:1494–1502.

Bodanapally UK, Shanmuganathan K, Mirvis SE, et al. MDCT diagnosis of penetrating diaphragm injury. *Eur Radiol*. 2009;19:1875–1881.

Burlew CC, Moore EE, Moore FA, et al. Western Trauma Association critical decisions in trauma: resuscitative thoracotomy. *J Trauma Acute Care Surg*. 2012;73:1359–1363.

Chapple C, Barbagli G, Jordan G, et al. Consensus statement on urethral trauma. *BJU Int*. 2004;93:1195–1202.

Co SJ, Yong-Hing CJ, Galea-Soler S, et al. Role of imaging in penetrating and blunt traumatic injury to the heart. *Radiographics*. 2011;31:E101–E115. http://dx.doi.org/10.1148/rg.314095177.

Como JJ, Bokhari F, Chiu WC, et al. Practice management guidelines for selective non-operative management of penetrating abdominal trauma. *J Trauma*. 2010;68:721–733.

Demetriades D, Velmahos G, Cornwell E III, et al. Selective non-operative management of gunshot wounds of the anterior abdomen. *Arch Surg*. 1997;132:178–183.

DuBose J, Inaba K, Demetriades D, et al. Management of post-traumatic retained hemothorax: a prospective, observational, multicenter AAST study. *J Trauma Acute Care Surg*. 2012;72:11–22.

Feliciano DV, Bitondo CG, Steed G, et al. Five hundred open taps or lavages in patients with abdominal stab wounds. *Ann Surg*. 1984;147:772–777.

Hanna WC, Ferri LE, Fata P, et al. The current status of traumatic diaphragmatic injury: lessons learned from 105 patients over 13 years. *Ann Thorac Surg*. 2008;85:1044–1048.

Hollerman JJ, Fackler ML, Coldwell DM, et al. Gunshot wounds, 1: bullet, ballistics, and mechanism of injury. *AJR Am J Roentgenol*. 1990;155:685–690.

Ivatury RR, Simon RJ, Stahl WM. A critical evaluation of laparoscopy in penetrating abdominal trauma. *J Trauma*. 1993;34:822–828.

Johnson JJ, Garwe T, Raines AR, et al. The use of laparoscopy in the diagnosis and treatment of blunt and penetrating abdominal injuries: 10-year experience at a level 1 trauma center. *Am J Surg*. 2013;205:317–321.

Keleman JJ, Martin RR, Obney JA, et al. Evaluation of peritoneal lavage in stable patients with peritoneal lavage. *Arch Surg*. 1997;132:909–913.

McAlvanah MJ, Shaftan GW. Selective conservatism in penetrating abdominal wounds: a continuing reappraisal. *J Trauma*. 1978;18:206–211.

Miller KS, McAninch JW. Radiographic assessment of renal trauma: our 15-year experience. *J Urol*. 1995;154:352–355.

Múnera F, Morales C, Soto JA, et al. Gunshot wounds of abdomen: evaluation of stable patients with triple-contrast helical CT. *Radiology*. 2004;231:399–405.

Navsaria PH, Nicol AJ, Krige JE, et al. Selective nonoperative management of liver gunshot injuries. *Ann Surg*. 2009;240:653–656.

Phillips T, Sclafani SA, Goldstein A, et al. Use of contrast-enhanced CT enema in the management of penetrating injuries trauma to the flank and back. *J Trauma*. 1986;26:593–600.

Powell BS, Magnotti LJ, Schroeppel TJ, et al. Diagnostic laparoscopy for the evaluation of occult diaphragmatic injury following penetrating thoracoabdominal trauma. *Injury*. 2008;39:530–534.

Renz BM, Feliciano DV. Gunshot wounds to the right thoracoabdomen: a prospective study of nonoperative management. *J Trauma*. 1994;37:737–744.

Salim A, Sangthong B, Martin M, et al. Use of computed tomography in anterior abdominal stab wounds: results of a prospective study. *Arch Surg*. 2006;141:745–750. discussion 750–752.

Santucci RA, Wessells H, Bartsch G, et al. Evaluation and management of renal injuries: consensus statement of the renal trauma subcommittee. *BJU Int*. 2004;93:937–954.

Schwab CW. Violence: American uncivil war. Presidential address, Sixth Scientific Assembly of the Eastern Association for the Surgery of Trauma. *J Trauma*. 1993;35:657–665.

Shanmuganathan K, Mirvis SE, Chiu WC, et al. Penetrating torso trauma: triple-contrast helical CT in peritoneal violation and organ injury—a prospective study in 200 patients. *Radiology*. 2004;231:775–784.

Soto JA, Morales C, Múnera F, et al. Penetrating stab wounds to the abdomen: use of serial US and contrast-enhanced CT in stable patients. *Radiology*. 2001;220:365–371.

Udobi KF, Rodriguez A, Chiu WC, et al. Role of ultrasonography in penetrating abdominal trauma: a prospective clinical study. *J Trauma*. 2001;50:475–479.

Voelzke BB, McAninch JW. Renal gunshot wounds: clinical management and outcome. *J Trauma*. 2009;66:593–600.

Wilson RF, Nichols RL. The EAST practice management guidelines for prophylactic antibiotic use in tube thoracostomy for traumatic hemopneumothorax: a commentary. Eastern Association for Trauma. *J Trauma*. 2000;48:758–759.

CHAPTER 13

Nontraumatic Abdominal Emergencies

Gastric and Duodenal Emergencies

Vincent M. Mellnick and Christine Menias

The upper gastrointestinal (GI) tract, including the esophagus, stomach, and duodenum, is a common but potentially overlooked site of disease that may prompt presentation to the emergency department (ED), including inflammation and infection, obstruction, and perforation. Although these organs have traditionally been evaluated by fluoroscopy, which offers mucosal detail, computed tomography (CT) is now the first-line imaging modality in most EDs, warranting knowledge of the appearance of these diseases on cross-sectional imaging as well. This section will discuss inflammation, infection, obstruction, and perforation of the esophagus, stomach, and duodenum. Of note, the topics of trauma, ischemia, and hemorrhage involving these organs will be discussed in other chapters.

■ NORMAL ANATOMY

The esophagus extends from the lower border of the cricoid cartilage to the stomach, passing through the diaphragmatic hiatus at T10. Spanning 25 to 30 cm in length, the esophagus deviates to the left in the neck, to the right in most of the thorax, and then back to the left as it joins the gastroesophageal junction. Normal esophageal wall thickness on CT is less than or equal to 5 mm. The esophageal wall has an adventitial layer, but no serosa, which permits esophageal diseases to more readily extend into the nearby neck, mediastinum, or upper abdomen.

■ ESOPHAGEAL EMERGENCIES

Esophageal Inflammation/Infection

Esophagitis

Esophagitis can arise from a number of causes, including infection, radiation, gastroesophageal reflux, and medications. Infectious esophagitis may have characteristic findings on barium fluoroscopy depending on the causative pathogen. *Candida* esophagitis manifests with raised mucosal plaques between which barium is trapped. Herpes esophagitis typically presents with multiple small ulcers represented by pooled barium. Larger ulcers are seen with cytomegalovirus and human immunodeficiency virus (HIV) esophagitis. Reflux esophagitis may manifest with strictures, as well as reticular-appearing mucosa distally, indicating Barrett esophagus. In contrast to the detailed mucosal evaluation afforded by barium fluoroscopy, CT findings of infectious esophagitis are nonspecific and insensitive, demonstrating a sensitivity of approximately 55% in one study. Computed tomography findings include long segment thickening of the esophageal wall (greater than 5 mm), as well as a "target" sign caused by mucosal hyperemia and submucosal edema (Fig. 13-1). There is a large overlap in the CT appearance of infectious and noninfectious esophagitis, such as from reflux or radiation. Complications of esophagitis include functional obstruction, aspiration, and perforation.

Esophageal Obstruction

Foreign Bodies

Esophageal foreign bodies are most often ingested by children and patients with cognitive defects. Commonly seen foreign bodies include impacted food boluses, fish and chicken bones, coins, and vinyl gloves. Although most esophageal foreign bodies pass spontaneously, 10% to 20% of cases require endoscopic removal and approximately 1% undergo surgery for treatment. Up to one third of affected adult patients with foreign body impaction have an underlying esophageal stricture contributing to their presentation. Diagnostic workup often starts with radiography, particularly if the ingested item is radiodense (e.g., metallic) or suspected to be lodged in the hypopharynx. Computed tomography is useful in select cases for definitive diagnosis and localization, and identifying suspected complications such as esophageal perforation (Fig. 13-2).

Esophageal Strictures

Although not an emergency per se, stricture of the esophagus can cause esophageal obstruction (including impaction of food boluses as discussed earlier) and presentation to the ED. Benign strictures have smooth borders and usually involve a longer segment of the esophagus. Possible causes of benign esophageal strictures include long-standing gastroesophageal reflux, radiation, chronic medication-induced esophagitis, nasogastric intubation, epidermolysis bullosa, and eosinophilic esophagitis. Barium studies can reliably characterize benign esophageal strictures, but those with equivocal or malignant features warrant further evaluation with endoscopy. Esophageal obstruction by a malignant stricture usually manifests with short segment involvement and mucosal shouldering on fluoroscopy. Corresponding submucosal soft tissue attenuation can be seen on CT, which may also demonstrate invasion into the adjacent mediastinum and mediastinal lymphadenopathy in advanced disease.

Esophageal Perforation

Mallory-Weiss Tears
The clinical presentation and imaging findings of esophageal perforation depend on the thickness of the

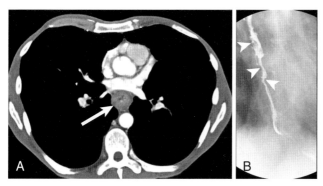

Figure 13-1 Candida esophagitis. Contrast-enhanced computed tomography (**A**) and barium esophagogram (**B**) images in a patient with *Candida* esophagitis show circumferential esophageal thickening on CT *(arrow)* with corresponding raised mucosal plaques on esophagography *(arrowheads)*. Upper endoscopy confirmed the presence of *Candida* infection.

esophageal tear. Superficial tears, or Mallory-Weiss tears, commonly result from repeated, forceful retching and may cause "coffee-ground" emesis caused by mucosal bleeding. These tears may have no imaging findings, particularly on CT. On barium studies they may manifest as linear collections of contrast, classically in the distal esophagus, corresponding to mucosal tears identified on endoscopy (Fig. 13-3).

Esophageal Dissection
Intermediate—or intramural—perforation is a rare form of esophageal perforation also referred to as *esophageal dissection*. This condition can be seen after instrumentation, foreign body impaction, or forceful vomiting. Imaging findings of intramural perforation include a "double-barrel esophagus" caused by an intraluminal flap separating the true and false lumens, which may be accentuated with oral contrast, creating what has been also been termed a *mucosal stripe sign*. The false lumen of esophageal dissection is often posterior to the true lumen and may be better demonstrated on coronal and sagittal reformatted images. There is considerable overlap between esophageal dissection and an intramural hematoma, which may be distinguished by visualization of contrast in the false lumen with a true dissection (Fig. 13-4).

Transmural Perforation
Similar to esophageal dissection, full-thickness esophageal perforation may be iatrogenic, such as from surgery, stricture dilatation, stenting, or thermal injury. In addition, full-thickness tears may occur from vomiting (Boerhaave syndrome), caused by incomplete cricopharyngeal relaxation and increased intraluminal pressure. On imaging, full-thickness perforation may result in pneumomediastinum, pleural effusions, and leak of oral contrast into the mediastinal and/or

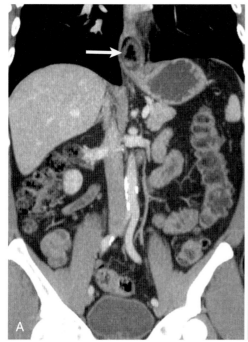

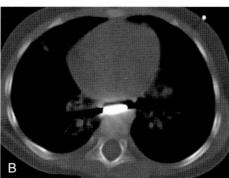

Figure 13-2 Esophageal foreign bodies. **A,** Coronal contrast-enhanced computed tomography shows a fat and soft tissue density food bolus impacted in the distal esophagus *(arrow)*. On upper endoscopy a Schatzki ring was discovered causing a focal stenosis at the site of impaction. **B,** Axial CT image from a child shows a coin lodged in the distal esophagus without CT findings to suggest perforation.

pleural spaces (Fig. 13-5). In addition to benign causes, primary or metastatic esophageal tumor may also perforate, particularly following palliative dilatation and/or stenting. Complications of esophageal perforation include mediastinitis, pneumonia (from direct spread of infection or from aspiration), and empyema/abscess formation.

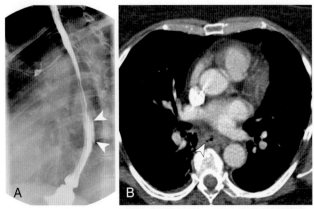

Figure 13-3 Mallory-Weiss tear. A, Water-soluble esophagogram in a patient with a recent episode of vomiting shows a linear collection of contrast *(arrowheads)*. B, Contrast-enhanced computed tomography demonstrates corresponding focus of submucosal gas *(arrowhead)*. These findings are consistent with a superficial mucosal tear, confirmed on endoscopy.

Aortoesophageal Fistulas

Chronically, esophageal perforation may result in fistula formation, including to the trachea, pleural space, and aorta. The majority of aortoesophageal fistulas result from aortic disease fistulizing to the esophagus, such as from rupture of a descending thoracic aortic aneurysm or an infected aortic graft. Primary esophageal disease may result in aortic fistulization as well: esophagitis, foreign body perforation, and advanced esophageal cancer have all been described as underlying causes. Clinically, patients with aortoesophageal fistulas present with the Chiari triad: midthoracic pain or dysphagia, a sentinel episode of hematemesis, and a symptom-free interval that gives way to massive upper GI bleeding. Imaging findings of aortoesophageal fistulas include a focal outpouching of the aorta toward the esophagus, adjacent esophageal wall thickening, and extraluminal gas within or abutting the aortic wall (Fig. 13-6). Oral contrast or angiographic studies may also demonstrate a luminal communication.

Gastric Emergencies

Normal Anatomy

The stomach is divided into five arbitrary segments: the cardia, fundus, body, antrum, and pylorus. The lesser curvature of the stomach is at the right, posterior aspect of the organ, whereas the greater curvature of

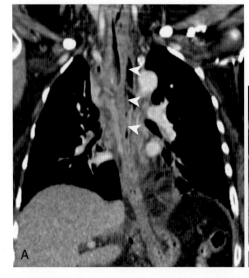

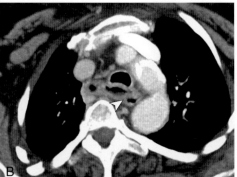

Figure 13-4 Esophageal dissection. Coronal (A) and axial (B) contrast-enhanced computed tomography images show a long segment intramural perforation or dissection in the thoracic esophagus, manifest by a mucosal flap *(arrowheads)* separating the true and false lumens. Note the "double-barrel" appearance on the axial image.

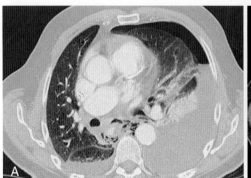

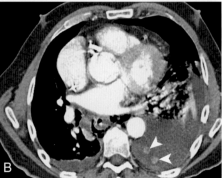

Figure 13-5 Transmural esophageal dissection. A, Contrast-enhanced computed tomography shows pneumomediastinum and a left hydropneumothorax. B, Note blushes of high-attenuation material *(arrowheads)* in the pleural fluid, which is extraluminal oral contrast, confirming esophageal perforation as the cause of these findings.

the stomach lies to the left and anteriorly. At the junction of the lesser curvature and antrum lies the incisura angularis. A line drawn from the incisura to the greater curvature of the stomach represents the transition zone from body-type to antral-type mucosa, which is a frequent site for gastric ulcers. Intraluminal rugal folds in the stomach are most prominent in the gastric fundus and body. The gastric antrum demonstrates a thicker wall on CT and can normally demonstrate mural stratification, owing to its greater muscular composition and increased peristalsis in this segment. The degree of distention within the gastric segment in question determines normal wall thickness on CT. The nondependent gastric body should be less than or equal to 5 mm in thickness when properly distended, whereas the antrum may normally measure up to 12 mm in thickness. The fundus is the most dependent portion of the stomach and is subsequently the most common site for layering intraluminal contents, notably blood products.

Gastric Inflammation and Infection

Gastritis
Gastritis has many potential underlying causes, including *Helicobacter pylori* infection, nonsteroidal antiinflammatory medications, and alcohol. Inflammation of the stomach is most commonly diffuse, but it can also be focal process. *H. Pylori* gastritis may be isolated to the antrum or greater curvature. On fluoroscopy, gastritis manifests with thickened rugal folds, erosions, and foci of ulceration, identified by persistent pooling of oral contrast. On CT, gastric inflammation appears as low-attenuation submucosal edema and mucosal hyperemia, which result in mural stratification. As previously discussed, attention to the degree of gastric distention helps discern true gastric wall thickening from artificial thickening resulting from collapsed lumen.

A subset of patients with gastritis can develop the emphysematous variant, an uncommon form with a high mortality rate. The underlying pathologic process in emphysematous gastritis is mucosal disruption and invasion of the gastric wall by a gas-producing organism, particularly *Escherichia coli*. On CT this condition presents with signs of gastritis (e.g., mural stratification), accompanied by gas bubbles in the stomach wall and potentially portal venous gas. Differentiation between emphysematous gastritis and more benign gastric emphysema may be difficult, but the latter is much more common, is typically seen in relatively asymptomatic patients, and appears with more linear intramural gas with no wall thickening to suggest gastritis (Fig. 13-7).

Peptic Ulcer Disease
Although the incidence of peptic ulcers has decreased since the advent of *H. pylori* treatment and proton pump inhibitors, they remain a potential cause for presentation to the ED. Whereas superficial ulcers can be seen only with endoscopy or with barium fluoroscopy, deeply penetrating ulcers may be identified on CT as a focal mucosal outpouching, submucosal edema, perigastric fat stranding, and in the case of perforation, extraluminal gas (Fig. 13-8). In patients who have undergone gastric surgery, particularly Billroth and Roux-en-Y gastric bypass procedures, marginal gastric ulcers may appear at the gastrojejunal anastomosis. These ulcers can be deeply penetrating, usually begin at the jejunal side of the anastomosis, and typically develop 2 to 4 years following surgery.

Crohn Disease
Gastroduodenal Crohn disease (CD) is rare, causing clinical symptoms in 0.5% to 4% of all patients with CD. Most of these patients have simultaneous involvement of the distal small bowel or the colon. The most common manifestation of gastroduodenal CD is contiguous involvement of the antrum, pylorus, and proximal duodenum, resulting in a nondistensible distal stomach and a characteristic "ram's horn" appearance. Other imaging findings include mucosal "cobblestoning," thickening folds, pseudopolyps, ulcers (including postbulbar ulcers in the duodenum), and strictures. Like CD elsewhere in the GI tract, gastroduodenal involvement may be complicated acutely by obstruction, perforation, abscess, and fistula formation.

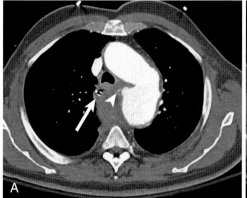 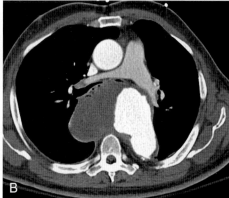

Figure 13-6 Aortoesophageal fistula. A and **B,** Contrast-enhanced computed tomography images reveal an irregular, saccular aneurysm arising from the descending thoracic aorta with associated hematoma. Note the loss of fat plane between the aneurysm and esophagus, which contains a nasogastric tube *(arrow)*. There is also a focus of extraluminal contrast arising from the superior portion of the aneurysm, indicating active bleeding *(arrowhead)*. A fistulous connection between the esophagus and the aorta was confirmed at surgery.

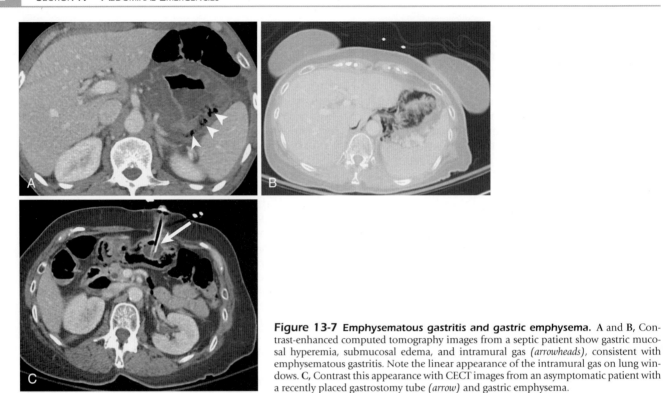

Figure 13-7 Emphysematous gastritis and gastric emphysema. A and **B,** Contrast-enhanced computed tomography images from a septic patient show gastric mucosal hyperemia, submucosal edema, and intramural gas *(arrowheads),* consistent with emphysematous gastritis. Note the linear appearance of the intramural gas on lung windows. **C,** Contrast this appearance with CECT images from an asymptomatic patient with a recently placed gastrostomy tube *(arrow)* and gastric emphysema.

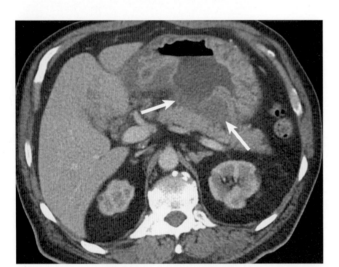

Figure   13-8 Penetrating   gastric   ulcer. Contrast-enhanced computed tomography shows a large crater in the lesser curvature posterior wall with associated wall thickening. Note the infiltration of the fat in the lesser sac *(arrows).* No free intraperitoneal gas was identified to suggest perforation. A large peptic ulcer was confirmed at endoscopy.

Gastric Obstruction

Gastric Volvulus

An uncommon cause of gastric obstruction, gastric volvulus presents clinically with Borchardt triad: sudden epigastric pain, intractable retching, and inability to pass a nasogastric tube. The two subsets of gastric volvulus are organoaxial and mesenteroaxial, although many are seen as a combination of these. Organoaxial gastric volvulus is the most common type and results from rotation about the long axis (line connecting the pylorus to the cardia) of the stomach with the antrum anterosuperiorly and the fundus posteroinferiorly (Fig. 13-9). This type of gastric volvulus is more commonly associated with diaphragmatic defects and vascular compromise. Mesenteroaxial gastric volvulus is less common and results from rotation of the stomach about its short axis, resulting in the antrum being positioned above the gastroesophageal junction (Fig. 13-10). These are more commonly chronic and less likely to be associated with diaphragmatic hernias.

On imaging, gastric volvulus presents with a distended stomach, nonpassage of oral contrast, and an abnormal lie to the stomach. Gastric volvulus requires at least 180 degrees of rotation and gastric outlet obstruction. Asymptomatic patients with large hiatal hernias may present with an abnormal lie, that is, organoaxial positioning of the stomach without volvulus. These patients are predisposed to both gastric volvulus and hiatal hernia incarceration, particularly when the fundus "redescends" into the abdomen, obstructing the mouth of the hernia sac.

Peptic Ulcer Disease

Similar to peptic ulcer disease in general, the incidence of gastric outlet obstruction due to peptic ulcer disease is decreasing. Acutely, obstruction from peptic ulcer disease occurs because of mucosal ulceration and submucosal edema. More commonly, in the chronically affected patient, fibrosis may also cause luminal narrowing and obstruction. On imaging this appears as narrowing of the affected segment with associated soft tissue thickening, most often the pylorus. However, because of its overlap with malignant causes of gastric outlet obstruction, exclusion of an underlying mucosal lesion is often warranted.

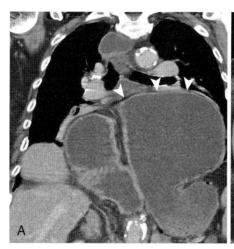

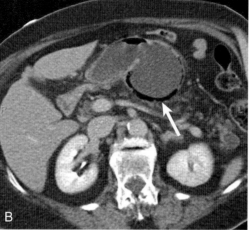

Figure 13-9 Organoaxial gastric volvulus. Coronal (A) and axial (B) contrast-enhanced computed tomography shows an obstructed hiatal hernia with the greater curvature situated superiorly *(arrowheads)*, consistent with organoaxial volvulus. Note the resulting gastric ischemia, evidenced by pneumatosis *(arrow)*.

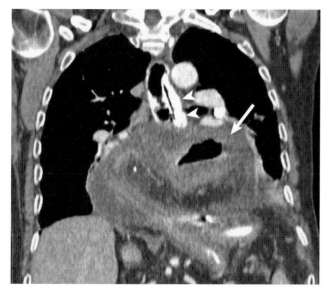

Figure 13-10 Mesenteroaxial gastric volvulus. Coronal contrast-enhanced computed tomography shows positioning of the pylorus *(arrow)* superior and to the left of the esophagus, which contains a nasogastric tube *(arrowheads)*. Note the thickening of the gastric wall with adjacent fluid, indicating inflammation. Gastric volvulus and ischemia were confirmed intraoperatively.

Malignancy

Primary tumors in or abutting the stomach may be associated with gastric outlet obstruction. This is most commonly seen with gastric adenocarcinoma but can be seen with pancreatic and biliary tumors, primary duodenal tumors, and rarely lymphoma. In the case of malignant duodenal obstruction, many such cases are generally classified as causing "gastric outlet obstruction," leading to ambiguity as to the precise level of obstruction. After gastric adenocarcinoma the second most common tumor to obstruct the stomach and/or duodenum is pancreatic head adenocarcinoma, which can cause gastric outlet obstruction in 15% to 25% of cases. Imaging clues to a malignant cause for gastric or duodenal obstruction include mucosal shouldering on barium studies, soft tissue thickening at the transition point of the obstruction on CT, and evidence of metastatic disease, such as enlarged lymph nodes, liver lesions, or omental deposits.

Bezoars

Ingested foreign bodies may be a cause of gastric or small bowel obstruction and often fall into two major categories: trichobezoars and phytobezoars. Trichobezoars are composed of hair and are most common in women and psychiatric patients, often those with long hair. When the hair extends from the stomach into the small and/or large bowel this has been termed *Rapunzel syndrome* (Fig. 13-11). Phytobezoars are composed of fruit or vegetable matter, commonly oranges and persimmons. Patients with decreased gastric motility, such as those who have undergone gastric surgery, are predisposed to formation of phytobezoars, which may also pass into the small bowel and cause obstruction more distally as well. Patients who have undergone organ transplantation also have an increased risk for developing bezoars, which is hypothesized to be secondary to decreased gastric motility, either due to vagus nerve injury or a side effect of cyclosporine.

Gastric Banding

The increasing rate of obesity in the United States has resulted in a rising number of bariatric surgery techniques, one of which is gastric banding. The gastric banding device is composed of the band itself, an access port, and connecting tube. The band is secured around the cranial portion of the stomach, approximately 2 cm from the gastroesophageal junction, forming a small pouch and limiting food intake. The port is usually placed outside the peritoneal cavity, either within the rectus abdominis muscles sheath or under the external thoracic fascia. If the band slips distally, it may surround a larger portion of the stomach and lead to gastric outlet obstruction. Normal gastric band orientation is assessed with the phi angle, which is increased with a slipped band. Measured in the anteroposterior dimension, the phi angle (angle between the spinal column and gastric band) has a normal range of 4 to 58 degrees.

Gastric Perforation

Peptic Ulcer Disease

Perforation complicates peptic ulcer disease in approximately 2% to 10% of affected patients. The imaging

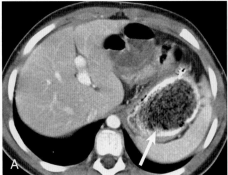
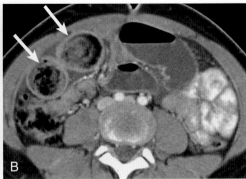

Figure 13-11 Gastric tricho-bezoar. A and **B,** Contrast-enhanced computed tomography images show a large, mottled mass in the gastric fundus *(arrow),* representing a trichobezoar that extends out of the stomach into the small bowel *(arrows),* causing obstruction, the "Rapunzel syndrome."

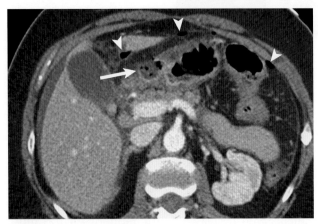

Figure 13-12 Perforated gastric ulcer. Contrast-enhanced computed tomography shows an ulcer crater in the gastric antrum *(arrow)* with associated gastric wall thickening, consistent with a peptic ulcer. Locules of free intraperitoneal gas *(arrowheads)* are diagnostic for perforation.

findings of perforation can vary depending upon the location of the perforated ulcer. Ulcers on the anterior wall and greater curvature perforate freely into the peritoneal space, whereas more posterior ulcers may have a relatively contained perforation into the lesser sac. Perforation of peptic ulcers within the duodenal bulb and stomach remains one of the most common causes of GI perforation, warranting close examination of the stomach and proximal duodenum for ulcers when free intraperitoneal gas is identified on CT (Fig. 13-12).

Malignancy

Gastric adenocarcinoma is complicated by perforation in 0.4% to 6.0% of cases and is more common in patients older than 65 years of age. Although typically found in locally advanced gastric cancer, a focal ulcerated malignancy may perforate if the ulcer crater is deeply penetrating. Perforation of GI lymphoma is most commonly seen in the small bowel, but gastric lymphoma may also perforate; perforation is seen in a higher percentage of T-cell lymphoma involving the GI tract than with B-cell lymphoma (Fig. 13-13). Clues to an underlying malignancy as a cause of gastric perforation include focal gastric wall thickening with soft tissue attenuation in the submucosa, as well as evidence of tumor outside of the stomach such as lymphadenopathy or metastases.

Gastric Banding

Perforation related to gastric banding can be seen acutely in 0.1% to 0.8% of patients and may have a varied clinical presentation. Computed tomography may demonstrate free or loculated extraluminal gas or abscess formation. Chronic perforation of the stomach complicates 1% to 3% of patients with gastric bands and results from erosion of the band into the stomach lumen. On fluoroscopy, demonstration of contrast outlining the band can confirm erosion, which may also manifest on CT with gas surrounding the band. In addition, CT may show inflammation or fluid tracking along the connector tubing and/or port; when seen, this should prompt evaluation of the band as the site of erosion or infection (Fig. 13-14).

Duodenal Emergencies

Normal Anatomy

The first segment of the small intestine, the duodenum is typically 25 to 38 cm in length and extends from the gastric pylorus to the duodenojejunal flexure (ligament of Treitz). The duodenum consists of four segments: the intraperitoneal bulb, followed by the retroperitoneal descending, transverse, and ascending portions. The second (descending) portion of the duodenum contains the ampulla of Vater and abuts the pancreas, forming the pancreaticoduodenal groove.

Duodenal Inflammation and Infection

Peptic Ulcer Disease

Duodenal peptic ulcers are more common than gastric ulcers, typically solitary, and located in the duodenal bulb in 5% to 11% of patients. In contrast to peptic ulcers in the stomach, duodenal ulcers have very low malignant potential and typically occur because of increased peptic acid secretion, including in the setting of chronic *H. pylori* infection. However, similar to their gastric counterparts, duodenal peptic ulcers show persistent pooling of oral contrast on fluoroscopy and on CT show a focal outpouching with mucosal hyperemia, submucosal edema, and adjacent fat stranding.

Zollinger-Ellison Syndrome

A subset of patients with duodenal ulcers will have Zollinger-Ellison syndrome, typically caused by a gastrin-secreting tumor in the gastrinoma triangle, an

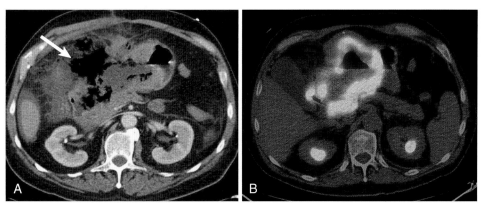

Figure 13-13 Perforated gastric lymphoma. A, Contrast-enhanced computed tomography shows a large amount of extraluminal gas *(arrow)*, with surrounding fluid and inflammatory stranding, consistent with perforation. The underlying stomach is diffusely thickened by lymphomatous involvement, demonstrated before perforation **B,** Fludeoxyglucose F 18 positron emission tomography/CT scan shows markedly increased tracer uptake in the stomach wall.

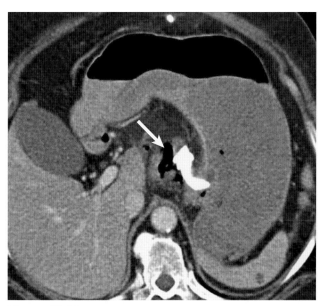

Figure 13-14 Eroded gastric band with perforation. Contrast-enhanced computed tomography shows changes from laparoscopic banding procedure. Note that the band has extraluminal gas surrounding it *(arrow)* with associated inflammatory fat stranding. Focal perforation of the stomach at the banding site was confirmed at surgery.

anatomic space defined by the junctions of the cystic and common bile ducts, the neck and body of the pancreas, and the second and third portions of the duodenum. The increased serum gastrin levels stimulate peptic acid secretion and lead to duodenal mucosal ulceration. Computed tomography findings of Zollinger-Ellison syndrome include reflux esophagitis, gastritis, and multiple duodenal ulcers, including distal to the duodenal bulb (Fig. 13-15). This conglomerate of findings should prompt a search for an adjacent hyperenhancing nodule representing a gastrinoma, although these may be difficult to identify on routine portal venous phase CT and may require multiphase phase CT, endoscopic ultrasonography (EUS), or octreotide scan to aid in detection.

Diverticulitis

Duodenal diverticula are very common, occurring in approximately 23% of patients, most common in the second portion and typically arising medially. Although a relative minority of duodenal diverticula cause symptoms, up to 1% of patients will have a complication from a duodenal diverticulum that requires treatment, including diverticulitis, perforation, and obstruction in the case of intraluminal diverticula. Computed tomography findings of duodenal diverticulitis resemble those seen in inflamed diverticula elsewhere in the GI tract: a focal, round outpouching from the duodenal lumen with wall thickening and adjacent fat stranding and fluid (Fig. 13-16). Treatment of duodenal diverticulitis may be operative or nonoperative (i.e., antibiotics), depending on the clinical condition and stability of the patient.

Groove Pancreatitis

A rare form of chronic pancreatitis, groove pancreatitis occurs because of inflammation in the pancreaticoduodenal groove, including the pancreatic head and pancreatic rests in the duodenal wall. Clinically patients may present with normal serum amylase and lipase levels. The focal inflammation in the duodenal wall may result in benign-appearing common bile duct strictures and duodenal obstruction. The imaging appearance of groove pancreatitis may overlap with pancreatic adenocarcinoma considerably, but groove pancreatitis classically manifests with low-attenuation cystic areas ("cystic degeneration") in the descending duodenal wall and soft tissue in the pancreaticoduodenal groove resulting from fibrosis. This disease can be particularly well characterized on magnetic resonance cholangiopancreatography (MRCP), which can demonstrate both the well-marginated T2-hyperintense cystic areas and biliary strictures without underlying mass lesion. These findings, along with a lack of vascular invasion, help differentiate between groove pancreatitis and adenocarcinoma of the pancreaticoduodenal groove (Fig. 13-17). Associated fibrosis, which can result from chronic inflammation, may demonstrate delayed contrast enhancement on CT and magnetic resonance imaging (MRI).

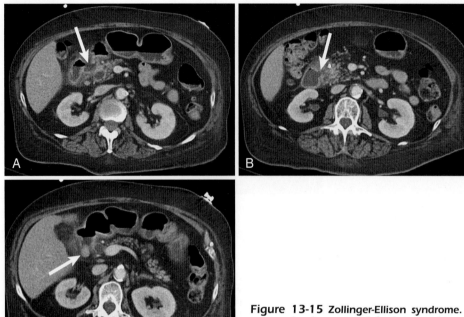

Figure 13-15 Zollinger-Ellison syndrome. A and **B,** Contrast-enhanced computed tomography shows several focal outpouchings with surrounding inflammation in the descending duodenum *(arrows)* representing peptic ulcers. **C,** Hyperenhancing nodule in the duodenal wall, consistent with a gastrinoma *(arrow),* causing Zollinger-Ellison syndrome with postbulbar ulcers.

Figure 13-16 Duodenal diverticulitis. A, Contrast-enhanced computed tomography shows a rounded, socklike outpouching *(arrow)* representing a diverticulum arising from the junction of the second and third portions of the duodenum. **B,** There is adjacent fat stranding *(arrows)* resulting from inflammation of the diverticulum.

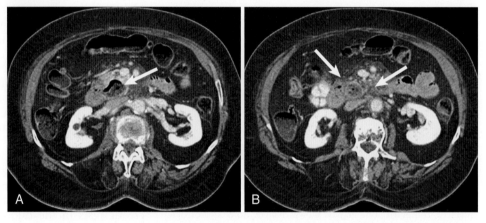

Duodenal Obstruction

Malrotation and Volvulus

Although malrotation is rare in adulthood—80% of patients will present in the first month of life and 90% within the first year—some cases remain quiescent for years and present later in life. Affected patients may present clinically with symptoms of proximal bowel obstruction, namely, severe abdominal pain and bilious vomiting. On imaging studies the findings of malrotation are the same as those seen in childhood: a duodenum that does not cross the spine, reversal of the relationship between superior mesenteric artery (SMA) and vein, colon situated on the left side of the abdomen, and small bowel on the right. When complicated by volvulus, CT shows a distended stomach and duodenum and an abrupt transition to decompressed bowel with a focal twist causing a "whirlpool" sign (Fig. 13-18). There may

also be occlusion of mesenteric vessels with associated bowel ischemia, indicated by bowel wall thickening, hypoenhancement, and/or pneumatosis with adjacent mesenteric edema and fluid.

Superior Mesenteric Artery Syndrome

Duodenal obstruction may result from compression of the transverse portion as it crosses between the aorta and SMA. Patients predisposed to this condition include those with prior surgery causing loss or distortion of normal retroperitoneal fat, rapid weight loss, or a lean body habitus. Superior mesenteric artery syndrome can be diagnosed with an abnormally acute aortomesenteric angle (normal range is 28 to 65 degrees) or a decreased aortomesenteric distance (normally 10 to 34 mm) resulting in extrinsic compression of the duodenum. Treatment can either be conservative, including nasogastric decompression and nutritional supplementation, or surgical such as duodenojejunostomy.

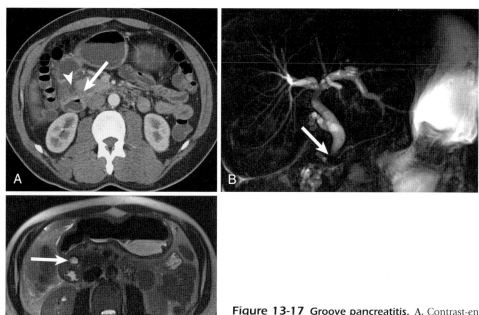

Figure 13-17 Groove pancreatitis. A, Contrast-enhanced computed tomography shows thickening within the pancreaticoduodenal groove *(arrow)* with focal low attenuation in the duodenal wall *(arrowhead)*. **B,** Magnetic resonance cholangiopancreatography (MRCP) shows a distal common bile duct stricture *(arrow),* and confirms cystic degeneration of the duodenal wall. **C,** Focally increased signal on axial T2-weighted imaging *(arrow)*.

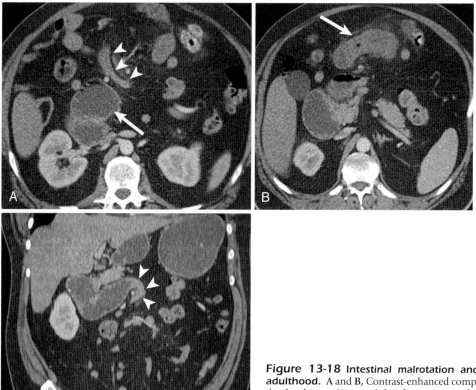

Figure 13-18 Intestinal malrotation and midgut volvulus presenting in adulthood. A and **B,** Contrast-enhanced computed tomography shows distention of the duodenum *(A, arrow)* that does not cross the spine *(arrow)*. **C,** Note the focal twist of the bowel *(A* and **C,** *arrowheads)* leading to a thickened loop of proximal jejunum *(B, arrow)* consistent with ischemia.

Gallstones

Gastric outlet obstruction due to gallstones, termed *Bouveret syndrome,* is a rare subset of gallstone ileus that presents classically with a triad of pneumobilia, an ectopic gallstone, and bowel obstruction (Fig. 13-19). Although the majority, approximately 85% of patients with cholecystenteric fistulas, have stones pass spontaneously, 15% of these patients will have a resulting bowel obstruction, most commonly in the terminal ileum and least commonly in the stomach and duodenum. Bouveret syndrome has a high mortality rate and is typically treated surgically.

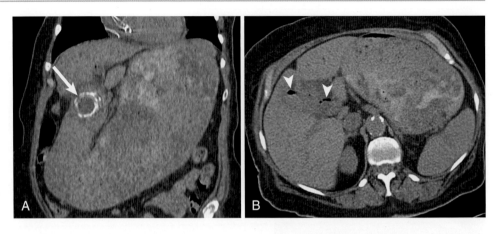

Figure 13-19 Bouveret syndrome. A, Contrast-enhanced computed tomography shows gastric outlet obstruction by a large, lamellated calcified structure *(arrow).* **B,** This appearance coupled with pneumobilia *(arrowheads)* is consistent with gastric outlet obstruction due to gallstones, also known as *Bouveret syndrome.*

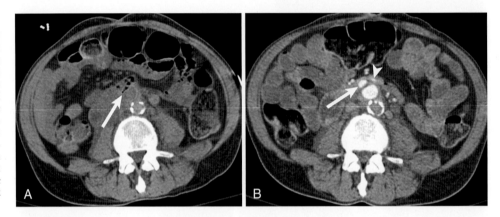

Figure 13-20 Aortoduodenal fistula A, Noncontrast computed tomography (CT) shows changes from open repair of an abdominal aortic aneurysm (AAA). There is ectopic gas in the graft *(arrow)* and loss of the fat plane between the graft and the duodenum. **B,** Arterial phase contrast-enhanced (CE) CT shows pseudoaneurysm formation *(arrow)* with extravasation of contrast into the duodenum *(arrowhead).* These findings are consistent with aortic bypass graft erosion into the duodenum.

Malignancy See Gastric Obstruction, Malignancy

Duodenal Perforation

Peptic ulcer disease, trauma, and iatrogenic causes lead the list of potential causes of duodenal perforation. The imaging appearance depends on the segment of duodenum affected: bulb perforations present with free intraperitoneal gas and/or fluid, whereas the remaining segments perforate into the retroperitoneum. As such, one important space to examine for extraluminal fluid and gas is the right anterior pararenal space, which immediately abuts the descending and proximal transverse duodenum. Although in some cases a focal wall discontinuity or extraluminal gas may be found, many times a duodenal perforation may simply present with an intramural hematoma and/or adjacent fluid. In such cases of equivocal findings for duodenal perforation, oral contrast, either for fluoroscopy or repeat CT, may be a useful adjunct because a delay in diagnosis may portend a poor outcome.

Aortoduodenal Fistulas

Chronic perforation of the duodenum, similar to that of the esophagus, may result in fistulization to nearby structures, including small and large bowel, bile ducts, kidneys and ureters, inferior vena cava (IVC), and aorta. These fistulas can result from primary duodenal perforation, such as from malignancy, ulcer disease, or trauma, or from an extrinsic source, as is often the case with aortoduodenal fistulas. The duodenum is the most common site for aortoenteric fistulas, owing to the proximity of these two structures in the retroperitoneum. This condition most frequently occurs in the setting of an abdominal aortic aneurysm (AAA), either arising as a primary event or a complication of surgical repair. Uncommonly, fistulas between the aorta and duodenum may result from vasculitis or radiation. Clinically patients may present with abdominal pain, GI bleeding, and a pulsatile mass. Similar to those with aortoesophageal fistulas, affected patients may have a "herald bleed" preceding life-threatening voluminous hemorrhage. Although diagnostic imaging options for aortoenteric fistulas include barium studies, aortography, and tagged red blood cell (RBC) scintigraphy, these options have limitations compared to CT. Computed tomography findings of aortoduodenal fistulas include focal tethering of the duodenum to the aortic wall with associated duodenal wall thickening, ectopic perigraft gas and fluid remote from the perioperative period, pseudoaneurysm formation, and possibly active contrast extravasation into the bowel lumen (Fig. 13-20).

Small Bowel Obstruction and Inflammation

Daniel Souza and Aaron Sodickson

Small bowel obstruction (SBO) and inflammation are common conditions, often presenting with non-specific signs and symptoms, similar to those seen in other acute abdominal disorders. Because an accurate clinical diagnosis remains challenging, imaging plays a central role in providing comprehensive information about bowel anatomy, the presence (and site) of the abnormality, distribution, severity, associated complications, and probable cause. The goal of this section is to provide an overview of the normal bowel anatomy, discuss the diagnostic approach, and describe common examples of SBO and inflammation. Acute disorders of vascular origin, such as acute hemorrhage, ischemia/infarction, and vasculitis are discussed in the nontraumatic vascular emergencies section.

■ ANATOMY OF THE SMALL BOWEL AND MESENTERY

The small bowel has always been a challenging organ for clinical and radiologic evaluation. It is a long and tortuous tube that extends for approximately 3 to 5 m from the pylorus to the ileocecal valve. The duodenum is the shortest segment, with retroperitoneal location and lacking a mesentery. It is a C-shaped structure that extends to the ligament of Treitz. The jejunum and ileum are mobile and intraperitoneal organs, attached to the posterior abdominal wall by the mesentery, which contains fat and provides the vasculature and lymphatics to the small bowel. The ileum has an abundance of lymphoid follicles, which are nearly absent in the jejunum. The layers of the visceral peritoneum encase the small bowel and associated mesentery. The visceral and parietal peritoneum enclose the large potential space referred to as the *peritoneal cavity*. The SMA supplies the jejunum and ileum. The venous return parallels the arterial supply, with drainage occurring to the superior mesenteric vein and then to the portal vein.

■ NORMAL IMAGING APPEARANCE OF THE SMALL BOWEL AND MESENTERY

The small bowel has a central location in the abdomen. There is no exact point of transition between the jejunum and ileum, but differences in their usual location, caliber, fold pattern, and degree of vascularity allow distinction between the two. The small bowel extends in a roughly clockwise direction from the right upper quadrant to the left upper and lower quadrants, tapering progressively from proximal to distal. The jejunum is located more proximal (and superior), with larger caliber, thicker folds, and greater vascularity than the jejunum. When the proximal small bowel is distended by pathologic processes, the mucosal folds (or valvulae conniventes) become visible. There is an inverse relationship between the normal bowel wall thickness and the degree of bowel distention. However, a bowel wall thickness greater than 5 mm should always be considered pathologic. In rare cases of midgut malrotation the third part of the duodenum is not visualized across the midline from the right to the left, there is reversal of the normal positions of the SMA and superior mesenteric vein, and the small bowel is completely right sided with a left-sided colon.

The vascular supply of the small and large bowel is supplied by the celiac trunk, which provides the blood supply from the distal esophagus to the descending duodenum; the SMA, which supplies the distal duodenum, jejunum, ileum, and the large bowel to the splenic flexure; and the inferior mesenteric artery (IMA), which supplies the more distal colon. There are important collateral pathways providing connection between these arteries, including between the celiac trunk and the SMA via the gastroduodenal artery and between the SMA and IMA via the marginal artery of Drummond and the arcade of Riolan.

■ IMAGING MODALITIES FOR SMALL BOWEL

Plain Radiography

Despite overall low diagnostic accuracy and specificity, the kidney, ureter, and bladder (KUB) radiographic examination is still sometimes used as an initial imaging examination in patients with abdominal symptoms. It is widely available, inexpensive, and reasonably sensitive for the diagnosis of high-grade bowel obstruction and radiopaque foreign bodies. Typical radiographic views include supine and upright views of the abdomen and an upright chest radiograph. The supine abdominal view demonstrates the bowel pattern to better extent, whereas air-fluid levels within the bowel are evident on the upright view. The upright view of the chest is best for the detection of free air under the diaphragm (pneumoperitoneum), which is an ominous sign of bowel perforation.

Although a fair amount of gas is normally seen within the stomach and colon, the small bowel should contain little gas. When bowel motility is affected by mechanical obstruction or nonobstructive adynamic ileus, gas accumulates within the small bowel. Small bowel obstruction is suspected when multiple gas- or fluid-filled loops of dilated small bowel are present. The presence of an unusual quantity of colonic gas in this setting usually indicates nonobstructive ileus, partial SBO, or early complete SBO. Common predisposing factors for ileus include sepsis, electrolyte disturbances, GI infection, and recent surgery. Differentiation between partial and early SBO can be challenging in the absence of clinical information. Although subjective, features favoring high-grade obstruction include (1) the presence of multiple air-fluid levels, particularly when discrepant levels are seen within the same loop, (2) dilated loops averaging more than 2.5 cm in diameter and/or exceeding 50% of the caliber of

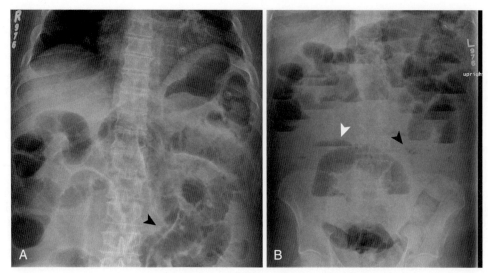

Figure 13-21 **A**, Supine abdominal radiograph demonstrates typical findings of complete small bowel obstruction (SBO). There is significant distention of a large number of loops of small bowel *(black arrowhead)*, with near complete absence of gas in the distal bowel, indicative of mechanical bowel obstruction with a probable distal transition point. **B**, The upright radiograph reveals numerous gas-fluid levels, some of which are broad-based, giving rise to the "tortoise-shell" sign *(white arrowhead)*, and the characteristic "string-of-pearls" sign *(black arrowhead)*, caused by bubbles of residual air at the top of fluid nearly completely filling adjacent distended bowel loops.

the largest visible colonic loop, and (3) a large number of distended loops of bowel. Although patients with SBO can present with normal KUB findings, a confident diagnosis can be made in 50% to 60% of cases when dilated gas or fluid-filled loops of small bowel are present in the setting of a gasless colon (Fig. 13-21).

Ultrasonography

The potential advantages of ultrasonography (US) include widespread availability, fast, dynamic real-time acquisition, low cost, and lack of ionizing radiation. Although US is often used in the diagnosis of intussusception in children, its role in the assessment of the small bowel in the adult population is very limited, particularly in the United States. Disadvantages include operator variability and incomplete evaluation of the small bowel due to intervening gas and obese habitus. However, it may be indicated in selected cases, such as in the follow-up of patients with inflammatory bowel disease (IBD) or critically ill patients.

Barium Contrast Studies

Although small bowel follow-through studies can provide spatial resolution in the evaluation of the mucosa that is superior to that of cross-sectional studies, and these studies have been performed in the past to triage patients with suspected SBO into surgical versus nonsurgical management, the widespread use of abdominal CT has largely replaced this practice. Rapid transit of contrast material within normal-caliber small bowel loops excludes SBO. However, in cases of SBO, the duration of the small bowel follow-through examination is lengthy, and retained fluid dilutes the barium, often limiting assessment of the point of obstruction, with delayed films needed if one wishes to identify the transition point or determine whether contrast passes distally.

Computed Tomography and Computed Tomography Enterography

The role of CT in the diagnosis of SBO cannot be overemphasized. It is fast and widely available, and it allows for the concurrent assessment of the mesentery, mesenteric vessels, and peritoneal cavity. In the setting of SBO, it can be performed without oral contrast administration, because the retained intraluminal fluid serves as a natural negative contrast agent (and delays transit of any ingested contrast). In the assessment of small bowel disease, CT enterography, with negative or neutral oral contrast material, can be used to achieve bowel distention and to improve evaluation of bowel wall morphologic characteristics, thickness, and enhancement. Multiplanar reformations (MPRs) and postprocessing techniques aid in a confident diagnosis and can be helpful to depicting findings. Coronal reformatted images are most intuitive because they are analogous to a frontal radiograph and the course of the bowel loops can be most readily followed in this plane. Maximum intensity projection images and other postprocessing techniques, such as volume-rendering techniques, can improve depiction of the vasculature and bowel anatomy and improve the communication of findings (Fig. 13-22).

Magnetic Resonance Imaging

Magnetic resonance imaging provides accurate anatomic and functional information about the small bowel without the use of ionizing radiation. A potential advantage over CT that has been proposed is the characterization of malignant versus benign strictures. In addition, because MR enterography can be used to monitor small-bowel filling in real time without radiation exposure, it is an alternative to CT enterography as a means of evaluating low-grade obstruction. It is an exceptional

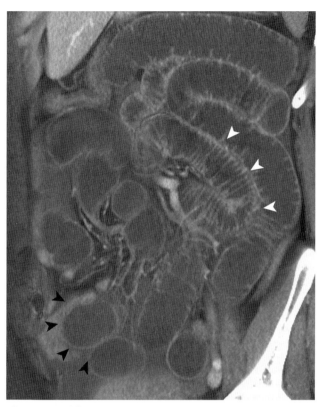

Figure 13-22 Coronal volume-rendered image obtained from computed tomography (CT) enterography in a patient with small bowel obstruction (SBO) depicts the small bowel anatomy and fold pattern. The patient was given neutral oral contrast to distend the bowel loops and to better depict the bowel wall and enhancement. Note the rich pattern of mucosal folds of the jejunum in the left upper quadrant *(white arrowheads)*, as opposed to the smoother appearance of the ileal loops in the right lower quadrant *(black arrowheads)*.

technique to evaluate patients with IBD because these patients are often young and require serial examinations due to acute exacerbations. Magnetic resonance imaging is more controversial in the setting of suspected SBO but may have a role in children and pregnant patients.

■ SMALL BOWEL OBSTRUCTION

Small bowel obstruction is common, accounting for 20% of surgical admissions and 4% of ED visits for abdominal pain. Although the diagnosis is often suspected based on clinical history, CT has become the primary modality in evaluation and management of patients with suspected bowel obstruction. Conservative management is preferred when possible, and surgery is performed much more selectively than in the past. As a result the radiologist plays a central role in answering specific questions to diagnose SBO and to guide conservative versus surgical management. These include (1) confirming (or excluding) SBO and elucidating alternative diagnoses in the absence of SBO; (2) assessing complexity/severity of the obstruction (simple versus closed-loop, complete versus partial, low-grade versus high-grade), and identifying the presence of complications (strangulation, perforation); (3) determining the presence and location of the transition point; and, whenever possible, (4) establishing the underlying cause (Box 13-1).

Box 13-1 Causes of Small Bowel Obstruction in Adults

Extrinsic Lesions
Adhesions
Hernias (external, internal)
Tumors (serosal disease)
Hematoma
Endometriosis

Intrinsic Lesions
Inflammatory diseases (Crohn, tuberculosis)
Neoplastic diseases (adenocarcinoma, gastrointestinal stromal tumor, lymphoma, metastatic disease)
Vascular lesions (radiation, ischemia)
Hematoma (anticoagulants, blood dyscrasia, trauma)
Intussusception

Intraluminal
Gallstones
Bezoars
Foreign bodies

Confirming the Presence and Severity of Obstruction

Typical findings of SBO include continuous loops of dilated (>2.5 cm) proximal small bowel, associated with normal caliber or collapsed bowel distal to a transition point. When oral contrast medium is used, the absence of contrast in distal loops of bowel is indicative of complete obstruction provided that enough time has been allowed for delayed passage. In selected cases, delayed scans can be performed to confirm complete obstruction, although this is rarely performed because the patient's clinical progression is the primary determinant of management approach in the absence of clear signs of high-grade or closed-loop obstruction.

Multiple conditions can result in small bowel dilatation (or abdominal distention) and be confused with SBO, particularly before clinical and radiologic information are integrated. Adynamic ileus is associated with bowel distention that may include the colon, in addition to the small bowel and stomach. Shock bowel can present with dilated loops of small bowel, but history, involvement of the colon, and other imaging findings such as a flattened IVC, and hyperenhancement of the adrenal glands, should help differentiate it from SBO. Bowel ischemia can likewise cause significant distention of atonic small bowel loops and simulate the appearance of obstruction, but ancillary findings of bowel thickening, segmental bowel perfusion abnormalities, and evidence of arterial atherosclerotic disease help suggest an ischemic cause for the dilatation.

Differentiation between partial low-grade or high-grade obstruction is subjective. High-grade obstruction should be suggested when there is a substantive caliber difference between proximal and distal loops of bowel (and absent passage of contrast material through the transition point if delayed imaging is performed). The diagnosis of partial low-grade obstruction is more challenging and considered a relative "blind spot" for CT because the degree of caliber change is generally less striking.

The use of oral contrast for the diagnosis of SBO is controversial. Potential advantages include the indirect assessment of bowel transit time, which may aid in the diagnosis of partial low-grade obstruction, and

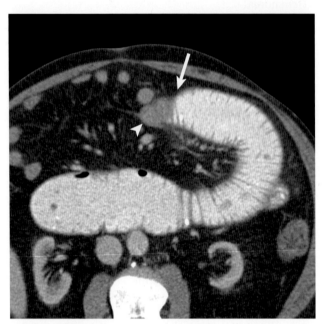

Figure 13-23 Axial computed tomography (CT) obtained after oral and intravenous contrast administration in a patient with history of treated lymphoma and suspected small bowel obstruction (SBO) shows evidence of complete bowel obstruction at the proximal jejunum, with absence of oral contrast beyond the transition point *(white arrow)*. Surgery confirmed the presence of small bowel obstruction at this level, caused by posttreatment fibrosis. There was no evidence of active lymphoma at pathologic examination.

the progressive dilution of contrast as the contrast column approaches the transition point, which may help to determine its location (Fig. 13-23). Delayed images can provide confirmation of a complete obstruction in the appropriate setting. However, oral contrast delays the diagnosis in the emergency setting and is generally not tolerated by obstructed patients presenting with nausea and vomiting. In addition, the fluid within the distended loops of bowel acts like a natural neutral oral contrast, as long as nasogastric tube decompression is not performed before imaging (Fig. 13-24).

Another helpful imaging feature in SBO is the "small bowel feces sign," or the presence of mottled, particulate matter and gas within the lumen that simulates the appearance of feces. It is often associated with high-grade obstruction but has been described in nonobstructed patients. When present, it is generally located immediately proximal to the transition point and is thus extremely helpful to locating the site of obstruction, which is the next step in the evaluation of SBO (Fig. 13-25).

Determining the Location and Cause

A transition zone or point is the region at which the bowel caliber changes and greatly increases confidence that a true mechanical obstruction is present by identifying the site of the obstruction. In the absence of a focal transition point, dilated loops are nonspecific and may be due to other conditions such as IBD, scleroderma, or ischemia. It is often easiest to identify a transition point by careful inspection of the course of the bowel loops, usually by an antegrade approach starting in the distended proximal loops. Distally located SBO can, however, be most readily evaluated by a retrograde approach starting at the decompressed

Figure 13-24 A, Coronal computed tomography (CT) image performed after intravenous and oral contrast administration demonstrates opacified stomach and jejunum in the left upper quadrant, as well as unopacified collapsed and distended loops of more distal small bowel, likely ileum *(white arrowheads)*. Limited bowel opacification by oral contrast due to delayed transit is typical in the setting of small bowel obstruction (SBO), particularly in cases of more distal obstruction. **B,** Sagittal CT image demonstrates significant focal narrowing at the transition point *(white arrowhead)*, without an extrinsic lesion. Despite suboptimal bowel opacification at this level, the diagnosis of the adhesive SBO could be made with confidence. The use of oral contrast in the setting of SBO is controversial.

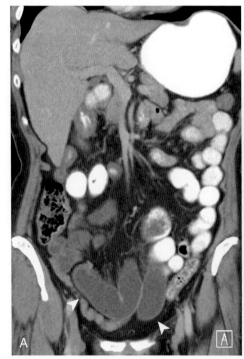

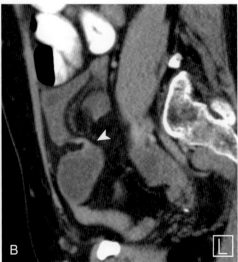

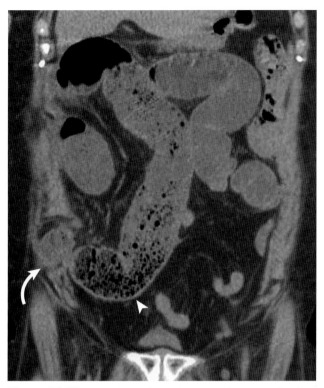

Figure 13-25 Coronal unenhanced computed tomographic (CT) image demonstrates mottled material within the obstructed loop of proximal small bowel ("small bowel feces" sign), adjacent to the transition point *(white arrowhead)*. There are decompressed loops of small bowel in the left lower quadrant. Although not pathognomonic for long-standing obstruction, it can help localize the transition point. There is a short C-shaped segment of small bowel within a spigelian hernia at the transition point *(curved white arrow)* consistent with a closed-loop obstruction. The presence of closed-loop obstruction predisposes to ischemia, and it is most often treated with surgery, because it will usually not resolve with conservative management such as nasogastric decompression.

terminal ileum. Careful and systematic travel through the bowel loops in multiple planes is the key to success. When the transition point is identified, a search for intraluminal, intrinsic, or extrinsic causes of obstruction should be performed. Intraluminal causes include foreign bodies, gallstones, and bezoar. Intrinsic bowel lesions typically manifest as mural or focal thickening. Extrinsic causes of obstruction, such as hernias and CD, are associated with other extraintestinal findings. It should be noted that adhesions, the most common cause of SBO in the United States, are typically not visible on CT and can be suggested in regions of an abrupt transition point when no clear cause is seen.

Determining the Presence of Closed-Loop Obstruction and Complications

In simple obstruction the bowel is occluded at one or more points along its course. The diagnosis of closed-loop obstruction is crucial because it carries a higher risk for strangulation and bowel infarction. Most often, an adhesion or hernia will cause partial or complete occlusion of a segment of bowel loop at two adjacent points. Computed tomography findings depend on the length, degree of distention, and orientation of the closed loop but include a characteristic fixed radial distribution of several dilated, usually fluid-filled bowel loops with stretched and prominent mesenteric vessels converging toward a point of torsion. The configuration is usually U shaped or C shaped. A narrow pedicle can be formed leading to torsion of the loops and producing a small bowel volvulus. A "beak" sign is seen at the site of the torsion as a fusiform tapering. Occasionally a "whirl" sign of the mesenteric vessels can be seen, reflecting the rotation of the bowel loops around the fixed point of obstruction. Strangulation is defined as closed-loop obstruction associated with intestinal ischemia, and

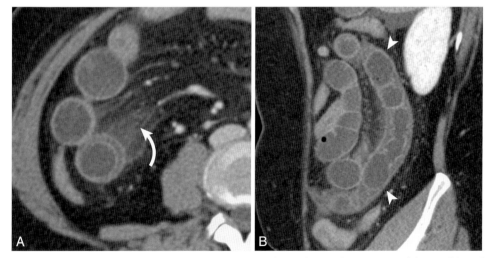

Figure 13-26 A, Axial contrast-enhanced computed tomographic image shows abnormal appearance of the small bowel in the right lower quadrant, associated with concentric mural thickening, submucosal edema, mucosal hyperenhancement, and mesenteric fat stranding *(curved white arrow)*. B, Sagittal CT image demonstrates a long segment of abnormal small bowel with C-shaped configuration *(white arrowheads)*, extensive fat stranding and mesenteric vascular engorgement. Given clinical deterioration and worrisome imaging findings, surgery was undertaken. The patient was found to have closed-loop obstruction of a long segment of ileum caused by adhesions.

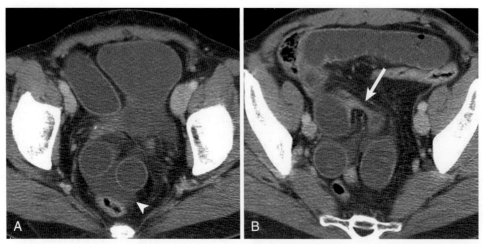

Figure 13-27 **A** and **B**, Axial computed tomographic (CT) images obtained after intravenous contrast administration, without oral contrast administration, shows multiple dilated loops of small bowel and significant narrowing at the level of the transition zone (**B**, *white arrow*) consistent with adhesion. There is free fluid in the cul-de-sac (**A**, *white arrowhead*), not an uncommon finding in the presence of uncomplicated small bowel obstruction (SBO), but it should prompt a search for findings of ischemia. Surgery confirmed the presence of SBO secondary to adhesions.

its occurrence depends on the time and degree of rotation of the incarcerated loops. The findings that indicate strangulation include bowel wall thickening and hyperattenuation, a halo or target sign, mesenteric fat stranding and/or fluid, pneumatosis intestinalis, and mesenteric or portal venous gas, but these findings are not entirely specific. More specific findings include absent, asymmetric, or delayed bowel wall enhancement, with or without focal mesenteric fluid or hemorrhage (Fig. 13-26).

■ CAUSES OF SMALL BOWEL OBSTRUCTION

Adhesions

Adhesions are the most common cause of SBO in the United States, ranging from 50% to 80% of cases. The diagnosis should not be excluded even in the absence of prior surgery because adhesions can occur as a result of prior peritonitis. Adhesions are typically not seen, and the diagnosis is one of exclusion. Computed tomography findings include an abrupt change in the caliber of the bowel, with focal kinking and tethering, in the absence of an underlying mass lesion, and significant inflammation or bowel wall thickening at the transition point (Fig. 13-27).

Hernias

Hernias are the most common cause of SBO in developing countries. An external hernia occurs as a result of a defect in the abdominal wall at sites of congenital weakness or previous surgery. Although the diagnosis can be obvious at clinical examination, it may be challenging in very obese patients (Fig. 13-28).

The less common internal hernia occurs when there is protrusion of the viscera through a defect in the peritoneum or mesentery into another compartment within the abdominal cavity. Closed-loop obstruction can result (Fig. 13-29). Early diagnosis in this scenario

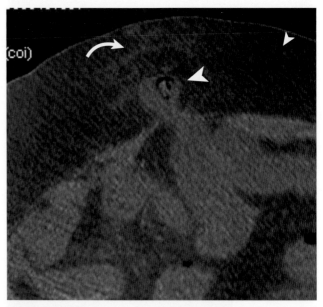

Figure 13-28 Unenhanced axial computed tomographic (CT) image obtained in an obese patient with abdominal pain and an unremarkable physical examination demonstrates a right paramedian ventral hernia containing a short segment of small bowel *(white arrowhead)*, associated with adjacent fat stranding *(curved white arrow)*. The findings are consistent with an incarcerated ventral hernia. The clinical diagnosis of external hernias, usually described as straightforward, can be challenging in the obese population. CT plays a major role in this setting.

becomes critical because these patients will often not benefit from conservative management because the involved segment will not be decompressed with nasogastric drainage, and bowel ischemia and necrosis can rapidly develop (Fig. 13-30).

Endometriosis

Endometriosis is common and underdiagnosed. It is estimated to affect approximately 5% of women of

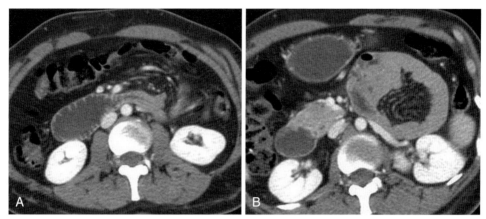

Figure 13-29 **A** and **B**, Axial contrast-enhanced computed tomographic images at the level of the kidneys demonstrate herniated loops of small bowel anterior to the aorta and left renal vein. There is twisting of the mesenteric vessels more inferiorly ("whirl" sign) with herniation of the bowel through a defect in the mesentery (internal hernia). Internal hernias can be congenital, as in this case (paraduodenal is the most common), or postoperative. They have similar imaging appearance and risk for ischemia as a closed-loop obstruction.

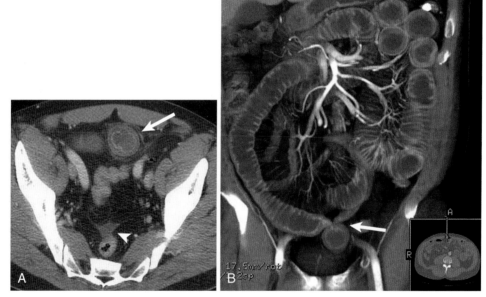

Figure 13-30 **A**, Axial postcontrast computed tomographic (CT) image obtained in a patient with suspected small bowel obstruction (SBO) shows a short segment of abnormal bowel above the bladder, with significant wall thickening, submucosal edema, and adjacent mesenteric fat stranding *(white arrow)*. There is a small amount of free fluid in the cul-de-sac *(white arrowhead)*. **B**, Coronal volume-rendered image shows the mesenteric vasculature, as well as multiple distended loops of proximal small bowel, with collapsed distal ileum and normal appearance of the colon. A transition zone is located in the pelvis *(white arrow)*, confirming the diagnosis of mechanical bowel obstruction. A short but viable segment of hyperemic small bowel was found at surgery. Early diagnosis and improved communication of the findings allowed for prompt surgical management in this patient.

reproductive age. Endometrial implants may manifest as contiguous or penetrating soft tissue nodules along the antimesenteric border of the bowel wall.

Malignancy

Metastatic involvement is far more common than primary disease. It can result in SBO by different mechanisms (intrinsic and extrinsic). It can be secondary to intraperitoneal seeding, hematogenous spread, or direct extension from an adjacent visceral malignancy. Although SBO can result from intrinsic obstruction from submucosal implants, such as from malignant melanoma and breast cancer, it most often occurs in the setting of peritoneal carcinomatosis, when extensive serosal disease will determine extrinsic compression and/or circumferential involvement at the transition point (Fig. 13-31).

Primary small bowel neoplasms are rare. Advanced cases of adenocarcinoma can present with SBO, with pronounced asymmetric and irregular mural

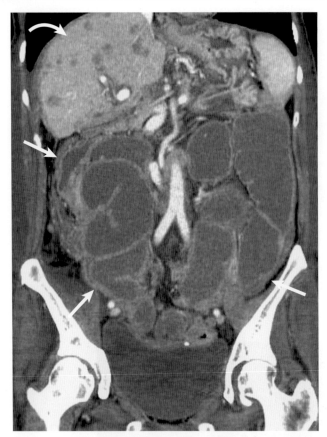

Figure 13-31 Coronal contrast-enhanced computed tomographic images performed in a middle-age woman with diagnosis of ovarian cancer show multiple liver metastases *(curved white arrow)*, a small amount of ascites, and extensive subcutaneous fat stranding consistent with widespread metastatic disease. Note the presence of multiple distended loops of small bowel, demonstrating wall thickening, but without a definite transition point *(white arrows)*. Findings are suspicious for partial small bowel obstruction (SBO) in the setting of advanced serosal disease, likely secondary to extrinsic compression.

thickening noted at the transition point (Fig. 13-32). Conversely, primary lymphoma of the small bowel, even when extensive or annular, is a soft tumor and does not generally cause obstruction unless it is associated with adhesions or posttreatment change (Fig. 13-33). Small bowel carcinoid is a relatively rare cause of SBO because the primary lesion is often occult, and it usually will manifest as spiculated mesenteric masses with calcification resulting from a desmoplastic reaction (Fig. 13-34).

Intussusception

Intussusception is a benign and common condition in children younger than 3 years old, but a rare cause of bowel obstruction in adults. When found in older children and adults, it should trigger a search for a lead point, such as an underlying neoplasm, inciting adhesion or foreign body. Computed tomography findings include the pathognomonic bowel-within-bowel configuration, with or without mesenteric fat and mesenteric vessels. The finding of a leading mass should be interpreted with caution because the intussusception itself can present as a pseudotumor (Fig. 13-35).

Functional disturbances that affect bowel motility, such as scleroderma, celiac disease, and cystic fibrosis, can cause transient intussusception. Clinical history can be helpful in these patients, and careful evaluation of the intussusception will confirm the absence of a neoplastic lead point. When multiphasic CT is performed, resolution of the intussusception can be often observed, confirming the transient nature of this phenomenon (Fig. 13-36).

Inflammation and Fibrosis

Acute and chronic inflammation, such as CD and radiation enteritis, can lead to fibrosis, strictures, and, in

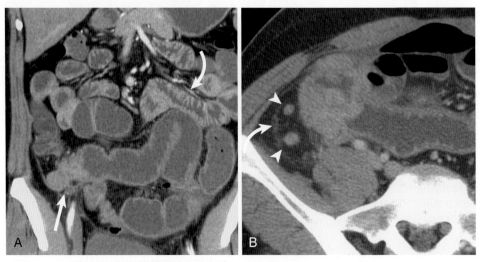

Figure 13-32 A, Coronal contrast-enhanced computed tomographic image shows an obstructing soft tissue mass at the level of the ascending colon *(white arrow)* invading the distal ileum. There are distended loops of ileum proximal to the obstruction. Note the normal prominent folds in the proximal jejunum *(curved white arrow)*. **B,** Axial CECT image shows multiple enlarged lymph nodes adjacent to the colonic mass *(white arrowheads)* associated with thickening of the peritoneal fascia *(curved white arrow)* and suspicion for regional metastases.

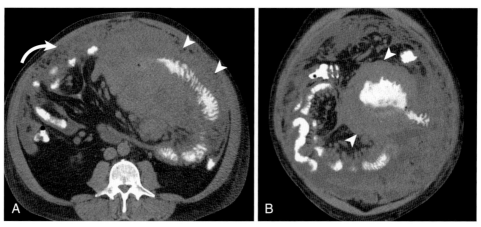

Figure 13-33 Axial (**A**) and coronal (**B**) computed tomographic (CT) images performed without intravenous contrast administration and after oral contrast administration in a patient with lymphoma demonstrates aneurysmal dilatation and significant bowel wall thickening involving the proximal jejunum *(white arrowheads)* surrounding the opacified lumen, without evidence of obstruction. There are multiple scattered regional lymph nodes, trace free fluid, and diffuse mesenteric and omental fat stranding *(curved white arrow)*, suspicious for peritoneal lymphomatosis. Even in cases of advanced disease, lymphoma is usually not associated with small bowel obstruction (SBO), unless due to development of fibrosis after treatment.

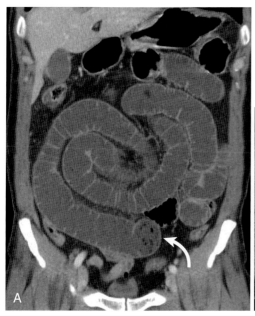

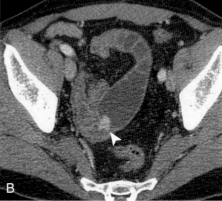

Figure 13-34 A, Coronal computed tomographic (CT) image shows significant fluid distention of multiple loops of small bowel, with collapsed loops of distal ileum and colon, consistent with high-grade bowel obstruction. Note the presence of the "small bowel feces" sign *(curved white arrow)*, suggesting that the transition point is likely located in the pelvis. **B,** Axial CT image shows an obstructing hypervascular submucosal mass at the transition point *(white arrowhead)*. The patient was found to have ileal carcinoid at surgery.

more severe cases, obstruction. Small bowel obstruction can occur during the acute phase of CD when the intense acute transmural inflammation causes narrowing of the bowel lumen, during the chronic phase due to fibrotic stenosis, postoperative adhesions, incisional hernias, and exacerbation of the inflammatory condition (acute flare). Small bowel obstruction occurs in the late phase of radiation enteritis, most often in the distal small bowel as a result of adhesive and fibrotic changes that develop several months after therapy. Radiation serositis can lead to narrowing of the lumen and abnormal peristalsis. Computed tomography findings include adhesions, narrowing of the lumen secondary to mural thickening, mesenteric retraction, and abnormal bowel enhancement within the radiation field.

Hematoma and Vascular Causes

Hematoma can mimic neoplasm and result in significant luminal narrowing. It is usually associated with anticoagulant therapy, iatrogenic intervention, or trauma. In the setting of severe stenosis or occlusion of the mesenteric arterial or venous supply, bowel ischemia can lead to significant bowel wall thickening, resulting in SBO. Although relatively benign, in advanced cases, pneumatosis and portomesenteric venous gas can signal the presence of infarction.

Gallstone Ileus

Gallstone ileus is a rare complication of chronic cholecystitis. It is the result of migration of a gallstone into the small bowel with subsequent impaction, most often at the ileocecal valve. The imaging features of the "Rigler triad" include SBO, an ectopic gallstone, and pneumobilia because a cholecystenteric fistula is needed for the migration of a large obstructing gallstone to occur (Fig. 13-37). In the event of proximal obstruction, at the level of the stomach or duodenum, gastric outlet obstruction may result (Bouveret syndrome).

Bezoar

Bezoar was considered a rare cause of SBO, but the number of reported cases is increasing in recent years as a result of gastric outlet surgery, because it prevents adequate digestion of vegetable fibers, which may become impacted. Computed tomography findings include an elongated and intraluminal mass demonstrating a mottled appearance at the transition point (Fig. 13-38).

Foreign Bodies

A wide range of foreign bodies can cause SBO with variable imaging appearances. Clinical history is very important in helping to establish preoperative diagnosis (Fig. 13-39). In children and, emotionally disturbed, or mentally disabled patients, foreign bodies should be suspected.

Iatrogenic SBO can occur as a result of endoscopic capsule retention because they have been used more often in the evaluation of the small bowel, particularly in patients with CD. Diagnosis is made by identifying an ovoid metallic object impacted at the transition point.

■ SMALL BOWEL INFLAMMATION

Infectious Enteritis

Infectious enterocolitis can cause mild symptoms resembling common viral gastroenteritis, but it can present with clinical findings that are indistinguishable from appendicitis and other surgical conditions. Although imaging findings are often nonspecific, including mural thickening, mesenteric fat stranding, and moderate mesenteric lymphadenopathy, the clinical history and distribution can be helpful in narrowing the differential diagnosis. *Giardia lamblia* is a protozoan known to cause severe diarrhea and malabsorption. The organism tends to inhabit the duodenum and jejunum. Imaging findings consist

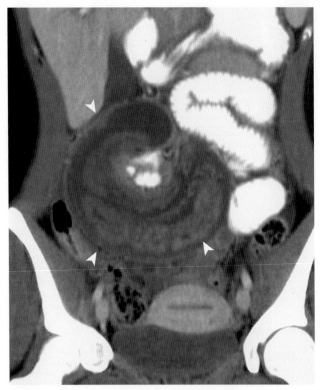

Figure 13-35 Coronal contrast-enhanced computed tomographic image obtained in a young woman with recurrent abdominal pain and gastrointestinal (GI) bleeding shows a long segment of jejuno-jejunal intussusception *(white arrowheads)*, with distended opacified proximal small bowel and collapsed loops of distal colon. There is no oral contrast distal to the intussusception consistent with complete small bowel obstruction (SBO). The presence of intussusception in an adult or older child should elicit the search for a lead point, although it is less common than intussusception without a lead point. Identification of an obstructing mass that is separate and distinct from bowel loops can be challenging, such as in this case, because the invaginated bowel can be edematous and simulate a mass.

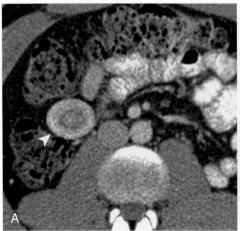
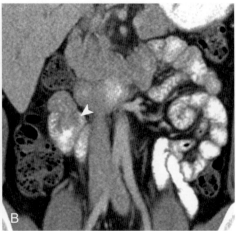

Figure 13-36 Axial (**A**) and coronal (**B**) contrast-enhanced computed tomographic images obtained for the workup of hematuria demonstrate incidental bowel-in-bowel appearance of a short segment of proximal jejunum without associated findings to suggest small bowel obstruction (SBO), consistent with transient intussusception (**A** and **B**, *arrowheads*).

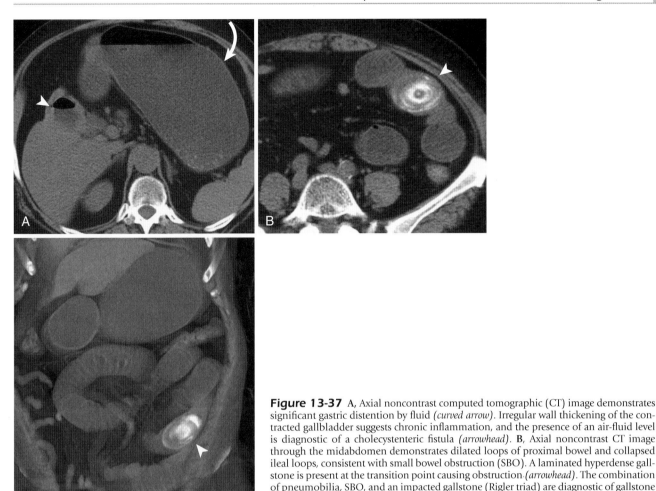

Figure 13-37 **A**, Axial noncontrast computed tomographic (CT) image demonstrates significant gastric distention by fluid *(curved arrow)*. Irregular wall thickening of the contracted gallbladder suggests chronic inflammation, and the presence of an air-fluid level is diagnostic of a cholecystenteric fistula *(arrowhead)*. **B**, Axial noncontrast CT image through the midabdomen demonstrates dilated loops of proximal bowel and collapsed ileal loops, consistent with small bowel obstruction (SBO). A laminated hyperdense gallstone is present at the transition point causing obstruction *(arrowhead)*. The combination of pneumobilia, SBO, and an impacted gallstone (Rigler triad) are diagnostic of gallstone ileus. **C**, Coronal volume-rendered image better demonstrates the findings of SBO and the impacted jejunal gallstone *(arrowhead)*.

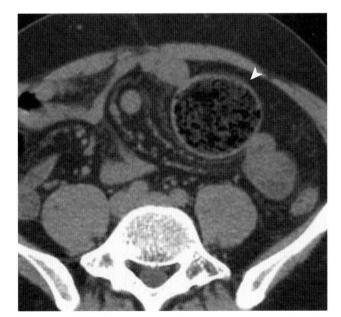

Figure 13-38 Unenhanced axial computed tomographic (CT) image obtained at the level of the pelvis in a patient with typical features of small bowel obstruction (SBO) show an intraluminal mottled-appearing density causing significant distention of the bowel lumen at the transition point, consistent with an obstructing bezoar *(arrowhead)*.

of mural thickening involving the proximal small bowel, increased luminal secretions, and disordered motility.

Immunocompromised patients can be affected with systemic infection with *Mycobacterium avium-intracellulare*. It affects multiple organs and has been called *pseudo-Whipple disease* because of clinical, histologic, and radiologic similarities. Computed tomography findings include thickened small bowel more pronounced in the jejunum, hepatomegaly, and splenomegaly. Focal, low-density lesions can be present in the spleen. Cytomegalovirus can be reactivated in the setting of immunosuppression and can result in hemorrhagic enteritis. Definitive diagnosis may require biopsy with immunohistochemical stains. *Cryptosporidium* is a GI parasite that results in watery diarrhea in patients with acquired immunodeficiency syndrome (AIDS). Clinical history is important in establishing the diagnosis. Computed tomography findings demonstrate wall thickening more often involving the proximal small bowel and stomach, similar to that of giardiasis. Other common pathogens that often affect the small bowel, typically the distal ileum and cecum, include *Yersinia*, *Campylobacter*, and *Salmonella* species (Fig. 13-40).

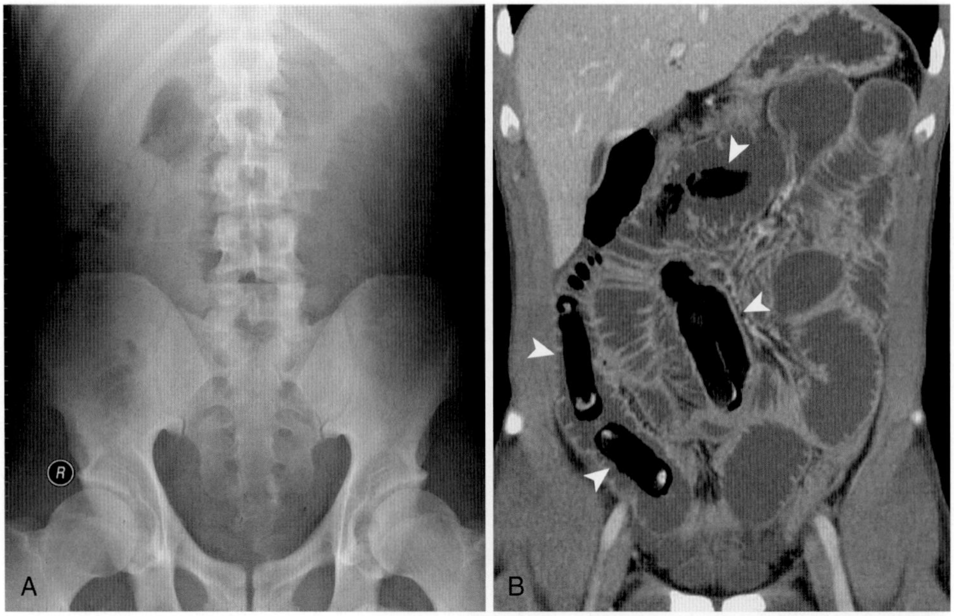

Figure 13-39 **A**, Supine abdominal radiograph performed in a suspected drug smuggler shows gaseous distention of small bowel loops, with a "stack of coins" appearance, with no gas within the transverse or descending colon or rectum, suspicious for high-grade small bowel obstruction (SBO). **B**, Coronal computed tomographic (CT) image demonstrates multiple intraluminal filling defects (*arrowheads*) throughout the entire length of the bowel, later confirmed as cocaine capsules. The patient was arrested.

Crohn Disease

Inflammatory bowel disease and infectious enteritis can have similar imaging findings, with distinction made based on the clinical history, as well as the distribution of findings within the bowel. Crohn disease is part of the IBD spectrum, characterized by chronic, relapsing inflammation of unknown cause. Despite abundant research in this field, it remains a diagnostic and therapeutic challenge. Crohn disease can affect any part of the GI tract but predominantly affects the small bowel (up to 80% of cases) and right colon. As opposed to ulcerative colitis (UC), rectal involvement is very rare in CD.

Crohn disease is characterized by the presence of granulomatous inflammation at histologic evaluation, with chronic erosions, ulceration, and transmural bowel inflammation, which predisposes to complications such as fistulas and abscess formation. The presence of "skip lesions" is one of the hallmarks of the disease. Crohn disease has a tendency toward remission and relapse, and acute and chronic changes often coexist within the same affected bowel segment. Fatty infiltration of the bowel wall may occur in chronic IBD and was thought to be pathognomonic of this disease. However, it has been demonstrated in healthy individuals, particularly in association with obesity.

Endoscopy and classic barium studies are critical in the initial diagnosis and staging of IBD in general because they are superior to cross-sectional imaging in the evaluation of the mucosa, particularly in early-stage disease. However, CT and MRI can depict several abnormalities that are associated with acute bowel inflammation, such as mural thickening and stratification, thickened folds and/or reduction or distortion of folds due to ulceration and cobblestoning. Additional findings include pseudosacculations or pseudodiverticulum formation, which occur as a consequence of relative sparing of the antimesenteric border within an affected segment. The

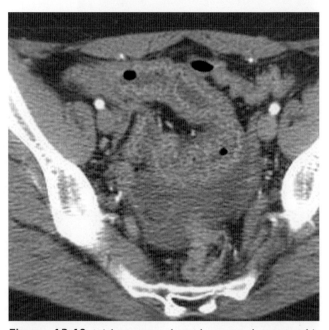

Figure 13-40 Axial contrast-enhanced computed tomographic image performed in a patient with 3-day history of low-grade fever, abdominal pain, and diarrhea demonstrates diffuse mural thickening of a long segment of distal ileum associated with mucosal hyperenhancement and submucosal edema, as well as a moderate amount of free fluid. Although the imaging findings are nonspecific, the self-limited nature of the infectious process can help make the distinction from other causes of bowel wall thickening. Common infectious agents that affect the distal small bowel include *Yersinia enterocolitica*, *Campylobacter jejuni*, and *Salmonella enteritidis*.

major advantage over endoscopy and classic barium studies is the assessment of extraenteric findings, which are relatively common in CD. In addition, cross-sectional imaging is reserved for the follow-up evaluation of established disease, assessment of treatment response, diagnosis of relapse, detection of complications, and assessment before surgical

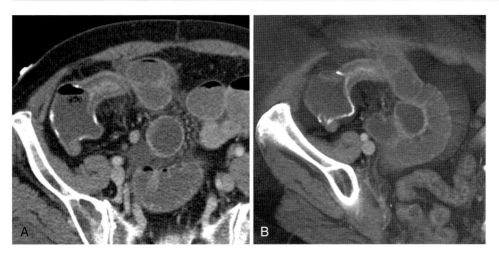

Figure 13-41 **A** and **B**, Axial volume-rendered image obtained in a patient with Crohn disease (CD) following ileocolectomy shows a short segment of wall thickening associated with mucosal hyperenhancement and submucosal edema adjacent to the surgical staple line. These findings are consistent with acute flare in the region of the ileocolic anastomosis. Recurrence is very common in these patients, and surgery is avoided whenever possible.

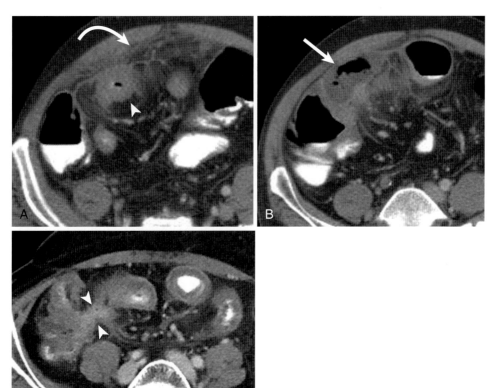

Figure 13-42 Spectrum of acute complications in Crohn disease (CD). **A** and **B**, Axial computed tomographic (CT) images obtained after oral and intravenous contrast administration demonstrate significant wall thickening of the distal ileum *(arrowhead)* associated with mucosal hyperenhancement and submucosal edema. There is extensive mesenteric fat stranding *(curved arrow)* and an encapsulated fluid collection containing debris and nondependent gas in the right lower quadrant *(straight white arrow)*, consistent with an abscess. **C**, Axial CT image obtained in another patient shows ill-defined soft tissue extending from the distal ileum to the colon with obliteration of the mesenteric fat, consistent with a fistula *(arrowheads)*. Given the transmural nature of the inflammatory process in Crohn disease, complications such as sinus tracts, fistulas, and abscesses are very common.

intervention. In the presence of abscesses, percutaneous drainage under CT guidance is favored over surgery.

Computed tomography findings of active inflammation in CD include significant mural enhancement and stratification due to submucosal edema (target or "double-halo" appearance), adjacent mesenteric fat stranding, and engorged vasa recta ("comb" sign). The presence of fibrofatty proliferation along the mesenteric border of the affected bowel is considered pathognomonic of this disease. Extraintestinal manifestations include mesenteric inflammatory changes and the presence of phlegmon, abscess, or lymphadenopathy. As described earlier, deformity of bowel loops, such

as pseudodiverticulum formation, is caused by asymmetric involvement by longitudinal ulcers and scars, both of which are well demonstrated on both axial and coronal images. Lymphadenopathy is not uncommon, and although controversial, it has been suggested that lymphadenopathy can allow differentiation between active inflammatory and chronic (fibrostenosing) disease. Nonetheless, lymph nodes larger than 10 mm in short axis should prompt evaluation for superimposed lymphoma or carcinoma (Figs. 13-41 and 13-42).

Magnetic resonance enterography is an attractive modality for the assessment of CD because it can offer dynamic evaluation of bowel motility, superior soft tissue contrast, and excellent depiction of fluid and edema, without associated ionizing radiation. Magnetic resonance enterography can be particularly useful in young patients that require serial examinations. Protocols are variable but generally include multiphasic coronal fluid-sensitive sequences. Optimal bowel distention is achieved by use of enteric contrast material, but the type of contrast material and method of administration are controversial. Most patients require a delay of at least 40 to 60 minutes from contrast material ingestion to imaging.

Magnetic resonance enterography can play an important role in the follow-up of patients with established IBD, or it can be used to exclude IBD in a young patient who presents with symptoms suggesting the disease. Although early changes, such as aphtoid ulceration, are beyond the resolution of MR, it can be useful in the evaluation of fixed stenoses and segmental dilatation and to detect adhesions. Because of high contrast, CT can better assess extent of fistulas in penetrating disease, mesenteric vascularity, and lymphadenopathy. Fistulas, sinus formation, and abscesses are features of penetrating disease. They are visible as wall-enhancing structures. Adhesions can be differentiated from fistulas because they are fibrotic and tend to be thinner and enhance later. Over time, chronic inflammation within the bowel wall leads to stricture formation, and bowel obstruction may develop. These findings are important to identify because they are not responsive to medical therapy and typically require surgical resection if associated with symptomatic bowel obstruction. On dynamic images, fibrotic strictures appear as aperistaltic bowel segments that often demonstrate fixed mural thickening and luminal narrowing. T2 hyperintensity is typically absent in these fibrotic regions, unless there is associated mural inflammation and edema (Fig. 13-43).

Radiation Enteritis

Radiation-induced enteropathy has distinct acute and chronic manifestations. Acute radiation enteritis occurs within the first few days or weeks after exposure. The most characteristic findings include mucosal hyperenhancement, submucosal edema, and bowel wall thickening. Chronic radiation enteritis is a transmural process that develops months to years after exposure in up to 16% of patients after radiation treatment to the pelvis. It is characterized by stricture formation and obstruction. Typical morphologic changes include diffuse bowel wall thickening, strictures and fistula formation, tethering, and impaired peristalsis.

Angioedema of the Bowel

Angioedema is not a true inflammatory disease, but it can mimic inflammation because it presents with bowel wall thickening. It is characterized by episodes of increased capillary permeability, with extravasation of intravascular fluid and subsequent edema of the skin, mucosa of the upper airways, or GI tract. Gastrointestinal involvement sometimes mimics an acute abdomen or rarely can cause life-threatening hypovolemic shock. Characteristic imaging features include reversible bowel and mesenteric edema, characterized by multiple dilated small-bowel loops with regular thickened mucosal folds, a stacked-coin appearance with bowel wall thickening, and thumb-printing. The small and large intestine may be involved, including jejunum, ileum, duodenum, and colon, in descending frequency of involvement. The findings are usually transient and segmental, returning to normal after an acute attack. A high degree of clinical suspicion is needed, particularly in patients using angiotensin-converting enzyme inhibitors and a variety of other medications, in the setting of typical imaging findings. A definite

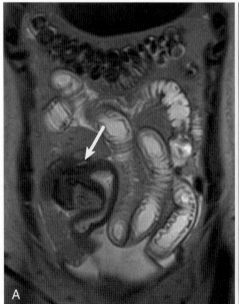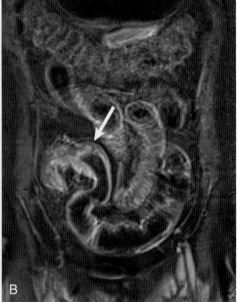

Figure 13-43 Coronal T2-weighted (**A**) and fat-suppressed contrast-enhanced T1-weighted (**B**) images performed in a patient with known Crohn disease (CD) demonstrate abnormal distal ileum, with relatively long segment of hyperenhancing wall thickening *(arrows)*. The lack of ionizing radiation and the need for serial examinations in these often young patients makes magnetic resonance imaging (MRI) an attractive alternative for the follow-up evaluation of patients with known inflammatory bowel disease (IBD). Computed tomography (CT) is the preferred modality in the emergency department (ED) setting for detection of acute complications.

diagnosis can be confirmed by elevated serum levels of C4 and C1 esterase inhibitor and C1 esterase inhibitor functional activity complement levels (Fig. 13-44).

Celiac Disease

Celiac disease in now recognized as a common but largely underdiagnosed disease, with typical diagnostic delay of more than 10 years from the onset of symptoms. It is a chronic autoimmune disorder induced in genetically susceptible individuals after ingestion of gluten proteins. The small bowel mucosa is primarily affected, resulting in progressive villus inflammation and destruction, with resulting induction of crypt hyperplasia. It may be asymptomatic or characterized by diverse symptoms of malabsorption with varying severity. Characteristic findings include duodenitis with dilution, slow transit, and flocculation of oral contrast, small bowel dilation, transient small bowel intussusception, villous atrophy and reversal of the fold pattern, with jejunization of the ileum, as reflected by a decrease in normal jejunal folds in contrast to the increasing fold pattern in the ileum.

Whipple Disease

Whipple disease is a rare multisystemic bacterial infection caused by the Whipple bacillus (*Tropheryma whipplei*), involving the small bowel (particularly the jejunum), lymph nodes, joints, and central nervous system. Barium studies can demonstrate to better extent the thickened, irregular folds and tiny nodules in the jejunum and, to a lesser degree, the ileum, due to accumulation of the Whipple bacilli and periodic acid-Schiff–positive macrophages in the submucosa and lamina propria. Characteristic imaging findings include mesenteric and retroperitoneal lymphadenopathy and fat-attenuation lymph nodes measuring between 10 and 20 HU. Whipple disease is an infectious condition, and these patients often demonstrate significant response to treatment with antibiotics.

Small Bowel Diverticulitis

Small bowel diverticulosis is far less common than colonic diverticulosis and characterized by the presence of multiple saclike mucosal herniations, or pseudodiverticula, through weak points in the intestinal wall. Duodenal diverticula are relatively common and have been found in up to 5% of the population undergoing barium studies. Jejunoileal diverticula are less common but usually multiple and localized to the proximal jejunum. They are frequently associated with disorders of intestinal motility such as scleroderma and visceral neuropathies. The major clinical manifestation of jejunoileal diverticula is malabsorption. Complications are more common in jejunoileal diverticula than duodenal diverticula and, similar to their colonic counterpart, include bleeding, intestinal obstruction, and diverticulitis.

Meckel diverticulum is the most common congenital anomaly of the GI tract, occurring in 2% of the population. It is a true diverticulum that contains all layers of the intestinal wall and has its own blood supply. It results from incomplete absorption of the omphalomesenteric duct and is frequently associated with heterotopic gastric or pancreatic mucosa in up to 50% of cases, with gastric heterotopia being most common. It is typically located in the distal ileum approximately 2 feet from the ileocecal valve. Although usually asymptomatic, approximately 2% of patients can present with complications, more common in children than adults. Inflammation (Meckel diverticulitis) is one of the most common complications, after hemorrhage and SBO. Computed tomography diagnosis relies on the identification of a blind-ending, tubular, round, or oval structure in the right lower quadrant or periumbilical region, with surrounding inflammation. The diverticulum can be associated with mural thickening and hyperenhancement, with focal calcifications at the base (enteroliths), and adjacent mesenteric fat stranding and fluid collections. In some instances the diverticulum will extend

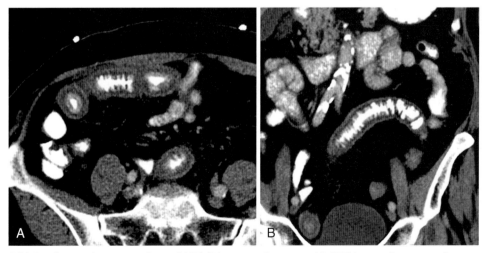

Figure 13-44 Axial (**A**) and coronal contrast-enhanced (CE) (**B**) computed tomographic (CT) images demonstrate long segment of concentric mural thickening of the ileum associated with submucosal edema and mildly engorged mesenteric vessels. The patient presented to the emergency department (ED) with right lower quadrant pain. Bowel angioedema was suggested because of the imaging appearance in combination with use of an angiotensin-converting enzyme inhibitor and a history of prior episodes of facial angioedema.

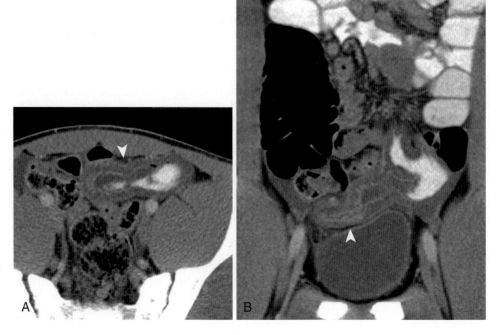

Figure 13-45 Axial (**A**) and coronal (**B**) contrast-enhanced computed tomographic images performed in a young patient with fever and abdominal pain demonstrates a blind-ending tubular fluid-filled structure arising from the distal ileum (**A** and **B**, *arrowheads*) and containing multiple layers ("gut signature"). Meckel diverticulitis was confirmed at surgery.

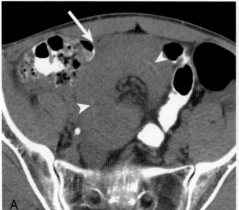
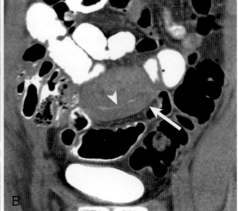

Figure 13-46 Axial (**A**) and coronal (**B**) contrast-enhanced computed tomographic images performed following oral administration in a young male patient with history of hemophilia and hematocrit drop demonstrates a relatively short segment of significant ileal wall thickening, of intermediate to high density (**A** and **B**, *white arrows*), causing significant narrowing of the lumen (**A** and **B**, *white arrowheads*), suggesting intramural hematoma, but no definite obstruction.

toward the umbilicus. The identification of a normal appendix can be very helpful because patients will often present with right lower quadrant pain. A Meckel scan can confirm the presence of gastric mucosa within the diverticulum in equivocal cases (Fig. 13-45).

Other Inflammatory Conditions of the Small Bowel

There are numerous additional inflammatory conditions of the small bowel that will present with nonspecific bowel wall thickening, including eosinophilic gastroenteritis, amyloidosis, Behçet syndrome, and primary lymphangiectasia. Differentiation will depend on the clinical history, distribution pattern, and often biopsy.

■ SMALL BOWEL HEMORRHAGE

Small bowel hemorrhage can be the result of ischemia, trauma, vasculitis, coagulopathies, and anticoagulation therapy. Bleeding usually occurs within the submucosal layer. It can cause bowel wall thickness of 1 cm or more, but it will often extend for less than 15 cm in length. The CT appearance of regular fold thickening, also known as the *picket fence* appearance on fluoroscopic studies, can be diffuse or segmental, depending on the underlying cause. It can present on CT as an intramural mass that narrows the lumen. If the hemorrhage is acute, the hematoma may have high density. Mesenteric fluid or hemoperitoneum is often associated with bowel wall hemorrhage or injury (Fig. 13-46).

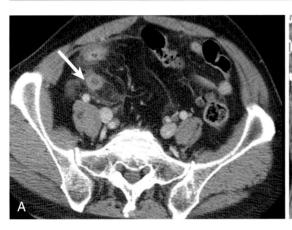 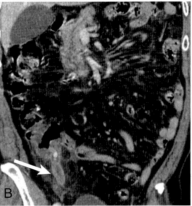

Figure 13-47 Axial (**A**) and coronal (**B**) contrast-enhanced computed tomographic images demonstrate a dilated, circumferentially thickened, fluid-filled structure with surrounding inflammatory changes *(arrows)* consistent with acute appendicitis. Two hyperdense appendicoliths are seen at the base of the appendix.

Colorectal Emergencies

Jennifer W. Uyeda, Jorge A. Soto, and Stephan W. Anderson

Rapid and accurate imaging and diagnosis is essential in the appropriate management of patients who present in the emergency setting with acute nontraumatic GI conditions. Appropriate diagnosis and subsequent treatment rely on accurate imaging diagnosis and radiologists' familiarity with the vast spectrum of GI diseases. This section will review the pathophysiology and pertinent imaging features of nontraumatic emergencies that affect the colon and the appendix.

■ ACUTE INFLAMMATION OF THE COLON AND APPENDIX

Acute Appendicitis

Acute appendicitis is the most common acute abdominal emergency requiring surgery and typically presents as periumbilical pain that migrates to the right lower quadrant with other characteristic clinical signs and symptoms, including nausea, anorexia, and fever, although the clinical presentation is highly variable. Initially the appendiceal lumen becomes obstructed by fecal material (appendicolith or fecalith), undigested material such as vegetables or seeds, hypertrophied Peyer patches, or neoplasm, and progressive accumulation of secretions leads to intraluminal distention and increased intramural pressure. The initial periumbilical abdominal pain represents referred pain from visceral innervation due to appendiceal luminal distention, and localized right lower quadrant pain is secondary to inflammation of the parietal peritoneum. Ongoing luminal distention and bacterial overgrowth result in lymphatic and venous obstruction leading to mucosal ischemia.

Plain abdominal radiographs have limited utility in the diagnosis of acute appendicitis. However, appendicoliths may be seen on abdominal radiographs and, in the appropriate clinical setting, are suggestive of acute appendicitis. In addition, free intra-abdominal air and bowel obstruction may readily be excluded on plain abdominal radiographs. In certain patients, such as

young women or generally thin patients, US of the right lower quadrant may be the first-line imaging modality. Acute appendicitis on US is seen as a noncompressible, thick-walled, dilated, blind-ending tubular structure in the right lower quadrant measuring 7 mm or more in diameter with graded compression, with or without a visible appendicolith. The utility of US for the diagnosis of acute appendicitis is highly operator dependent, and this modality is limited in obese patients and in the presence of gas-filled bowel. Typically, in cases of ongoing clinical suspicion, negative or inconclusive US examination results warrant a subsequent CT examination. In the majority of patients, CECT represents the first-line imaging modality of choice and is the most accurate imaging study with well-demonstrated sensitivity, specificity, and diagnostic accuracy exceeding 95% for the diagnosis of acute appendicitis. On CT, acute appendicitis is seen as a distended, circumferentially thickened, fluid-filled structure with mucosal hyperenhancement and surrounding fat stranding consistent with periappendiceal inflammation (Fig. 13-47). Although a strict size limit for normal appendices, similar to ultrasonographic imaging, is not applicable to CT given the lack of compression, acutely inflamed appendices are typically dilated and approach or exceed 1 cm in diameter. Furthermore, CECT is the imaging modality of choice to detect complications of acute appendicitis such as appendiceal perforation and periappendiceal abscess formation. On unenhanced CT examinations, a thickened appendix with surrounding inflammatory changes, with or without a calcified appendicolith (see Fig. 13-47), is diagnostic of acute appendicitis. In cases in which positive oral contrast agents are administered, opacification of the appendiceal lumen with oral contrast effectively excludes a diagnosis of appendicitis. However, the converse does not hold true, and a lack of appendiceal opacification with oral contrast material does not definitively indicate a diagnosis of acute appendicitis because this is often the case with normal appendices.

In cases of suspected acute appendicitis in pregnant women, an abdominal US is often the initial imaging study obtained to evaluate for possible appendicitis. However, because the sensitivity of this modality for the detection of acute appendicitis is limited, especially in pregnant women, a noncontrast MRI of the abdomen is often employed after an inconclusive US. With a reported sensitivity and specificity comparable to that of CT, with the benefits of a lack of ionizing radiation exposure to the fetus, MRI has gained wide acceptance for this application. With the use of MRI, the need for CT in cases of suspected acute appendicitis may be markedly decreased or eliminated altogether. Typically MRI examinations in cases of suspected appendicitis include multiplanar T1- and T2-weighted sequences. In pregnancy, intravenous gadolinium should not be administered for this application and the utility of oral contrast is a subject of ongoing investigation. Appendicitis on MRI is readily depicted on T2-weighted sequences acquired with and without fat suppression. The inflamed and edematous appendix is dilated and fluid filled and exhibits surrounding periappendiceal edema and fat inflammation (Fig. 13-48).

Appendectomy is the treatment of choice in simple acute appendicitis, and laparoscopic appendectomy is increasingly common. Antibiotic treatment for small abscesses is feasible, whereas image-guided percutaneous drainage may be performed for larger abscesses.

Acute Colonic Diverticulitis

Acute diverticulitis results from the obstruction and subsequent perforation of a colonic diverticulum. Colonic diverticula are small, focal outpouchings that occur at weak areas of the bowel wall, typically between the mesenteric and antimesenteric teniae where the vasa recta penetrate the circular muscle layer of the bowel wall. Diverticular disease is the most common pathologic process that involves the colon, with the sigmoid colon most commonly affected in up to 90% of the population. Initially the neck of a colonic diverticulum becomes obstructed by stool, undigested food particles such as seeds, or inflammation, eventually resulting in microscopic or macroscopic perforation and inflammation, contamination, and infection of the pericolic fat. Patients with acute diverticulitis typically present with left lower quadrant pain and fever. Less common signs and symptoms include nausea, vomiting, constipation, and urinary symptoms. Importantly, the location of the abdominal pain varies depending on the segment of colon that is affected.

On imaging, acute diverticulitis may yield abnormalities on abdominal radiographs, including pneumoperitoneum, bowel obstruction, or the presence of a focal region of increased soft tissue density related to the presence of an abscess. Although rarely employed currently, barium enema with water-soluble contrast may demonstrate extravasation of contrast material, as well as the presence of an intramural sinus tract or

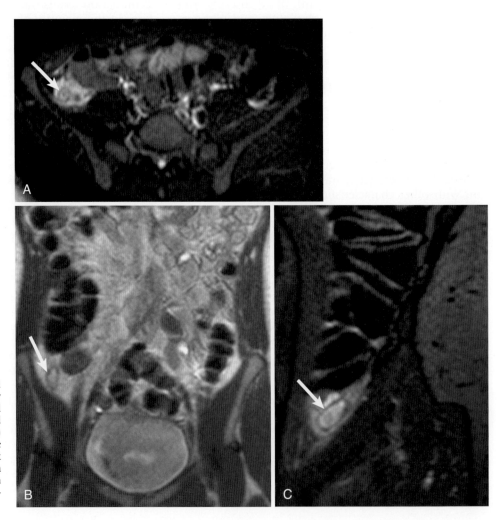

Figure 13-48 Axial T2-weighted short tau inversion recovery (STIR; **A**), coronal T2-weighted without fat saturation (**B**), and sagittal T2-weighted with STIR (**C**) sequences in a pregnant female demonstrate findings consistent with acute appendicitis, noting a dilated fluid-filled appendix with hyperintense signal in the surrounding fatty tissues (*arrows*).

a fistula. Contrast-enhanced CT of the abdomen and pelvis is currently the study of choice in patients with suspected acute diverticulitis, which manifests with pericolic inflammation, engorgement of the adjacent mesenteric vasculature, and focal colonic wall thickening with or without abscess formation (Fig. 13-49). In many cases the offending diverticulum may be directly visualized on CT, further increasing reader confidence in the diagnosis of acute diverticulitis.

Complications, including diverticular perforation with frank abscess formation, fistulas, (e.g., vesicocolonic or colocolonic among others), pyelophlebitis, or liver abscesses, may also be readily visualized with CT. A pericolic abscess appears as a hypoattenuating, pericolic collection with peripheral enhancement, often containing air or an air-fluid level. Acute diverticulitis represents the most common cause of vesicocolonic fistulas, which often occur along the left posterolateral aspect of the bladder in cases of sigmoid diverticulitis and may be suspected based on the presence of intravesicular air and focal bladder wall thickening adjacent to an inflamed diverticulum.

Treatment options in cases of acute diverticulitis range from conservative management with antibiotics and bowel rest to emergent surgery in cases of complications. Computed tomography-guided percutaneous abscess drainage is a viable treatment option in patients with abscesses related to diverticulitis in which CT readily depicts the anatomy and may be used to guide catheter placement.

An important differential diagnostic consideration in patients with focal colonic wall thickening includes colon carcinoma, which may have similar imaging findings to that of acute diverticulitis. Marked wall thickening out of proportion to the degree of pericolic inflammation, obliteration of the expected mural enhancement pattern of the colon, the presence of mesenteric lymphadenopathy, and acute bowel obstruction are imaging findings that are suggestive of colonic carcinoma. In contradistinction, the presence of fluid within the root of the sigmoid mesentery, visualization of an offending diverticulum, preservation of the expected mural enhancement pattern, and a relatively long segment of circumferential colonic wall thickening favor the diagnosis of acute diverticulitis.

Infectious Colitis

Infectious colitis refers to colonic inflammation caused by a variety of bacterial, viral, fungal, or protozoan infections. Presenting symptoms typically include acute onset of crampy abdominal pain and tenderness and watery or bloody diarrhea. Additional signs and symptoms include fever, rash, nausea, vomiting, headache, malaise, and weight loss. Patients with infectious colitis may be found to have electrolyte imbalances and leukocytosis.

Bacterial causes of infectious colitis include *Salmonella, Shigella, Campylobacter, Yersinia, Staphylococcus, E. coli* (O157:H7), *Staphylococcus,* and *Clostridium difficile.* Viral organisms known to cause colitis include herpes, cytomegalovirus, Norwalk virus, and *Rotavirus,* and associated fungal organisms include *Histoplasma* and *Mucor.* Finally, parasitic infections known to cause colitis include *Entamoeba histolytica, Schistosoma, Strongyloides, Trichuris,* and *Anisakis,* all of which are more commonly seen in underdeveloped countries. Some of the more commonly encountered causes of infectious colitis include *Campylobacter jejuni, Yersinia enterocolitica, Salmonella typhi,* and *Clostridium difficile. C. jejuni* is one of the most common causes of infectious diarrhea in the United States and is the leading cause of infectious colitis worldwide. *Y. enterocolitica* typically involves the ileocecal valve and usually affects infants, young children, and young adults. *S. typhi* causes enterocolitis, usually involving the cecum and ascending colon, and is the cause of typhoid fever. *Salmonella* may penetrate the mucosa and submucosa of bowel, thereby resulting in the release of endotoxins into the bloodstream leading to severe septicemia. Complications of *Salmonella* infection include bowel perforation, toxic megacolon, gangrenous cholecystitis, and massive lower GI bleeding. *C. difficile* overgrowth is normally suppressed by colonic bacteria; however, antibiotic use suppresses normal bowel flora, enabling the overgrowth of *C. difficile.* Therefore *C. difficile* colitis often occurs 4 to 9 days after the initiation of antibiotics.

The clinical diagnosis of infectious colitis is based on visualizing the organisms in stool cultures, blood cultures, and/or serologic studies. Proctoscopy or flexible sigmoidoscopy may demonstrate inflamed mucosa, and endoscopic biopsies may be used to establish the

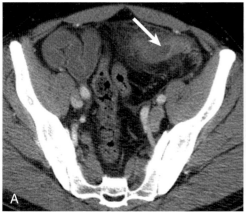
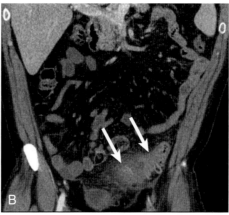

Figure 13-49 Axial (A) and coronal (B) contrast-enhanced computed tomographic images show a sigmoid diverticulum that has perforated with surrounding inflammatory changes in the surrounding fat *(arrow)*. There is also engorgement of the mesenteric vessels and colonic wall thickening *(arrows)*.

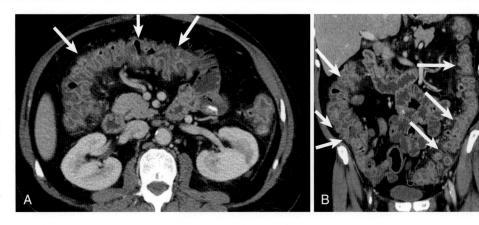

Figure 13-50 Mucosal hyperenhancement of the colon with pericolic inflammation and diffuse thickened mucosal folds secondary to edema, so called thumbprinting (arrows), are seen on axial (**A**) and coronal (**B**) contrast-enhanced computed tomographic images in a patient with Clostridium difficile colitis.

diagnosis. Imaging is reserved for cases in which blood and stool cultures are negative and in cases of failed colonoscopies. Imaging may also used in cases of infectious colitis to assess for complications such as colonic strictures, bowel gangrene, and perforation.

Although CT has largely replaced barium enema, imaging findings that have been well described on barium studies include a narrowed bowel lumen and focal or diffuse bowel wall thickening. Thumbprinting, nodules, inflammatory polyps, and ulcers are additional findings that may be identified in cases of infectious colitis on barium enema. On CT, abnormally increased mucosal and serosal enhancement of affected colonic segments, bowel wall thickening, and ascites are suggestive of infectious colitis (Fig. 13-50). In addition, depending on the underlying cause, air-fluid levels, pericolic inflammation, and mesenteric lymphadenopathy may also be visualized on CT in cases of infectious colitis.

The treatment for infectious colitis varies depending on the organism; however, most cases are self-limiting. Bacterial-induced colitis, which typically persists for 1 to 2 weeks and up to 1 month, may require antibiotic treatment. Viral causes are self-limited; however, fungal and parasitic organisms are typically treated with antifungal and antihelminthic drugs, respectively.

Typhlitis (Neutropenic Colitis)

Typhlitis, also known as *neutropenic colitis*, is seen in profoundly neutropenic and severely immunocompromised patients. Patients with typhlitis typically present with abdominal pain, fever, nausea, and diarrhea. Patients susceptible to typhlitis most commonly are receiving chemotherapy for acute leukemia; however, typhlitis may occur in the setting of AIDS, aplastic anemia, bone transplantations, and multiple myeloma. Bacteria, viruses, and fungi may penetrate the damaged colonic mucosa and proliferate in the setting of a compromised immune system and neutropenia, leading to subsequent colonic edema and inflammation. In the absence of appropriate treatment, there may be progressive colonic inflammation with transmural necrosis, perforation, and even death. Although the pathophysiologic process is not fully understood, typhlitis is likely secondary to a combination of ischemia, infection, and mucosal hemorrhage.

On radiography, ileocecal dilatation can be seen with thumbprinting secondary to edema. Computed tomography is the imaging study of choice. Findings in typhlitis include circumferential mural thickening, predominantly of the cecum and ascending colon. Hypoattenuation secondary to submucosal edema, pericolic inflammatory stranding, and ascites are also frequently identified on CT. Pneumatosis intestinalis may be present in severe cases, presumably related to disruption of mucosal integrity. Computed tomography may be employed to confirm a suspected diagnosis of typhlitis, to monitor disease progression based on the mural thickness, and to detect complications such as pneumoperitoneum in cases of silent perforation or necrosis. Direct visualization with endoscopy or the use of barium enema is typically contraindicated in cases of suspected typhlitis given the high risk for bowel perforation. Complications related to typhlitis include the formation of abscesses or fluid collections, bowel perforation, bowel necrosis, and sepsis.

The treatment of patients with typhlitis typically includes high doses of antibiotics and intravenous fluids to prevent transmural necrosis and perforation. Surgical resection may be indicated when complications such as transmural necrosis, intramural necrosis, abscess, uncontrolled sepsis, and/or GI hemorrhage are present.

Toxic Megacolon

Toxic megacolon represents acute transmural fulminant toxic colitis resulting in colonic dilatation greater than 6 cm in a patient with clinical signs of toxicity. Patients with toxic megacolon are typically quite ill with abdominal pain and tenderness, fever, leukocytosis, dehydration, altered mental status, and tachycardia. The inflammation involves the mucosa, but unlike uncomplicated colitis, in cases of toxic megacolon the inflammation extends through the submucosa and serosa of the bowel wall. The nitrous oxide created from the inflammation is believed to inhibit smooth muscle tone, resulting in bowel distention. Toxic megacolon may be a complication of infectious colitis such as C. difficile colitis, IBD, ischemic colitis, radiation colitis, and colonic volvulus. Medications such as anticholinergics, chemotherapy, and opiates have been associated with the development

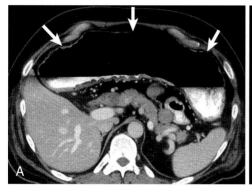
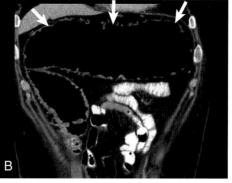

Figure 13-51 Axial (**A**) and coronal (**B**) computed tomographic (CT) images show a distended transverse colon *(arrows)* with a thickened and nodular bowel wall in a septic patient.

of toxic megacolon, and various procedures, including colonoscopies and barium enemas, have been implicated as causes. Overall the most common causes of toxic megacolon are *C. difficile* and UC.

On plain abdominal radiographs, marked focal or diffuse colonic dilatation, commonly of the transverse colon, greater than 6 cm (mean dilatation is 8 to 9 cm) in a patient exhibiting signs of sepsis is diagnostic of toxic megacolon. Although colonic dilatation is nonspecific, additional imaging findings that may be identified in patients with toxic megacolon include thickened bowel wall and markedly edematous haustra. Pseudopolyps, which are nodular masses of inflamed mucosa, may be seen projecting into the lumen of affected colon. On CT a distended colon with a markedly thickened and nodular bowel wall and submucosal edema may be seen (Fig. 13-51). Furthermore, the complications of toxic megacolon, including abscess formation, pneumoperitoneum, and pneumatosis intestinalis, may be readily identified on CT. In addition, imaging findings of septic thrombophlebitis may be visualized on CT, including thrombus in mesenteric and portal veins.

Treatment in patients with toxic megacolon may include operative intervention with colectomy and treatment of associated complications. Ultimately the prognosis varies and is highly dependent on the presence of complications, including frank bowel perforation and abscess formation.

Epiploic Appendagitis

Epiploic appendagitis represents acute inflammation or infarction of an epiploic appendage. Located on the antimesenteric side of the colon, the epiploic or omental appendages are small, lobulated masses containing adipose tissue and blood vessels, arising from the serosal surface of the colon. The epiploic appendages may become inflamed or torsed, resulting in infarction. Other reported causes of epiploic appendagitis include incarcerated hernia or bowel obstruction. Patients with epiploic appendagitis typically present with an acute onset of abdominal pain with localized tenderness over the portion of the affected colon with the left lower quadrant being the most commonly affected site. Marked abdominal tenderness to palpation with significant rebound tenderness is elicited on physical examination. Both a normal white blood cell count and body temperature are commonly found, and constitutional symptoms such as nausea, vomiting, and anorexia are uncommon.

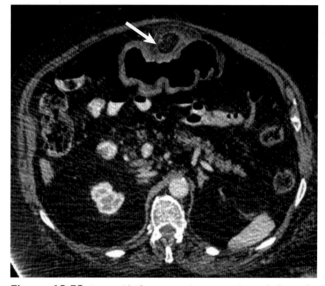

Figure 13-52 An ovoid, fat-attenuating mass situated along the transverse colon *(arrow)* along the antimesenteric border with surrounding inflammation consistent with epiploic appendagitis.

Computed tomography is the imaging modality of choice to diagnose acute epiploic appendagitis, which is visualized as an ovoid, fat-attenuating pericolic mass situated along the antimesenteric border of the colon, ranging in size from 1 to 4 cm (Fig. 13-52). In addition, surrounding inflammatory changes with a thin hyperattenuating rim due to thickening of the visceral peritoneum may be identified. Finally, a central "dot" of increased attenuation within the inflamed appendage may be identified and represents an engorged or thrombosed central vein. On US a targeted evaluation of the area of pain may reveal a noncompressible, hyperechoic mass adherent to the colon without central vascularity. Finally, MRI and T1- and T2-weighted images demonstrate a small pericolic mass that exhibits fat signal. Similar to CT, a hypointense central dot with a thin, surrounding rim of edema and inflammation, as well as peripheral enhancement, may be appreciated on MRI.

Acute epiploic appendagitis is usually self-limited with resolution of symptoms in 1 week, and conservative management with analgesics is the treatment of choice. Although rare, complications occasionally occur and include the formation of adhesions, bowel obstruction, peritonitis, and intraperitoneal abscesses.

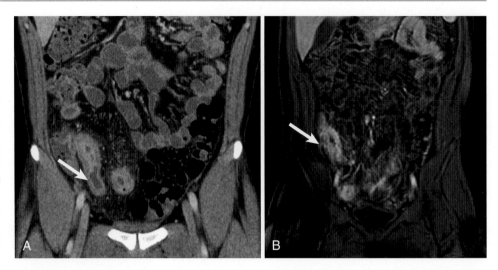

Figure 13-53 Coronal images from computed tomography (CT) enterography (**A**) and magnetic resonance (MR) enterography (**B**) demonstrate colonic wall thickening of the cecum and ascending colon (*arrows*) with mural stratification and trilaminar appearance of the bowel. There is mesenteric fibrofatty proliferation and engorgement of the vasa recta ("comb" sign) and mesenteric vessels in the right lower quadrant, best seen on the CT enterogram (**A**).

Acute Presentations of Inflammatory Bowel Disease

Crohn Disease

Crohn disease is one of the major forms of IBD and represents a chronic and recurrent granulomatous inflammatory disease. Acute presentations and exacerbations of this disease are common source of symptoms seen in ED patients. Crohn disease is more common in white and Jewish populations and in northern Europe and North America and typically occurs in the second and third decades of life, affecting both sexes equally. The cause is unknown, but recent advances in knowledge revolve around multiple factors, including genetics with a familial predisposition, intestinal microbial flora and infection, nutritional factors, and immunologic factors.

The most common presenting symptoms in patients with CD include chronic diarrhea and abdominal pain. Weight loss, malabsorption, and perianal fistulas and fissures are also frequently observed. Extraintestinal manifestations are common, particularly when the colon is involved, and they include abnormalities of the skin, joints, eyes, kidneys, and liver and biliary tree. Crohn disease, unlike UC, is patchy and segmental with skip lesions and transmural involvement. Any part of the GI tract may be involved, from the mouth to the anus, and the disease process is commonly discontinuous.

Colonoscopy with the retrieval of multiple biopsy specimens is the first-line study for diagnosing this disease. Aphthous ulcers with a target appearance, deep fissuring ulcers, and lymphoid hyperplasia are characteristic findings on colonoscopy. The role of CT and MRI in CD has expanded with recent advances in technology allowing for rapid acquisition of high-resolution images of the bowel. Computed tomography and MRI may identify disease, localize and characterize the severity and extent of disease, indicate the presence of acute complications, assess the severity of inflammation, and monitor disease progression. In the acute stage, bowel wall thickening greater than 3 mm is the most consistent cross-sectional imaging finding (Fig. 13-53). Mural stratification with a target appearance consisting of intense enhancement of the mucosa, hypoattenuation of the submucosa, and an outer enhancing muscularis propria may be identified (see Fig. 13-53). Mucosal hyperenhancement reflects inflammation, and the degree of enhancement correlates with the degree of inflammation. Mesenteric fibrofatty proliferation, comb sign (engorgement of the vasa recta), and mesenteric lymphadenopathy are additional findings (see Fig. 13-53). Complications of CD include abscesses, fistula formation, anal fissures, and colon cancer. Many of these complications are first diagnosed in the ED setting.

Ulcerative Colitis

Ulcerative colitis, another form of IBD, represents a chronic, idiopathic, diffuse inflammatory process in the colon. Ulcerative colitis typically affects patients between 15 and 25 years of age with women slightly more frequently affected than men. Similar to CD, UC is more common in white and Jewish populations and in northern Europe and North America. Although the cause is not entirely clear, genetic susceptibility, host immunity, and environmental factors have been implicated. Patients with UC usually present with bloody diarrhea, passage of mucus, abdominal pain, tenesmus, and urgency of defecation. Ulcerative colitis is also associated with extraintestinal manifestations, similar to those seen in CD. Not uncommonly, UC is first diagnosed when patients present with these symptoms to the ED. Acute exacerbations also require emergent medical attention.

At presentation a majority of patients (>95%) are found to have rectosigmoid involvement, which not uncommonly progresses to pancolitis and rarely affects the small bowel. In UC the inflammation is limited to the mucosa and typically ends at the muscularis mucosae, which is in contradistinction to the transmural involvement in CD. Continuous and symmetrical involvement is the hallmark of UC with distinct transitions between diseased and unaffected segments of colon, which again is in contrast to CD, in which the entire digestive tract may be affected in a discontinuous manner with transmural involvement. In early disease, mucosal edema and hyperemia are encountered, and with disease progression the mucosa develops punctate ulcers that enlarge and may extend into the lamina propria. The epithelium regenerates between acute inflammatory attacks, resulting in the formation of pseudopolyps, usually seen in long-standing disease. In chronic UC the colon becomes foreshortened, and featureless, with the loss of haustral folds, and exhibits luminal narrowing. In 15% to 20% of patients with UC a fulminant form of the disease may develop that is characterized by extensive inflammation with severe symptoms and colonic dilatation.

On abdominal radiography there is bowel wall thickening and colonic distention. In cases of fulminant UC severe colonic dilatation or toxic megacolon may be seen. As in all cases of IBD, CT (and increasingly MRI) is employed for determining disease activity. On CT a target or double-halo appearance due to mural stratification is commonly identified. However, this imaging finding is nonspecific and may be seen in patients with CD, pseudomembranous colitis, ischemic and radiation enterocolitis, infectious colitis, and bowel edema. With disease progression the bowel wall thickens and becomes featureless due to the loss of haustral folds.

Acute complications of UC that are particularly relevant in the ED setting include toxic megacolon, perforation with peritonitis and abscess formation, and venous thrombosis. Urgent surgery may be necessary when these complications develop. More chronic complications include colorectal cancer and stricture formation.

Perirectal Fistula and Abscess

Perirectal abscess and fistulization are inflammatory conditions of the rectum and anus that can cause severe perirectal pain and sinus discharge, often sending patients to seek emergency medical attention. A fistula results from an abscess derived from an infection originating in the anal canal glands at the dentate line. Sepsis from a perirectal abscess usually resolves after antibiotic treatment and surgical drainage; however, in approximately 25% of patients the abscess cavity does not resolve completely, and the infection decompresses to the skin. There is often a skin opening with erythema and focal granulation tissue with purulent or serosanguineous discharge. An inflammatory tract develops between a primary internal opening in the anal crypt at the dentate line and extends to a secondary external opening in the perianal skin. The tract decompresses in the anatomic plane of least resistance, the most common being the plane located between the internal and external sphincters, extending into the ischiorectal fascia and to the perineal skin. The fistulous tract may also extend circumferentially in the ischiorectal fossa with the tract passing into the contralateral fossa through the posterior rectum, forming a horseshoe fistula. Perirectal fistulas are classified into four types based on the anatomic relation of the tract to the sphincter muscles. However, a precise definition of the specific type of fistula requires a dedicated MRI examination with high-resolution imaging and is seldom necessary in the emergency setting.

Computed tomography is the imaging study typically requested in the ED. Computed tomography should be performed with intravenous contrast. The use of rectal contrast may be necessary for proper detection of perianal fistulas. Abscesses are identified as loculated low-attenuation fluid collections, possibly containing foci of air or an air-fluid level, with peripheral enhancement. Magnetic resonance imaging is the imaging modality of choice to depict the anatomy of the anal sphincter and perianal structures. However, as mentioned previously, emergent MRI is usually not required for this indication.

■ ACUTE COLONIC OBSTRUCTION

Large bowel obstructions are less common than SBOs and account for approximately 20% of all obstructions. Acute colonic obstructions are emergencies requiring early detection to prevent complications such as perforation or ischemia. The most common cause of acute colonic obstruction is malignancy, usually occurring in the sigmoid colon (Fig. 13-54). Other causes of large bowel obstruction include acute sigmoid diverticulitis and colonic volvulus. Abdominal pain, failure to pass stool or gas, and abdominal distention are common presenting symptoms of acute colonic obstruction. Differentiating between mechanical obstruction and Ogilvie syndrome, also known as *colonic pseudo-obstruction*, has therapeutic implications and should be accomplished with barium enema. A false diagnosis of colonic obstruction, particularly in patients with obstructive symptoms, may lead to inappropriate surgical exploration.

Imaging, particularly CT, is essential in assessing crucial information that has therapeutic implications. Computed tomography can help determine whether small or large bowel is affected, assess the location and severity of obstruction, and identify the cause and potential complications. On plain radiography, dilated colon (dilation being a caliber greater than 6 cm and 9 cm in the cecum) is seen. The presence of free air is indicative of bowel perforation. On CT the cause can be identified, and imaging appearances vary depending on whether colonic malignancy, acute diverticulitis, volvulus, or other pathologic process is present. Large bowel obstruction usually warrants surgical exploration, particularly when complications such as perforation or ischemia are present.

Sigmoid Volvulus

Sigmoid volvulus represents torsion or twisting of the sigmoid colon around the mesenteric axis. Patients typically present with acute or insidious onset of abdominal pain, nausea, abdominal distention, and obstipation. Vomiting usually occurs in late stages of disease when abdominal distention is severe. The presence of tachycardia, rebound tenderness, and severe abdominal pain are predictors of poor outcome. Patients with sigmoid volvulus are at increased risk for developing bowel ischemia by two mechanisms: arterial occlusion from mesenteric arterial torsion and mural ischemia due to increased wall tension of distended bowel. Colonic volvulus is associated with a high morbidity, particularly in cases of late presentation.

Sigmoid volvulus accounts for up to 75% of cases of volvulus of the bowel but accounts for less than 10% of all cases of intestinal obstruction in the United States. Predisposing factors for sigmoid volvulus include chronic constipation, obstipation from medications, high-fiber diet resulting in bulky stool causing elongation of bowel, and prior abdominal surgeries. Comorbidities include psychiatric conditions, advanced age, and institutionalization in medical facilities.

Imaging is particularly useful in diagnosing colonic volvulus. Abdominal radiographs are diagnostic in a majority of cases when classic findings of a distended, inverted U-shaped loop of sigmoid colon is seen, along with an absence of haustral markings (Fig. 13-55). The

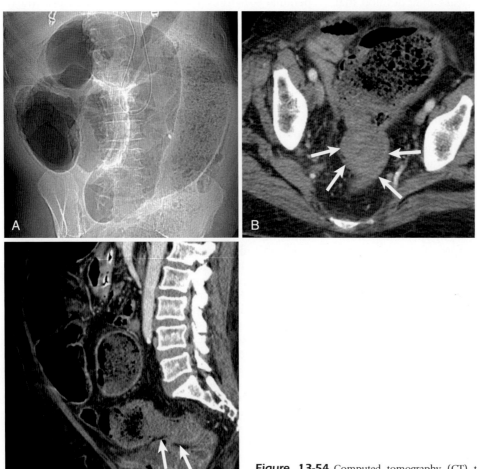

Figure 13-54 Computed tomography (CT) topogram (**A**) demonstrates multiple dilated loops of colon exceeding 6 cm in diameter. Axial (**B**) and sagittal (**C**) CT images show a large sigmoid mass *(arrows)* with proximal colonic dilatation causing large bowel obstruction. The mass was found to be a sigmoid adenocarcinoma.

Figure 13-55 Computed tomography (CT) topogram (**A**) shows the "coffee bean" sign referring to the inverted U shape of the sigmoid colon with a dense white line formed by the apposed colonic wall directed from the pelvis to the right upper quadrant. Coronal (**B**) contrast-enhanced (CE) CT image demonstrates a "whirl" sign whereby the sigmoid colon and mesentery twist *(arrow)*.

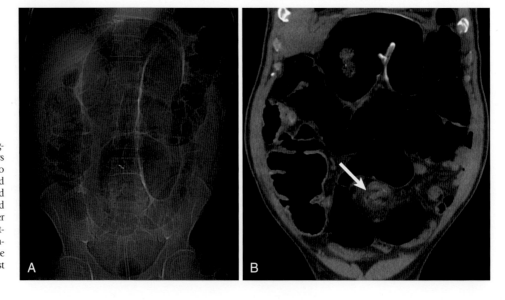

"coffee bean" sign refers to the inverted U shape of the sigmoid colon with a dense white line formed by the apposed colonic walls, which is directed from the pelvis to the right upper quadrant. A single contrast enema typically reveals a smoothly tapered narrowing of the rectosigmoid junction at the distal aspect of the volvulus, resulting in a "bird beak" appearance. On CT a whirl sign may be visualized in which twisting of the sigmoid colon (see Fig. 13-55) and the mesentery is present and "beaking" due to tapered narrowing of the afferent and efferent bowel loops may be seen. Computed tomography may readily identify complications of sigmoid volvulus, including bowel ischemia or perforation.

Sigmoid volvulus may be treated nonoperatively with proctoscopic/colonoscopic decompression with a high success rate. In some cases nonoperative treatment of sigmoid volvulus may be followed with an elective sigmoidectomy. In cases of sigmoid volvulus with complications such as bowel ischemia or perforation, emergent surgery is often performed.

Cecal Volvulus

Cecal volvulus refers to torsion or twisting of the cecum around a fixed and twisted mesenteric axis, resulting in massively dilated bowel with the tip pointing to the left upper quadrant. Patients present with abdominal pain of acute or insidious onset, nausea, and vomiting. Like sigmoid volvulus, patients are at increased risk for developing bowel ischemia, and cecal volvulus is associated with a high morbidity, especially in cases of late presentation.

As opposed to sigmoid volvulus, in which the cause is usually acquired, the most common predisposing factor to cecal volvulus is an abnormal embryologic connection of the right colon to retroperitoneum resulting in increased mobility of the cecum. Other causes of cecal volvulus include cecal bascule with anterior folding of the cecum, postpartum ligamentous laxity, colonic distention, and chronic constipation. Cecal bascule refers to abnormal positioning of the cecum in the midabdomen

secondary to loose mesenteric attachment, which results in folding of the cecum.

On abdominal radiographs, cecal volvulus has a characteristic appearance with a dilated loop of inverted U-shaped bowel eccentrically located in the left upper quadrant that is directed from the pelvis to the left upper quadrant. The diagnosis of cecal volvulus may be confirmed on contrast enema or CT. On contrast enema examination a beaklike tapering of the cecum is seen at the level of the volvulus, and contrast usually does not pass into the proximal colon or small bowel. On CT the cecum is abnormally positioned in the mid and left abdomen (Fig. 13-56). Progressive narrowing of the afferent and efferent limbs of colon is seen, leading to a whirl sign, which represents a tight twisting of the mesentery and "beaking" due to tapered narrowing of the afferent and efferent bowel loops. Computed tomography may readily identify complications, including bowel ischemia or perforation. Colonoscopy can be performed to reduce the volvulus, but surgical intervention, including cecopexy or resection, is indicated in complicated cases.

Intussusception

Colonic intussusception refers to invagination or telescoping of a proximal loop of bowel (intussusceptum) into the lumen of an adjacent, distal segment of bowel (intussuscipiens). Intussusception may be intermittent, particularly in the absence of a lead point. Patients typically present with abdominal pain, nausea, and vomiting, and in patients with an underlying malignancy, weight loss, palpable abdominal mass, melena, and constipation may be seen.

The cause and pathophysiologic process of intussusception are not well understood, particularly intussusception without a lead point. Dysrhythmic bowel contractions have been implicated. Intussusceptions may be caused by lesions within the intestinal wall, or, alternatively, intraluminal lesions may act as lead points. Large bowel intussusception is commonly associated with lead points. Benign lesions such as lipomas, adenomatous polyps, colitis, epiploic appendagitis, and

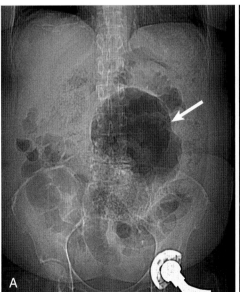
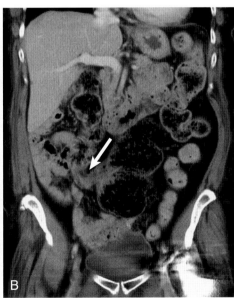

Figure 13-56 Computed tomography (CT) topogram (**A**) shows a markedly dilated loop of bowel (*arrow*) located slightly to the left of the midline. **B,** Thin-section maximum intensity projection (MIP) reformation confirms the abnormal location of the cecum, which is markedly distended and filled with stool, as well as the site of twisting and a "beak" sign (*arrow*).

postoperative adhesions, as well as malignant lesions such as metastatic disease, primary malignancy, and lymphoma, may act as lead masses causing intussusception.

Four major forms of intussusception have been described, including enteroenteric, ileocolic, ileocecal, and colocolic. The majority of cases involve the small bowel. Ileocolic or ileocecal intussusception is often associated with small bowel metastatic disease; the most common primary malignancies include melanoma, breast, and lung. The most common benign causes of colocolic intussusception are lipomas, followed by adenomatous polyps, whereas colonic adenocarcinoma is the most common malignant cause.

Contrast-enhanced CT is the imaging modality of choice to evaluate the bowel in cases of suspected intussusception. The appearance of the bowel on CT varies widely depending on various factors such as the presence and configuration of the lead mass, presence of bowel dilatation and degree of obstruction, degree of bowel wall edema, and amount of invaginated mesenteric fat and blood vessels. Intussusceptions on CT typically demonstrate a targetlike appearance, with or without the presence of mesenteric fat or vessels, with the outer layer representing the intussuscipiens and the inner layer representing the intussusceptum (Fig. 13-57). Typically the cross-sectional diameter of an intussusception with a lead mass is greater than that of normal bowel. In addition, signs of obstruction may also be seen, including proximal bowel dilatation with distally collapsed loops. A relatively short length of intussusception and the absence of proximal obstruction, typically in the small bowel, support the diagnosis of a transient, nonobstructive intussusception.

Treatment for transient, nonobstructive intussusception is conservative, whereas surgical reduction or resection is the usual treatment for obstructive intussusception and for malignant lead masses.

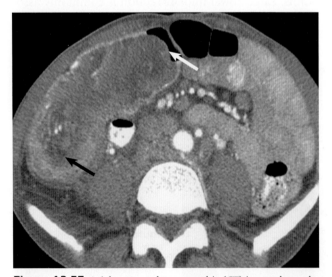

Figure 13-57 Axial computed tomographic (CT) image shows the characteristic signs of ileocolic intussusception. The lead point *(white arrow)* is a mass lesion subsequently diagnosed as lymphoma; this is the intussusceptum. Intraluminal gas outlines the surface of the mass and separates the intussusceptum from the outer intussuscipiens. Note the mesenteric fat *(black arrow)* and vessels, also a characteristic sign of intussusceptions.

Ogilvie Syndrome

Ogilvie syndrome, also known as *colonic pseudo-obstruction*, is characterized by colonic dilatation with obstructive symptoms in the absence of a true mechanical obstruction. Patients present with obstructive symptoms of abdominal pain and distention, nausea, vomiting, and failure to pass stool. Although no underlying mechanical obstruction exists, Ogilvie syndrome is a significant cause of morbidity and death with possible progression to bowel ischemia and perforation. Although the pathogenesis of colonic pseudo-obstruction is not fully understood, abnormal parasympathetic autonomic regulation of the colon and intramural ganglion damage are among proposed mechanisms. A false diagnosis of colonic obstruction, particularly in patients with obstructive symptoms, may lead to inappropriate surgical exploration. The term *Ogilvie syndrome* has been applied to both the acute and chronic forms of colonic pseudo-obstruction, though some authors believe this term applies to the acute form, which represents a reversible condition, associated with major surgery or severe medical illness. The chronic form of pseudo-obstruction is characterized by repeated episodes of bowel dilatation and obstructive symptoms.

On imaging, marked dilatation of the colon is seen on abdominal radiography with the cecum and ascending and transverse colons more severely affected. In patients with Ogilvie syndrome, CT readily demonstrates marked colonic distention with a long segment of relative transition to more collapsed bowel occurring in the absence of an obstructing lesion. This relative transition often occurs at the splenic flexure where the parasympathetic bowel innervation changes from the vagal nerve to the sacral nerve, lending support to the hypothesis that transient impairment of the sacral plexus leads to functional obstruction of the proximal colon. Computed tomography also is useful for accurately depicting the degree of colonic distention that may warrant surgical decompression. In addition, complications of pseudo-obstruction, including bowel ischemia and perforation, may be assessed with CT. The treatment of Ogilvie syndrome is based on the clinical and imaging assessment and includes supportive treatment, endoscopic decompression, and surgical decompression. The presence of bowel ischemia and perforation typically warrant surgical intervention.

■ ACUTE COLONIC ISCHEMIA AND PNEUMATOSIS

Ischemic Colitis

Ischemic colitis is the most common vascular disorder of the GI tract and is caused by compromise of the mesenteric vascular supply. Ischemic colitis commonly occurs in the so-called watershed areas supplied by the SMA and IMA at the splenic flexure and decreased perfusion between the IMA and hypogastric artery at the rectosigmoid junction. The rectum is typically spared secondary to extensive collateral blood supply. In older adults, left-sided ischemic colitis is more typical secondary to hypoperfusion, whereas right-sided ischemic colitis due to hemorrhagic shock is more common in younger patients.

Presenting signs and symptoms in patients with acute ischemic colitis include the acute onset of mild to severe crampy abdominal pain, nausea, and vomiting; bloody diarrhea and rectal bleeding may also occur several hours after the onset of abdominal pain. Predisposing factors to ischemic colitis include, among others, hypotension from hemorrhagic or septic shock, cardiogenic shock, arrhythmias, congestive heart failure, vasculitis, mechanical bowel obstruction, and certain medications.

The degree of bowel wall involvement ranges from isolated mucosal to transmural pathologic process depending on the severity and duration of ischemia. Because the mucosa receives a majority of the vascular supply to the colonic wall, it is most susceptible to ischemia. The sequelae of acute ischemic colitis include reversible ischemic colitis, chronic ulcerative ischemic colitis, ischemic colonic stricture, or colonic necrosis with perforation and sepsis.

Abdominal radiographs demonstrate thumbprinting in up to 75% of patients with ischemic colitis. This sign reportedly appears within 24 hours of the onset of ischemia. Thumbprinting manifests as smooth, round, polypoid, and scalloped filling defects projecting into the colonic lumen, which correspond to thickened mucosal folds related to submucosal edema or hemorrhage. Additional radiographic findings that may be appreciated in patients with acute ischemic colitis include the presence of a nonspecific ileus, loss of haustral folds, pneumatosis intestinalis, and luminal narrowing. Contrast-enhanced CT has become the imaging modality of choice in cases of suspected ischemic colitis with imaging features of circumferential bowel wall thickening and pericolic inflammation (Fig. 13-58). A target sign resulting from hyperenhancement of the mucosa and serosa secondary to hyperemia and relative submucosal hypoattenuation related to edema may be identified. Following reperfusion, hypoattenuation of the bowel wall due to edema or hyperattenuation of the bowel wall due to hemorrhage may be seen. In cases of continued occlusion of the colonic vasculature without reperfusion, the bowel wall may remain hypodense with nonenhancement of the bowel wall after intravenous contrast administration. In cases of suspected ischemic colitis the mesenteric vessels should be closely scrutinized for obstructing arterial or venous thrombi. In the setting of ischemic colitis, pneumatosis intestinalis or the presence of portomesenteric venous air is highly suggestive of frank bowel wall necrosis.

In cases of acute ischemic colitis, patients with nonocclusive mural ischemia may be treated conservatively, whereas patients with transmural infarction typically require urgent operative intervention and surgical resection.

Pneumatosis Coli

Primary pneumatosis coli is rare, accounting for 15% of cases, whereas secondary causes are associated with benign as well as clinically worrisome, life-threatening causes. Bowel necrosis from infarction or caustic ingestion is the most common cause of secondary pneumatosis coli (see Fig. 13-58). Mucosal defects from iatrogenic causes such as endoscopy, ulcers, IBD, surgery, collagen vascular diseases, and increased mucosal permeability from steroids, chemotherapy, and immunodeficiency states represent additional reported causes. Pulmonary diseases, including chronic obstructive pulmonary disease, asthma, cystic fibrosis, positive end-expiratory pressure, and bronchitis, may cause pneumatosis.

There are various mechanisms thought to cause pneumatosis coli. The bacterial theory proposes that gas-forming bacteria gain access to the bowel wall through a wall defect. The mechanical theory, another proposed mechanism of pneumatosis, purports that increased intraluminal pressure results in gas tracking into the bowel wall. Finally, the pulmonary theory suggests that alveolar rupture causes gas to track into the mesentery and eventually into the bowel wall.

Pneumatosis coli is an imaging sign, as opposed to a disease or diagnosis, and the significance of this imaging sign is dependent on the underlying cause and on the patient's clinical status. Benign pneumatosis is self-limiting and is usually incidentally diagnosed in the asymptomatic patient. If presenting symptoms include abdominal pain with rebound tenderness, abdominal distention, melena, fever, or vomiting, clinically worrisome or life-threatening causes requiring appropriate medical or even surgical treatment must be considered.

On imaging the morphologic characteristics of the intramural gas have been evaluated in an attempt to differentiate benign, self-limiting causes from the

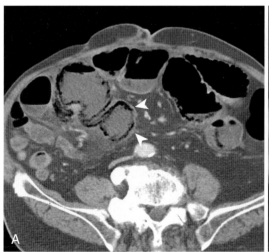
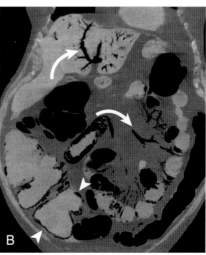

Figure 13-58 Axial (**A**) computed tomographic (CT) image demonstrates intramural air in a curvilinear distribution (*arrowheads*) within loops of bowel. Coronal (**B**) CT image shows intramural air in multiple loops of small bowel and cecum (*arrowheads*) and portomesenteric venous gas (*curved arrows*).

life-threatening causes that require subsequent management. A cystic appearance of the intramural gas, consisting of either single cysts or clusters of cysts (pneumatosis cystoides coli [PCC]), is thought to correlate with a benign cause compared to a more curvilinear appearance. However, life-threatening causes of pneumatosis coli may have a cystic appearance, and the substantial overlap in imaging appearances makes correlation with the patient's clinical status, signs and symptoms, and laboratory values imperative. On CT, PCC is best seen with lung windows to detect clusters of rounded or cystic intramural gas-filled structures and, in some cases, the presence of portomesenteric venous gas. In PCC caused by ischemic bowel, additional CT findings include a thickened bowel wall, dilated bowel loops, and abnormal enhancement. On abdominal radiographs, radiolucencies in a cystic or linear distribution along the periphery of the bowel wall may be seen. Similarly, on fluoroscopic barium enema images, bubbly intramural lucencies may be identified. Imaging pitfalls for the diagnosis of PCC include the presence of intraluminal gas surrounding stool, which may mimic intramural air. In addition, on CT colonography, PCC may simulate a colonic polyp on three-dimensional (3-D) CT images; however, two-dimensional CT images readily reveal the air-filled intramural cyst.

■ CONCLUSION

In summary, the causes of colonic emergencies are diverse, but in all cases timely and accurate diagnosis is critical in delivering successful clinical care. Fortunately, the imaging technologies in the modern radiologist's armamentarium are powerful tools that may be leveraged in the diagnostic evaluation of this patient population. With an awareness of the clinical features and the pertinent imaging manifestations described earlier, radiologists may serve an integral role in the clinical management of patients with acute colonic emergencies.

Abdominal Vascular Emergencies

Russ Kuker, Anthony M. Durso, Gary Danton, Kim Caban, and Felipe Munera

■ NONTRAUMATIC EMERGENCIES OF THE MESENTERIC AND VISCERAL VASCULATURE

Acute Small Bowel Mesenteric Ischemia

Acute mesenteric ischemia is a life-threatening condition with high morbidity and mortality that requires early diagnosis and treatment. Angiography has been the reference standard for diagnostic evaluation; however, the role of CT in this setting continues to expand,

and CT offers advantages over angiography by showing abnormalities of the bowel wall and mesentery in addition to the vasculature. With advancements in scanning capability and (3-D) data acquisition, the ability of CT to diagnose mesenteric ischemia has been reported to have a sensitivity of approximately 90%. It can also provide alternative diagnoses for patients in whom mesenteric ischemia is suspected.

The CT findings in acute mesenteric ischemia vary widely depending on the cause and underlying pathophysiologic process. When interpreting studies, it is important to assess the thickness and attenuation of the bowel wall, the degree of luminal dilatation, the mesentery, and the mesenteric vessels. The normal bowel wall measures 0.3 to 0.5 cm in thickness depending on the degree of distention. Although nonspecific, bowel wall thickening is a frequently observed CT finding in acute mesenteric ischemia and is caused by mural edema, hemorrhage, or superinfection. The degree of thickening is typically 0.8 to 0.9 cm and does not correlate with the severity of ischemia. Bowel wall thickening is often observed in mesenteric venous occlusion, strangulation, ischemic colitis, and mesenteric arterial occlusion after reperfusion. In exclusively arterial occlusive mesenteric ischemia, however, the bowel wall becomes thinner because there is no arterial flow and neither mural edema nor hemorrhage occurs.

The attenuation of the bowel wall should be assessed on both enhanced and unenhanced CT images. Pneumatosis intestinalis or air within the bowel wall can be seen in the setting of mesenteric ischemia and often indicates transmural infarction, particularly if it is associated with portal venous gas. On unenhanced CT images, low attenuation of the bowel wall indicates mural edema, which typically occurs in mesenteric arterial occlusion after reperfusion, mesenteric venous occlusion, strangulation, and ischemic colitis. High attenuation of the bowel wall is caused by intramural hemorrhage and hemorrhagic infarction.

On CECT a highly specific but insensitive finding for acute mesenteric ischemia is absent or diminished enhancement of the bowel wall. A halo or target appearance is also indicative of mesenteric ischemia, representing mural edema with surrounding hyperemia and hyperperfusion, and can be seen in arterial occlusion after reperfusion, nonocclusive and venoocclusive bowel ischemia, strangulation, and ischemic colitis. Although it seems paradoxical, hyperenhancement of the bowel wall may also be observed in cases of mesenteric ischemia caused by hyperemia (mesenteric venous occlusion), hyperperfusion (reperfusion after arterial occlusion), or prolonged enhancement due to reduction of arterial perfusion and venous outflow (strangulation, nonocclusive bowel ischemia, or shock bowel). The bowel lumen is often dilated because of interruption of normal bowel peristalsis (adynamic ileus).

The mesenteric vessels can be evaluated on CECT images for filling defects that may indicate emboli or thrombi in the mesenteric arteries and veins. Engorgement of the mesenteric veins caused by congestion of venous outflow is typically seen in venoocclusive bowel ischemia or strangulating bowel obstruction. Mesenteric fat stranding and ascites appear with transudation of fluid in the mesentery or the peritoneal cavity caused by

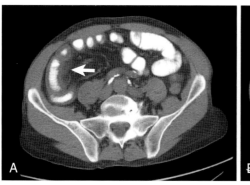
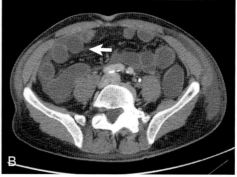

Figure 13-59 A 61-year-old man with acute thrombosis of the superior mesenteric artery (SMA) from an embolic source likely arising from a large thrombus in the left atrial appendage (not shown). **A,** Initial computed tomographic (CT) image without contrast shows diffuse small bowel wall thickening *(arrow),* possibly reflecting reperfusion. **B,** CT angiographic examination, which was done several days later, shows progressive ischemic changes in the small bowel with a paper-thin hypoenhancing wall *(arrow)* and new ascites.

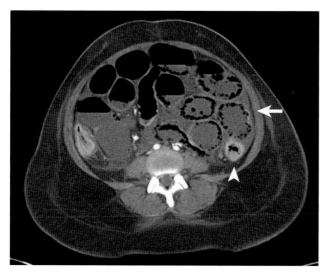

Figure 13-60 A 26-year-old woman with status epilepticus found to have late stages of bowel ischemia. Computed tomography (CT) with contrast shows pneumatosis intestinalis *(arrow)* and ascites. Also note thickening and hyperenhancement of the colonic wall *(arrowhead).*

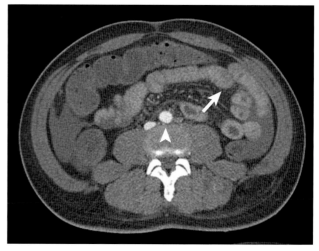

Figure 13-61 A 60-year-old man with shock bowel from hypoperfusion demonstrated on computed tomography (CT) with diffuse thickening and hyperenhancement of the bowel wall *(arrow).* Note the small caliber of the abdominal aorta *(arrowhead)* and collapsed inferior vena cava (IVC). Ascites is present in paracolic gutters.

elevation of mesenteric venous pressure. These findings are more common in venous occlusive than in arterial mesenteric ischemia.

Arterial Inflow—Occlusive

The most common cause of acute mesenteric arterial occlusion is thromboembolism from cardiovascular sources, followed by arterial thrombosis. Most emboli wedge at branching points around or distal to the middle colic artery, whereas thrombosis typically occurs at or near the origin of the mesenteric arteries. Although the severity may vary, bowel ischemia is usually followed by infarction, perforation, and peritonitis unless reperfusion occurs. On CECT images, emboli or thrombi can be seen as filling defects in the SMA and its branches. The thickness of the bowel wall of the involved segments is the same or thinner than the healthy segments unless reperfusion occurs. The lumen of the bowel may be filled with fluid, gas, or both; however, the bowel seldom contains a large amount of fluid. The classic appearance is

paper-thin bowel loops distended with air (Fig. 13-59). Contrast enhancement of the involved bowel is absent or diminished. Pneumatosis can typically be observed in cases with transmural infarction with or without associated portal venous gas (Fig. 13-60). Coexisting embolism of other organs may also be observed on CECT, which supports the diagnosis of mesenteric ischemia.

Arterial Inflow—Nonocclusive

Nonocclusive mesenteric ischemia occurs when bowel perfusion is reduced despite patent mesenteric vessels. It can be a difficult diagnosis to make clinically and with imaging because symptoms are nonspecific and it is much easier to see a thrombosed vessel than infer disease from either the clinical history or secondary imaging findings. Bowel findings are no different than what may be seen in occlusive mesenteric ischemia, but the patent vessels should suggest the diagnosis. Findings include dilated bowel, focal or diffuse bowel wall thickening, and abnormal bowel wall enhancement (Fig. 13-61).

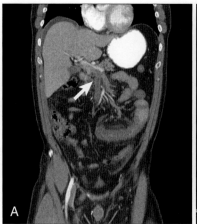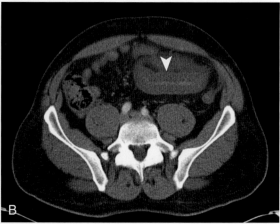

Figure 13-62 A, A 36-year-old man with thrombosis of the superior mesenteric vein partially extending into the main portal vein *(arrow)*. B, There are ischemic changes in the small bowel with a target appearance on computed tomography angiography (CTA) *(arrowhead)*. The patient subsequently underwent thrombolysis using tissue plasminogen activator infusion.

Low Flow

Low-flow states causing acute mesenteric ischemia are best demonstrated in the critical care postsurgical setting, in which low cardiac output, episodes of hypotension, use of vasopressors, or intra-abdominal hypertension leading to abdominal compartment syndrome is most likely to occur. Abdominal pain with nonspecific bowel findings on imaging suggests ischemia in these patients. Low-flow nonocclusive ischemia also occurs in patients who are very aggressively resuscitated. Development of ascites and bowel wall thickening post resuscitation leads to intra-abdominal hypertension, abdominal compartment syndrome, a low-flow state, and ischemia. Nontrauma emergency patients with decreased cardiac output are also susceptible to suffering nonocclusive mesenteric ischemia. Combinations of factors such as a low-flow state along with vascular stenosis likely facilitate development of ischemia.

Vasculitis

Vasculitis is another cause of nonocclusive mesenteric ischemia. Diagnosis relies on either an appropriate clinical history or the imaging findings of vasculitis in addition to imaging signs of mesenteric ischemia. Specific types of vasculitis that can cause bowel ischemia include Takayasu arteritis ("pulseless" disease), polyarteritis nodosa, microscopic polyangiitis, Wegener granulomatosis, Churg-Strauss vasculitis, systemic lupus erythematosus, and Henoch-Schönlein purpura. In the ED setting it is probably not critical to diagnose the specific type, but rather to be able to recognize that a patient with findings of bowel ischemia and patent vessels could potentially have a vasculitis. Suggesting the diagnosis may get the right team members involved earlier, leading to prompt diagnosis and intervention.

Venous Outflow—Occlusive

Restriction of venous outflow is another cause of bowel ischemia and most commonly results from venous thrombosis (primary or secondary causes) or bowel obstruction (either mechanical obstruction of mesenteric veins or bowel distention with increased intraluminal pressures). Bowel ischemia and infarction caused by closed-loop obstruction are discussed in detail in Chapter 13, section 2.

Mesenteric venous thrombosis accounts for approximately 5% to 15% of all mesenteric ischemia cases. The symptoms are subtle and not usually associated with characteristic laboratory abnormalities or distinct physical examination findings. Early identification of the condition allows for conservative treatment with anticoagulation and improved outcomes. The most common causes include hypercoagulable states such as primary hematologic diseases, oral contraceptive use, pregnancy, and malignancy; intra-abdominal inflammatory conditions (pancreatitis, diverticulitis, appendicitis, peritonitis, or IBD); the postoperative state; and cirrhosis/portal hypertension. The clinical manifestations include abdominal pain, diarrhea, GI hemorrhage, perforation, and peritonitis.

Computed tomography is generally the imaging modality of choice due to its high sensitivity (90% to 100%) and wide availability. An acute thrombus is evident as a central filling defect in the mesenteric vein (Fig. 13-62). Other CT findings include enlargement of the vessel and a sharply defined wall with a rim of increased density. Persistent enhancement of the bowel wall, pneumatosis intestinalis, and portal vein gas are late findings. Abdominal radiographs are abnormal in 50% to 75% of patients, but specific findings of bowel ischemia (thumbprinting, pneumatosis intestinalis, or portal venous gas) are found in only 5%. Ultrasonography with color Doppler analysis has also been used with success but is generally less sensitive (73% to 80%) and can be technically difficult to perform.

■ NONTRAUMATIC VISCERAL ARTERIAL EMERGENCIES

Nontraumatic visceral arterial emergencies encompass both hemorrhagic and ischemic conditions that can involve nearly all organ systems below the diaphragm. In the abdomen, causes include aneurysms, both aortic and visceral arterial, visceral organ neoplasms, and coagulopathy. Ischemic and hemorrhagic disorders of the GI tract will be discussed in separate sections within this chapter. Spontaneous hemorrhage from gynecologic causes, most commonly ruptured cysts and ectopic pregnancy, will not be discussed in this chapter.

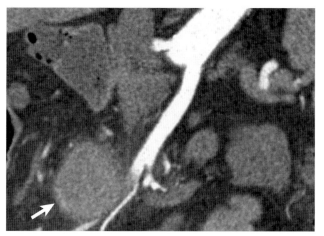

Figure 13-63 A 55-year-old man with a saccular mycotic aneurysm *(arrow)* of the superior mesenteric artery (SMA) evidenced by a thick wall and adjacent fat stranding on curved multiplanar reformation (MPR) image from computed tomography angiography (CTA).

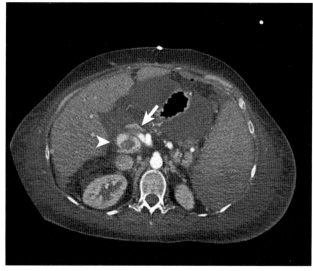

Figure 13-64 A 44-year-old woman following liver transplant with thrombosis of the common hepatic artery and pseudoaneurysm formation *(arrow)* seen on computed tomography angiography (CTA). Note also partial thrombosis of the main portal vein *(arrowhead)*.

Rupture of Nontraumatic Aneurysms of the Visceral Arteries

Aneurysms can occur in any of the visceral branches of the aorta. Although initially thought to be uncommon, because of the increasing use of cross-sectional imaging, particularly CT, visceral arterial aneurysms are being detected more frequently. The arteries most commonly affected are the splenic artery, the hepatic artery, and the renal arteries.

Most splenic artery aneurysms are found incidentally and are asymptomatic. They have a strong female predilection and associations with pregnancy and portal hypertension. Left upper quadrant pain can be a symptom of impending rupture. A ruptured splenic artery aneurysm can be a life-threatening event presenting with pain, hypotension, and hemoperitoneum. In particular, splenic artery aneurysm rupture in pregnancy is associated with high mortality. Indications for treatment of splenic artery aneurysms include symptomatic aneurysms, rupture, and pregnancy. Other considerations for intervention include enlargement, size greater than 2.5 to 3 cm, and portal hypertension.

In contrast to splenic artery aneurysms, hepatic artery aneurysms are more commonly symptomatic and have a male predilection. Patients can present with pain, hemobilia, or symptoms of rupture; the latter can occur into either the peritoneum or GI tract.

Renal artery aneurysms are also more commonly asymptomatic. They can develop because of atherosclerosis, fibromuscular dysplasia, vasculitis, trauma, or iatrogenic causes. In addition to rupture, other potential complications include arterial thrombosis and distal embolization. As with splenic artery aneurysms, young, pregnant women are at higher risk for rupture (Fig. 13-63).

Acute End Organ Ischemia

Like mesenteric ischemia, infarcts of the visceral organs can result from insults to either the arterial supply or venous drainage. They occur across a wide range of demographics and can be due to a wide range of causes. Visceral organ infarcts resulting from arterial insults are usually the result of thrombus or embolus, whereas venous insults are usually the result of thrombosis. The unique blood supply of each organ determines its susceptibility to infarction. The spleen and kidneys are more susceptible to infarction due to their single blood supply and relative lack of collaterals compared to the liver and pancreas. The liver with its dual arterial and portal venous blood supply is relatively protected from infarction, as is the pancreas because of its rich collateral circulation.

Generally infarction manifests as wedge-shaped areas of hypoattenuation with the base at the periphery of the organ and the apex toward hilum of the organ or as complete devascularization of the organ manifest by complete loss of enhancement on CECT (Fig. 13-64).

Bleeding Caused by Anticoagulants

Hemorrhage is a recognized risk factor of anticoagulation therapy with subdiaphragmatic spontaneous bleeding not an uncommon presentation. But coagulopathy in any form, either drug induced or due to bleeding diatheses, can present with spontaneous hemorrhage. Most physicians will be familiar with retroperitoneal hemorrhage due to coagulopathy, but coagulopathy-related hemorrhage can occur in nearly any compartment in the abdomen. Body wall muscular compartments, such as the rectus sheath and iliopsoas muscles, are fairly common sites for such bleeding, but other locations of hemorrhage, including the perirenal space, within the collecting systems, and within the bowel wall, are known to occur. Abdominal CT has long been accepted as the examination to evaluate for retroperitoneal hemorrhage, and the interpreting radiologist should consider these relatively more rare locations. On noncontrast CT the "hematocrit sign," a cellular-fluid level, is both a highly sensitive and specific sign for coagulopathy-related

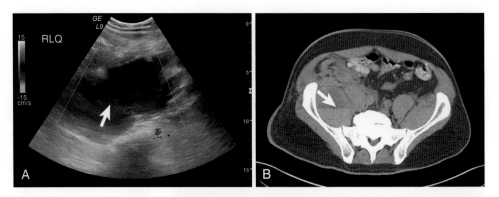

Figure 13-65 A 52-year-old man on anticoagulation with large spontaneous right retroperitoneal hematoma. **A,** "Hematocrit" sign seen on ultrasonography (US) *(arrow)*. **B,** Noncontrast computed tomography (CT) with layering hyperattenuating blood products displacing the right iliopsoas muscle medially *(arrow)*.

hemorrhage (Fig. 13-65). Contrast enhanced CT is not necessary to make the diagnosis but will aid in the detection of active extravasation, which, if present, is usually venous.

One potential diagnostic dilemma is the presentation of retroperitoneal hemorrhage in a patient with an AAA and on anticoagulant therapy, where it is necessary to determine if the hemorrhage is coagulopathy related or due to a ruptured aneurysm. Some authors have suggested that the presence of the hematocrit sign is the most useful indicator that coagulopathy is the source with additional signs favoring coagulopathy including isolated iliopsoas hemorrhage or concomitant rectus sheath hemorrhage. In this particular case, CECT may also aid in differentiating the two by allowing more complete assessment of the aorta for the classic signs of rupture, to be discussed in the next section. If detected on CECT, the location of active extravasation is also useful, with coagulopathy-related extravasation usually remote from the aorta, whereas active extravasation from a ruptured aortic aneurysm is usually seen at the site of rupture/leak.

■ RUPTURE OF NONTRAUMATIC ANEURYSMS OF THE ABDOMINAL AORTA AND ILIAC ARTERIES

Ruptured AAA is the fourteenth leading cause of death in the United States. Most AAAs are usually asymptomatic and detected incidentally. They are four to six times more common in men than women. Risk for AAA rupture has been associated with smoking, hypertension, and size and expansion rate of the aneurysm. The Joint Council of the American Association for Vascular Surgery and Society for Vascular Surgery estimates the following AAA annual rupture risks: less than 4.0 cm, 0%; 4 to 4.9 cm, 0.5% to 5%; 5 to 5.9 cm, 3% to 15%; 6 to 6.9 cm, 10% to 20%; 7 to 7.9 cm, 20% to 40%; and greater than or equal to 8 cm, 30% to 50%. Other acute complications of AAA include peripheral embolization of plaque causing ischemia and acute aortic occlusion.

Most AAAs occur between the renal arteries and above the iliac arteries. A diameter of 2.9 cm or a diameter 1 to 1.5 times the diameter of the aorta at the renal artery level (usually 2.0 cm) is diagnostic of an AAA. The American Heart Association and the American College of Cardiology recommend ultrasonographic monitoring of AAAs under 4 cm every 2 to 3 years and for those that are 4 to 5.4 cm, US or

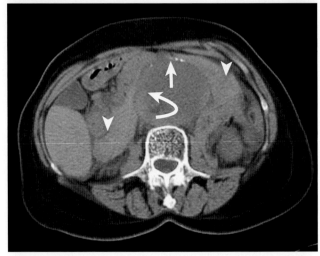

Figure 13-66 An 82-year-old woman with a ruptured abdominal aortic aneurysm (AAA) larger than 7cm with discontinuous intimal calcifications *(arrow)*, intramural hematoma *(curved arrow)*, and large retroperitoneal hematoma *(arrowheads)* on noncontrast computed tomography (CT).

CT every 6 to 12 months. Surgery is recommended for symptomatic aneurysms of any size and for asymptomatic AAAs greater than or equal to 5.5 cm. Abdominal aortic aneurysms that expand 0.5 cm or more in 6 months should also be repaired because they are associated with a high risk for rupture.

Patients with rupture complain of abdominal and/or back pain and have a pulsatile abdominal mass on examination. Fifty percent of patients that have suffered a ruptured AAA reach the hospital alive, but of those, 50% will not survive repair. The imaging modality of choice for patients with suspected ruptured AAA is noncontrast CT; intravenous contrast is administered if the diagnosis is not established on the noncontrast study. Abdominal aortic aneurysms rupture into the retroperitoneum (Fig. 13-66), mostly commonly in the posterolateral aspect of the aorta; hematomas are usually large and accumulate in the pararenal space, perirenal space, or both. Less commonly, the rupture causes intraperitoneal bleeding and exsanguination. Signs of impending aneurysm rupture include acute expansion and intramural bleeding (seen as a hyperattenuating crescent in the wall of the aneurysm). Other suspicious signs of contained rupture include poor definition of the posterior aortic wall and an interrupted ring of calcification in the aortic wall.

Endovascular Repair of Abdominal Aortic Aneurysm

Endovascular stent grafting of the aorta has become a good option for poor surgical candidates, replacing open repair. Endovascular aneurysm repair (EVAR) has a lower mortality than open repair of an AAA. The goal of EVAR, similar to open repair, is to exclude the aneurysm from circulation, preventing enlargement and therefore decreasing the risk for rupture. A transfemoral approach is usually used for EVAR. The criteria to stent an AAA and obtain adequate seal are as follows: less than 4 cm aortic diameter, less than 3 cm aneurysm neck diameter, and neck length of at least 1 cm.

Many imaging modalities have been proven useful in diagnosing the complications of EVAR. Ultrasonography generally requires the use of contrast air bubbles to diagnose an endoleak. Plain films are useful in the evaluation of stent-graft migration, component separation, and structural abnormalities. Computed tomography angiography with intravenous but no oral contrast should be performed in symptomatic patients who previously underwent EVAR. With dual energy–dual source CT, virtual nonenhanced images may be generated from the CE delayed-phase images, decreasing radiation exposure to the patient. Noncontrast CT images help identify areas of increased attenuation before the administration of contrast that may mimic a complication of EVAR. Magnetic resonance imaging offers the additional ability to evaluate patients suffering from renal disease and CT contrast allergies. Magnetic resonance angiography time-resolved techniques can be used to characterize endoleaks. Digital subtraction angiography is usually reserved for therapeutic interventions.

Nontraumatic Iliac Artery Aneurysm

Ten percent to 20% of AAAs involve the iliac arteries. Isolated iliac artery aneurysms (IAAs) are rare. Iliac artery aneurysms are usually asymptomatic and found incidentally. They tend to be symptomatic when they are large and result in mass effect on adjacent structures. Seventy percent occur in the common segment, 20% are internal, and 10% are seen in the external artery. Repair is recommended for symptomatic IAA of any size and asymptomatic aneurysm of greater than or equal to 4 cm. It has been shown that it is rare for an IAA less than 3 cm in diameter to rupture, but there is a high risk for rupture with an IAA greater than or equal to 5 cm. Acute IAA rupture causes acute severe abdominal pain and shock. Treatment of symptomatic IAA can be performed via open or endovascular repair. Complications after endovascular repair of IAAs are similar to those after EVAR. The same imaging modalities and protocols used for AAAs, preoperatively and postoperatively, can be used to evaluate IAAs.

■ COMPLICATIONS ENCOUNTERED WITH ENDOVASCULAR ANEURYSM REPAIR AND USE OF IMAGING FOR DIAGNOSIS

Many complications can occur after EVAR for AAA, including stent-graft migration, endoleak, aortoduodenal

fistula, aortovenous fistula, wound problems, graft infection, embolism, pseudoaneurysm, stent-graft thrombosis, iliac artery injury, branch occlusion causing ischemia, and structural defects of the stent-graft. Wound problems such as hematoma, infection, necrosis, and lymph fistulas occur commonly. Complications during EVAR placement can also occur, the most lethal being vessel rupture leading to exsanguination. Any of these can cause a patient to seek emergency medical attention.

Graft infections, which are rare but difficult to manage, usually present as sepsis (acute or chronic) or as GI bleeding. Imaging of an infected graft will demonstrate periaortic fluid collections, perigraft soft tissue thickening, and surrounding or internal gas. Infection may spread to involve the adjacent spine, paraspinal musculature, adjacent bowel, and even lead to pseudoaneurysm formation. Secondary aortoduodenal fistulas are also rare. Most occur in the third portion of the duodenum just proximal to the graft typically 3 to 5 years after surgery. These patients may present with GI bleeding, which may be intermittent or acute and fatal. On CT or MRI, intravenous contrast filling of the duodenum and periaortic free air are suggestions of a fistula. Aortovenous fistulas may also develop after EVAR. These require prompt repair to prevent irreversible hyperdynamic (high output) heart failure. Patients present with tachycardia, heart failure, lower extremity edema, abdominal thrill, renal failure, pelvic venous hypertension, and peripheral ischemia. On CECT, aortoenteric and arteriovenous fistulas (AVFs) are generally easy to diagnose: there is periaortic inflammation and abnormal accumulation of contrast in the duodenum or early filling of the IVC.

■ ACUTE GASTROINTESTINAL BLEEDING

Acute GI hemorrhage is an important cause of emergency hospital admissions, with substantial mortality ranging from 8% to 16%. Bleeding may originate from the upper or lower GI tract depending on the location proximal or distal to the ligament of Treitz. Peptic ulcer disease accounts for more than 50% of upper GI bleeding, whereas colonic diverticula and angiectasia are the most common causes of lower GI bleeding. The clinical presentation is often misleading. For example, melena can come from the upper GI tract in cases with rapid bleeding. Conversely, melena can be found in patients with lower GI bleeding because of slow peristalsis. Rapid identification of the source and cause of bleeding is essential in the initial evaluation of patients presenting with acute GI bleeding. The main diagnostic modalities used in the evaluation of patients with acute GI hemorrhage are endoscopy, CT angiography, radionuclide scintigraphy, and conventional angiography.

Endoscopy

Upper endoscopy is the diagnostic modality of choice for acute upper GI bleeding. Endoscopy has a high sensitivity and specificity for locating and identifying sites of bleeding in the upper GI tract. In addition, once a bleeding lesion has been identified, therapeutic interventions can achieve hemostasis and prevent recurrent bleeding in most patients. Early endoscopy (within 24 hours) is recommended for most patients with acute upper GI bleeding, although whether early endoscopy affects outcomes and resource use is uncertain.

A colonoscopy is generally required for patients with hematochezia and normal upper endoscopy finding unless there is an alternative source for the bleeding. Despite the relatively low yield, colonoscopies are routinely performed in patients with melena and a normal upper endoscopy findings because many right-sided colonic lesions may present with melena. Even if bowel preparation is adequate, urgent colonoscopy in the evaluation of acute lower GI bleeding is more difficult given potential poor visibility of the colon due to the presence of intraluminal blood clots.

Computed Tomography Angiography

Computed tomography angiography is an accurate, rapid, noninvasive diagnostic alternative in the initial evaluation of patients presenting to the ED with acute GI bleeding, and it is increasingly being used in this setting. The examination can be performed when endoscopy fails to reveal the bleeding source or may also be used as an initial diagnostic method in the evaluation of acute GI hemorrhage, particularly in patients presenting with an acute episode of lower GI bleeding. Computed tomography angiography can demonstrate the presence and location of active bleeding or recent hemorrhage, as well as the potential cause, in the majority of patients. In a recent meta-analysis the sensitivity of CT angiography for detecting active acute GI hemorrhage was 85.2%, and the overall specificity was 92.1%.

Technique

No oral contrast or fluid is administered. The anatomic coverage includes from the diaphragm to the inferior pubic ramus to encompass the entire rectum. A preliminary unenhanced examination is performed to depict any preexisting intraluminal hyperattenuating material. These unenhanced scans are obtained using a low-dose radiation technique. The initial scan is followed by a biphasic acquisition in the arterial and portal phases. The patient is injected intravenously with 100 to 120 mL of contrast media (350 mg of iodine per millimeter or higher) at 4 mL/sec, followed immediately by a 40 mL 0.9% saline bolus at 4 mL/sec through an 18- or 20-gauge catheter located in an antecubital vein. An automated triggering device is used with the region of interest placed in the proximal abdominal aorta and a threshold to start the injection of 150 HU. The isotropic data set obtained in current-generation multidetector CT (MDCT) scanners allows the routine generation of MPRs and (3-D) reconstructions.

Imaging Findings

Active extravasation of contrast is seen as an intraluminal focal collection or linear "jet" visible in the arterial and/or portal phase but not in the unenhanced scan (Fig. 13-67). Hyperattenuating material in the noncontrast scan usually indicates recent, nonactive bleeding. However, care should be taken to differentiate these hyperattenuating areas from potential pitfalls, including suture material, clips, foreign bodies, orally administered pharmaceutical drugs, cone beam artifacts, and fecaliths or retained contrast material within a diverticulum.

Nuclear Scintigraphy

Radionuclide imaging can be used for the diagnosis of GI bleeding and for guiding angiographic intervention. Either technetium Tc 99m sulfur colloid or tagged RBCs can be used as the radiotracer. Sulfur colloid imaging is very sensitive and can detect bleeding rates as low as 0.05 to 0.1 mL/min (angiography realistically requires a bleeding rate of about 1 mL/min). However, the imaging time is markedly limited at no more than 10 minutes because of rapid clearance from the intravascular space by the reticuloendothelial system. Unless the patient is actively bleeding at the time of the study, the site of hemorrhage will likely not be detected.

The main advantage of using tagged RBCs is that the agent remains in the intravascular space for at least 24 hours and thus is excellent for imaging intermittent or slow bleeds. Liver and spleen activity is visualized but to a lesser degree than with sulfur colloid imaging and rarely obscures a bleeding focus. The tagged RBC examination can detect bleeding rates as low as 0.1 to 0.5 mL/min and has a reported sensitivity of 91% and a specificity of 95% for GI bleeding. The tagged RBC

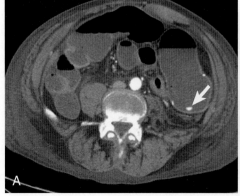
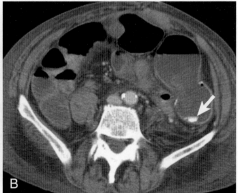

Figure 13-67 *Patient following colectomy presenting with acute hematochezia.* **A,** Computed tomography (CT) angiography shows a linear jet of active bleeding at the anastomosis with contrast pooling on the portal venous phase *(arrow).* **B,** Subsequently confirmed with angiography *(arrow)* and treated with embolization (not shown). (Courtesy Jorge A. Soto, MD.)

study is considered positive if there is a focus of activity that changes in location and increases in intensity over time (Fig. 13-68). Small bowel bleeds frequently show only brief accumulation with rapid dissipation because of marked small bowel motility. Glucagon may sometimes be useful in aiding detection of small bowel bleeding by producing smooth muscle relaxation. One study suggested a prognostic value of the tagged RBC examination: those patients with normal scan results or delayed positive scan with abnormal localization after 1 hour of imaging did not require surgery or excessive blood transfusions. Although it is widely accepted that scintigraphy has high sensitivity for detecting moderate or severe bleeding, it has some limitations such as the inability to localize the precise source of bleeding and to determine its cause.

Angiography

In the majority of patients with upper or lower GI bleeding, the bleeding either resolves spontaneously or can be controlled by medical and/or endoscopic therapy. However, persistent or recurrent bleeding occurs in 7% to 16% of patients with upper GI bleeding and in up to 25% of patients with lower GI bleeding. Such patients may require angiographic intervention to locate and treat the source of bleeding. Arterial GI bleeding can be controlled by the selective arterial infusion of vasoconstrictive drugs, embolization of the bleeding vessel, or a combination of these techniques.

Locating the site of bleeding usually begins with the evaluation of the celiac artery or SMA for upper GI bleeding, whereas the SMA or IMA is evaluated when lower GI bleeding is suspected. Contrast extravasation into the bowel lumen is considered definitive evidence of a bleeding site. Indirect evidence includes visualization of an aneurysm or pseudoaneurysm, filling of spaces outside the bowel lumen (diverticula), early draining vessels (angiodysplasia), neovascularity (tumors), AVFs, and hyperemia (colitis).

Once the site of bleeding is identified, angiographic therapy can be delivered. Vasopressin causes generalized vasoconstriction and produces a rapid reduction in

local blood flow that gradually returns to normal several hours after the infusion has been terminated. The goal is to decrease the perfusion pressure and permit stable clot formation at the bleeding site. However, rebleeding once vasopressin has been stopped is common, and its use can be associated with significant ischemic events. Embolization works by mechanically occluding the arterial blood supply to the bleeding site. Materials used for embolization are either temporary (Gelfoam) or permanent (microcoils). Embolization is mainly indicated for patients in whom vasopressin infusion failed or who have active bleeding occurring at a rate greater than 0.5 mL/min visible angiographically and amenable to percutaneous access, pyloric or duodenal sources of bleeding, hemobilia, bleeding into pancreatic pseudocysts or from visceral artery aneurysms, underlying coagulopathy, or bleeding after attempted endoscopic intervention.

■ ACUTE VENOUS THROMBOSIS

This section will focus mainly on the imaging findings and end-organ manifestations associated with IVC thrombosis. Acute renal vein thrombosis is discussed in Chapter 13, section 5, "Renal and adrenal emergencies"; acute hepatic vein thrombosis and portal/mesenteric vein thrombosis are discussed in Chapter 13, section 8, "hepatic inflammation and infections".

Inferior Vena Cava

Although there are different causes of IVC thrombosis, the wide variety of these conditions all relate in one or more ways to Virchow's classic description. Inferior vena cava thrombosis can result from malignancies, extrinsic compression, hypercoagulable states, and propagation of a deep venous thrombosis or iatrogenic causes related to the presence of a central venous catheter, placement of an IVC filter, or liver transplantation. Membranous obstruction (partial or complete) of the IVC and/or the hepatic veins is an unusual but potentially treatable cause in the United States but is much more common in South Africa, India, and Asia. These weblike lesions

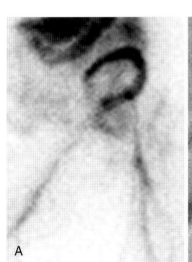

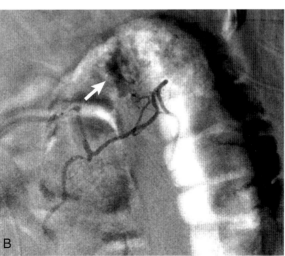

Figure 13-68 A 63-year-old woman with acute lower gastrointestinal (GI) bleed. **A,** Radionuclide scan is positive in the region of the splenic flexure. **B,** Angiogram performed subsequently shows extravasation from a third-order branch of the inferior mesenteric artery (IMA) *(arrow)*.

are usually found just cephalad to the entrance of the right hepatic vein into the IVC and may be the result of a congenital anomaly. However, they are more often attributable to an acquired thrombotic process such as a myeloproliferative disorder.

Renal and Adrenal Emergencies

Suzanne T. Chong, Ania Z. Kielar, Peter S. Liu, and Michael B. Mazza

The adrenal glands and kidneys are paired retroperitoneal organs that serve critical physiologic functions. When the physiologic functions of either the adrenal glands or kidneys are disrupted, the results can be catastrophic and life threatening. In evaluating the adrenal glands and kidneys in the acute but nontraumatic setting, it is important to be aware of conditions that need to be urgently addressed and simultaneously be able to recognize conditions that do not necessarily constitute emergencies but may result in harm to the patient if not communicated to the ordering physician. With this in mind, this chapter will address adrenal and renal diseases that represent acute emergencies and those that are nonemergent but are commonly identified in ED settings and that require further evaluation.

■ ADRENAL NONTRAUMATIC EMERGENCIES

Situated along the superior aspect of the kidneys, the adrenal glands are inverted Y- or V-shaped organs composed of a body and two limbs with an outer layer cortex and inner medulla. The body of the adrenal gland is made up of mostly cortical tissue that produces glucocorticoids and mineralocorticoids, whereas the limbs are mostly medullary tissue and produce norepinephrine and epinephrine. The adrenal glands are important endocrine organs that produce hormones that help the body cope with infections, hypotension, and stresses such as surgery. The most common nontraumatic emergencies that affect the adrenal glands are hemorrhage and infection, and both can result in acute primary adrenal insufficiency. Adrenal tumors do not typically need to be emergently addressed but need to be communicated to the ordering physician.

Adrenal Insufficiency

Primary adrenal insufficiency is a life-threatening condition that may result in severe hypotensive crisis and decreased mentation and represents the most catastrophic of all possible nontraumatic adrenal emergencies. Timely diagnosis is critical so that replacement glucocorticoids and mineralocorticoids can be immediately started to avert hemodynamic collapse. If time permits, a corticotropin simulation test may be

administered to confirm the diagnosis; serum cortisol levels fail to increase normally in response to the challenge when primary adrenal insufficiency is present. In cases of suspected acute primary adrenal insufficiency, diagnostic imaging can be performed to evaluate patients for adrenal hemorrhage and infection, the two most common causes.

Adrenal Hemorrhage

Bilateral adrenal hemorrhage is the most frequent cause of acute adrenal insufficiency. This is most commonly due to Waterhouse-Friderichsen syndrome, a syndrome related to overwhelming sepsis, classically from meningococcal infection although other pathogens have been implicated (including *Staphylococcus* species), and anticoagulation therapy (heparin, warfarin). Thrombocytopenia is a complication of heparin therapy that can cause adrenal vein thrombosis, leading to the leakage or rupture of numerous small venous channels in the adrenal glands with resultant adrenal hemorrhage and subsequent hemodynamic collapse. Antiphospholipid antibody syndrome is caused by circulating antibodies to a plasma glycoprotein and is characterized by recurrent arterial and venous clots that can lead to adrenal venous thrombosis and resultant adrenal hemorrhage. Patients with antiphospholipid antibody syndrome may also rarely develop adrenal infarctions that can lead to acute primary adrenal insufficiency, in the absence of adrenal hemorrhage.

Acute or subacute adrenal hemorrhage results in enlargement of the adrenal glands (Fig. 13-69). Hemorrhage can appear quite masslike, mimicking other adrenal masses. On CT, acute hemorrhage is hyperattenuating, measuring approximately 45 to 70 HU. This characteristic high attenuation is easiest to recognize on non–contrast-enhanced CT, where the attenuation-altering effects of iodinated contrast material are absent. On MRI, which is only occasionally performed in the emergency setting, subacute hemorrhage (hemorrhage imaged approximately 7 days to 7 weeks after onset) is typically hyperintense relative to the liver on T1- and T2-weighted images due to the presence of methemoglobin (see Fig. 13-69). After 7 weeks the MRI appearance of blood becomes peripherally hypointense, reflecting hemosiderin deposition and formation of a fibrous capsule. Over time, adrenal calcifications may form, often easier to recognize on CT than MRI.

Post-contrast images with CT or MRI are used to detect an underlying mass as the cause of hemorrhage. Although adrenal tumors can hemorrhage, these are unlikely to result in acute adrenal insufficiency. Most (80%) adrenal tumors are unilateral, and greater than 90% of adrenal tissue needs to be destroyed in order for the symptoms of adrenal insufficiency to become manifest.

Adrenal Infection

Adrenal infections are the second most common cause of primary adrenal insufficiency in the United States.

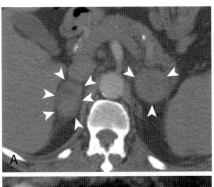
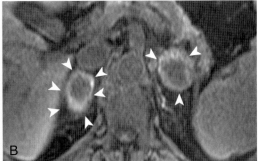
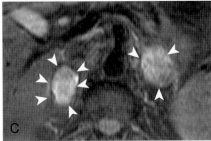

Figure 13-69 A to C, Masslike enlargement of the adrenal glands *(arrowheads)* due to spontaneous hemorrhage. Some of the increased attenuation on the nonenhanced computed tomographic (CT) image has corresponding hyperintensity. T1-weighted image (**B**) and T2-weighted image (**C**) are consistent with subacute hemorrhage.

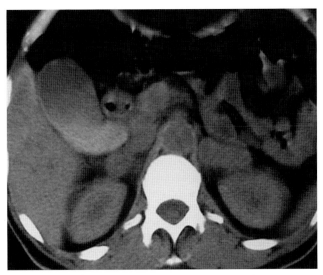

Figure 13-70 Axial contrast-enhanced computed tomography (delayed phase) demonstrates bilateral enlargement of the adrenal glands in a patient with adrenal insufficiency. Tuberculous adrenalitis was diagnosed with culture of a CT–guided aspirate. (Case courtesy Jorge A. Soto, MD.)

With infection the onset of adrenal insufficiency is usually insidious rather than acute. Causative infections include tuberculosis, histoplasmosis, and blastomycosis. Tuberculous adrenalitis has seen resurgence because of AIDS. Cytomegalovirus adrenalitis can also affect patients with advanced AIDS and may be lethal. Acute adrenal abscesses are rare but have also been reported in patients with AIDS.

On CT and MRI, adrenalitis usually results in adrenal enlargement with peripherally enhancing, low-attenuation lesions representing areas of caseous necrosis (Fig. 13-70). Adrenalitis typically involves both adrenal glands in an asymmetric fashion. There may be associated inflammatory changes or edema in the adjacent fat. Calcifications may form over time but are not specific for adrenal infection.

Adrenal Tumors

Adrenal tumors are commonly encountered in daily practice, with adrenal nodules detected incidentally on 5% of all abdominal CT scans in patients without known malignancy or endocrine dysfunction. Thus basic familiarity with the imaging characteristics of the most common adrenal tumors and appropriate follow-up imaging recommendations is essential for any radiologist practicing in the ED. Although most adrenal nodules found incidentally will represent benign adenomas, lesions that are of soft tissue attenuation, irregular, heterogeneous, and exceed 4 cm in diameter must be considered suspicious for malignancy, and the appropriate workup should be recommended. Recommendations for follow-up management of an incidental adrenal nodule can be found at the American College of Radiology (ACR) website according to the ACR Appropriateness Criteria for an incidentally discovered adrenal mass (http://www.acr.org/Quality-Safety/Appropriateness-Criteria).

■ RENAL NONTRAUMATIC EMERGENCIES

The kidneys are composed of an outer layer cortex and an inner layer medulla and surrounded by a capsule. The perinephric space refers to the anterior and posterior perinephric fat that surrounds the kidney and is demarcated from the pararenal space by the Gerota fascia. The kidneys are highly specialized organs that serve filtration, endocrine, and excretory functions by maintaining electrolyte and acid-base balance; secreting key hormones such as erythropoietin, calcitriol, and renin; and removing waste products from the blood. Renal nontraumatic emergencies can be divided into four main categories: (1) acute obstruction (urolithiasis), (2) inflammatory/infectious processes, (3) vascular abnormalities (including renal artery dissection and renal infarctions), and (4) renal tumors that present urgently (usually due to hemorrhage) or that are detected incidentally in patients being imaged for other reasons in the emergency setting.

Urolithiasis

Urolithiasis is commonly encountered in the ED. It is a significant health problem, costing approximately $2.1 billion annually in the United States. Approximately 2% to 3% of the population will develop urinary tract calculi, with up to 12% experiencing an obstructing urinary tract stone in their lifetime. Recurrence rates in this subset of patients with renal stones approach 50%. Men are three times more likely to be affected than women. Urgent intervention is required when patients with obstructing stones have intractable pain, infected hydronephrosis, or high-grade obstruction of a solitary or transplant kidney (which can result in anuria and azotemia). Patients with urolithiasis classically present with acute, colicky flank pain that may radiate to the groin. As the obstructing stone descends toward the ureterovesical junction, the pain can radiate toward the urethra and symptoms may then include dysuria and urinary urgency and frequency, mimicking cystitis. On physical examination, patients with obstructing stones may have tenderness along the costovertebral angle or in a lower quadrant of the abdomen. Although hematuria is present in the majority of patients with acute renal stones, it is not infrequently absent. Therefore the absence or presence of hematuria is generally not used to determine whether a stone may be present.

Noncontrast CT is the best imaging test for the detection of renal stones with sensitivities, specificities, and accuracies reported from various studies of 97% to 100%, 94% to 98%, and 96% to 98%, respectively, clearly outperforming conventional radiography and replacing intravenous urography, the preferred test in the past. Abdominal radiographs detect only 45% to 59% of urinary tract stones. Gray-scale US is inadequate for the detection of ureteral stones, with reported sensitivities of 11% to 24%. On color Doppler, the "twinkling" artifact, described as a focus of alternating colors with or without a comet tail observed when insonating certain rough surfaces, improves the sonographic sensitivity for the detection of renal stones to approximately 90%. Computed tomography is rapid, does not require intravenous contrast material administration, can detect nonstone causes of flank pain, and is cost-effective. Recent improvements in CT hardware and software have helped to minimize patient exposure to ionizing radiation, an important improvement because many patients with urolithiasis are young and some patients will undergo multiple CT examinations in their lifetimes because of recurrent symptoms (see discussion on radiation reduction methods in Chapter 1).

The most specific CT sign of urolithiasis is direct visualization of the stone in the ureter. Thin-section CT (images less than 5-mm thickness reconstructed at less

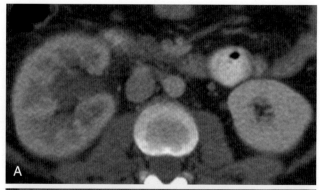

Figure 13-71 **A** and **B,** Contrast-enhanced computed tomography demonstrates prominent right renal enlargement, perinephric fat infiltration, urothelial thickening and enhancement, and a delayed nephrogram because of an obstructing calculus at the ureterovesical junction (**B,** *arrow*). CECT was performed in this patient who presented with nonspecific abdominal symptoms of suspected gastrointestinal (GI) origin. No other CT abnormalities were identified.

than 5-mm intervals) allows the radiologist to track the ureter confidently along its entirety and detect renal calculi as small as 2 to 3 mm. Obstructing ureteral calculi tend to lodge at the three points of anatomic ureteral narrowing: the ureterovesical junction (most commonly), the ureteropelvic junction, and the pelvic brim. Thus these regions should be evaluated carefully. The vast majority of renal stones are hyperattenuating on CT, making them easily visible. Dual-energy CT can help distinguish stone composition (calcium, uric acid, struvite, and cystine) with high accuracy, which can be important for clinical management; for example, uric acid stones can be managed with oral medications, whereas struvite stones are amenable to fragmentation by lithotripsy, but calcium-based cystine calculi are relatively resistant to lithotripsy. In very rare instances, urease-producing bacteria can lead to the production of matrix stones of soft tissue attenuation (isodense to the kidney and ureter) and therefore difficult or impossible to visualize. Indinavir, a protease inhibitor used to treat HIV, can accumulate in the urinary tract and produce soft tissue attenuation stones but is currently used very rarely. A more popular protease inhibitor today, atazanavir, can crystallize in the urinary tract and also result in soft tissue attenuation stones. Secondary signs are often extremely helpful in making the diagnosis and include renal collecting system and ureteral dilatation, perinephric and/or periureteral edema, and enlargement and decreased attenuation of the obstructed kidney (Fig. 13-71). Urothelial thickening may also be present but is nonspecific, usually indicating concomitant inflammation or infection. Urine in the obstructed collecting system is usually of water attenuation. Pus and/or hemorrhage, when present, may increase the attenuation of the urine in the obstructed collecting

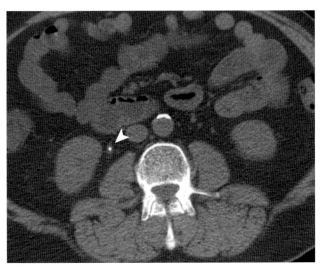

Figure 13-72 A hyperdense calcification (calculus) surrounded by a rim of soft tissue (ureter) referred to as the *rim sign (arrowhead)*.

system and ureter and should be noted when present. One of the biggest challenges of interpreting renal stone CT images is differentiating renal stones from calcified phleboliths, the latter being benign venous calcifications that may occur in veins anywhere in the abdomen but are most frequently observed in the pelvis near the distal portions of the ureters. Although coronal reconstructions may be helpful for differentiating ureteral calculi from phleboliths in some patients, even these images may not be diagnostic, especially in patients in whom the distal ureters cannot be identified. This is a particular problem in patients who do not have ureteral dilatation or have minimal retroperitoneal fat. In problematic cases, two other signs have been used: the rim sign and the comet-tail sign. The rim sign refers to a rim of soft tissue surrounding the calcification, a finding only seen around some small ureteral calculi (Fig. 13-72). The comet-tail sign is a triangular or tubular area of soft tissue attenuation, with its apex oriented toward or away from a calcification, a finding representing a venous structure and indicating that the associated calcification is a phlebolith. Unfortunately, both signs are neither highly sensitive nor specific, and they are rarely able to assist the radiologist in determining whether a pelvic calcification is within or merely adjacent to a ureter.

Another problem in interpreting renal stone CT examinations relates to instances in which secondary signs are present, but no obstructing stone is visualized. In these cases, several diagnoses must be considered: a recently passed calculus, an alternative cause of urinary tract obstruction (such as a urothelial cancer), infection, renal vein thrombosis, acute renal emboli, infarction and, most rarely, a low-attenuation stone. Follow-up enhanced CT may be helpful in these instances.

Finally, all stones, especially those with high attenuation, can be obscured by excreted contrast material on CECT that is obtained on a delayed basis, after contrast material has been excreted into the renal collecting systems and ureters as is often the case during CT urography.

The likelihood of stone passage and treatment options depends upon the size and location of urinary tract stones. In general, the smaller the stone and the more distally the stone is located, the sooner and more likely it will pass spontaneously. Approximately two thirds of renal stones measuring less than 5 mm on CT will pass spontaneously within 4 weeks. Many ureteral stones can be extracted ureteroscopically; however, some stones may require shock wave lithotripsy.

Nonstone causes of flank pain are present in 12% to 45% of the unenhanced CT studies performed for flank pain due to suspected renal stone. The shared innervation of the genitourinary and GI systems can result in overlap of clinical symptoms, with symptoms from one system referred to the other. Acute pelvic or abdominal conditions may present with symptoms of colicky, flank pain mimicking a renal calculus. Renal capsular distention from hydronephrosis may result in nausea and vomiting. The most common alternative diagnoses made on renal stone CT examinations are adnexal masses, appendicitis, and diverticulitis. Occasionally patients with suspected urinary tract calculi may instead have AAAs (which may be in the process of rupturing) or aortic dissections; the latter may not be apparent on non–contrast-enhanced CT. For this reason, follow-up CECT may be necessary for further evaluation in some patients.

Renal Inflammatory and Infectious Disorders

Acute Pyelonephritis

In most cases, acute pyelonephritis is due to bacterial infections ascending from the bladder and involving the renal parenchyma. Acute pyelonephritis is usually diagnosed based on clinical presentation (flank pain and fevers) and laboratory test results (pyuria and leukocytosis). Imaging is generally reserved for patients with acute pyelonephritis who do not respond well to appropriate antibiotic therapy, such as persistent fevers after 72 hours or rapid recurrence of symptoms. Complications such as urinary tract obstruction or abscess should be suspected in these cases. Factors that predispose patients to developing complications include advanced age, diabetes, and immunosuppression. These complications usually can be easily identified on any cross-sectional imaging study. Imaging may also help guide subsequent percutaneous interventions.

Acute pyelonephritis is usually unilateral but within the kidney can be diffuse or focal, resulting in different imaging manifestations. At some institutions US is used as the initial imaging test. However, CECT is generally preferred because it has higher sensitivity for the detection of complicated pyelonephritis. On CECT, diffuse acute pyelonephritis produces a classic "striated nephrogram," in which linear bands of low attenuation, representing the poorly enhancing tubules, alternate with more normally enhancing renal parenchyma (Fig. 13-73). Diffuse acute pyelonephritis may also merely manifest as an enlarged, edematous kidney on either imaging modality. Perinephric infiltration, suggesting inflammation or spread of infection, may be present. Urothelial thickening and enhancement can occur (Fig. 13-74). Uncomplicated pyelonephritis can easily be overlooked on noncontrast CT. Careful inspection of the images may

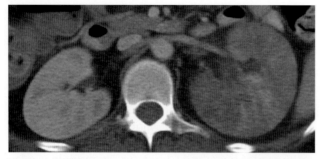

Figure 13-73 Alternating bands of decreased attenuation representing poorly enhancing renal tubules with normally enhancing renal parenchyma in the left kidney consistent with a striated nephrogram on contrast-enhanced computed tomography due to acute pyelonephritis.

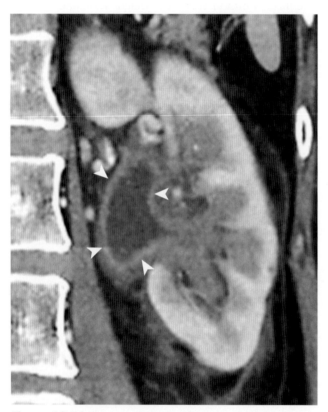

Figure 13-74 Contrast-enhanced computed tomography showing urothelial thickening of the left kidney *(arrowheads)* secondary to acute pyelonephritis in a young woman who presented with fever after having symptoms of a urinary tract infection for an undisclosed period of time.

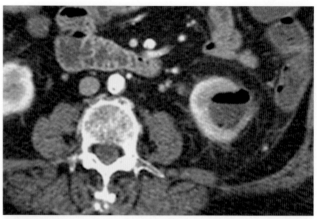

Figure 13-75 Air within a preexisting renal cyst is due to superimposed infection of the cyst rather than air within a renal abscess in a patient with pyelonephritis and perinephric infiltration. The cyst was partially ruptured, with gas and inflammatory changes extending into the perinephric space.

demonstrate subtle perinephric standing, fascial and/or urothelial thickening, or renal enlargement. Occasionally, wedge-shaped or linear areas of high attenuation, which likely represent foci of hemorrhage, may be observed. Focal pyelonephritis appears as a rounded or wedge-shaped area of decreased attenuation in the CE renal parenchyma. The appearance may also be masslike and mimic a solid renal neoplasm.

A complicating renal abscess appears as a focal hypoechoic area without color Doppler flow on US and as a rim-enhancing low-attenuation lesion on CECT. Gas may be present in the abscess in rare instances (Fig. 13-75). Calyceal or collecting system rupture may occur (Fig. 13-76). Pyelosinus extravasation allows the infection to spread into the perinephric, paranephric, and retroperitoneal spaces.

One of the challenges in establishing the diagnosis of pyelonephritis is that CT findings are nonspecific. Glomerulonephritis and interstitial nephritis due to noninfectious causes such as sarcoidosis or medications or immune or metabolic-related conditions may have similar appearances, with areas of low attenuation in the renal parenchyma. Renal enlargement may be caused by lymphoma. Perinephric infiltration may be seen with prior infection, recent trauma, or vascular diseases, including renal vein thrombosis and vasculitides. Thus correlation of the imaging findings with clinical presentation and laboratory values is critical for limiting the diagnostic possibilities.

Acute Pyelitis, Ureteritis, and Pyonephrosis

Pyelitis and ureteritis refer to infections of the renal collecting system and ureter, respectively. These processes produce discernible urothelial thickening on US and CT. Computed tomography may also demonstrate contrast enhancement of the urothelium. Pyonephrosis refers to the accumulation of purulent material in the renal collecting systems and/or ureters. Pyonephrosis usually requires immediate drainage to prevent permanent renal parenchymal destruction and life-threatening sepsis. Obstructing renal calculi are the most common underlying cause of pyonephrosis, but iatrogenic strictures and retroperitoneal fibrosis should be considered as well. On imaging studies, patients with pyonephrosis usually have dilated renal collecting systems and/or ureters with associated urothelial thickening. The infected urine contains echogenic material on US and appears hyperattenuating (relative to sterile urine) on CT. The renal parenchyma may or may not be involved (i.e., concomitant pyelonephritis).

Emphysematous Pyelonephritis

Emphysematous pyelonephritis refers to infection of the renal parenchyma by a gas-producing organism, usually

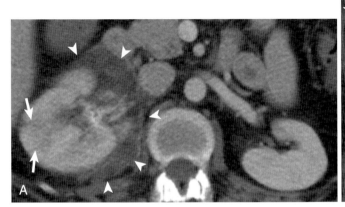

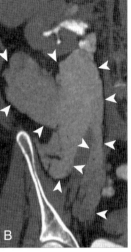

Figure 13-76 A, Enlarged and edematous right kidney with a striated nephrogram *(arrows)* on contrast-enhanced computed tomography in a 28-year-old woman presenting with fever and flank pain. There is a rim-enhancing fluid collection along the medial aspect of the kidney *(arrowheads)*. A defect was identified in the renal pelvis consistent with collecting system rupture. B, Coronal delayed CT image demonstrates a large volume of excreted contrast in the right retroperitoneum *(arrowheads)*, consistent with a large urinoma.

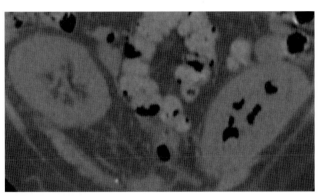

Figure 13-77 Coronal non–contrast-enhanced computed tomography demonstrates gas in the collecting system of the left transplant kidney consistent with emphysematous pyelitis. The right transplant kidney is normal.

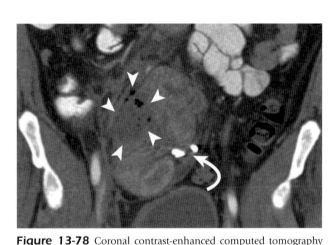

Figure 13-78 Coronal contrast-enhanced computed tomography of focal emphysematous pyelonephritis in a pelvic kidney *(arrowheads)* with gas bubbles that extend beyond the renal capsule into the perinephric space. A ureteral stent is present *(curved arrow)*.

E. coli (70%), *Klebsiella pneumoniae*, or *Proteus mirabilis*. The end result of such infection is parenchymal necrosis. Emphysematous pyelonephritis is usually unilateral and occurs more frequently in women and almost exclusively (80% to 100%) in patients with uncontrolled diabetes. On physical examination a flank mass, representing the affected kidney, can be palpated in 50% of patients with emphysematous pyelonephritis. Crepitus over the flank or thigh may also be present. Rapid progression to overwhelming septicemia is common.

Several classification systems have been proposed to correlate imaging findings with subsequent prognosis and management. The mildest forms of emphysematous pyelonephritis are confined to the collecting system (emphysematous pyelitis) (Fig. 13-77) or form loculated air-fluid collections in or adjacent to the kidneys. These may be amenable to percutaneous drainage. The more severe infections are characterized by spread of gas into the renal parenchyma and can extend into the perinephric and paranephric spaces and often require emergency nephrectomy.

On imaging studies, emphysematous pyelonephritis has a characteristic and often diagnostic appearance.

Conventional radiographs may demonstrate a cluster of mottled lucencies within the kidneys. Ultrasonography shows echogenic foci with "dirty" shadowing within the kidneys. On CT the collections of gas are seen directly as hypoattenuating foci in the renal parenchyma (Fig. 13-78).

Xanthogranulomatous Pyelonephritis

Xanthogranulomatous pyelonephritis (XGP) is a rare chronic infection, typically occurring in middle-age women. Diabetes is a predisposing factor. XGP results from long-standing obstruction of the collecting system, usually from a staghorn calculus, and superimposed chronic bacterial infection that provokes an atypical immune response with accumulation of lipid-laden macrophages (xanthoma cells), eventually causing permanent destruction of renal tissue. The most common bacteria are *E. coli* and *P. mirabilis*. XGP is usually diffuse but can also have focal involvement, resulting in localized renal swelling that may be mistaken for a solid renal mass ("tumefactive" or "pseudotumoral"). Although most patients with XGP have long-standing symptoms, often consisting of low-grade fevers, pain, and weight loss, acute presentations in the ED are not uncommon.

The diagnosis of XGP can often be suggested on imaging studies. Obstructing calculi are usually identified in the affected renal collecting system, often of the staghorn type (Fig. 13-79). The renal pelvis and calyces are dilated, sometimes massively, from a combination of urinary tract obstruction with accumulation of pus and debris in the renal collecting system. The affected kidney is diffusely enlarged but preserves its reniform contour with diffuse parenchymal thinning. Impaired renal function causes delayed or absent excretion of contrast material. Infected loculated fluid collections are frequently found in the adjacent tissues, including in the perinephric space, the anterior and posterior pararenal spaces, and even the psoas muscles. Rarely, renocolic or renocutaneous fistulas may develop.

Human Immunodeficiency Virus–Related Renal Conditions

HIV can affect every organ system in the body, either from the virus directly, from the opportunistic infections or malignancies for which HIV patients are at increased risk, or from side effects of HIV therapy. HIV-associated nephropathy is caused directly by HIV. The relevance of HIV nephropathy in the ED results from the resulting renal failure that precludes administration of intravenous contrast material in many of these patients. Kidneys affected by HIV nephropathy appear enlarged at imaging, with markedly echogenic renal cortex on US and a striated pattern of enhancement at CECT.

Opportunistic fungal infections caused by *Candida* or *Aspergillus* show focal hypoechoic areas on US (hypoattenuating on CT). Fungus balls (mycetomas) can develop in the renal collecting systems and ureters and can obstruct the collecting system. These are seen as filling defects on both US and CT. Multifocal infections need to be differentiated from renal and perirenal neoplasms, especially high-grade non-Hodgkin lymphoma, which are also common in patients infected with HIV. AIDS-related tuberculosis causes asymmetric calcification of the renal cortex and medulla resulting in "partial nephrocalcinosis."

Patients undergoing therapy with highly activated antiretroviral medications have an increased incidence of urolithiasis and can present with acute urinary tract obstruction and flank pain. As previously mentioned,

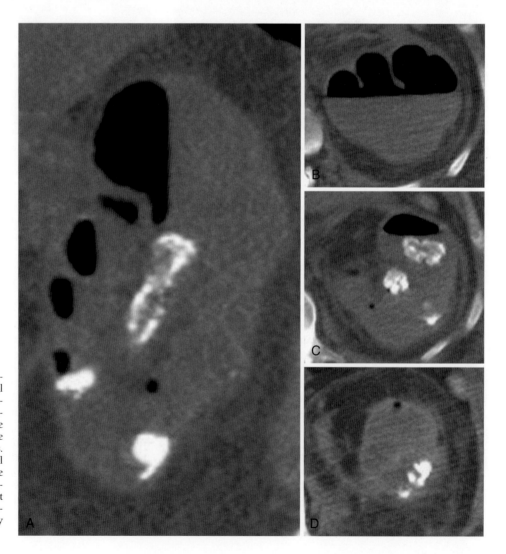

Figure 13-79 A, Staghorn calculus is best seen on the coronal contrast-enhanced computed tomographic image with additional calculi in the lower pole. A to C, Large pockets of gas are present as are perinephric inflammatory changes. Low-attenuation areas in the renal parenchyma are best seen in the lower pole. D, The presence of lipid-laden xanthoma cells in this patient with xanthogranulomatous pyelonephritis (XGP) complicated by emphysematous pyelonephritis.

these stones are composed of drug crystals and may not be hyperattenuating.

Other Renal Infections

Other infections that can involve the kidneys include tuberculosis from hematogenous dissemination, fungal infections such as aspergillosis or candidiasis (usually from colonization of chronic indwelling catheters rather than systemic infections) in which mycetomas can form and potentially obstruct the collecting systems, and echinococcus infection, which is extremely rare. There should be greater suspicion for renal tuberculosis and fungal causes of pyelonephritis in patients who are immunocompromised or immunosuppressed.

Renal Vascular Disorders

Vascular abnormalities of the kidneys that can present acutely include critical renal artery stenosis/occlusion, infarction, spontaneous hemorrhage, vasculitis, renal artery aneurysm, arteriovenous malformations (AVMs), renal artery dissections, and renal vein thrombosis. Acute flank pain, mimicking that of renal calculi, is a common presenting symptom. Cross-sectional imaging with US, CT, and MRI can often identify the specific cause.

Renal Infarction

The most common cause of renal infarction is an acute embolus, usually from a cardiac source in patients with endocarditis or atrial fibrillation. Infarction can also be caused by arterial occlusion from acute dissection, underlying critical artery stenosis caused by atherosclerosis, fibromuscular dysplasia, or vasculitis. Venous infarctions also occur, usually in patients who are in a hypercoagulable state, but are less common.

Patients with acute renal infarction often present with nonspecific symptoms of abdominal pain, flank pain, nausea/vomiting, fever, and leukocytosis. These symptoms overlap with those of renal infection and acute renal obstruction from calculi. Thus, if unenhanced CT does not reveal a calculus in a patient with flank pain, and symptoms cannot be explained, a CECT is usually indicated to assess the renal parenchyma fully.

The typical appearance of a renal infarct on CECT is a geographic or wedge-shaped area of absent or reduced enhancement in an otherwise normal-appearing kidney. Rare variations include global renal infarction and acute cortical necrosis. In global renal infarction, the renal parenchyma fails to enhance, but capsular enhancement is maintained via collateral vessels (Fig. 13-80). Acute cortical necrosis is a form of acute renal failure that can be associated with complications of pregnancy such as septic abortion and placental abruption, as well as other clinical disorders (e.g., sepsis, transfusion reaction, severe dehydration) in which there is ischemic necrosis of the cortex but medullary enhancement is preserved. Nephrographic phase CT is preferred because renal infarcts may be undetectable or indistinguishable from the unenhanced medulla during the early corticomedullary phase of imaging. In the early subacute phase the imaging appearance of

an infarct can be misleading, particularly if an inflammatory reaction occurs causing mass effect in the renal parenchyma and perinephric fat stranding. In such instances the CT appearance can mimic that of focal pyelonephritis or in some instances a renal neoplasm. The cortical rim sign can be a useful imaging feature of infarction distinguishing infarction from infection or neoplasm, although it is not always present. This appearance is caused by contrast enhancement of a thin rim of functioning renal parenchyma supplied by preserved collateral vessels from the renal capsular, peripelvic, and periureteric vessels to the outer rim of the renal cortex. The cortical rim sign is not seen in patients with pyelonephritis or renal masses. Over time, infarcted tissue becomes atrophic, leading to renal parenchymal scars and defects. Other less common sequelae of renal infarction include loss of renal function and hypertension.

Spontaneous Renal Hemorrhage

Spontaneous (nontraumatic) renal hemorrhage may occur because of a number of causes but is usually the result of a ruptured tumor, most commonly a renal cell carcinoma, a simple renal cyst (Table 13-1), or an angiomyolipoma. A renal hematoma occurring after minimal trauma should raise suspicion of a preexistent renal cyst (Fig. 13-81). Spontaneous hemorrhage occurs more commonly in angiomyolipomas, benign fat-containing renal tumors (Fig. 13-82). Large angiomyolipomas (> 4 cm) are at higher risk for spontaneous rupture, and it is recommended that these patients undergo prophylactic transarterial embolization (see Fig. 13-82).

Other causes of spontaneous renal hemorrhage include vascular diseases, such as vasculitis, aneurysm, and anticoagulation. Spontaneous hemorrhage may occur in the subcapsular and perinephric spaces. In anticoagulated patients, hemorrhage may also occur in the suburothelium and renal sinus. Patients with large spontaneous bleeds typically experience acute flank pain mimicking renal colic from a stone.

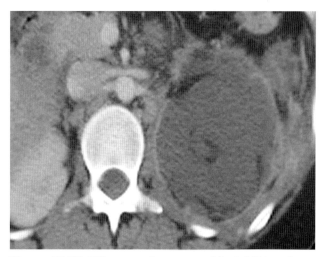

Figure 13-80 Diffuse nonenhancement of the left kidney due to global infarction in a patient with factor V Leiden deficiency. Capsular enhancement is preserved.

Table 13-1   Bosniak Renal Cyst Classification System

Grade	Description	Likelihood of Malignancy	Follow-up Recommendation
I	Well-defined, thin-walled simple cyst measuring < 20 HU; no septa, calcifications, or enhancing soft tissue components	Benign	No further evaluation needed
II	Few, thin septa with perceived enhancement; thin calcification; short segment of slightly thickened calcification; small (<3 cm) cyst that measures above water attenuation (usually 40-90 HU) but otherwise has features diagnostic of a simple cyst	Nearly always benign	No further evaluation needed
IIF	Thin wall, more numerous hairline septa with perceived enhancement; smooth thickened wall or septa; thick, irregular, nodular calcifications; no soft tissue components	Up to 25% are malignant	Initial follow-up at 6 months then annual surveillance for a minimum of 5 years is generally recommended
III	Multiloculated; thickened walls or septa with measurable enhancement	Approximately half are malignant	Most are surgically removed or ablated
IV	Features of grade III plus enhancing soft tissue components adjacent to or separate from the wall or septa	Nearly all are malignant	All are surgically removed or ablated

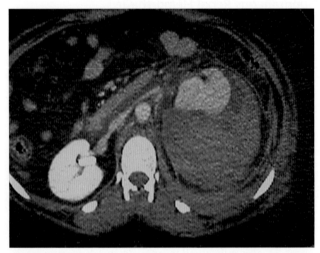

Figure 13-81 Contrast-enhanced computed tomography shows a large left perinephric fluid collection that is a combination of urinoma and hematoma. This was due to a ruptured renal calyx from an obstructing ureteral calculus with subsequent spontaneous hemorrhage in a patient on anticoagulation medication. The patient eventually developed hypertension due to renal compression from the fluid collection (Page kidney). Note the delayed nephrogram in the left kidney, indicating impaired renal function.

Ultrasonography, CT, and MRI may all be used to demonstrate renal hemorrhage. Careful evaluation for an underlying mass lesion is necessary because renal cell carcinoma may be found in half of patients with spontaneous renal hemorrhage. As such, if no immediate cause of renal hemorrhage is apparent, follow-up imaging is warranted. Constrained by the overlying capsule, the reniform contour is characteristically preserved with subcapsular hemorrhage, and the parenchyma may be indented by the blood. Perinephric hematomas are bounded by the Gerota fascia and, when large enough, can indent upon the reniform contour and may displace and rotate the kidney, most often anteromedially. Acute renal hemorrhage appears as echogenic (US) or hyperattenuating (CT) fluid in the subcapsular or perinephric spaces (see Fig. 13-82) that becomes progressively hypoechoic

or hypoattenuating as it ages. On MRI, subacute renal hemorrhage is hyperintense on T1-weighted images and either hypointense or hyperintense on T2-weighted images depending on the age of the subacute hemorrhage. Page kidney is a rare complication of subcapsular fluid collections, most commonly hematomas, in which extrinsic compression of the renal parenchyma causes activation of the renin-angiotensin-aldosterone system and results in systemic hypertension (Fig. 13-83).

Vasculitis
Vasculitis, which refers to leukocytic infiltration of the vessel wall that often leads to necrosis, can involve any vessel in the body. It is usually classified according to the size of the involved vessels as large, medium, or small vessel disease. Small vessel vasculitis, which includes glomerulonephritis, is the most frequent renal vasculitis. This subtype of small vessel vasculitis is usually diagnosed with US-guided core needle biopsy. Polyarteritis nodosa is a progressive vasculitis of medium and small arteries that commonly affects the kidneys and can cause renal ischemia and progressive renal failure. A characteristic finding of polyarteritis nodosa is the presence of multiple small aneurysms and renal infarctions, which can be identified on CT or MRI. Large vessel vasculitis, such as Takayasu arteritis, only rarely affects the kidney directly.

Renal Artery Aneurysm
Renal artery aneurysms have a prevalence of up to 1% in the general population. Most isolated renal artery aneurysms are small, detected incidentally by US, CT, or MRI, and require no treatment. Larger (> 2 cm) aneurysms have a higher risk for spontaneous rupture and emergent presentation with acute flank pain. The risk for rupture is also higher in pregnant patients.

On gray-scale US, renal artery aneurysms may mimic a simple cyst in the renal sinus, but color Doppler interrogation demonstrates characteristic turbulent arterial flow patterns that are absent in simple cysts. On MRI examinations, renal artery aneurysms will demonstrate flow void

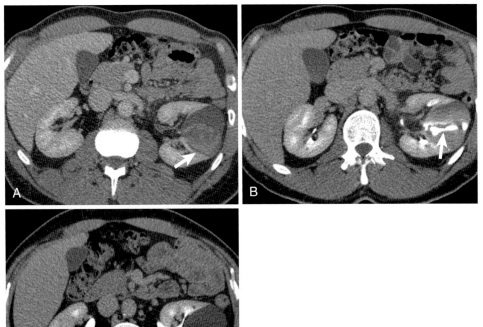

Figure 13-82 Contrast-enhanced computed tomography in the nephrographic (**A**) and urographic (**B**) phases obtained on a patient who presented with pain and gross hematuria after sustaining minor trauma. There is a cystic lesion with high-attenuation dependent clot (**A**, *arrow*) with accumulation of concentrated contrast on the delayed image (**B**, *arrow*). This finding indicates rupture into the collecting system, which explains the gross hematuria. The patient was treated conservatively. **C**, Follow-up CT obtained 2 months later demonstrates a simple cyst and resolution of the hemorrhagic component. (Case courtesy Brian Lucey, MD.)

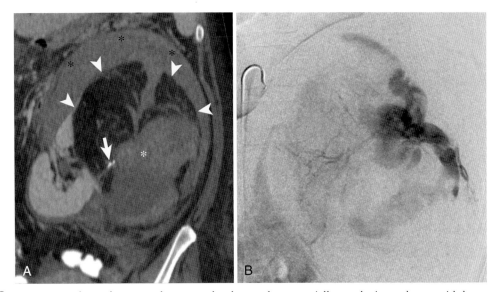

Figure 13-83 **A**, Contrast-enhanced computed tomography shows a large, partially exophytic renal mass with large areas of fat *(white arrowheads)* consistent with an angiomyolipoma that had ruptured. There is a heterogenous area of intratumoral hemorrhage *(white asterisk)* and a perinephric hematoma *(black asterisks)*. Tiny foci of increased attenuation *(white arrow)* are embolism coils, not calcifications. **B**, Catheter angiography shows the large rupture and contrast extravasation. The extensive tumor vascularity is evidenced by the presence of multiple small vessels.

on spin-echo sequences and brisk enhancement with gadolinium-based contrast material. The CT appearance of renal artery aneurysms can be more problematic in some instances. On unenhanced CT, renal artery aneurysms are usually small, rounded, soft tissue attenuation masses. They demonstrate brisk enhancement after

contrast-material administration, a feature that could lead to the misdiagnosis of these lesions as hypervascular renal cancers that project into the renal sinus. Differentiation of renal artery aneurysms from solid masses on CT can be made if the radiologist is careful to consider the possibility of aneurysm when an enhancing spherical lesion is noted in the renal sinus. Also, the presence of peripheral curvilinear calcification in the wall of the aneurysm is a common distinguishing feature. Finally, unlike solid renal masses, renal artery aneurysms will enhance to precisely the same degree as the patent abdominal aortic lumen. In difficult cases US or MRI can resolve the dilemma. Ruptured aneurysms will demonstrate evidence of recent hemorrhage on imaging tests.

Renal Arteriovenous Fistulas and Malformations

Renal AVMs and AVFs account for approximately one quarter of all renal vascular abnormalities, with the latter being more common (usually a result of renal biopsy). Acute clinical presentations include hematuria and flank pain due to rupture. Systolic hypertension and high-output heart failure also occur in patients with larger shunts.

Arteriovenous malformations are often easily detected by US. Color Doppler identifies areas of abnormal blood flow. The arterial phase of CECT is valuable in distinguishing AVMs from hypervascular solid renal masses because the vast majority of AVMs will demonstrate brisk arterial enhancement whereas renal malignancies usually do not enhance to the same degree on arterial phase imaging. Additional useful imaging features of AVMs are diminished focal renal enhancement or cortical atrophy distal to the AVM due to chronic vascular shunting, and early enhancement of the ipsilateral renal vein and IVC. Both CT and MR angiography may identify tangles of vessels. On MRI, flow voids on flow-sensitive sequences also indicate the presence of abnormal blood vessels.

Renal Artery Dissection

Isolated renal artery dissection is rare and most often secondary to trauma when it does occur. The renal artery may be secondarily involved when aortic dissection extends to involve the renal artery (Fig. 13-84). In select cases with acute ischemia or poor renal function, stenting and surgical intervention may be required. Renal artery dissections are usually best depicted on CT. Arterial phase CECT can demonstrates the presence of a dissection flap, often with associated aneurysmal dilation and/or thrombosis of the false lumen. Thin-section, multiplanar reconstructed images during the arterial phase are also helpful in depicting the morphologic changes and extent of the dissection and branch vessel involvement.

Renal Vein Thrombosis

Renal vein thrombosis is a rare cause of acute flank pain. Predisposing conditions include chronic hypercoagulable conditions (e.g., antiphospholipid syndrome, protein S deficiency) and severe, unremitting nephrotic syndrome (e.g., membranous glomerulonephritis). Proteinuria, reduced renal function, and hematuria can also be found at presentation. Two thirds of patients with renal vein thrombosis have bilateral involvement. Anticoagulant therapy is the mainstay of treatment, but invasive procedures, including thrombectomy and catheter-directed thrombolysis, can be attempted. Ultrasonography or

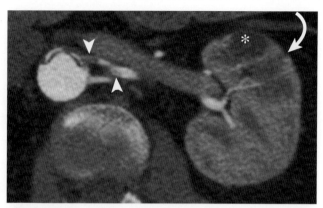

Figure 13-84 Left renal artery dissection caused by propagation of the intimal flaps *(arrowheads)* from the aortic dissection. A small renal infarct *(curved arrow)* is present, as is an incidental renal cyst *(asterisk)*.

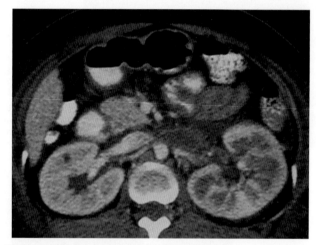

Figure 13-85 Low-attenuation thrombus enlarges and occludes the left renal vein resulting in a delayed nephrogram, which suggests impaired renal function in a patient with nephrotic syndrome. (Case courtesy Jorge A. Soto, MD.)

CECT is used for diagnosing renal vein thrombosis. The affected kidney is generally larger as a result of congestion due to venous outflow obstruction. On US, in the acute phase the kidney is echogenic with loss of corticomedullary differentiation. After the first week there is increasing heterogeneity of the parenchyma due to hemorrhage and either edema or maturation of blood products. Visualization of the thrombus within the renal vein and absent flow on Doppler interrogation are characteristic findings. Lack of collateral venous circulation may lead to renal infarction. Characteristic imaging findings on CT include renal vein enlargement with intraluminal clot, absent or delayed opacification of the renal collecting system, thickening of the renal fascia, and perinephric fat stranding (Fig. 13-85).

■ CONCLUSION

Many nontraumatic conditions can affect the adrenal glands and kidneys, some of which require immediate attention whereas others require further evaluation. A number of imaging modalities can be used to identify and characterize these conditions. Familiarity with the clinical presentation and imaging manifestations of these conditions can help to expedite appropriate patient management.

Acknowledgments

The authors would like to acknowledge with gratitude Sian Jones, MD, for her expert input regarding HIV-related conditions, and Richard H. Cohan, MD, and James H. Ellis, MD, for their generous help with reviewing the manuscript.

Spleen, Peritoneum, and Abdominal Wall

Michael N. Patlas, Mariano Scaglione, Luigia Romano, and Jorge A. Soto

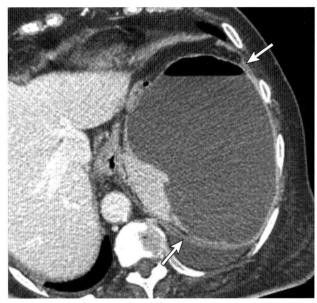

Figure 13-86 Axial contrast-enhanced computed tomographic image shows a large intrasplenic collection with an air-fluid level *(arrows)*. Ultrasonography (US)-guided drainage confirmed the diagnosis of abscess caused by *Staphylococcus aureus.*

■ SPLEEN

Splenic Abscess and Other Acute Infections

Splenic abscess is a rare entity, with an incidence in autopsy series ranging from 0.14% to 0.7%. Splenic abscesses usually develop in patients with sepsis, immunosuppression, poorly controlled diabetes, as a complication of splenic injury, or from contiguous spread of an abdominal infection. Bacterial abscesses are most common, but the prevalence of specific pathogens depends on regional patterns. A review of 67 cases of splenic abscess at a single center in Taiwan reported that 55% of abscesses were caused by gram-negative bacteria. The most common pathogens in immunocompetent patients are *K. pneumoniae*, *E. coli*, and *Enterococci*, followed by gram-positive *Staphylococcus aureus* and *Streptococcus viridans*. Mycobacteria, fungi, and protozoa are encountered less often, predominantly in immunosuppressed patients.

The clinical presentation includes fever, left upper quadrant pain, diffuse abdominal pain, left chest wall pain, and dyspnea. Given the rarity of splenic abscesses and the nonspecific signs and symptoms, the diagnosis is challenging. Therefore imaging plays a crucial role. Chest radiographs show left lower lobe atelectasis or air space disease and left pleural effusion in the majority of cases. The specific diagnosis requires cross-sectional abdominal imaging. At most institutions, evaluation of patients with fever of unknown origin with a suspected abdominal cause starts with US or CT, with MRI (and occasionally nuclear scintigraphy with radiolabeled leukocytes) reserved for patients with equivocal findings on other imaging modalities. US and CT typically demonstrate solitary or multiple splenic lesions. Septic collections in the spleen can be located in the parenchyma, in the subcapsular space, or in both. Ultrasonography shows purely cystic or complex hypoechoic splenic lesions. The appearance on CT is that of a hypoattenuating lesion(s) with thick, enhancing walls after injection of intravenous contrast and internal debris. The walls can be smooth or nodular, and thus differentiation from splenic tumors often requires biopsy or percutaneous drainage. Gas within the cavity of the abscess is a specific but very uncommon finding (Fig. 13-86). On MRI the abscess appears as a lesion of fluid signal intensity, hypointense on T1-weighted images and hyperintense on T2-weighted images. There is peripheral enhancement after administration of gadolinium chelates.

Candidiasis is the most common opportunistic infection involving the spleen in immunocompromised patients (Fig. 13-87). On CT, *Candida* lesions are multiple, hypoattenuating, ring enhancing, and typically less than 1 cm in diameter. Magnetic resonance imaging has been shown to be superior to CT in the detection of microabscesses secondary to candidiasis.

The number of patients diagnosed with abdominal tuberculosis is increasing in both immunocompetent and immunocompromised individuals. Splenic involvement occurs via hematogenous dissemination of primary tuberculosis. Splenic tuberculosis may be micronodular (miliary) or macronodular. Miliary splenic disease appears as multiple tiny low-attenuation foci at CT. The macronodular form is rare and manifests as diffuse splenic enlargement with multiple low-attenuation lesions or as a single tumorlike mass. On CE images, early-stage lesions may demonstrate central enhancement, whereas liquefaction develops over time. More chronic lesions may develop calcifications.

Traditionally antibiotics and splenectomy were the mainstay of treatment of splenic abscesses. Image-guided interventional procedures such as catheter drainage were not widely performed because of the perceived high risk for complications. However, more recently image-guided percutaneous drainage is progressively gaining acceptance as an efficacious alternative to splenectomy, with minimal risks in well-selected patients. Successful percutaneous drainage avoids the immediate and long-term morbidity and mortality of laparoscopic or open surgery and splenectomy-associated infections.

Atraumatic Splenic Rupture

Atraumatic splenic ruptures are uncommon. A recent systematic review analyzed all published cases from 1980 to 2008 and identified only 845 cases. Most patients with atraumatic rupture have significant splenomegaly. Spontaneous rupture of a normal-size spleen is highly unusual; only 59 such cases were reported during the past 29 years in the same review. The most common causes of splenic enlargement causing spontaneous rupture are hematologic malignancies and infections such as mononucleosis and malaria. Primary and secondary splenic neoplasms and complications of pancreatitis are other, less common, potential causes. There is a direct correlation between the degree of splenomegaly and the likelihood of rupture. Patients typically present with acute abdominal, pleuritic, or left shoulder pain caused by diaphragmatic irritation. Historically the majority of spontaneous rupture cases

were diagnosed at laparotomy. Currently the preoperative diagnosis is made on CT or US. Both modalities show an enlarged and abnormal spleen with perisplenic clot and free hemoperitoneum. An underlying splenic mass or masses may be seen in some cases (Fig. 13-88). A precise diagnosis of the underlying cause is crucial for making appropriate decisions regarding treatment. The majority of patients still undergo emergency splenectomy because the abnormal, dysfunctional spleen is unlikely to generate adequate hemostasis. In addition, the specific diagnosis can usually be made only via pathologic evaluation of the involved splenic parenchyma. However, select groups of patients with spontaneous rupture in whom the diagnosis of the underlying cause is established may respond to conservative medical treatment, such as those with infectious mononucleosis or malaria. Some patients may also benefit from embolization of the splenic artery as adjuvant therapy.

Splenic Infarct

Splenic infarcts are typically caused by underlying hematologic diseases and thromboembolic conditions. The clinical presentation varies from sharp left upper quadrant pain, fever, and chills to an incidental finding on imaging studies. Patients with nonmalignant hematologic conditions often develop asymptomatic splenic infarcts. The number and size of splenic infarcts is highly variable and can be single or multiple.

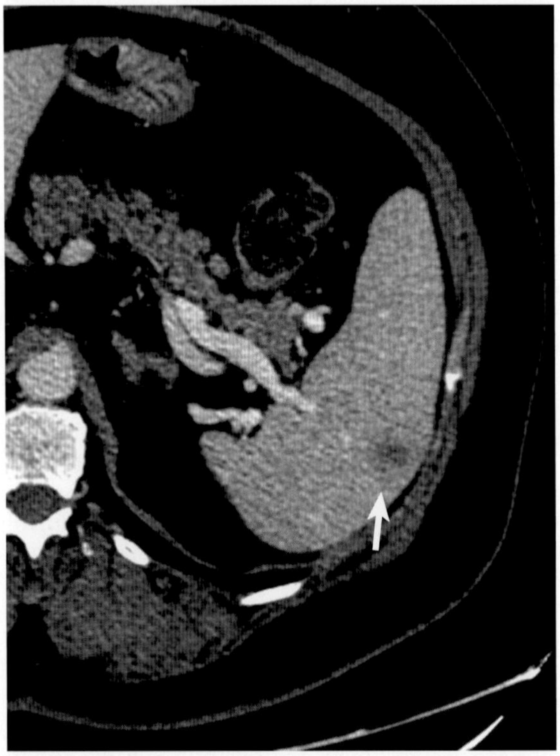

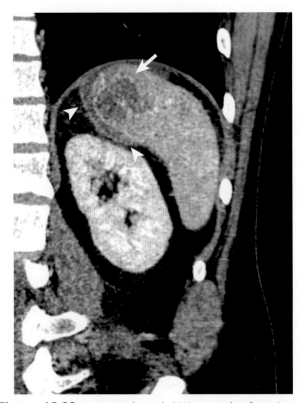

Figure 13-87 Axial contrast-enhanced computed tomographic image demonstrates an ill-defined low-attenuation lesion in the periphery of the spleen *(arrow)* confirmed to represent an abscess caused by *Candida* in an immunocompromised patient receiving chemotherapy for leukemia.

Figure 13-88 Contrast-enhanced (CE) coronal reformation of computed tomographic (CT) data shows a necrotic mass with a rim of enhancement in the upper pole of the spleen *(arrow)*, with a subcapsular fluid collection hematoma *(arrowheads)*. This lesion was confirmed to represent metastatic colon cancer with spontaneous splenic rupture.

On US, acute infarcts are wedge-shaped or round hypoechoic lesions, whereas older infarcts are more echogenic. The appearance on CT also varies with infarct age. Acute infarcts are well defined, peripheral, and hypoattenuating. In the subacute phase the lesions may appear more cystlike (Fig. 13-89). Chronic infarcts undergo fibrosis and produce parenchymal volume loss. Magnetic resonance imaging demonstrates triangular lesions with low signal intensity on T1-weighted imaging and high signal on T2-weighted images, with no appreciable enhancement on postgadolinium images. Superimposed

infection or impending rupture should be considered when follow-up scans show progressive liquefaction or expansion. Splenic abscesses and rupture usually occur in patients with infarcts caused by thromboembolic disorders. Patients with impending rupture usually report sharp abdominal pain. Secondary infection of a splenic infarction remains a difficult diagnosis and requires a high index of suspicion. Image-guided aspiration should be performed when an infected splenic collection is considered.

Splenic Torsion

Imaging evaluation of patients with severe intermittent or acute abdominal pain, especially if located in the left flank, may demonstrate a spleen that has migrated inferiorly; this condition is called a *wandering spleen*. This hypermobility predisposes the spleen to acute or intermittent torsion. Splenic torsion is more common in the pediatric age-group and is caused by congenital absence or maldevelopment of the splenic ligaments. Predisposing causes in adults include postpartum laxity, splenomegaly, previous abdominal surgery, and trauma. Torsion of an orthotopic spleen has been also described (Fig. 13-90). Complications of splenic torsion include splenic congestion, compression of nearby organs, and complete infarction. Abdominal radiographs may show absence of the normal splenic outline in the left upper quadrant and a soft tissue mass in the mid-abdomen. Cross-sectional imaging is usually confirmatory: malpositioned spleen along with splenic engorement and enlargement. Sonographic findings include heterogeneous splenic echotexture with diminished or absent Doppler flow. Doppler interrogation of the proximal splenic artery will demonstrate low diastolic velocity with an elevated resistive index. Computed tomography depicts heterogeneous attenuation of the splenic parenchyma with minimal or absent enhancement. A whirled appearance of the splenic hilum, caused by twisting of the vascular pedicle is a characteristic, though uncommon, finding (see Fig. 13-90). Splenic torsion complicated by infarction usually requires splenectomy. If the spleen is found to be viable at laparotomy, splenopexy is an option to preserve splenic function.

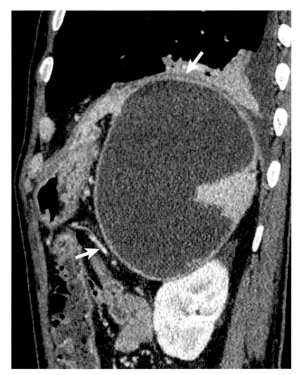

Figure 13-89 Sagittal reformation of axial contrast-enhanced computed tomography depicts a large hypoattenuating splenic infarction with a cystic appearance *(arrows)* in a patient with partial thrombosis of splenic artery. The thrombosis was caused by cardiac emboli related to recent myocardial infarction.

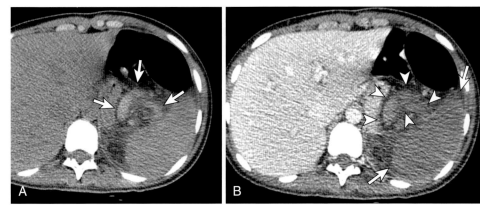

Figure 13-90 Axial unenhanced (**A**) and portal phase contrast-enhanced (CE) (**B**) computed tomographic (CT) images demonstrate torsion of an orthotopic spleen. The unenhanced image shows whirled appearance of the splenic hilum with a hyperattenuating acute splenic vein thrombus *(arrows)*. The CE image confirms complete infarction of the spleen *(arrows)* and splenic vein thrombosis *(arrowheads)*.

■ PERITONEAL AND MESENTERIC EMERGENCIES

Nontraumatic Hemoperitoneum

Spontaneous hemoperitoneum is uncommon. Possible causes include bleeding from vascular tumors (hepatocellular carcinoma [HCC], hepatic adenoma), spontaneous splenic rupture, ruptured ectopic pregnancy, leaking arterial aneurysm, and anticoagulation therapy. Patients typically present with severe abdominal pain or distention, decreased hematocrit, or hypovolemic shock. Computed tomography is the modality of choice for evaluating patients with suspicion of spontaneous hemoperitoneum due to its speed and ability to assess all peritoneal recesses, regardless of body habitus. As in trauma patients it is important to identify the source of active bleeding . Evidence for active bleeding should lead to immediate clinical assessment with prompt decision regarding endovascular or surgical intervention. If active bleeding is excluded, a meticulous search should try to locate the sources of bleeding. The pouch of Douglas should be carefully assessed in every patient with suspected abdominal bleeding because blood from the upper abdomen extends caudally and forms a "hematocrit level." The amount of blood present in the pouch of Douglas is a good indication of the severity of bleeding. A meticulous search of the viscera should include evaluation of the liver to exclude bleeding from a ruptured vascular hepatic tumor and the spleen to rule out a spontaneous splenic rupture (Fig. 13-91). Rupture of a splenic artery aneurysm or pseudoaneurysm is an uncommon but life-threatening condition. Large leaking AAAs can also be the source of intraperitoneal bleeding. In cases of suspicion of bleeding originating from the female reproductive organs, additional evaluation with US is advised. Gynecologic conditions, such as ruptured ovarian cysts and ruptured ectopic pregnancies, are the most common sources of spontaneous hemoperitoneum in women of childbearing age.

Peritonitis and Peritoneal Abscess

Causes of peritonitis can be infectious and noninfectious. Patients with infectious peritonitis usually have a history of recent abdominal surgery, bowel perforation, appendicitis, diverticulitis, CD, or perforated peptic ulcer. Primary bacterial peritonitis occurs in patients with cirrhosis or nephrotic syndrome. Causes of noninfectious peritonitis include chemical peritonitis in patients with pancreatitis due to irritation of the peritoneum by leaked pancreatic juice and sclerosing peritonitis in individuals on continuous ambulatory peritoneal dialysis.

Peritonitis appears on CT and MRI as diffused thickening and enhancement of the peritoneal surface and mesentery (Fig. 13-92). Computed tomography is ideal for detecting intra-abdominal abscesses. Ultrasonography shows loculated ascites and echogenic debris within the ascitic fluid. Peritonitis can be complicated by intra-abdominal abscess. The main limitation of US for diagnosis of intra-abdominal infected fluid collections is the difficulty differentiating fluid and/or gas-containing abscess from similarly appearing bowel loops. Ultrasonography can also be a challenging examination in obese or postoperative patients who cannot tolerate compression with the transducer. However, US has an important role in bedside assessment of critically ill patients with suspected abscess for guidance of percutaneous drainage procedures and for follow-up of patients with a previously diagnosed abscess.

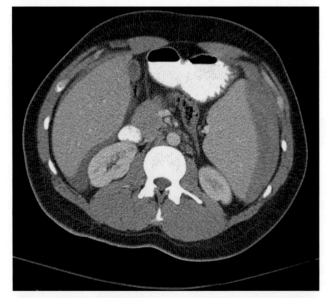

Figure 13-91 Axial contrast-enhanced computed tomographic image in a patient with infectious mononucleosis who presented to the emergency department (ED) with left upper quadrant pain. CT demonstrated perisplenic clot and hemoperitoneum. The diagnosis of splenic rupture was confirmed at laparotomy.

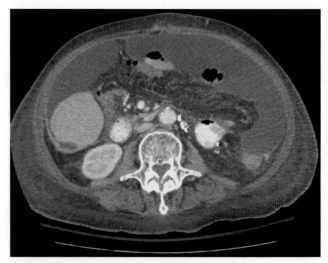

Figure 13-92 Axial contrast-enhanced computed tomographic image shows thickened and hyperenhancing peritoneum in a patient with bacterial peritonitis after laparotomy due to perforated ischemic bowel.

Omental Infarction

Patients with acute right upper or right lower quadrant pain are often referred to imaging for exclusion of cholecystitis, appendicitis, or diverticulitis. One important mimic of these conditions is omental infarction, which cannot be reliably diagnosed on the basis of clinical findings alone. Imaging plays a crucial role in the accurate diagnosis and avoidance of unnecessary antibiotic therapy and laparotomy. Although the omentum has a rich blood supply, perfusion of the right lateral edge is tenuous. Therefore the right inferior omentum is more prone to suffering infarction than the left side. Secondary causes of omental infarction include trauma, incarcerated hernias, surgery, and inflammation. Computed tomography shows a large encapsulated fatty mass located anterior to the ascending or transverse colon (Fig. 13-93). Milder cases demonstrate only subtle haziness of the omental fat. Swirling of the omental vessels is observed in cases of torsion. Colonic wall thickening can develop secondary to omental inflammation, such that differentiation from acute diverticulitis may be difficult. Follow-up imaging with CT or US is required in these cases to demonstrate the predominant extracolonic fatty mass. Omental infarctions manifest on US as an echogenic, noncompressible mass. The location of the mass corresponds precisely to the point of maximal tenderness. This inflammatory mass does not move with respiration during dynamic scanning.

Mesenteric Adenitis

Mesenteric adenitis should be considered in the differential diagnosis of patients presenting to the ED with right lower quadrant pain, malaise, and fever, especially when the appendix is clearly normal in appearance. The timely imaging diagnosis of mesenteric adenitis avoids unnecessary surgery. Although this is a diagnosis of exclusion,

certain CT criteria have been described to suggest mesenteric adenitis as the cause of acute abdominal pain (Fig. 13-94). Mesenteric adenitis has been defined as the presence of three or more right lower quadrant mesenteric lymph nodes, each measuring 5 mm or greater. Mesenteric adenitis is divided into primary and secondary types. Secondary adenitis is associated with specific inflammatory abdominal conditions (CD, appendicitis, celiac disease). In cases of primary mesenteric adenitis an underlying inflammatory process is not evident on imaging. Infectious terminal ileitis is considered to be the cause of primary adenitis. When cross-sectional imaging demonstrates mild thickening of the terminal ileum and mesenteric adenitis in patients with acute right lower quadrant pain, infection with *Y. enterocolitica* should be considered.

Mesenteric Panniculitis

Mesenteric panniculitis is a nonspecific inflammation and fibrosis of the fatty tissue of the bowel mesentery. The majority of cases of mesenteric panniculitis are discovered incidentally on abdominal CT examinations performed for unrelated indications. However, some patients present with abdominal pain, fever, and vomiting related to the inflammation and/or mass effect. There is predominant involvement of the jejunal mesentery. Therefore the most common locations for the findings of mesenteric panniculitis are on the left side and middle of the abdomen. The inflamed mesentery envelops the superior mesenteric

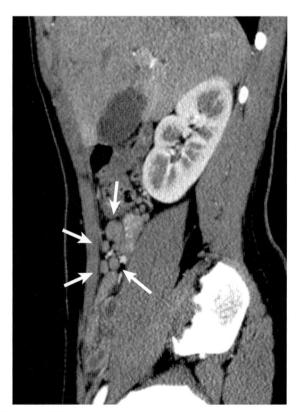

Figure 13-94 Sagittal reformation of contrast-enhanced computed tomography in a patient with acute right lower quadrant pain demonstrates a cluster of multiple enlarged mesenteric lymph nodes at the right lower quadrant *(arrows)*. The appendix (not shown) was normal. The patient was diagnosed with mesenteric adenitis.

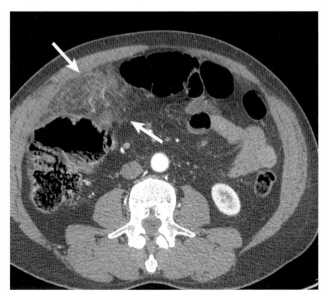

Figure 13-93 Axial Contrast-enhanced computed tomography shows a large mixed fatty and soft tissue attenuation mass *(arrows)* located anterior to the ascending colon. This appearance is characteristic of an omental infarct.

vessels and displaces adjacent bowel loops (Fig. 13-95). The mass may be surrounded by a thin pseudocapsule of slightly higher attenuation. There are usually multiple small (less than 5 mm in diameter) mesenteric lymph nodes within the mass. The "fat halo" sign refers to low-density fat surrounding the higher-density inflamed fat, vessels, and nodules and represents relatively preserved mesentery. Although it was originally thought that the fat halo sign helps differentiate mesenteric panniculitis from malignant conditions involving the mesentery, more recent papers described this sign in patients with lymphoma. Mesenteric panniculitis diagnosed on CT scans obtained in the ED requires clinical and imaging follow-up to rule out the uncommon progression to retractile mesenteritis, which causes SBO and vascular narrowing.

ABDOMINAL WALL

Hernias

Spontaneous abdominal wall hernias are very common, with a lifetime risk in the general population of approximately 5%. Many patients are asymptomatic or complain only of mild discomfort. Complications of abdominal wall hernias are common causes of acute abdominal pain in the ED. The most important complications are incarceration, bowel obstruction, and strangulation. Approximately 80% of abdominal wall hernias are inguinal hernias, 5% are femoral hernias, and 15% are miscellaneous hernia types. Diagnosis is usually made on physical examination. However, clinical diagnosis can be challenging, especially in obese patients or patients with prior inguinal surgery. Various imaging modalities have been used to confirm the diagnosis of hernia and rule out complications. In experienced hands, US is a valuable tool for assessment of the neck and contents of the hernia sac and exclusion of several mimics (lymphadenopathy, undescended testicle, enlarged vessels). However, in the emergency setting, MDCT is the imaging test of choice. Multidetector CT is used for accurate characterization of the exact type of hernia and its contents and for prompt diagnosis of complications that require urgent surgery. The preoperative differentiation between inguinal and femoral hernias is important due to the higher risk for strangulation in patients with femoral hernias (40%). Therefore all femoral hernias, including nonincarcerated cases, require surgical repair. Clinical examination is often unreliable for differentiation between the various types of hernias. Compression of the femoral vein by the hernia sac is seen in the majority of patients with a femoral hernia on MDCT and allows for a quick and elegant preoperative diagnosis.

Abdominal wall hernias are the second most common cause of SBO, after postoperative adhesions. Most cases of bowel obstruction develop in patients with incarceration or strangulation (Fig. 13-96). Multidetector CT affords the ability to diagnose obstruction, show the transition point at the level of hernial sac, and assess viability of the bowel wall. Incarceration refers to a nonreducible hernia. Narrowing of the hernia neck at MDCT suggests incarceration, but this is mainly a clinical diagnosis. Bowel strangulation is the most severe complication of abdominal wall hernias, with a fatality rate of 6% to 23%. Strangulation occurs when blood supply to the herniated bowel wall is compromised,

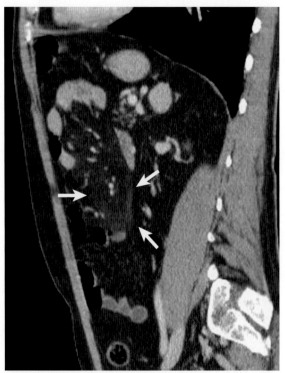

Figure 13-95 Sagittal reformation of contrast-enhanced computed tomography obtained in the portal venous phase depicts a mesenteric mass with fatty attenuation *(arrows)* displacing loops of small bowel. This appearance is characteristic of mesenteric panniculitis.

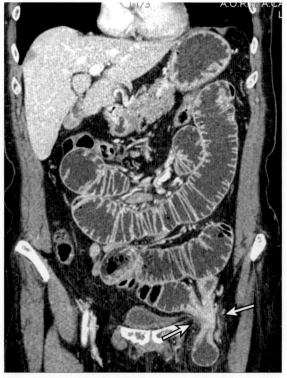

Figure 13-96 Coronal reformation of contrast-enhanced computed tomography shows small bowel obstruction (SBO) caused by an incarcerated direct inguinal hernia *(arrows)*.

with subsequent development of ischemia and infarction. Strangulation occurs when the afferent and efferent bowel loops are obstructed at the hernia neck, with creation of a closed loop. Loculated fluid within the hernia sac and thickening of herniated loops should raise suspicion for impending strangulation and should lead to a recommendation for urgent surgery. U- or C-shaped closed loops within the sac, lack of bowel wall enhancement, intestinal pneumatosis, and mesenteric vessel engorgement are signs of established strangulation, a surgical emergency.

Spontaneous Hemorrhage

Spontaneous rectal sheath hematomas may occur secondary to coagulopathies or blood dyscrasias. The most frequent cause of spontaneous rectal sheath hematoma is anticoagulation therapy. The hematoma most commonly results from spontaneous rupture of the inferior epigastric artery. The characteristic location is the inferior abdominal wall, below the arcuate line where only the fascia transversalis and peritoneum support the rectus sheath. Strong aponeurotic sheaths above the arcuate line prevent cephalad expansion of the hematoma. Patients present with painful tender swelling mimicking an intra-abdominal mass or abdominal wall hernia. Imaging evaluation is frequently required because of the ambiguity of the clinical picture.

Ultrasonography shows a solid or complex cystic lesion. Sonography cannot differentiate hematoma from an abdominal wall tumor in some cases. Multidetector CT confirms the correct diagnosis of abdominal wall hematoma and excludes intraperitoneal abnormalities (Fig. 13-97). In addition, CE MDCT

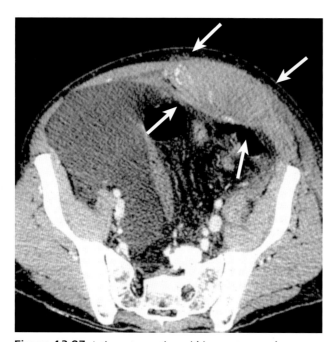

Figure 13-97 Active extravasation within spontaneous hematoma of the left rectus sheath *(arrows)* in a patient receiving anticoagulation therapy. The hematoma was demonstrated on axial contrast-enhanced computed tomographic image. Note ascites related to chronic liver disease.

may show findings of active bleeding. Conservative management is the most common approach due to the self-limited nature of rectal sheath hematomas. Surgical ligation or transarterial embolization of bleeding epigastric vessels is required only in cases of uncontrollable hemorrhage.

Acute Pancreatitis

Leena Tekchandani, Ritu Bordia, Lewis K. Shin, Giovanna Casola, James H. Grendell, Bruce R. Javors, and Douglas S. Katz

■ DEFINITION AND EPIDEMIOLOGY

Acute pancreatitis is an acute inflammation of the pancreas with variable involvement of local tissues and remote organ systems. It has a highly variable clinical course, ranging from mild and self-limited to severe and life threatening. Acute pancreatitis occurs more often in men than in women. The most common cause in men is alcohol abuse, and gallstones are the most common cause in women. The median age at onset depends on cause, with alcohol-related pancreatitis occurring around 40 years of age, and biliary tract–related pancreatitis occurring around 70 years of age.

■ CAUSES/PATHOGENESIS

There are many causes of acute pancreatitis, which can be easily identified in about 80% of patients. Choledocholithiasis (38%) and alcohol abuse (36%) are the most common causes. However, only an estimated 3% to 7% of patients with gallstones eventually develop acute pancreatitis. With obstruction of the common bile duct the pancreatic duct pressure increases, and bile refluxes into the pancreatic duct, causing trypsin activation and pancreatic autodigestion (Fig. 13-98). The exact pathogenesis of alcohol-induced pancreatitis is less clear. Alcohol may increase the amount of digestive and lysosomal enzymes produced by pancreatic acinar cells. Also, alcohol may cause hypersensitivity of acini to cholecystokinin. Genetic and environmental factors also influence development of pancreatitis in alcoholics because only a relatively small percentage of alcoholics develop pancreatitis (Fig. 13-99).

Medications, hypercalcemia, and severe hypertriglyceridemia are uncommon causes of pancreatitis. Serum triglyceride concentrations usually need to be above 1000 mg/dL (11 mmol/L) to potentially cause acute pancreatitis. Post–endoscopic retrograde cholangiopancreatography (ERCP) pancreatitis occurs in 3% of patients undergoing the procedure and in approximately 5% of patients undergoing therapeutic ERCP. Asymptomatic hyperamylasemia occurs in 35% to 70% of patients after the procedure. Acute pancreatitis is diagnosed if these elevated levels are accompanied by abdominal pain (Fig. 13-100). Pancreatitis

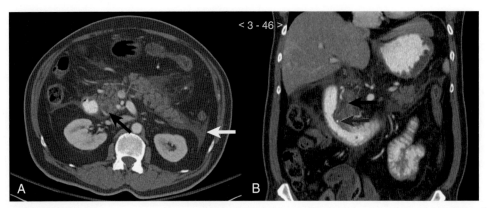

Figure 13-98 Gallstone pancreatitis. A 62-year-old man presented with abdominal pain and a serum lipase level of 900. Axial (**A**) and coronal (**B**) images from computed tomography (CT) with oral and intravenous contrast demonstrate interstitial edematous pancreatitis (IEP) caused by obstruction of the common bile duct by a small stone *(red arrow)* at its distal end. Note that the common bile is dilated *(black arrows)*. There is an acute peripancreatic fluid collection associated with the IEP *(white arrow)*.

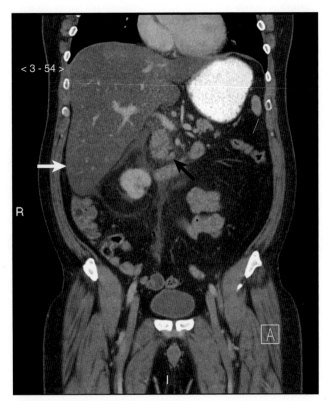

Figure 13-99 Alcoholic pancreatitis. A 47-year-old man with a history of alcoholism presented with diffuse abdominal pain and fever. This coronal computed tomographic (CT) image of the abdomen with oral and intravenous contrast demonstrates interstitial edematous pancreatitis (IEP) *(black arrow)*, which was caused by alcohol abuse. Note fatty infiltration and edema of the liver *(white arrow)*, which is much lower in attenuation compared to the spleen *(red arrowhead)*. These latter findings are also related to the patient's alcohol abuse.

is also associated with various infections from viruses (mumps, coxsackievirus, hepatitis B, cytomegalovirus, varicella-zoster, herpes simplex, HIV), bacteria (*Legionella*, *Leptospira*, *Salmonella*), fungi (*Aspergillus*), and parasites (*Toxoplasma*, *Cryptosporidium*, *Ascaris*). A venomous bite from certain arachnids and reptiles, trauma, and vascular disease are other rare causes of pancreatitis.

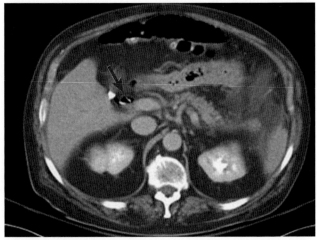

Figure 13-100 Post–endoscopic retrograde cholangiopancreatography (ERCP) pancreatitis. A 69-year-old man underwent ERCP with stenting of the common bile duct. This axial computed tomographic (CT) image of the abdomen with intravenous contrast demonstrates a stent and air within the common bile duct, which is dilated *(red arrow)*, related to the recent ERCP. There are inflammatory changes around the tail of the pancreas, representing interstitial edematous pancreatitis.

In up to 30% of patients, initial history, laboratory tests, and gallbladder/biliary tract ultrasonographic results fail to reveal a specific cause of acute pancreatitis. Even after more extensive workup with MRCP, EUS, ERCP, analysis of bile for microlithiasis, and sphincter of Oddi manometry, upwards of 15% to 25% of patients will still have an idiopathic cause.

■ CLINICAL PRESENTATION AND DIAGNOSIS

Acute pancreatitis is an important cause of upper abdominal pain, but its clinical features are similar to many other acute illnesses. Making an accurate diagnosis based only on symptoms and signs can be challenging, particularly in the absence of prior documented episodes of acute pancreatitis. Patients tend to present with the key symptom of dull, steady pain that usually has a sudden onset and progressively intensifies into a constant ache. The pain is commonly located in the epigastric region but can be more severe on one side depending on which portion of the pancreas is most involved. In about one half of patients the pain radiates to the back. Accompanying symptoms of nausea, vomiting, diarrhea, anorexia, and shortness of breath are common in more severe cases. The pain usually has been present for more than 24 hours, and the severity and persistence of pain often cause the patient to seek medical attention. In mild pancreatitis, physical examination may only reveal slight epigastric tenderness. In more severe pancreatitis, tenderness is more intense with guarding, often accompanied by tachycardia, fever, and even shock. Respirations may be shallow and rapid due to diaphragmatic irritation.

According to the revised Atlanta classification of acute pancreatitis, the diagnosis of acute pancreatitis is made if at least two of the following three features are present:
1. Abdominal pain characteristic of acute pancreatitis, as described earlier.
2. Serum amylase and lipase levels three or more times above normal.
3. Characteristic findings on CT, MRI, or US.

■ SEVERITY

Clinical Systems for Predicting Severity

Because clinical features of severe pancreatitis develop relatively late in the course of the disease, clinicians can predict a severe attack of pancreatitis in only 34% to 39% of patients at the time of admission. Also, elevated serum lipase and amylase levels, although useful diagnostic indicators, correlate poorly with the severity of pancreatitis. In fact, no individual laboratory or clinical parameter is adequately sensitive or specific for categorizing patients with severe pancreatitis. Therefore, the Ranson criteria, the Acute Physiology and Chronic Health Evaluation II (APACHE II) score, the bedside index of severity in acute pancreatitis (BISAP) score, and the Glasgow system all use a combination of laboratory and clinical parameters to help identify patients with severe pancreatitis by evaluating its systemic effects.

Computed Tomography Severity Index

Although clinical systems for predicting severe pancreatitis evaluate the systemic effects of pancreatitis, they only infer the presence and amount of pancreatic necrosis and local complications. Pancreatic necrosis is a critical prognostic factor because more than 80% of deaths associated with acute pancreatitis occur in patients with pancreatic necrosis. In addition, the extent of necrosis is very important. In a 1985 study by Balthazar and colleagues the severity of pancreatitis was graded from A to E based on the appearance on noncontrast CT of the pancreas and of the

Table 13-2   Noncontrast Computed Tomography Grade of Acute Pancreatitis

Grade	Computed Tomography Findings
A	Normal pancreas
B	Enlargement of pancreas
C	Inflammation of pancreas and/or peripancreatic fat
D	Single peripancreatic fluid collection
E	Two or more fluid collections and/or retroperitoneal air

Table 13-3   Computed Tomography Severity Index

Computed Tomography Grade	Points	Percentage Necrosis	Additional Points	Severity Index
A	0	0	0	0
B	1	0	0	1
C	2	<30	2	4
D	3	30-50	4	7
E	4	>50	6	10

Severity index = (Points allotted for computed tomography grade) + (Points allotted for percentage necrosis).

peripancreatic fat, as well as the presence and number of fluid collections (Table 13-2). Correlation between this CT grade and the morbidity/mortality of these patients was then measured. It was found that patients with one or more pancreatic fluid collections (grades D and E) had the highest mortality (14%) and morbidity (54%). In contrast, patients without pancreatic fluid collections (grades A, B, and C) had no mortality and a much lower morbidity (4%).

With the enhancements in CT technique the early prognostic value of CT for acute pancreatitis significantly improved. In the 1990 series by Balthazar and colleagues, patients with less than 30% pancreatic necrosis had no mortality and less than 50% morbidity. Patients with more than 30% necrosis had a morbidity rate of greater than 75% and a mortality of 11% to 25%. Balthazar modified his scoring system by incorporating the presence and amount of pancreatic necrosis on IV contrast-enhanced CT, thereby giving the patient a score from 0 to 10. He called this new system of scoring the CT Severity Index (CTSI) (Table 13-3). Increasing morbidity and mortality of the patients significantly correlated with increasing CTSI scores. Patients with a CTSI of 0 or 1 had 0% mortality and morbidity. Patients with a CTSI of 2 had a mortality of 0% and a morbidity of 4%. On the other hand, patients with a CTSI of 7 to 10 had a mortality of 17% and a morbidity of 92% (see Table 13-3). A modified CT severity index was proposed by Mortele and coworkers in 2004, which was reported to have improved correlation with patient outcome, particularly length of hospitalization and organ failure. This index involves a simplified evaluation of fluid collections and pancreatic necrosis and addition of extrapancreatic complications in the scoring system.

Revised Atlanta Classification for Acute Pancreatitis

According to the revised Atlanta classification, there are two phases of acute pancreatitis. The early phase occurs within the first week of onset. The late phase occurs after the first week of onset and may extend for weeks to months. Note: The onset of acute pancreatitis is defined as the moment the symptoms start, not the time at which the patient presents to the hospital.

Severity is determined during the early phase primarily by clinical parameters because morbidity and mortality are largely due to organ failure caused by the systemic inflammatory response syndrome (Fig. 13-101). Mild pancreatitis is defined as acute pancreatic inflammation without organ failure, local complications, or systemic complications. A patient with moderately severe acute pancreatitis may have transient organ failure, which resolves within 48 hours, or has local or systemic complications without persistent organ failure. Severe pancreatitis is defined as organ failure lasting longer than 48 hours or resultant death.

Though local complications can be demonstrated during the early phase, it is generally not necessary to determine their presence by imaging at this time because during the first week pancreatic and peripancreatic necrosis may be underestimated. These complications are best assessed at least 72 hours after onset of symptoms. Also, necrosis and other morphologic changes do not always correlate well with clinical severity and organ failure during this period. Finally, there are no treatment requirements for pancreatic necrosis and peripancreatic fluid collections during the early phase.

On the other hand, treatment is largely determined by morphologic criteria during the late phase, when morbidity and mortality are often due to infection and sepsis. Only patients with moderately severe and severe pancreatitis progress to the late phase. It is important to define and differentiate the various morphologic

characteristics of local complications because these may require different interventions to avoid further sequelae and in particular death.

■ IMAGING

Indications for Imaging

According to the revised Atlanta classification of acute pancreatitis, CECT is the imaging examination of choice for assessing acute pancreatitis due to its widespread availability and high accuracy. If the diagnosis of acute pancreatitis can be made by using the first two criteria mentioned earlier, a CECT is not indicated. However, mildly elevated serum amylase and lipase levels and/or vague abdominal pain are not specific for acute pancreatitis and may also be seen in cholecystitis, bowel obstruction, bowel infarction, perforated ulcer, and other abdominal emergencies. Therefore, if alternative diagnoses are being considered, early imaging is recommended to confirm a diagnosis of acute pancreatitis and/or to exclude other causes of abdominal pain.

Imaging is also used to help determine the cause of acute pancreatitis, stage the severity of disease, assess local and extrapancreatic complications, and monitor treatment response through follow-up examinations. In addition, if a patient is older than 40 years of age and has a first-time diagnosis of pancreatitis without an identifiable cause, CECT should be used to help exclude an underlying neoplasm. Finally, imaging can guide interventional procedures.

Technical Considerations

There is no longer an important role for radiography and fluoroscopic GI studies in the evaluation of disease severity of acute pancreatitis. Visualization of the pancreas by US is sufficient in only 60% to 70% of cases, compromised by overlying bowel gas caused by peripancreatic ileus. Also, US cannot reliably depict pancreatic necrosis. Therefore its role in the diagnosis and assessment of the severity of acute pancreatitis is usually limited to detection of cholelithiasis, choledocholithiasis, and fluid collections.

Contrast-enhanced CT, on the other hand, is the imaging modality of choice for acute pancreatitis because it depicts and permits quantification of pancreatic parenchymal necrosis, demonstrates fluid collections, and may aid in establishing a cause. Computed tomography is 100% specific and sensitive for necrosis if more than 30% of the pancreas is nonenhancing. Thin-section CT (thinner than 5 mm) should be used to evaluate the pancreas in cases of suspected acute pancreatitis. The use of positive oral contrast is generally discouraged because it may obscure hemorrhage or calculi and does not usually add diagnostic value; therefore either no oral contrast or neutral oral contrast may be used instead. A monophasic protocol of the entire abdomen and pelvis with intravenous contrast in the early portal venous phase (60 to 70 seconds after administration of 100 or more mL iodinated contrast at a rate of 3 mL/sec) can be administered. Alternatively, initial assessment can be

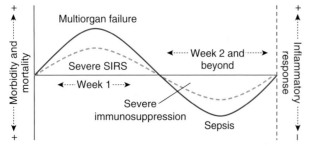

Figure 13-101 Graph of inflammation and mortality versus time. During the first week of acute pancreatitis there is a proinflammatory response, causing systemic inflammatory response syndrome (SIRS). During this early phase, sepsis or infection rarely occurs. Severe SIRS will lead to early multiple organ failure. After the first week there is a transition from a proinflammatory to an antiinflammatory response, during which the patient experiences severe immunosuppression. The patient is at risk for the translocation of intestinal flora, which can infect necrotic tissue and fluid collections. The ensuing sepsis may result in late multiple organ failure. (Modified from www.radiologyassistant.nl.)

performed with a three-phase intravenous contrast CT protocol, which consists of a low-radiation-dose non-contrast examination, a pancreatic parenchymal phase examination (at about 40 seconds), and a portal venous phase examination. The noncontrast examination is useful for visualizing hemorrhagic collections and common duct stones. The pancreatic parenchymal phase is ideal for assessment of necrosis because normal pancreatic parenchyma enhances the most during this phase, making nonenhancing necrotic regions more evident. Follow-up imaging can usually be performed with a monophasic early portal venous protocol, and radiation dose reduction techniques can be employed, particularly in younger patients.

Magnetic resonance imaging scans of acute pancreatitis are generally comparable to those of CT. In general, MRI should be performed with a fat-suppressed T1-weighted sequence, a fast spin-echo T2-weighted sequence, and T1-weighted gradient-echo sequences before and during late arterial and portal venous phases of intravenous gadolinium enhancement. A heavily T2-weighted MRCP sequence should also generally be performed.

Modality-Based Imaging Findings

Ultrasonography

Ultrasonography may reveal a normal-appearing gland in milder cases of acute pancreatitis. Focal or diffuse enlargement of the gland, with heterogeneous or low echogenicity may alternatively be present in more severe pancreatitis. The findings of pancreatic and peripancreatic collections range from anechoic, simple-appearing fluid to more complex fluid mixed with solid components. Ultrasonography can be used to diagnose and monitor these collections, as well as guide percutaneous or endoscopic drainage as needed. Ultrasonography is superior to CT for the identification of cholelithiasis, which helps deduce a cause for the acute pancreatitis and allows appropriate patients to receive therapeutic ERCP in a timely manner.

Computed Tomography

In patients with interstitial edematous pancreatitis (IEP) there is diffuse or localized enlargement of the pancreas due to inflammatory edema. The gland enhances completely, though sometimes heterogeneously. The peripancreatic fat may show inflammatory changes of fat stranding or haziness. Variable amounts of peripancreatic fluid may also be present (Fig. 13-102).

There are three types of necrotizing pancreatitis. The most common type of necrosis involves both the pancreas and peripancreatic tissues and is seen in 75% to 80% of patients with acute necrotizing pancreatitis. An uncommon form of necrotizing pancreatitis is necrosis of only the peripancreatic tissue, occurring in 20% of patients. The rarest type of pancreatic necrosis is necrosis of only the pancreas, occurring in less fewer than 5% of patients. All three of these types of necrotizing pancreatitis can be sterile or infected. Necrosis progresses and evolves over several days; thus early CECT may lead to underestimation of the extent of necrosis.

Pancreatic parenchymal necrosis appears as a homogeneous nonenhancing region of variable attenuation in the first week, which progresses to a more heterogeneous nonenhancing region later in the course of disease. Peripancreatic necrosis appears as heterogeneous areas of nonenhancement with nonliquified components, often located in the retroperitoneum and lesser sac (Fig. 13-103).

Fluid Collections

An important component of the revised Atlanta classification of acute pancreatitis is its new, more objective terms for describing pancreatic and peripancreatic collections, with a clear distinction made between purely liquid collections, which are associated with IEP, and collections containing nonliquified components, which are associated with all forms of necrotizing pancreatitis. As previously noted, all collections can be either sterile or infected.

An acute peripancreatic fluid collection (APFC) is a purely liquid, homogeneous, low-attenuation collection, which is confined to the retroperitoneum

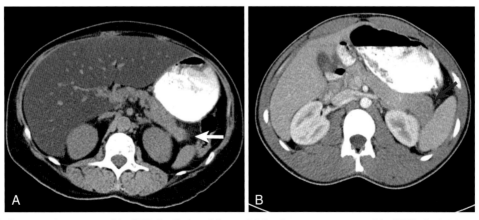

Figure 13-102 Computed tomographic (CT) findings of interstitial edematous pancreatitis (IEP). A, A 59-year-old woman with abdominal pain and vomiting. An axial view of the abdomen from CT with oral contrast only demonstrates mild fullness of the pancreas with mild peripancreatic fat stranding *(white arrow),* consistent with IEP. **B,** A 23-year-old man who presented with abdominal pain. On this axial contrast-enhanced (CE) CT image of the abdomen, the tail of the pancreas is prominent with slightly heterogeneous enhancement *(red arrow),* which is due to IEP.

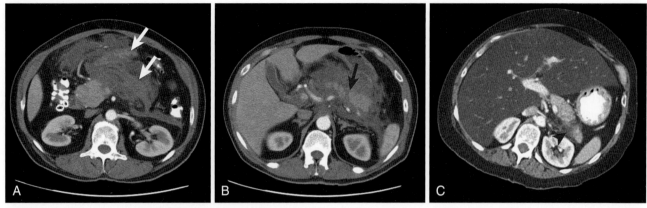

Figure 13-103 *Computed tomographic (CT) findings of necrotizing pancreatitis.* **A** and **B**, Axial views from a contrast-enhanced (CE) CT demonstrating both peripancreatic and pancreatic necrosis. Note the nonenhancing portion of the pancreas *(red arrow).* Also note the large peripancreatic collection with nonliquefied components *(white arrows).* **C**, A 58-year-old woman who presented with hepatomegaly, abdominal pain, and elevated serum amylase (294 units/L) and lipase (>900 units/L) levels. This axial CECT image of the abdomen demonstrates a nonenhancing portion of the pancreatic tail *(red arrowhead).*

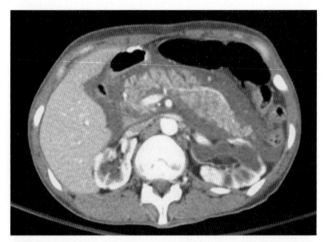

Figure 13-104 *Computed tomographic (CT) findings of an acute peripancreatic fluid collection (APFC).* A 31-year-old woman presented with epigastric pain and elevated serum lipase level (>900 units/L). Axial image from contrast-enhanced (CE) CT of the abdomen demonstrates a low-attenuation, homogeneous peripancreatic collection immediately adjacent to the pancreas, representing an APFC.

and is immediately adjacent to the pancreas (Fig. 13-104). These collections occur in patients with IEP during the first 4 weeks of the disease course. This peripancreatic fluid is reactionary to the pancreatic and peripancreatic inflammation and/or is a result of peripheral pancreatic duct side branch rupture. These collections are self-limited with spontaneous reabsorption within the first few weeks. They usually do not become infected and therefore usually do not require intervention.

A pseudocyst is a well-circumscribed, round or ovoid peripancreatic purely liquid collection of homogeneously low attenuation with an enhancing capsule, which evolves from an APFC after the first 4 weeks of onset of IEP (Fig. 13-105, *A*). Pseudocysts are caused by leakage from the pancreatic ductal system. Many pseudocysts seal off this communication to the pancreatic ductal system and spontaneously resorb.

An acute necrotic collection (ANC) is a heterogeneous collection that occurs in the first 4 weeks

after the onset of necrotizing pancreatitis. It contains both fluid and nonliquified necrotic material. Acute necrotic collections may involve both the peripancreatic and pancreatic tissue (Fig. 13-106, *A*). Any collection that replaces the pancreatic parenchyma in the first 4 weeks should be considered an ANC, and not a pseudocyst.

Walled-off necrosis (WON) is an ANC that develops a thickened, nonepithelialized wall after the first 4 weeks of the disease course (Fig. 13-106, *B*). Just as an ANC, WON may also involve pancreatic and peripancreatic tissue. Any collection that replaces the pancreatic parenchyma after the first 4 weeks is called *WON*.

Magnetic Resonance Imaging/Magnetic Resonance Cholangiopancreatography

Interstitial edematous pancreatitis is depicted as an enlarged pancreas, often with heterogeneous hypointensity and peripancreatic inflammation on T1-weighted, fat-suppressed, CE images. Necrotizing pancreatitis is best identified as nonenhancing regions on the CE images and is most visible on the arterial-phase images.

APFCs and pseudocysts are homogeneously hyperintense on T2-weighted images (see Fig. 13-105, *B*) and hypointense on T1-weighted images. Solid necrotic components of ANCs and WON are often better depicted on MRI than CT, with low T2 signal of these components before they liquefy. Though MRI may demonstrate large pockets of gas or air-fluid levels, CT is more sensitive for depicting small pockets of gas.

MRCP and other T2-weighted images are useful for evaluating the integrity of the biliary system and pancreatic duct. On these sequences, gallstones and common duct stones will appear hypointense within a background of hyperintense bile (Fig. 13-107, *A* and *B*). MRCP accurately depicts biliary/pancreatic ductal anatomy and abnormalities (see Fig. 13-107, *C*). MRCP is also very valuable for detecting communication of peripancreatic and pancreatic collections with the pancreatic ductal system.

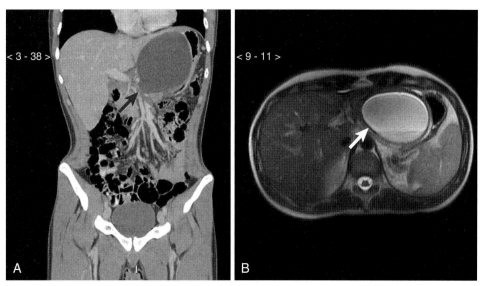

Figure 13-105 Computed tomography (CT) and magnetic resonance imaging (MRI) findings of a pseudocyst. These images are of a 19-year-old man who fell onto the handlebars of his bike several weeks earlier, with injury to his epigastric region and resultant pancreatitis. **A,** This contrast-enhanced (CE) coronal CT image of the abdomen and pelvis demonstrates a well-circumscribed, ovoid peripancreatic liquid collection of homogeneously low attenuation, with an enhancing capsule *(red arrow)*, which represents a pseudocyst. **B,** Axial T2-weighted MRI of the abdomen of the same patient demonstrates the pseudocyst as a hyperintense peripancreatic collection with a relatively thin hypointense capsule *(white arrow)*.

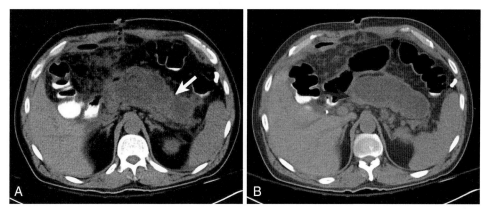

Figure 13-106 Computed tomographic (CT) findings of acute necrotic collection (ANC) and walled-off necrosis (WON). These images are of a 45-year-old man who presented with abdominal pain. **A,** Axial CT image of the abdomen with oral contrast only, performed at the time of admission, demonstrates a heterogeneous collection that contains both fluid and nonliquefied necrotic material in the pancreatic and peripancreatic tissues *(white arrow)*, representing an ANC. More than 4 weeks later the patient was reimaged (**B**). This axial CT image of the abdomen with oral contrast only demonstrates a collection with a thick wall *(red arrow)* that developed from the ANC. This is now a focus of WON.

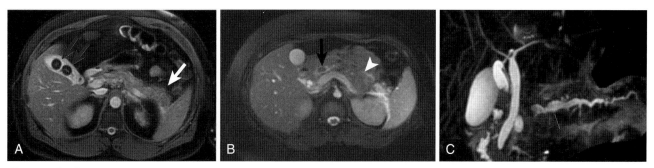

Figure 13-107 T2-weighted magnetic resonance imaging (MRI) and magnetic resonance cholangiopancreatography (MRCP) findings in gallstone pancreatitis. **A,** Axial image from a T2-weighted MR sequence in a 37-year-old man, demonstrating heterogeneity of the pancreas *(white arrow)*, which is due to interstitial edematous pancreatitis (IEP). There are stones in the gallbladder *(red arrows)*, which strongly suggest underlying gallstone pancreatitis. **B,** T2-weighted axial image of the abdomen from a 20-year-old woman with recurrent pancreatitis and right upper quadrant pain demonstrates a slightly heterogeneous pancreas, representing IEP *(white arrowhead)*. This is caused by the hypointense stone within the distal pancreatic duct *(black arrow)*. **C,** An MRCP from the same patient shows resultant pancreatic ductal dilatation *(red arrowhead)*.

Endoscopic Ultrasonography

Endoscopic ultrasonography provides a high-spatial-resolution view of the distal common bile duct, which on conventional transabdominal US is often more difficult to evaluate. However, the distal common bile duct is commonly the location of an obstructing stone or other cause of bile duct obstruction, including tumors. Pancreas divisum may also be identified on EUS. Endoscopic ultrasonography is also useful for depicting sludge or microlithiasis in patients with idiopathic acute pancreatitis and otherwise normal transabdominal ultrasonographic results.

Imaging Appearance of Complications

Local complications of pancreatitis include infection, vascular complications, and hemorrhage. An infected pseudocyst, ANC, or WON may contain gas. Without the presence of gas, an aspiration with Gram stain and culture is usually required to diagnose clinically suspected infection.

Vascular complications, particularly pseudoaneurysm formation and mesenteric/portal venous thrombosis, can be identified on US, CT, and MRI. Pseudoaneurysms are caused by weakening of the arterial wall by proteolytic enzymes released by the damaged pancreas. They usually affect the pancreaticoduodenal, splenic, or gastroduodenal artery. Contrast-enhanced CT and MR images show enhancement of an arterial outpouching, which is similar in attenuation to that of adjacent arteries. Venous thrombosis is the most common vascular complication of acute pancreatitis, affecting mainly the splenic vein and, less commonly, the portal and superior mesenteric veins. Thrombus is well visualized on CE cross-sectional imaging as a filling defect (Fig. 13-108). Over time, associated varices may develop, especially adjacent to the stomach and the spleen.

Hemorrhage can occur in severe necrotizing pancreatitis, and appears as a relatively high density fluid collection on CT in its acute phases (Fig. 13-109). On MRI, acute hemorrhage will be hyperintense on T1-weighted images and hypointense on T2-weighted images. These signal abnormalities on MRI persist for a longer period than the attenuation abnormalities on CT.

Potential Imaging Pitfalls—False Positives and False Negatives

Potential imaging pitfalls include an underestimation of the presence or degree of pancreatic necrosis, false-positive diagnosis of superinfected pancreatitis and pancreatic necrosis, groove pancreatitis, autoimmune pancreatitis, and underlying malignancy.

One potential pitfall is an underestimation of necrosis on an early CECT. Necrosis develops between 24 and 48 hours after onset, with zones of liquefaction becoming better defined 2 to 3 days after onset. Therefore premature CT imaging may not depict the true extent of disease.

A potential cause of a false-positive diagnosis of superinfected pancreatitis is spontaneous drainage of a peripancreatic or pancreatic collection into the GI tract. This process allows gas to migrate into these collections, which can be misinterpreted as infection with a gas-forming

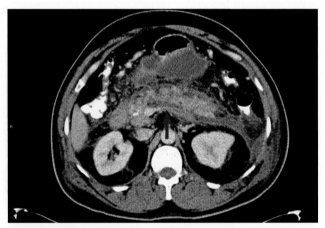

Figure 13-108 Mesenteric venous thrombosis. A 44-year-old man presented with abdominal pain. On this axial contrast-enhanced computed tomographic image of the abdomen, the pancreas is heterogeneous and there are severe peripancreatic inflammatory changes. Though the portal splenic confluence is well opacified, there is a filling defect within the splenic vein (*red arrow*), which is splenic vein thrombosis.

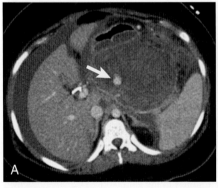
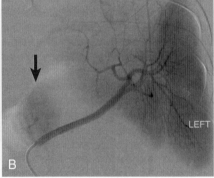
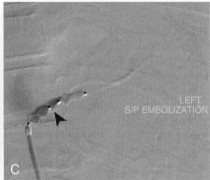

Figure 13-109 Hemorrhagic pancreatitis and subsequent intervention. A, Axial contrast-enhanced computed tomographic image of the abdomen demonstrates a large heterogeneous peripancreatic collection with a region of active bleeding (*white arrow*), which is hemorrhagic pancreatitis. A conventional angiogram of the splenic artery (**B**) shows a region of blush (*red arrow*), which represents the site of active hemorrhage. This was repaired (**C**) with a vascular plug (*red arrowhead*).

organism. Pancreatic necrosis can be overestimated because of the intrinsic regional enhancement differences of the pancreas; however, these differences typically manifest as attenuation coefficient variations of less than 30 HU. Also, otherwise healthy patients with fatty infiltration of the pancreas may have low enhancement values. Finally, there may be low enhancement values in patients with IEP, due to parenchymal edema. These entities should not be confused with necrosis of the pancreas. In true necrosis the texture of the gland will be abnormal.

Another important potential imaging pitfall is failure to diagnose underlying pancreatic malignancy. Pancreatic tumors obstructing the ampulla can rarely present as acute pancreatitis (1% to 2% of cases) and may be masked by the acute inflammatory process, delaying the correct diagnosis. Intraductal papillary mucinous tumor, and rarely lymphoma and metastases, can also cause acute pancreatitis. These masses likely cause acute pancreatitis by mass effect on the ductal system with resultant ductal obstruction. Intraductal papillary mucinous tumor also causes pancreatitis by plugging the pancreatic ductal system with mucin or by releasing enzymes that activate trypsinogen.

Significant dilatation of the pancreatic duct with acute pancreatitis with a disproportionately larger pancreatic head compared to the pancreatic body may be a clue to suspect underlying malignancy on imaging. Also, peripancreatic and upper abdominal lymphadenopathy, metastases, and vascular encasement/invasion may be seen, which more readily lead to the correct underlying diagnosis. The underlying pancreatic mass may be seen only on follow-up imaging examinations, after inflammation has subsided.

Variants of Pancreatitis

Groove pancreatitis is focal inflammation of the pancreatoduodenal groove. The groove is located between the head of the pancreas and the second portion of the duodenum and contains the distal common bile duct. Groove pancreatitis may mimic pancreatic carcinoma or other masses. Its pathogenesis is controversial but may be related to/associated with biliary disease, peptic ulcers, gastric resection, duodenal wall or pancreatic head cysts, and/or pancreatic heterotopia within the duodenum. There is chronic inflammatory involvement of the duodenum, with fibrotic changes leading to various levels of stenosis. There may also be involvement of the pancreatic head, with predominance of the inflammatory process located in the groove.

On CT, soft tissue with variable delayed enhancement will be seen in the pancreatoduodenal groove. There may also be small cystic lesions along the medial aspect of the duodenum (Fig. 13-110). On MRI, a T1-hypointense mass in the pancreatoduodenal groove may be demonstrated, with variable T2 intensity. A subacute process will be higher in signal on T2, and chronic processes will appear more hypointense.

Autoimmune pancreatitis is a form of chronic pancreatitis caused by lymphoplasmacytic infiltration and fibrosis of the pancreas and is another entity that may be mistaken for pancreatic malignancy. A number of extrapancreatic manifestations of an autoimmune nature may coexist, facilitating the diagnosis on imaging and on clinical/laboratory evaluation.

Computed tomography, the modality of choice for imaging this disorder, characteristically demonstrates generalized enlargement of the pancreas with loss of its normal lobular architecture ("sausage" or "featureless" pancreas) (Fig. 13-111). The gland is homogeneously hypoattenuating with a nondilated or narrowed pancreatic duct. In a minority of cases there may be a peripancreatic "halo" of relatively low density. However, depending on the extent of fibrosis and inflammation, the imaging appearance of autoimmune pancreatitis can vary widely. When the

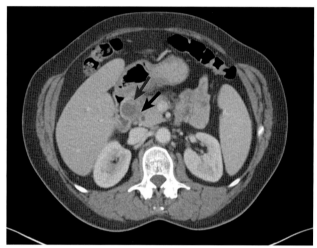

Figure 13-110 Groove pancreatitis. A 49-year-old woman presented with pleuritic back and abdominal pain. An axial view of the abdomen from contrast enhanced computed tomography demonstrates soft tissue in the pancreatoduodenal groove *(black arrow)*, with a cystic lesion along the medial aspect of the duodenum *(red arrow)*, in this patient with groove pancreatitis.

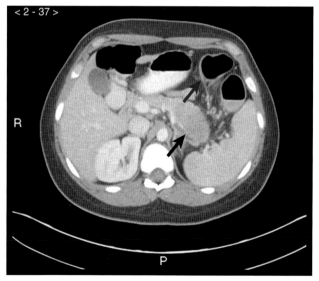

Figure 13-111 Autoimmune pancreatitis. A 27-year-old woman presented with acute abdominal pain and established diagnoses of autoimmune pancreatitis and inflammatory bowel disease (IBD). Note the characteristic sausage-shaped pancreatic tail with loss of its normal lobular architecture and generalized enlargement *(black arrow)*. There is also relatively mild peripancreatic fat stranding. Also note the transverse colon wall thickening and pericolic stranding *(red arrow)*, as well as the mild proliferation of the adjacent fat and blood vessels.

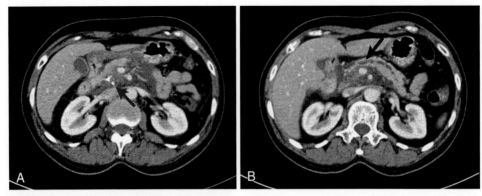

Figure 13-112 Acute upon chronic pancreatitis. A 52-year-old woman with a history of alcohol abuse, presented with midabdominal pain radiating to the back. **A** and **B**, Axial images from contrast-enhanced computed tomography showing characteristic features of chronic pancreatitis, including pancreatic atrophy, pancreatic calcifications *(red arrow)*, and pancreatic ductal dilatation *(black arrow)*. There are also features of acute pancreatitis, including peripancreatic inflammatory changes and fluid.

disease takes a focal form, most commonly in the head of the pancreas, it may appear as a pancreatic mass and can be particularly difficult to differentiate from pancreatic necrosis based on CT findings alone. Magnetic resonance imaging also characteristically demonstrates generalized gland enlargement. There is variable T2 signal and either heterogeneous or homogeneous enhancement in autoimmune pancreatitis. MRCP may show pancreatic duct narrowing, biliary strictures, and other biliary abnormalities.

Diagnostic criteria for autoimmune pancreatitis include elevated serum IgG4 levels and/or the presence of autoantibodies, although not all patients have these laboratory abnormalities. The standard treatment of autoimmune pancreatitis is corticosteroid therapy. There is a significant decrease in prominence of the pancreas and a normalization of the pancreatic duct caliber approximately 4 to 5 weeks post therapy.

Superimposed acute pancreatitis on underlying chronic pancreatitis is yet another potential imaging pitfall. Acute inflammatory changes can be present on CT concurrently with chronic pancreatitis findings of pancreatic atrophy, calcifications, and/or pancreatic ductal dilatation (Fig. 13-112).

TREATMENT
Conservative Management

Mild pancreatitis is generally self-limited and amenable to supportive therapy. This treatment involves pain control, correction of electrolyte and metabolic abnormalities, and administration of intravenous fluids. These patients usually resume an oral diet within 1 week, but for those who do not, nasojejunal feeding is preferred over total parenteral nutrition.

Percutaneous Intervention/ Interventional Radiology

APFCs and most pseudocysts regress spontaneously over time, but about 25% of pseudocysts become symptomatic and/or infected and need to be drained. A sterile symptomatic pseudocyst can be drained via percutaneous drainage.

In general, a retroperitoneal approach through the flank is preferred to avoid solid organs, bowel, and the spread of infectious material into the peritoneal cavity. In patients with pancreatic and/or peripancreatic collections and a worsening clinical status, without imaging signs strongly suggestive of infection (i.e., extraluminal gas), an image-guided fine-needle aspiration for Gram stain and culture should be performed. Also, patients with sterile necrotizing pancreatitis who do not improve clinically may have a disrupted pancreatic duct; in this setting, percutaneous drainage should be strongly considered as well.

Though infected pancreatic necrosis usually requires surgical débridement in conjunction with antibiotic therapy, some studies have shown that percutaneous drainage alone can be successful as long as all collections are drained. Patients with infected pancreatic necrosis who are poor surgical candidates can undergo percutaneous catheter drainage of the more liquefied portion of the collection to help stabilize the patient before surgery.

Interventional radiologic treatments are also used for pseudoaneurysm repair, most commonly with coil embolization. In aneurysms with larger necks or where coil embolization is too risky, a covered stent can be placed. Emergency embolization of a hemorrhaging vessel caused by pancreatitis can also be performed.

Endoscopic Treatments and Surgical Interventions

Transgastric drainage of uninfected pseudocysts, usually guided by EUS, should be limited to pseudocysts that cannot be accessed by other routes to avoid superinfection of sterile collections. The pseudocyst should also have a mature wall before drainage. Endoscopic approaches are generally not suitable for draining infected pseudocysts. Surgical débridement is generally reserved for patients with infected pancreatic necrosis.

PROGNOSIS

Acute pancreatitis is mild and self-resolving in 80% of patients, but has complications and causes significant morbidity and mortality because of severe pancreatitis in about 20% of patients. Mortality in the first week is most commonly due to the systemic inflammatory response syndrome and organ failure. Mortality after the first week is typically caused by sepsis and its complications. Overall mortality in patients with acute pancreatitis is 5% (1.5% in patients with mild acute pancreatitis and 17% in patients with severe acute pancreatitis). The mortality rate is approximately 12% with sterile necrotizing pancreatitis, 30% with infected necrotizing pancreatitis, and 47% with multisystem organ failure caused by necrotizing pancreatitis.

■ CONCLUSION

Imaging, especially CT, plays an integral role in the management of acute pancreatitis. Early in the disease process, imaging can help confirm the diagnosis of acute pancreatitis and can aid in determining its cause. Later in the course of disease, as was established by the revised Atlanta classification of acute pancreatitis, CT is useful for detecting necrosis and characterizing various pancreatic and peripancreatic collections. This helps determine the severity of disease, the patient's prognosis, and the best treatment options. Finally, imaging is an excellent way to monitor treatment response and to guide interventional procedures.

Hepatic Emergencies

Shamir Rai, Patrick McLaughlin, and Savvas Nicolaou

■ ACUTE HEPATITIS (Box 13-2)

Acute hepatitis, defined as an acute nonspecific inflammation of the liver parenchyma, has multiple causes with the most common being viral infection and alcohol. In the acute setting, imaging is often requested because hepatitis sometimes presents with symptoms that mimic an acute abdomen. The typical patient would be a young or a middle-age individual presenting with a history of fever, undefined pain in the upper right quadrant, jaundice, and elevations in liver function test results.

Acute Viral Hepatitis (Table 13-4)

Several viruses have been associated with acute liver failure (ALF), including hepatitis A, B, C, D, and E. Acute liver failure has also been seen with herpes simplex, varicella-zoster, Epstein-Barr virus (EBV), adenovirus, and cytomegalovirus; however, these viral infections are very rare causes of ALF. Although these viruses can be distinguished by their molecular and antigenic properties, all types of viral hepatitis produce clinically similar illnesses.

Acute liver failure is estimated to develop in 0.35% percent of patients with hepatitis A (fulminant hepatitis A) and in 0.1% to 0.5% of patients with acute hepatitis B. Acute hepatitis C causes ALF in Asia, but not Western countries. Hepatitis C virus alone does not appear to be a significant cause of ALF but requires coinfection with hepatitis B. Infection with hepatitis D virus can lead to ALF in patients with hepatitis B infection. A patient may

> **Box 13-2   Causes of Acute Hepatitis**
>
> **Infectious**
> Viral hepatitis type A-E
> Herpes simplex virus
> Varicella-zoster virus
> Epstein-Barr virus
> Cytomegalovirus
> Adenovirus
>
> **Vascular**
> Budd-Chiari syndrome
> Venoocclusive disease
> Ischemic hepatopathy
> HELLP syndrome
> Systemic hypoperfusion
>
> **Toxic**
> Alcohol
> Acetaminophen
> Halothane
> Idiosyncratic drug reaction
> Food-borne toxins, including mushroom poisoning
> Reye syndrome
>
> **Other**
> Sepsis
> Heat stroke
> Autoimmune
> Therapeutic embolization
> Radiation hepatitis (including external beam and yttrium 90)
> Wilson disease

HELLP, Hemolytic anemia, elevated liver enzyme levels, low platelet count.

either acquire both viruses at the same time (coinfection) or acquire hepatitis D in the setting of preexisting chronic hepatitis B (superinfection). The risk for ALF appears to be higher among patients who are coinfected than in those with hepatitis D superinfection or with acute hepatitis B alone. Hepatitis E virus is a significant cause of liver failure in countries where it is endemic, such as Russia, Pakistan, Mexico, and India. Overall, the case-fatality rate for hepatitis E is 0.5% to 3%, but for pregnant women mortality increases to 5% with a risk for fulminant liver failure of 15% to 25%. EBV hepatitis is generally regarded as a complication of infectious mononucleosis, but recently EBV hepatitis and jaundice have been described in patients without clinical features of infectious mononucleosis. Cholestatic jaundice due to EBV has also been documented.

Alcoholic and Toxic Hepatitis

Excessive alcohol consumption is associated with a spectrum of hepatic injury ranging from steatosis to acute hepatitis to end-stage liver disease. The majority of patients who present with symptomatic acute alcoholic hepatitis have a history of chronic alcohol abuse defined as consumption of greater than 100 g of ethanol per day for greater than two decades. Although obtaining an accurate clinical history may be difficult

Table 13-4   Hepatitis Viruses: Characteristics, Incubation Period, and Main Modes of Transmission

	A	B	C	D	E
Virus type	Picornaviridae	Hepadnaviridae	Flaviviridae	Deltaviridae	Hepeviridae
Nucleic acid	RNA	DNA	RNA	RNA	RNA
Mean (range) incubation period (days)	30 (15-50)	80 (28-160)	50 (14-160)	Variable	40 (15-45)
Main modes of transmission	Orofecal, sexual	Sexual, blood	Blood	Sexual, blood	Orofecal

in many alcoholic patients, the pattern of liver function test results derangement may be helpful. The majority of infective, vascular, and toxic causes of hepatocellular injury are associated with an aspartate aminotransferase (AST) level that is lower than the alanine aminotransferase (ALT) level; however, an AST-to-ALT ratio of 2:1 or greater is highly suggestive of alcoholic liver disease.

Acetaminophen poisoning has become the most common cause of ALF in the United States. Although repeated therapeutic dosages may lead to acute hepatitis in susceptible individuals, such as alcoholics, the vast majority of cases of hepatotoxicity result from overdosage, defined in adults as greater than 250 mg/kg or greater than 12 g over a 24-hour period. Acetaminophen is rapidly and completely absorbed from the GI tract with peak serum concentrations occurring approximately 4 hours after dosage. An overdose causes saturation of normal hepatic pathways in which acetaminophen is metabolized. Excess quantities of acetaminophen are subsequently metabolized to a toxic intermediate. This intermediate is converted via the cytochrome P-450 pathway, leading to depletion of hepatic glutathione stores and ultimately to hepatocellular injury. Patients who are taking medications that induce cytochrome P-450 enzymes, such as trimethoprim-sulfamethoxazole, carbamazepine, phenytoin, isoniazid, and rifampin may be at increased risk for hepatotoxicity following acetaminophen overdosage.

Liver function abnormalities peak from 72 to 96 hours after ingestion and are accompanied by clinical symptoms such as diaphoresis, pallor, lethargy, and nausea. Patients may be jaundiced and demonstrate symptoms and signs of hepatic encephalopathy. Up to half of patients with hepatic failure may also develop acute renal failure, and a large proportion of patients may also become coagulopathic. Mortality also peaks during this time window and is typically due to multiorgan failure. Patients who survive enter a recovery phase, and complete hepatic function is usually regained after 3 months.

Imaging (Table 13-5)
The imaging features of acute hepatitis are nonspecific, and the diagnosis is primarily based on clinical history and serologic and virologic findings. The most important role of imaging in patients with acute hepatitis is to evaluate for acute vascular complications and unexpected patterns of other diseases that produce similar clinical and biochemical abnormalities,

Table 13-5   Summary of Imaging Findings for Acute Hepatitis

Imaging Modality	Imaging Features
Ultrasonography	Starry-sky appearance (increased echogenicity of the portal-venous wall against a hypoechoic liver) Periportal edema Hepatomegaly Reduced hepatic echogenicity Gallbladder wall thickening Ascites
Computed tomography	Hepatomegaly Heterogenous parenchymal enhancement Periportal edema Ascites Gallbladder wall thickening Lymphadenopathy along hepatoduodenal ligament
Magnetic resonance imaging	Consistent findings with CT and US Periportal edema appears as high-signal intensity areas on T2-weighted images Involved parenchyma may demonstrate reduced signal intensity on T1-weighted images and increased signal intensity on T2-weighted images

CT, Computed tomography; *US*, ultrasonography.

such as extrahepatic cholestasis, diffuse metastatic disease, and cirrhosis.

Frequently encountered US findings in acute hepatitis include the "starry-sky" appearance, which is created by echogenic portal triads superimposed on a hypoechoic liver (Fig. 13-113). In addition, periportal lucency (hypoechoic or anechoic) is frequently encountered, which is suggestive of periportal edema due to hydropic swelling of hepatocytes. Hepatomegaly and a diffusely hypoechoic liver may often be the only manifestations of acute viral or acute alcoholic hepatitis. Ascites may be present, and in some cases of acute hepatitis the gallbladder wall is thickened (see Fig. 13-113). Computed tomography findings correlate well with ultrasonographically detected pathologic processes.

With CECT, heterogeneous parenchymal enhancement patterns may be present. In chronic disease, lymphadenopathy is frequently seen along the hepatoduodenal ligament. On MRI periportal edema appears as high-signal-intensity areas on T2-weighted images, and heterogeneous parenchymal enhancement patterns may also be found after the administration of gadolinium-based intravenous contrast agents (Fig. 13-114).

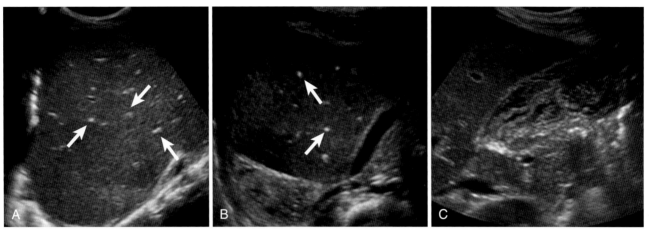

Figure 13-113 **A** and **B,** Ultrasonography (US) demonstrating a "starry-sky" appearance of the liver in a case of acute hepatitis, which describes an increased echogenicity of the portal-venous wall (**A** and **B,** *arrows*) against a hypoechoic liver. **C,** US demonstrating marked thickening of the gall bladder wall in a case of acute hepatitis.

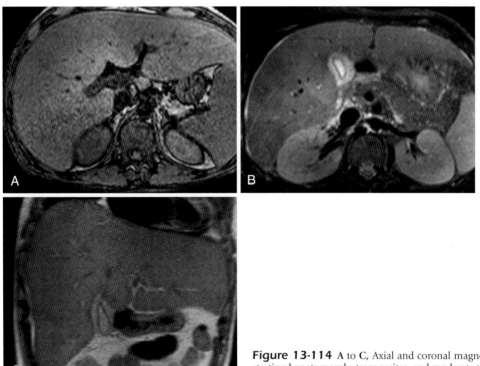

Figure 13-114 **A** to **C,** Axial and coronal magnetic resonance images (MRI) demonstrating hepatomegaly, trace ascites, and moderate to severe thickening and edema of the gall bladder wall (**B**) in a male patient with acute viral hepatitis.

■ PERIHEPATITIS (FITZ-HUGH-CURTIS SYNDROME)

Fitz-Hugh–Curtis syndrome (FHCS) is characterized by perihepatic inflammation secondary to transcoelomic dissemination of pelvic inflammatory disease (PID). This condition almost always involves women of childbearing age, but higher rates have been seen in adolescents, which may be attributed to differences in genital tract anatomy between adolescents and adults. Patients typically present with right upper quadrant pain that is often pleuritic in nature. Associated symptoms include fever, nausea, vomiting, and, in fewer cases, pain in the left upper quadrant. *Chlamydia trachomatis* and Neisseria gonorrhoeae are the most common pathogens associated with FHCS.

Perihepatitis specifically refers to secondary inflammation of the liver capsule and adjacent peritoneal surfaces. Perihepatitis is reported in 5% to 15% of cases of PID. The pathogenesis of this entity is not fully understood but may involve either direct extension of infected material from the cul-de-sac through the peritoneum and/or lymphatics or an immunologically mediated mechanism.

Imaging

Computed tomography features of FHCS include thickening of the parietal peritoneum, hepatic capsule, or more frequently, small loculated collections of subcapsular fluid. Hepatic capsular enhancement on CECT or MRI is present due to increased blood flow or inflammation of the hepatic capsule and is considered a characteristic feature of the acute phase of FHCS (Fig. 13-115). Definitive diagnosis is obtained by laparoscopic evaluation of the abdomen demonstrating "violin-string" adhesions. Ultrasonography images of the gallbladder, bile ducts, and liver parenchyma should be normal, although in the presence of ascites thin, stringy adhesions between the liver capsule and the anterior abdomen have been described. Ultrasonography is useful in excluding cholelithiasis and cholecystitis, although a thorough look at the ovaries for tubo-ovarian abscesses could substantiate a clinical diagnosis of PID. Ultrasonography may demonstrate the violin-string adhesions, but widening of the right anterior renal space and loculation of fluid in the hepatorenal space are typical findings.

■ HEPATIC ABSCESS

Abscesses of the liver most commonly are pyogenic or amebic in origin. They are defined as localized collection of pus with concomitant destruction of hepatic parenchyma and stroma. Pyogenic abscesses account for up to 88% of liver abscesses. In developing countries, liver abscesses are mostly due to parasitic infection. Imaging with US and CT provide the foundation for detection of intra-abdominal fluid collections and abscesses. Radionuclide imaging still plays a limited role, where intra-abdominal sepsis is suspected, but no definite abnormality is identified on US or CT. Ultrasonography and CT provide guidance for needle aspiration of fluid collections, making them ideal modalities for initial evaluation of patients with suspected abdominal sepsis.

Pyogenic Abscess

Pyogenic abscess, especially when multiple, may be caused by biliary infection (ascending cholangitis), hematogenous dissemination (GI infection via portal vein or disseminated sepsis via hepatic artery), or superinfection of necrotic tissue. Other causes for pyogenic abscess include direct extension from contiguous organs, such as a perforated gastric or duodenal ulcer,

lobar pneumonia, pyelonephritis, and subphrenic abscess. Before the advent of antibiotics, phlebitis of the portal vein secondary to appendicitis and diverticulitis was the most common cause of hepatic abscess. With portal-venous infection the right liver lobe is most commonly affected. With a biliary genesis, both lobes are involved equally. Abscesses are also observed subsequent to surgery and after blunt or penetrating trauma, most commonly during conservative treatment of severe liver injury. Pyogenic liver abscesses may also result from benign or malignant obstruction of the biliary tract or as a complication of biliary tract infection.

Patients usually present with fever and pain, guarding, and/or rocking tenderness localized to the upper right quadrant. *E. coli* and *K. pneumoniae* are two of the most important pathogens causing pyogenic liver abscess in adults. *S. aureus* is commonly isolated from pyogenic liver abscesses in children. Less commonly, isolated organisms include *Streptococcus faecalis, Clostridium,* and *Bacteroides.* It should be noted, however, that most pyogenic liver abscesses are polymicrobial. Mixed enteric facultative and anaerobic species are the most commonly reported pathogens. Anaerobes are probably underreported because they are difficult to culture and characterize. Studies have determined that approximately one quarter of pyogenic abscesses in Western countries are due to *K. pneumoniae.* Treatment with intravenous antibiotics and application of catheter drainage (under the guidance of imaging techniques) are principal therapies. Surgical intervention is indicated for medical treatment failure and abscess rupture. Mortality rates have decreased substantially over the past several decades, with recent studies reporting rates of 11% to 31%.

Imaging (Table 13-6)

Computed tomography and US are the imaging modalities of choice for detection of pyogenic abscesses, both demonstrating high sensitivity. Pyogenic abscesses may be classified as either microabscesses, if they are less than 2 cm, or macroabscesses when greater than 2 cm. Typically, initially small hypodense lesions with wall enhancement progress to form large, partially septated, sharply defined liquefied masses. When abscesses are multiple, they have a clustered appearance that coalesces into a single large cavity creating a "cluster"

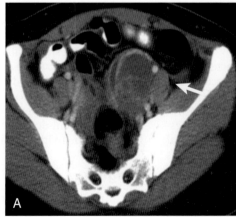
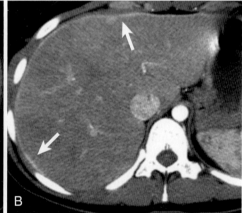

Figure 13-115 **A,** Axial contrast-enhanced computed tomographic scan demonstrating a complex tubo-ovarian abscess *(white arrow)* in a patient with *Chlamydia trachomatis.* **B,** Enhancement of the hepatic capsule *(white arrows)* was demonstrated, consistent with perihepatitis (Fitz-Hugh–Curtis syndrome).

sign (Fig. 13-116). By US most abscesses are anechoic; however, in about 30% echogenicity varies according to the amount and nature of debris contained within (Fig. 13-117). Gas locules contained within an abscess can be seen as a brightly echogenic foci with posterior reverberation artifact. Intralesional gas formation is more consistent with *Klebsiella* infection (Fig. 13-118).

Table 13-6   Summary of Imaging Findings of Pyogenic Abscess

Imaging Modality	Imaging Features
Radiography	Right lower lobe atelectasis Pleural effusion Hepatomegaly Intrahepatic gas Air-fluid level
Ultrasonography	Most abscesses are anechoic; about 30% have marked hyperechogenicity, dependent on the amount of debris Gas in an abscess can be seen as a brightly echogenic foci with posterior reverberation artifact
Computed tomography	Cluster sign: cluster of microabscesses coalesce into a single large cavity Hypodense, round, well-defined abscess Rarer (<20% cases): abscess with central gas—more consistent with *Klebsiella* infection Rim and septations show contrast enhancement Double target sign (present in only 30% of cases)
Magnetic resonance imaging	Cluster sign: cluster of microabscesses coalesce into a single large cavity On T1-weighted image the abscesses will typically appear as hypointense; however, on T2-weighted image the abscesses will appear as a hyperintense mass with perilesional edema (characterized by subtly increased signal intensity) Restricted diffusion

Borders may be well defined to irregular on US, with more acute lesions having a tendency to be less well demarcated.

The rim and septations of the abscess can show marked contrast enhancement on CT and MRI. Rim enhancement and perilesional edema are findings that help differentiate pyogenic abscesses from hepatic cysts. A double target sign consisting of a hypodense central area surrounded by a hyperdense ring and a more peripheral hypodense zone can sometimes be seen on CT, but this finding is not a common sign, documented in only 30% of patients. Very small abscesses will sometimes show more homogenous peripheral enhancement, which renders differentiation from a small hemangioma difficult. Atelectasis and pleural effusion are often demonstrated at the right lung base. On MRI, distinct perilesional edema

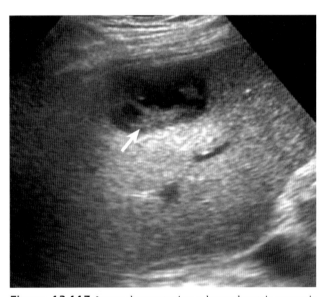

Figure 13-117 Image demonstrating a hypoechogenic pyogenic abscess with complex fluid collection *(white arrow)*.

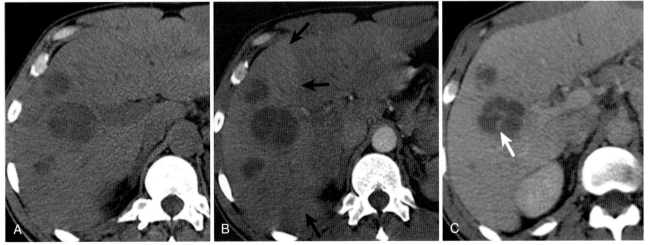

Figure 13-116 Noncontrast (**A**), arterial phase (**B**), and portal venous phase (**C**) contrast-enhanced computed tomographic images demonstrating the cluster sign in a patient with pyogenic hepatic abscesses. A cluster of microabscesses coalesce into a single large cavity *(white arrow)* with visible septations containing density content that is slightly higher than water. Of important note is the hyperemia *(black arrows)* surrounding the pyogenic hepatic abscess, noted only in the arterial phase (**B**).

and a characteristic pattern of dynamic enhancement of the abscess wall and perilesional liver tissue allows one to differentiate between infective and noninfective processes. Abscesses typically appear hypointense on T1-weighted images and variably hyperintense on T2-weighted images related both to internal fluid content and perilesional edema (Fig. 13-119). Diffusion is often restricted, and one published series of 18 patients found that apparent diffusion coefficient values in hepatic abscesses were lower than those in cystic and necrotic metastases ($0.67 \pm 0.35 \times 10^{-3}$ mm^2/sec in hepatic abscesses versus $2.65 \pm 0.49 \times 10^{-3}$ mm^2/sec in cystic and necrotic tumors). The perilesional liver tissues often show increased enhancement on both arterial and intermediate-phase CE MRIs.

Historically radiography showed signs of right lower lobe atelectasis, right hemidiaphragm elevation, right

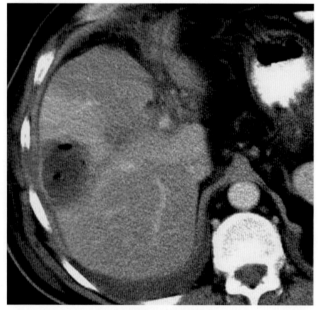

Figure 13-118 Computed tomographic (CT) image demonstrating a pyogenic abscess containing fluid and gas with perilesional edema. The gas is consistent with, but not exclusive, to a gram-negative bacterial infection—most commonly *Klebsiella pneumoniae*.

pleural effusion, and a focal hepatic air fluid level secondary to gas-producing pyogenic organisms. On abdominal radiography signs of hepatomegaly, intrahepatic gas, and air-fluid levels can also be detected.

Amebic Abscess

Amebiasis is defined by the World Health Organization and Pan American Health Organization as infection with the protozoan *Entamoeba histolytica*. The disease is global but most prevalent in developing countries and countries where poor sanitary conditions predominate. *E. histolytica* is most prevalent in India, the Far East, Africa, and Central and South America. In developed countries, infection with *E. histolytica* is typically seen in travelers and immigrants from endemic areas.

Amebic liver abscess is the most common extraintestinal complication of invasive amebiasis, occurring in 8.5% of cases, in which trophozoites from the colon invade the portal vein and subsequently the liver parenchyma. Amebic liver abscess is 7 to 10 times more common among adult men, despite equal gender distribution of intestinal *E. histolytica* infection. It is most frequently observed in individuals in their fourth or fifth decade of life. Amebic liver abscess can be life threatening. Patients typically present with right upper quadrant abdominal pain and fever for 1 to 2 weeks. The pain may radiate to the epigastrium, right thorax, or right shoulder. The pain is typically dull but can be pleuritic or aching. Other symptoms may include cough, sweating, malaise, weight loss, anorexia, and hiccup. Disease can occur months to years after exposure but most often occurs within 8 to 20 weeks after travel to endemic areas. In comparison to patients with pyogenic abscess, patients are usually younger and more acutely ill.

Imaging (Table 13-7)

Both CT and US are sensitive for detection of amebic abscess. In many patients it can be difficult to differentiate amebic from pyogenic abscess by imaging alone; however, in conjunction with the clinical and epidemiologic context a diagnosis can usually be made. On US, amebic abscesses typically present as peripherally located, round, sharply

Figure 13-119 A, Axial T1-weighted magnetic resonance image (MRI) demonstrating hypointense discrete pyogenic abscess pocket. **B,** Axial T2-weighted MRI demonstrating hyperintense discrete pyogenic abscess pocket with perilesional edema (*white arrow*).

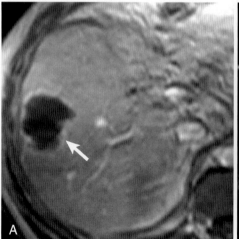
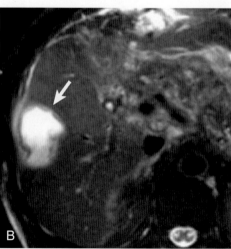

defined hypoechoic mass with low-level internal echoes and absence of significant wall echoes. The abscess can be anywhere from a few millimeters to a few centimeters in size. Amebic abscesses are more frequently found on the right lobe of liver (approximately 72% of the time). On CECT, amebic abscesses appear as round, well-defined unilocular or multilocular cystic lesions with an attenuation profile that suggests the presence of complex fluid (>10 to 20 HU) (Fig. 13-120). Amebic abscesses often demonstrate a peripheral zone or "halo" of edema and an enhancing wall that can range from 3 mm to 15 mm in thickness (see Fig. 13-120). On MRI, amebic liver abscesses are spherical and usually solitary lesions with a hyperintense center on T2-weighted images and a hypointense center on T1-weighted images. The abscess wall is usually thick, ranging from 5 mm to 10 mm. As with CT imaging, a characteristic finding of amebic abscess is a peripheral halo. The peripheral halo appears hypointense on T1-weighted and hyperintense on T2-weighted MRI.

■ VASCULAR PATHOLOGIC PROCESSES

Portal Vein Thrombosis/Occlusion (Box 13-3)

Acute portal vein thrombosis typically manifests with abdominal pain, fever, and nausea. Patients may be asymptomatic or have nonspecific symptoms. Portal vein thrombosis is defined as a condition resulting from formation of a blood clot in the extrahepatic portion of the portal vein. The portal vein accounts for 75% of blood flow to the liver. Many factors have been implicated in portal vein thrombosis ranging from local processes to systemic prothrombic factors. Cirrhosis is an important predisposing factor. The incidence of thrombosis in patients with liver cirrhosis varies from 0.6% to 11%. The incidence is much higher in individuals with HCC, in which it can reach

as high as 35%. Other important entities in the differential diagnosis, unrelated to hepatic disease, include acute appendicitis, cholecystitis, acute necrotizing pancreatitis, cholangitis, diverticulitis, and perforated peptic ulcers.

Imaging (Table 13-8)

Ultrasonography with Doppler imaging remains the modality of choice for portal vein occlusion or thrombosis. Doppler US allows determination of the direction and velocity of blood flow. On gray-scale imaging, hyperechoic material may be present within the portal vein, sometimes extending into the mesenteric veins. Doppler US can demonstrate absent flow, reversed flow in splenic veins, tumor vessels, and/or continuous flow in collaterals. Collaterals can be identified by the lack of respiratory variation in spectral Doppler velocities. Normal color Doppler imaging has a negative predictive value of 98%. Computed tomography and MRI often provide more detailed information about the extent of portosystemic collaterals and may better predict the origin and cause of thrombus. Chronic rather than acute portal vein occlusion is characterized by the presence of cavernous transformation or a portal cavernoma, which appears as a serpiginous network of small veins passing along the porta hepatis.

Budd-Chiari Syndrome

Budd-Chiari syndrome (BCS) is characterized by hepatic venous outflow obstruction either at the level of the hepatic veins, the IVC, or the right atrium. Diagnosis is primarily radiologic. Causes of BCS include hypercoagulable states such as pregnancy and oral contraceptive

Table 13-7 Summary of Imaging Findings of Amebic Abscess

Imaging Modality	Imaging Features
Radiography	Right lower lobe atelectasis Pleural effusion Elevation of right hemidiaphragm
Ultrasonography	Ovoid or round sharply defined hypoechoic mass with low-level internal echoes and absence of significant wall echoes
Computed tomography	Ovoid or round well-defined hypoattenuating lesion Thick enhancing wall that can range from 3 mm to 15 mm Peripheral zone of edema May be unilocular or multilocular
Magnetic resonance imaging	Hyperintense center on T2-weighted images and a hypointense center on T1-weighted images Thick enhancing wall Peripheral halo that is hypointense on T1-weighted and hyperintense on T2-weighted magnetic resonance images

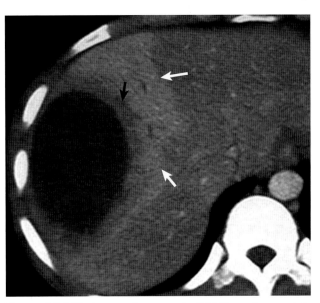

Figure 13-120 Computed tomography (CT) illustrating a peripherally located, sharply defined, round hypodense amebic abscess in the right lobe of the liver. A zone of peripheral low-density edema can be seen, which is characteristic of an amebic abscess *(black arrow)*. Hyperperfusion of the surrounding normal parenchyma can be seen *(white arrows)* due to increased arterial blood flow induced by the abscess.

Box 13-3   Causes of Portal Vein Occlusion and Thrombosis

Systemic
Cirrhosis
Portal venous hypertension
Pancreatitis
Peptic ulcer perforation
Surgical procedures, including liver transplantation, cholecystectomy
Splenectomy
Inflammatory bowel disease
Posttraumatic

Infectious
Cholangitis Cholecystitis
Appendicitis
Diverticulitis
Omphalitis
Sepsis and/or bacteremia

Malignant
Cholangiocarcinoma
Hepatocellular cancer
Gastric cancer
Pancreatic cancer
Lymphoma

Prothrombotic (Inherited)
Antithrombin III deficiency
Factor V Leiden
Prothrombin gene mutation
Protein C and S deficiency

Prothrombotic
Oral contraceptive use
Pregnancy
Myeloproliferative disorders: polycythemia vera, essential thrombocythemia
Antiphospholipid syndrome
Paroxysmal nocturnal hemoglobinuria

Table 13-8   Summary of Imaging Findings of Portal Vein Thrombosis/Occlusion

Imaging Modality	Imaging Features
Ultrasonography	Hyperechoic material within portal vein lumen Nonvisualized portal vein Chronic: cavernous transformation May see soft tissue mass or findings of pancreatitis if portal vein occlusion secondary to these causes
Doppler imaging	Absent flow in portal vein Reversed flow in splenic veins Tumor vessels Continuous flow in collaterals (no respiratory variation)
Computed tomography	Extensive portosystemic collaterals Small amount of ascites Contrast enhanced computed tomography can demonstrate a filling defect in the lumen of the portal vein Cause of portal vein occlusion (eg, pancreatitis/tumor)

use, tumor obstruction, and trauma. Hypercoagulable states alone accounted for 75% of all cases on BCS in the United States in 2006. About one third of patients present with acute symptoms ranging from sudden abdominal pain to ascites and liver failure. Jaundice and encephalopathy may be seen in the fulminant form of BCS. This entity represents a true nontraumatic hepatic emergency. If not treated promptly and appropriately the outcome is often fatal, secondary to liver failure.

Imaging

On US the key diagnostic finding is lack of blood flow or thrombus within the hepatic veins. The caudate lobe can be hypertrophied because of its independent venous drainage to the IVC. Visualization of a caudate lobe vein that is greater than or equal to 3 mm in diameter is strongly suggestive of the diagnosis of BCS. Color Doppler US has been demonstrated to have a sensitivity and specificity of 85% or greater and a negative predictive value of 98%. Spectral Doppler US may show a loss of variation of IVC phasicity during respiration, especially prominent in the distal IVC, hepatofugal blood flow, and bidirectional blood flow varying during the cardiac cycle from hepatofugal to hepatopetal. Computed tomography in the acute setting may demonstrate hepatomegaly with reduced peripheral subcapsular enhancement. Other findings include an enlarged caudate lobe that shows increased contrast enhancement relative to the rest of the liver, ascites, failure of opacification of the hepatic veins, and patchy enhancement of the hepatic hilum. Chronic BCS is associated with a spiderweb pattern of enhancement related to hepatic venous collaterals and also peripheral liver atrophy with relative sparing of the caudate lobe.

Hepatic Infarction

Hepatic infarctions are uncommon, because the liver has a dual blood supply from the hepatic artery and the portal vein and extensive collateral pathways. Hepatic infarction typically occurs from occlusion of a single intrahepatic arterial branch. This should be differentiated from ischemic hepatitis, in which ischemia is due to a systemic decrease in perfusion or oxygenation. Studies have shown that certain segments of the liver (segments IV and VIII) are more susceptible to infarctions especially following liver transplant. Other regions such as segment I have been shown to be at a lower risk. It has been hypothesized that some regions are more susceptible to infarctions post transplant because there is a variable distribution of a third hepatic blood supply termed the *parabiliary system*.

Spontaneous occlusion of the hepatic artery is typically related to trauma, aortic dissection, or cocaine toxicity. Iatrogenic causes include ligation of the hepatic artery after laparoscopic cholecystectomy, intimal injury or dissection related to chemoembolization of hepatic tumors, and thrombosis of the hepatic artery after transplantation. Rarely, hepatic infarction can be caused by nonocclusive circulatory disorders such as hypovolemia, sepsis, and other causes of shock. HELLP syndrome (hemolytic anemia, elevated liver enzyme levels, low platelet count) is an important cause of hepatic infarction in pregnant patients and other acute hepatic disorders of pregnancy discussed later.

Imaging (Table 13-9)

The classic finding of hepatic infarction is a geographic hypoenhancing focus within the liver with wedge-shaped borders (Fig. 13-121). As revascularization occurs, wedge-shaped infarcts have the potential to form round or oval-shaped lesions over a period of 48 hours after presentation. Acute infarcts are often not as well demarcated as subacute lesions. Gas may be seen within both sterile and infected infarcts. Hepatic infarcts often appear hypoechogenic on US and, similar to CT, commonly have indistinct margins in the acute setting. Doppler US is used to assess the patency of the hepatic artery and to assess for portosystemic shunting and collateral blood flow. Features on US, CT, and MR images are summarized in Table 13-9.

Nontraumatic Hemorrhagic Hepatic Lesions

In the absence of trauma or anticoagulant therapy, spontaneous hepatic bleeding is a rare condition. The most common causes of nontraumatic hepatic hemorrhages are HCC and hepatic adenoma, discussed later. Acute hemorrhage related to focal nodular hyperplasia, hemangiomas, and metastases are rarer entities. As mentioned previously, HELLP can be associated with hepatic infarction, but has also been associated with spontaneous hepatic hemorrhage as discussed in the following sections.

Hepatocellular Carcinoma

Ruptured HCC is an acute emergency associated with a high mortality that should be immediately suspected in any patient with a history of cirrhosis who presents with acute abdominal pain. Rupture is a reported complication in approximately 3% to 15% of HCC. Rupture is more likely to occur in the case of large primaries that are located toward the hepatic periphery, particularly in tumors that have extended beyond the capsule into the peritoneal cavity.

Imaging

Contrast-enhanced CT is the most effective method of diagnosing hepatic hemorrhage and has the additional benefit of determining the underlying cause. In addition to an enucleation sign, foci of active extravasation may be found on CECT. An enucleation sign is characterized by a low-attenuation mass with peripheral rim enhancement and focal discontinuity of the hepatic surface and is named after the expected appearance of a globe enucleated from the orbit. Hepatocellular carcinoma rupture is typically accompanied by hemoperitoneum (Fig. 13-122). Foci of parenchymal hemorrhage would appear hyperechoic on US, hyperattenuating on noncontrast CT, and of high signal on T1-weighted MRI (Fig. 13-123). It should be noted that the imaging appearances could vary significantly depending on the timing of imaging and the contrast bolus.

Hepatocellular Adenoma

Hepatocellular adenoma is a rare and benign liver tumor with a natural history of central necrosis, internal hemorrhage, and occasionally rupture. Hepatocellular adenomas are most commonly seen in young women with a history of oral contraceptive use but are also recognized in patients with glycogen storage disease, diabetes mellitus, or iron overload. Similar to HCC these lesions have an arterial blood supply, and

Table 13-9   Imaging Findings in Hepatic Infarction

Imaging Modality	Imaging Features
Ultrasonography	Hypoechogenic wedge-shaped areas Absence of flow in hepatic artery Portosystemic shunting and collateral blood flow (Doppler) Bile duct cysts or larger bile duct lakes (subacute finding)
Computed tomography	Hypoenhancing, geographic, wedge-shaped lesion with ill-defined borders (acute) Round or oval low-attenuation lesions located centrally within the liver with sharp borders (subacute) Atrophic capsular retraction (subacute) Bile duct cysts or larger bile duct lakes (subacute)
Magnetic resonance imaging	Well-defined wedge-shaped hypointense region as compared with normal parenchyma on T1-weighted MR images Heterogenously increased parenchymal signal on T2-weighted MR images.

MR, Magnetic resonance.

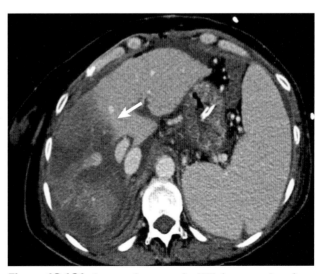

Figure 13-121 Computed tomography (CT) demonstrating a large region of hypoattenuation within the right lobe with a linear wedge-shaped border *(white arrow)* in a patient with hepatic infarction.

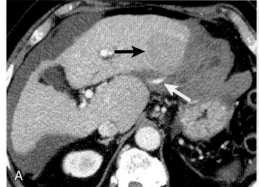
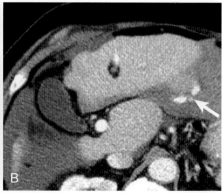

Figure 13-122 A and **B**, Contrast-enhanced computed tomographic scan demonstrates a subtle low-attenuation subcapsular mass in segment II *(black arrow)* of cirrhotic liver with surrounding hemoperitoneum. The *white arrow* denotes a small, but brisk focus of active contrast extravasation that can be seen pooling slightly inferiorly in **B**.

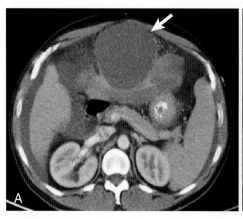
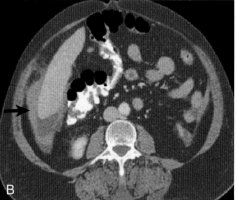

Figure 13-123 A, Computed tomography (CT) demonstrating a well-circumscribed exophytic, predominantly low-attenuation mass, low in segment II *(white arrow)* of a normal liver. **B**, *Black arrow* denotes a small collection of high-density fluid in the right subhepatic space consistent with acute hemoperitoneum.

spontaneous rupture and hemorrhage of a hepatocellular adenoma can be severe enough to produce hemorrhagic shock.

Imaging

Hepatocellular adenomas are often large and heterogenous in appearance. Ultrasonography may demonstrate a hypoechoic mass with internal echogenic regions. Doppler US may demonstrate large vessels in the periphery of the tumor. These features are replicated on CT and MRI. In addition, macroscopic fat or calcification may be seen within the mass lesion on CT. The presence of an acute subcapsular and/or intralesional and peritoneal hematoma can also be detected on CT or MRI.

■ HEPATIC EMERGENCIES—A FOCUS ON PREGNANCY

The two most common hepatic disorders in later pregnancy associated with preeclampsia are acute fatty liver and hepatic infarction as part of the HELLP syndrome. Because of the prothrombotic state of pregnancy, the risk for BCS increases, as discussed earlier. Hepatic infarction is associated with HELLP syndrome, which may subsequently lead to secondary rupture of the Glisson capsule, resulting in fatal intra-abdominal hemorrhage.

HELLP Syndrome

HELLP is an acronym that refers to a syndrome characterized by hemolysis (with a microangiopathic blood smear), elevated liver enzyme levels (serum AST > 70 units/L and serum lactate dehydrogenase value > 600 units/L or total bilirubin level > 1.2 mg/dL), and a low platelet count (< 100×10^9/L). HELLP syndrome is thought to occur as a result of obstruction of blood flow in the hepatic sinusoids and most likely is the result of a placenta-instigated disordered immunologic process. HELLP occurs in approximately 10% to 20% of pregnant women who present with severe preeclampsia/eclampsia and is a true nontraumatic hepatic emergency because it can be associated with hepatic infarction, hemorrhage, and spontaneous hepatic rupture.

Imaging (Table 13-10)

Computed tomography is not recommended because of the risks of radiation exposure to the fetus. Ultrasonography is useful for detecting acute hematomas, infarcts, and hepatic enlargement and for narrowing the differential diagnosis in ambiguous cases. Spontaneous rupture, if present, is most frequently observed involving the right hepatic lobe, in about 75% of cases (Fig. 13-124). Other findings include marked fatty infiltration and ascites and an irregular or wedge-shaped infarcted area or hematoma with increased echogenicity.

Table 13-10 Summary of Imaging Findings of HELLP Syndrome

Imaging Modality	Imaging Features
Ultrasonography	Irregular or wedge-shaped infarcted area or hematoma with increased echogenicity Periportal tracking Periportal halo sign
Computed tomography	Heterogenous areas of low attenuation that can be wedge shaped Enhanced vessels coursing through low-attenuation areas Hyperattenuating hematomas—most often found present in right lobe of the liver Marked fatty infiltration Signs of infarction (wedge-shaped, low-attenuation, peripheral lesion typically) Ascites

HELLP, Hemolytic anemia, elevated liver enzyme levels, low platelet count.

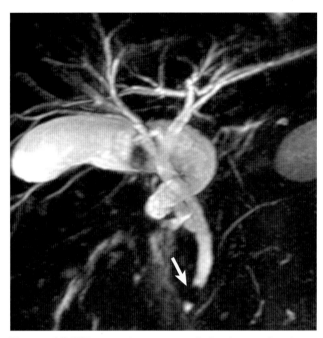

Figure 13-125 Magnetic resonance cholangiogram (maximum intensity projection [MIP] reformation of a three-dimensional [3-D] fast spin-echo data set) demonstrates a hypointense stone *(arrow)* in the distal common bile duct.

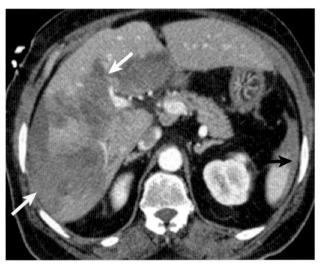

Figure 13-124 Axial contrast-enhanced computed tomographic scan demonstrating well-defined geographic low-attenuation regions within the anatomic right lobe of liver *(white arrows)* with associated small-volume acute hemoperitoneum *(black arrow)*. No focal mass was found, and a diagnosis of spontaneous hepatic rupture was confirmed at laparotomy.

Biliary Tract Emergencies

Jorge A. Soto and Stephanie L. Coleman

■ INTRODUCTION AND IMAGING TECHNIQUES

Acute diseases of the biliary system are common and often suspected as the cause of abdominal pain and other symptoms that bring patients to the ED. Thus considerable resources and effort are devoted to diagnosing these conditions accurately and avoiding potentially devastating delay. Advances in imaging technology have improved our ability to assess the biliary tract and gallbladder noninvasively in the vast majority of patients and increase diagnostic certainty.

Ultrasonography is the test used most often for initial evaluation. A complete US examination requires a thorough evaluation of the gallbladder, biliary ducts, and pancreas in multiple positions. Color Doppler adds relevant information about the status of vascular flow to the gallbladder wall. Computed tomography has become the workhorse imaging modality in the ED. Computed tomography is a very powerful diagnostic tool, with very high accuracy for detecting acute diseases, including those that affect the biliary tract. Although concerns about radiation exposure have brought increased scrutiny to the use of CT, a rational use ensures that in the vast majority of cases the expected benefits outweigh the largely theoretical risks derived from a single CT examination. A proper CT technique includes minimizing radiation exposure, as described in other sections of this book. Intravenous contrast (100 to 120 mL) is indicated. In most patients a single series acquired in the portal venous phase (60 to 75 seconds after the beginning of contrast administration) is sufficient. Noncontrast, arterial (25 to 30 seconds after the initiation of the contrast bolus injection) and delayed (5 to 7 minutes) phase images are seldom necessary in the emergency setting. Oral contrast material is typically not necessary for patients with suspected biliary tract pathologic processes. However, patients who are unable to receive intravenous contrast should undergo a complete preparation with oral contrast material.

MRCP is an accurate, noninvasive, test for evaluating the biliary tract (Fig. 13-125). MRCP has virtually replaced ERCP for diagnosis. As the number of MRI scanners installed worldwide continues to grow steadily, so has the number of legitimate indications for MRI for

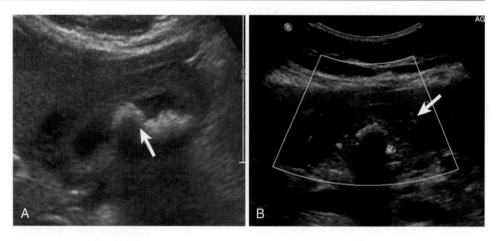

Figure 13-126 Ultrasonographic (US) images (**A**, longitudinal and **B**, transverse with color Doppler) of the gallbladder demonstrate characteristic findings of acute cholecystitis. There are multiple stones in the gallbladder (**A**, *arrow*), with associated diffuse wall thickening and wall hyperemia (**B**, *arrow*). The patient also complained of exquisite pain over the gallbladder (positive US Murphy sign).

evaluating acute abdominal conditions, including those affecting the gallbladder and biliary tract.

Other diagnostic tests that are used in the emergency setting for evaluating the gallbladder and biliary tract include nuclear biliary scintigraphy (mostly hepatobiliary iminodiacetic acid [HIDA] scans), ERCP, and percutaneous transhepatic cholangiography (both used almost exclusively for therapeutic purposes given their invasive nature), EUS, and, in some countries, CT cholangiography.

In the remaining sections a detailed description of the diseases affecting the biliary tract that are often seen in clinical emergency practice is provided. Emphasis is placed on the relative merits and weaknesses of each imaging technique for the diagnosis of the various diseases.

■ GALLBLADDER

Calculous Cholecystitis

The vast majority of cases of acute cholecystitis occur secondary to an impacted stone in the neck of the gallbladder or in the cystic duct (acute calculous cholecystitis). The stone precludes drainage of bile into the extrahepatic ducts and duodenum, causing progressive gallbladder dilatation and increased intraluminal pressure. Progressive wall ischemia and infiltration with inflammatory cells develop, followed by superimposed bacterial infection, hemorrhage, and necrosis. Occasionally, cystic duct patency is reestablished, and the cascade of events that leads to acute cholecystitis is halted. Cholecystitis can also occur in the absence of associated cholelithiasis (acute acalculous cholecystitis). When acute cholecystitis is not diagnosed and treated promptly, the complications that follow are the same for the calculous and acalculous varieties. These include gangrenous and emphysematous cholecystitis, which are discussed in detail later.

Gallstones and calculous cholecystitis are more common in women than men. Patients with acute cholecystitis often describe having suffered multiple prior episodes of biliary-type pain, which typically begin in the epigastrium and then localize focally in the right upper quadrant. Although the pain may initially be colicky, it eventually becomes constant in virtually all patients with acute cholecystitis. Constant pain lasting for more than 6 hours should raise the clinical suspicion of acute

cholecystitis. Fever, chills, leukocytosis, and other laboratory evidence of acute infection are present once acute inflammation is established. Approximately 10% to 15% of patients with acute cholecystitis have mild hyperbilirubinemia or jaundice. In elderly and diabetic patients the clinical presentation is often atypical and nonspecific, with minimal or no pain and fever. On physical examination there is tenderness in the right subcostal area that worsens considerably with deep inspiration (Murphy sign). A distended, painful gallbladder may be palpated in some patients. The Murphy sign can also be elicited during the US examination by asking the patient to take a deep inspiration with the ultrasonographic probe located over the gallbladder; this sign is present in 40% to 50% of patients with confirmed acute cholecystitis.

Ultrasonography is the primary method used when the clinical presentation suggests a biliary pathologic process. Characteristic findings of acute calculous cholecystitis on US include cholelithiasis, diffuse wall thickening with surrounding fluid and hyperemia (determined with color Doppler), gallbladder distention, and a positive Murphy sign (Fig. 13-126). These findings are suggestive, but none is diagnostic of acute cholecystitis; thus careful correlation with the patient's clinical status is critical. For patients with diffuse or nonlocalized abdominal pain, unexplained liver enzyme level elevation, or unexplained fever or leukocytosis, CT may be preferable to US as the initial imaging test. Computed tomography also depicts the gallbladder changes characteristic of acute inflammation. In addition to changes of acute inflammation in the gallbladder wall, CT shows abnormalities in the gallbladder fossa and pericholecystic fat (Fig. 13-127). Computed tomography is also preferred if a difficult US examination is anticipated, such as in obese patients or in the presence of distended loops of bowel. Magnetic resonance imaging with MRCP may be indicated to exclude coexisting choledocholithiasis in patients with known or suspected acute calculous cholecystitis. Magnetic resonance imaging demonstrates similar findings of acute inflammation in the gallbladder wall and surrounding fat as CT (Fig. 13-128). Biliary scintigraphy is a highly sensitive test for diagnosing acute cholecystitis (Fig. 13-129) but is currently being used mostly as a problem-solving tool in patients with questionable or inconclusive US findings. It is important

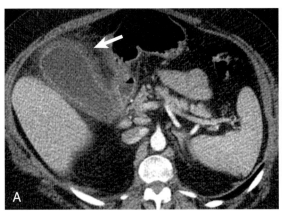
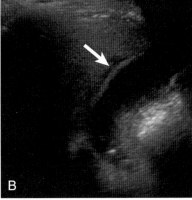

Figure 13-127 A, Axial contrast-enhanced computed tomographic image shows a distended gallbladder with wall thickening *(arrow).* These findings are characteristic of acute cholecystitis. **B,** Transverse ultrasonographic (US) image of the same patient shows subtle hypoechogenicity adjacent to the gallbladder wall. However, the degree of pericholecystic fat inflammation is underestimated on the US examination *(arrow).*

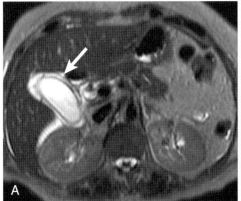
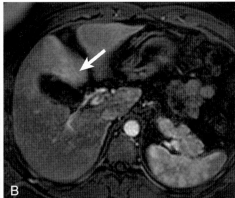

Figure 13-128 Axial heavily T2-weighted magnetic resonance image (MRI) **(A)** and axial fat-uppressed T1-weighted MRI **(B)** obtained in the arterial phase after the administration of intravenous contrast demonstrate characteristic changes of acute calculous cholecystitis. The gallbladder is distended with wall thickening and pericholecystic fluid **(A,** *arrow).* There is also hepatic parenchymal hyperenhancement in the gallbladder fossa **(B,** *arrow).*

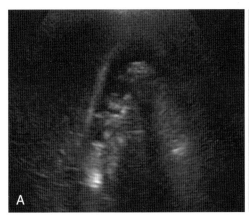
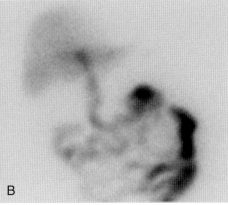

Figure 13-129 A, Ultrasonographic (US) image demonstrates findings suspicious for acute cholecystitis: multiple gallstones and associated gallbladder wall thickening. **B,** The hepatobiliary iminodiacetic acid (HIDA) scan confirms acute cholecystitis. The image was acquired 60 minutes after injection of the radiotracer. There is adequate filling of the extrahepatic bile ducts and passage of the tracer to the duodenum and small bowel, but no filling of the gallbladder. In the proper clinical setting these findings are highly consistent with acute cholecystitis.

to bear in mind that all imaging tests have pitfalls that can lead to a false-negative or false-positive diagnosis of acute cholecystitis. Close correlation with the clinical information available increases diagnostic certainty.

Acute Acalculous Cholecystitis

Acute acalculous cholecystitis is caused by prolonged fasting and decreased gallbladder contractions, leading to bile stasis, luminal overdistention, and secondary wall ischemia. Acalculous cholecystitis occurs most commonly after a prolonged hospitalization in debilitated patients with comorbidities such as diabetes, sepsis,

coronary artery disease, or multitrauma and in patients receiving total parenteral nutrition or mechanical ventilatory support in intensive care units. Acalculous cholecystitis causes approximately 5% to 10% of all cases of acute cholecystitis. The mortality rate (10% to 50%) is considerably higher than that of calculous cholecystitis (1% to 2%). Compared to cholecystitis caused by stone disease, acalculous cholecystitis is also associated with a higher incidence of complications such as gangrene, emphysema, and perforation.

Results of routine laboratory tests are nonspecific and include an elevated white blood cell count and altered liver function test results. Blood cultures may isolate a microorganism but do not localize the focus of the infection. Thus the diagnostic evaluation of these severely ill patients with unexplained sepsis or leukocytosis eventually leads to the request for imaging tests, especially CT. Findings include a distended gallbladder with thickened walls (>3 to 4 mm), with or without pericholecystic fluid. Intraluminal sludge may be present but without stones (Fig. 13-130). These findings are not specific for cholecystitis and can be mimicked by other diseases and conditions, such as hepatitis, cirrhosis, heart failure, and hypoalbuminemia. Nuclear scintigraphy with HIDA can be used to confirm a suspected diagnosis of acalculous cholecystitis (see Fig. 13-130). Unfortunately, scintigraphy also has numerous potential pitfalls leading to false-negative and especially false-positive results. In this setting, nonfilling of the gallbladder on a HIDA scan is highly suggestive of acute cholecystitis, but not diagnostic. Definitive therapy is achieved with cholecystectomy (open or laparoscopic). Nonsurgical candidates may undergo percutaneous cholecystostomy tube placement under imaging guidance. This procedure also has a diagnostic role in complex or questionable cases. Bile cultures are positive in only 50% of patients with confirmed acalculous cholecystitis.

Complicated Acute Cholecystitis

As untreated acute cholecystitis progresses, various complications can develop, including gallbladder empyema, gangrenous and emphysematous cholecystitis, gallbladder perforation with pericholecystic abscess, hemorrhage, and bilioenteric fistula. These complications occur more commonly in elderly and debilitated patients, as well as in patients with significant comorbidities. An infected gallbladder in the setting of cystic duct obstruction progresses to gallbladder empyema and eventually to wall gangrene and/or perforation.

Gangrenous Cholecystitis

Gangrenous cholecystitis is a surgical emergency because these patients rapidly become toxic and develop septicemia and septic shock. On US a gangrenous gallbladder wall has a striated, multilayered appearance (Fig. 13-131), with decreased or absent flow on Doppler evaluation. On CT or MRI the wall is indistinct, with no enhancement in the foci of gangrene (see Fig. 13-131). This decrease in wall enhancement has been shown to be highly predictive of wall gangrene. Intramural or intraluminal hemorrhage is another manifestation of wall ischemia. The presence of blood contents is also a highly specific sign of gangrenous cholecystitis.

Gallbladder Perforation

A defect in the wall of the gallbladder is a sign of perforation. Perforations usually result in extraluminal fluid that can be localized (intramural or pericholecystic abscess) or free, causing peritonitis. The inflamed gallbladder wall may also adhere to the wall of the colon or

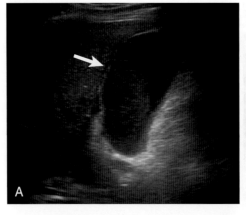
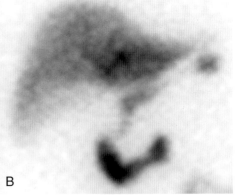

Figure 13-130 A, Transverse ultrasonographic (US) image shows a distended gallbladder containing biliary sludge, but no stones. There is a halo of pericholecystic hypoechogenicity *(arrow)*. **B,** Hepatobiliary iminodiacetic acid (HIDA) scan static image obtained 60 minutes after injection of the radiotracer shows patent bile ducts, but no filling of the gallbladder, confirming the clinical diagnosis of acute acalculous cholecystitis.

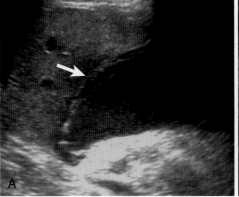
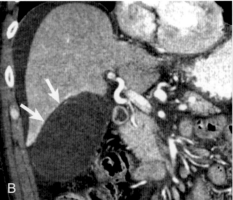

Figure 13-131 A, Longitudinal ultrasonographic (US) image demonstrates a distended gallbladder with echogenic sludge and a striated appearance of the wall *(arrow)*, consistent with gangrenous cholecystitis. **B,** Coronal reformation of a computed tomographic (CT) examination performed with intravenous contrast shows areas of absent enhancement in the gallbladder wall *(arrows)*.

duodenum and subsequently create a free communication between the gallbladder lumen and these hollow viscera. This fistulous communication allows passage of infected bile and gallstones into the bowel lumen and eventually causes gallstone ileus (impaction of a gallstone in the ileocecal valve with bowel obstruction) or rarely Bouveret syndrome (impaction of a stone in the duodenum).

Emphysematous Cholecystitis

Emphysematous cholecystitis develops when ischemia of the gallbladder wall is complicated by infection with gas-forming organisms and gas accumulates within the gallbladder lumen and gallbladder wall. Emphysematous cholecystitis can occur in patients with acute calculous or acalculous cholecystitis. Diabetes predisposes to the development of emphysematous cholecystitis; 40% to 60% of patients are diabetic. The mortality rate of emphysematous cholecystitis can be as high as 15% to 20%, but clinical symptoms can be deceptively mild. On imaging the defining finding is the presence of intramural or intraluminal gallbladder gas. Gas is seen on US as nondependent echogenic foci in the lumen or as curvilinear echogenic foci in the wall of the gallbladder, but CT may be necessary to confirm the diagnosis (Fig. 13-132). However, other potential causes of intraluminal gas in the gallbladder, such as recent ERCP, indwelling biliary stent, or prior biliary-enteric anastomosis must be excluded to make a definitive diagnosis.

■ ACUTE BILIARY DUCTAL OBSTRUCTION

The clinical presentation of patients with acute biliary obstruction varies with the severity of the obstruction and with the presence or absence of complicating ascending cholangitis. Abnormal laboratory test results,

such as elevated bilirubin, alkaline phosphatase, and γ-glutamyl transpeptidase levels, are common but are nonspecific. If there is associated leukocytosis, ascending cholangitis needs to be considered and excluded because emergent biliary drainage will be necessary (see later discussion of ascending cholangitis).

Choledocholithiasis

Choledocholithiasis is the most common cause of acute biliary obstruction. Ten percent to 15% of patients with cholelithiasis develop bile duct stones, either at the time of cholecystectomy or following removal of the gallbladder. The frequency is higher in elderly patients. The majority of cases of choledocholithiasis are secondary to the passage of stones from the gallbladder through the cystic duct into the common bile duct. Primary choledocholithiasis (i.e., de novo formation of stones within the common bile duct) is much less common. Because the presence of stones in the bile ducts increases the morbidity and mortality associated with gallstone disease, the clinical suspicion of choledocholithiasis complicates the workup and management of cholelithiasis and results in the need for additional diagnostic and therapeutic procedures.

The clinical presentation of patients with choledocholithiasis is highly variable. Bile duct stones are an incidental finding in 7% to 10% of patients who undergo routine cholecystectomy for symptomatic cholelithiasis. Approximately 50% eventually develop symptoms such as right upper quadrant or epigastric pain and dyspepsia. Laboratory test result abnormalities include elevated bilirubin and alkaline phosphatase levels. Confirmation of the diagnosis requires visualizing the stones on imaging. Ultrsonography is an excellent modality for detecting biliary ductal dilatation, but direct visualization of stones in the bile ducts as echogenic foci with acoustic shadowing (Fig. 13-133) surrounded by anechoic bile is

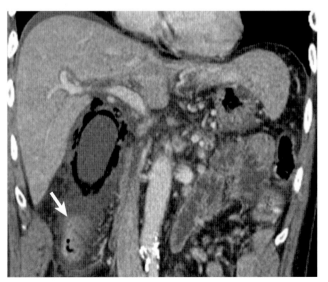

Figure 13-132 Coronal contrast-enhanced computed tomographic image demonstrates concentric intramural gas in the gallbladder. This finding is diagnostic of emphysematous cholecystitis. In addition, there is infiltration of the surrounding fat and wall thickening in the adjacent colon (*arrow*).

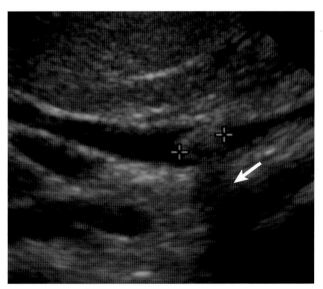

Figure 13-133 Ultrasonographic (US) image obtained along the long axis of the common bile duct demonstrates an echogenic intraductal focus (*calipers*) with distal acoustic shadowing (*arrow*), representing a stone.

frequently suboptimal. The literature reports sensitivity rates of US for detecting stones in the common bile duct varying between 15% and 70%. Bowel gas and abdominal fat often hinder visualization of the more distal common bile duct (Fig. 13-134).

Computed tomography is also sensitive for depicting ductal dilatation and is more accurate than US for determining the exact site and likely nature of the obstructing lesion. Sensitivity of CT for detecting choledocholithiasis varies between 60% and approximately 90%. High-spatial-resolution images acquired with multidetector technology and high-quality MPRs enhance the ability to detect smaller stones. The appearance of biliary stones on CT is dependent upon stone composition and is generally divided into three types: predominantly cholesterol, predominantly pigment, and mixed cholesterol and pigment. The calcium content varies proportionally with the pigment content; thus a homogeneously hyperattenuating appearance on CT is indicative of a predominantly pigment composition (Fig. 13-135). Conversely, stones composed primarily of cholesterol stones tend to be lower in attenuation (see Fig. 13-135). Most stones contain both pigment and cholesterol, and consequently their appearance on CT is variable. Computed tomography exposure parameters, especially the kilovolts peak, also have a direct effect on the attenuation of biliary stones on CT. Although enhancement of the pancreatic glandular parenchyma and periductal tissues may obscure small intraductal stones, the clinical indication for performing the CT usually calls for the administration of intravenous contrast.

MRCP is the definitive noninvasive test for diagnosing bile duct stones. MRCP has very high sensitivity and specificity (approximately 95% to 98%, comparable to ERCP). All stones, regardless of their composition, are markedly hypointense on heavily T2-weighted MR images and appear as low-signal-intensity intraductal foci, outlined by high-signal-intensity bile (see Fig. 13-125). With the use of state-of-the-art MRI equipment, ultrafast pulse sequences, and high-performance coils, excellent quality MRCP images can be acquired during short breath-hold periods. ERCP confirms the diagnosis of choledocholithiasis and serves as the preferred means of therapy for retained bile duct stones. The role of EUS and choledochoscopy in the preinterventional diagnosis of choledocholithiasis is limited.

Mirizzi Syndrome

Mirizzi syndrome occurs in the setting of acute or chronic calculous cholecystitis, when a stone becomes fixed in the gallbladder neck or cystic duct and the inflammation extends to the hepatoduodenal ligament, secondarily involving and obstructing the common hepatic duct. This leads to proximal biliary ductal dilatation. A fistulous

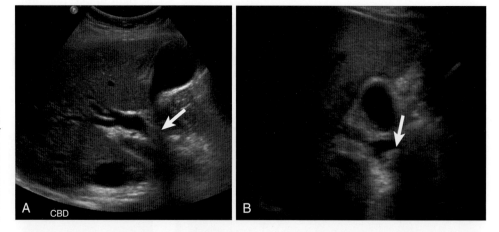

Figure 13-134 A, The shadow arising from the duodenum *(arrow)* precludes visualization of the distal common bile duct on this ultrasonographic (US) image obtained along the long axis of the duct. **B,** Transverse image obtained a few hours later demonstrates an echogenic dependent intraductal focus, representing a stone *(arrow)*.

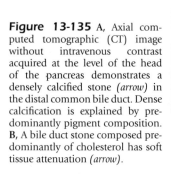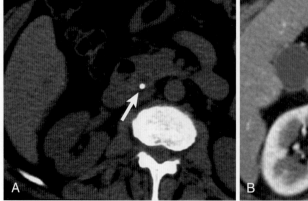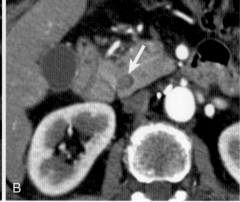

Figure 13-135 A, Axial computed tomographic (CT) image without intravenous contrast acquired at the level of the head of the pancreas demonstrates a densely calcified stone *(arrow)* in the distal common bile duct. Dense calcification is explained by predominantly pigment composition. **B,** A bile duct stone composed predominantly of cholesterol has soft tissue attenuation *(arrow)*.

communication between the cystic duct and the common hepatic duct may be created as well. Patients present clinically with pain and other symptoms of acute biliary tract obstruction. Certain anatomic variants, such as a long cystic duct that courses parallel to the common hepatic duct or a cystic duct that inserts low into the common bile duct are associated with a higher risk for developing Mirizzi syndrome. Accurate presurgical diagnosis of Mirizzi syndrome directly affects patient prognosis. Chronic inflammation with formation of adhesions can lead to serious surgical complications if the diagnosis is not suggested before intervention. Adhesions may severely limit the ability of the surgeon to properly assess the biliary anatomy in the hepatoduodenal ligament, especially at laparoscopic cholecystectomy. The common bile duct may be mistaken for the cystic duct, not uncommonly leading to ligation or permanent injury. Therefore, when the diagnosis of Mirizzi syndrome is entertained, a traditional ("open") approach to cholecystectomy should be considered.

The diagnosis of Mirizzi syndrome can be made, or at least suggested, on carefully interpreted imaging studies. Ultrasonography may demonstrate the stone in the cystic duct or gallbladder neck, along with dilatation of the intrahepatic and common hepatic ducts and a normal-caliber distal common bile duct. Computed tomography shows similar findings, but direct visualization of the impacted stone may be difficult. On MRCP the impacted stone in the gallbladder neck or distal cystic duct is usually very well seen, along with the dilated proximal common hepatic duct and intrahepatic ducts (Fig. 13-136). The gallbladder may be distended as well. On direct cholangiography (ERCP or percutaneous transhepatic cholangiography), the impacted calculus appears as a rounded filling defect or a smooth extrinsic compression of the common hepatic duct.

Acute Cholangitis

Acute ascending cholangitis occurs when the obstructed and dilated biliary tree becomes secondarily infected with bacteria. Bacteria reach the bile ducts directly from the duodenum (ascending) or via the portal venous system (hematogenous). Bacterial colonization of a properly draining biliary system usually does not result in acute cholangitis. However, with obstruction the increasing intraductal pressures push the infection proximally into the intrahepatic ducts, hepatic veins, and perihepatic lymphatics. This sequence eventually causes bacteremia and sepsis. Pyogenic liver abscesses and microabscesses, originating in the infected bile ducts, are a common finding in ascending cholangitis.

The underlying cause of the obstruction is most often a stone, followed by neoplasms and benign strictures. Ascending cholangitis can also occur as a complication of ERCP, when pressure is applied to inject contrast material into a dilated and obstructed biliary tree. The clinical presentation varies widely, from mild and nonspecific symptoms such as malaise and low-grade fever to overwhelming and sometimes fatal sepsis. The Charcot triad (right upper quadrant pain, fever, and jaundice) occurs in up to 25% of patients; the Reynolds pentad adds mental status changes and sepsis. In the past, mortality approached 100%, but increased awareness leading to more timely diagnosis and aggressive therapy have improved prognosis. Current mortality rates vary between 5% and 10%. Emergent therapeutic interventions that are often necessary include ERCP with sphincterotomy, stone extraction, and biliary stent or nasobiliary drain placement.

On imaging, findings of biliary obstruction and acute infection/inflammation are demonstrated. Pneumobilia is a common ancillary finding because there is often history of recurrent biliary disease and prior interventions. Imaging studies show ductal dilatation, pneumobilia, and possibly stones in the common bile duct. Additional findings seen on CT and MRI include signs of bile duct inflammation, such as wall thickening, hyperenhancement, and periductal fat stranding. When a stone is suspected as the underlying cause of acute obstruction, MRI/MRCP has advantages in accuracy over US and CT, as described earlier. Multiphasic CT and MRI scans may also demonstrate a characteristic sign of ascending cholangitis: early (arterial phase) hyperenhancement of the

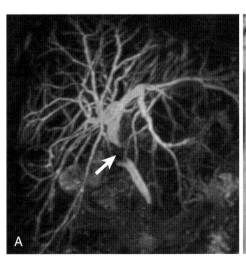
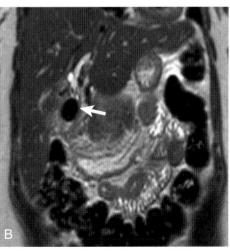

Figure 13-136 Mirizzi syndrome demonstrated with magnetic resonance imaging (MRI). A, Magnetic resonance cholangiopancreatography (MRCP) (three-dimensional [3-D] fast spin-echo sequence) demonstrates dilated intrahepatic ducts and common hepatic duct, with a normal-caliber common bile duct. There is a low-signal-intensity focus *(arrow)* at the junction of the cystic duct and common hepatic duct. **B,** Coronal T2-weighted image shows the large impacted hypointense stone *(arrow)*.

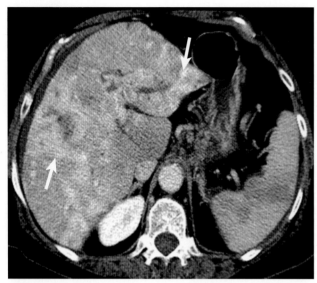

Figure 13-137 Contrast-enhanced computed tomographic image obtained in the arterial phase demonstrates multiple ill-defined foci of hyperenhancement in the liver parenchyma *(arrows)* surrounding dilated intrahepatic bile ducts. These foci represent hyperemia and are caused by infection of the obstructed biliary tree (ascending cholangitis).

hepatic parenchyma surrounding the infected bile ducts (Fig. 13-137). Intrahepatic abscesses of variable size are a common finding seen as well. These abscesses communicate with the dilated intrahepatic ducts, as demonstrated on ERCP.

Recurrent Pyogenic Cholangitis

Recurrent pyogenic cholangitis is a type of infectious cholangitis that occurs most commonly in people from Southeast Asia. Chronic infection with the parasites *Ascaris lumbricoides* or *Clonorchis sinensis* and malnutrition are predisposing factors, by promoting the calcium formation of pigmented stones. Bacterial superinfection ensues, and affected patients present with recurrent episodes of ascending cholangitis. Recurrent inflammation leads to the development of chronic complications such as fibrosis with strictures, parenchymal disruption and cirrhosis, hepatic abscesses, portal hypertension, and cholangiocarcinoma.

Ultrasonography, CT, and MRI show biliary ductal dilatation with casts of sludge and stones filling the ducts. Calculi and pneumobilia are both frequent findings, but differentiation of the two on US may be difficult because both can produce acoustic shadowing. Periportal hyperechogenicity is a common sonographic finding as well. On CT, pigment stones are typically hyperattenuating relative to the unenhanced liver parenchyma. Magnetic resonance imaging and MRCP show all the characteristic findings of recurrent pyogenic cholangitis: segmental duct dilatation, ductal strictures, and calculi. The main advantage of MRCP over ERCP is the ability to depict ducts proximal to stenotic segments without the risk for causing or worsening biliary sepsis. Noncalcified calculi are better visualized with MRI than CT but, as on US, differentiating between stones and gas on MRI may be

difficult because both are hypointense intraductal foci. Imaging surveillance of patients with recurrent pyogenic cholangitis focuses on the detection of complications: abscess formation, intrahepatic bilomas, portal vein thrombosis, and cholangiocarcinoma.

Nontraumatic Pelvic Emergencies

Refky Nicola, Daniel Kawakyu-O'Connor and Jennifer W. Uyeda

■ NONOBSTETRIC PELVIC EMERGENCIES

Adnexal Torsion

Adnexal torsion is defined as the twisting of the adnexa, including the ovary, on its ligamentous support. The ligamentous support is composed of the lymphatic, veins, and arteries. Initially there is an obstruction of the lymphatic supply, which causes an increase in capillary pressure and massive edema of the ovaries. If left untreated, this will progress to hemorrhagic infarction of the ovary. Ovarian torsion is most prevalent during the reproductive years. Risk factors include pregnancy, dermoid cyst, hemorrhagic cyst, and ovarian hyperstimulation syndrome. Some studies have hypothesized that the right ovary is more susceptible to torsion due to the fact that the sigmoid colon forms a protective barrier on the left side.

The clinical presentation of ovarian torsion is nonspecific, and the condition is generally included in the differential diagnosis of acute abdominal and pelvic pain. Symptoms include nausea, vomiting, sharp right or left lower abdominal pain, and tenderness. Patients may complain of constant or intermittent abdominal pain depending on whether there is complete torsion or a torsion/detorsion of the adnexa.

Ultrasound (transvaginal and transabdominal) is the primary modality used for the evaluation of patients with adnexal torsion. On gray-scale US examination, the most common finding is marked enlargement of the ovary, which may measure up to 12 to 20 times the normal size. Because of the venous congestion and lymphatic obstruction, the US image will also demonstrate multiple cysts along the periphery of the engorged ovary (Fig. 13-138). In addition, there is associated free fluid within the cul-de-sac in almost 90% of cases. In addition to evaluating the symptomatic side, an examination of the contralateral side is recommended for comparison. On color Doppler imaging the classic appearance is the complete absence of arterial flow, but this is present in only a minority of cases. Ovaries without arterial flow are usually found to be infarcted at surgery. The most frequent findings is a decrease or complete absence of venous flow due to collapse of the more compliant venous walls (Fig. 13-139). Lee and colleagues described a finding, which incorporates both the gray-scale and color Doppler ultrasonographic features, that is known as the *twisted pedicle* or the *whirlpool* sign. The twisted

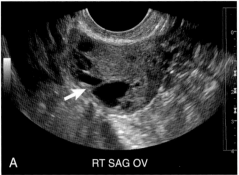

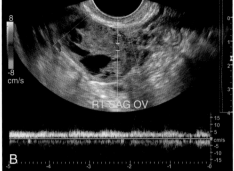

Figure 13-138 A, Transvaginal gray-scale ultrasound (US) image of the right ovary demonstrates an enlarged ovary with multiple follicles along the periphery in a partially torsed ovary. This is known as the "string of pearls" sign. B, Spectral Doppler images of the right adnexa demonstrate dampening of the venous waveforms, which is consistent with a torsion-detorsion of the right ovary.

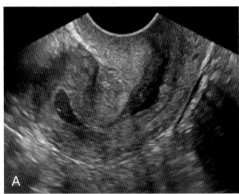

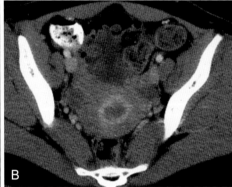

Figure 13-139 A, Sagittal ultrasonographic image of the uterus demonstrates a small volume of hypoechoic fluid within the endometrial cavity and increased echogenicity of adjacent pelvic fat. B, Axial postcontrast computed tomography (CT) image of the pelvis demonstrates low-attenuation fluid within the endometrial cavity and mild endometrial enhancement. The findings are suggestive of endometritis.

pedicle represents the vascular pedicle rotated upon itself and is typically seen as an echogenic round or beaked mass with multiple concentric hypoechoic, targetlike stripes. On color Doppler US the twisted vascular pedicle is visualized as a series of circular or coiled vessels.

Pelvic Inflammatory Disease

Pelvic inflammatory disease (PID) refers to a spectrum of infectious disease states involving the upper genital tract. The CDC estimates that more than 750,000 women experience acute PID annually, which results in approximately 50,000 hospitalizations. The chronic sequelae of PID can result in significant morbidity, including infertility, ectopic pregnancy, ovarian and pelvic vein thrombosis and thrombophlebitis, and chronic pelvic pain.

In most cases of PID the microorganisms in the lower genital tract pass through the endocervical canal and cause infection of the endometrium, which may progress to involve the fallopian tubes, ovaries, adjacent pelvic structures, and peritoneal surfaces.

The most common organism is *Chlamydia trachomatis;* others include *Neisseria gonorrhoeae, Haemophilus influenzae, Gardnerella vaginalis,* enteric gram-negative rods (e.g., *Escherichia coli*), *Mycoplasma* species, streptococci, and anaerobes. Tubo-ovarian abscesses are often polymicrobial and may involve both anaerobic and coliform bacteria. Viruses, including herpes simplex virus 2 and cytomegalovirus, have also been found to sometimes be implicated in the process.

Signs and symptoms of acute PID are nonspecific. Sometimes the presence of cervical, uterine, or adnexal tenderness is sufficient evidence to warrant therapy if there is no other probable cause for the patient's symptoms. Additional signs of lower genital tract infection that increase specificity of diagnosis include cervical friability, vaginal or cervical discharge, fever, elevated erythrocyte sedimentation rate or C-reactive protein level, or laboratory evidence of presence of *C. trachomatis* or *N. gonorrhoeae* in secretions. Fitz-Hugh-Curtis syndrome, a complication of PID, presents as right upper quadrant and/or right-sided pleuritic pain secondary to perihepatitis.

There are limited data supporting the routine use of imaging tests for the diagnosis of PID; empiric therapy is effective and widely accepted. Imaging of PID is more commonly used when the clinical diagnosis is equivocal or complications are suspected. Imaging findings suggestive of PID also may be incidentally noted in the evaluation of acute abdominal or pelvic pain.

Endometritis is a presentation of PID involving the endometrial cavity. Ultrasonographic findings of endometritis may include mild enlargement of the uterus, thickening of the endometrium, endometrial fluid, and/or increased echotexture of the adjacent pelvic fat (Fig. 13-140). Computed tomography may depict endometrial enhancement and fluid (see Fig. 13-138) and increased volume of intraperitoneal fluid. The presence of gas within the endometrial cavity, a common nonspecific finding in postpartum patients and often present in postpartum endometritis, is uncommon in patients with PID.

Salpingitis represents the next level of disease progression, with involvement of one or both fallopian tubes. Findings on imaging may be subtle and limited to thickening and hyperemia of the tubal walls. Advanced

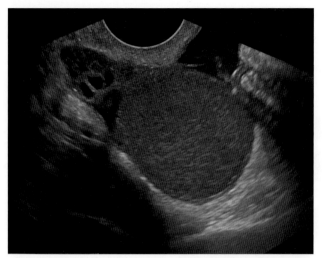

Figure 13-140 Sonographic image demonstrates the distended fallopian tube with echogenic material and posterior acoustic enhancement. The findings are consistent with pyosalpinx.

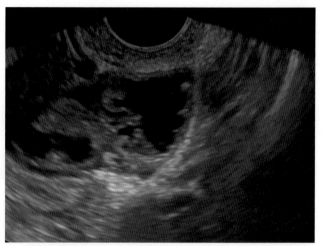

Figure 13-142 Ultrasonographic image of the fallopian tube in cross section demonstrates distension of the lumen with anechoic fluid and peripheral corrugated appearance representing thickening of the lining of the fallopian tubes. The findings are consistent with the cogwheel sign.

Tubo-ovarian complex and tubo-ovarian abscess occur when the infection extends beyond the fallopian tube to involve the ovary and regional pelvic structures. In addition to the imaging findings associated with salpingitis or pyosalpinx, tubo-ovarian complex demonstrates an adherent adjacent ovary, which is no longer freely mobile under transvaginal transducer probe pressure. In contrast, a tubo-ovarian abscess represents the clinical and imaging findings of advanced PID with additional loss of architecture of the adnexa and ill-defined or completely obscured ovarian tissue due to the distribution and degree of inflammation (Fig. 13-144). The term *abscess* is a misnomer because in most cases of tubo-ovarian abscess the fluid and debris are predominantly contained within a distended but anatomically intact space (the fallopian tube) and do not represent the organization of infectious fluid and debris seen in a typical abscess.

Ovarian Hyperstimulation Syndrome

Ovarian hyperstimulation syndrome (OHSS) is a potentially serious (occasionally life-threatening) complication that occurs in approximately 20% to 30% of patients undergoing therapy with exogenous gonadotropins, particularly during the luteal phase. The hallmark of OHSS is an increase in capillary permeability resulting in fluid shift from the intravascular space to third space compartments. Patients typically present with diffuse abdominal pain, abdominal distention, ascites, moderate to large pleural effusions, and hemoconcentration. Severe OHSS (seen in up to 2% of patients undergoing exogenous administration of gonadotropins) is associated with hypercoagulability causing arterial or venous thrombosis, renal failure, and hepatic dysfunction.

The ultrasonographic findings of OHSS include bilateral enlarged ovaries containing multiple variably sized cystic lesions resulting from enlarged follicles or corpus luteal cysts with ascites. The location of the follicles is mostly peripheral and is described as a "wheel spoke"

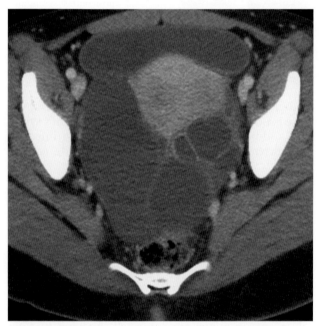

Figure 13-141 Axial computed tomography (CT) image demonstrates bilateral thin-walled fluid-filled tubular structures adjacent to the uterus in an asymptomatic patient consistent with bilateral hydrosalpinx.

salpingitis may progress to pyosalpinx, in which the fimbrial end of the fallopian tube becomes occluded and the tube is distended with fluid and debris (Fig. 13-141). The "beads-on-a-string" or cogwheel sign may be present, representing the thickened endosalpingeal folds with incomplete septations projecting into a fluid-filled lumen (Fig. 13-142). Following resolution of the acute infection, a hydrosalpinx may form in which the fallopian tube remains distended with sterile watery fluid following proteolysis of pus. Hydrosalpinx may be distinguished from pyosalpinx by the presence of thin walls, lack of hyperemia, and simple or anechoic appearance of tubal contents in a patient without signs of symptoms of acute PID (Fig. 13-143).

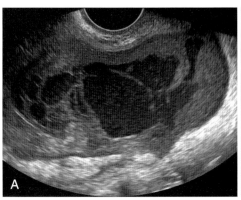
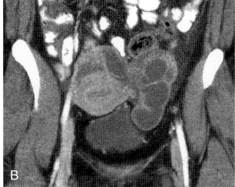

Figure 13-143 A, Ultrasonographic image of adnexal region demonstrates thickened, fluid-filled appearance of the fallopian tube with increased echogenicity of the adjacent pelvic fat. B, Coronal computed tomography (CT) image of same patient demonstrates thickened, enhancing, fluid-filled appearance of the left fallopian tube without identifiable left ovary. The findings are consistent with tubo-ovarian abscess.

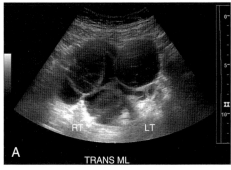
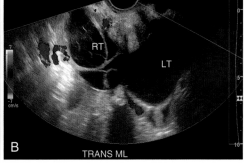

Figure 13-144 A, Ultrasound (US) images of the right (A) (gray scale) and left (B) (color Doppler) adnexa demonstrate markedly enlarged ovaries with multiple follicles with internal echoes and a reticular pattern consistent with ovarian hyperstimulation syndrome (OHSS).

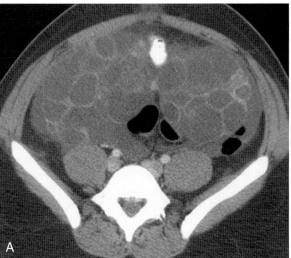
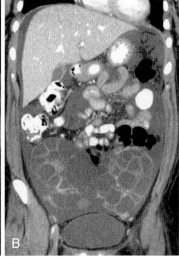

Figure 13-145 Axial (A) and coronal (B) contrast-enhanced computed tomography (CT) images of the abdomen and pelvis demonstrate markedly enlarged right and left ovaries with multiple follicles in both ovaries and a moderate amount of free fluid in the abdomen and pelvis. (Courtesy Jorge Soto, MD, Boston University Medical Center.)

appearance with thin septa separating the cysts. The cysts are typically anechoic but may be complicated with hemorrhage (see Fig. 13-144). On CT the central ovarian stroma is relatively higher in attenuation than the surrounding water-attenuation cysts (Fig. 13-145). There is also free fluid, which may be simple ascites but can be higher in attenuation due to a ruptured hemorrhagic cyst. On MRI the cysts are predominantly T1 hypointense and T2 hyperintense, although they may demonstrate high T1 signal intensity due to internal hemorrhage.

■ ECTOPIC PREGNANCY

A woman of reproductive age who presents to the ED with pelvic pain and vaginal bleeding must be evaluated for an ectopic pregnancy. Differential considerations for pelvic pain in a pregnant woman include normal early intrauterine pregnancy, spontaneous abortion, and ectopic pregnancy. Ectopic pregnancy is the leading cause of first-trimester pregnancy-related mortality. Predisposing risk factors that increase the risk for ectopic pregnancy include a personal history of a prior ectopic pregnancy; prior tubal surgery; use of an intrauterine device; a tubal pathologic condition, including PID; and use of infertility treatments. The overall incidence of ectopic pregnancies was 2% in 1992 and has since increased to approximately 4.5 %, primarily because of an increase in the use of in vitro fertilization. Early diagnosis and treatment are crucial because the risk for rupture increases as the ectopic pregnancy enlarges. Ultrasound

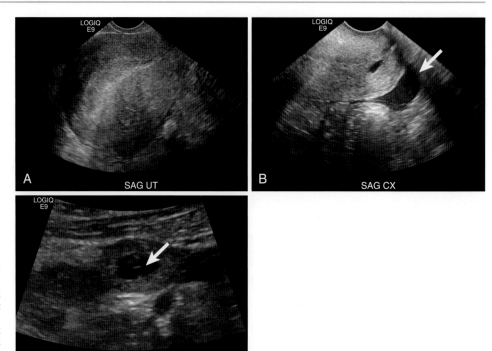

Figure 13-146 A, Sagittal ultrasonography (US) of the uterus does not demonstrate an intrauterine pregnancy. B, Complex free fluid is seen in the cul-de-sac *(arrow)* on the sagittal US image. C, Right adnexal mass with a yolk sac *(arrow)* is visualized, consistent with an ectopic pregnancy with hemoperitoneum.

is the imaging modality of choice, both from a diagnostic standpoint and a management perspective. Triaging a patient to surgical versus nonsurgical management, guiding percutaneous treatments of ectopic pregnancies, and following patients who are medically or expectantly managed are additional indications for US.

Serum human chorionic gonadotropin (HCG) is a glycoprotein that consists of α and β subunits. The β-HCG levels increase in a curvilinear fashion in early pregnancy before reaching a plateau at 9 to 11 weeks. Typically β-HCG levels double approximately every 48 hours in a viable pregnancy, whereas levels rise much more slowly in an ectopic pregnancy. If the β-HCG level increases by less than 50% during a 48-hour period, there is almost always a nonviable pregnancy, either intrauterine or extrauterine.

In a normal intrauterine pregnancy, the first ultrasonographic sign is the intradecidual sign, typically seen at 4 menstrual weeks. It manifests on US as a well-defined, small collection of fluid that is completed surrounded by an echogenic ring. At 5 weeks, a double-decidual sac sign can be visualized that manifests as two concentric hyperechoic rings surrounding an anechoic gestational sac. The double-decidual sac sign must be differentiated from a pseudogestational sac, which is a focal intrauterine fluid collection surrounded by decidual reaction located centrally in the endometrial cavity. The double-decidual sac sign can be seen in up to 20% of ectopic pregnancies. At around 5.5 weeks, when the gestational sac measures 10 mm, a yolk sac may be seen within the gestational sac. Fetal cardiac activity is typically seen at 5 to 6 weeks, when the gestational sac measures 18 to 20 mm or when the fetal pole measures at least 5 mm. If an intrauterine pregnancy cannot be identified in a pregnant patient with vaginal bleeding, and no ultrasonographic signs of an ectopic pregnancy are seen, close

surveillance with serial serum β-HCG levels and serial US examinations is necessary.

On imaging, ectopic pregnancies have varying appearances depending on the location. Locations of ectopic pregnancies include tubal, interstitial, ovarian, scar, cervical, intra-abdominal, and heterotopic. Tubal pregnancies account for a majority (approximately 95%) of ectopic pregnancies and occur in the ampulla (75% to 80%), isthmus (10%), and fimbria (5%). On US an adnexal mass separate from the ovary is typically seen in up to 90% to 100% of cases, and the most specific (100% specificity) sign is a live extrauterine embryo (Fig. 13-146). Another sign of tubal ectopic pregnancy is the "ring of fire" seen as peripheral hypervascularity in color Doppler evaluation of the extraovarian adnexal mass, related to high-velocity, low-impedance flow. Although this can be seen in tubal ectopic pregnancies, the ring of fire is not specific because it can also be seen in corpus luteum cysts. Additional intrauterine findings include the previously mentioned pseudogestational sac and decidual cysts. Decidual cysts are thin-walled, simple cysts located at the junction of the myometrium and endometrium and tend to be multiple. Extrauterine findings seen in ectopic pregnancy include free fluid (Fig. 13-147), hemoperitoneum, and hematosalpinx. The presence of hemoperitoneum in a patient with a positive β-HCG has a positive predictive value of 86% to 93% for the diagnosis of ectopic pregnancy.

Interstitial ectopic pregnancies are rare, accounting for 2% to 4% of all ectopic pregnancies. They occur when the blastocyst implants in the intramyometrial segment of the fallopian tube. Interstitial ectopic pregnancies carry higher mortality and morbidity rates because of later presentation in pregnancy and the potential for massive hemorrhage given the close proximity of the uterine artery. On US, interstitial ectopic pregnancies appear as a gestational

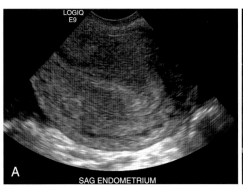
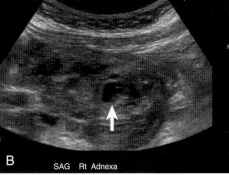

Figure 13-147 **A**, No intrauterine pregnancy is identified within the uterus on the sagittal ultrasonographic image. **B**, On the sagittal image of the right adnexa, a gestational sac *(arrow)* is seen adjacent to the right ovary in a patient with a positive β-HCG level, which was diagnostic of a fallopian tube ectopic pregnancy.

sac that is eccentrically located and surrounded by a layer of myometrium that is less than 5 mm thick in all planes.

■ SCROTAL EMERGENCIES

Testicular Torsion

Testicular torsion is a source of pain for men of all ages, but the most common presentation is acute scrotal pain in a young male. The most common predisposing condition is the bell clapper deformity, which is a congenital anomaly in which the testicle and epididymis are nearly completely surrounded by the tunica vaginalis, leaving the support structures and epididymis prone to twisting. Gray-scale US with color or power Doppler is the imaging study of choice for the evaluation of acute scrotal pain, for which the differential diagnosis includes testicular torsion, epididymitis/orchitis, infarction, incarcerated inguinal hernia, torsion of the appendix, and trauma. Testicular torsion is a surgical emergency. The rate of testicular salvage is inversely proportional to the duration of ischemia, and delays in appropriate treatment increase the risk for infarction.

On gray-scale US the affected testicle will be enlarged and hypoechoic. However, in early acute torsion the testicle may show no ultrasonographic changes or appreciable enlargement (Fig. 13-148). Color Doppler is a very useful adjunct in diagnosing testicular torsion, in which the most common and specific finding is absence of testicular blood flow (see Fig. 13-148). In cases where there has been detorsion, increased testicular blood flow from postischemic hyperemia can be seen and can be misinterpreted as epididymo-orchitis. Correlation with the patient's clinical history and the time of onset of symptoms is essential to accurately diagnosing testicular torsion in the setting of hyperemia.

Epididymo-orchitis

The most common cause of acute scrotal pain is epididymo-orchitis, which accounts for 75% of all scrotal inflammatory processes. Epididymo-orchitis most commonly results from bacterial seeding or ascending infection of the genitourinary tract. In younger males the most common organisms are *N. gonorrhoeae* and *Chlamydia*, whereas urinary tract infections from urinary retention are the most common causes in older males, with *E. coli* being the most common organism. Because the route of spread is ascending from the genitourinary

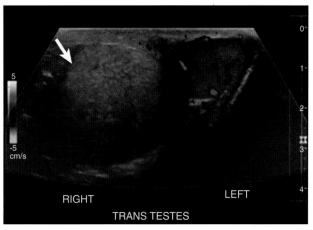

Figure 13-148 Color Doppler of the right and left testes demonstrates an enlarged and heterogeneous right testis with complete absence of flow. Patient was found to have a complete testicular torsion, and orchiectomy was necessary.

tract, the tail of the epididymis is initially affected with spread of infection through the tail into the testicle, resulting in orchitis. Isolated orchitis is rare but can be seen in mumps infection.

On gray-scale US images the epididymis is enlarged and thickened, up to two to three times the normal size, and the testicle may be normal or heterogeneous with hypoechoic areas and linear striations secondary to edema along the blood vessels. With color Doppler the epididymis and testicle are hyperemic (Fig. 13-149), with increased blood flow seen in the capsular and centripetal arteries of the testicles. The contralateral epididymis and testis can be used as direct comparison of size, echogenicity, and vascularity. If left untreated, abscesses can form in the epididymis and/or testis, which appear on US as complex fluid collections or hypoechoic testicular lesions with peripheral hypervascularity. Another potential complication is testicular infarct or ischemia (Horstman). Complex hydroceles may also be seen.

Accurately differentiating between acute testicular torsion and epididymo-orchitis has important therapeutic implications, and it is imperative to prevent potential complications in both diagnoses. Although gray-scale and color Doppler US can differentiate the two diagnoses, there are overlapping imaging appearances. Magnetic resonance imaging may be helpful for an accurate diagnosis, and dynamic contrast-enhanced images can provide information about testicular perfusion.

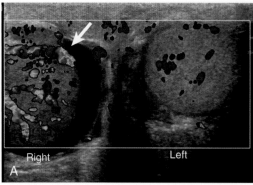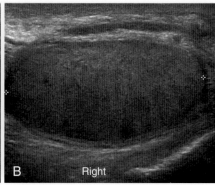

Figure 13-149 A, Patient presented with acute right scrotal pain, and the transverse ultrasonographic image with color Doppler demonstrates increased vascular flow in the right testicle (arrow) compared with the left testicle, with overlying asymmetric right scrotal wall thickening. B, Longitudinal image of the right testicle shows heterogeneity of the parenchyma. The patient was treated for epididymo-orchitis.

Selected Reading

http://www.aast.org/library/traumatools/injuryscoringscales.aspx#liver.

http://www.aast.org/library/traumatools/injuryscoringscales.aspx#spleen.

Afgha FP. Intussusception in adults. AJR Am J Roentgenol. 1986;146:527–531.

Aguirre DA, Santosa AC, Casola G, et al. Abdominal wall hernias: imaging features, complications, and diagnostic pitfalls at multi–detector row CT. Radiographics. 2005;25:1501–1520.

Albashir S, Stevens T. Endoscopic ultrasonography to evaluate pancreatitis. Cleve Clin J Med. 2012;79:202–206. http://dx.doi.org/10.3949/ccjm.79a.11092.

Almeida AT, Melao L, Viamonte B, et al. Epiploic appendagitis: an entity frequently unknown to clinicians—diagnostic imaging pitfalls and look-alikes. AJR Am J Roentgenol. 2009;193:1243–1251.

Alsaif HS, Venkatesh SK, Chan DS, et al. CT appearance of pyogenic liver abscesses caused by Klebsiella pneumoniae. Radiology. 201;260:129–138.

Anderson SW, Rho E, Soto JA. Detection of biliary duct narrowing and choledocholithiasis: accuracy of portal venous phase multidetector CT. Radiology. 2008;247:418–427.

Badea R. Ultrasonography of acute pancreatitis—an essay in images. Rom J Gastroenterol. 2005;14:83–89.

Balci NC, Sirvanci M. MR imaging of infective liver lesions. Magn Reson Imaging. 2002;10:121–135.

Balthazar EJ. Acute pancreatitis: assessment of severity with clinical and CT evaluation. Radiology. 2002;223:603–613.

Balthazar EJ, Robinson DL, Megibow AJ, et al. Acute pancreatitis: value of CT in establishing prognosis. Radiology. 1990;174:331–336.

Banks PA, Bollen TL, Dervenis C, et al. Classification of acute pancreatitis—2012: revision of the Atlanta classification and definitions by international consensus. Gut. 2013;62:102–111. http://dx.doi.org/10.1136/gutjnl-2012-302779.

Barie PS, Eachempati SR. Acute acalculous cholecystitis. Gastroenterol Clin North Am. 2010;39:343–357.

Baron R, Koehler RE, Gutierrez FR, et al. Clinical and radiographic manifestations of aortoesophageal fistulas. Radiology. 1981;141:599–605.

Barton JR, Sibai BM. Hepatic imaging in HELLP syndrome (hemolysis, elevated liver enzymes, and low platelet count). Am J Obstet Gynecol. 1996;174:1820–1827.

Berkovich GY, Levine MS, Miller Jr WT. CT findings in patients with esophagitis. AJR Am J Roentgenol. 2000;175:1431–1434.

Blake M, Cronin CG, Boland GW. Adrenal imaging. AJR Am J Roentgenol. 2010;194:1450–1460.

Blasbalg R, Baroni RH, Costa DN, et al. MRI features of groove pancreatitis. AJR Am J Roentgenol. 2007;189:73–80.

Bollen TL. Imaging of acute pancreatitis: update of the revised Atlanta classification. Radiol Clin North Am. 2012;50:429–445. http://dx.doi.org/10.1016/j.rcl.2012.03.015.

Bollen TL, van Santvoort HC, Besselink MG, et al. Update on acute pancreatitis: ultrasound, computed tomography, and magnetic resonance imaging features. Semin Ultrasound CT MR. 2007;28:371–383.

Bornstein SR. Predisposing factors for adrenal insufficiency. N Engl J Med. 2009;360. 2328.

Bradbury MJ, Kavanagh PV, Bechtold RE, et al. Mesenteric venous thrombosis: diagnosis and noninvasive imaging. Radiographics. 2002;22:527–541.

Braude P, Rowell P. Assisted conception, III: problems with assisted conception. BMJ. 2003;327(7420):920–923.

Brook OR, Kane RA, Tyagi G, et al. Lessons learned from quality assurance: errors in the diagnosis of acute cholecystitis on ultrasound and CT. AJR Am J Roentgenol. 2011;196:597–604.

Brown DL, Doubilet PM. Transvaginal sonography for diagnosing ectopic pregnancy: positivity criteria and performance characteristics. J Ultrasound Med. 1994;13(4):259–266.

Brown RFJ, Meehan CP, Colville J, et al. Transitional cell carcinoma of the upper urinary tract: spectrum of imaging findings. Radiographics. 2005;25:1609–1627.

Buckley O, O'Brien J, Snow A, et al. Imaging of Budd-Chiari syndrome. Eur Radiol. 2007;17:2071–2078.

Burks DD, Markey BJ, Burkhard TK, et al. Suspected testicular torsion and ischemia: evaluation with color Doppler sonography. Radiology. 1990;175:815–821.

Caoili EM, Korobkin M, Francis IR, et al. Adrenal masses: characterization with combined unenhanced and delayed enhanced CT. Radiology. 2002;222:629–633.

Casillas VJ, Amendola MA, Gascue A, et al. Imaging of nontraumatic hemorrhagic hepatic lesions. Radiographics. 2000;20:367–378.

Chang KC, Chuah SK, Changchien CS, et al. Clinical characteristics and prognostic factors of splenic abscess: a review of 67 cases in a single medical center of Taiwan. World J Gastroenterol. 2006;21(12):460–464.

Chang HC, Bhatt S, Dogra VS. Pearls and pitfalls in diagnosis of ovarian torsion. Radiographics. 2008;28(5):1355–1368.

Connor R, Jones B, Fishman EK, et al. Pneumatosis intestinalis: role of computed tomography in diagnosis and management. J Comput Assist Tomogr. 1984;8:269–275.

Cura M, Haskal Z, Lopera J. Diagnostic and interventional radiology for Budd-Chiari syndrome. Radiographics. 2009;29:669–681.

Cura M, Suri R, Bunone A, et al. Vascular malformations and arteriovenous fistulas of the kidney. Acta Radiol. 2010;51:144–149.

Demertzis J, Menias CO. State of the art: imaging of renal infections. Emerg Radiol. 2007;14:13–22.

Desser TS, Gross M. Multidetector row computed tomography of small bowel obstruction. Semin Ultrasound CT MR. 2008;29:308–321.

Dogra V, Paspulati RM, Bhatt S. First trimester bleeding evaluation. Ultrasound Q. 2005;21(2):69–85. quiz 149-150, 153-144.

Duda JB, Bhatt S, Dogra VS. Utility of CT whirl sign in guiding management of small-bowel obstruction. AJR Am J Roentgenol. 2008;191:743–747.

Dunnick NR, Sandler CM, Newhouse JH, et al. Textbook of Uroradiology. ed 4. Philadelphia: Lippincott Williams & Wilkins; 2008.

Dyer R, DiSantis DJ, McClennan BL. Simplified imaging approach for evaluation of the solid renal mass in adults. Radiology. 2008;247:331–343.

Eisenberg RL. Gastrointestinal Radiology: A Pattern Approach. ed 2. Philadelphia, PA: Lippincott; 1990. xiv, 1053.

Elsayes KM, Al-Hawary MM, Jagdish J, et al. CT enterography: principles, trends, and interpretation of findings. Radiographics. 2010;30:1955–1970.

Elsayes KM, Menias CO, Harvin HJ, et al. Imaging manifestations of Meckel's diverticulum. AJR Am J Roentgenol. 2007;189:81–88.

Fan CM, Rafferty EA, Geller SC, et al. Endovascular stent-graft in abdominal aortic aneurysms: the relationship between patent vessels that arise from the aneurysmal sac and early endoleak. Radiology. 2001;218:176–182.

Federle MP, Pan KT, Pealer KM. CT criteria for differentiating abdominal hemorrhage: anticoagulation or aortic aneurysm rupture? AJR Am J Roentgenol. 2007;188:1324–1330.

Fidler J. Small bowel disease: CT imaging. Abdom Imaging. 2009;34:281.

Fishman EK, Urban BA, Hruban HR. CT of the stomach: spectrum of disease. Radiographics. 1996;16:1035–1054.

Frauenfelder T, Wildermuth S, Marincek B, et al. Nontraumatic emergent abdominal vascular conditions: advantages of multi-detector row CT and three-dimensional imaging. Radiographics. 2004;24:481–496.

Furlan A, Fakhran S, Federle MP. Spontaneous abdominal hemorrhage: causes, CT findings and clinical implications. AJR Am J Roentgenol. 2009;193:1077–1087.

Furukawa A, Kanasaki S, Kono N, et al. CT diagnosis of acute mesenteric ischemia from various causes. AJR Am J Roentgenol. 2009;192:408–416.

Furukawa A, Saotome T, Yamasaki M, et al. Cross-sectional imaging in Crohn disease. Radiographics. 2004;24:689–702.

García-Blázquez V, Vicente-Bártulos A, Olavarria-Delgado A, et al. Accuracy of CT angiography in the diagnosis of acute gastrointestinal bleeding: systematic review and meta-analysis. Eur Radiol. 2013;23:1181–1190.

Garcia-Sancho Tellez L, Rodrigues-Montes JA, Fernandes LS, et al. Acute emphysematous cholecystitis: report of twenty cases. Hepatogastroenterology. 1999;46:2144–2148.

Gaspary MJ, Auten J, Durkovich D, et al. Superior mesenteric vein thrombosis mimicking acute appendicitis. West J Emerg Med. 2011;12:262–265.

Ghanem N, Altehoefer C, Springer O, et al. Radiological findings in Boerhaave's syndrome. *Emerg Radiol.* 2003;10:8–13.

Goerg C, Schwerk WB. Splenic infarction: sonographic patterns, diagnosis, follow-up, and complications. *Radiology.* 1990;174:803–807.

Gradison M. Pelvic inflammatory disease. *Am Fam Physician.* 2012;85(8):791–796.

Granberg S, Gjelland K, Ekerhovd E. The management of pelvic abscess. *Best Pract Res Clin Obstet Gynaecol.* 2009;23(5):667–678.

Grayson DE, Abbott RM, Levy AD, et al. Emphysematous infections of the abdomen and pelvis: a pictorial review. *Radiographics.* 2002;22:543–561.

Ha HK, Lee SH, Rha SE, et al. Radiologic features of vasculitis involving the gastrointestinal tract. *Radiographics.* 2000;20:779–794.

Hammond NA, Nikolaidis P, Miller FH. Infectious and inflammatory diseases of the kidney. *Radiol Clin North Am.* 2012;50:259–270.

Hanau LH, Steigbigel NH. Acute (ascending) cholangitis. *Infect Dis Clin North Am.* 2000;14:521–546.

Hanbidge AE, Lynch D, Wilson SR. US of the peritoneum. *Radiographics.* 2003;23:663–684. discussion 684–685.

Hanbidge AE, Lynch D, Wilson SR. US of the peritoneum. *Radiographics.* 2003;23:663–684.

Hara AK, Leighton JA, Sharma VK, et al. Imaging of small bowel disease: comparison of capsule endoscopy, standard endoscopy, barium examination, and CT. *Radiographics.* 2005;25:697–711.

Hauser SC. Clinical manifestations, diagnosis, and treatment of the Budd-Chiari syndrome. In: Basow DS, ed. Waltham, MA; September 2, 2013. In: UpToDate, Basow DS (Ed), UpToDate, Waltham, MA. Accessed on September 2, 2013.

Hauser SC. Etiology of Budd-Chiari syndrome. In: Basow DS, ed. Waltham, MA; September 2, 2013. In: UpToDate, Basow DS (Ed), UpToDate, Waltham, MA. Accessed on September 2, 2013.

Henry M, Amor M, Henry I, et al. Endovascular treatment of internal iliac artery aneurysms. *J Endovasc Surg.* 1998;5:345–348.

Holber BL, Baron RL, Dodd GD. Hepatic infarction caused by arterial insufficiency: spectrum and evolution of CT findings. *AJR Am J Roentgenol.* 1996;166:815–820.

Horrow MM, Rodgers SK, Naqvi S. Ultrasound of pelvic inflammatory disease. *Ultrasound Clin.* 2007;2:297–309.

Horton KM, Cori FM, Fishman EK. CT evaluation of the colon: inflammatory disease. *Radiographics.* 2000;20:399–418.

Horton KM, Fishman EK. Uncommon inflammatory diseases of the small bowel: CT findings. *Am J Roentgenol.* 1998;170:385–388.

Horton KM, Fishman EK. Current role of CT in imaging of the stomach. *Radiographics.* 2003;23:75–87.

Hussain HK, Korobkin M. MR imaging of the adrenal glands. *Magn Reson Imaging Clin N Am.* 2004;12:515–544.

Jain M, Agarwal A. MRCP findings in recurrent pyogenic cholangitis. *Eur J Radiol.* 2008;66:79–83.

Jeffrey RB, Laing FC, Wong W, et al. Gangrenous cholecystitis: diagnosis by ultrasound. *Radiology.* 1983;148:219–221.

Joo SH, Kim M, Lim J, et al. CT diagnosis of Fitz-Hugh and Curtis syndrome: value of the arterial phase scan. *Korean J Radiol.* 2007;8:40–47.

Kamaya A, Federle MP, Desser TS. Imaging manifestations of abdominal fat necrosis and its mimics. *Radiographics.* 2011;31:2021–2034.

Karch LA, Hodgson KJ, Mattos MA, et al. Adverse consequences of internal iliac artery occlusion during endovascular repair of abdominal aortic aneurysms. *J Vasc Surg.* 2000;32:676–683.

Kawashima A, Sandler KM, Ernst RD, et al. CT evaluation of renovascular disease. *Radiographics.* 2000;20:1321–1340.

Kaza R, Platt J, Cohan RH, et al. Dual-energy CT with single- and dual-source scanners: current applications in evaluating the genitourinary tract. *Radiographics.* 2012;23:353–369.

Kefalas CH. Gastroduodenal Crohn's disease. *Proc (Bayl Univ Med Cent).* 2003;16:147–151.

Kielar AZ, Shabana W, Vakili M, et al. Prospective evaluation of Doppler sonography to detect the twinkling artifact versus unenhanced computed tomography for identifying urinary tract calculi. *J Ultrasound Med.* 2012;31:1619–1625.

Kim YH, Blake MA, Harisinghani MG, et al. Adult intestinal intussusception: CT appearances and identification of a causative lead point. *Radiographics.* 2006;26:733–744.

Koo BC, Chinogureyi A, Shaw AS. Imaging acute pancreatitis. *Br J Radiol.* 2010;83:104–112. http://doi.org/10.1259/bjr/13359269.

Kumar S, Sarr MG, Kamath PS. Mesenteric venous thrombosis. *N Engl J Med.* 2001;345:1683–1688.

Lassandro F, Romano S, Ragozzino A, et al. Role of helical CT in diagnosis of gallstone ileus and related conditions. *AJR Am J Roentgenol.* 2005;185:1159–1165.

Lee EJ, Kwon HC, Joo HJ, et al. Diagnosis of ovarian torsion with color Doppler sonography: depiction of twisted vascular pedicle. *J Ultrasound Med.* 1998;17(2):83–89.

Lee MJ, Wittich GR, Mueller PR. Percutaneous intervention in acute pancreatitis. *Radiographics.* 1998;18:711–724. discussion 728.

Leung K, Stamm M, Raja A, et al. Pheochromocytoma: the range of appearances on ultrasound, CT, MRI and functional imaging. *AJR Am J Roentgenol.* 2013;200:370–378.

Leyendecker JR, Bloomfeld RS, DiSantis DJ, et al. MR enterography in the management of patients with Crohn disease. *Radiographics.* 2009;29:1827–1846.

Low G, Dhliwayo H, Lomas DJ. Adrenal neoplasms. *Clin Radiol.* 2012;67:988–1000.

Lozeau AM, Potter B. Diagnosis and management of ectopic pregnancy. *Am Fam Physician.* 2005;72(9):1707–1714.

Lubner M, Menias C, Rucker C, et al. Blood in the belly: CT findings of hemoperitoneum. *Radiographics.* 2007;27:109–125.

Lucey BC, Stuhlfaut JW, Soto JA. Mesenteric lymph nodes seen at imaging: causes and significance. *Radiographics.* 2005;25:351–365.

Macari M, Hines J, Balthazar E, et al. Mesenteric adenitis: CT diagnosis of primary versus secondary causes, incidence, and clinical significance in pediatric and adult patients. *AJR Am J Roentgenol.* 2002;178:853–858.

Mak SY, Roach SC, Sukumar SA. Small bowel obstruction: computed tomography features and pitfalls. *Curr Probl Diagn Radiol.* 2006;35:65–74.

Marti M, Artigas JM, Garzon G, et al. Acute lower intestinal bleeding: feasibility and diagnostic performance of CT angiography. *Radiology.* 2012;262:109–116.

Maturen KE, Feng MU, Wasnik AP, et al. Imaging effects of radiation therapy in the abdomen and pelvis: evaluating "innocent bystander" tissues. *Radiographics.* 2013;33:599–619.

Méndez RJ, Schiebler ML, Outwater EK, et al. Hepatic abscesses: MR imaging findings. *Radiology.* 1994;190:431–436.

Menke J. Diagnostic accuracy of multidetector CT in acute mesenteric ischemia: systematic review and meta-analysis. *Radiology.* 2010;256:93–101.

Merine D, Fishman EK, Jones B. Pseudomembranous colitis: CT evaluation. *J Comput Assist Tomogr.* 1987;11. 1917–1020.

Middleton WD, Siegel BA, Melson GL, et al. Acute scrotal disorders: prospective comparison of color Doppler US and testicular scintigraphy. *Radiology.* 1990;177:177–181.

Miller FH, Keppke AL, Dalal K, et al. MRI of pancreatitis and its complications: part 1, acute pancreatitis. *AJR Am J Roentgenol.* 2004;183:1637–1644.

Morris J, Spender JA, Ambrose NS. MR imaging classification of perianal fistulas and its implications for patient management. *Radiographics.* 2000;20:623–635.

Mortele KJ. A modified CT severity index for evaluating acute pancreatitis: improved correlation with patient outcome. *AJR Am J Roentgenol.* 2004;183:1261–1265.

Mortele KJ, Segatto E, Ros PR. The infected liver: radiologic-pathologic correlation. *Radiographics.* 2004;24:937–955.

Nicolaou S, Kai B, Ho S, et al. Imaging of acute small-bowel obstruction. *AJR Am J Roentgenol.* 2005;85:1036–1044.

Nosher JL, Chung J, Brevettis LS, et al. Visceral and renal artery aneurysms: a pictorial essay on endovascular therapy. *Radiographics.* 2006;26:1687–1704.

O'Connor OJ, Buckley JM, Maher MM. Imaging of the complications of acute pancreatitis. *AJR Am J Roentgenol.* 2011;197:W375–W381. http://dx.doi.org/10.2214/AJR.10.4339.

O'Connor OJ, McWilliams S, Maher MM. Imaging of acute pancreatitis. *AJR Am J Roentgenol.* 2011;197:W221–W225. http://dx.doi.org/10.2214/AJR.10.4338.

Okino Y, Kiyosue H, Mori H, et al. Root of the small-bowel mesentery: correlative anatomy and CT features of pathologic conditions. *Radiographics.* 2001;21:1475–1490.

Parikh S, Shah R, Kapoor P. Portal vein thrombosis. *Am J Med.* 2010;123:111–119.

Pear MS, Hill MC, Zeman RK. CT findings in duodenal diverticulitis. *AJR Am J Roentgenol.* 2006;187:W392–W395.

Pedrosa I, Guarise A, Goldsmith J, et al. The interrupted rim sign in acute cholecystitis: a method to identify the gangrenous form with MRI. *J Magn Reson Imaging.* 2003;18:360–363.

Pedrosa I, Levine D, Eyvazzadeh AD, et al. MR imaging evaluation of acute appendicitis in pregnancy. *Radiology.* 2006;238:891–899.

Pedrosa I, Rofsky NM. MR imaging in abdominal emergencies. *Radiol Clin North Am.* 2003;41:1243–1216.

Pereira JM, Sirlin CB, Pinto PS, et al. Disproportionate fat stranding: a helpful CT sign in patients with acute abdominal pain. *Radiographics.* 2004;24:703–715.

Perks FJ, Gillespie I, Patel D. Multidetector computed tomography imaging of aortoenteric fistula. *J Comput Assist Tomogr.* 2004;28:343–347.

Peterson CM, Anderson JS, Hara AK, et al. Volvulus of the gastrointestinal tract: appearances at multimodality imaging. *Radiographics.* 2009;29:1281–1293.

Philpotts LE, Heiken JP, Westcott MA, et al. Colitis: use of CT findings in differential diagnosis. *Radiology.* 1994;190:445–449.

Pickhardt PJ, Bhalla S. Intestinal malrotation in adolescents and adults: spectrum of clinical and imaging features. *AJR Am J Roentgenol.* 2002;179:1429–1435.

Pickhardt PJ, Bhalla S, Balfe DM. Acquired gastrointestinal fistulas: classification, etiologies, and imaging evaluation. *Radiology.* 2002;224:9–23.

Podolsky DK. Inflammatory bowel disease. *N Engl J Med.* 2002;347:417–429.

Pooler BD, Lawrence EM, Pickhardt PJ. Alternative diagnoses to suspected appendicitis at CT. *Radiology.* 2012;265:733–742.

Pritt BS, Clark CG. *Amebiasis Mayo Clin Proc.* 2010;83:1154–1160.

Radin DR, Philip PW, Colletti PM, et al. CT of amebic liver abscess. *AJR Am J Roentgenol.* 1988;150:1297–1301.

Rahimian J, Wilson T, Oram V, et al. Pyogenic liver abscess: recent trends in etiology and mortality. *Clin Infect Dis.* 2004;39:1654–1658.

Raman SP, Hruban RH, Fishman EK. Beyond renal cell carcinoma: rare and unusual renal masses. *Abdom Imaging.* 2012;37:873–884.

Raman SP, Neyman EG, Horton KM, et al. Superior mesenteric artery syndrome: spectrum of CT findings with multiplanar reconstructions and 3-D imaging. *Abdom Imaging.* 2012;37:1079–1088.

Raza SA, Sohaib SA, Sahdev A, et al. Centrally infiltrating renal masses on CT: differentiating intrarenal transitional cell carcinoma from centrally located renal cell carcinoma. *AJR Am J Roentgenol.* 2012;198:846–853.

Reinhold C, Taourel P, Bret PM. Choledocholithiasis: evaluation of MR cholangiography for diagnosis. *Radiology.* 1998;209:435–442.

Renzulli P, Hostettler A, Schoepfer AM, et al. Systematic review of atraumatic splenic rupture. *Br J Surg.* 2009;96:1114–1121.

Rha SE, Ha HK, Lee SH, et al. CT and MR imaging findings of bowel ischemia from various primary causes. *Radiographics.* 2000;20:29–42.

Riddell AM, Khalili K. Sequential adrenal infarction without MRI-detectable hemorrhage in primary antiphospholipid-antibody syndrome. *AJR Am J Roentgenol.* 2004;183:220–222.

Ripolles T, Garcia-Aquayo J, Martinez MJ, et al. Gastrointestinal bezoars: sonographic and CT characteristics. *AJR Am J Roentgenol.* 2001;177:65–69.

Rizk MK, Gerke H. Utility of endoscopic ultrasound in pancreatitis: a review. *World J Gastroenterol.* 2007;47:6321–6326.

Romano S. Diagnostic imaging of intestinal ischemia and infarction. *Radiol Clin North Am.* 2008;48:845–956.

Ros PR, Huprich JE. ACR Appropriateness Criteria on suspected small-bowel obstruction. *J Am Coll Radiol.* 2006;3:838–841.

Rosado Jr WM, Trambert MA, Gosink BB, et al. Adnexal torsion: diagnosis by using Doppler sonography. *AJR Am J Roentgenol.* 1992;159(6):1251–1253.

Rubesin SE, Furth EE, Levine MS. Gastritis from NSAIDS to *Helicobacter pylori.* *Abdom Imaging.* 2005;30:142–159.

Rubesin SE, Levine MS, Laufer I. Double-contrast upper gastrointestinal radiography: a pattern approach for diseases of the stomach. *Radiology.* 2008;246:33–48.

Rucker CM, Menias CO, Bhalla S. Mimics of renal colic: alternative diagnoses at unenhanced helical CT. *Radiographics.* 2004;24:S11–S33.

Sakamoto I, Sueyoshi E, Hazama S, et al. Endovascular treatment of iliac artery aneurysms. *Radiographics.* 2005;25:213–227.

Saltzman JR. Approach to acute upper GI bleeding in adults. In: Basow DS, ed. Waltham, MA; 2013. In: UpToDate, Basow DS (Ed), UpToDate, Waltham, MA. Accessed on September 5, 2013.

Santillan CS. Computed tomography of small bowel obstruction. *Radiol Clin North Am.* 2013;51:17–27.

Sanyal AJ. Acute portal vein thrombosis in adults: clinical manifestations, diagnosis, and management. In: Basow DS, ed. Waltham, MA; 2013. UptoDate.

Sawhney R, Kerlan RK, Wall SD, et al. Analysis of initial CT findings after endovascular repair of abdominal aortic aneurysm. *Radiology.* 2001;220:157–160.

Scholz FJ, Afnan J, Behr SC. CT findings in adult celiac disease. *Radiographics.* 2011;31:977–992.

Schueller G. Liver and bile ducts. In: *Emergency Radiology of the Abdomen: Imaging Features and Differential Diagnosis for a Timely Management Approach.* In: Scaglione M, Linsenmaier U, Schueller G, eds. Milano: Springer; 2012:31–54.

Sebastia C, Quiroga S, Espin E, et al. Portomesenteric vein gas: pathologic mechanisms, CT findings, and prognosis. *Radiographics.* 2000;20:1213–1224.

Servaes S, Zurakowski D, Laufer MR, et al. Sonographic findings of ovarian torsion in children. *Pediatric Radiol.* 2007;37(5):446–451.

Shakespear JS, Shaaban AM, Rezvani M. CT findings of acute cholecystitis and its complications. *AJR Am J Roentgenol.* 2010;194:1523–1529.

Shanbhogue AK, Fasih N, Surabhi VR, et al. A clinical and radiologic review of uncommon types and causes of pancreatitis. *Radiographics.* 2009;29:1003–1026.

Siddiki H, Fidler J. MR imaging of the small bowel in Crohn's disease. *Eur J Radiol.* 2009;69:409–417.

Sidhu R, Lockhart ME. Imaging of renovascular disease. *Semin Ultrasound CT MRI.* 2009;30:271–288.

Silva AC, Pimenta M, Guimaraes LS. Small bowel obstruction: what to look for. *Radiographics.* 2009;29:423–439.

Silverman S, Israel G, Herts B, et al. Management of the incidental renal mass. *Radiology.* 2008;249:16–31.

Singh AK, Gervais DA, Hahn PF, et al. Acute epiploic appendagitis and its mimics. *Radiographics.* 2005;25:1521–1534.

Singh AK, Sagar P. Gangrenous cholecystitis: prediction with CT imaging. *Abdom Imaging.* 2005;30:218–221.

Singh AK, Shankar S, Gervais DA, et al. Image-guided percutaneous splenic interventions. *Radiographics.* 2012;32:523–534.

Smith AD, Remer EM, Cox KL, et al. Bosniak category IIF and II cystic renal lesions: outcomes and associations. *Radiology.* 2012;262:152–160.

Sonavane SK, Menias CO, Kantawala KP, et al. Laparoscopic adjustable gastric banding: what radiologists need to know. *Radiographics.* 2012;32:1161–1178.

Stavropoulos SW, Charagundla SR. Imaging techniques for detection and management of endoleaks after endovascular aortic aneurysm repair. *Radiology.* 2007;243:641–655.

Stolzmann P, Frauenfelder T, Pfammatter T, et al. Endoleaks after endovascular abdominal aortic aneurysm repair: detection with dual-energy dual-source CT. *Radiology.* 2008;249:682–691.

Strate L. Approach to resuscitation and diagnosis of acute lower GI bleeding in the adult patient. In: Basow DS, ed. Waltham, MA; September 7, 2013. In: UpToDate, Basow DS (Ed), UpToDate, Waltham, MA. Accessed on September 7, 2013.

Symeonidou C, Hameeduddin A, Hons B, et al. Imaging features of renal pathology in the human immunodeficiency virus-infected patient. *Semin Ultrasound CT MRI.* 2009;30:289–297.

Teichman JMH. Acute renal colic from ureteral calculus. *N Engl J Med.* 2004;350:684–693.

Theofanakis CP, Kyriakidis AV. Fitz-Hugh–Curtis syndrome. *J Gynecol Surg.* 2010;8:129–134.

Thoeni RF. The revised Atlanta classification of acute pancreatitis: its importance for the radiologist and its effect on treatment. *Radiology.* 2012;262:751–764. http://dx.doi.org/10.1148/radiol.11110947.

Timpone VM, Lattin Jr GE, Lewis RB, et al. Abdominal twists and turns: part 2, solid visceral torsions with pathologic correlation. *AJR Am J Roentgenol.* 2011;197:97–102.

Tkacz JN, Anderson SA, Soto JA. MR imaging in gastrointestinal emergencies. *Radiographics.* 2009;29:1767–1780.

Torabi M, Hosseinzadeh K, Federle MP. CT of nonneoplastic hepatic vascular and perfusion disorders. *Radiographics.* 2008;28:1967–1982.

Trambert MA, Mattrey RF, Levine D, et al. Subacute scrotal pain: evaluation of torsion versus epididymitis with MR imaging. *Radiology.* 1990;175:53–56.

Trowbridge RL, Rutkowski NK, Shojania KG. Does this patient have acute cholecystitis? *JAMA.* 2003;289:80–86.

Ubee SS, McGlynn L, Fordham M. Emphysematous pyelonephritis. *BJU Int.* 2010;102:1474–1478.

Valla DC. Hepatic vein thrombosis (Budd-Chiari syndrome). *Semin Liver Dis.* 2002;22:5–14.

Vinholt Schiødt F. Viral hepatitis-related acute liver failure. *Am J Gastroenterol.* 2003;98:448–453.

Wang GJ, Gao CF, Wei D, et al. Acute pancreatitis: etiology and common pathogenesis. *World J Gastroenterol.* 2009;15:1427–1430.

Washburn ZW, Dillman JR, Cohan RH, et al. Computed tomographic urography update: an evolving urinary tract imaging modality. *Semin Ultrasound CT MRI.* 2009;30:233–245.

Watanabe Y, Nagayama M, Okumura A, et al. MR imaging of acute biliary disorders. *Radiographics.* 2007;27:477–495.

Webb EM, Green GE, Scoutt LM. Adnexal mass with pelvic pain. *Radiol Clin North Am.* 2004;42(2):329–348.

Wei SC, Fitzgerald K, Maglinte DD. CT findings in small bowel angioedema: a cause of acute abdominal pain. *Emerg Radiol.* 2007;13:281–283.

Yikilmaz A, Karahan OI, Senol S, et al. Value of multislice computed tomography in the diagnosis of acute mesenteric ischemia. *Eur J Radiol.* 2011;80:297–302.

Young CA, Menias CO, Bhalla S, et al. CT features of esophageal emergencies. *Radiographics.* 2008;28:1541–1553.

Zhang H, Prince MR. Renal MR angiography. *Magn Reson Imaging Clin N Am.* 2004;12:487–503.

Zissin R, Ellis M, Gayer G. The CT findings of abdominal anticoagulant-related hematomas. *Semin Ultrasound CT MR.* 2006;27:117–125.

Zissin R, Osadchy A, Gayer G, et al. Pictorial review. CT of duodenal pathology. *Br J Radiol.* 2002;75:78–84.

Zissin R, Yaffe D, Fejgin M, et al. Hepatic infarction in preeclampsia as part of the HELLP syndrome: CT appearance. *Abdom Imaging.* 1999;24:594–596.

Musculoskeletal Emergencies

CHAPTER 14

Upper Extremity

Shoulder

Hamid Torshizy, Tudor H. Hughes,
and Christine B. Chung

The *shoulder girdle* is a general term describing a complex network of soft tissue and osseous structures, demarcated by numerous joints, which serve to both suspend and connect the upper extremity to the torso. Injuries of the shoulder girdle are common, with sites of injury varying with the age of the patient. In general, whereas fractures of the clavicle are the most common cause of skeletal injury in younger populations, glenohumeral and acromioclavicular joint dislocations predominate between 20 and 40 years of age, and proximal humeral fractures prevail in older adults. This section will emphasize common mechanisms of injury, common patterns of injury, classification of injury types, variations of injury, and common pitfalls to diagnosis.

■ ANATOMY

The osseous structures constituting the shoulder girdle are the clavicle, the scapula, and the proximal humerus (Fig. 14-1). The scapula is further divided into the acromion, coracoid, scapular body, neck proper, and glenoid. Interposed between these structures are three joints, the acromioclavicular, sternoclavicular, and glenohumeral.

The clavicle is an S-shaped bone that is more tubular medially, gradually becoming flatter at its lateral extent. It connects the manubrium to the scapula, forming a diarthrodial joint proximally (sternoclavicular) and distally (acromioclavicular). Several ligaments act as key stabilizers of the clavicle. The coracoclavicular ligament, consisting of the conoid (medial) and trapezoid (lateral) portions, acts to bind the clavicle to the scapula. The acromioclavicular ligament links the clavicle to the acromion. Several muscles insert on the clavicle, including the pectoralis major, deltoid, sternocleidomastoid, and trapezius.

The scapula is a flat, triangular bone that is often divided into two parts, the body and the neck. The body is composed of several osseous prominences. These include the spine dorsally which terminates in the acromion process, the superior lateral angle which forms the glenoid fossa, and the superior and inferior angle. The coracoid process arises just medial to the glenoid fossa along its superior edge. The neck refers to the flared portion of the scapula that forms the glenoid fossa.

The proximal humerus is anatomically divided into the head, anatomic neck, surgical neck, and the lesser and greater tuberosities. The anatomic neck refers to the constricted portion of the humeral head circumference. The surgical neck is the constricted osseous portion arising below the tuberosities. The greater tuberosity is an osseous prominence arising from the head laterally, serving as insertion primarily for the supraspinatus, infraspinatus, and teres minor tendons. The lesser tuberosity is an osseous prominence arising from the anterior humerus below the anatomic neck, serving as attachment for the subscapularis tendon. The tuberosities are separated by an osseous concavity, the bicipital groove, which houses the long head of the biceps tendon.

■ OSSEOUS EMERGENCIES

Clavicle Fractures

Fractures of the clavicle are one of the most common injuries of the shoulder girdle, with the majority occurring during childhood and 50% occurring in children under 10 years of age. Fractures occur as a result of falls with direct trauma or from falls on an outstretched arm. In childhood, fractures are often either a greenstick or bowing variety. In adults, fractures have been traditionally categorized using the Allman classification, with injuries divided anatomically into those affecting the

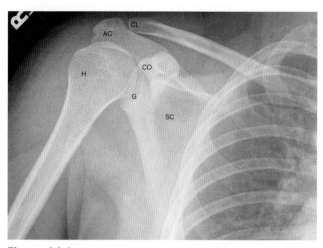

Figure 14-1 Normal shoulder. Frontal radiograph of the shoulder shows the normal osseous anatomy. *AC,* Acromion; *CL,* clavicle; *CO,* coracoid; *G,* glenoid; *H,* humerus; *SC,* scapula.

proximal third, middle third, and distal third of the clavicle (Fig. 14-2).

Injuries involving the middle third are most common, accounting for nearly 80% of fractures. Patterns can be transverse and complete or comminuted. Frequently the distal fragment is depressed due to the weight of the upper extremity and the proximal fragment is elevated due to the pull of the sternocleidomastoid muscle. A more exaggerated pattern involves overriding of edges, where the distal fragment underlies the proximal.

Fractures of the outer third account for 15% of injuries and can be associated with fractures through the base of the coracoid process. Unlike fractures involving the middle or inner one third, fractures of the outer third can be associated with disruption of the coracoclavicular ligaments, which include the conoid and trapezoid ligaments. Commonly this can lead to superior displacement of the medial fragments and an increase in the distance between the coracoid and clavicle, caused by the unopposed pull of the sternocleidomastoid muscle attachment to the clavicle. However, this may not be readily apparent on standard views. Therefore, whenever a fracture of the outer third is encountered, it is recommended that stress views be obtained to accentuate possible ligamentous injury.

Lastly, fractures of the medial or inner third account for 5% of injuries. These fractures are difficult to identify owing to overlapping ribs and spine. Fractures are best identified on steeply angled lordotic anteroposterior (AP) projection and/or on computed tomography (CT).

Pitfalls of diagnosis include lack of adequate technique for evaluation of undisplaced fractures of the middle third, which requires 15 degrees cephalic angulation of the beam. In addition, episternal ossicles, accessory ossification centers located posterior or cephalad to the manubrium, may be mistaken for fracture (Fig. 14-3). Fractures of the clavicle are infrequently associated with injury to the underlying subclavian artery and brachial plexus in the setting of severe trauma.

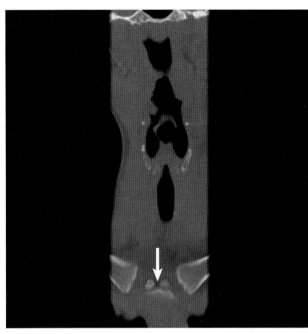

Figure 14-3 Episternal ossicles. Coronal computed tomographic (CT) image at the level of the sternoclavicular joints demonstrates bilateral episternal ossicles *(arrow)*, a variant not to be confused with fracture.

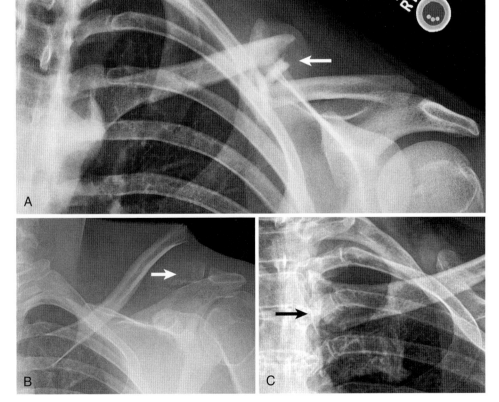

Figure 14-2 Clavicle fractures. A, Frontal radiograph demonstrates a displaced, comminuted fracture of the midthird of the clavicle *(arrow)* with depression of the distal fracture fragment and elevation of the proximal fracture fragment. **B,** Shoulder radiograph in a different patient shows a displaced fracture of the distal third of the clavicle *(arrow)*. There is superior migration of the proximal clavicle and an abnormal coracoclavicular distance, suggesting tear of the coracoclavicular ligaments. **C,** Coneddown radiograph in a third patient shows a minimally displaced fracture of the medial third of the clavicle *(arrow)*.

An important cause of pain in the area of the acromioclavicular joint is distal clavicular osteolysis. Most instances are caused by overuse, particularly from weight lifting, although it may also occur as a consequence of traumatic joint separation. The radiographic manifestation is focal osteopenia in the distal 2 cm of the clavicle, as well as loss of the articular cortical margin (Fig. 14-4).

Scapular Fractures

The scapula is protected by overlying soft tissues, thus injuries of the scapula occur infrequently, accounting for 3% to 5% of all shoulder girdle injuries. The mean age of patients who present with injuries ranges from 35 to 45 years. Common mechanisms include axial loading on an outstretched arm (scapular neck, glenoid), direct high-energy trauma (body), direct trauma (acromion, coracoid), glenohumeral joint dislocation (glenoid, coracoid), or traction by ligaments (avulsion fractures). Overall, the majority of injuries are caused by severe high-impact trauma, with vehicular accidents accounting for 75% of them. Fractures are generally described according to anatomic area: acromion, coracoid, body, and neck/glenoid, with glenoid

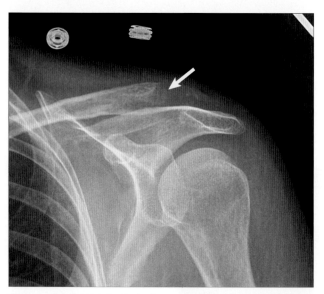

Figure 14-4 Distal clavicular osteolysis. Frontal radiograph shows marked lysis of the distal clavicle *(arrow)* from overuse.

fractures further dividing into extra-articular and intra-articular. Fractures of the scapular neck (10% to 60%) and the body (49% to 89%) are most common.

Fractures involving the acromion process are most often transverse in orientation and affect the acromial base. Kuhn and coworkers classified acromial fractures into three types, with surgery reserved for type III injuries. Type I are nondisplaced and subdivided into an avulsive type IA or direct trauma type IB (Fig. 14-5); type II fractures are displaced laterally, anteriorly, or superiorly and do not reduce the subacromial space; and type III fractures reduce the subacromial space by an inferiorly displaced acromial fracture or an acromial fracture associated with an ipsilateral superiorly displaced glenoid neck fracture. The os acromiale, a secondary ossification center identified at the level of the acromioclavicular joint, may persist into adult life and be mistaken for a fracture (Fig. 14-6). It is present in 2.7% of randomly selected adults and when present, occurs bilaterally in 60% of cases. Distinction from fracture is made by its typical location, recognizing its well-corticated borders and/or symmetry.

Coracoid fractures are characterized into two types based upon the fracture location with respect to the coracoclavicular ligaments. Type I fractures occur proximal to the coracoclavicular ligament attachment (Fig. 14-7) and may require surgical correction because they are often associated with acromioclavicular separation, clavicular fracture, superior scapular fracture, and/or glenoid fracture. Type II fractures occur distal to the coracoclavicular ligament attachment and are treated conservatively (Fig. 14-8). These fractures are very difficult to identify on standard AP views and are best demonstrated by 25- to 45-degree cephalic angulation of the beam in the frontal projection. Stress fractures of the base of the coracoid, a less common pattern of injury, have been described in trapshooters. A small secondary ossification center located on the surface of the coracoid, often presenting as a fine shelf of bone, should not be confused with fracture.

Glenoid fractures either involve or spare the articular surface. Extra-articular glenoid fractures are classified according to the presence or absence of concomitant acromioclavicular separation or clavicular fracture. Unlike their extra-articular counterparts, intra-articular fractures of the glenoid are more complex. Ideberg and coworkers classified fractures into five types, with a sixth type added

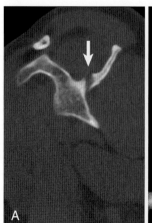
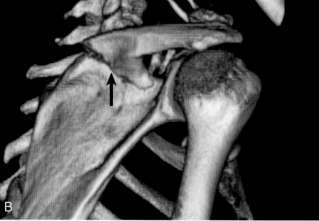

Figure 14-5 Type IB acromial fracture. A, Sagittal computed tomographic (CT) image shows a fracture of the acromion *(arrow).* **B,** three-dimensional (3-D) CT reconstruction shows the orientation of the acromion fracture *(arrow).*

by Goss and colleagues. Type I involves the glenoid rim with type IA affecting the anterior and type IB the posterior surfaces; type II are transverse or oblique fractures through the glenoid fossa with inferior fragment displaced; type III are oblique fractures of the glenoid exiting at the mid to superior scapular border, often associated with acromio-clavicular fracture and/or dislocation; type IV are horizontal fractures exiting through the medial scapular border; type V are a type IV fracture pattern with separation of the inferior half of the glenoid; and type VI is a comminuted fracture.

Fractures of the scapular body are generally categorized as being vertical or horizontal. Numerous classifications exist in the literature. The classification system introduced by Zdravkovic and Damholt is a system most used by orthopedic surgeons in the clinical setting. This classification divides injuries into three types: type I are fractures of the body (Fig. 14-9); type II are fractures of the apophyses, including the acromion and coracoid; and type III are fractures of the superolateral angle, including the glenoid neck. Nutrient canals or foramina can mimic fractures, most commonly in the body and spine (Fig. 14-10). They are usually oriented horizontally, paralleling the superior border of the scapula, and demonstrate a well-corticated margin. In addition, a persistent ossification center at the inferior angle of the scapula can also simulate a pathologic process. Scapular fractures are commonly associated with important findings, including pulmonary injury, brachial plexus injury, clavicle fractures, rib fractures, and other fractures of the axial and appendicular skeleton.

Atypical Injuries of the Shoulder Girdle

Avulsion injuries of the shoulder girdle represent a less common pattern of injury, with failure occurring at insertion of ligaments. The most common sites of injury include the inferolateral margin of the glenoid at the insertion of the long head of the triceps tendon (Fig. 14-11) and the lateral scapular margin at the insertion of the teres

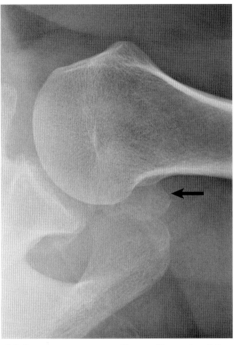

Figure 14-6 Os acromiale. Axillary radiograph of the shoulder demonstrates a secondary ossification center of the acromion *(arrow).*

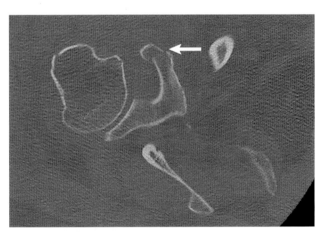

Figure 14-8 Type II coracoid fracture. Axial computed tomographic (CT) image shows a fracture of the coracoid occurring distal to the attachment of the coracoclavicular ligament *(arrow).*

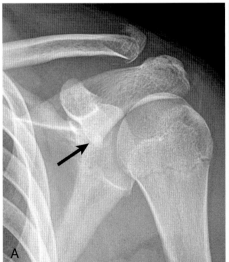

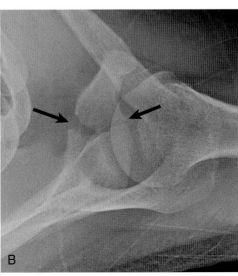

Figure 14-7 Type I coracoid fracture. A, Frontal radiograph shows disruption of the cortex of the coracoid process *(arrow).* **B,** Axillary view demonstrates that the fracture is proximal to the coraco-clavicular ligament *(arrows).*

minor muscle. Lastly, insufficiency fractures of the scapula represent a rare pattern of injury seen most commonly with mineralization disorders such as encountered in osteomalacia.

Fractures of the Proximal Humerus

Fractures of the proximal humerus are biphasic in occurrence, most commonly occurring in people in their second decade of life and in people over 50 years of age. Patients presenting from 20 to 50 years of age are less common, and their injuries are the result of high-impact trauma. Fractures in patients younger than 20 years often result in separation of the proximal humeral epiphysis, whereas fractures in patients over the age of 50 years are often associated with osteoporosis.

Fractures of the proximal humerus can be classified using an anatomic basis. In general, isolated fractures of a single region are uncommon. Fractures of the surgical neck are most common and often associated with fractures of the greater tuberosity. There is often anterior and medial displacement of the shaft owing to the pull of the pectoralis major muscle. Fractures of the anatomic neck, though less common, have a higher potential for complication with avascular necrosis because of disruption of the blood supply to the humeral head. Atypical patterns of injury include isolated fractures of the tubercles and should elicit a search for signs of shoulder dislocation.

Alternatively, the Neer classification takes into account the number of fragments and degree of angulation and/or displacement. Fractures are classified as being one-, two-, three-, or four-part in nature. One-part fractures account for 80% of cases and are nondisplaced and stable injuries occurring most often at the surgical neck. Two-part injuries constitute 10% of all fractures, with the most common pattern being anterior and

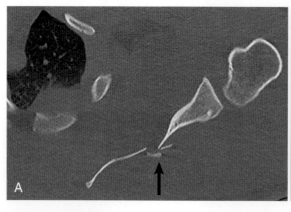
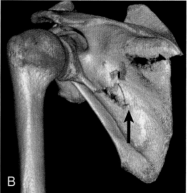

Figure 14-9 Scapular fracture. A, Axial computed tomographic (CT) image of the scapula shows a comminuted fracture of the body of the clavicle *(arrow)*. **B,** Three-dimensional (3-D) coronal CT reconstruction of shoulder shows the extent of comminution *(arrow)*.

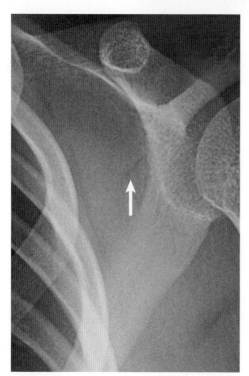

Figure 14-10 Nutrient foramen. Coned-down frontal radiograph of the shoulder demonstrates a nutrient foramen of the scapula *(arrow)*.

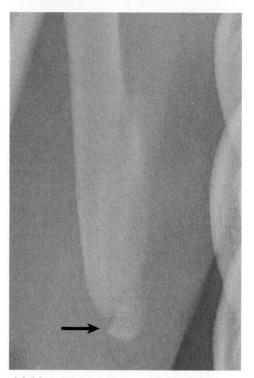

Figure 14-11 Scapular fracture, inferior angle. Coned-down radiograph of the scapula demonstrates a minimally displaced fracture of the inferior scapula *(arrow)*.

medial displacement of the shaft and fracture extension to the tubercles. Three-part fractures account for 3% of cases and are characterized by displaced fractures of the surgical neck associated with displaced fractures of either the lesser or greater tuberosity. Rotator cuff tears are common with this pattern of injury, requiring open reduction and repair of both the cuff and the fracture fragment. Lastly, four-part fractures account for about 4% of injuries and are characterized as severely comminuted fractures that may be associated with dislocation (Fig. 14-12). These fractures often result in avascular necrosis. When fractures of the proximal humerus occur, they may be associated with other soft tissue injuries to the brachial plexus, axillary artery, and joint capsule.

JOINT EMERGENCIES

Acromioclavicular Joint

The acromioclavicular (AC) joint is the second most commonly dislocated joint in the shoulder, accounting for nearly 12% of all dislocations. The glenohumeral joint constitutes 85% of shoulder dislocations, and the sternoclavicular joint makes up the remaining 2% to 3% of dislocations. Dislocations of the AC joint most commonly occur between the ages of 15 and 40 years, usually precipitated by a fall onto an outstretched hand or directly by a fall on the point of the shoulder.

The Tossy and Allman classification is the most widely used classification describing injuries to the AC joint (Fig. 14-13). In a type I separation, conventional radiographs appear normal or may show some soft tissue swelling over the joint. In a type II injury, there is disruption of the AC ligament and partial disruption of the coracoclavicular ligaments so that the clavicle migrates superiorly less than 5 mm or 50% of the width of the clavicle on weight-bearing views. In type III injuries the AC and coracoclavicular ligaments are completely disrupted, and there is clavicular migration exceeding 5 mm or 50% of the bone width. Rockwood and coworkers proposed three additional grades to the classification. In type IV injuries the clavicle displaces posteriorly into or through the trapezius

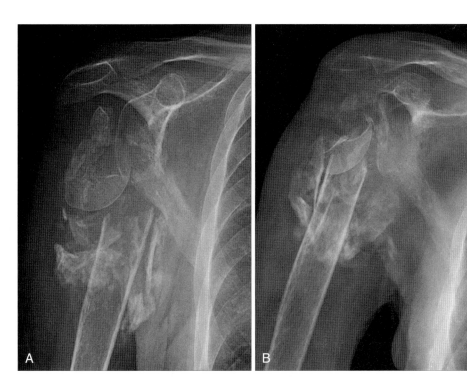

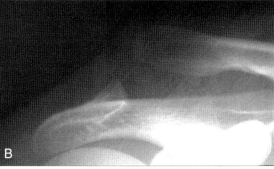

Figure 14-12 Humerus fracture, Neer four-part. A and B, Radiographs of the shoulder show a markedly comminuted impacted fracture of the proximal humerus with bisection of the head, fragmentation of both tuberosities, and displacement of the shaft. This fracture has a high incidence of osteonecrosis.

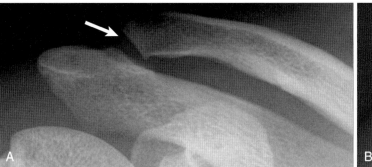

Figure 14-13 Acromioclavicular (AC) joint separation. A, Coned-down radiograph shows a slight offset of the joint consistent with a type II separation *(arrow)*. B, This patient shows complete dislocation of the joint typical of a type III separation.

muscle. In type V injuries, superior clavicle migration is more pronounced than in a type III separation. In type VI injuries the clavicle dislocates inferiorly below the coracoid or acromion process, often with associated rib fractures. Types IV to VI are extremely rare injury patterns.

Sternoclavicular Joint

Dislocation of the sternoclavicular joint is uncommon but an important diagnosis. Dislocations are classified as either anterior or posterior, with anterior being more common. Anterior dislocations are caused by trauma to the anterior shoulder. With the clavicle acting essentially as a lever and the sternoclavicular joint as a fulcrum, the impact force is transmitted to the sternoclavicular joint, resulting in dislocation. Rarely, spontaneous dislocations may occur in patients with osteoarthrosis. Injuries of the sternoclavicular joint are often difficult to diagnose on standard AP radiographs, particularly with the overlapping mediastinal and spinal contours. The only clue to injury may be an offset of the medial ends of the clavicles appearing at different levels on standard frontal radiographs, but the direction of dislocation may be impossible to ascertain without CT. When using radiography, it is important to image both joints because comparison with the contralateral side is essential. Posterior dislocations are important because of associated soft tissue injuries (Fig. 14-14).

Complications include trauma to the vascular structures, hematoma formation, fractures of the regional skeleton, injury to the trachea and/or esophagus, and development of pneumomediastinum and/or pneumothorax.

Glenohumeral Joint

The glenohumeral joint is the most commonly dislocated joint in the body. The joint is anatomically predisposed to dislocation owing to the discrepancy between the large surface area of the humeral head and the significantly smaller surface area of the glenoid fossa. It is this configuration that allows for the large dynamic range of this joint. Dislocations are classified as anterior (subcoracoid, subglenoid, subclavicular, intrathoracic), posterior, inferior (luxatio erecta), and superior.

Anterior glenohumeral joint dislocations account for nearly 95% of glenohumeral joint injuries and are the result of an external rotation and abduction injury of the upper extremity. The most common type is a subcoracoid dislocation, which is characterized by anterior, inferior, and medial displacement of the humeral head beneath the coracoid process (Fig. 14-15). Subglenoid dislocation is characterized by anterior, inferior, and more medial displacement with the humeral head resting beneath the inferior rim of the glenoid. Subclavicular anterior dislocation results in anterior, inferior, and even more

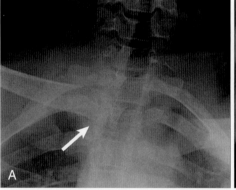
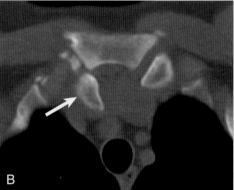

Figure 14-14 Sternoclavicular joint dislocation, posterior. A, Frontal radiograph shows that the right clavicular head is located more superiorly than the left *(arrow)*. The intercostal spaces are a good measure of the displacement. **B,** Axial computed tomographic (CT) image shows that the head of the clavicle does not articulate the manubrium but is also dislocated posteriorly *(arrow)*.

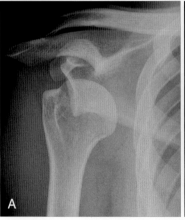
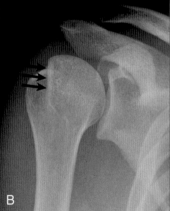
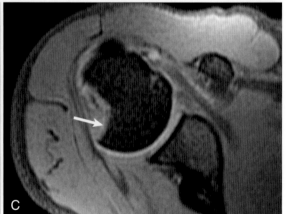

Figure 14-15 Anterior glenohumeral dislocation, subcoracoid type. A, Frontal radiograph of the shoulder shows that the humeral head has dislocated beneath the coracoid process. **B,** Upon reduction, a linear defect indicating a Hill-Sachs lesion is shown in the internal rotation view *(arrows)*. **C,** Axial gradient-recalled echo (GRE) magnetic resonance image (MRI) shows the wedge-like defect. The linear defect in the prior radiograph is caused by the back edge of the Hill-Sachs lesion *(arrow)*.

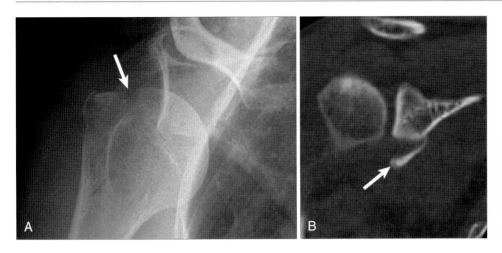

Figure 14-16 Anterior glenohumeral joint dislocation, associated fractures. A, Frontal radiograph shows a greater tuberosity fracture *(arrow)*. B, Coronal reformatted computed tomographic (CT) image in another patient shows an osseous Bankart lesion *(arrow)*.

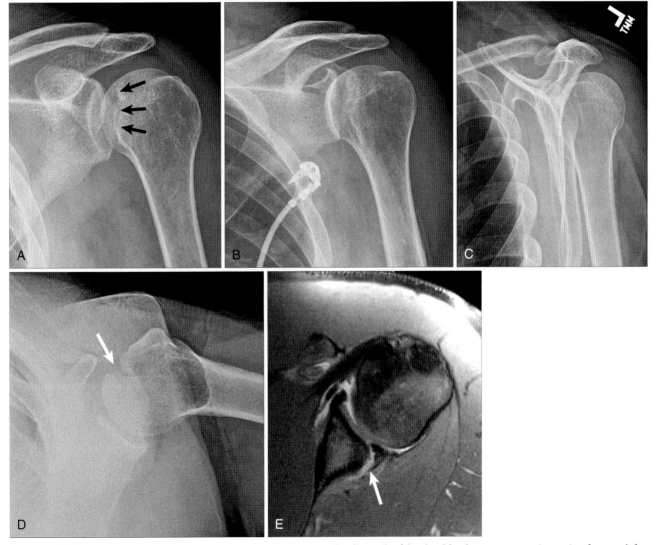

Figure 14-17 Posterior glenohumeral joint dislocation. A, Frontal radiograph of the shoulder demonstrates an impaction fracture deformity of the anterior humeral head *(arrows)* compatible with a "trough" sign (reverse Hill-Sachs) deformity. B, Grashey radiograph shows the overlapping cortical surfaces of the humerus and glenoid fossa. C, Lateral radiograph confirms the posterior location of the humeral head with respect to the glenoid margin. D, After reduction the impaction fracture in the anterior humeral head is conspicuous on the axillary view *(arrow)*. E, Axial fluid-sensitive magnetic resonance image (MRI) shows a reverse Bankart lesion with a tear through the base of the posterior labrum and disruption of the posterior periosteum *(arrow)*.

medial displacement so that the humeral head terminates beneath the clavicle. Lastly, intrathoracic anterior dislocation occurs when the humeral head penetrates the intercostal space. Anterior glenohumeral joint dislocations are most commonly associated with impaction fractures in the posterosuperior aspect of the humeral head (Hill-Sachs deformity), occurring in as many as 75% of cases, and to the anterior/anteroinferior glenoid margin (Bankart lesion), seen in about 5% to 8% of cases. In addition, 15% of dislocations are associated with fractures of the greater tuberosity of the humerus (Fig. 14-16).

Posterior glenohumeral dislocations are uncommon, accounting for 2% to 4% of glenohumeral joint dislocations. The mechanism of injury is either a fall on an outstretched hand or a direct trauma to a flexed, adducted, and internally rotated shoulder, which forces the internally rotated humeral head posteriorly. When this occurs, the anterior aspect of the humeral head can impact the posterior glenoid margin. Classically associated with convulsive seizures, bilateral patterns of injury are common. Posterior dislocations are subtle

and can be more challenging to diagnose. Nearly 50% to 60% of injuries are still missed on initial evaluation. Radiographic signs of injury include the arm remaining fixed in internal rotation ("lightbulb" sign), linear sclerosis of the medial humeral head with impaction deformity ("reverse Hill-Sachs deformity"; Fig. 14-17), and an injury to the posterior labrum ("reverse Bankart lesion"). Additional signs include loss of the normal overlap of the humeral head and glenoid margin on standard AP views ("crescent" sign), widening of the glenohumeral joint space more than 6 mm on standard AP views ("rim" sign), disrupted scapulohumeral arch, and a posteriorly dislocated humeral head on axillary views (Fig. 14-18). There are two other fractures that are important in posterior dislocations. When a posterior glenoid rim fracture or a lesser tuberosity fracture is identified, a prior dislocation should be considered (Fig. 14-19).

Inferior glenohumeral dislocations (luxatio erecta) occur as a result of headfirst fall onto a fully abducted outstretched arm, which causes impingement of the

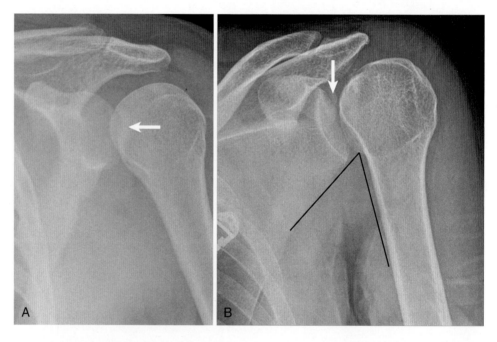

Figure 14-18 Posterior glenohumeral dislocation. Important indicators of a posterior dislocation include the rim sign, a joint space wider than 6 mm; absent half-moon sign, showing the lack of overlap between humeral head and glenoid (*arrow* in **A** and **B**); and a broken arch sign (*black lines* in **B**), depicting the absence of a scapulohumeral arch normally formed by the lateral cortex of the scapula and medial cortex of the humerus.

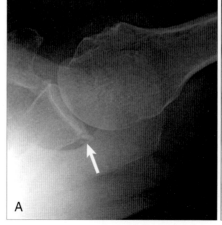

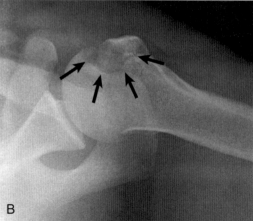

Figure 14-19 Posterior glenohumeral joint dislocation, associated fractures. A, Axillary radiograph shows a fracture of the posterior glenoid rim (*arrow*). **B,** Axillary radiograph in another patient shows a lesser tuberosity fracture (*arrows*) adjacent to a trough lesion (*arrow*).

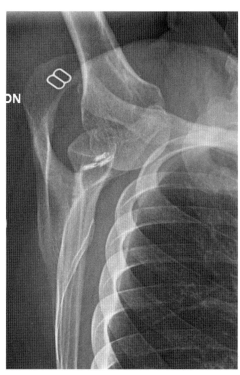

Figure 14-20 Luxatio erecta. Inferior glenohumeral joint dislocation with the humeral head perched against the glenoid so that the upper extremity is fixed in abduction.

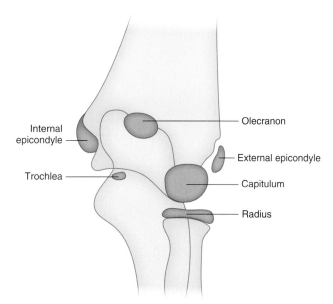

Figure 14-21 Diagram of a pediatric elbow. The mnemonic CRITOE is useful to recall the sequence of ossification in the skeletally immature elbow: *C*, capitellum (1 year); *R*, radial head (3 to 6 years); *I*, internal or medial epicondyle (5 to 7 years); *T*, trochlea (9 to 10 years); *O*, olecranon (6 to 10 years); and *E*, external or lateral epicondyle (9 to 13) years.

humerus against the acromion and levers the humeral head out from the glenoid fossa (Fig. 14-20). Patients present with the upper extremity fixed in severe abduction, with their arm straight up as if asking a question. The radiographic appearance is pathognomonic, with the upper extremity fixed in abduction, the humeral head dislocated inferiorly to the glenoid, and the humeral shaft pointing superiorly and laterally. Associated injuries include tearing of the inferior capsule, tearing of the rotator cuff, injury to the brachial plexus, injury to the adjacent vasculature, and fractures of the surrounding regional skeleton (clavicle, coracoid, glenoid rim, greater tuberosity of the humerus).

Superior glenohumeral dislocations are a result of trauma to a flexed elbow while the arm is in adduction, resulting in superior dislocation of the humeral head, with the humeral head resting beneath the acromion process. Associated injuries include tearing of the joint capsule, tearing of the rotator cuff tendons, and fracture of the regional skeleton.

Elbow

Jason E. Payne and Joseph S. Yu

■ ANATOMIC CONSIDERATIONS AND MECHANICS

The elbow consists of three articulations confined within a single joint capsule: the ulnotrochlear,

radiocapitellar, and proximal radioulnar joints. Each articulation allows a specific range of motion and provides a certain degree of stability. The ulnotrochlear articulation serves as the primary static stabilizer of the elbow, and its principal action is flexion-extension with a normal range of motion of approximately 0 to 140 degrees. The semispherical capitellum of the humerus articulates with the discoid radial head resulting in an axial-rotational joint. The radiocapitellar joint in conjunction with the proximal radioulnar articulation allows supination and pronation of the forearm ranging from 0 to 180 degrees.

Soft tissues also contribute to the stability of the elbow with the collateral ligament complexes representing important stabilizers of the elbow joint. The ulnar collateral ligament (UCL) is composed of the anterior, posterior, and transverse bands that originate on the medial epicondyle. The anterior band of the UCL is the most important resistor to valgus stress. The radial collateral ligament (RCL), lateral UCL, annular ligament, and accessory lateral collateral ligament compose the lateral collateral ligament complex. The RCL arises from the lateral epicondyle, blending with the annular ligament at the radial neck, and serves to prevent radial head displacement from the lesser sigmoid notch. The lateral UCL inserts on the supinator crest of the ulna preventing posterolateral rotatory instability.

Fractures around the elbow account for approximately 5% of all skeletal fractures. The majority of fractures around the elbow are closed fractures. The patient's age and sex may be predictive in the injury pattern. Many elbow injuries occur in skeletally immature patients. It is therefore important to recall the sequence of ossification in the pediatric elbow (Fig. 14-21).

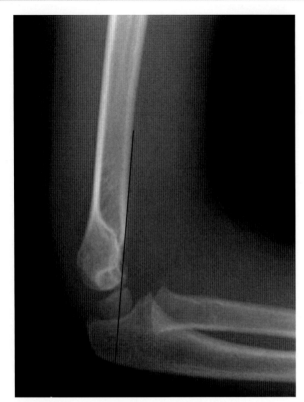

Figure 14-22 The anterior humeral line sign. In the lateral projection a line drawn along the anterior cortex of the humeral shaft to the elbow should traverse the middle third of the capitellum.

■ DISTAL HUMERUS FRACTURES

About 80% of distal humeral fractures occur in children. However, fractures of the distal humerus in adults account for 10% of all elbow fractures. The most common mechanism of injury is a fall on a flexed elbow, which transmits a force from the trochlear groove of the ulna to the distal humerus. The degree of flexion or extension at the time of injury will determine whether anterior or posterior angulation of the distal humerus will occur. A thorough evaluation of the articular surface should be performed because 95% of fractures are intercondylar fractures that violate the articular surface. The other fractures in adults can be divided into supracondylar and transcondylar fractures. About one half of fractures demonstrate a T- or Y-shaped pattern arising at or near the trochlea and extend proximally to involve one or both humeral epicondyles. The anterior humeral line sign is useful particularly in the pediatric population, in which fracture lines tend to be more subtle (Fig. 14-22). In supracondylar fractures the line crosses the anterior third of the capitellum owing to posterior displacement or angulation of the distal fragment. The most common pitfall preventing diagnosis is an inadequate lateral projection of the elbow.

Multiple classification schemes exist for distal humeral fractures. The most commonly used is the AO/ASIF classification system proposed by Mueller, which divides the fractures into three primary groups, each with three subgroups (Fig. 14-23). Surgical repair of distal humerus fractures focuses on restoration of the valgus tilt and external rotation of the trochlea and

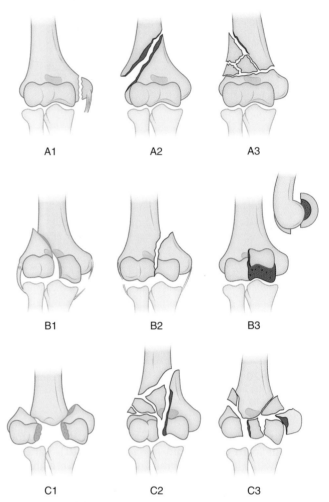

Figure 14-23 Mueller (AO/ASIF) classification of distal humerus fractures. Fractures are divided into three groups each containing three subgroups. Type A fractures are extra-articular. A1 is medial epicondyle avulsion. A2 is a transcondylar or supracondylar fracture. A3 is a comminuted supracondylar fracture. Type B fractures are unicondylar, intra-articular fractures. B1 involves lateral condyle, B2 involves medial condyle, and B3 the capitellum. Type C fractures are intra-articular, bicondylar fractures. C1 is a Y- or T-shaped fracture. C2 is intercondylar with comminution of the humeral shaft. C3 is comminuted, intercondylar involving articular surface and distal shaft.

congruency of the medial and lateral columns to restore full range of elbow motion.

Pediatric distal humeral fractures are distinct from those that occur in the adult population. Sixty percent of elbow fractures in the pediatric population are in the supracondylar region. Whereas 15% to 20% involve the lateral condyle, 10% are avulsions of the medial epicondylar ossification center (Fig. 14-24). In cases of elbow dislocation the ossification center avulses inferiorly and may become trapped in the joint upon reduction (Fig. 14-25). This appearance can simulate the trochlear ossification center; however, it is important to recall that the trochlear ossification center should not be present before the medial epicondyle ossification center.

Capitellar fractures account for approximately 1% of all elbow fractures and approximately 10% of distal humeral fractures. The mechanism of injury is typically

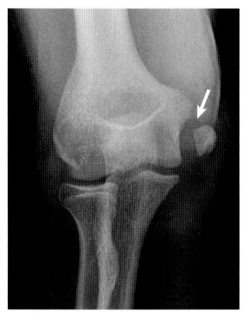

Figure 14-24 Little Leaguer's elbow. Frontal radiograph in a pediatric patient shows displacement of the medial epicondylar epiphysis *(arrow)* from the rest of the humerus and an abnormally widened growth plate. The ulnar nerve can be traumatized as well.

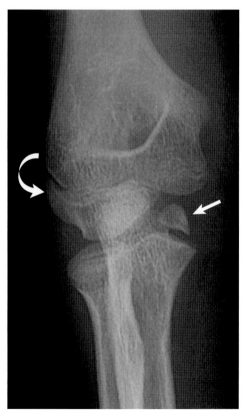

Figure 14-25 Entrapped medial epicondylar ossification center. Frontal radiograph in a 12-year-old after reduction of a dislocation shows that the medial epicondylar ossification center has displaced inferiorly and become entrapped in the medial joint space *(arrow)*. Both lateral epicondylar center *(curved arrow)* and medial epicondylar center should be present in a patient of this age.

a fall on an outstretched hand so that a shearing force transmitted through the radial head produces an intra-articular fracture, displacing the articular portion of the capitellum at the lateral margin of the trochlea. Close attention should be paid to the radius to avoid missing a second fracture. The pseudodefect of the capitellum marks the posterior margin of the articular cartilage and can be easily mistaken for an osteochondral defect.

Bryan and Morrey classified capitellar fractures into three different types. In type I the fracture involves most or all of capitellum; in type II a shearing injury produces an osteochondral defect; and in type III a comminuted fracture of the capitellum occurs, often associated with a radial head fracture. Type I fractures are conspicuous on the lateral view due to a characteristic displaced and rotated fragment giving the appearance of an igloolike density adjacent to the radial head (Fig. 14-26). A common pitfall is to misdiagnose the fragment as an intra-articular body, but an important observation is the absence of the articular cortex of the capitellum in the frontal projection, which is observed in the intact capitellum. Type II fractures are most optimally depicted on magnetic resonance imaging (MRI), although intra-articular contrast may be required if the defect is purely cartilaginous. Condylar fractures of the humerus are uncommon and result from a fall on an outstretched hand with either valgus or varus forces on the elbow, producing a combination of shearing and avulsion. The most common classification system that describes condylar fractures is the Milch classification (Fig. 14-27).

■ PROXIMAL RADIUS FRACTURES

Fractures of the radial head and neck are the most common type of fracture encountered in the adult elbow, whereas isolated radial neck fractures are more common in children. These fractures also typically result from a fall on an outstretched hand. Associated injuries may include a capitellar fracture, rupture of the UCL, rupture of the triceps tendon, and an elbow dislocation. Often the only indicator of a nondisplaced radial head fracture is the presence of a joint effusion on the lateral radiograph secondary to hemarthrosis (Fig. 14-28). Close inspection of the lateral margin of the radial head may reveal a nondisplaced vertical fracture that may only be seen with a radiocapitellar projection. Any angular deformity of the cortex at the head-neck junction should raise suspicion of a nondisplaced radial neck fracture (Fig. 14-29). Mason initially classified radial head fractures into three types. Type I fractures demonstrate less than 2 mm of displacement, type II fractures demonstrate greater than 2 mm of displacement, and comminution of the articular surface defines type III fractures. The classification system was later modified to include a fourth type that is associated with an elbow dislocation.

Comminuted distal radius fractures can involve injury to the interosseous membrane, producing disruption of the distal radioulnar joint (DRUJ), a constellation of findings referred to as the *Essex-Lopresti fracture-dislocation complex*. Severe injuries to the distal

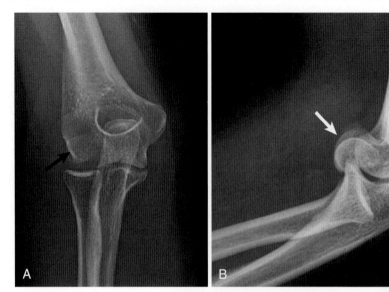

Figure 14-26 Capitellar fracture. A, Frontal radiograph shows a large, rounded bone fragment above the joint *(arrow)*. Note the absence of the lateral articular cortical surface. B, Lateral radiograph shows a volarly rotated capitellar fragment forming the shape of an igloo *(arrow)*, characteristic of a Bryan and Morrey type I fracture.

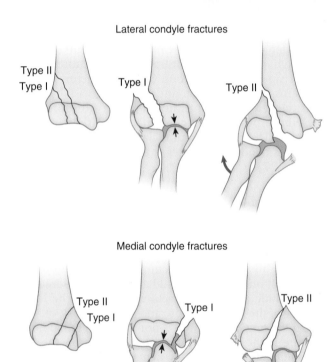

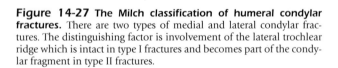

Figure 14-27 The Milch classification of humeral condylar fractures. There are two types of medial and lateral condylar fractures. The distinguishing factor is involvement of the lateral trochlear ridge which is intact in type I fractures and becomes part of the condylar fragment in type II fractures.

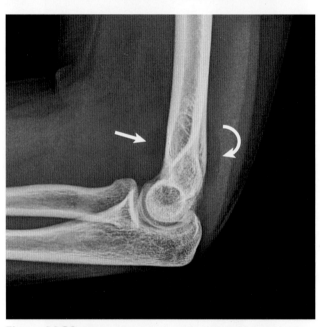

Figure 14-28 Elbow fat pads. Lateral radiograph shows displacement of the anterior coronoid fossa *(arrow)* and posterior olecranon fossa *(curved arrow)* fat pads by an effusion. The angle subtended by the anterior cortex of the distal humerus and the anterior margin of the anterior fat pad should not exceed 30 degrees, and the posterior fat pad is not normally seen.

radius should include thorough evaluation of the wrist for this injury pattern in addition to fractures of the carpus. Appropriate treatment of proximal radial fractures is imperative given the importance of the radiocapitellar and proximal radioulnar joints for both flexion/extension and supination/pronation of the forearm.

PROXIMAL ULNA FRACTURES

Coronoid Process Fractures

Most fractures of the coronoid process are associated with a posterior dislocation of the elbow. Fractures that involve more than 50% of the surface of the coronoid process result in a marked decrease in stability. The coronoid is an important location for the soft tissue stabilizers, including the anterior band of the UCL, which inserts on the sublime tubercle, the brachialis muscle, and the anterior capsule. Regan and Morrey classified coronoid fractures into three types based on the location of the fracture on the coronoid process as seen on

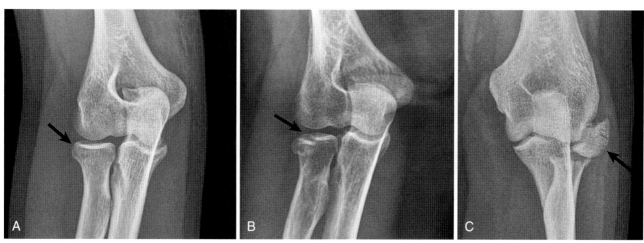

Figure 14-29 Radial head fractures. A, Frontal radiograph shows a subtle angular deformity *(arrow)* of the lateral margin of the radial head consistent with a Mason type I nondisplaced radial head fracture. B, A type II fracture *(arrow)* has greater than 2 mm of displacement. C, A type III fracture shows comminution with rotation of the articular surface in this patient *(arrow)*.

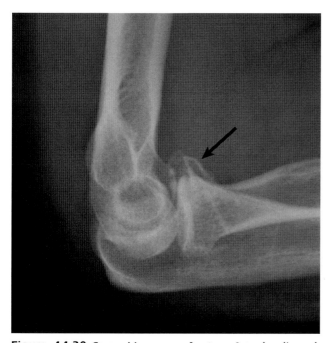

Figure 14-30 Coronoid process fracture. Lateral radiograph shows a comminuted fracture of the coronoid process involving greater than 50% of the coronoid *(arrow)*, a type III Regan and Morrey fracture.

the lateral radiograph. Type I fractures involved the tip of the coronoid, type II fractures involve less than 50% of the coronoid, and type III fractures involve more than 50% of the coronoid (see Fig. 14-30). Classification schemes have been subsequently refined to include more specificity regarding anatomic location and morphologic characteristics. It is important to recall that in posterior dislocations the coronoid fragment may become an intra-articular fragment.

Olecranon Fractures

Olecranon fractures account for 20% of elbow injuries in adults and are common in older adults. Fractures are caused by direct trauma with a force directed to the point of the olecranon, a fall on a flexed elbow, hyperextension, or indirect trauma due to forceful contraction of the triceps against a flexed elbow. Most fractures are oriented perpendicular to the long axis of the ulna. Distraction of the proximal fragment may occur owing to tension by the triceps tendon. Fractures oriented more longitudinally with respect to the ulnar shaft may be difficult to visualize, but swelling of the olecranon bursa should prompt a careful search. These fractures arise when a valgus or varus force is applied to a fully extended elbow. Avulsion fractures of the tip of the olecranon occur most commonly in older patients. The Mayo Clinic classification takes into account stability, displacement, and comminution. Type I fractures are nondisplaced. Type II fractures are displaced more than 3 mm, but the ligamentous structures remain intact, preventing dislocation. Type III are fracture-dislocation complexes. Each fracture type can be placed into subclass A (noncomminuted) or B (comminuted) (Fig. 14-31). Displaced fractures typically require surgical reduction and fixation.

■ DISLOCATIONS

The elbow is the most commonly dislocated articulation in children and the third most commonly dislocated joint in adults after the AC and glenohumeral joints of the shoulder. The most common mechanism of injury is hyperextension so that the olecranon is forced into the olecranon fossa, which acts as a fulcrum to dislocate the joint. In nearly all cases both the radius and ulna displace in the same direction, but occasionally the radius and ulna displace in opposite directions, resulting in a divergent dislocation. Dislocations are classified based on the direction of the displaced forearm bones with respect to the humerus. Dislocations in adults typically occur in combination with a fracture of the ulna. Isolated radial head dislocation or subluxation is common in children.

The majority of elbow dislocations occur in the posterior or posterolateral directions (Fig. 14-32). The remaining dislocations are equally divided into lateral,

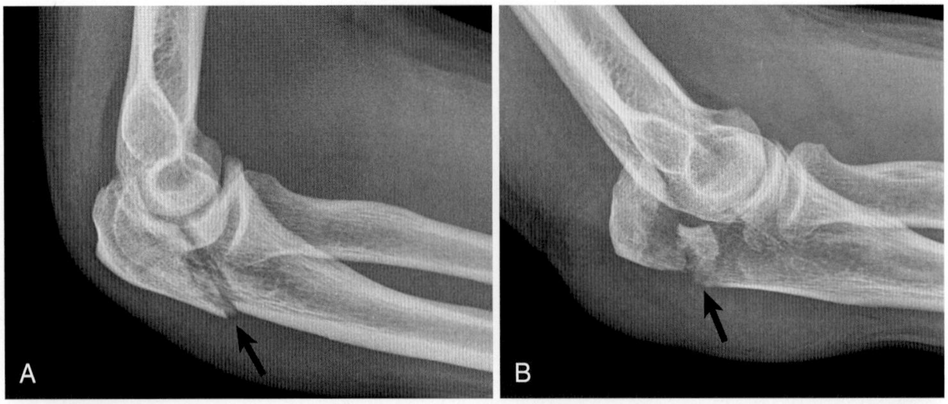

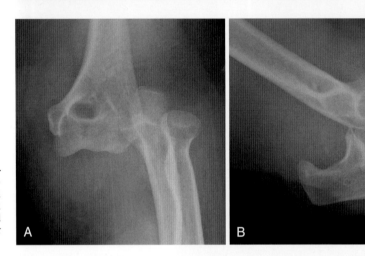

Figure 14-31 Olecranon fractures. A, Lateral radiograph demonstrates a nondisplaced, linear Mayo Clinic IA fracture of the olecranon process *(arrow)*. B, Lateral radiograph shows a comminuted Mayo Clinic IIB fracture with greater than 3 mm of displacement *(arrow)*.

Figure 14-32 Elbow dislocation. Frontal (**A**) and lateral (**B**) radiographs show posterolateral dislocation of the elbow. A careful inspection should be performed upon reduction for intra-articular fractures.

anterior, and medial/posteromedial types. Dislocations are often associated with fractures, particularly involving the medial epicondyle, radial head/neck, and coronoid process. A common indicator of elbow dislocation is disruption of the radiocapitellar line. In a normal elbow a line that bisects the proximal shaft of the radius passes through the capitellum on every radiographic projection. An important pitfall is improper drawing of the line. Inclusion of only the proximal end of the radius without the radial tuberosity will shift the line more laterally and anteriorly than expected, whereas if the line is extended too far distally it may not extend to the proximal end of the radius. In children an overly pronated elbow will result in a similar pitfall.

■ LIGAMENT INJURIES

The UCL provides resistance to valgus stress. Injuries are often the result of repetitive throwing motion as seen in baseball pitchers, which results in tremendous valgus force during the late-cocking and acceleration phases. Small tears in the ligament begin to develop, which may progress to a complete rupture when there is continued activity, although a tear can occur from a single traumatic episode. The majority of UCL tears involve the anterior band and are complete disruptions. Magnetic resonance imaging is the modality of choice for evaluating the integrity of the UCL. When torn, the anterior UCL band may depict abnormal signal within or around the ligament, discontinuity, and/ or changes in its morphologic characteristics (Fig. 14-33).

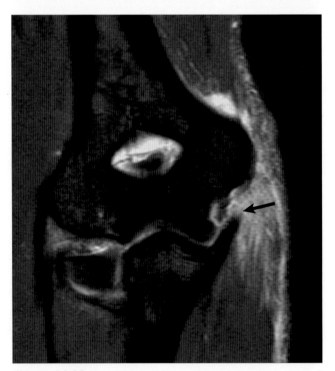

Figure 14-33 Tear of the ulnar collateral ligament. Coronal short tau inversion recovery (STIR) magnetic resonance image (MRI) shows complete proximal disruption of the anterior band of the ulnar collateral (UCL) ligament from a valgus injury *(arrow)*. There is edema in the adjacent flexor musculature.

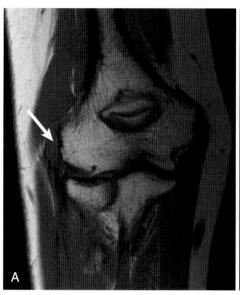
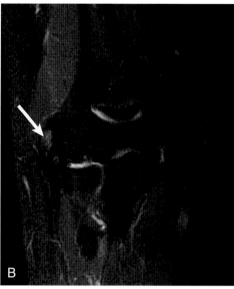

Figure 14-34 Lateral epicondylitis. A, Coronal T1-weighted image shows thickening of the common tendon of the extensor muscle group with increased intermediate signal *(arrow)* characteristic of tendinosis of the common extensor tendon (lateral epicondylitis). **B,** Coronal T2-weighted image shows increased fluid signal within the tendon *(arrow)*, indicating a partial tear.

The RCL is less susceptible to isolated injuries. Rupture is typically related to posterior dislocation and if not repaired may lead to chronic subluxation. A complete tear of the ulnar bundle of the lateral collateral ligament can result in posterolateral rotatory instability. A severe varus stress to the elbow produces this injury. In this situation the radial head subluxes with secondary rotatory subluxation of the ulnohumeral joint. On MRI the RCL appears as a linear, low-signal structure along the lateral margin of the joint. Abnormalities are best depicted in the coronal plane and include complete absence of the ligament fibers, increased signal in or around the ligament, or changes in morphologic characteristics.

▪ TENDON INJURIES

Epicondylitis

Lateral and medial epicondylitis are pathologically identical entities that appear on opposite sides of the elbow. The more frequently encountered lateral epicondylitis affects the origin of the common tendon of the extensor muscle group on the lateral humeral epicondyle, whereas medial epicondylitis affects the common flexor tendon that attaches to the medial epicondyle. Radiographs may show enthesopathy of the common tendons in both medial and lateral epicondylitis. Lateral epicondylitis, or "tennis elbow" due to its prevalence in racquet sport athletes, is much more frequent in non-athletes between the ages of 40 and 60 years. Patients typically present with chronic lateral elbow pain exacerbated by activities that involve extension of the wrist. The cause is repetitive microtears of the tendon cycled with insufficient healing, particularly of the extensor carpi radialis brevis tendon. On MRI, thickening and increased signal at the origin on T1- and T2-weighted images is characteristic (Fig. 14-34). A focus of increased T2 signal within the tendon is consistent with either partial or complete macroscopic tear. Medial epicondylitis occurs most frequently in athletes who are involved in activities that produce chronic valgus stress, such as racquetball players and golfers.

Biceps Tendon Injuries

The biceps brachii muscle originates from the supraglenoid tubercle and the coracoid process and inserts on the radial tuberosity of the proximal radius. It is frequently bifid with the short head initially medial to the long head but rotating to become more superficial at the insertion. Distal biceps tendon rupture occurs most commonly in the dominant arm of men between the ages of 40 and 60 years. Tendinosis is a frequent finding at the enthesis. Injury almost always occurs during eccentric contraction, with forceful extension of the elbow while the muscle is flexing. Patients feel a tearing sensation and pain in the antecubital space at the time of injury. Ecchymosis and tenderness in the antecubital fossa are characteristic physical findings. Most tears occur at the insertion on the radial tuberosity. Radiographs may show masslike swelling. Magnetic resonance imaging is optimal for evaluating patients with biceps injuries. A gap in the tendon accompanied by a hematoma may be observed between the retracted tendon and the radial tuberosity (Fig. 14-35). T2-weighted images show edema in and around the tendon. Axial images are particularly useful in differentiating between true partial tears and complete tears that involve one limb of a bifid tendon. The integrity of the biceps aponeurosis determines the amount of tendon retraction. If the gap is less than 2 cm, the aponeurosis is likely to be intact.

Triceps Tendon Injuries

Triceps tendon rupture is an uncommon injury. An avulsion of the olecranon tip may be visible on a lateral radiograph (Fig. 14-36). Intratendinous rupture occurs in individuals with predisposing conditions such as diabetes or a history of exogenous steroid administration. Rupture is almost always secondary to a single traumatic event such as fall on an outstretched hand. In weight lifters it is the culmination of repetitive injuries with microtears

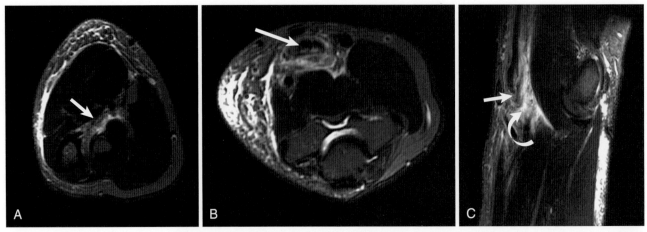

Figure 14-35 Biceps brachii tendon tear A, Axial short tau inversion recovery (STIR) image at the level of the radial tuberosity shows absence of the biceps tendon, consistent with complete avulsion *(arrow)*. Soft tissue edema is present in the anterior subcutaneous tissues. **B,** Axial STIR image more proximally shows a retracted biceps tendon surrounded by edema *(arrow)* and the lacertus fibrosus. **C,** Sagittal STIR image shows the end of the tendon *(arrow)* and hemorrhage in the gap *(curved arrow)*.

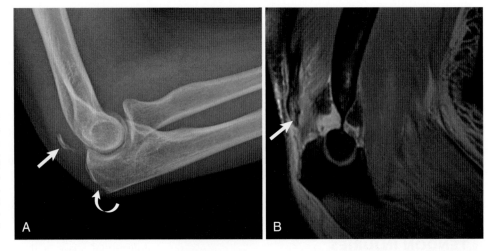

Figure 14-36 Triceps tendon tear. A, Lateral radiograph shows a displaced bone fragment from the olecranon process *(arrow)* and the olecranon donor site *(curved arrow)*, consistent with a triceps tendon avulsion. **B,** Sagittal proton density magnetic resonance image (MRI) shows retraction of the triceps tendon with interstitial edema *(arrow)*.

that precede ultimate tendon failure. Magnetic resonance imaging can distinguish between partial and complete triceps tendon tears. Triceps tears are depicted on sagittal images as a focus of fluid signal intensity within a tendon defect, although axial images are more useful for characterizing partial tears.

Bursitis and Infection

The superficial olecranon bursa resides in between the olecranon process and subcutaneous tissues and is the most common location for bursitis in the elbow. The radiographic findings of olecranon bursitis are distinctive (Fig. 14-37). Depending on the cause, calcium deposits or loose bodies may be apparent. Trauma is the most common cause of olecranon bursitis, although less common causes include infection, rheumatoid arthritis, and crystal deposition arthropathies. When a patient presents with bilateral olecranon bursitis, it is likely caused by gout. When there is surrounding cellulitis, infection is an important consideration. The superficial location of the bursa and the exposure to trauma place the bursa at high risk for the introduction of bacteria. The infected bursa

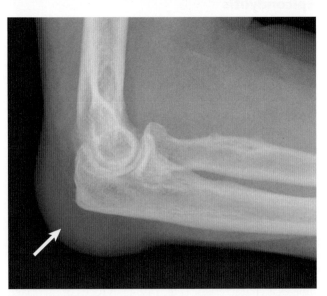

Figure 14-37 Olecranon bursitis. Lateral radiograph shows the characteristic features of superficial olecranon bursitis with focal soft tissue protuberance posterior to the olecranon process *(white arrow)* from distention of the bursa by fluid.

presents with increasing fluid, redness, and pain. Because septic olecranon bursitis can progress to osteomyelitis, prompt diagnosis should be performed (Fig. 14-38).

■ FOREARM

Most fractures of the forearm are the result of a fall on an outstretched hand. Occasionally a direct blow may fracture one or both forearm bones such as a nightstick fracture. In addition, several fracture-dislocation complexes that involve the elbow, forearm, and wrist are noteworthy because they require inspection of the elbow and wrist.

■ FRACTURE-DISLOCATION COMPLEXES

Monteggia

A Monteggia fracture-dislocation complex is a fracture of the proximal third of the ulna that is associated with

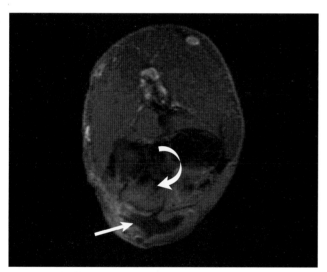

Figure 14-38 Infected olecranon bursa. Axial T1-weighted fat-saturated contrast-enhanced magnetic resonance image (MRI) shows distention of the olecranon bursa with enhancement of the thickened bursal wall *(arrow)*. There is also enhancement of the ulna indicative of osteomyelitis *(curved arrow)*.

dislocation of the radial head, typically from a fall on an outstretched hand. Bado classified the injury complex into four types. A type I lesion accounts for 60% of fracture-dislocations in this group and is characterized by anterior angulation of the ulnar fracture and anterior dislocation of the radial head (Fig. 14-39). A type II lesion results in posterior dislocation of the radial head with posterior angulation of the ulnar fracture, accounting for 10% to 15% of cases. A type III lesion results in lateral or anterolateral dislocation of the radial head, usually associated with fracture of the ulna just distal to the coronoid process. This type is most commonly seen in children between the ages of 5 and 9 years. The least common type IV lesion results in fracture of the proximal ends of both the radius and ulna with anterior dislocation of the radial head. When a fracture of the ulna is apparent, close inspection of the proximal radius should be performed. A pitfall to remember is that if a fracture is located in the mid or distal forearm, initial radiographs should include both the elbow and the wrist, particularly if the shaft fracture is angulated.

Galeazzi

A Galeazzi fracture-dislocation is another forearm injury that involves both bones. It is a fracture of the diaphysis of the radius associated with subluxation or dislocation of the ulnar head (Fig. 14-40). This complex is likely the result of a fall on an outstretched hand with pronation of the forearm. The radial fracture is typically displaced and angulated, but dislocation of the DRUJ may be easily overlooked because there may only be widening of the DRUJ on the AP view or an overlap of the distal ulna and radius if the arm is rotated.

Essex-Lopresti

The Essex-Lopresti fracture is characterized by a markedly comminuted and displaced fracture of the radial head and dislocation/subluxation of the DRUJ. Displaced fractures of the radial head and neck can propagate a rupture of the interosseous membrane of the forearm that produces disruption of the DRUJ. As with

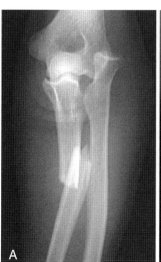

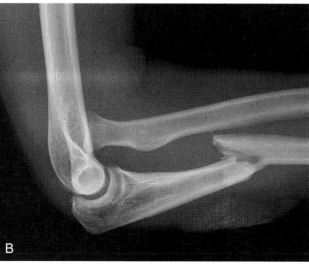

Figure 14-39 Monteggia fracture-dislocation complex. A, Frontal radiograph shows an angulated and displaced fracture of the ulnar shaft and dislocation of the radial head. **B,** Lateral radiograph shows anterior angulation of the fracture and anterior dislocation of the radial head consistent with a Bado type I lesion.

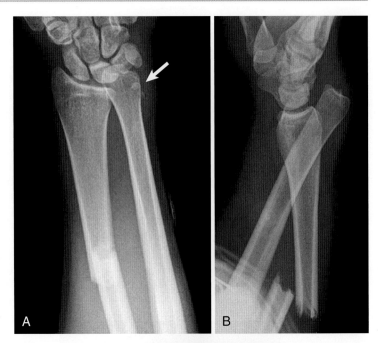

Figure 14-40 Galeazzi fracture-dislocation complex. **A,** Frontal radiograph shows an angulated, displaced radial shaft fracture and dislocation of the ulnar head consistent with a Galeazzi fracture-dislocation. Note the comminuted, displaced ulnar styloid fracture *(arrow).* **B,** Lateral radiograph depicts the disruption of the distal radioulnar joint.

the Galeazzi complex, any severe injury to the elbow should prompt a close inspection of the wrist for associated abnormalities.

■ COMPARTMENT SYNDROME

The forearm is divided into three fascial compartments: dorsal (extensor), volar (flexor), and lateral, each containing several muscles. The interosseous membrane separates the volar and dorsal compartments. Compartment syndrome may be caused by a fracture of the forearm, muscle injury, crush injury, or improper casting/splinting. It occurs when the perfusion pressure falls below the compartment pressure. If left untreated, it may result in nerve and muscle ischemia that can become permanent. The volar compartment is most frequently affected. Clinically the pain is out of proportion to the injury. Magnetic resonance imaging is the modality of choice. Enlargement of the affected muscle group from edema is characteristic. Fluid-sensitive sequences show diffuse hyperintensity in the affected muscles. As the process progresses, intravenous administration of gadolinium often shows nonperfused areas that represent areas of myonecrosis, which requires surgical fasciotomy for decompression.

Hand and Wrist

Felix S. Chew and Rachel F. Gerson

■ FRACTURES OF THE PHALANGES

The ends of the fingers and thumb are very common sites of musculoskeletal trauma. Direct injury such as a hammer blow or entrapment in a car door may result

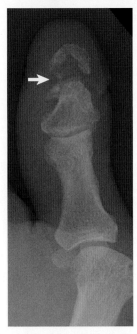

Figure 14-41 Comminuted fracture *(arrow)* of the distal phalanx of the thumb from direct crushing trauma, disrupting the thumbnail.

in comminuted fractures of the distal phalangeal tuft or shaft, often with concomitant injury of the nail and soft tissues (Fig. 14-41). Fractures of the distal phalanx associated with nail injuries are considered to be open fractures. Therefore in skeletally immature patients the growth plate should also be closely inspected for involvement. The phalanges are also vulnerable to amputation.

Axially directed trauma to the extended fingertips, as in a jammed finger, may result in transmission of the force from the distal phalanx to the middle phalanx, causing oblique fractures. These fractures may be intra-articular and involve the distal articular condyles at the distal interphalangeal (DIP) joint (Fig. 14-42), or they may be extra-articular and involve

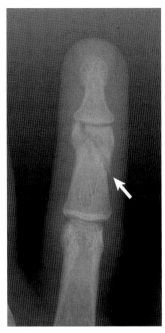

Figure 14-42 Comminuted oblique intra-articular fracture *(arrow)* of the middle phalanx of the ring finger at the distal interphalangeal (DIP) joint from indirect axial loading.

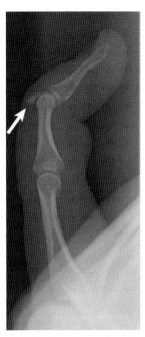

Figure 14-44 Proximally distracted avulsion fracture *(arrow)* of the distal phalanx of the little finger at the insertion of the extensor tendon, with flexion deformity (mallet finger).

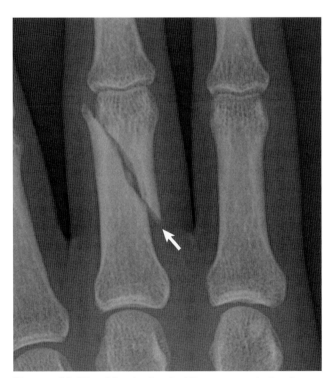

Figure 14-43 Mildly displaced oblique extra-articular fracture *(arrow)* of the shaft of the proximal phalanx of the middle finger from indirect axial loading.

■ INJURIES OF THE INTERPHALANGEAL AND METACARPOPHALANGEAL JOINTS

The IP joints of the fingers and thumb normally have motion in flexion and extension that is mediated through mutually opposed extensor and flexor tendons. An injury of the extensor mechanism at the DIP joint, either through avulsion fracture of the insertion at the dorsal aspect of the distal phalanx (Fig. 14-44) or through rupture of the tendon itself, will result in asymmetrically opposed flexor action and mallet finger deformity (Fig. 14-45). At the DIP, injury of the extensor mechanism is much more common than injury of the flexor mechanism.

The flexor mechanism of the proximal interphalangeal (PIP) joint attaches to the middle phalanx through the volar plate. Avulsion fractures at this site are often difficult to identify because the fracture fragment may be very small (Fig. 14-46). At the PIP joint, injury of the flexor mechanism is much more common than injury of the extensor mechanism.

At the IP and MCP joints, ulnar (medial) and radial (lateral) collateral ligaments are static stabilizers against valgus and varus stresses, respectively. Avulsion fractures at the medial or lateral margins of the distal phalanx at the DIP joints, of the middle phalanx at the PIP joints, and of the proximal phalanx at the MCP joints correspond to collateral ligament injuries (Fig. 14-47).

A UCL injury at the MCP joint of the thumb is called a *gamekeeper's thumb* or *skier's thumb*, names that reflect activities leading to the injury through excessive valgus stress. These injuries may manifest either as an avulsion fracture of the ulnar aspect of the proximal phalanx (Fig. 14-48) or as a rupture of the ligament without fracture. If there is no fracture, stress views may demonstrate the resultant insta-

only the shaft (Fig. 14-43). If the fist is partially closed at impact (flexion of the interphalangeal [IP] joints with extension at the metacarpophalangeal [MCP] joint), the distal end of the proximal phalanx becomes exposed to the impact and it may be fractured. A blow with a fully closed fist exposes the metacarpals to injury.

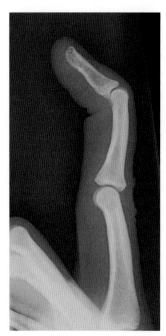

Figure 14-45 Traumatic rupture of the extensor tendon from the distal phalanx without fracture, resulting in flexion deformity at the distal interphalangeal (IP) joint (mallet finger).

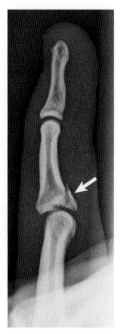

Figure 14-46 Volar plate avulsion fracture *(arrow)* of the middle phalanx at the proximal interphalangeal (PIP) joint.

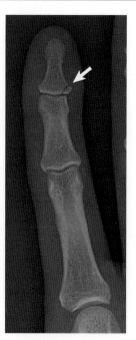

Figure 14-47 Ulnar collateral ligament (UCL) avulsion fracture *(arrow)* of the distal phalanx of the index finger distal interphalangeal (DIP) joint.

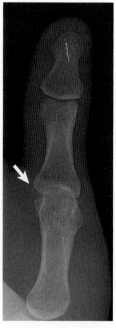

Figure 14-48 Ulnar collateral ligament (UCL) avulsion fracture *(arrow)* of the proximal phalanx of the thumb at the metacarpophalangeal (MCP) joint (gamekeeper's thumb).

bility but should be carefully performed. Magnetic resonance imaging is preferred for demonstrating ligament tears either with or without MCP arthrography because stress views increase the risk for converting a ruptured UCL into a Stener lesion, in which the adductor aponeurosis is interposed between the bone and the retracted ligament (Fig. 14-49).

Dorsal dislocations of the DIP or PIP joints (Fig. 14-50) are much more common than volar dislocations (Fig. 14-51). Following relocation, lateral radiographs should be obtained to look for associated avulsion fractures.

Dislocations at the MCP joint are much less common than dislocations at the IP joints because they are less exposed and vulnerable. Multiple simultaneous dislocations may occur in high-energy trauma (Fig. 14-52).

■ FRACTURES OF THE METACARPALS

The most common metacarpal fracture is the boxer's fracture, a volarly angulated fracture of the metacarpal neck sustained when a blow is struck with the closed fist. The

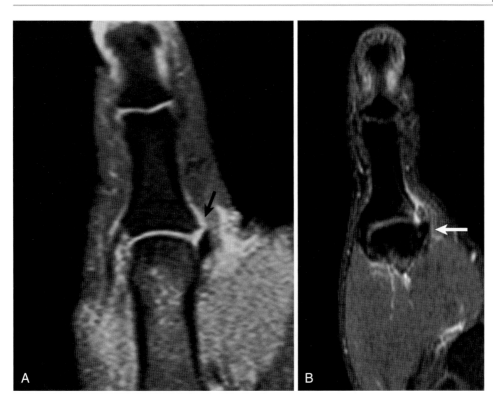

Figure 14-49 A, Tear of the distal attachment of the ulnar collateral ligament (UCL) from the base of the first proximal phalanx on a coronal gradient-recalled echo magnetic resonance image (MRI). B, MR fluid-sensitive image shows a retracted UCL tear *(arrow)* superficial to the adductor aponeurosis (Stener lesion).

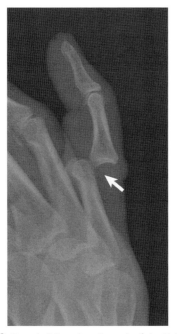

Figure 14-50 Dorsal dislocation *(arrow)* of the little finger at the proximal interphalangeal (PIP) joint.

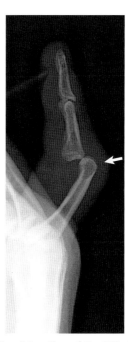

Figure 14-51 Volar dislocation of the little finger at the proximal interphalangeal (PIP) joint. A small avulsion fragment *(arrow)* is present dorsal to the distal end of the proximal phalanx, which may indicate an extensor mechanism injury.

fifth metacarpal is most commonly involved, but depending on the forces involved, other metacarpals may be involved at the same time or in succession (Fig. 14-53).

In gunshot wounds to the hand the projectile often passes completely through because of the thinness of the extremity. Fractures along the path of the projectile will be seen, often with metal fragments (Fig 14-54, A). Digits may be traumatically amputated (see Fig. 14-54, B).

Blast injuries may occur in a variety of settings, typically the premature detonation of a celebratory

firework. When severe, these injuries may consist of combinations of burns, open soft tissue injuries, fractures, dislocations, and amputations. Because the firework is often being held in the hand, the soft tissues of the first web space may be split open and the thumb may be dislocated (Fig. 14-55).

Industrial injuries to the hand may result from exposure to cutting or crushing machinery. These are often open fractures or amputations in dirty environments

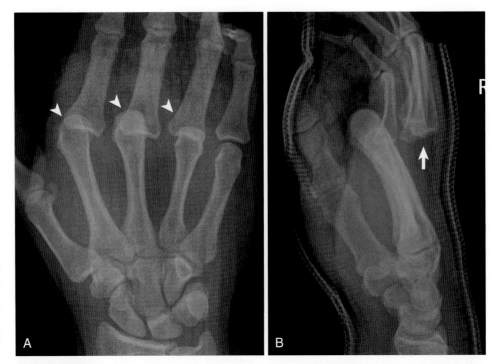

Figure 14-52 A, Multiple meta-carpophalangeal (MCP) dislocations involving the index, middle, and ring fingers are demonstrated on the posteroanterior radiograph as overlapping of the proximal phalanges *(arrowheads)* and metacarpal heads. A fiberglass cast is in place. B, Dorsal dislocations of the index, middle, and ring MCP joints *(arrow)* shown on lateral radiograph.

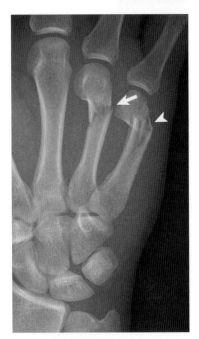

Figure 14-53 Comminuted fractures *(arrow and arrowhead)* of the necks of the fourth and fifth metacarpals, with volar angulation (boxer's fractures).

with extensive soft tissue damage (Fig. 14-56). Any portion of the hand may be involved. In the case of traumatic amputation the amputated part should be recovered for possible surgical replantation.

■ INJURIES OF THE CARPOMETACARPAL JOINTS

Extra-articular fractures of the first metacarpal that do not involve the joint are often treated with closed methods

(Fig. 14-57). There are two types of intra-articular fractures at the first carpometacarpal (CMC) joint. The Bennett fracture is a two-part avulsion fracture of the ulnar aspect of the base of the first metacarpal. The avulsed fracture fragment retains its ligamentous attachment to the trapezium through the anterior oblique ligament, while the remaining metacarpal may be subluxated or dislocated from the trapezium from the pull of the abductor pollicis longus muscle (Fig. 14-58). The Rolando fracture is a T- or Y-shaped intra-articular fracture (Fig. 14-59, *A*). Because the treatment and prognosis of these fractures is different, CT may be used to characterize the position and alignment of the fragments (see Fig. 14-59, *B*).

The most common CMC injuries involving the fingers occur at the articulations of the fourth and fifth metacarpals with the hamate. The most common pattern is fracture of the body of the hamate with dorsal dislocation of the metacarpal. Because of the interlocking geometry of the second and third CMC joints, multiple CMC dislocations are rare injuries that require high energy (Fig. 14-60). Because of their rarity and the frequent presence of other injuries, they may be initially overlooked.

■ FRACTURES OF THE CARPAL BONES

The most commonly fractured carpal bone is the scaphoid. As an elongated bone that bridges the proximal and distal rows, it is vulnerable to injury during falls. Scaphoid fractures may occur not only in isolation but also as one component of more complex carpal injuries. Fractures of the scaphoid waist are at increased risk for osteonecrosis of the proximal fragment because the blood supply enters the bone distally and flows proximally. The oblique orientation of the scaphoid relative to the remainder of the carpus may make fractures difficult to

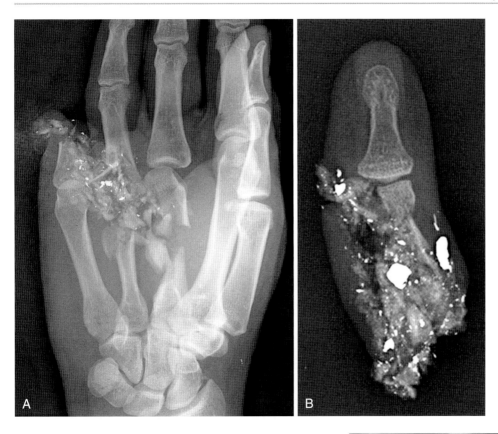

Figure 14-54 A, Gunshot wound to the hand with open fractures of the third metacarpal, ring metacarpophalangeal (MCP) joint, and little finger. **B,** Traumatic amputation of the little finger resulting from gunshot wound.

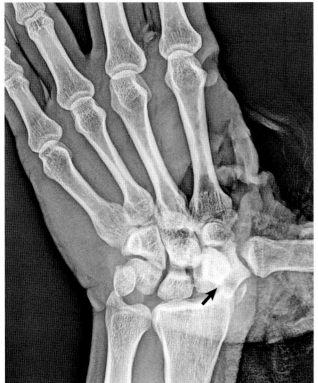

Figure 14-55 Severe degloving blast injury of the hand and carpus with fracture-dislocation of the trapezium *(arrow)* and thumb, the result of the premature explosion of a handheld firework.

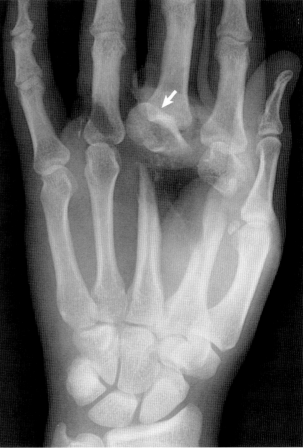

Figure 14-56 Comminuted open fractures of the second and third metacarpals *(arrow)* with displacement, dislocation, and degloving, caused by an accident with power machinery.

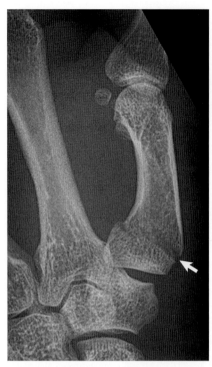

Figure 14-57 Transverse extra-articular fracture *(arrow)* of the proximal shaft of the first metacarpal.

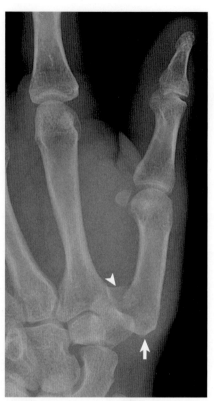

Figure 14-58 Intra-articular avulsion fracture *(arrowhead)* of the medial portion of the first metacarpal with carpometacarpal (CMC) dislocation *(arrow)* (Bennett fracture-dislocation).

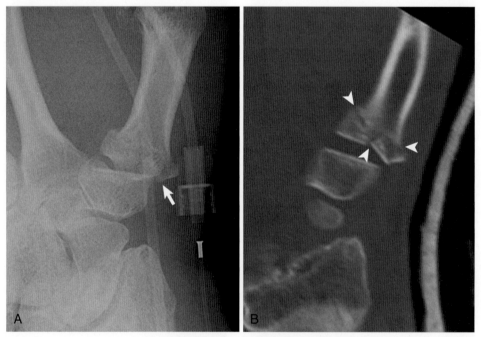

Figure 14-59 **A,** T-shaped comminuted intra-articular fracture *(arrow)* of the first metacarpal is partially obscured by intravenous tubing on posteroanterior radiograph (Rolando fracture). **B,** Coronal computed tomographic (CT) reformation shows impacted T-shaped comminuted intra-articular fracture *(arrowheads)* of the first metacarpal at the carpometacarpal (CMC) joint (Rolando fracture).

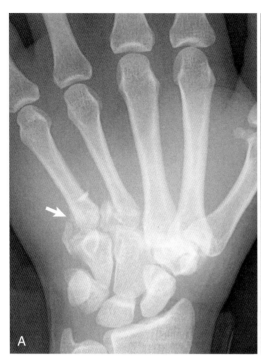
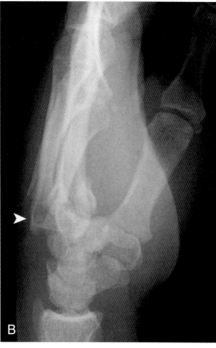

Figure 14-60 A, Multiple carpometacarpal (CMC) fracture-dislocations manifested as multiple fractures of the bases of the metacarpals *(arrow)* with overlap of the metacarpal bases and the proximal carpal row. **B,** Multiple dorsal CMC fracture-dislocations *(arrowhead)* demonstrated on lateral radiograph.

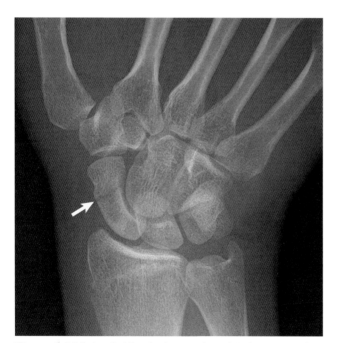

Figure 14-61 Scaphoid waist fracture *(arrow)* is demonstrated on angled, ulnar deviation radiograph.

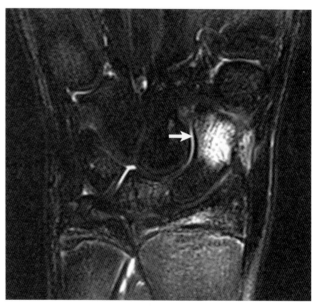

Figure 14-62 Coronal magnetic resonance imaging (MRI) of the wrist performed at 3 T shows T2 high signal *(arrow)* in the distal pole of the scaphoid.

see unless a special scaphoid view (ulnar deviation of the hand, angulation of the x-ray beam perpendicular to the plane of the scaphoid) is obtained (Fig. 14-61). Even with dedicated scaphoid views, some scaphoid fractures may require CT or even MRI (Fig. 14-62) for visualization. Surgical indications include displacement by more than 1 mm, angulation, dorsal intercalated segmental instability, and movement with ulnar deviation.

Most fractures of the triquetrum are sustained in falls. The fragment is typically displaced dorsally and may be visible only on the lateral view (Fig. 14-63). Stick-

handling sports may cause fractures of the pisiform and hamate. Fractures of the hook of the hamate may sometimes be demonstrated on radiographs positioned to demonstrate the carpal tunnel (Fig. 14-64). More often CT is required to demonstrate hook of the hamate fractures (Fig. 14-65). Fractures of the body of the hamate may also require cross-sectional imaging for diagnosis.

■ INJURIES OF THE CARPUS

Injuries of the carpus tend to occur in younger adults; in children the open growth plate is more vulnerable, and

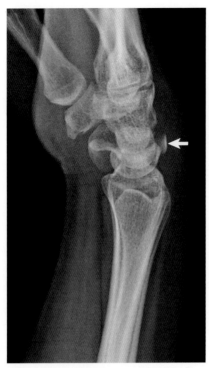

Figure 14-63 Dorsally displaced fragment *(arrow)* from triquetral fracture is shown on lateral radiograph.

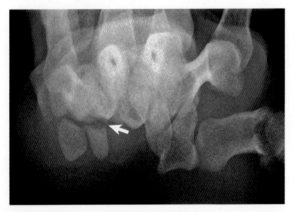

Figure 14-64 Distracted hook of hamate fracture *(arrow)* demonstrated on carpal tunnel radiograph.

in older adults the osteopenic distal radius is more vulnerable. Most fracture-dislocations of the carpal bones can be described using a progressive perilunar instability model. There are four specific injuries resulting from increasing severity of the same mechanism. The least severe is rotatory subluxation of the scaphoid (also called *scapholunate dissociation*), followed by perilunate dislocation, midcarpal dislocation, and lunate dislocation. In perilunate dislocation the carpus is disrupted on the lateral side, typically by a scaphoid fracture, and the carpus rotates dorsally with the ulnar side as a hinge until the capitate dislocates from the lunate (Fig. 14-66); the lunate retains its articulation with the radius. In lunate dislocation the carpal bones completely dislocate from around the lunate and then eject it from the radial fossa anteriorly, so that the capitate comes to rest in the radial fossa (Fig. 14-67). The soft tissue damage associated

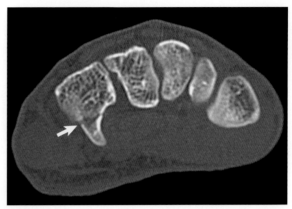

Figure 14-65 Minimally displaced hook of hamate fracture *(arrow)* demonstrated on axial computed tomography (CT).

with these injuries may be extensive, and if there are associated scaphoid fractures, the risk for osteonecrosis is heightened because of the severe displacement. High-energy trauma in uncontrolled circumstances such as motorcycle or all-terrain vehicle crashes may result in complex and unique combinations of carpal fractures and dislocations. After initial reduction and splinting, CT may be helpful in identifying the full extent of such injuries (Fig. 14-68).

■ INJURIES OF THE DISTAL RADIUS AND ULNA

In patients with open physes the growth plate is often the weakest link in a fall on an outstretched hand, typically resulting in Salter-Harris type II fracture, which is easily recognizable by the presence of a metaphyseal fragment. Less commonly the fracture plane extends through the physis without involving the metaphysis, referred to as a *Salter-Harris type I fracture* (Fig. 14-69). When nondisplaced, this injury may be recognized radiographically by widening of the physis.

Distal radius fractures sustained in low-energy ground-level falls onto an outstretched hand increase in prevalence with age, becoming the most prevalent extremity fracture in older adults. The typical fracture has dorsal and radial impaction and angulation, commonly extending from the metaphysis to the articular surface; ulnar styloid process fractures are often present (Fig. 14-70). High-energy distal radius fractures sustained in falls from a height or motor vehicle accidents may be highly comminuted and associated with soft tissue injury and neurovascular damage. Radial styloid fractures may occur in isolation as a result of low-energy falls or as a component of complex carpal, radial, or radiocarpal injuries that result from high-energy trauma (Fig. 14-71).

Radiocarpal fracture-dislocations are uncommon high-energy injuries typically sustained in motorcycle or other motor vehicle crashes, with shearing or rotational forces that disrupt the radiocarpal ligaments (Fig. 14-72). In addition to fractures of the radial and ulnar styloid processes, DRUJ injuries and neurovascular injuries may be associated with radiocarpal dislocations.

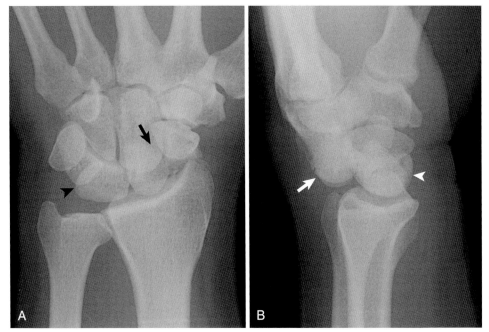

Figure 14-66 A, Transscaphoid perilunate dislocation of the carpus with displaced fracture of the scaphoid waist *(arrow)* and overlap *(arrowhead)* of the proximal and distal carpal rows shown on posteroanterior radiograph. **B,** Perilunate dislocation with dorsal dislocation of the capitate *(arrow)* from the lunate, but normal location of the lunate *(arrowhead)* within the radial fossa shown on lateral radiograph.

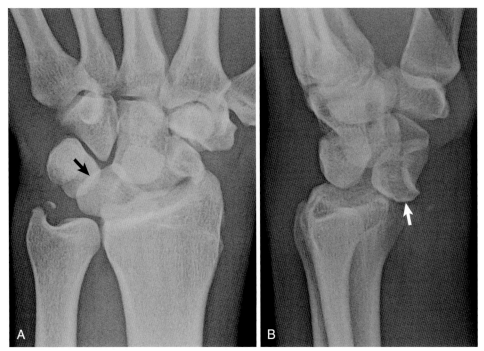

Figure 14-67 A, Transscaphoid lunate dislocation with displaced scaphoid waist fracture, complete overlap of the lunate *(arrow)* with the carpus and distal radius, and ulnar styloid process avulsion fracture, demonstrated on posteroanterior radiograph. **B,** Transscaphoid lunate dislocation with anterior ejection and 90-degree rotation of the lunate *(arrow)* from the carpus while the capitate remains aligned with the distal radius, demonstrated on lateral radiograph.

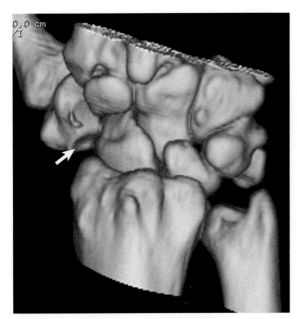

Figure 14-68 The proximal articular surface of the trapezium *(arrow)* is shown to be dislocated from the scaphoid on three-dimensional (3-D) computed tomographic (3-D CT) reformation.

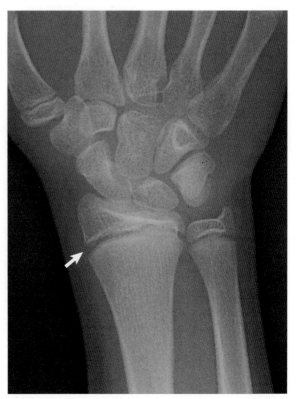

Figure 14-69 There is widening of the distal radial physis *(arrow)* without evident fracture, indicative of Salter-Harris type I fracture of the distal radius.

Figure 14-70 A, Comminuted intra-articular fracture of the distal radius *(arrow)* with dorsal impaction and angulation, shown on posteroanterior radiograph. There is also an avulsion fracture of the tip of the ulnar styloid process *(arrowhead)*. **B,** Distal radial fracture with dorsal impaction and angulation *(arrow)* shown on lateral radiograph.

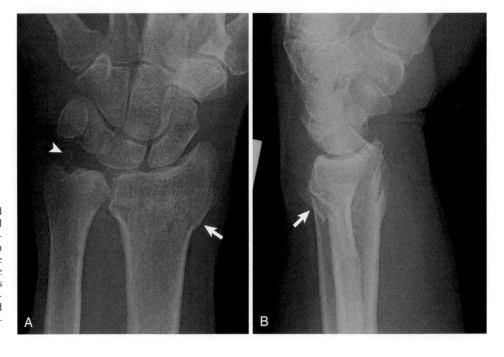

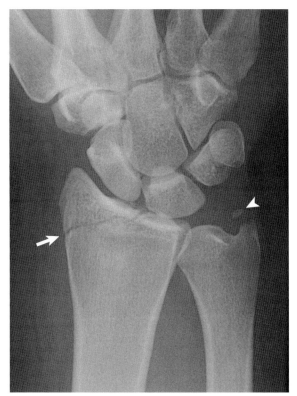

Figure 14-71 Minimally displaced intra-articular fracture *(arrow)* of the radial styloid process with an accompanying avulsion fracture of the tip of the ulnar styloid process *(arrowhead)*.

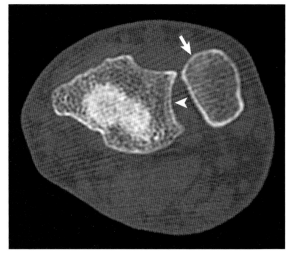

Figure 14-73 Axial computed tomographic (CT) image through the distal radioulnar joint with the wrist positioned in pronation shows severe dorsal subluxation of the head of the ulna *(arrow)* relative to the sigmoid notch of the distal radius *(arrowhead)*.

Disruption of the DRUJ is usually associated with fractures of the distal radius. The ulnar head is normally located within an articular fossa on the ulnar aspect of the radius called the *sigmoid notch*. A lesion of the triangular fibrocartilage complex, the major stabilizer of the DRUJ, is typically the underlying cause of DRUJ instability. The position of the ulnar head relative to the sigmoid notch is often difficult to determine on radiographs, so CT is the imaging method of choice for the diagnosis of DRUJ abnormalities (Fig. 14-73). Sometimes subluxation or dislocation of the DRUJ occurs only in certain positions, so CT in both supination and pronation may be appropriate. Poor outcomes of distal radius fractures may be the result of untreated or unrecognized DRUJ injuries.

Selected Reading

Armstrong CP, Van Der Spuy J. The fractured scapula: importance and management based on a series of 62 patients. *Injury.* 1984;15:324–329.

Calfee RP, Sommerkamp TG. Fracture-dislocation about the finger joints. *J Hand Surg Am.* 2009;34:1140–1147. http://dx.doi.org/10.1016/j.jhsa.2009.04.023.

Carlsen BT, Moran SL. Thumb trauma: Bennett fractures, Rolando fractures, and ulnar collateral ligament injuries. *J Hand Surg Am.* 2009;34(5):945–952. http://dx.doi.org/10.1016/j.jhsa.2009.03.017.

Cisternino SJ, Rogers LF, Stufflebam BC, et al. The trough line: a radiographic sign of posterior shoulder dislocation. *AJR Am J Roentgenol.* 1978;130:951–954.

Downey EP Jr, Curtis DJ, Brower AC. Unusual dislocations of the shoulder. *AJR Am J Roentgenol.* 1983;140:1207–1210.

Ennis O, Miller D, Kelly CP. Fractures of the adult elbow. *Curr Orthop.* 2008;22:111–131.

Farber JM, Buckwalter KA. Sports-related injuries of the shoulder: instability. *Radiol Clin North Am.* 2002;40:235–249.

Freiberg A, Pollard BA, Macdonald MR, et al. Management of proximal interphalangeal joint injuries. *Hand Clin.* 2006;22:235–242.

Frick MA, Murthy NS. Imaging of the elbow: muscle and tendon injuries. *Semin Musculoskelet Radiol.* 2010;14:430–437.

Gove N, Ebraheim NA, Glass E. Posterior sternoclavicular dislocations: a review of management and complications. *Am J Orthop.* 2006;35:132–136.

Grayson DE. The elbow: radiographic imaging pearls and pitfalls. *Semin Roentgenol.* 2005;40:223–247.

Ilyas AM, Mudgal CS. Radiocarpal fracture-dislocations. *J Am Acad Orthop Surg.* 2008;16:647–655.

Jones NF, Jupiter JB, Lalonde DH. Common fractures and dislocations of the hand. *Plast Reconstr Surg.* 2012;130:722e–736e. http://dx.doi.org/10.1097/PRS.0b013e318267d67a.

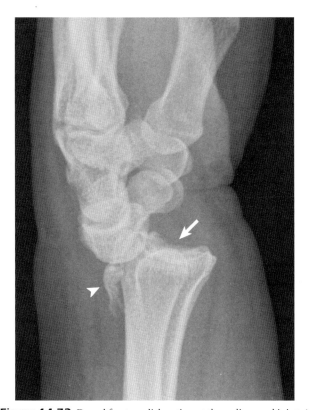

Figure 14-72 Dorsal fracture-dislocation at the radiocarpal joint. A fragment *(arrowhead)* consisting of the radial styloid process has displaced with the dislocated carpus. The radial fossa is empty *(arrow)*.

Kennedy SA, Hanel DP. Complex distal radius fractures. *Orthop Clin North Am.* 2013;44:81–92. http://dx.doi.org/10.1016/j.ocl.2012.08.008.

Kijowski R, Tuite M, Sanford M. Magnetic resonance imaging of the elbow, 1: normal anatomy, imaging technique, and osseous abnormalities. *Skeletal Radiol.* 2004;33:685–697.

Kijowski R, Tuite M, Sanford M. Magnetic resonance imaging of the elbow, 2: abnormalities of the ligaments, tendons, and nerves. *Skeletal Radiol.* 2005;34: 1–18.

Neer II CS. Displaced proximal humeral fractures, I: classification and evaluation. *J Bone Joint Surg Am.* 1970;52:1077–1089.

Neuhaus V, Jupiter JB. Current concepts review: carpal injuries—fractures, ligaments, dislocations. *Acta Chir Orthop Traumatol Cech.* 2011;78:395–403.

Neviaser RJ. Injuries to the clavicle and acromioclavicular joint. *Orthop Clin North Am.* 1987;18:433–438.

O'Shea K, Weiland AJ. Fractures of the hamate and pisiform bones. *Hand Clin.* 2012;28:287–300. http://dx.doi.org/10.1016/j.hcl.2012.05.010. viii.

Pavlov H, Freiberger RH. Fractures and dislocations about the shoulder. *Semin Roentgenol.* 1978;13:85–96.

Reichel LM, Bell BR, Michnick SM, et al. Radial styloid fractures. *J Hand Surg Am.* 2012;37:1726–1741. http://dx.doi.org/10.1016/j.jhsa.2012.06.002.

Richards RD, Sartoris DJ, Pathria MN, et al. Hill-Sachs lesion and normal humeral groove: MR imaging features allowing their differentiation. *Radiology.* 1994;190:665–668.

Ridpath CA, Wilson AJ. Shoulder and humerus trauma. *Semin Musculoskelet Radiol.* 2000;4:151–170.

Ritting AW, Baldwin PC, Rodner CM. Ulnar collateral ligament injury of the thumb metacarpophalangeal joint. *Clin J Sport Med.* 2010;20:106–112. http://dx.doi.org/10.1097/JSM.0b013e3181d23710.

Rosas HG, Lee KS. Imaging acute trauma of the elbow. *Semin Musculoskelet Radiol.* 2010;14:394–411.

Sanders T, Morrison W, Miller M. Imaging techniques for the evaluation of glenohumeral instability. *Am J Sports Med.* 2000;28:414–434.

Sawardeker PJ, Kindt KE, Baratz ME. Fracture-dislocations of the carpus: perilunate injury. *Orthop Clin North Am.* 2013;44:93–106. http://dx.doi.org/10.1016/j.ocl.2012.08.009.

Sendher R, Ladd AL. The scaphoid. *Orthop Clin North Am.* 2013;44:107–120. http://dx.doi.org/10.1016/j.ocl.2012.09.003.

Shah SS, Techy F, Mejia A, et al. Ligamentous and capsular injuries to the metacarpophalangeal joints of the hand. *J Surg Orthop Adv.* 2012;21(3): 141–146.

Sonin A. Fractures of the elbow and forearm. *Semin Musculoskelet Radiol.* 2000;4: 171–191.

Taljanovic MS, Karantanas A, Griffith JF, et al. Imaging and treatment of scaphoid fractures and their complications. *Semin Musculoskelet Radiol.* 2012;16:159–173. http://dx.doi.org/10.1055/s-0032-1311767. Epub 2012 May 30.

Tuttle HG, Olvey SP, Stern PJ. Tendon avulsion injuries of the distal phalanx. *Clin Orthop Relat Res.* 2006;445:157–168.

Zyluk A, Piotuch B. Distal radioulnar joint instability: a review of literature. *Pol Orthop Traumatol.* 2013;78:77–84.

CHAPTER 15

Lower Extremity

Hip/Proximal Femur

Alan Rogers and Joseph S. Yu

The hip is a common site of trauma and when injured can have a significant impact on the patient's well-being. Worldwide the total number of hip fractures is expected to exceed 6 million by the year 2050. In 2003 over 300,000 patients were hospitalized with hip fractures in the United States, accounting for 30% of all hospitalized patients according to data from the U.S. Agency for Healthcare Research and Quality. The cost of treatment of hip fractures is estimated at $10 billion to $15 billion per year in this country alone.

The hip is a large spheroidal (ball and socket) synovial joint. The relationships between the acetabulum, femoral head, labrum, and joint capsule make the hip an extremely stable joint. The acetabulum is formed at the union of the ilium, ischium, and pubic bones and is partially covered by a horseshoe-shaped lining of hyaline cartilage. The acetabular labrum is a fibrocartilaginous structure that is firmly adhered to the acetabular rim and transverse ligament that serves to effectively deepen the socket, increasing the coverage of the femoral head and adding stability. The synovial-lined capsule surrounds the hip joint with focal condensations forming the iliofemoral, pubofemoral, and ischiofemoral ligaments providing further stability to the joint.

The femoral head is a partial sphere articulating with the acetabulum. It is largely covered by cartilage except for a central depression termed the *fovea capitis*. The ligamentum teres attaches to the femoral head at the fovea and attaches to the transverse ligament and margins of the acetabular notch. The foveal artery courses through the ligamentum teres, providing a small contribution to the vascular supply of the femoral head. The main vascular supply to the femoral head arises from an extracapsular vascular ring around the base of the femoral neck. The greater and lesser trochanters serve as attachment sites for the gluteus medius and minimus muscles and iliopsoas, respectively.

Acetabular fractures are discussed in Chapter 16. Fractures of the proximal femur can be broadly categorized as intracapsular—those involving the femoral head or neck—or extracapsular—those involving the greater or lesser trochanters, the intertrochanteric or subtrochanteric regions. Intracapsular fractures are more susceptible to complications of nonunion, malunion, or avascular necrosis (AVN) of the femoral head due to the tenuous nature of the blood supply.

■ BONE AND JOINT

Intracapsular Fractures

Femoral Head Fractures

Fractures of the femoral head are relatively uncommon but often are associated with a poor functional outcome. They are typically seen in the setting of high-velocity trauma that results in a hip dislocation, such as a motor vehicle accident. In a dashboard injury the hip is vulnerable to dislocation due to its flexed and adducted position. The fracture occurs either from impaction or shearing. Reportedly, femoral head fractures occur in 7% to 15% of posterior hip dislocation injuries and as high as 68% of anterior hip dislocations. Associated complications include injuries to the sciatic nerve, AVN of the femoral head, periarticular heterotopic ossification, and secondary osteoarthritis.

Although several classifications exist, the Pipkin classification, which is based on the location of the femoral head fracture and the presence of associated acetabular or femoral neck fractures, is most widely used. A type I fracture involves the femoral head inferior to the fovea capitis, and type II fractures involve the femoral head superior to the fovea capitis. A type III fracture is a type I or II injury associated with a fracture of the femoral neck. A type IV fracture is a type I or II fracture with an associated acetabular fracture (Fig. 15-1). The Pipkin scheme does not differentiate the type of hip dislocation injury. A more comprehensive classification that includes anterior and central hip dislocations has been proposed by Brumback and colleagues. This scheme divides fractures into one of five categories with A and B subsets incorporating the position of the femoral head with respect to the acetabulum (Fig. 15-2).

Radiographically an alteration in the normal contour of the femoral head denotes a femoral head fracture (but this may require computed tomography [CT] for diagnosis). Any fracture that creates a step-off greater than 2mm constitutes a surgical lesion. It is also essential to evaluate for a concurrent femoral neck fracture. Additional observations on CT that may be seen in patients with a femoral head fracture include the presence of intra-articular fragments, congruency of the articular surfaces, and the integrity of the acetabulum.

Femoral Neck Fractures

Femoral neck fractures occur most commonly in older adults. Several theories related to the mechanism of these fractures have been postulated, including direct

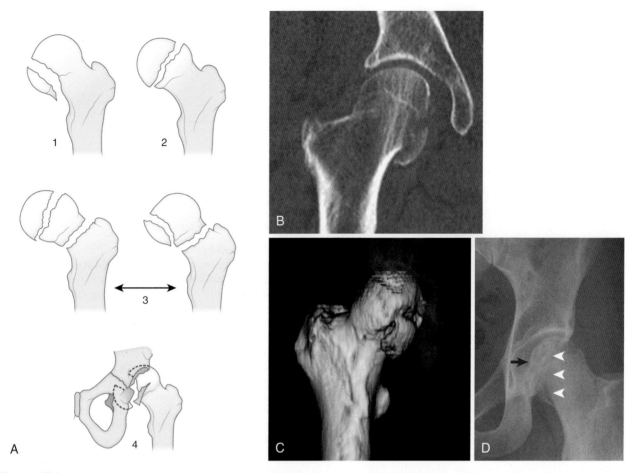

Figure 15-1 **A,** Pipkin classification. Type 1, fracture inferior to the fovea capitis. Type 2, fracture extending superior to fovea capitis. Type 3, any femoral head fracture with concurrent femoral neck fracture. Type 4, any femoral head fracture with concurrent acetabular fracture. **B,** Coronal computed tomographic (CT) reconstruction of Pipkin I fracture. The fracture does not involve the weight-bearing portion of the femoral head. **C,** Three-dimensional (3-D) CT reconstruction of the same fracture viewed from an anteroposterior (AP) direction. **D,** Radiograph of Pipkin II fracture. Note the fracture line *(white arrowheads)* extends superior to the fovea capitis *(red arrow).*

trauma to bone that is weakened by osteoporosis, rotational forces incurred on the femoral neck at the time of a fall, or the completion of a fatigue fracture that subsequently causes a fall. Femoral neck fractures in patients under 50 years of age are relatively rare and are typically the result of high-energy trauma such as a motor vehicle accident or fall from height. Most femoral neck fractures occur just below the femoral head at the junction of the femoral head and neck (subcapital), although fractures may also occur through the midportion of the femoral neck (transcervical) or at the base of the femoral neck (basicervical). The medial and lateral femoral circumflex arteries supply 75% of the blood to the femoral head by way of the medial and lateral epiphyseal arteries and the inferior metaphyseal artery. Additional blood supply comes from the obturator internus artery and the artery of the ligamentum teres. The circumflex vessels may be disrupted when femoral neck fractures become displaced, resulting in AVN of the femoral head.

Evaluation of a patient suspected of having a hip fracture begins with radiographs. Proper technique is

critical to accurately detecting femoral neck fractures. Anteroposterior radiographs of the pelvis should be performed with the hip in internal rotation when possible. Oblique frog-leg or cross-table lateral views are useful for delineating displacement of a fracture. As in pelvis fractures, it is useful to compare symmetry with the contralateral hip. When radiographs are negative or inconclusive for a fracture but there remains high clinical suspicion (i.e., unwillingness to bear weight), then magnetic resonance imaging (MRI) is the modality of choice for further study. The reported sensitivity and specificity of MRI for detection of radiographically occult fractures is nearly 100%, and it also has the added benefit of surveying the surrounding soft tissues for additional injuries.

Subcapital femoral neck fractures may be complete or incomplete. In addition, complete fractures may be impacted or displaced. There are numerous available classification systems for describing subcapital fractures, but the Garden classification, which consists of four stages, is perhaps the most recognizable. A stage I fracture is an incomplete (or occasionally complete)

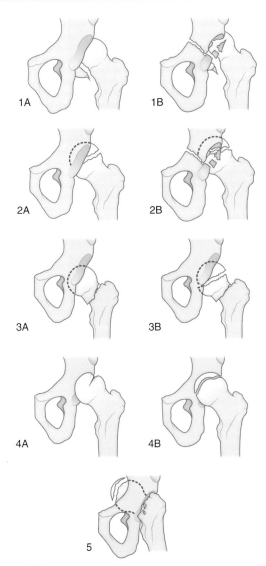

line caused by trabecular overlap, cortical buckling or irregularity, and trabecular angulation should suggest this diagnosis.

True transcervical femoral neck fractures are rare and are treated in the same way as patients with subcapital fractures. Basicervical fractures occur at the base of the femoral neck at its junction with the trochanters (Fig. 15-4). When a basicervical fracture occurs, the possibility of a completed stress fracture or a pathologic fracture should be considered.

There are two types of stress fractures, fatigue and insufficiency. Fatigue stress fractures result from abnormally increased stress placed on normal bone, which occurs frequently in athletes and military recruits. Insufficiency stress fractures are the result of normal stress placed on abnormal bone occurring, for instance, in the settings of osteoporosis, renal osteodystrophy, or chronic steroid use. In the femoral neck, stress fractures may affect the compressive side or the tensile side. The majority of stress fractures are compressive, involving the inferomedial cortex of the femoral neck. Radiographically the appearance of these fractures is a linear area of sclerosis perpendicular to the cortex with or without an associated linear lucency through the cortex. Surrounding endosteal sclerosis and periosteal reaction may be observed as well (Fig. 15-5). Tensile stress fractures typically are insufficiency type of fractures occurring in the superolateral cortex of the femoral neck just inferior to the femoral head. The characteristic radiographic appearance is an ill-defined linear area of sclerosis or simply a break in the cortex (Fig. 15-6). These fractures may progress to a complete subcapital fracture if left untreated.

Extracapsular Fractures

Trochanteric and Intertrochanteric Fractures

Intertrochanteric fractures are common in older adults. Isolated trochanteric fractures are less common and can affect people in any age-group. Isolated greater trochanteric fractures are often the result of a fall or direct trauma (Fig. 15-7). They may be difficult to detect radiographically, particularly in osteoporotic or thin patients. The treatment of greater trochanteric fractures is conservative unless the greater trochanter is severely displaced. It is important to characterize the fracture as not part of a more extensive intertrochanteric fracture. If the radiographic findings are equivocal, MRI is recommended to accurately define the extent of the fracture. In skeletally immature patients, avulsion fractures of the greater trochanter may occur owing to sudden forceful contraction of the gluteal muscles on the apophysis. These are treated conservatively if displacement is less than 1 cm and displacement does not increase on sequential follow-up radiographs. Isolated fractures of the lesser trochanter are usually the result of tension by the iliopsoas tendon on the enthesis and characteristically occur in children or adolescent athletes. In skeletally mature people, isolated lesser trochanteric fractures often are pathologic fractures, indicative of an underlying bone neoplasm or metastasis (Fig. 15-8).

Figure 15-2 Brumback classification. Type 1, posterior dislocation with fracture of the inferomedial aspect of the femoral head. 1A, stable hip joint with minimal or no fracture of the acetabular rim. 1B, significant acetabular rim fracture and joint instability. Type 2, posterior dislocation with fracture of the superomedial aspect of the femoral head. A and B subsets are divided the same way as type I on the basis of acetabular involvement and joint stability. Type 3, dislocated hip (in any direction) with a femoral neck fracture. 3A, no femoral head fracture. 3B, with an associated femoral head fracture. Type 4, anterior dislocation with a femoral head fracture. 4A, femoral head fracture is an impaction fracture. 4B, femoral head fracture is a shearing-type fracture. Type 5, central fracture-dislocation with a femoral head fracture.

fracture with lateral impaction resulting in a valgus angulation. A type II fracture is a complete nondisplaced fracture that is impacted along the entire length of the fracture. A type III fracture is a complete fracture with partial displacement, usually with varus angulation. A type IV fracture is a completely displaced fracture with displaced fragments caused by proximal migration of the femoral shaft (Fig. 15-3). Subcapital fractures may be extremely subtle, and a combination of a sclerotic

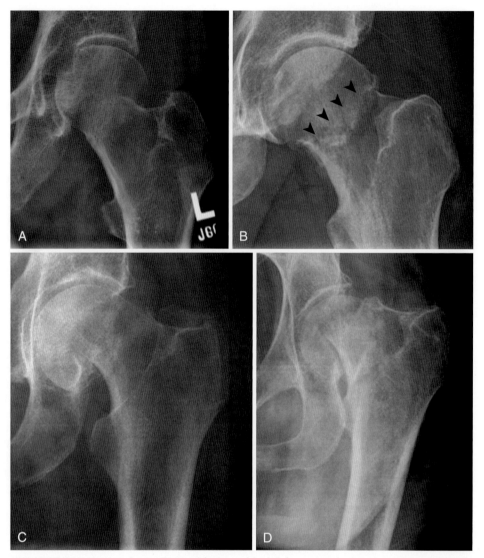

Figure 15-3 Garden classification. A, Garden I, subcapital fracture of the left femoral neck. There is no displacement, but there is impaction laterally, resulting in valgus angulation at the fracture site. **B,** Garden II, fracture of the left femoral neck. There is a complete fracture with impaction along the entire length of the fracture *(black arrowheads)*. **C,** Garden III, fracture with partial displacement and varus angulation at the fracture site. **D,** Garden IV. There is complete displacement of the fracture with proximal migration of the femoral shaft. The Shenton line is disrupted.

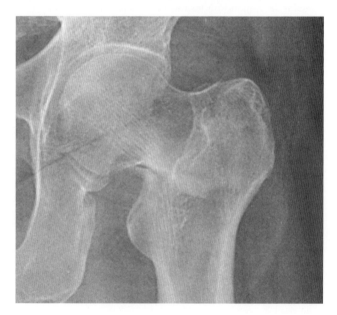

Figure 15-4 Femoral neck fracture. Basicervical fracture at the base of the femoral neck near the junction with the trochanters. Note that these fractures mimic intertrochanteric fractures.

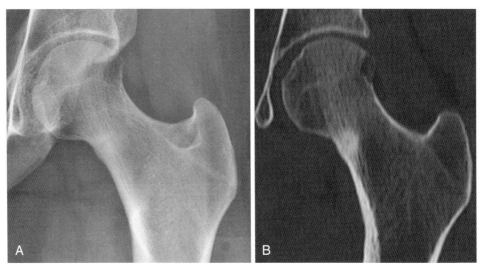

Figure 15-5 Compressive side femoral neck stress fracture. **A,** Focal linear sclerosis in the inferomedial aspect of the femoral neck denotes a compressive stress fracture. There are associated endosteal and periosteal reactive changes. **B,** Coronal computed tomographic (CT) reconstruction of the same fracture clearly demonstrates the unicortical nature of the fracture.

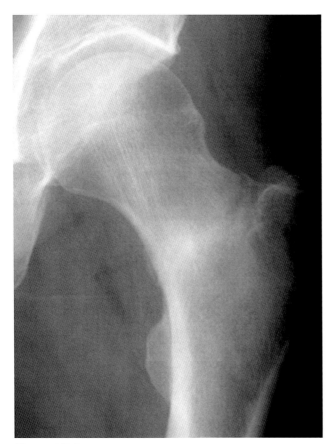

Figure 15-6 Tensile side femoral neck stress fracture. Incomplete lucent fracture line in the inferolateral aspect of the femoral neck denotes a tensile stress fracture.

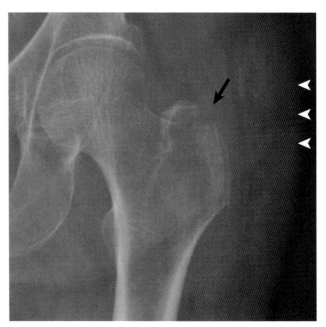

Figure 15-7 Greater trochanteric fracture. There is soft tissue swelling lateral to the hip *(white arrowheads)*. Avulsion fracture of the greater trochanter *(black arrow)* is slightly displaced. This fracture occurred after a fall.

Intertrochanteric fractures extend from the superolateral aspect of the greater trochanter to the inferomedial aspect of the lesser trochanter along the intertrochanteric ridge. Comminution is common, and as many as 50% are considered unstable. The integrity of the calcar femorale, posterior and medial cortices, number of fragments, and displacement determine stability.

There are several classifications available for characterizing intertrochanteric fractures. A common method employed is the Evans classification, which subdivides intertrochanteric fractures into six types (Fig. 15-9). A type I is a simple two-part nondisplaced fracture that parallels the intertrochanteric line. A type II is a two-part fracture that is displaced. Both of these are considered stable. A type III fracture is a three-part fracture with displacement of the greater trochanter, resulting

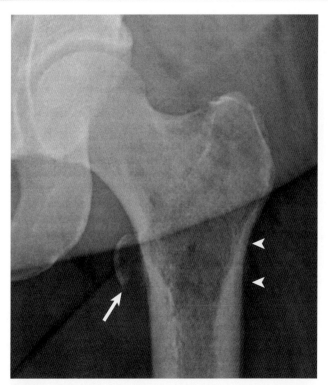

Figure 15-8 Lesser trochanter fracture. There is a distracted fracture of the lesser trochanter *(arrow)* with medial and superior displacement of the fragment caused by an avulsion of the insertion of the iliopsoas. This fracture was a pathologic fracture. Note the permeative appearance of the bone in the intertrochanteric region, as well as periosteal reaction along the lateral cortex *(white arrowheads)*.

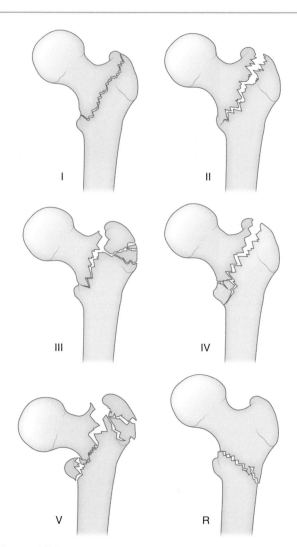

Figure 15-9 Evans classification. Type I, two-part nondisplaced fracture. Type II, two-part displaced fracture. Type III, three-part fracture with displacement of the greater trochanter. Type IV, three-part fracture with displacement of the lesser trochanter. Type V, four-part fracture with displacement of both the greater and lesser trochanters. Type R, fracture with reversed obliquity. Type I and type II fractures are considered stable.

in loss of posterolateral support. A type IV fracture is also a three-part fracture but with displacement of the lesser trochanter, resulting in loss of medial support. Both type III and type IV Evans fractures are considered unstable and difficult to reduce. A type V fracture is a four-part fracture with displacement of both the greater and lesser trochanters. The final type is termed *R* and denotes a fracture with reversed obliquity, with the fracture line beginning in the lesser trochanter medially and extending inferolaterally to exit below the lesser trochanter. These fractures are inherently unstable due to the unopposed traction of the abductors on the greater trochanter and adductors on the lesser trochanter and femoral shaft. It is noteworthy, however, that these fractures may be nondisplaced at presentation (Fig. 15-10).

Subtrochanteric Fractures

Subtrochanteric fractures occur between the lesser trochanter and the proximal 5 to 7 cm of the femoral shaft and account for about 10% to 34% of all hip fractures. These fractures have a bimodal age distribution. In younger patients they are typically the result of high-energy trauma resulting in comminution and significant soft tissue injuries. In older patients the fractures are often the result of low-energy trauma, and diminished overall bone density is an important contributing factor. Radiographically, fractures in older adults tend to be linear or spiral and only minimally displaced.

Numerous classifications for subtrochanteric fractures have been proposed. The AO classification is a complicated three-part scheme with multiple subtypes often used in research. The Seinsheimer classification consists of eight subgroups based on stability of the medial cortex. The Russell-Taylor classification is useful in determining the mode of fixation required based on involvement of the piriformis fossa. Type I fractures do not involve the piriformis fossa. Type I fractures are subdivided into type IA, which occur below the lesser trochanter, and type IB, which involve the lesser trochanter. Type II fractures involve the piriformis fossa. Type IIA fractures demonstrate a stable medial cortex, and type IIB denotes involvement of the piriformis fossa with lack of stability of the medial femoral cortex. Management is determined by the extent of the fracture, with type I fractures being treated with intramedullary devices whereas type II fractures require open reduction and internal fixation (Fig. 15-11). The Fielding classification

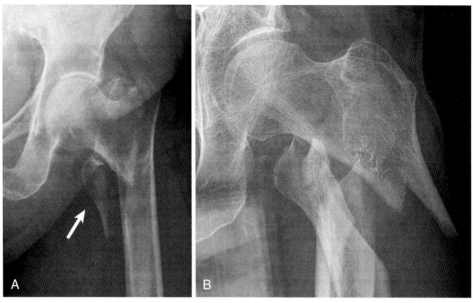

Figure 15-10 Intertrochanteric fractures in two different patients. A, Three-part fracture with displacement of the lesser trochanter *(white arrow)* results in loss of medial support and instability of the fracture. This would be considered an Evans type IV fracture. **B,** Reversed obliquity fracture with the fracture line oriented from the superomedial to inferolateral cortex. There is medial displacement of the femoral shaft due to the action of the adductor muscles, and the greater trochanter is displaced superolaterally by unopposed action of the abductor muscles.

divides subtrochanteric fractures into three zones. Zone 1 includes fractures that involve the lesser trochanter, zone 2 occurs 1 to 2 inches distal to the lesser trochanter, and zone 3 occurs 2 to 3 inches distal to the lesser trochanter (Fig. 15-12).

Hip Dislocation

Hip dislocations are severe injuries caused by high-energy trauma and account for 5% of all joint dislocations. Dislocation of the femoral head is dictated by the position of the lower extremity and hip at time of injury, as well as the vector or direction of force. There are three types—central, posterior and anterior—based on the terminal position of the dislocated femoral head.

Although assessment of hip dislocations begins with radiographs, CT is critical in the management of hip dislocations. Long-term disability may be caused by an injury to the sciatic nerve; AVN, which occurs in up to 17% of hip dislocations; and osteoarthritis. The risk for AVN increases proportionally with the length of time that the hip is dislocated. Osteoarthritis is the most common complication, occurring in 16% of dislocations without associated fractures and up to 80% when there is a concomitant acetabular fracture. Computed tomography is ideal for determining congruency of the joint after reduction, identifying other fractures of the acetabulum or femoral head, and detecting trapped intra-articular fracture fragments. The role for MRI is currently reserved for chronic or persistent pain that may be caused by underlying injuries to the ligamentum teres, acetabular labrum, or articular cartilage.

Central dislocations occur in patients with acetabular fractures that disrupt the quadrilateral plate, produced when a lateral force strikes an adducted femur. In this injury the femoral head displaces medially and the joint space may narrow medially, superiorly, or in both directions. Computed tomography is critical for preoperative planning because the acetabular fracture is often complex. Most surgeons advocate that CT be performed within the first 10 days of the injury for optimal results (Fig. 15-13).

Posterior dislocations account for 80% to 85% of all hip dislocations. The most common mechanism of injury is an anterior-to-posterior force directed to the lower extremity with the hip held in flexion (i.e., a dashboard injury). In this dislocation the femoral head displaces superiorly to the acetabulum and the femur rotates internally (Fig. 15-14). Associated fractures of the posterior wall of the acetabulum are common and should be evaluated with CT because fractures that affect greater than 60% of the articular surface are likely unstable (Fig. 15-15). Fractures of the femoral head are relatively less common and are the result of impaction or a shearing when the femoral head strikes the posterior wall of the acetabulum. Note that posterior dislocations may also occur with fractures of the ipsilateral femoral shaft.

Anterior dislocations account for 10% to 15% of hip dislocation injuries. The dislocation occurs when a posteriorly directed force is applied to the inner aspect of the knee while the hip is abducted and externally rotated. There are two types, obturator and subspinous, and the degree of hip flexion determines the type of dislocation that will occur. An obturator dislocation is more common, with the femoral head displacing inferomedially while the femur abducts and externally rotates (Fig. 15-16). In a subspinous dislocation the femoral head displaces superiorly beneath the spine of the iliac bone, and the femur extends and abducts. The terminal position of the femoral head, which is superior and lateral, may be

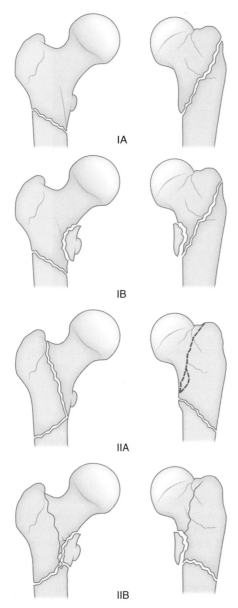

IA

IB

IIA

IIB

Figure 15-11 Russell-Taylor classification of subtrochanteric fractures. Type I fractures do not involve the piriformis fossa, and type II fractures involve the piriformis fossa. A and B subsets are divided on the basis of stability of the medial cortex determined by involvement of the lesser trochanter.

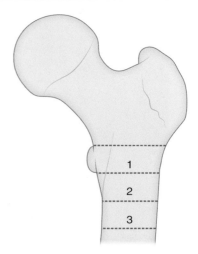

1
2
3

Figure 15-12 Fielding classification. This classification divides subtrochanteric fractures on an anatomic basis, describing the position of the fracture in relation to the lesser trochanter.

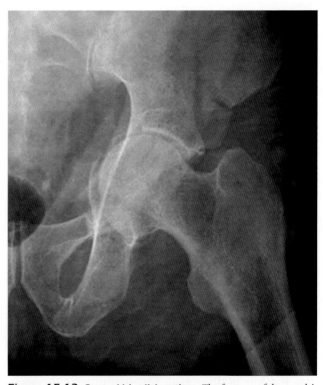

Figure 15-13 Central hip dislocation. The fracture of the quadrilateral plate allows medial displacement of the femoral head.

confused for a posterior dislocation injury. The key to differentiating between these dislocations is the femoral position. In an anterior dislocation the femur is locked in external rotation, and the femur will also be abducted or neutral in position. In a posterior dislocation the femur is adducted and fixed in internal rotation (Fig. 15-17).

Septic Arthritis
Septic arthritis of the hip is more prevalent in children than adults. Adult populations at increased risk include intravenous drug abusers; patients with chronic liver disease or kidney disease, diabetes, or rheumatoid

arthritis; and patients requiring long-term corticosteroid use. Patients with joint replacements are also at increased risk.

Radiographically, early findings tend to be relatively nonspecific, but as the infection progresses, the joint space narrows because of destruction of the cartilage. Periarticular osteopenia, marginal erosion, and osteolysis of the cortex are also important observations (Fig. 15-18). Synovial inflammatory arthropathies

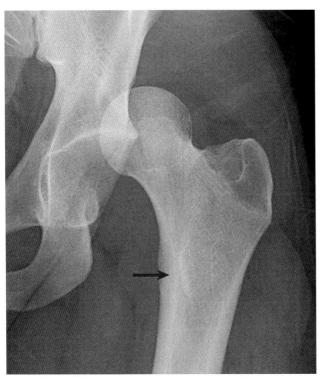

Figure 15-14 Posterior hip dislocation. The femoral head projects superior and lateral to the acetabulum. Note that the femur is internally rotated so that the lesser trochanter overlaps the femoral shaft *(red arrow)*.

share some similar findings, but rapidly progressive destructive changes should prompt an expeditious search for an infectious cause. Joint aspiration is useful in confirming the diagnosis and providing critical information regarding the source.

■ SOFT TISSUE EMERGENCIES

Bursitis

A bursa is a fluid-filled sac lined with synovial cells located in areas of friction between tendons or against bony surfaces. Repetitive friction and overuse, infection, direct trauma, and arthritis can cause inflammation of various bursae, which then fill with fluid. Common presenting symptoms include regional pain and tenderness. Clinically bursitis may mimic joint-, tendon-, or muscle-related pain. The main bursae in the hip region are the iliopsoas, obturator externus, ischial, and trochanteric bursae. The iliopsoas bursa, located between the anterior hip capsule and the distal iliopsoas tendon, is the largest bursa in the hip. It communicates with the joint in 10% to 15% of people. The obturator externus bursa is located between the obturator externus and the ischium and may also communicate with the joint in up to 10% of people. A bursa exists between the greater trochanter and each of the gluteal tendons. The largest of these is the trochanteric or subgluteus maximus bursa located lateral and superior to the greater trochanter. The ischial bursa is

situated between the hamstring tendons and the adjacent ischium.

Magnetic resonance imaging or ultrasonography is the preferred modality for evaluating bursitis because radiographs are usually normal. The sonographic appearance of a distended bursa is an anechoic fluid-filled structure lined by a hyperechoic wall. On MRI, bursitis characteristically appears as lobulated fluid-containing (T1 hypointense, T2 hyperintense) structure (Fig. 15-19) that demonstrates a thin rim of peripheral enhancement after intravenous contrast administration. Enhancement extending beyond the bursa into the surrounding soft tissues is atypical and could indicate an infectious cause.

Tendon Injuries

Injuries of the proximal thigh musculature and/or tendons are painful conditions that may mimic other pathologic processes. The quadriceps, hamstrings, adductors, or gluteal muscles are frequent injury locations among young athletes. Most acute injuries are diagnosed clinically; however, imaging can be useful in cases in which the history and physical examination are inconsistent. Radiographs can confirm pathologic conditions in the bones such as stress fractures, neoplasia, or avulsion injuries. Ultrasonography provides a way to dynamically evaluate the muscles and tendons and is useful in detecting intramuscular hematomas. Avulsion occurs in predictable locations in the pelvis (Fig. 15-20). Computed tomography is particularly useful for avulsion fractures that are radiographically occult. Magnetic resonance imaging is both sensitive and specific for diagnosis of muscular and tendinous injuries due to superior spatial resolution and optimal contrast between soft tissues. Contusions, hematomas, and partial or complete tendon ruptures are readily characterized as well.

The severity of tendon injury can be ascertained on MRI. Generally a grade 1 injury demonstrates an intact tendon with interstitial edema and hemorrhage at the injury site characterized by high-signal intensity around the tendon on fluid-sensitive sequences. There may be a feathery appearance in the adjacent muscle. A grade 2 injury is partial disruption of the tendon. A hematoma may be present in the acute setting. A grade 3 injury is a complete disruption of the tendon, which may be retracted because of muscle spasm. An avulsion fracture is characterized by edema at the enthesis of the tendon with a donor defect in the adjacent bone. Most soft tissue injuries are treated conservatively; however, complete tendon ruptures and osseous avulsions are indications for surgical intervention, particularly in active people and athletes. Surgical intervention may be required to evacuate a large hematoma in the muscle and to treat compartment syndrome. Avulsion of the hamstring tendon from the ischium is an important injury. It is caused by abrupt tensile forces that overload the enthesis or musculotendinous junction during eccentric contraction of the muscle. Important observations include the length of the tendon gap, presence of a hematoma, and perineural edema around the sciatic nerve (Fig. 15-21).

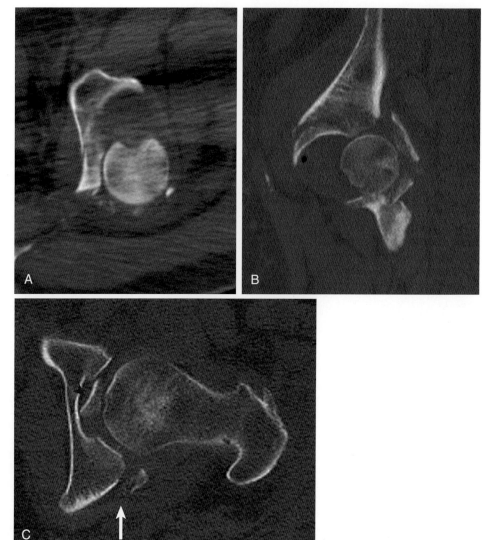

Figure 15-15 Posterior hip dislocation. **A,** Axial computed tomography (CT) of posterior hip dislocation with concomitant acetabular fracture. **B,** Sagittal CT reconstruction of a different patient with a posterior hip dislocation. There is also a comminuted fracture of the acetabulum involving the posterior wall and roof. **C,** Axial CT image after reduction of left hip dislocation in a third patient. A trapped intra-articular fracture fragment is present in the medial joint space *(red arrowhead)*, as well as a concomitant fracture of the posterior acetabular rim *(white arrow)*.

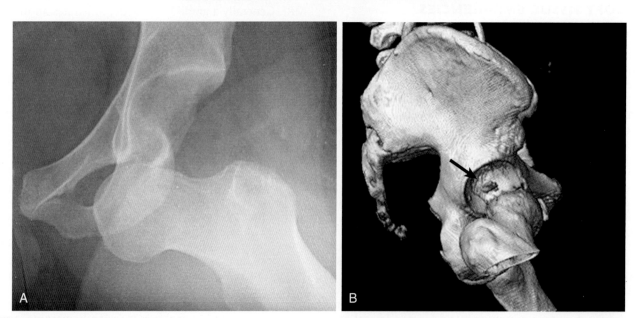

Figure 15-16 Anterior hip dislocation. **A,** The femoral head displaces inferomedially beneath the anterior column in the obturator type of dislocation. Note that the femur is abducted and externally rotated. **B,** Computed tomographic (CT) three-dimensional (3-D) reconstruction in a different patient demonstrating the anterior displacement of the femoral head from the acetabulum. There is a fracture of the femoral head with an intra-articular fragment *(black arrow)*.

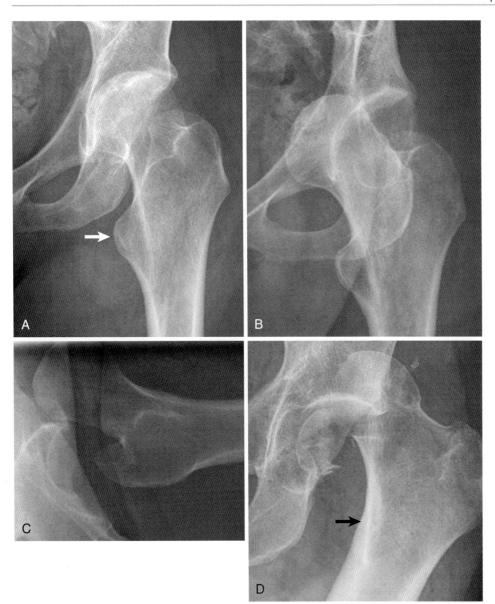

Figure 15-17 Anterior hip dislocation. A, In the subspinous type the femoral head superiorly displaces beneath the spine of the iliac bone. The femur is abducted and externally rotated, profiling the lesser trochanter *(white arrow).* **B** and **C,** Left posterior oblique Judet and cross-fire lateral views confirm anterior dislocation of the femoral head from the acetabulum. **D,** In a posterior dislocation the femur is adducted and fixed in internal rotation with the lesser trochanter overlying the femoral shaft *(black arrow).* (From Fuller M. Radiography of hip dislocations. Applied radiography. Case 1, Figs. 1 to 3. *wikiRadiography.* 2010.)

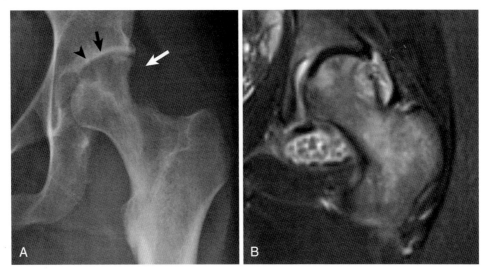

Figure 15-18 Septic arthritis. A, Anteroposterior (AP) radiograph of the left hip shows narrowing of the joint space *(black arrowheads),* periarticular osteopenia, and osteolysis of the lateral aspect of the femoral head *(white arrow).* **B,** Coronal short tau inversion recovery (STIR) magnetic resonance image (MRI) shows marked edema within the bones on both sides of the joint. Note the erosion on the lateral aspect of the femoral head from bone lysis *(red arrow).* There is also a large joint effusion containing proteinaceous debris.

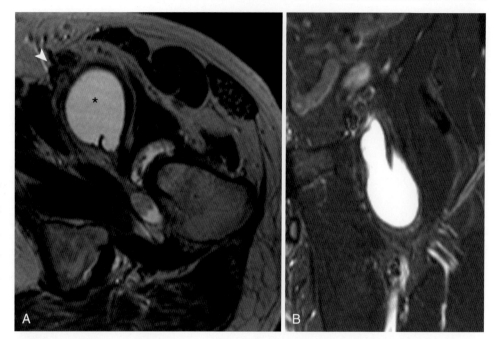

Figure 15-19 Distended iliopsoas bursa. A, Axial T2-weighted image of the left hip demonstrating a fluid collection (*) in the iliopsoas bursa. The bursa is located anterior to the hip joint and lateral to the femoral vessels *(white arrowhead).* **B,** Coronal short tau inversion recovery (STIR) image demonstrating the typical teardrop configuration of the distended iliopsoas bursa when visualized in the coronal plane.

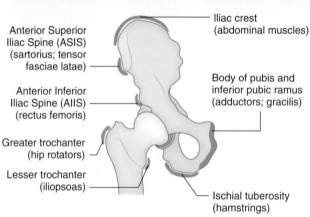

Anterior Superior Iliac Spine (ASIS) (sartorius; tensor fasciae latae)

Anterior Inferior Iliac Spine (AIIS) (rectus femoris)

Greater trochanter (hip rotators)

Lesser trochanter (iliopsoas)

Iliac crest (abdominal muscles)

Body of pubis and inferior pubic ramus (adductors; gracilis)

Ischial tuberosity (hamstrings)

Figure 15-20 Common pelvic avulsion fractures. These fractures are associated with the insertions of the proximal thigh and pelvic musculature. They are common in skeletally immature patients but also may also occur in adults.

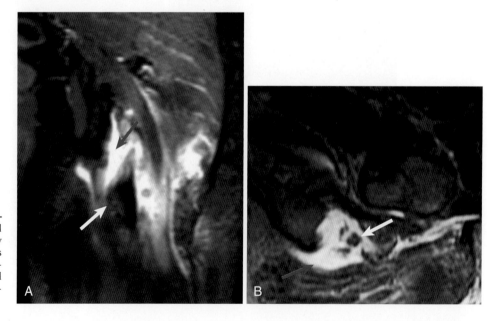

Figure 15-21 Hamstring tendon tear. Coronal (**A**) and axial (**B**) short tau inversion recovery (STIR) magnetic resonance images (MRIs) demonstrate a right hamstring avulsion injury with retracted tendon *(white arrow)* and hematoma *(red arrow).*

Knee

David M. Melville and Jon A. Jacobson

Knee radiography is the most common radiographic study performed for trauma in the emergency department, with nearly 75% of patients with acute knee injury undergoing evaluation with radiographs; however, radiographs obtained for acute knee trauma do not consistently depict all important injuries, and 25% of radiographic findings do not correlate with clinical presentation. Twisting injuries are responsible for three quarters of all knee injuries, but the majority of knee fractures result from blunt trauma. Knee radiographs should be carefully scrutinized for features suggestive of acute knee injury and further evaluation with cross-sectional imaging, including CT and MRI, should be recommended in cases with suggestive history or findings.

■ KNEE JOINT EFFUSION

Knee joint effusion may result from a variety of causes, including infection, inflammation, and trauma. The presence of a knee joint effusion should prompt a search for an underlying cause. Conventional radiographs may detect as little as 4 to 5 mL of fluid. An effusion may be detected radiographically by increased density in the suprapatellar recess located between the anterior suprapatellar and prefemoral fat pads on a lateral projection with slight knee flexion (Fig. 15-22).

Posttraumatic hemarthrosis is considered an indicator of serious ligamentous injury, but there are no typical radiographic features to distinguish acute hemorrhage from simple knee joint effusion. The time course of effusion development may suggest cause because an effusion developing within the first several hours following a traumatic event is typically related to hemarthrosis, whereas reactive effusions appear 12 to 24 hours following injury. The presence of fat within a joint effusion, termed *lipohemarthrosis*, is a reliable indicator of intra-articular fracture because it represents the sequelae of cortical disruption and extrusion of marrow fat, although occasionally it may also be seen with cartilage, ligamentous, or synovial injury in the absence of fracture (Fig. 15-23).

■ INDICATORS OF LIGAMENTOUS INJURY

Radiographs often show normal findings in the setting of internal derangement of the knee joint, but there are several characteristic fractures that are indicative of significant ligamentous injuries. These fractures are often subtle but may be accurately identified with careful attention to frequent injury sites and understanding of injury patterns. Correct diagnosis of these fractures allows recommendation of additional imaging evaluation with MRI.

Segond Fracture

A Segond fracture is an avulsion fracture arising from the rim of the lateral tibia just distal to the plateau.

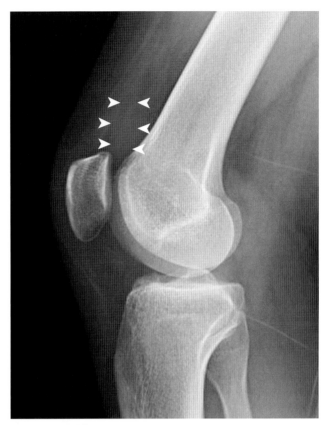

Figure 15-22 Knee joint effusion. Lateral knee radiograph shows moderate knee joint effusion as increased lenticular density *(arrowheads)* in the suprapatellar recess between the relatively radiolucent anterior suprapatellar and prefemoral fat pads.

The mechanism of injury is internal rotation and varus stress of the knee. Tears of the anterior cruciate ligament (ACL) occur in 75% to 100% of cases, as well as meniscal tears. Classically the insertion of the middle third of the lateral capsular ligament at the lateral aspect of the proximal tibia was believed to be the source of injury, but recent anatomic investigations suggest involvement of the iliotibial tract and anterior oblique band of the fibular collateral ligament in Segond fracture pathogenesis. The avulsion fracture usually manifests on frontal radiographs as a small, often subtle, linear or elliptic ossific fragment immediately adjacent to the lateral aspect of the tibia just distal to the tibial plateau with minimal displacement (Fig. 15-24). Cortical irregularity at the donor site may be present.

Anterior Cruciate Ligament Avulsion Fracture

Forced flexion with internal rotation may cause the ACL to avulse from the tibia. Anterior cruciate ligament avulsion fractures with intact ACL fibers are more common in the pediatric population and are usually seen in isolation without additional injury. In adults the avulsion may be caused by severe hyperextension and be associated with bone contusions, posterior cruciate ligament (PCL), and medial collateral ligament (MCL) tears, manifesting as an ossific fragment of varying size located in the anterior aspect of the intercondylar notch (Fig. 15-25). The Meyers and McKeever classification describes four subtypes of tibial eminence fractures (type I, minimally displaced; type II, anterior elevation of fracture fragment; type III, complete fragment separation from tibia; and type IV, complete separation with rotation). Arthroscopy is recommended for type II to

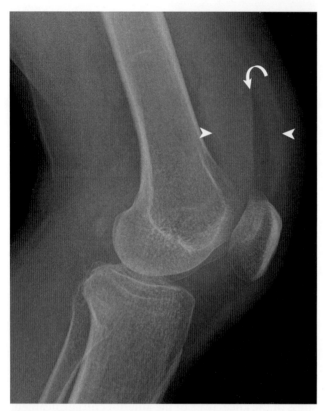

Figure 15-23 Lipohemarthrosis. Cross-table lateral view shows suprapatellar recess distention *(arrowheads)* containing low-density fat layering over high-density blood products with discrete fat-fluid level *(curved arrow)* from lipohemarthrosis in patient with tibial plateau fracture (not depicted).

IV, and type III and IV injuries require internal fixation to ensure stability. Magnetic resonance imaging may be used to identify the fracture site and associated injuries.

Deep Notch Sign

Anterior cruciate ligament tears resulting from the pivot shift mechanism, which consists of valgus force applied to externally rotated tibia (or internally rotated femur), may produce an impaction fracture of the lateral femoral condyle. On lateral radiographs a wedge-shaped or deep concave defect occurs at or near the condylopatellar sulcus, termed the *deep notch sign* or *deep lateral femoral sulcus sign* (Fig. 15-26). The depth of the lateral sulcus can be measured by drawing a line tangential to the articular surface of the lateral femoral condyle and the depth of the lateral sulcus is measured perpendicular to this tangent line. A depth greater than 1.5 mm is considered abnormal and highly associated with ACL tear, whereas a measurement equal to or greater than 2 mm is definitive.

Magnetic resonance imaging is considered the preferred modality for confirming an ACL tear. Several important indirect signs of an ACL tear include a positive ACL angle sign, which is defined as an angle subtended by the anteromedial ACL bundle and the Blumensaat line exceeding 15 degrees; the exposed lateral meniscus sign, when the posterior edge of the lateral meniscus hangs over the posterior edge of the tibia by more than 3.5 mm; a buckled PCL sign; and an anterior drawer sign (Fig. 15-27).

Reverse Segond Fracture

An avulsion fracture involving the medial tibial rim corresponds to the attachment of the deep capsular component of the MCL and is referred to as a *reverse Segond fracture*. These injuries are associated with midsubstance PCL tears, PCL avulsions, and medial meniscal tears and have also been identified in the setting of traumatic knee dislocation. This fracture is best appreciated on frontal

Figure 15-24 Segond fracture. A, Anteroposterior (AP) radiograph shows a displaced elliptical avulsion fracture fragment *(curved arrow)* arising from the lateral tibial plateau in a patient with an anterior cruciate ligament (ACL) tear. B, Fat-saturated coronal magnetic resonance image (MRI) shows a fracture fragment attached to the iliotibial band *(arrow)* and a rupture of the ACL *(curved arrow)*. Note the marrow edema in the lateral femoral condyle.

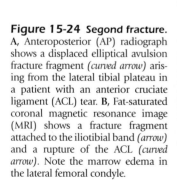

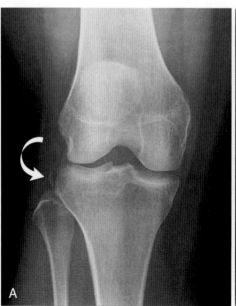

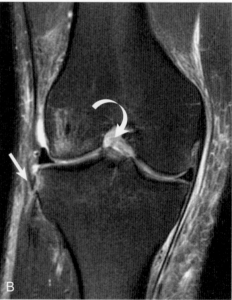

radiographs as an elliptic ossific fragment, similar to a Segond, but it occurs on the opposite side of the knee adjacent to the medial aspect of the proximal tibia from forced flexion with internal rotation.

Posterior Cruciate Ligament Avulsion

Avulsion fractures affect the PCL tibial insertion site less frequently than with the ACL, but it does represent the most common form of isolated PCL disruption. The two common mechanisms of injury are severe hyperextension and a classic dashboard injury in which there is direct impaction on the anterior tibia in a knee that is flexed. On a lateral view a displaced fragment of bone occurs posteriorly with disruption of the articular surface (Fig. 15-28). Clinical assessment of the PCL is challenging, and unrecognized injuries can result in chronic instability.

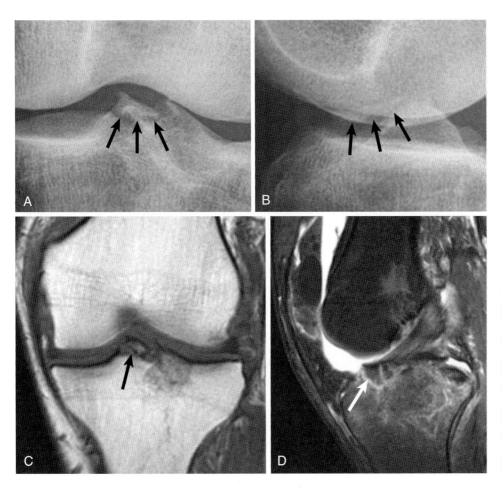

Figure 15-25 Anterior cruciate ligament (ACL) avulsion fracture. Anteroposterior (AP) (**A**) and lateral (**B**) radiographs show an ossific fragment in the anterior aspect of the intercondylar notch (*arrows*) corresponding to the ACL insertion site at the tibial eminence. **C**, Coronal T1-weighted magnetic resonance image (MRI) shows the avulsed fragment of bone (*arrow*). **D**, Sagittal T2-weighted MRI shows the separation of the fragment of bone still attached to the ACL from the rest of the tibia (*arrow*) surrounded by intense bone marrow edema.

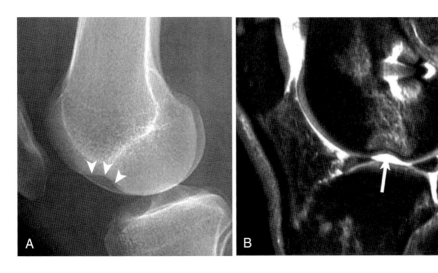

Figure 15-26 Deep notch sign. **A**, Lateral radiograph shows a deep notch sign (*arrowheads*) at the midaspect of the lateral femoral condyle, representing an impaction fracture in a patient with an anterior cruciate ligament (ACL) tear. **B**, Sagittal T2-weighted magnetic resonance image (MRI) shows marrow edema surrounding the impaction fracture (*arrow*).

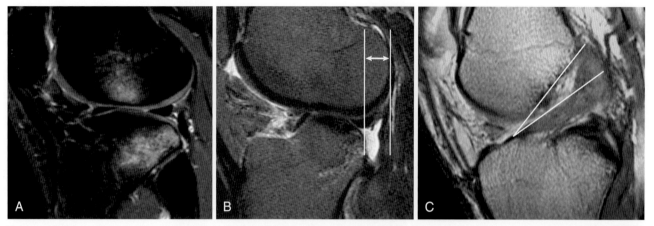

Figure 15-27 Indirect magnetic resonance imaging (MRI) signs of anterior cruciate ligament (ACL) tear. A, Sagittal fluid-sensitive MRI shows a classic "kissing" contusion pattern of a pivot shift rotational injury involving the lateral femoral condyle and posterolateral tibia. **B,** The anterior drawer sign occurs when the tibia translates anteriorly by more than 5 mm *(arrows between lines)*. **C,** This patients shows a positive ACL angle sign. When intact, the anteromedial bundle of the ACL is more vertically oriented than the roof of the intercondylar notch.

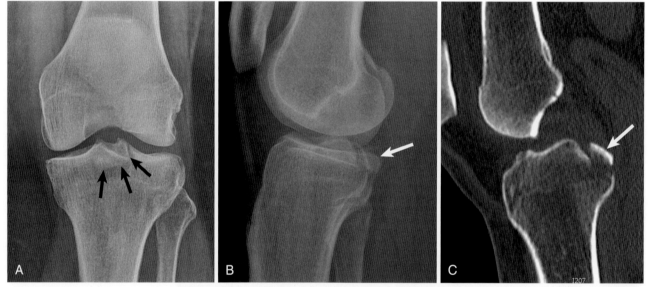

Figure 15-28 Posterior cruciate ligament (PCL) avulsion fracture. A, Frontal radiograph shows a lucency in the region of the tibial eminence *(arrows)*. **B,** Lateral radiograph shows a fracture in the posterior tibia where the PCL attaches *(arrow)*. **C,** Sagittal computed tomographic (CT) reformatted image shows the relationship of the fragment with the ligament *(arrow)*.

Arcuate Sign

The arcuate complex consists of the fabellofibular, popliteofibular, and arcuate ligaments and is critical in maintaining stability. An avulsed ossific fragment at the tip of the fibular styloid, termed the *arcuate sign*, occurs most commonly from a direct blow to the anteromedial tibia with knee extension. The avulsion fracture produces a variably sized, curvilinear, horizontally oriented bone fragment at the fibular styloid process (Fig. 15-29). This fracture has a high association with injury to other stabilizing ligamentous structures, particularly the PCL. Failure to diagnose and treat posterolateral corner injury may result in

chronic instability and lead to a failed cruciate ligament reconstruction.

Biceps Femoris Tendon Avulsion Fracture

The biceps femoris tendon and lateral collateral ligament (LCL) have a conjoined attachment on the lateral margin of the fibular head. An avulsion fracture involving this conjoined attachment is located at the lateral aspect of the fibular head, which is in contrast to the arcuate sign, which occurs more proximally on the fibular styloid (Fig. 15-30). Magnetic resonance imaging may be used

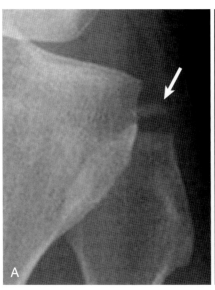
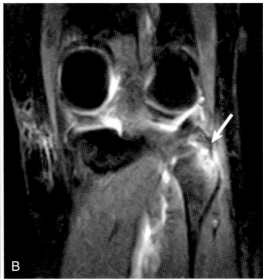

Figure 15-29 Arcuate sign. A, Frontal radiograph shows a transverse fracture of the fibular styloid producing a small elliptical bone fragment *(arrow)*. **B,** Coronal short tau inversion recovery (STIR) image shows the retracted arcuate ligament *(arrow)* and intense bone marrow edema in the fibular head.

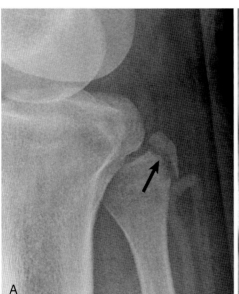
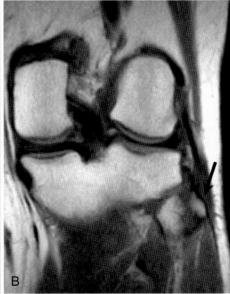

Figure 15-30 Biceps femoris avulsion fracture. A, Lateral radiograph shows an oblique fracture *(arrow)* arising from the lateral aspect of the fibular head, consistent with biceps femoris avulsion. Note larger size and origin of fracture fragment compared to arcuate avulsion. **B,** Coronal T1-weighted magnetic resonance image (MRI) shows relationship with the conjoined portion of the distal biceps tendon *(arrow)*.

to verify the origin of the fracture in ambiguous cases. Often due to varus stress, these fractures are associated with LCL injury owing to its shared attachment.

■ EXTENSOR MECHANISM AND PATELLA

Patellar Fracture and Dislocation

Patellar fractures are the most common injury of the extensor mechanism, and these fractures may be transverse, vertical, or comminuted. The mechanism of injury is either a direct blow to the patella or opposing tensile forces generated by the quadriceps muscles and patellar tendon. Transverse fractures typically occur in the midportion of the patella and are readily apparent, whereas vertical fractures often require additional sunrise or Merchant

patellar views for diagnosis. When high-energy trauma results in a comminuted fracture, CT is recommended for further evaluation before surgery.

Patellar sleeve fracture is a subtype of patellar fracture occurring in the pediatric population. It occurs during jumping activities where there is forced knee hyperextension, creating an osteochondral fracture that avulses the inferior patellar pole. Magnetic resonance imaging is recommended to search for osteochondral injuries (Fig. 15-35). If a small osseous bone fragment near the inferior patellar pole is visualized in a skeletally immature patient with patella alta, the diagnosis is unequivocal; however, in the absence of an avulsed fracture fragment, the injury is occult, and the extent of cartilage abnormality may be severely underestimated. Further evaluation with MRI may be useful to more optimally demonstrate the cartilage defect.

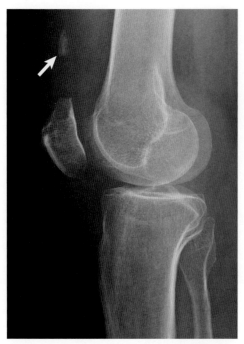

Figure 15-31 Quadriceps avulsion fracture. Lateral radiograph shows displaced, retracted quadriceps tendon avulsion fracture *(arrow)* with associated irregularity of the superior patellar pole.

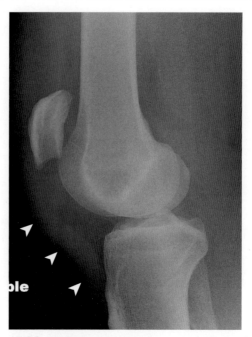

Figure 15-32 Patellar tendon rupture. Lateral radiograph shows superior displacement of the patella with marked soft tissue thickening in the expected location of the patellar tendon *(arrow)*.

Transient patellar dislocation is unsuspected clinically in 73% of patients with magnetic resonance (MR) evidence of dislocation. These injuries occur from a twisting injury in which the femur internally rotates upon a fixed tibia when the knee joint is in slight flexion. Few patients actually present with persistent dislocation. Magnetic resonance imaging is recommended to search for osteochondral injuries. A sliver sign may be depicted in patients who experience lateral dislocations, with linear or curvilinear bone fragment(s) that are the sequela to the intra-articular fracture.

Quadriceps and Patellar Tendon Rupture

Quadriceps tendon rupture may result from acute trauma or sports injury or may be due to underlying tendinosis. Quadriceps tendon rupture may be inferred by loss of the tendon contour, soft tissue swelling, and a low-lying patella, referred to as *patella baja*. The most widely accepted objective method for determining patellar position is the Insall-Salvati ratio, which is calculated by dividing the patellar tendon length by the length of the patella as measured on the lateral projection. Normal is defined as 0.8 to 1.2, and patellar baja is less than 0.8. Less commonly, an avulsion fracture from the superior patellar pole may occur when rapid deceleration results in sudden contraction of the quadriceps muscle with knee flexion (see Fig. 15-31).

Patellar tendon ruptures occur less frequently than tears of the quadriceps tendon. The diagnosis is suggested by patella alta, an abnormally high position of the patella defined by an Insall-Salvati ratio greater than 1.2. Other important observations include soft tissue swelling, loss of the margins of the patellar tendon, and distension of the prepatellar bursa (Fig. 15-32). Patellar tendon rupture occurs from eccentric quadriceps contraction with the foot firmly planted and the knee in a flexed position.

Knee Dislocations

Most knee joint dislocations are the product of high-energy trauma, such as falls or motor vehicle collisions, but some may be related to low-energy athletic injuries. Knee dislocations may be anterior, posterior, lateral, medial, or rotary based on the terminal position of the tibia. Anterior or posterior knee joint dislocations constitute three fourths of dislocations (Fig. 15-33). Many dislocations are reduced at the time of injury, thus radiographic findings of a prior dislocation may include widened or incongruent joint spaces or residual joint malalignment. Absence of an effusion should not discourage this diagnosis because many occur with capsular rupture. Other important concomitant findings include ligamentous and meniscal tears, as well as bone contusions and frank fractures. A dislocation constitutes an orthopedic emergency owing to neural (5%) or vascular (20%) injury, particularly when it follows a high-velocity mechanism. Posterior knee dislocation is associated with a vascular injury in approximately 30% of patients, leading to amputation in up to 20% of these patients.

■ DISTAL FEMUR

Supracondylar Fracture

Blunt trauma that causes axial loading on a flexed knee may result in a supracondylar fracture. This fracture has

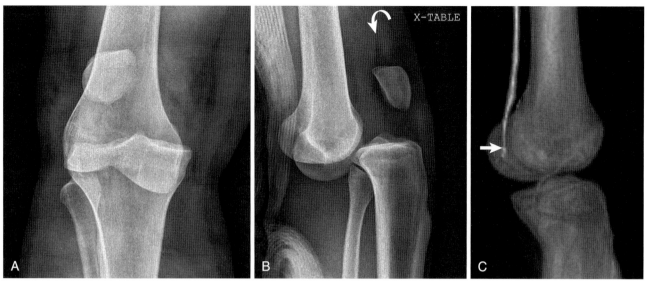

Figure 15-33 Anterior knee joint dislocation. Anteroposterior (AP) radiograph (**A**) shows overlap of the distal femur and proximal tibia with marked anterior dislocation of the proximal tibia on cross-table lateral radiograph (**B**). Note lipohemarthrosis *(curved arrow)* on cross-table lateral. **C,** Three-dimensional computed tomographic (3-D CT) rendering after intravenous contrast administration shows abrupt cutoff of the popliteal artery at the knee joint *(arrow)*, consistent with traumatic occlusion.

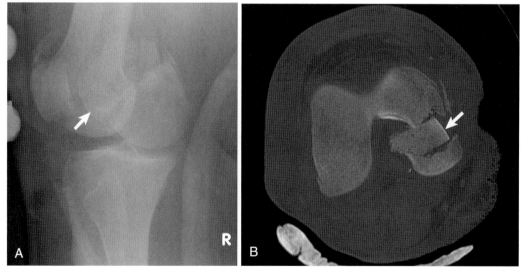

Figure 15-34 Hoffa fracture. A, Oblique lateral radiograph shows severely comminuted distal femoral fracture with disruption and displacement of the articular surface of the medial femoral condyle. **B,** Axial computed tomography (CT) shows a fracture in the coronal plane, representing a Hoffa fracture, with rotation of the articular surface *(arrow)*.

a bimodal distribution, occurring from high-energy trauma in young patients, such as a motor vehicle collision, and occurring from low-energy trauma in older adults, often osteoporotic patients, such as a fall. Supracondylar femoral fractures are classified as extra-articular, unicondylar, or bicondylar and may demonstrate intercondylar and intra-articular extension. A Hoffa fracture is an intercondylar fracture with an associated fracture in the coronal plane, typically in the lateral femoral condyle (Fig. 15-34). Computed tomography is recommended for evaluating complex fractures so that the appropriate operative management is performed.

Subchondral Insufficiency Fracture

Older, osteoporotic patients presenting with acute-onset, atraumatic knee pain may have a subchondral insufficiency fracture, most commonly involving the medial femoral condyle. This condition may be suggested when an eccentric lucency with slight flattening or irregularity involving the subchondral bone is observed. More advanced lesions may demonstrate peripheral sclerosis, and chronic fractures show cortical impaction. Because radiographs frequently show normal results, MRI is preferred for diagnosis. The characteristic appearance

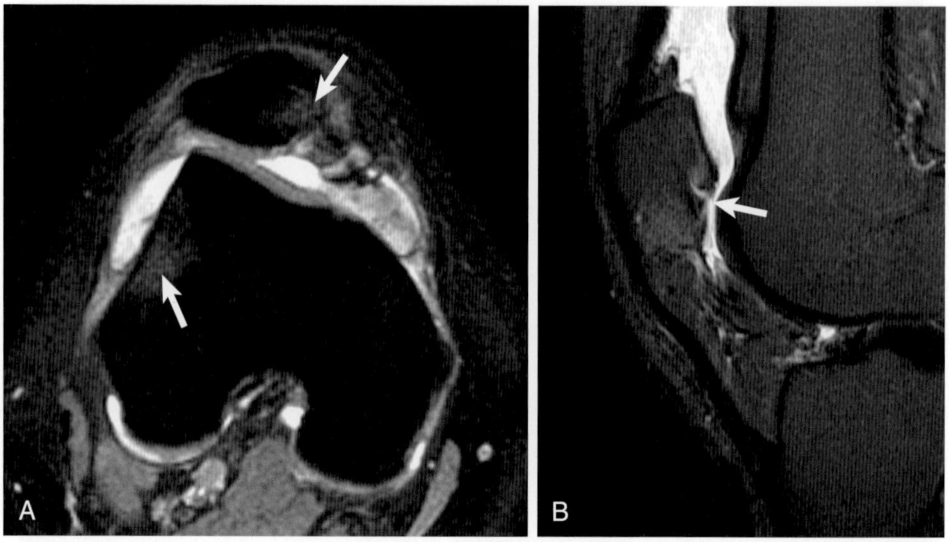

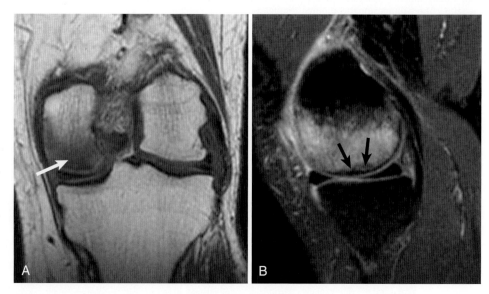

Figure 15-35 Lateral patellar dislocation. A, Axial fat-saturated proton-density magnetic resonance image (MRI) shows "kissing" contusion *(arrows)* characteristic of a lateral patellar dislocation. B, Sagittal fluid-sensitive MRI shows a defect in the patellar cartilage *(arrow)*.

Figure 15-36 Insufficiency fracture. A, Coronal T1-weighted magnetic resonance image (MRI) shows a large area of marrow edema involving the medial femoral condyle *(arrow)*. B, Sagittal T2-weighted MRI shows an arcuate linear low–signal intensity defect in the subchondral bone *(arrows)* corresponding to the insufficiency fracture.

is that of a short, linear low–signal intensity defect paralleling the articular cortex surrounded by intense bone marrow edema (Fig. 15-36). The term *spontaneous osteonecrosis of the knee* (SONK) is generally no longer used.

Osteochondral Injury

When traumatic, an osteochondral injury involves the articular cartilage and subchondral bone. An in situ form occurs in young people, termed *osteochondritis dissecans*, and is likely caused by repetitive overloading of the bone. Nearly 80% involve the medial femoral condyle. Unstable injuries appear as a well-defined crescentic lucency involving the articular surface with a bone fragment within the concavity of the defect (Fig. 15-37). Magnetic resonance imaging is useful to further evaluate a lesion's stability by characterizing fluid imbibition within the cartilage defect and the presence of bone cysts.

■ PROXIMAL TIBIA

Tibial Fractures

Tibial plateau fractures range from minimally displaced impacted fractures to markedly disorganized bicondylar fractures. Accurate assessment of these fractures is important because the tibial plateau is critical in maintaining knee alignment and stability. Expeditious repair can reduce the risk for posttraumatic osteoarthritis.

The Schatzker classification is the most widely used method for characterizing tibial plateau fracture (Fig. 15-38). This scheme divides tibial plateau fractures into six types (Fig. 15-39): lateral tibial plateau split without depression (<4 mm depression or displacement; I), lateral tibial plateau split with depression (>4 mm depression or displacement; II), lateral (IIIa) or central (IIIb) plateau depression, medial plateau depression (IV), bicondylar fracture (V), and tibial plateau fracture with diaphyseal involvement (VI). Types I to III fractures

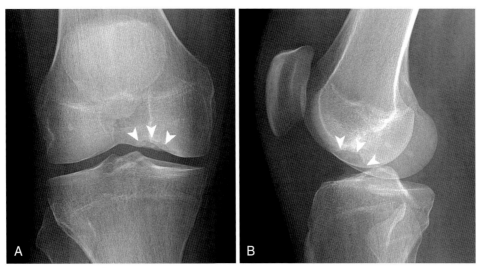

Figure 15-37 Osteochondral defect. Anteroposterior (AP) (**A**) and lateral (**B**) radiographs show a crescentic lucency *(arrowheads)* involving the medial articular surface of the medial femoral condyle with irregular, sclerotic margins. No in situ or intra-articular fragment is identified. Compare the appearance and location of this abnormality to the deep notch sign.

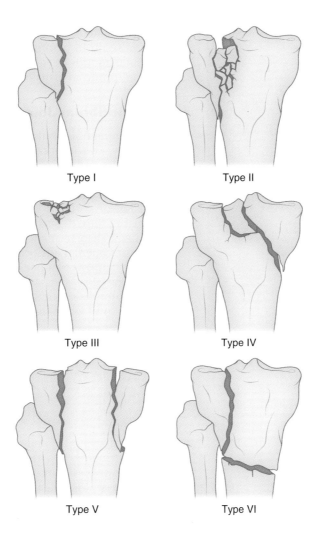

Figure 15-38 Schatzker classification of tibial plateau fractures (sequentially labeled from type I to type VI in panel diagram).

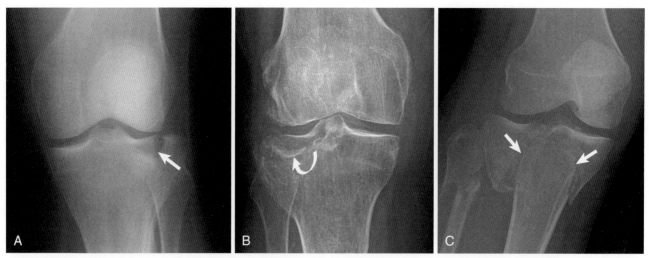

Figure 15-39 Tibial plateau fractures. **A,** Anteroposterior (AP) radiograph shows Schatzker type I split fracture *(arrow)* of the lateral tibial plateau without impaction. **B,** AP radiograph in a different patient shows impaction fracture *(curved arrow)* of the lateral tibial plateau without split, a Schatzker type III fracture. **C,** Oblique AP radiograph of a third patient shows bicondylar fractures *(arrows)* involving the medial and lateral tibial plateaus with splitting, a Schatzker type V fracture. Also note comminuted proximal fibula in this patient, who was involved in a high-speed motor vehicle collision.

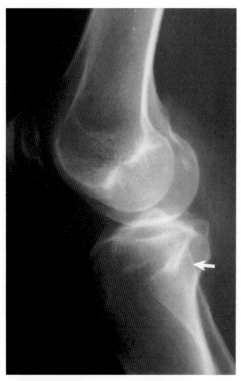

Figure 15-40 Tibiofibular joint dislocation. Lateral knee radiograph shows anterior displacement of proximal fibula *(arrow)* with respect to the posterior tibial plateau in a patient with clinically apparent tibiofibular joint dislocation. Compare fibular position to other lateral knee radiographs in this chapter.

may undergo immediate repair, whereas types V and VI fractures typically require external fixation with delayed repair because of extensive soft tissue involvement.

Fractures of the tibial tubercle usually affect adolescent males who participate in athletic activities that involve jumping. It is the result of violent contraction of the quadriceps muscle. Chronic stress injury at the distal patellar tendon in active and growing adolescents can result in painful swelling and irregular or fragment tibial apophysis (termed *Osgood-Schlatter disease*) which can mimic an avulsion fracture.

Tibiofibular Joint Dislocation

Proximal tibiofibular joint dislocation is an uncommon injury. This injury may occur as an isolated injury from a direct impact resulting in anterolateral or posteromedial displacement. These injuries are easily overlooked. Anterolateral dislocations are most common, caused by a fall on a flexed knee with the foot in inversion and plantar flexed. Such injuries may be detected by anterolateral displacement of the fibular head (Fig. 15-40). Posteromedial dislocations occur from direct trauma (i.e., auto-versus-pedestrian accidents) and have an increased incidence of peroneal nerve injury. Tibiofibular joint dislocations are frequently subtle, and CT may be helpful when there is high clinical suspicion.

Ankle and Foot
Nidhi Gupta and Joseph S. Yu

The tibia, fibula, and talus form the ankle joint, which acts primarily as a hinge joint. Stability of the ankle joint depends on the integrity of a ring formed by these three bones and the ligaments that unite them. The medial malleolus includes the anterior colliculus, onto which the superficial deltoid ligament attaches, and the posterior colliculus, which anchors the deep deltoid ligament. The fibula functions as a barrier to resist lateral translation of the talus. The posterior malleolus restrains the talus from posterior translation, and fractures involving

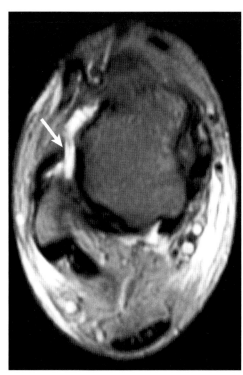

Figure 15-41 Ankle sprain. Axial T2-weighted magnetic resonance image (MRI) shows disruption of the anterior talofibular ligament *(arrow)* and diffuse soft tissue swelling

(in which the talus is displaced internally, or medially), abduction (in which the talus is displaced laterally without significant rotation), adduction (in which the talus is displaced medially without significant rotation), and dorsiflexion (in which the talus is dorsiflexed on the tibia).

Supination-External Rotation

The supination-external rotation injury is the most common mechanism, accounting for 60% to 75% of all ankle injuries. The external rotation of the talus impacts against the lateral malleolus forcing it in the posterior direction producing the characteristic abnormalities. There are four stages in this group. In stage I the anterior tibiofibular ligament ruptures. A stage II injury is characterized by an oblique distal fibular fracture and an anterior tibiofibular ligament tear. A stage III injury is a progression of the injury vector with findings of stage I and stage II with a tear of the posterior tibiofibular ligament or a posterior malleolus fracture. Finally, a stage IV injury includes those of stages I to III plus a transverse medial malleolus fracture.

Supination-Adduction

Supination-adduction is the second most common mechanism, accounting for 20% of ankle injuries. There are two stages in this group. In stage I injury either there is rupture of the LCL or a transversely oriented avulsion fracture of the lateral malleolus. In stage II continued talar adduction and supination causes it to impact with the medial malleolus, producing an oblique fracture of the medial malleolus (Fig. 15-44).

Pronation-Abduction

In the pronation-abduction injury mechanism the lateral surface of the talus impacts the lateral malleolus, forcing it laterally. There are three stages in this group. In stage I there is either rupture of the deltoid ligament or a transverse fracture of the medial malleolus. In stage II continued abduction produces findings of stage I plus rupture of the anterior and posterior tibiofibular ligaments, with or without a posterior malleolar fracture. In stage III the fibula breaks, producing a characteristic oblique fracture above the level of the syndesmosis.

Pronation-External Rotation

In the pronation-external rotation mechanism the foot is pronated, and external rotation causes the talus to impact against both the anterior and medial surfaces of the lateral malleolus, producing an injury pattern that is similar to those of pronation-abduction. There are four stages. In stage I there is either rupture of the deltoid ligament or a transverse avulsion fracture of the medial malleolus. In stage II the anterior tibiofibular ligament ruptures in addition to findings of stage I. In stage III a high fibular fracture, usually 6 to 8 cm above the joint line, occurs in addition to findings of stages I and II. Stage IV represents findings of stages I to III plus a tear

more than 25% of the articular surface of the plafond will result in posterior instability. A single break in the ring, whether in the form of a fracture or ruptured ligament, does not allow subluxation of the talus in the mortise (Fig. 15-41). Two or more breaks in the ring allow abnormal talar motion that may be evident radiographically, but application of stress often is required to confirm the diagnosis of instability.

Low-energy trauma often results in fractures that are easily overlooked. Localizing the epicenter of soft tissue swelling is important in the identification of acute fractures. Yu and coworkers have devised a simple search strategy for rapid inspection of the ankle that identifies commonly occurring avulsion fractures, chip fractures, and shearing injuries of the ankle and hind foot (Fig. 15-42). Major axial load (crush) or direct impaction typically produces fractures that are complex and although conspicuous radiographically do require cross-sectional imaging for further characterization.

■ ANKLE FRACTURES AND SUBLUXATION/DISLOCATION

Ankle fractures have been classified most widely using either the Lauge-Hansen or Danis-Weber classifications. The Lauge-Hansen classification is devised on the basis of the mechanism of injury (Fig. 15-43). The first term depicts supination (inversion) or pronation (eversion). The second term reflects the direction in which the talus is displaced or rotated relative to the ankle mortise. Five directions of talar displacement are possible in the classification system: external rotation (in which the talus is displaced externally, or laterally), internal rotation

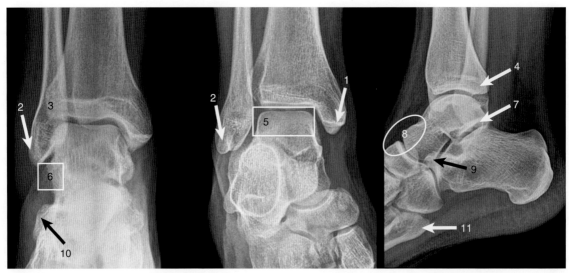

Figure 15-42 Search template for ankle injuries. There are 11 target sites that represent vulnerable areas where fractures occur, including the medial (1) and lateral (2) malleoli, anterior tibial tubercle (3) and posterior tibial malleolus (4), talar dome (5), lateral talar process (6), tubercles of the posterior talus process (7), dorsal to the talonavicular joint (8), anterior calcaneus process (9), calcaneal insertion of the extensor digitorum brevis (10), and the base of the fifth metatarsal bone (11). (Used with permission from Yu JS, Cody ME. A template approach for detecting fractures in low energy ankle trauma. *Emerg Radiol.* 2009;16:309-318.)

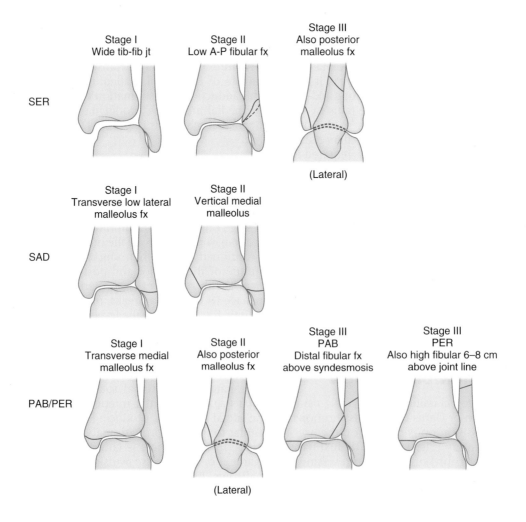

Figure 15-43 Diagram of Lauge-Hansen classification of distal tibial and fibula fractures.

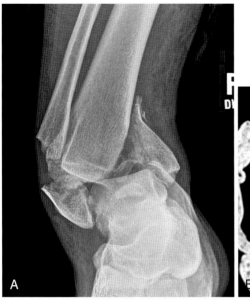 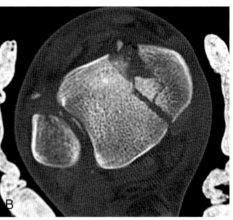

Figure 15-44 Bimalleolar ankle fractures. A, Frontal radiograph shows medial subluxation of the talus and a displaced and distracted medial malleolus fracture. The transverse fibular fracture is distracted. **B,** Axial computed tomographic (CT) images shows comminution of both fractures.

Table 15-1 Important Characteristics of Lauge-Hansen and Danis-Weber Type of Fractures

	Fibula Fracture Location	Fracture Type/ Orientation	Radiographic Projection	Syndesmosis	Treatment for Fibula Fracture*
SA (Danis-Weber A)	Below joint line	Transverse	AP	Intact	Closed reduction
SE (Danis-Weber B)	At joint line	Oblique P → A	Lateral	Intact	Closed reduction
PA (Danis-Weber C1)	Just above syndesmosis	Oblique M → L	AP	Disrupted	Surgical
PE (Danis-Weber C2)	Well above syndesmosis	Oblique A → P	AP/Lateral	Disrupted	Surgical

A → P, Anterior to posterior; *AP*, anteroposterior; *M → L*, medial to lateral; *P → A*, posterior to anterior; *PA*, pronation-abduction; *PE*, pronation–external rotation; *SA*, supination-adduction; *SE*, supination-external rotation.
*Preferred or usual treatment.

of the posterior tibiofibular ligament or a fracture of the posterior malleolus.

The Danis-Weber classification has also been widely used for describing ankle fractures because it is a good predictor of severity and therefore management (Table 15-1). In Type A the lateral malleolar fracture occurs below the ankle joint level. The deltoid ligament and distal tibiofibular syndesmosis are intact, but there may be an oblique medial malleolar fracture. In Type B the distal fibular fracture begins at the tibiotalar joint level and courses obliquely as it extends proximally. There may be an associated deltoid ligament tear or a transverse medial malleolar fracture. The distal tibiofibular syndesmosis may be intact or partially torn. In type C the fibular fracture occurs above the ankle joint and is associated with deltoid ligament rupture or medial malleolar fracture (Fig. 15-45). There is complete disruption of distal tibiofibular syndesmosis. Type C has been classified into C1, C2, and C3. Type C1 refers to a simple distal fibular fracture without interosseous membrane injury, and type C2 refers to a complex fibular fracture higher up in the fibula associated with interosseous membrane injury at the fracture site. Type C3 is a proximal fibular fracture associated with rupture of the interosseous membrane causing instability of fibula or a Maisonneuve fracture. Injuries affecting the interosseous membrane may result in its ossification, limiting motion.

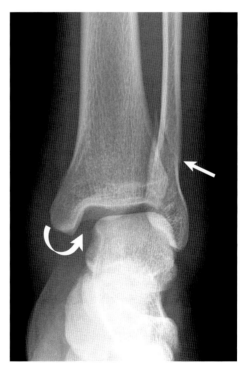

Figure 15-45 Weber C1 fracture. There is widening of the medial clear space between the talus and medial malleolus (*curved arrow*) and an oblique distal fibular fracture (*arrow*). This corresponds to a Lauge-Hansen pronation-abduction stage III.

Pilon Fracture

A pilon fracture is an intra-articular fracture of the plafond of the distal tibia caused by axial loading, often extending to the metaphysis. It occurs from high-energy trauma. Dorsiflexion on the pronated foot produces impaction of the distal tibia with the talus, often resulting in extensive comminution of the tibia, although the medial malleolus usually maintains its relationship with the talus. Computed tomography is advocated to evaluate for displacement, comminution, and impaction at the articular surface. The fibula may fracture in 15% of the cases. Several classifications have been used to describe pilon fractures. The AO classification classifies fractures into three groups: extra-articular, partial articular, and complete articular fracture groups (Fig. 15-46). The Ruedi-Allgower classification describes three intra-articular types that vary depending on the articular congruity and degree of comminution (Fig. 15-47).

Maisonneuve Fracture

The Maisonneuve fracture is a high-fibular fracture that occurs above the midshaft level and often at the fibular neck (Fig. 15-48). It is caused by external rotation of the ankle with a tear of the interosseous membrane at the level of the fibular fracture. It can occur with either pronation or supination. Ankle radiographs that show an isolated fracture of either the medial or posterior malleolus should be followed with tibia/fibula radiographs to search for the injury.

Increased tension within the posterior tibiofibular ligament can cause an avulsion fracture of the posterior tibial malleolus. When small, it has the appearance of an arcuate sliver of bone adjacent to the posterior tibial lip on the lateral radiograph. When larger, it assumes a triangular shape and involves the posterior articular surface of the tibial plafond (Fig. 15-49). An avulsion fracture of the anterior tibial tubercle, the Tillaux fracture,

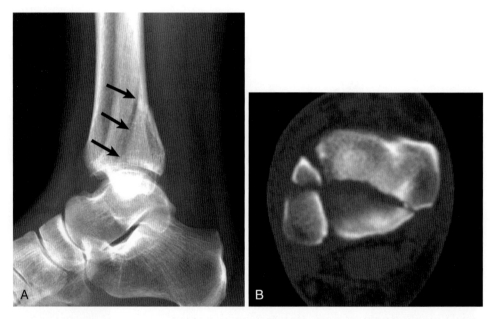

Figure 15-46 Pilon fracture. A, The tibial fracture is difficult to visualize. The fibular fracture is more conspicuous *(arrows)*. **B,** Axial and sagittal reformatted computed tomographic (CT) images show the orientation of the intra-articular fracture.

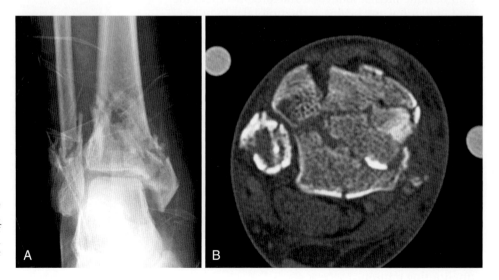

Figure 15-47 Comminuted pilon fracture. A, Frontal radiograph shows extensive comminution of the tibial fracture. **B,** Axial computed tomographic (CT) image more clearly depicts the fracture planes.

occurs when a tensile force on the anterior tibiofibular ligament caused by external rotation of the foot overwhelms the bone (Fig. 15-50).

Juvenile Tillaux and Triplane Fracture

A juvenile Tillaux fracture occurs in adolescents and represents a Salter-Harris III injury caused by external rotation force. The fracture line typically extends horizontally along the physeal plate and then turns 90 degrees vertically to the articular surface because the medial part of the growth plate has fused while the lateral part has not. The triplane fracture is similar to a juvenile Tillaux fracture, but it also extends into the

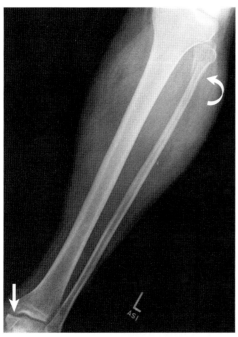

Figure 15-48 Maisonneuve fracture. There is a medial malleolus fracture *(arrow)* and a proximal fibular fracture *(curved arrow)*, with traumatic disruption of the interosseous membrane.

posterior tibial metaphysis. The fracture lines are oriented in three geometric planes, which include a horizontal fracture through the lateral tibial physeal plate, a vertical fracture in the sagittal plane through the epiphysis, and a vertical fracture in the coronal plane through the posterior tibial metaphysis (Fig. 15-51). There are two types of triplane fractures depending on whether there are two (most common type) or three fragments. Both types occur as a result of plantar flexion and external rotation and may occur with or without an associated fracture of the distal fibula.

Tibiotalar and Subtalar Dislocations

The tibiotalar joint is inherently stable, so a dislocation requires high-energy trauma to produce disarticulation. The most common ankle dislocation is a posterior dislocation with the talus disarticulating to a terminal position posterior to the tibial plafond. Anterior, lateral, and superior dislocations are relatively less common.

Subtalar dislocations are uncommon. They involve simultaneous dislocation of the talus at the talonavicular and talocalcaneal joints while maintaining normal tibiotalar alignment (Fig. 15-52). This dislocation occurs as a result of fall from height, motor vehicle accident, or severe twisting of the ankle. Dislocation can occur medially, constituting about 80% of subtalar dislocations, or laterally in about 20% of cases. It is important to make this distinction because the method of reduction will be different. In a medial dislocation the calcaneus and foot displace medially. In a lateral dislocation the calcaneus displaces laterally and the foot may appear pronated. Anterior and posterior subtalar dislocations are rare. When there is combined tibiotalar and subtalar dislocation, it is considered a total talar dislocation. Midfoot dislocation is rare.

Talus Fractures

Osteochondral Defects

Impaction/shearing injuries of the distal tibia or fibula can result in osteochondral lesions of either the medial

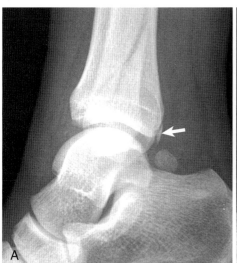
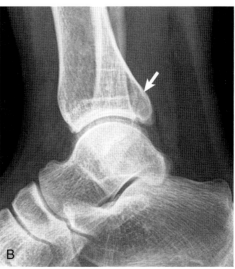

Figure 15-49 Fractures of the posterior malleolus. A, Lateral radiograph shows a linear cortical fragment arising from the posterior tibia corresponding to an avulsion of the posterior tibiofibular ligament *(arrow)*. **B,** Another patient shows a larger triangular posterior malleolus fragment from a coronally oriented fracture *(arrow)* caused by vertical impaction of the talus against the posterior tibia.

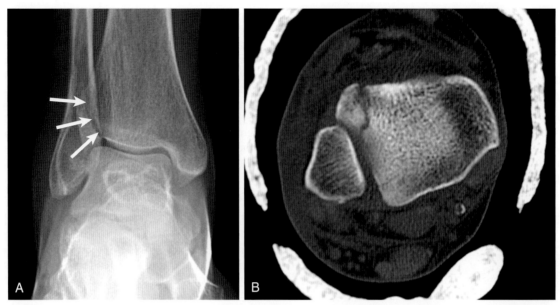

Figure 15-50 Anterior tubercle (Tillaux) fracture. A, Radiograph shows a linear fracture *(arrows)* of the anterior tibial tubercle. **B,** Axial computed tomographic (CT) image shows slight rotation of the fragment from the pull of the anterior tibiofibular ligament.

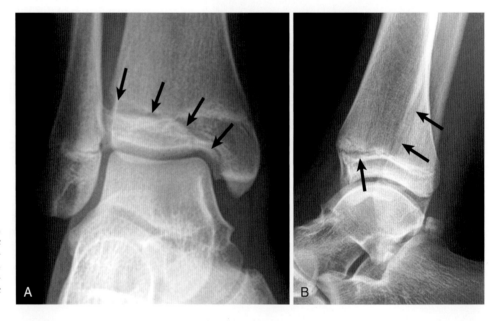

Figure 15-51 Triplane fracture. A, Frontal radiograph shows the fracture of the horizontal and sagittal fracture planes *(arrows).* **B,** Lateral radiograph shows the horizontal and coronal (third) fracture planes *(arrows).*

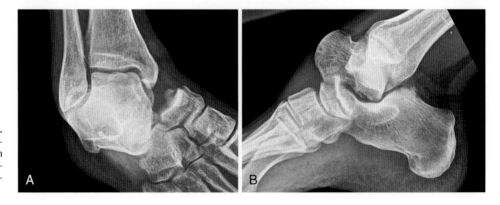

Figure 15-52 Talar dislocation. A and **B,** Frontal and lateral radiographs show complete dislocation of the talus. Note that the talonavicular, calcaneocuboid, and subtalar joints are disarticulated.

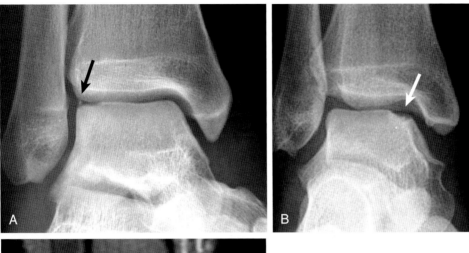

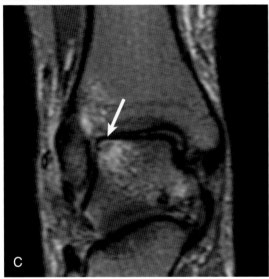

Figure 15-53 **Talar osteochondral defect.** A, Radiograph shows a shallow defect of the lateral talar dome. A free osseous fragment is consistent with an unstable osteochondral fragment *(arrow)*. B, Radiograph in a different patient shows a craterlike defect in the medial talar dome *(arrow)*. The fragment was disengaged and free in the joint. C, Magnetic resonance imaging (MRI) is ideal when occult lesions are encountered such as this lateral osteochondritis dissecans with surrounding bone marrow edema *(arrow)*.

or lateral talar dome (Fig. 15-53). The mechanism of injury differs depending on the location of the defect. Lesions that affect the lateral dome are typically due to dorsiflexion and inversion, with the defect developing when the talus strikes the inside of the lateral malleolus. Lesions of the medial dome are the result of plantar flexion and inversion so that the talus strikes the articular surface of the tibial plafond. Talar dome fractures have been described in the Berndt and Harty classification (Fig. 15-54).

Talar Neck/Body Fractures

Although less common than calcaneal fractures, talar fractures are common injuries. About 75% of talar fractures occur in the neck or body of the talus, and 25% are part of a fracture-dislocation injury. Most occur from an axial-loading mechanism with the force driving the neck of the talus against the anterior lip of the tibia. The vascular supply of the proximal pole is tenuous; therefore fractures that occur proximal to the middle of the talus are more susceptible to developing AVN.

The Hawkins classification discusses three types that are predictive for the risk for developing AVN. In type I fractures the talar neck fracture is not displaced and

BERNDT-HARTY CLASSIFICATION FOR TALAR DOME OCDS

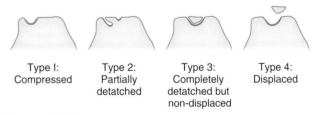

| Type I: Compressed | Type 2: Partially detatched | Type 3: Completely detatched but non-displaced | Type 4: Displaced |

Figure 15-54 **Berndt-Harty classification for talar dome osteochondral defects.**

has a low risk for developing AVN (less than 10%) (Fig. 15-55). Type II fractures are displaced talar neck fractures with subluxation or dislocation of the subtalar joint that disrupts the talocalcaneal ligament. The tibiotalar joint remains anatomically aligned. The incidence of AVN in this type is reported to be as high as 40%. Type III fractures are displaced talar neck fractures that are associated with complete dislocation of the talus, disarticulating the subtalar and tibiotalar joints. Avascular necrosis develops in 90% to100% cases. When there is subchondral lucency along the cortex of the talar dome related to bone resorption, it implies an intact blood supply and is a useful radiographic observation that excludes AVN. This is referred to as the *Hawkins sign*.

Lateral and Posterior Talar Fractures

Lateral talar process fractures are commonly from snowboarding injury, with eversion and dorsiflexion of the ankle so that the superolateral surface of the calcaneus strikes the lateral talar process (Fig. 15-56). An important observation is that soft tissue swelling has its epicenter inferior to the lateral malleolus. The fracture may be difficult to visualize, and CT is often required for better depiction and assessment of the extent of involvement of the subtalar joint.

Fractures involving the posterior talar process may be extremely subtle and should be differentiated from an os trigonum (Fig. 15-57). Injuries that cause dorsiflexion and pronation of the ankle may avulse the medial tubercle of the posterior talar process. Displacement of the os trigonum may occur with fractures of the posterior talus.

Avulsion Fractures of the Dorsal Talus

Avulsion fractures are most common at the dorsal talar neck. Linear bone fragments seen at the capsular attachment should be considered an avulsion when there is acute soft tissue swelling. Similar fractures may be related to an avulsion of the dorsal talonavicular ligament attachment site.

Calcaneal Fractures

The calcaneus is the most frequently fractured tarsal bone, accounting for 60% of all foot fractures. Calcaneal fractures are classified as either intra-articular or extra-articular depending on whether the fracture extends to the subtalar joint. Extra-articular calcaneal fractures account for about 25% of calcaneal fractures and spare the subtalar joint. They are classified into three types: type A involves the anterior calcaneal process, type B involves the body, and type C involves the posterior tuberosity and medial tubercle. Many are avulsion type of fractures (Fig. 15-58). Avulsion fractures can occur in the calcaneus at the enthesis of the Achilles tendon or at the attachment of the extensor digitorum brevis in the lateral cortex adjacent to the peroneal tubercle. Avulsion fractures at the calcaneocuboid ligament attachment result in small flakes of bone adjacent to the joint. Anterior calcaneal process fractures may be caused by an avulsion of the bifurcate ligament or by compression from forced dorsiflexion of the foot producing a "nutcracker" mechanism (Fig. 15-59).

Approximately 75% of fractures are intra-articular fractures caused by axial loading or compression forces, like those that occur from fall from a height. When evaluating the calcaneus, it is important to assess the Böhler angle and the critical angle of Gissane. Computed tomography is advocated to assess a calcaneal fracture

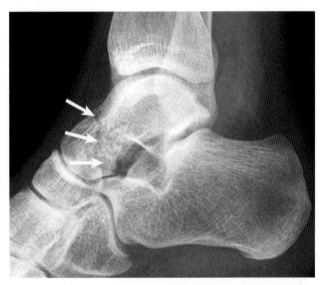

Figure 15-55 Talar neck fracture. Lateral radiograph shows a nondisplaced fracture *(arrows)*.

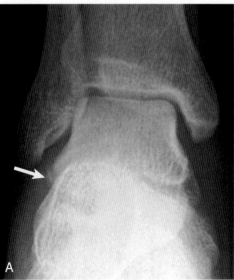
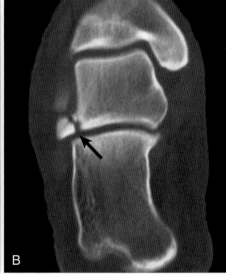

Figure 15-56 Lateral talar process fracture. A, Frontal radiograph shows a bone fragment in the lateral aspect of the talus *(arrow)*. B, Coronal computed tomographic (CT) image through the talus shows a fractured lateral talar process *(arrow)*.

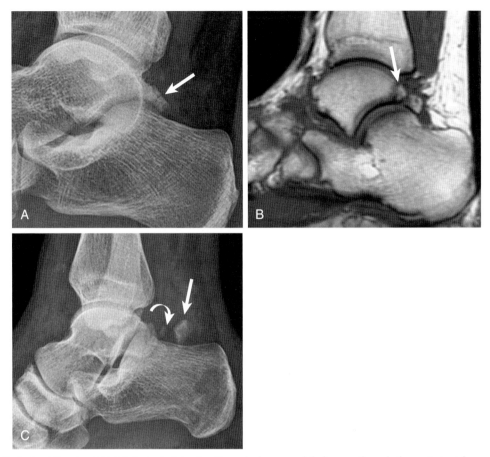

Figure 15-57 **Posterior talar process fracture.** **A,** Lateral radiograph shows a subtle lucency through the posterior talar process *(arrow)*. This appearance can mimic an os trigonum but is differentiated from the ossicle by a lack of cortex at the fracture side. **B,** Sagittal T1-weighted magnetic resonance image (MRI) in a different patient with an os trigonum shows a similar fracture *(arrow)*. **C,** Displacement of an os trigonum *(arrow)* can herald a posterior talar fracture *(curved arrow)*.

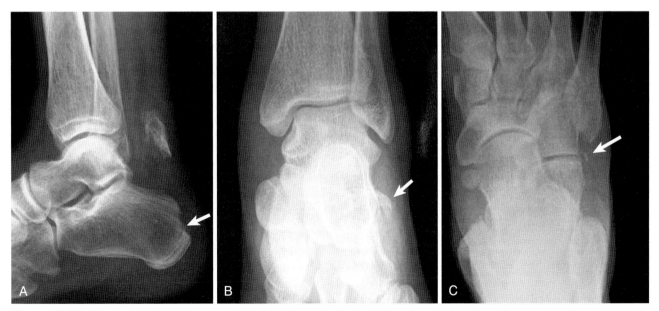

Figure 15-58 **Calcaneal avulsion fractures.** **A,** Avulsion fractures of the posterior tuberosity *(arrow)* may be posttraumatic or neuropathic. **B,** Soft tissue swelling laterally in the hindfoot may be an indicator of avulsion of the extensor digitorum brevis attachment *(arrow)*. **C,** Another subtle fracture is avulsion occurring at the calcaneocuboid ligament attachments *(arrow)*. These are generally much smaller bone fragments than os peroneum.

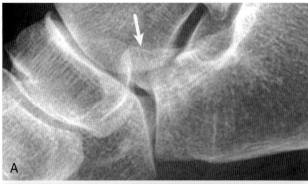

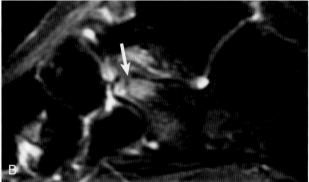

Figure 15-59 Anterior calcaneal process fracture. A, There is a subtle lucency through the anterior calcaneal process *(arrow).* **B,** The sagittal short tau inversion recovery (STIR) magnetic resonance image (MRI) shows the marrow edema surrounding the fracture *(arrow).*

and for preoperative planning when there is a collapse. In intra-articular fractures there is a primary compression fracture line and often secondary shearing fracture lines. Most primary fracture lines involve the posterior facet. The Sanders classification is useful for these types of calcaneal fractures (Fig. 15-60). It is based on the degree of comminution and location of fractures in the posterior calcaneal facet. Computed tomography images performed parallel to the posterior facet of the subtalar joint are most optimal for categorizing these fractures. Type I fractures are nondisplaced. Type II fractures (with two articular pieces) involve the posterior facet and are further subdivided into subtypes A (lateral), B (middle), and C (medial), depending on the location of the fracture line (Fig. 15-61). Type III fractures (three articular pieces) include an additional depressed middle fragment and are subdivided into types AB, AC, and BC, depending on the position and location of the fracture lines (Fig. 15-62). Type IV fractures (four or more articular fragments) are highly comminuted fractures. It is important to consider that patients with intra-articular calcaneal fractures often have fractures elsewhere, including the tibia, contralateral foot, and the spine. About 10% of calcaneal fractures are bilateral as well.

Navicular Fractures

Navicular avulsion fractures are common. Dorsal navicular avulsion fractures are caused by tension on the dorsal talonavicular ligament and/or joint capsule during forced plantar flexion (Fig. 15-63). This injury is characterized by a linear flake of bone arising from the proximal posterior cortex of the navicular on the lateral radiograph with adjacent soft tissue swelling. Avulsion of the tuberosity occurs with an eversion injury, causing the posterior tibialis tendon to separate from its attachment along with the tibionavicular ligament, and should not be mistaken for an os naviculare.

Navicular body fractures are the result of axial loading and may be associated with other midfoot fractures. The Sangeorzan classification is useful for characterizing these fractures. In type I fracture there is a coronal fracture that involves less than 50% of the bone, and there is no angulation of the forefoot. In type II fracture there is an oblique dorsolateral to plantar-medial fracture and associated medial forefoot adduction. In a type III fracture there is a comminuted fracture with lateral forefoot abduction (Fig. 15-64). All navicular body fractures with 1 mm or more of displacement require open reduction and internal fixation.

Stress fractures involving the navicular may be a source of midfoot pain in athletes. These injuries are a result of chronic overload and often are difficult to detect radiographically and may require MRI for diagnosis (Fig. 15-65). These affect basketball players and other jumping athletes relatively more frequently because this activity compresses the navicular between the talus and the cuneiform bones, creating a nutcracker effect. The fracture is oriented in the sagittal plane, usually at the junction of the middle and lateral thirds of the bone because its blood supply comes from the medial side. If the fracture becomes complete, AVN may develop in the lateral fragment if the diagnosis is delayed and the patient remains weight bearing.

Lisfranc Fracture-Dislocation

The Lisfranc joint collectively refers to the tarsometatarsal joints. About 20% of injuries of these joints go undetected. They are the result of either plantar flexion of the midfoot or axial loading in the longitudinal axis of the foot. The tarsometatarsal joints are stabilized by intermetatarsal ligaments that exist between the second to the fifth metatarsal bases and by the dorsal and plantar tarsometatarsal ligaments. The first and second tarsometatarsal joints are different from the other joints in that there is no substantial intermetatarsal ligament between the first and second metatarsal bases. Instead, an oblique Lisfranc ligament extends between the base of the second metatarsal and the medial cuneiform. The alignment of the medial cortices of the metatarsal bones corresponds to their respective tarsal bones. On the lateral view the dorsal cortex of every metatarsal base should be contiguous with the dorsal cortex of the corresponding tarsal bone.

A Lisfranc fracture-dislocation accounts for 0.2% of all fractures (Fig. 15-66). There are two types of Lisfranc injuries, homolateral and divergent. In homolateral dislocations, there is lateral subluxation/dislocation of any of the second to fifth metatarsal bases with respect to the corresponding tarsal bone (Fig. 15-67). When the first metatarsal base is also laterally subluxed, the injury pattern is considered a complete homolateral configuration. Divergent dislocation occurs when

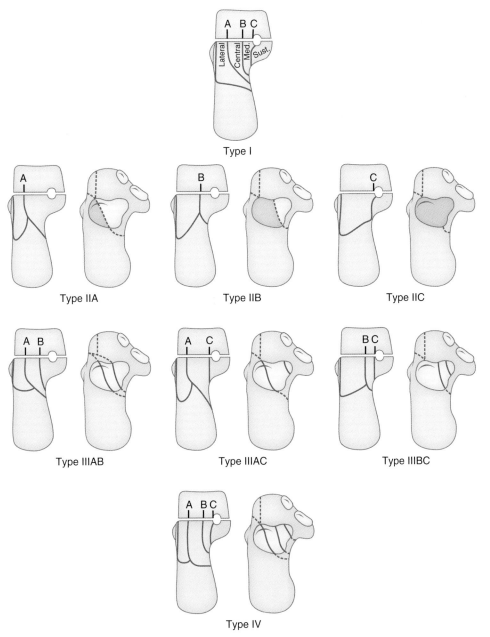

Type I

Type IIA   Type IIB   Type IIC

Type IIIAB   Type IIIAC   Type IIIBC

Type IV

Figure 15-60 Diagram of Sanders classification for intra-articular calcaneal fractures.

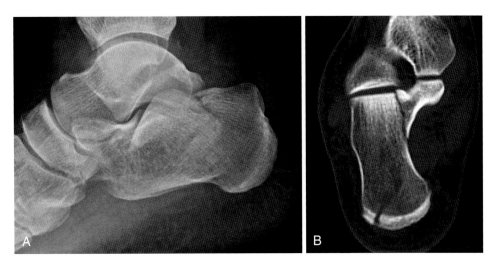

Figure 15-61 Type II Sanders fracture. A, Lateral view shows depression of the Böhler angle and disruption of the angle of Gissane. **B,** Axial computed tomographic (CT) image shows partial disruption of the posterior facet consistent with a IIB fracture.

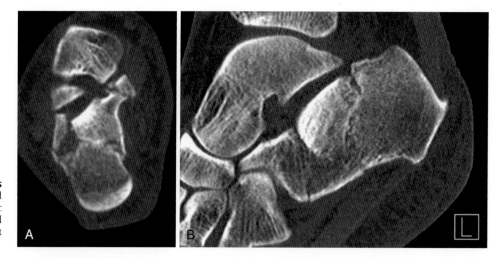

Figure 15-62 Type III Sanders fracture. A and **B,** Axial and sagittal reformatted computed tomographic (CT) images show a comminuted fracture of the calcaneus consistent with a IIIAC fracture.

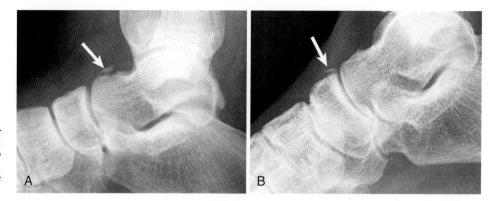

Figure 15-63 Dorsal talonavicular ligament avulsion fractures. A, A sliver of bone has been lifted up from the head of the talus *(arrow)*. **B,** A similar fracture arises from the navicular in a different patient.

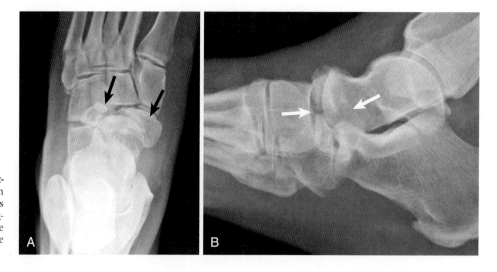

Figure 15-64 Comminuted navicular fracture. A, Frontal radiograph shows two large distracted fragments *(arrows)*, as well as several smaller fragments. **B,** The lateral view shows the fracture plane *(arrows)* created by the nutcracker effect.

there is a lateral subluxation/dislocation of the second to fifth metatarsal bases with medial subluxation/dislocation of the first metatarsal base or the medial cuneiform, creating a larger space between the first and second rays than typically seen in the homolateral types of Lisfranc injuries (Fig. 15-68). Weight-bearing views may be necessary to demonstrate subluxation either dorsally or laterally if initial radiographs show normal results but the injury is suspected clinically. Both frontal and lateral projections are recommended when weight bearing. If the diagnosis is equivocal, both CT and MRI are useful. Computed tomography has the capability of demonstrating fractures and small bone fragments, whereas MRI can directly depict the integrity of the ligament and show edema and any bone contusions that are present.

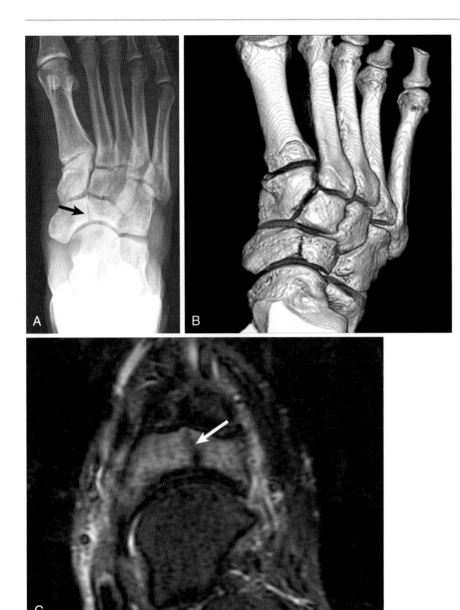

Figure 15-65 Navicular stress fracture. Frontal radiograph (**A**) and three-dimensional (3-D) reconstructed computed tomographic (CT) image (**B**) show a fracture in the sagittal plane of the navicular at the junction between the middle and lateral thirds of the bone *(arrow)*, the vascular watershed area. **C**, Axial short tau inversion recovery (STIR) magnetic resonance image (MRI) shows marrow edema surrounding the stress fracture *(arrow)*.

Metatarsal Fractures

There are several common fractures that involve the fifth metatarsal (Fig. 15-69). The Jones fracture classically occurs approximately 1.5 to 2 cm distal to the tuberosity and is transversely oriented. It can be the result of a single traumatic episode or from repeated chronic overload. Delayed union may require surgical fixation to avert the development of nonunion. Tubercle fractures are caused by the tensile forces that occur when the foot plantar flexes and inverts, resulting in avulsion of either the insertion of the peroneus brevis tendon, lateral cord of the plantar fascia, or both. In children with an immature skeleton, this fracture should be differentiated from the normal apophysis, which has a longitudinal orientation.

Metatarsal shaft fractures may result from direct or indirect forces. Fractures involving the metatarsal head (turf toe) are uncommon and usually result from a direct impaction injury from either hyperextension

or hyperflexion of the toe (Fig. 15-70). Defects in the articular cartilage may predispose the metatarsophalangeal joint to osteoarthritis later in life. Isolated fractures of the shaft and neck of the bone often are from direct trauma from a heavy object falling on the foot.

Sesamoids of the first metatarsophalangeal joint are located within the flexor hallucis brevis tendon and are vulnerable to compressive forces. The diagnosis of a fracture requires close inspection, and often additional views or CT imaging may be performed for confirmation (Fig. 15-71). The sesamoids are also susceptible to developing stress-induced injuries from repetitive tensile forces, and MRI is the preferred modality for diagnosis. Dislocations at the metatarsophalangeal and interphalangeal joints may be associated with a fracture (Fig. 15-72). If the joint appears asymmetric after reduction, it is important to exclude an entrapped bone fragment.

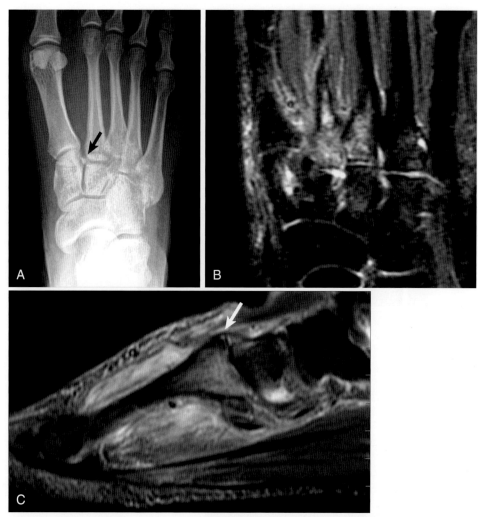

Figure 15-66 Lisfranc fracture-dislocation. A, Frontal radiograph shows a bone fragment from the base of the second metatarsal *(arrow)* associated with widening of the intermetatarsal space between the first and second metatarsal bones. B, Axial short tau inversion recovery (STIR) magnetic resonance image (MRI) shows extensive bone marrow edema at the tarsometatarsal joints throughout the Lisfranc joint. C, Sagittal T2-weighted MRI shows dorsal subluxation of the second metatarsal base with respect to the middle cuneiform *(arrow)*.

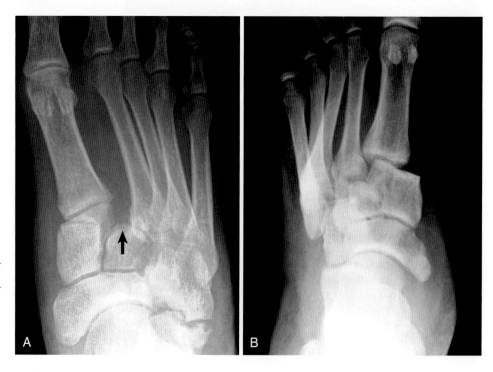

Figure 15-67 Homolateral Lisfranc injury A, Frontal radiograph shows an incomplete homolateral injury pattern with subluxation of the second to fifth metatarsal bases. Note the bare articular surface of the middle cuneiform *(arrow)*. B, This radiograph in a different patient shows a complete homolateral pattern with lateral subluxation of all of the metatarsal bases.

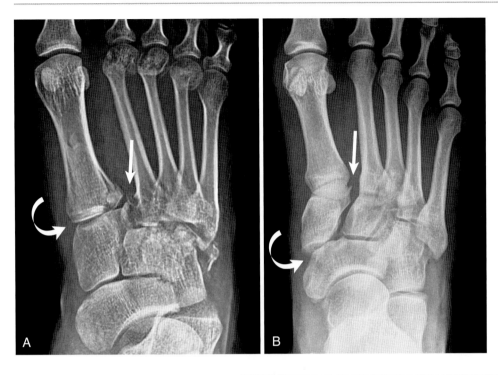

Figure 15-68 Divergent Lisfranc injury A, Frontal radiograph shows widening of the intermetatarsal space *(arrow),* as well as numerous fractures, including the base of the both the first and second metatarsal bones. The first metatarsal (MT) is medially subluxed *(curved arrow),* while the second to fifth MT bases are subluxed laterally. **B,** Radiograph in a different patient shows widening of the intermetatarsal space *(arrow)* as medial subluxation of the medial cuneiform with respect to the navicular *(curved arrow).*

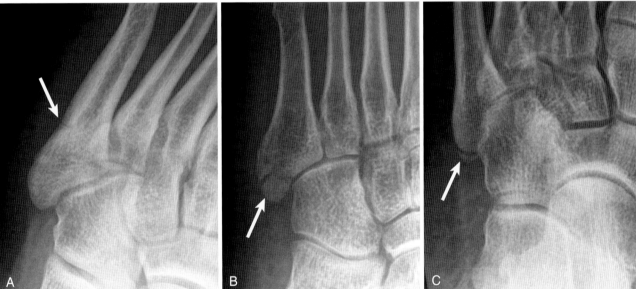

Figure 15-69 Fifth metatarsal fractures. A, A classic Jones fracture occurs about 2 cm from the tubercle *(arrow).* **B** and **C,** Smaller fragments at the base are often caused by avulsion of either the peroneus brevis tendon *(arrow in* **B**) or the lateral cord of the plantar fascia *(arrow in* **C**). The latter injury typically produces very small bone fragments.

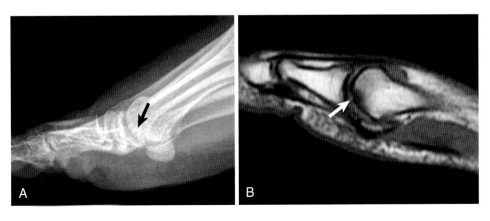

Figure 15-70 Turf toe A, Lateral view of the forefoot shows some sclerosis in the head of the first metatarsal bone *(arrow).* **B,** Sagittal T1-weighted magnetic resonance image (MRI) shows the impaction defect of the articular surface *(arrow).*

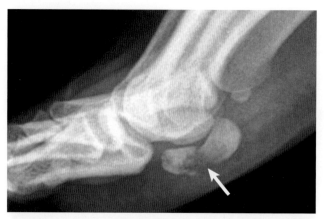

Figure 15-71 Sesamoid fracture. Lateral view shows a sesamoid fracture *(arrow)*. Fractures are differentiated from bipartite sesamoid by the lack of a cortical margin that is typical of all ossicles.

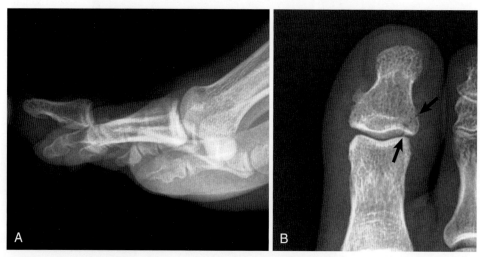

Figure 15-72 Interphalangeal joint dislocation. **A,** Lateral view shows dorsal dislocation of the distal phalanx of the great toe. **B,** Frontal radiograph after reduction shows a subtle intra-articular fracture of the base *(arrows)*.

Selected Reading

Arimoto HK, Forrester DM. Classification of ankle fractures: an algorithm. *AJR Am J Roentgenol.* 1980;135(5):1057-1063.

Ashman C, Klecker R, Yu JS. Forefoot pain involving the metatarsal region: differential diagnosis with MR imaging. *Radiographics.* 2001;21:1425-1440.

Badillo K, Pacheco JA, Padua SO, et al. Multidetector CT evaluation of calcaneal fractures. *Radiographics.* 2011;31(1):81-92.

Bahel A, Yu JS. Lateral plantar pain: diagnostic considerations. *Emerg Radiol.* 2010;17(4):291-298.

Campos JC, Chung CB, Lektrakul N, et al. Pathogenesis of the Segond fracture: anatomic and MR imaging evidence of an iliotibial tract or anterior oblique band avulsion. *Radiology.* 2001;219:381-386.

Cannon J, Silvestri S, Munro M. Imaging choices in occult hip fracture. *J Emerg Med.* 2009;37:144-152.

Cavaglia HA, Osorio PQ, Comando D. Classification and diagnosis of intracapsular fractures of the proximal femur. *Clin Orthop Relat Res.* 2002;399:17-27.

Droll KP, Broekhuyse H, O'Brien P. Fracture of the femoral head. *J Am Acad Orthop Surg.* 2007;15:716-727.

Gottsegen CJ, Eyer BA, White EA, et al. Avulsion fractures of the knee: imaging findings and clinical significance. *Radiographics.* 2008;28:1755-1770.

Haramati N, Staron RB, Barax C, et al. Magnetic resonance imaging of occult fractures of the proximal femur. *Skeletal Radiol.* 1994;23:19-22.

Harley JD, Mack LA, Winquist RA. CT of acetabular fractures: comparison with conventional radiography. *AJR Am J Roentgenol.* 1982;138:413-417.

Huang GS, Yu JS, Munshi M, et al. Avulsion fracture of the head of the fibula (the "arcuate" sign): MR imaging findings predictive of injuries to the posterolateral ligaments and posterior cruciate ligament. *AJR Am J Roentgenol.* 2003;180:381-387.

Jensen JS. Classification of trochanteric fractures. *Acta Orthop Scand.* 1980;51:803-810.

Kirsch MD, Fitzgerald SW, Friedman H, et al. Transient lateral patellar dislocation: diagnosis with MR imaging. *AJR Am J Roentgenol.* 1993;161:109-113.

Koulouris G, Morrison WB. Foot and ankle disorders: radiographic signs. *Semin Roentgenol.* 2005;40(4):358-379.

Laorr A, Greenspan A, Anderson MW, et al. Traumatic hip dislocation: early MRI findings. *Skeletal Radiol.* 1995;24:239-245.

Lundy DW. Subtrochanteric femoral fractures. *J Am Acad Orthop Surg.* 2007;15:663-671.

Mack LA, Harley JD, Winquist RA. CT of acetabular fractures: analysis of fracture patterns. *AJR Am J Roentgenol.* 1982;138:407-412.

Markhardt BK, Gross JM, Monu JU. Schatzker classification of tibial plateau fractures: use of CT and MR imaging improves assessment. *Radiographics.* 2009;29:585-597.

Miller L, Yu JS. Radiographic indicators of acute ligament injuries of the knee: a mechanistic approach. *Emerg Radiol.* 2010;17:435-444.

Mulligan ME. Ankle and foot trauma. *Semin Musculoskeletal Radiol.* 2000;4:241-253.

Norfray JF, Feline RA, Steinberg RI, et al. Subtleties of Lisfranc fractures-dislocations. *AJR Am J Roentgenol.* 1981;137:1151-1156.

Okanobo H, Khurana B, Sheehan S, et al. Simplified diagnostic algorithm for Lauge-Hansen classification of ankle injuries. *Radiographics.* 2012;32(2):E71-E84.

Pascarella R, Maresca A, Reggiani LM, et al. Intra-articular fragments in acetabular fracture-dislocation. *Orthopedics.* 2009;32:402. http://dx.doi.org/10.3928/01477447-20090511-15.

Pavlov H, Torg JS, Freeberger RH. Tarsal navicular stress fractures. *Radiology.* 1983;148:641-645.

Pipkin G. Treatment of grade IV fracture-dislocation of the hip: a review. *J Bone Joint Surg.* 1957;39A:1027-1042.

region: differential diagnosis with MR imaging. *Radiographics.* 2001;21:1425-1440.

Remer EM, Fitzgerald SW, Friedman H, et al. Anterior cruciate ligament injury: MR imaging diagnosis and patterns of injury. *Radiographics*. 1992;12:901-915.

Sangeorzan BJ, Benirschke SK, Mosca V, et al. Displaced intra-articular fractures of the tarsal navicular. *J Bone Joint Surg Am*. 1989;71(10):1504-1510.

Sonin AH, Fitzgerald SW, Friedman H, et al. Posterior cruciate ligament injury: MR imaging diagnosis and patterns of injury. *Radiology*. 1994;190:455-458.

Tuite MJ, Daffner RH, Weissman BN, et al. ACR appropriateness criteria(®) acute trauma to the knee. *J Am Coll Radiol*. 2012;9:96-103.

Verbeeten KM, Hermann KL, Hasselqvist M, et al. The advantages of MRI in the detection of occult hip fractures. *Eur Radiol*. 2005;15:165-169.

Yu J, Cody Y. A template approach for detecting fractures in low energy ankle trauma. *Emerg Radiol*. 2009;16(4):309-318.

Yu JS. Hip and femur trauma. *Semin Musculoskeletal Radiol*. 2000;4:205-220.

Yu JS, Petersilge C, Sartoris D. MR imaging of injuries of the extensor mechanism of the knee. *Radiographics*. 1994;14:541-551.

CHAPTER 16

Pelvis

Pelvic Fractures

Howard J. O'Rourke and
Georges Y. El-Khoury

■ OSSEOUS EMERGENCIES

Mechanisms and Patterns of Fractures of the Pelvis

The pelvis is a complex series of articulations supported by a strong ligamentous network. The posterior ligaments are the strongest (Fig. 16-1). The sacroiliac joint has thin anterior and thick posterior ligaments. The sacrospinous and sacrotuberous ligaments are additional posterior ligaments that primarily serve to resist rotational deformity of the pelvis. The pubic symphysis is supported by a series of comparably weaker ligaments.

Pelvic fractures are a potentially devastating injury encountered in emergency medicine with an overall mortality reported between 8% and 17%. Fractures of the pelvis may be classified as stable or unstable; with unstable fractures the pelvic ring is disrupted, particularly posteriorly. The most common cause of mortality is hemorrhage, which may be arterial, venous, or bleeding from fractured cancellous bone. The most widely used classification system is the Young-Burgess system, which seeks to classify fractures based on the vector of force at the time of injury.

Radiology plays a central role in the classification and management of pelvic ring disruption. A strict approach to the pelvic radiograph will help in identifying and classifying fracture patterns. One's search pattern in a trauma patient should evaluate the iliopectineal and ilioischial lines as well as the obturator and pelvic rings (Figs. 16-2 and 16-3). The sacroiliac joints and pubic symphysis should also be evaluated for widening and craniocaudal displacement.

According to the classification system proposed by Young and colleagues, fractures are defined as lateral

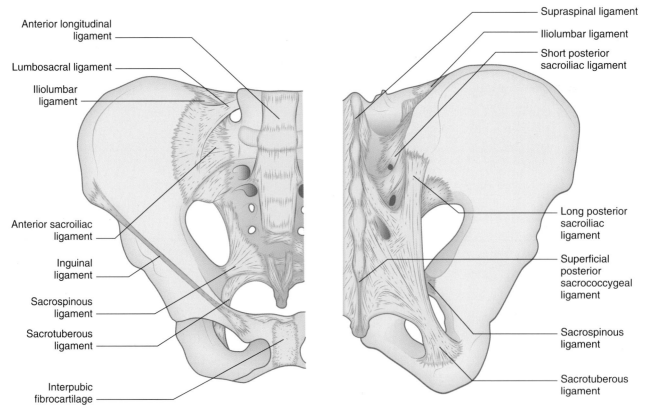

Anterior longitudinal ligament
Lumbosacral ligament
Iliolumbar ligament
Anterior sacroiliac ligament
Inguinal ligament
Sacrospinous ligament
Sacrotuberous ligament
Interpubic fibrocartilage

Supraspinal ligament
Iliolumbar ligament
Short posterior sacroiliac ligament
Long posterior sacroiliac ligament
Superficial posterior sacrococcygeal ligament
Sacrospinous ligament
Sacrotuberous ligament

Figure 16-1 Pelvic ligaments.

compression, anteroposterior compression, vertical shear, and combined mechanical injury. Lateral compression and anteroposterior injuries are further subdivided into types I to III depending on severity of injury (Table 16-1).

Lateral compression (LC) injuries represent the most common type of pelvic ring fracture. So named for the direction of force, there is resultant internal rotation of the iliac bone (Fig. 16-4). In LCI fractures the fractures of the rami are horizontal and overlapping. The posterior ring injury most often is a buckle fracture of the sacrum. Given the stability of the sacrospinous and sacrotuberous ligaments, the pelvis remains vertically stable (Fig. 16-5). In LCII fractures the iliac wing fractures, and the fracture may extend posteriorly to the sacroiliac joint. LCIII fractures are LCI or LCII on the side of injury and a contralateral open-book injury. The mechanism is internal rotation on the side of injury and external rotation on the contralateral side. The contralateral side may show partial or complete disruption of the sacroiliac joint. LCIII injuries are rotationally and possibly vertically unstable.

Anteroposterior compression (APC) injuries account for 15% to 20 % of all pelvic ring injuries. The vector of force leads to diastasis of the symphysis pubis with or without diastasis of the sacroiliac joint or fracture of the iliac bone. APCI injuries show less than 2 cm widening at the pubic symphysis and little to no widening of the sacroiliac joint. Vertical rami fractures may be seen. More severe APC injuries cause disruption of the sacroiliac joint, ranging from either anterior widening to disruption of the entire joint (Fig. 16-6). Complete separation of the hemipelvis precludes the tamponade of vascular injury. The proximity of the superior gluteal arteries and internal pudendal arteries to the sacroiliac joint contributes to the incidence of significant hemorrhage with APC injuries (Figs. 16-7 and 16-8).

Vertical shear injuries occur because of axial loading of the pelvis, as with a fall from height on an extended leg (Fig. 16-9). Characteristic radiographic findings include vertical rami fractures or diastasis of the symphysis and dislocation of the sacroiliac joint or sacral fracture. Furthermore, the hemipelvis displaces superiorly and posteriorly. In combined mechanical injuries, a combination of two or more vectors results in complex pelvic fractures (Fig. 16-10).

Sacral Fractures

Sacral fractures are an important yet difficult-to-recognize injury. Mechanistically injuries can be associated with high-energy trauma or simply normal stress on insufficient bone. The most widely used system for describing sacral fractures was created by Denis and coworkers in 1988 (Fig. 16-11). The sacrum is divided into three zones. Zone 1 fractures involve the region of the sacral ala; L5 is occasionally injured with zone 1 fractures. Zone 2 fractures involve the region of the sacral foramina. These frequently cause sciatica and rarely bladder dysfunction. Zone 3 fractures occur more centrally, and the patients experience saddle anesthesia and sphincter dysfunction.

Radiographs are relatively insensitive in detecting sacral fractures due to significant overlying soft tissues

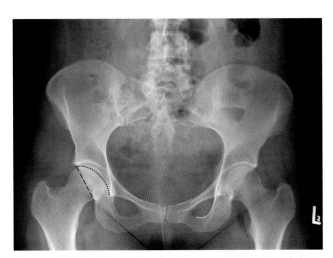

Figure 16-2 Pelvic landmarks. The normal iliopectineal *(green line)* and the ilioischial *(blue)* lines represent the anterior and posterior columns of the acetabulum, respectively. The anterior rim line *(dotted line)* and posterior rim line *(dashed line)* are also shown.

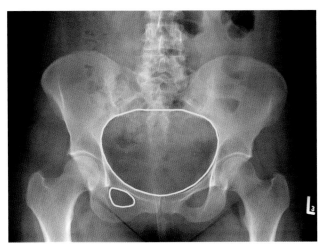

Figure 16-3 Both sides of the pelvis should appear symmetric. The normal pelvic *(larger circle)* and obturator *(smaller circle)* rings are shown.

Table 16-1   Classification of Pelvic Fractures

Fracture Type	Description
Lateral compression—internal rotation injuries	I—Compression fracture of sacrum
	II—Iliac wing fracture
	III—Contralateral open-book injury
Anteroposterior compression—external rotation injuries*	I—Stretched but intact anterior sacroiliac, sacrospinous, and sacrotuberous ligaments
	II—Torn anterior sacroiliac ligaments with intact posterior ligaments
	III—Complete ligamentous disruption
Vertical shear	Diastasis of symphysis or vertical rami fractures with vertical displacement at either sacroiliac joint, iliac fracture, or sacral fracture
Combined mechanism	Combined other patterns

*Arterial bleeding most prevalent.

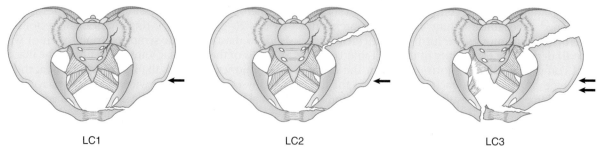

Figure 16-4 Diagram of lateral compression fracture. The lateral compressive forces cause horizontal pubic rami fractures, internal rotation of the ipsilateral iliac bone, and a compression fracture of the sacrum. (Used with permission from Hunter JC, Brandser EZ, Tran KA. Pelvic and acetabular trauma. *Radiol Clin North Am.* 1997; 35[3]:559-590.)

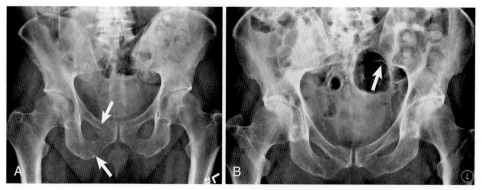

Figure 16-5 **A,** Lateral compression fractures. Anteroposterior (AP) view of the pelvis shows overlapping right rami fractures *(arrows)*, indicative of a lateral compression mechanism. **B,** Inlet view shows the displaced fracture in the right pubis and disruption of the left second arcuate line of the sacrum, indicative of a sacral fracture *(arrow)*.

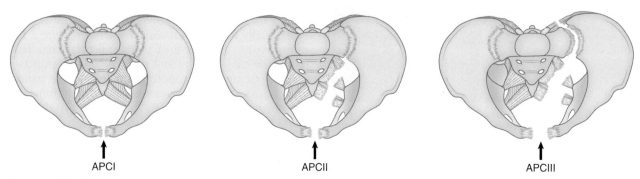

Figure 16-6 Diagram of anteroposterior compression (APC) fractures. The pubic ligaments are disrupted, but with increasing force, the sacroiliac and pelvic floor ligaments become disrupted as well. Posterior disruption may be either unilateral or bilateral.

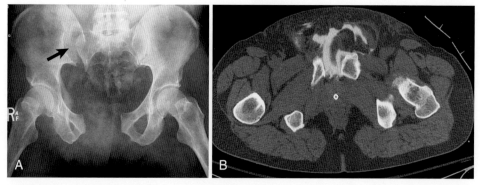

Figure 16-7 Anteroposterior compression (APC) injury. A, Anteroposterior (AP) pelvic radiograph shows diastasis of the symphysis pubis and right sacroiliac joint *(black arrow)*. **B,** Vascular and visceral injuries are common. Computed tomographic (CT) scan demonstrates extravasation of contrast material from a rupture of the urethra.

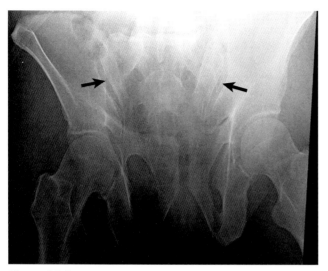

Figure 16-8 Anteroposterior compression (APC) injury. Outlet view shows mild diastasis of the symphysis pubis and both sacroiliac joints *(arrows)*.

and bowel gas. Radiologists should be sensitive to the disruption of sacral ala on anteroposterior (AP) pelvis radiographs. A bone scan is very sensitive to the presence of a sacral insufficiency fracture (Fig. 16-12). Fractures are optimally characterized at computed tomography (CT). Traumatic sacral injuries frequently occur in association with other pelvic fractures.

Sacral insufficiency fractures are common in osteoporotic women. On magnetic resonance imaging (MRI), the appearance on a T2-weighted image may occasionally be mistaken for a primary or metastatic tumor. When observed, this should prompt a search for a low–signal intensity fracture line on the corresponding T1-weighted sequence (Fig. 16-13).

Sacroiliac Joint

The sacroiliac joint is an amphiarthrodial joint and consists of a true synovial joint and ligamentous attachments. The synovial joint is located in the anteroinferior

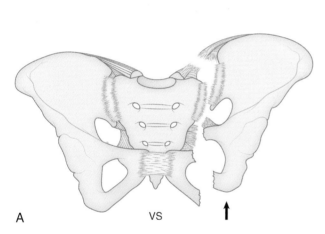

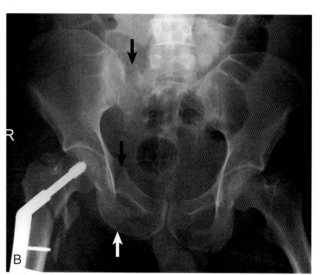

Figure 16-9 **A,** Diagram of vertical shear fractures. The vector of force causes vertical rami fractures and dislocation through the sacroiliac joint or fracture through the sacrum. **B,** Anteroposterior radiograph of the pelvis shows vertical inferior and superior *(white arrows)* rami fractures and vertical fracture through the sacrum *(black arrow)*. (**A** used with permission from Hunter JC, Brandser EZ, Tran KA. Pelvic and acetabular trauma. *Radiol Clin North Am.* 1997; 35[3]:559-590.)

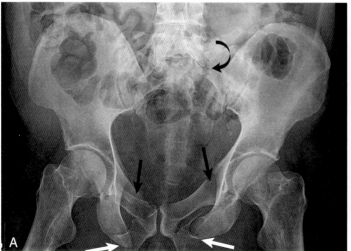

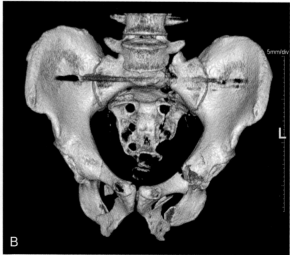

Figure 16-10 Malgaine fracture. **A,** This vertical shear injury results in bilateral superior and inferior pubic rami fractures *(straight arrows)*, as well as fracture of the sacrum *(curved arrow)*. **B,** Three-dimensional computed tomographic (3-D CT) reconstructed images optimally demonstrate all of the fractures.

one third of the joint. This iliac side has fibrous cartilage measuring 1 mm thick, and the sacral side has hyaline cartilage measuring 3 to 5 mm thick. Therefore, any inflammatory process affecting the sacroiliac joint will first be detectable on the iliac side.

Infection

In a patient presenting with nontraumatic acute pelvic pain and fever, particular attention should be paid to the sacroiliac joint on the AP pelvic radiograph. The thin white cortical line on both the sacral and iliac sides should be intact. The joints should also be evaluated for widening and sclerosis. Unfortunately, the sacroiliac joint can be exceedingly difficult to evaluate

on a standard AP pelvic radiograph, and early signs of inflammation may go undetected.

Radiographic manifestations of infection include erosions, widening of the sacroiliac joint, and evidence of reactive sclerosis. Magnetic resonance imaging is more sensitive for cases of early infection. The MR findings of infection include bone marrow edema, enhancement, surrounding inflammation, fluid within the joint, and bone destruction. Computed tomography, however, is superior for demonstrating small erosions. The distribution of sacroiliac joint inflammation is critical to narrowing the differential. Sacroiliac joint infection is almost always unilateral (Fig. 16-14).

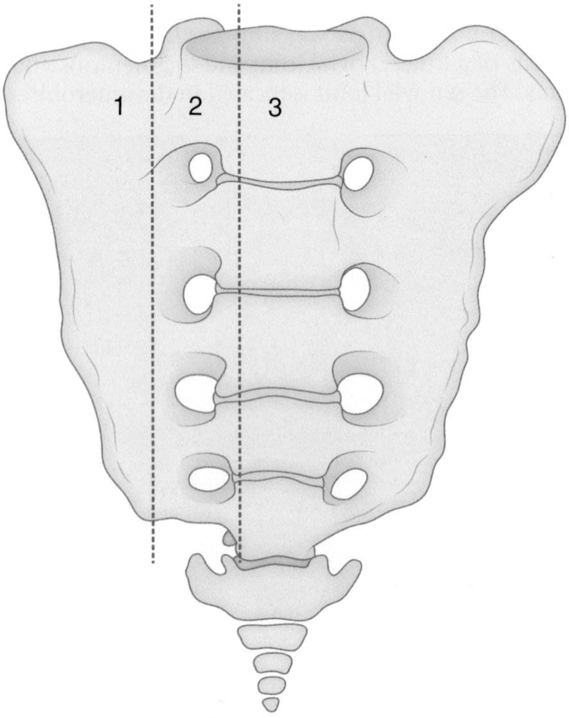

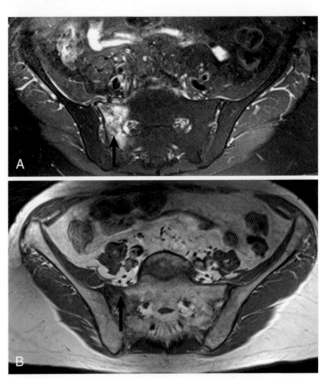

Figure 16-13 Sacral insufficiency fracture. **A,** Axial T2-weighted magnetic resonance image (MRI) of a different patient shows increased signal intensity in the right sacrum *(black arrow).* **B,** Axial T1-weighted MRI highlights the low–signal intensity line, compatible with a diagnosis of sacral insufficiency fracture.

Figure 16-11 Zones of Denis. Anatomy of the sacrum, highlighting zones 1, 2, and 3.

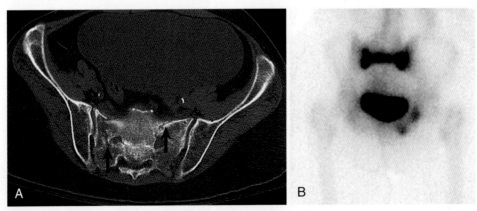

Figure 16-12 Sacral insufficiency fracture. **A,** Axial computed tomographic (CT) scan in an osteopenic patient showing bilateral sacral insufficiency fractures *(black arrows).* Note that the left fracture extends to the neural foramen, compatible with a zone 2 fracture. Also note the distended bladder due to autonomic dysfunction secondary to fracture. **B,** Planar image from nuclear medicine bone scan shows the "Honda sign" of sacral insufficiency fractures, as well as pubic rami insufficiency fractures on the left side.

When the disease is identified in an adult patient, one should interrogate the patient's history for predisposing factors. Along with the spine and sternoclavicular joints, sacroiliac joint infections are common among intravenous drug users.

Sacroiliitis

Although not generally in the domain of emergency medicine, the seronegative spondyloarthropathies are a group of diseases that are included in the differential diagnosis of sacroiliac joint inflammation. Classically, ankylosing spondylitis and inflammatory bowel disease show bilateral and symmetric involvement (Fig. 16-15). Psoriasis and reactive arthritis will present with asymmetric disease (Fig. 16-16).

Acetabular Fractures
Sarah M. Yu and Joseph S. Yu

■ FRACTURES OF THE ACETABULUM

Acetabular fractures constitute about one fourth of all pelvic fractures. These fractures typically occur as a result of high-energy trauma, and patients tend to be younger than those who sustain fractures of the femoral neck. As such, fractures of the acetabulum often have complex morphological changes and

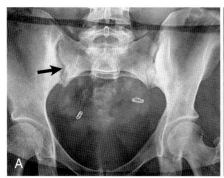
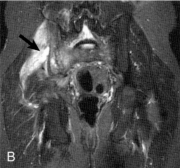
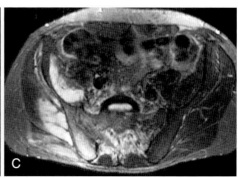

Figure 16-14 Infectious sacroiliitis. A, Anteroposterior (AP) radiographs shows cortical disruption affecting the iliac and sacral side of the right sacroiliac joint *(arrow)*. **B,** Coronal T2-weighted magnetic resonance image (MRI) shows bone marrow edema surrounding the right sacroiliac joint and infectious myositis involving the right gluteal musculature *(arrow)*. **C,** Axial T1-weighed fat-saturated MRI after intravenous gadolinium shows enhancement of the affected sacrum, ilium, and gluteal and iliacus muscles.

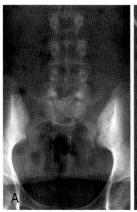
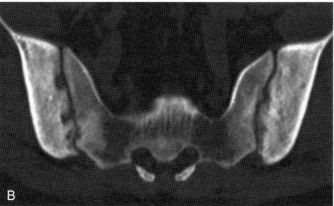

Figure 16-15 Bilateral sacroiliitis. A, Anteroposterior (AP) radiograph show sclerosis and irregularity of both sacroiliac joints, predominating on the iliac side. **B,** Computed tomography (CT) confirms the presence of bilateral symmetric sacroiliitis, illustrating erosions and marked subchondral sclerosis.

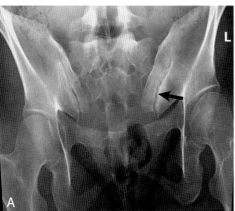
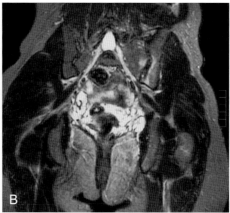

Figure 16-16 Unilateral sacroiliitis. A, Anteroposterior (AP) radiograph show erosions of the left sacroiliac joint, predominating on the iliac side *(arrow)*. **B,** Coronal T2-weighted magnetic resonance image (MRI) highlights the subchondral edema and fluid within the joint, compatible with sacroiliitis.

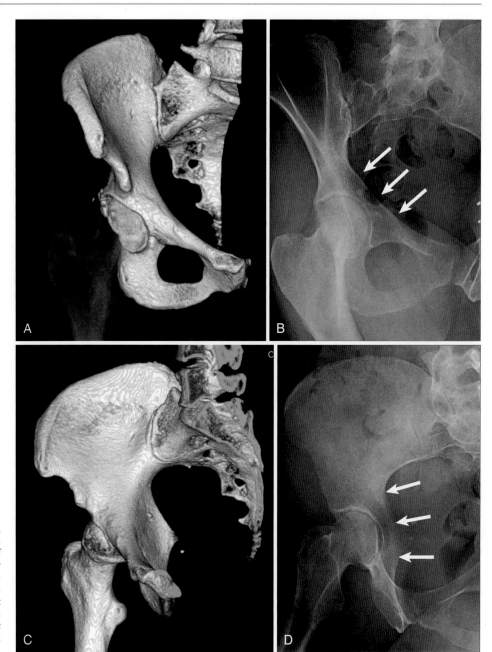

Figure 16-17 Judet views. **A** and **B,** The obturator oblique projection, obtained with the hip of interest rotated 45 degrees away from the film, allows more complete inspection of the anterior column *(arrows).* **C** and **D,** In the iliac oblique projection, obtained with the hip rotated toward the film, the entire posterior column is shown *(arrows).*

numerous fragments, so it becomes critical to assess the orientation of the fracture lines, number and relationship of large fragments, and the integrity of the articular surface. Judet views, radiographs performed with 45 degrees of obliquity, show more of the acetabular geometry than standard frontal radiographs (Fig. 16-17). Complex fractures, however, require CT for optimal evaluation. Patients with persistent incongruity of the articular surface may develop subsequent posttraumatic osteoarthritis.

The Judet classification of acetabular fractures, later modified by Letournel, is the most widely recognized surgical classification, and the fracture type is based on the involvement of either one or both acetabular columns, one or both acetabular walls, or the bone between both columns (Fig. 16-18). The classification defines five elementary (simple) acetabular fractures with a single dominant fracture line and five associated (complex) types that are formed by a combination of different simple fracture types. The simple fracture types, which constitute 30% of acetabular fractures, include posterior acetabular wall, posterior column, anterior acetabular wall, anterior column, and transverse acetabular fractures. The five associated fracture types, which constitute the other 70% of fractures, include transverse and posterior acetabular wall, T-shaped, anterior column and posterior hemitransverse, posterior column and posterior acetabular wall, and both-column fractures. The advent of multidetector CT has allowed rapid scanning in the emergency setting (Fig. 16-19). The application of two-dimensional multiplanar reformation (MPR) and three-dimensional (3-D) image reconstruction also has become indispensable for diagnosis of these fractures, as well as preoperative planning.

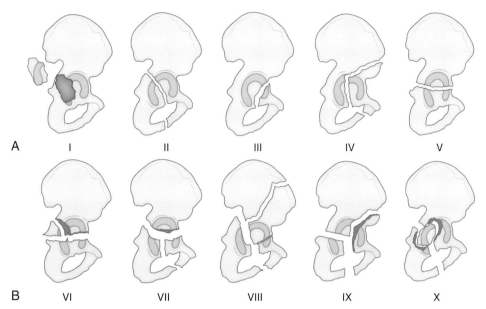

Figure 16-18 Diagram of the Judet and Letournel classification of acetabular fractures. A, Simple fractures types. I, Posterior wall fracture; II, posterior column fracture; III, anterior wall fracture; IV, anterior column fracture; V, transverse fracture. **B,** Associated fracture types. VI, Associated transverse and posterior wall fracture; VII, T-shaped fracture; VIII, Fracture of both columns; IX, Associated anterior column and posterior hemitransverse fracture; X, Associated posterior column and posterior wall fracture. (Used with permission from Yu JS. Hip and femur trauma, *Semin Musculoskelet Radiol.* 2000;4:205.)

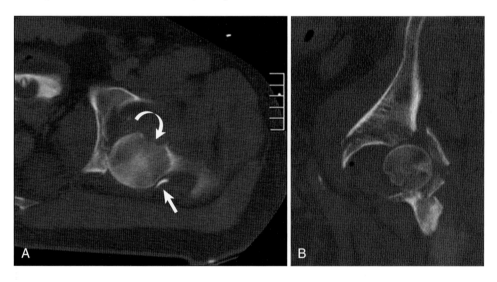

Figure 16-19 Computed tomography (CT). A, Small entrapped osseous fragments *(arrow)* and occult fractures *(curved arrow)* can be problematic because they often are radiographically occult but can have an impact on patient outcome. **B,** Sagittal reformatted image in another patient shows the extent of articular disruption, incongruity, number of osseous fragments, and the relative orientation of fracture lines. These features are easily and rapidly evaluated on CT.

With regard to these fractures it is useful to remember that five fracture types contribute over 90% of acetabular fractures. These include both-column (28% to 33%), transverse and posterior wall (20% to 24%), posterior wall (17% to 23%), T-shaped (5% to 14%), and transverse (4% to 10%) fractures. The other Judet and Letournel types contribute the remaining 10% of acetabular fractures.

When evaluating acetabular fractures, it important to fully inspect the osseous landmarks that define the margins of the acetabulum (Fig. 16-20). The main radiographic elements that define the fracture type are disruption of the iliopectineal line defining involvement of the anterior column, disruption of the ilioischial line defining involvement of the posterior column, disruption of the rim lines defining involvement of either the anterior or posterior acetabular walls or both, and extension into the obturator ring. On CT the important elements

ANATOMY OF THE HIP

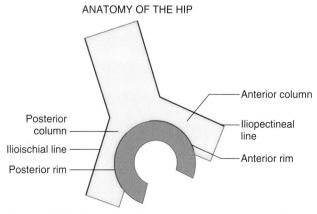

Figure 16-20 Diagram of the osseous landmarks. The relationship of the osseous landmarks to their respective structures is shown. The iliopectineal and ilioischial lines demarcate the columns, whereas the anterior and posterior rim lines demarcate the acetabular walls.

include involvement of the iliac wing, the fracture orientation at the dome of the acetabulum, the integrity of the columns, and the involvement of the obturator ring (Fig. 16-21).

Wall Fractures

The most common elementary type of acetabular fracture is a posterior wall fracture (Fig. 16-22). Often the result of a posterior hip dislocation, this fracture may affect the posterior acetabular rim, a portion of the retroacetabular surface, and a variable segment of the articular cartilage. One or multiple bone fragments may be observed. Oblique views are optimal for demonstrating this fracture, but when there are large or numerous fragments, CT is preferred for complete evaluation because instability occurs when a large percentage of the posterior surface is disrupted. When less than 34% of the posterior acetabular surface remains intact, the hip joint becomes unstable, whereas fractures that preserve greater than 55% of the posterior surface are generally stable. A posterior wall fracture can extend to involve the

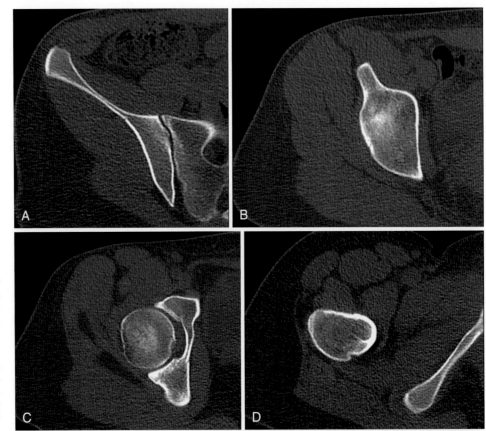

Figure 16-21 Assessment of an acetabular fracture on computed tomography (CT). There are four key areas to evaluate when assessing an acetabular fracture. **A,** Iliac wing. **B,** Acetabular dome. **C,** Anterior and posterior columns. **D,** Obturator ring. Remember that the iliac wing is affected in only anterior column or both-column fractures and that the obturator ring is involved in column and T-shaped fractures.

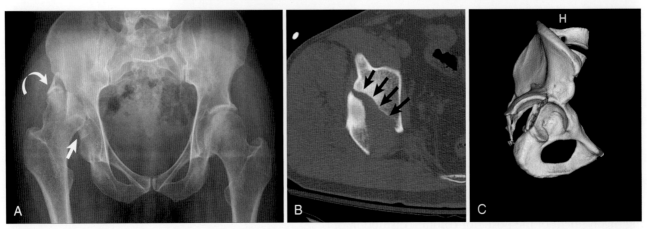

Figure 16-22 Posterior wall fracture. A, Radiograph shows posterior dislocation of the right femoral head with disruption of the posterior wall *(arrow)* and a displaced bone fragment *(curved arrow).* **B,** Axial computed tomographic (CT) image through the dome shows characteristic oblique projection of the fracture *(arrows).* **C,** Three-dimensional (3-D) image shows the relationship of the entire fragment with the native acetabulum with the femoral head subtracted from the image.

sciatic notch and/or quadrilateral plate and thus resemble a posterior column fracture. However, radiographically only the posterior rim line is disrupted, while the iliopectineal and ilioischial lines, as well as the obturator ring, remain intact. These fractures have an oblique orientation on CT. Occasionally, subtle subluxation of the femoral head may occur.

An anterior wall fracture is the least common type of acetabular fracture. It usually is associated with an anterior hip dislocation. This fracture may extend inferiorly to disrupt the obturator ring. With this fracture the iliopectineal and anterior rim lines become disrupted, while the ilioischial and posterior rim lines remain intact.

Transverse Fractures

A transverse fracture of the acetabulum is the second most common elementary fracture type, and it is often associated with a central dislocation of the femoral head. In this fracture type the innominate bone is bisected into two halves, a superior iliac component and an inferior ischiopubic component with a portion of the acetabular roof that remains attached to the ilium. Radiographically there is disruption of the iliopectineal, ilioischial, and both acetabular rim lines, but the obturator ring remains intact because the fracture plane is through the acetabulum. On CT these transverse type of fractures show a characteristic AP (vertical) fracture plane (Fig. 16-23).

Posterior wall fractures frequently occur with a transverse type of fracture of the acetabulum (Fig. 16-24). This fracture type is the second most common associated type of fracture in the Judet and Letournel classification. In nearly all cases the femoral head dislocates either posteriorly (80%) or anteriorly (20%). In transverse acetabular and posterior wall fractures there is disruption of the iliopectineal, ilioischial, and both acetabular rim lines. The obturator ring, however, remains intact.

The T-shaped fracture is another common associated type of fracture of the acetabulum (Fig 16-25). In this

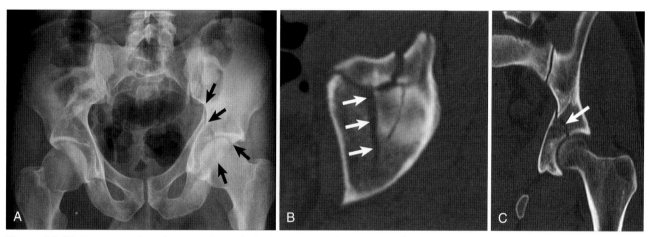

Figure 16-23 Transverse fracture. A, Radiograph shows a transverse fracture of the left acetabulum with disrupted iliopectineal, ilioischial, anterior rim, and posterior rim lines *(arrows)*. **B,** Axial computed tomographic (CT) image through the dome shows comminution, but a characteristic anterior-to-posterior orientation of the primary fracture *(arrows)*. This CT finding is present in all isolated and associated transverse fractures. **C,** Coronal reformatted image shows bisection of the left innominate bone into iliac and ischial components by the fracture *(arrow)*.

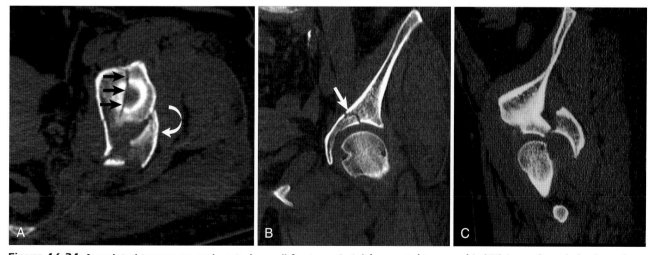

Figure 16-24 Associated transverse and posterior wall fracture. A, Axial computed tomographic (CT) image through the dome shows the characteristic anterior-to-posterior orientation of a transverse acetabular fracture *(arrows)* and displaced posterior wall fragment *(curved arrow)*. **B,** Coronal reformatted image shows bisection of the left innominate bone by the fracture *(arrow)*. **C,** Sagittal reformatted image shows displaced posterior wall fragment.

fracture the top half of the fracture connects to the axial skeleton by an intact strut of bone that extends from the sacroiliac joint to the articular surface of the acetabular dome. In a T-shaped fracture two fractures converge; a transverse fracture bisects the acetabulum, and a second perpendicular fracture extends inferiorly from the transverse fracture. As a result, the obturator ring divides into two halves. A portion of the acetabular roof remains attached to the ilium. Radiographically the iliopectineal and anterior rim lines remain intact, while the ilioischial and posterior rim lines become disrupted.

Column Fractures

There are two elementary column fracture types, anterior and posterior. An anterior column fracture may be associated with an anterior dislocation of the hip. Severe comminution of the innominate bone can cause separation of the anterior column from the remainder of the pelvis. Low fractures involve the superior pubic ramus and pubic portion of the acetabulum, whereas high fractures involve the entire anterior border of the innominate bone (Fig. 16-26). In this fracture there is disruption of the iliopectineal and occasionally the anterior rim lines depending on where the fracture occurs. The obturator ring, however, is always disrupted.

A fracture involving the posterior column usually begins above the acetabulum and courses inferiorly through the posterior acetabulum and into the ischium. It involves the entire retroacetabular surface, extending inferiorly either into the obturator foramen or more posteriorly, splitting the ischial tuberosity into two pieces. The posterior column usually rotates along its longitudinal axis as it displaces. Because this fracture often accompanies a central dislocation, medial displacement of the posterior column fragment may also be seen. In this fracture the iliopectineal and anterior rim lines remain intact, but the ilioischial and posterior rim lines become disrupted. The dome of the acetabulum usually remains intact.

Computed tomography images of column fractures show a distinctive horizontal pattern with the fracture plane oriented from medial to lateral, dividing the acetabulum into anterior and posterior segments. Depending on the type, one or both columns will be dissociated from the axial skeleton. The fracture line extends above the acetabulum into the iliac wing in anterior column fractures and is at or inferior to the level of the dome for posterior column fractures.

The most common associated fracture type involving the columns in the Judet and Letournel classification is a both-column fracture (Fig. 16-27). In this fracture the spur sign is nearly pathognomonic when present.

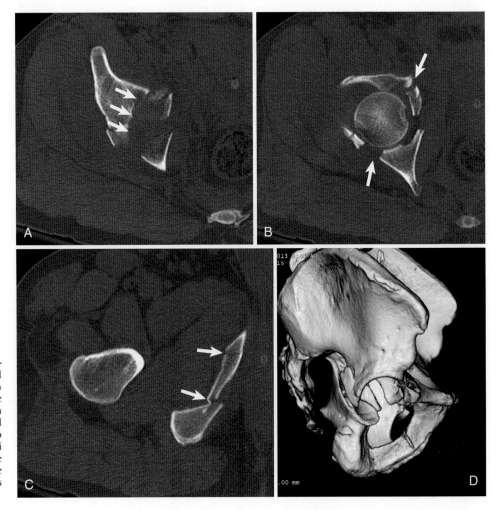

Figure 16-25 T-shaped fracture. A and **B,** Axial computed tomographic (CT) images through the dome and columns show the transverse fracture orientation *(arrows).* **C,** Axial image at the level of the obturator ring shows two fractures of the inferior pubic rami *(arrows).* **D,** The main difference between an elementary transverse fracture and a T-shaped fracture is involvement of the obturator ring.

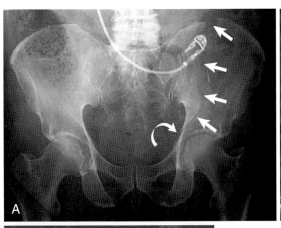

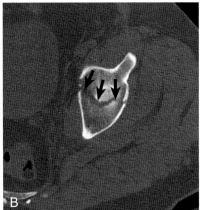

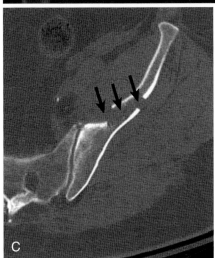

Figure 16-26 Anterior column fracture. A, Radiograph shows disruption of the iliopectineal line *(curved arrow)* and displaced vertical fracture of the left iliac wing *(arrows).* **B** and **C,** Axial computed tomographic (CT) images through the dome and left ilium show the characteristic medial-to-lateral orientation of a column fracture *(arrows).* Involvement of the left iliac wing makes this a high anterior column fracture.

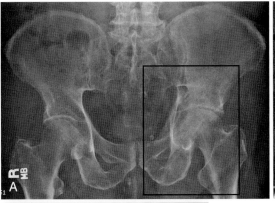

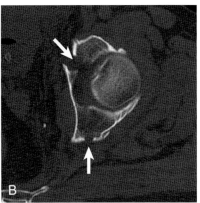

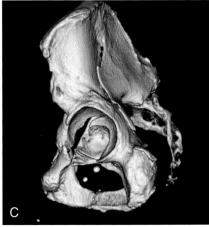

Figure 16-27 Both-column fracture. A, Radiograph shows a complex left acetabular fracture with displacement and comminution *(open box).* **B,** Axial computed tomographic (CT) image through the columns shows fractures involving both the anterior and posterior columns *(arrows).* **C,** Three-dimensional (3-D) image shows the degree of distraction and the relationship of the fracture fragments.

A triangular fragment of iliac bone remains attached to the sacroiliac joint and is conspicuous when the more anterior acetabular fragments displace medially. The femoral head often dislocates centrally. In both-column fractures the iliopectineal, ilioischial, and posterior rim lines usually are disrupted as is the obturator ring.

There are two other associated fracture types involving the columns that are relatively uncommon. An anterior column and posterior hemitransverse fracture has two components, an anterior column fracture and a second transversely oriented fracture that arises from the column fracture and is directed posteriorly. In this fracture the iliopectineal, ilioischial, anterior rim, and posterior rim lines are all disrupted. A posterior column and posterior wall fracture is the least common type of associated fracture. In this fracture there is a posterior wall fracture fragment that is displaced because the femoral head typically dislocates posteriorly. The posterior column, however, usually is not displaced. In this fracture the ilioischial and posterior rim lines become disrupted, while the anterior landmarks remain intact.

Selected Reading

Burgess AR, Eastridge BJ, Young JW, et al: Pelvic ring disruption: effective classification system and treatment protocols, *J Trauma* 30(7):848–856, 1990.

Chong KH, DeCoster T, Robinson B: Pelvic fractures and mortality, *Iowa Orthop J* 17:110–114, 1997.

Denis F, Davis S, Comfort T: Sacral fractures: an important problem. Retrospective analysis of 236 cases, *Clin Orthop Relat Res.* 227:67–81, 1988.

El-Khoury GY, Daniel WW, Kathol MH: Acute and chronic avulsive injuries, *Radiol Clin North Am* 35:747–766, 1997.

Harley JD, Mack LA, Winquist RA: CT of acetabular fractures: comparison with conventional radiography, *AJR Am J Roentgenol* 138:413–417, 1982.

Hunter JC, Brandser EZ, Tran KA: Pelvic and acetabular trauma, *Radiol Clin North Am* 35:559–590, 1997.

Judet R, Judet J, Letournel E: Fractures of the acetabulum: classification and surgical approaches for open reduction, *J Bone Joint Surg* 46A:1615–1646, 1964.

Laorr A, Greenspan A, Anderson MW, et al: Traumatic hip dislocation: early MRI findings, *Skeletal Radiol* 24:239–245, 1995.

Letournel E: Acetabular fractures: classification and management, *Clin Orthop* 151:81–106, 1980.

Mack LA, Harley JD, Winquist RA: CT of acetabular fractures: analysis of fracture patterns, *AJR Am J Roentgenol* 138:407–412, 1982.

Quinn SF, McCarthy JL: Prospective evaluation of patients with suspected hip fracture and indeterminate radiographs: use of T1-weighted MR images, *Radiology* 187:469–471, 1993.

Richardson P, Young JWR, Porter D: CT detection of cortical fracture of the femoral head associated with posterior hip dislocation, *AJR Am J Roentgenol* 155:93–94, 1990.

Buckholz RW, Heckman JD, Court-Brown C, editors: *Rockwood and Green's Fractures in Adults*, ed 6, Philadelphia, Lippincott, 2006.

Saks BJ: Normal acetabular anatomy for acetabular fracture assessment: CT and plain film correlation, *Radiology* 159:139–145, 1986.

Saterbak AM, Marsh JL, Turbett T, et al: Acetabular fractures classification of Letournel and Judet: a systematic approach, *Iowa Orthop J* 15:184–196, 1995.

Scott WW, Fishman EK, Magid D: Acetabular fractures: optimal imaging, *Radiology* 165:537–539, 1987.

Stambaugh L, Blackmore CC: Pelvic ring disruptions in emergency radiology, *Eur J Radiol* 48:71–87, 2003.

Stevens M, El-khoury GY, Kathol M, et al: Imaging features of avulsion injuries, *Radiographics* 3:655–661, 1999.

Young JWR, Burgess AR, Brumback RJ, et al: Pelvic fractures: value of plain radiography in early assessment and management, *Radiology* 160:445–451, 1986.

CHAPTER 17

Emergent Soft Tissue Conditions

Joseph S. Yu

Acute inflammatory and infectious soft tissue disorders are important conditions that affect nearly 2 million people in the United States every year. Inflammation versus infection of the skin, subcutaneous tissues, and muscles is often difficult to differentiate clinically, and early detection and accurate diagnosis have a significant impact on the immediate course of treatment and on the magnitude of any subsequent complication and morbidity. Although many of these conditions present with similar clinical symptoms, the recognition of key laboratory and constitutional findings can aid in the diagnosis of specific diseases and determine whether surgical intervention is required. In many situations, important differentiating characteristics on imaging enable diagnosis.

■ CELLULITIS

Cellulitis is a localized infectious process that affects the dermal layers and subcutaneous fat. The infection often begins with minor disruption of the skin that allows the invasion of microorganisms into the subcutaneous tissues. There is an increased risk in patients with diabetes mellitus, peripheral vascular disease, human immunodeficiency virus (HIV) infection, immune deficiency from other disease processes, or a retained foreign body. The most common organism involved is *Staphylococcus aureus*. Typically patients present with fever, focal pain and swelling, erythema and warmth, and leukocytosis.

Radiographically cellulitis manifests with soft tissue swelling causing induration of the subcutaneous fat. On computed tomography (CT), swelling may focal or diffuse, with altered soft tissue attenuation that enhances variably with intravenous administration of iodinated contrast. Skin thickening can accompany the underlying inflammation. Although magnetic resonance imaging (MRI) rarely is required for diagnosis of cellulitis, this modality is indicated when the character of the disease is atypical, either because of suspected abscess formation, neoplastic disorder, or a rapidly progressive nature that can compromise a limb or become life threatening. Foreign bodies are frequently the nidus of infection in the foot and hand. Ultrasonography is the preferred modality for identifying retained foreign bodies, particularly those of wooden composition.

On MRI, cellulitis is characterized by focal or diffuse regions in the subcutaneous fat of low signal intensity on T1-weighted images with corresponding striated high signal intensity on fluid-sensitive sequences (Fig. 17-1). Enhancement occurs after administration of intravenous gadolinium, differentiating these findings from nonspecific soft tissue edema. The adjacent fascia may also enhance.

■ ABSCESS

A focal soft tissue infection may become diffuse and evolve into a phlegmon or become more localized into an abscess. A phlegmon is a purulent inflammatory process that may either spread or become walled off into an inflammatory mass, often occurring without a bacterial infection. An abscess is a well-demarcated collection

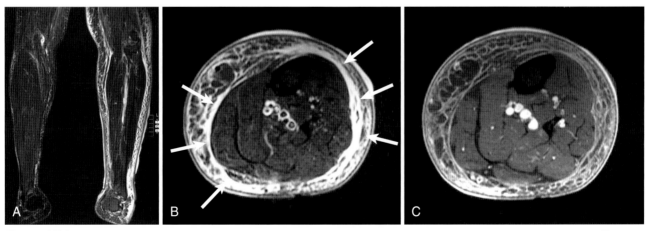

Figure 17-1 Cellulitis. A, Short tau inversion recovery (STIR) coronal magnetic resonance image (MRI) of both calves shows diffuse subcutaneous fat edema in the left calf from the thigh to the ankle. **B,** Axial T2-weighted image shows striated areas of increased signal intensity and perifascial fluid accumulation *(arrows).* **C,** Fat-saturated T1-weighted axial image after intravenous administration of contrast shows diffuse enhancement of the infected dermal and subcutaneous soft tissues.

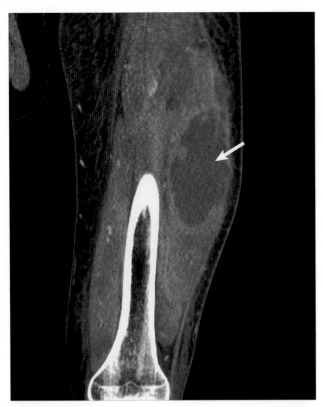

Figure 17-2 Abscess. Contrast-enhanced coronal computed tomographic (CT) image shows a fluid collection in the vastus lateralis muscle with rim enhancement *(arrow)*.

of purulent fluid that has accumulated as a result of an infectious process. It is differentiated from a phlegmon by the formation of a capsule in an attempt to contain the infected fluid from adjacent structures. The clinical presentation of both processes may be similar to that of cellulitis. An abscess, however, requires drainage in addition to appropriate antibiotic treatment. Frequently *S. aureus* is isolated as the infectious agent, and as many of 51% of infections may be methicillin resistant.

Unless gas is conspicuous, an abscess may be difficult to identify on radiographs. An abscess has a distinctive appearance on contrast-enhanced CT, with a brightly rim-enhancing fluid collection with an irregularly thickened wall (Fig. 17-2). Internal attenuation is variable and influenced by the amount of cellular debris and protein in the fluid. The hallmark of an abscess is gas within the fluid collection. On MRI an abscess is characterized by a localized fluid collection with intermediate to low signal intensity on T1-weighted images and bright signal intensity on fluid-sensitive sequences. The developed wall is often irregular and thick and enhances peripherally after intravenous administration of gadolinium contrast material.

■ NECROTIZING FASCIITIS

One of the most serious complications of a soft tissue infection is necrotizing fasciitis, an infectious process that has spread to the deep fascial layers. This rare disorder is a life-threatening condition characterized by progressive necrosis of the subcutaneous tissue and fascia and frequently accompanied by severe systemic

toxicity. Clinically, early necrotizing fasciitis mimics cellulitis with fever, pain, tenderness, swelling, and erythema. An important observation is severe pain at onset that is out of proportion to local findings. It may be difficult to discern between necrotizing fasciitis and diffuse cellulitis, but necrotizing fasciitis is a rapidly progressive infection that requires surgical débridement of the infected tissues. Intermediate skin changes include a serous-filled blister or bullae formation with skin fluctuance and induration. Late findings include hemorrhagic bullae, skin anesthesia, crepitus, and skin necrosis with discoloration.

The prevalence of necrotizing fasciitis is increasing owing to a larger population of patients with immune deficiency, including HIV infection, diabetes, organ transplantation, cancer, alcoholism, and chronic liver or renal disease. Intravenous drug abusers particularly are at risk for developing necrotizing fasciitis in the upper extremity. Necrotizing fasciitis is classified into four categories according to the causative microorganism. Type 1 necrotizing fasciitis is a polymicrobial infection with both aerobic and anaerobic bacteria occurring in individuals with chronic diseases. Type 2 necrotizing fasciitis is usually a monomicrobial infection with group A β-hemolytic streptococcus. It can affect people at any age and with no preexisting medical condition. Type 3 necrotizing fasciitis is an infection with a gram-negative monomicrobial infection with a marine-related organism or *Clostridium* species and is most prevalent in patients suffering from liver cirrhosis and alcoholism. Type 4 necrotizing fasciitis is a fungal infection usually affecting immunocompromised patients.

Early surgical intervention has been associated with improved survival. The current recommendation is wide, extensive débridement of all tissues that can be easily elevated off the fascia with gentle pressure, a characteristic of necrotic and poorly perfused tissue. Hyperbaric oxygen may be a useful adjunctive therapy. Today the reported mortality rate ranges from 22% to 30%, although some studies still report a mortality rate as high as 80%. High mortality rate is directly related to delayed diagnosis, as well as the type of necrotizing fasciitis. Common causes of death are sepsis, respiratory failure, renal failure, and multiorgan failure.

The diagnosis of necrotizing fasciitis is difficult on radiographs because only 13% of patients present with soft tissue gas. Computed tomography demonstrates induration of the subcutaneous fat, but when there is fluid and gas dissecting along the fascial planes, the diagnosis is apparent. Magnetic resonance imaging is the preferred modality for diagnosis, but it should not delay treatment if it is not readily available. The early findings of necrotizing fasciitis are similar to cellulitis (Fig. 17-3). On T1-weighted images, necrotizing fasciitis is depicted by areas of soft tissue edema and enhancement with administration of intravenous gadolinium. Infected deep and intramuscular fascia is characterized by increased signal intensity on both sides of the fascia on fluid-sensitive images, representing purulent perifascial fluid (liquefaction necrosis) and edema, and this finding is not typical of uncomplicated cellulitis. The appearance of a thickened fascia greater than 3 mm thick should increase the index of suspicion (Fig. 17-4).

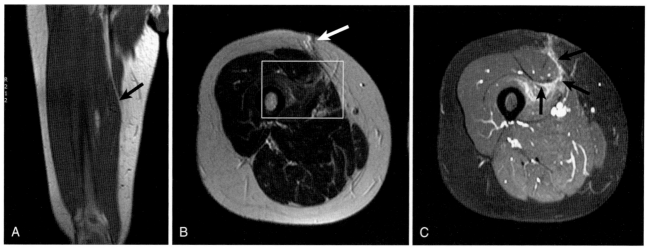

Figure 17-3 **Necrotizing fasciitis.** **A,** Coronal T1-weighted magnetic resonance image (MRI) shows a collection of gas within the soft tissues of the midthigh *(arrow).* **B,** Axial T2-weighted image shows localized muscle edema in the vastus intermedius and medialis and rectus femoris muscles *(open box).* There is a penetrating injury in the adjacent subcutaneous fat *(arrow).* **C,** Fat-saturated T1-weighted axial image after intravenous contrast shows enhancement along the superficial fascia and the involved intermuscular fascia *(arrows).*

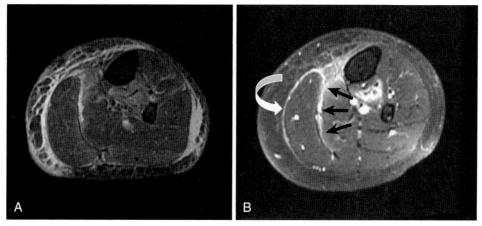

Figure 17-4 **Necrotizing fasciitis.** **A,** T2-weighted axial image of the left calf shows areas of cellulitis and increased signal intensity in the superficial fascia and in the fascia between the soleus and gastrocnemius muscles. There is muscular edema in the soleus and deep posterior compartment muscles. **B,** Fat-saturated T1-weighted axial image after intravenous administration of contrast shows enhancement of the deep fascia *(arrows),* as well as the perifascial fluid surrounding the superficial fascia *(curved arrow).*

Early in the disease there is enhancement of the deep fascia, but as necrosis progresses, diminished enhancement of the fascia is observed. Low signal intensity on fat-saturated T2-weighted images is characteristic of necrotizing fasciitis, indicating formation of gas (Fig. 17-5). Bandlike edema in the periphery of adjacent muscles indicates progressive disease. Loculation into an abscess indicates progression of the disease. A lack of fascial enhancement is associated with frank necrosis and is a manifestation of advanced necrotizing fasciitis, characteristically involving three or more compartments in the affected extremity.

■ PYOMYOSITIS

A suppurative bacterial infection of skeletal muscle is termed *pyomyositis.* Over three fourths of cases are caused by the organism *S. aureus.* Of these, about 25% are methicillin resistant. The average mortality rate of pyomyositis is reported to be as high as 10%. *Streptococcus* is the second most common organism identified, but

infection with this microbe tends to be very aggressive and lead to extensive muscle destruction and an 85% mortality rate in some studies. Healthy striated muscle is inherently resistant to infection, and bacteremia alone is not sufficient to cause pyomyositis. In the United States, the increased prevalence of HIV infection accounts for nearly one half of cases of bacterial myositis. Other risk factors include muscle trauma with a hematoma serving as the initial source of infection, diabetes, connective tissue disorders, malnutrition, and conditions that produce immune deficiency, including cancer.

Clinically, pyomyositis has three stages. The early or invasive stage occurs within 1 to 2 weeks of the initial infection, with edema giving way to localized pain, leukocytosis, and erythema (Fig. 17-6). The patient may also be febrile. As the disease progresses, the patient develops the second or purulent stage, characterized by fever, chills, and rigors as the myositis evolves to suppuration and abscess formation. About 90% of patients present with this stage, typically occurring 10 to 21 days after the

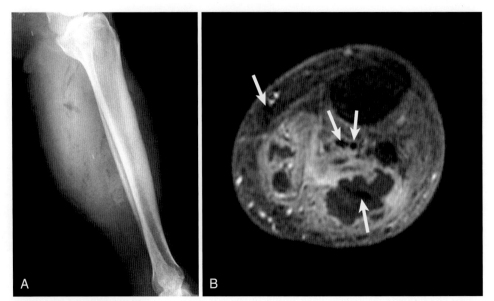

Figure 17-5 Necrotizing fasciitis, late. A, Lateral radiograph of the calf shows an abundance of gas in the muscles, as well as diffuse soft tissue swelling. **B,** Fat-saturated T1-weighted axial image after intravenous administration shows enhancing tissue surrounding large areas of devitalized muscles and the presence of gas seen as foci of signal void *(arrows)*.

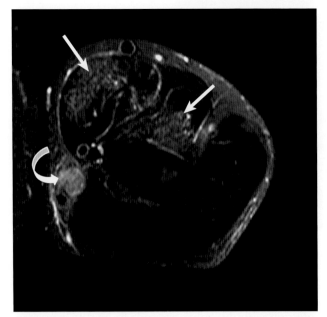

Figure 17-6 Pyomyositis, early. T2-weighted axial image of the left arm shows interstitial edema in the anterior compartment during the first stage of this disorder, manifested by focal areas of increased signal intensity *(arrows)*. There is minimal edema in the superficial fascia anteriorly, but note the absence of cellulitis. An enlarged lymph node is evident *(curved arrow)*.

onset of symptoms. If the condition is not treated, sepsis and life-threatening systemic toxicity can lead to death as the infection spreads into the surrounding structures. Bacteremia may be complicated with septic embolization, with seeding of the heart, brain, lung, and other vital organs. Generally one muscle is involved, but multiple sites can be affected in up to 40% of patients. Radiographic evaluation may show generalized swelling and occasionally gas in the soft tissues. Periostitis of the bone may occur if the infection is deep. Osteomyelitis may complicate a long-standing infection.

Computed tomography is useful in diagnosis of pyomyositis. Early in the disease the muscle enlarges and

shows heterogeneous attenuation. Administration of intravenous contrast at this stage shows normal enhancement or hyperemia. In the second stage, intravenous contrast administration shows rim enhancement and variable attenuation in developing abscesses. On MRI the affected muscle may appear enlarged with loss of the architectural definition with diffuse, heterogeneous areas of low signal intensity on T1-weighted images. In the absence of an abscess, edema may be the only finding, manifested by corresponding high signal intensity on fluid-sensitive sequences. On T2-weighted images, disorganized phlegmonous collections herald the development of abscess formation (Fig. 17-7). The abnormal signal intensity within the muscle may be poorly marginated, and heterogeneous enhancement may be seen as suppuration develops. After intravenous administration of a gadolinium contrast agent, characteristic rim enhancement and central liquefaction are observed (Fig. 17-8). However, if the abscess is long-standing, it may contain areas of intermediate signal intensity surrounded by a low–signal intensity rim of fibrous tissue. The preferred treatment of pyomyositis is surgical débridement and administration of antibiotics.

■ DIABETIC MUSCLE INFARCTION

A serious complication in diabetic patients with poorly controlled disease is spontaneous muscle infarction, typically affecting the lower extremities. The thighs are involved in 80% of cases, followed by the calf region in nearly another 20%. Patients present with severe, acute pain and tenderness and often a palpable mass. The clinical presentation may be similar to patients presenting with pyomyositis or an intramuscular abscess, except that the entire muscle is usually edematous and the process is bilateral in almost 40% of cases. Clinically, swelling is an early finding. The patient may have either a normal temperature or a low-grade fever, but there is absence of leukocytosis. Blood or muscle cultures are typically negative, and the creatine kinase levels may be mildly elevated. The pathogenesis of this disorder is likely extensive throm-

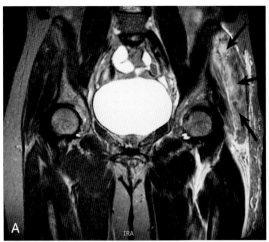

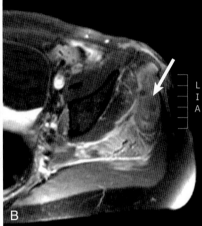

Figure 17-7 Pyomyositis. A, Coronal T2-weighted image of the pelvis shows extensive edema in the left side of the pelvis involving the gluteal muscles *(arrows)*. Overlying cellulitis was evident, as well as intermuscular edema. **B,** Fat-saturated T1-weighted axial image after intravenous administration of contrast shows phlegmonous changes in the gluteus medius muscle *(arrow)*.

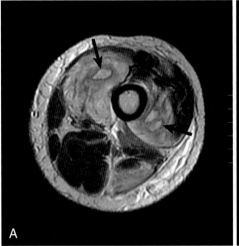

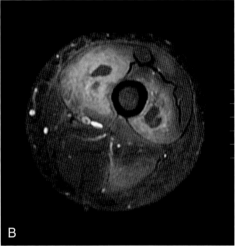

Figure 17-8 Pyomyositis, late. A, T2-weighted axial image of the right distal thigh shows interstitial edema in the quadriceps and biceps femoris muscles, diffuse soft tissue swelling, and fluid cavities in the vastus medialis (VM) and lateralis (VL) muscles *(arrows)*. **B,** Fat-saturated T1-weighted axial image after intravenous administration of contrast shows heterogeneous enhancement of the VM and VL around the developing abscesses.

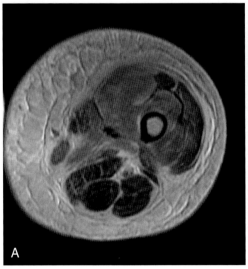

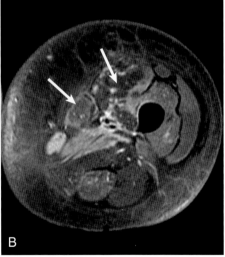

Figure 17-9 Diabetic muscle infarction. A, T2-weighted axial image of the distal thigh shows marked edema in the quadriceps and adductor muscles. **B,** Fat-saturated T1-weighted axial image after intravenous administration of contrast shows devitalized ischemic muscles *(arrows)*. The serum white blood cell count was normal.

bosis of medium and small arterioles, although embolic thrombosis may be a contributing cause, resulting in decreased blood flow. Patients with this condition typically present with other complications of severe diabetes, including nephropathy (60% to 70%), neuropathy (30% to 60%), and retinopathy. The mortality rate associated with this condition reflects the severity of the disease and ranges from 14% to 20%.

On MRI, muscle infarction is characterized by muscle edema, manifested by loss of normal muscle architecture and intense interstitial high signal intensity on T2-weighted images (Fig. 17-9). Subcutaneous and sub-

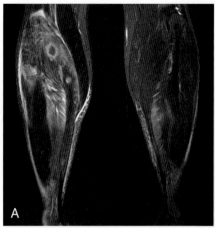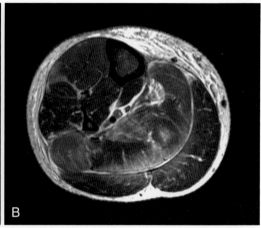

Figure 17-10 Rhabdomyolysis.
A, Short tau inversion recovery (STIR) coronal image of both calves shows extensive interstitial edema in the muscles bilaterally after a strongman contest. **B,** T2-weighted axial image of the right calf shows marked edema in the soleus and gastrocnemius muscles and mild edema in the anterior calf compartment. There is diffuse subcutaneous edema. The creatine kinase level in this patient reached 80,000 units/L with subsequent involvement of the thigh muscles.

fascial edema are common associated findings. There may be diffuse muscular enhancement after intravenous contrast administration acutely, but as the muscle tissue becomes devitalized, sites of peripheral rim enhancement with central low signal intensity develop in areas where there is actual myonecrosis and infarction. The diagnosis of diabetic muscle infarction remains a clinical diagnosis because MRI findings are not specific and may be similar to pyomyositis and other causes of focal myositis. Occasionally diagnosis may be confirmed with a biopsy, but ultimately areas of necrosis will not require aspiration, in contradistinction to an abscess.

RHABDOMYOLYSIS

Rhabdomyolysis is a potentially life-threatening syndrome resulting from the breakdown of skeletal muscle fibers caused by the loss of integrity of the muscle cell membranes, releasing cellular contents into the circulation. Common causes are excessive physical activity, seizure, prolonged muscle compression, hyperthermia, hypothermia, coma, drug overdose, toxins, alcohol abuse, and autoimmune inflammation. Clinically, patients may complain of myalgia, weakness, and pain, and diffuse muscle swelling may be notable. Tea-colored urine may be an early sign of rhabdomyolysis. An elevated creatine kinase level, frequently by at least five times the normal serum level, and serum potassium level are typical findings, and a positive urine myoglobin test is definitive. Complications are classified as early or late. Early complications from hyperkalemia include cardiac arrhythmia and arrest. The most serious late complication is transient renal failure from myoglobinuria, occurring in 15% of patients with rhabdomyolysis. This complication is particularly prevalent in HIV-infected patients. Full recovery is expected with early diagnosis, and treatment is directed toward preserving renal function. Dialysis is a therapeutic alternative that may be required. Critically ill patients with acute renal failure may develop multiorgan failure which increases mortality. Other late complications include disseminated intravascular coagulation and compartment syndrome.

On MRI, homogeneous to heterogeneous increased signal intensity on fluid-sensitive sequences is characteristically observed with either homogeneous enhancement with intravenous contrast administration or rim enhancement around areas of devitalization (Fig. 17-10). Two important complications include development of frank myonecrosis in severe injuries and progression to a compartment syndrome, which may necessitate surgical intervention.

Acute compartment syndrome occurs when there is prolonged increase in intramuscular pressure within a fascial compartment. Clinically, compartment syndrome is characterized by swelling, edema, ischemia, and pain. It most commonly affects the anterior and lateral compartments of the lower extremity. Increased intramuscular pressures above 30 mm Hg are diagnostic, producing ischemic changes to the muscle. Treatment is aimed at reducing the effects of nerve damage and rhabdomyolysis and involves a fasciotomy of the affected compartment. Delay in treatment may result in muscle fibrosis and contracture. On MRI the characteristic finding is diffuse increase in signal intensity on T2-weighted images in one compartment of a limb. Focal muscle herniation is not uncommon. If early in the process, contrast administration shows variable but often intense muscular enhancement. Delayed muscle soreness occurring after strenuous exercise may have a similar MRI appearance but often involves more than one compartment.

PITFALLS

Two traumatic conditions may mimic an inflammatory condition, myositis ossificans and Morel-Lavallée lesion. Myositis ossificans is a self-limiting, nonneoplastic soft tissue mass in skeletal muscle occurring as a consequence of trauma. The pathogenesis of this benign condition is unknown, and its imaging appearance corresponds to its stage. Early myositis ossificans is manifested by an enlarging soft tissue mass distorting the architecture of the muscle. Calcification begins at the periphery and works toward the center of the lesion. Radiographs and CT show faint peripheral calcification within 2 to 4 weeks of the onset of symptoms

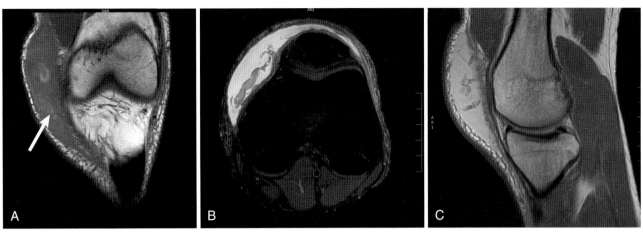

Figure 17-11 Morel-Lavallée lesion. **A,** Coronal T1-weighted image shows a complex fluid collection with blood and fat globules within it *(arrow).* **B,** Axial fluid-sensitive image shows that the fluid tapers at the edges and is not the prepatellar bursa. **C,** Sagittal proton density–weighted image demonstrates debris often seen in these lesions.

and a sharply delineated ossified rim by 6 to 8 weeks, and the mass eventually becomes smaller by 5 to 6 months. The MRI manifestation of early myositis ossificans is a well-defined mass with heterogeneous signal intensity surrounded by edema. Central areas of increased signal intensity on fluid-sensitive sequences correspond to extremely cellular regions of proliferating myofibroblasts. Administration of intravenous gadolinium frequently shows early enhancement of the lesion. As the lesion matures, the signal intensity in the periphery decreases, corresponding to areas of mineralization. Mature lesions are avascular and demonstrate no enhancement.

Morel-Lavallée lesion is a traumatic degloving injury that occurs when the skin and subcutaneous fat is sheared away from the underlying fascia, often occurring during a fall, which causes disruption of the perforating vessels and nerves. This creates a potential space that fills with blood, lymph, and fat. Radiographically, soft tissue swelling predominates, but MRI is necessary for confirmation of the diagnosis. Most often these lesions occur over the greater trochanters, gluteal regions, flank, lumbar spine, shoulder, and knee. Clinically, pain occurs over a fluctuant area of soft tissue, often with concomitant skin paresthesia. On MRI a well-defined fluid collection in the subcutaneous space, occasionally with fluid-fluid levels, is surrounded by a hypointense capsule (Fig. 17-11). Floating fat globules are nearly pathognomonic of this lesion. Treatment is usually conservative with a pressure bandage when acute, but more chronic lesions may be drained and sclerosed with talc or doxycycline.

Selected Reading

Chason DP, Fleckenstein JL, Burns DK, et al: Diabetic muscle infarction: radiologic evaluation, *Skeletal Radiol* 25:127–132, 1996.

Christian S, Kraas J, Conway WF: Musculoskeletal infections, *Semin Roentgenol* 42:92–101, 2007.

Fayad LM, Carrino JA, Fishman EK: Musculoskeletal infection: role of CT in the emergency department, *Radiographics* 27:1723–1736, 2007.

Fugitt JB, Puckett ML, Quigley MM, et al: Necrotizing fasciitis, *Radiographics* 24:1472–1476, 2004.

Gordon BA, Martinez S, Collins AJ: Pyomyositis: characteristics at CT and MR imaging, *Radiology* 197:279–286, 1995.

Jelinek JS, Murphey MD, Aboulafia AJ, et al: Muscle infarction in patients with diabetes mellitus: MR imaging findings, *Radiology* 211:241–247, 1999.

Loh NN, Chen IY, Cheung LP, et al: Deep fascial hyperintensity in soft-tissue abnormalities as revealed by T2-weighted MR imaging, *AJR Am J Roentgenol* 168:1301–1304, 1997.

Lu CH, Tsang YM, Yu CW, et al: Rhabdomyolysis: magnetic resonance imaging and computed tomography findings, *J Comput Assist Tomogr* 31:368–374, 2007.

Mellado JM, Perez del Palomar L, Diaz L, et al: Long-standing Morel-Lavallee lesions of the trochanteric region and proximal thigh: MRI features in five patients, *AJR Am J Roentgenol* 182:1289–1294, 2004.

Peterson JJ, Bancroft LW, Kransdorf MJ: Wooden foreign bodies: imaging appearance, *AJR Am J Roentgenol* 178:557–562, 2002.

Rahmouni A, Chosidow O, Mathieu D, et al: MR imaging in acute infectious cellulitis, *Radiology* 192:493–496, 1994.

Restrepo CS, Lemos DF, Gordillo H, et al: Imaging findings in musculoskeletal complications of AIDS, *Radiographics* 24:1029–1049, 2004.

Revelon G, Rahmouni A, Jazaerli N, et al: Acute swelling of the limbs: magnetic resonance pictorial review of fascial and muscle signal changes, *Eur J Radiol* 30:11–21, 1999.

Rominger MB, Lukosch CJ, Bachmann GF: MR imaging of compartment syndrome of the lower leg: a case control study, *Eur Radiol* 14:1432–1439, 2004.

Schmid MR, Kossman T, Duewell S: Differentiation of necrotizing fasciitis and cellulitis using MR imaging, *AJR Am J Roentgenol* 170:615–620, 1998.

Soler R, Rodriguez E, Aguilera C, et al: Magnetic resonance imaging of pyomyositis in 43 cases, *Eur J Radiol* 35:59–64, 2000.

Struk DW, Munk L, Lee MJ, et al: Imaging of soft tissue infections, *Radiol Clin North Am* 39:277–303, 2001.

Verleisdonk EJMM, van Gils A, van der Werken C: The diagnostic value of MRI scans for the diagnosis of chronic exertional compartment syndrome of the lower leg, *Skeletal Radiol* 30:321–325, 2001.

Index

Page numbers followed by "f" indicate figures, "t" indicate tables, and "b" indicate boxes.